Benign and Reactive Conditions of Lymph Node and Spleen

ATLAS OF NONTUMOR PATHOLOGY

ARP PRESS™

Editorial & Production Manager: Mirlinda Q. Caton
Production Editor: Dian S. Thomas
Editorial Assistant: Melanie J. De Boer
Editorial Assistant: Magdalena C. Silva
Copyeditor: Audrey Kahn

ATLAS OF NONTUMOR PATHOLOGY

First Series
Fascicle 7

Benign and Reactive Conditions of Lymph Node and Spleen

Dennis P. O'Malley, MD

Tracy I. George, MD

Attilio Orazi, MD, FRCPath

Susan L. Abbondanzo, MD

Published by the
American Registry of Pathology
Washington, DC
in collaboration with the
Armed Forces Institute of Pathology
Washington, DC

2009

ATLAS OF NONTUMOR PATHOLOGY

Available from the American Registry of Pathology
Armed Forces Institute of Pathology
Washington, DC 20306-6000
www.afip.org
ISBN: 1-933477-06-7
978-1-933477-06-0

INTRODUCTION TO SERIES

This is the seventh Fascicle of the Atlas of Nontumor Pathology, a complementary series to the Armed Forces Institute of Pathology (AFIP) Atlas of Tumor Pathology, first published in 1949.

For several years, various individuals in the pathology community have suggested the formation of a new series of monographs concentrating on this particular area. In 1998, an Editorial Board was appointed and outstanding authors chosen shortly thereafter.

The purpose of the atlas is to provide surgical pathologists with ready expert reference material most helpful in their daily practice. The lesions described relate principally to medical non-neoplastic conditions. Many of these lesions represent complex entities and, when appropriate, we have included contributions from internists, radiologists, and surgeons. This has led to some increase in the size of the monographs but the emphasis remains on diagnosis by the surgical pathologist.

Previously, the Fascicles have been available on CD-ROM format as well as in print. In order to provide the widest possible advantages of both modalities, we have formatted the print Fascicle on the World Wide Web. Use of the Internet allows cross-indexing within the Fascicles.

Our goal is to continue to provide expert information at the lowest possible cost. Therefore, marked reductions in pricing are available to residents and fellows as well as to pathology faculty and other staff members purchasing the Fascicles on a subscription basis.

We believe that the Atlas of Nontumor Pathology will serve as an outstanding reference for surgical pathologists as well as an important contribution to the literature of other medical specialties.

Donald West King, MD
William A. Gardner, MD
Leslie H. Sobin, MD
J. Thomas Stocker, MD
Bernard Wagner, MD

INTRODUCTION

This Fascicle on benign and reactive conditions of lymph node and spleen has developed over a long period of time. Without doubt, it was a vast undertaking: quite simply, to cover everything that could possibly occur in lymph nodes or spleens that was not a malignant neoplasm. This, of course, is an impossible charge. We were compelled, however, to try to accomplish several tasks in this book. First, to live up to the standards set by previous authors of the excellent books of this series. Next, to provide a book that is both useable, but still fairly comprehensive; the delicate balance of providing a book that is at the same time encyclopedic and a manageable size is quite a challenge! Finally, we attempted to provide numerous excellent quality photographs and photomicrographs to illustrate the lesions.

An eminent hematopathologist once said, "The study of malignant lymphomas is boring compared to that of benign proliferations of the immune system, which are very complex and very interesting." This statement lies at the heart of our motivation for this book. Although malignant processes garner the majority of our attention, it is the benign processes that have an underlying complexity that is often an illustration of the delicate interplay of many components of the active immune system. In diagnosing the pathologic specimen, a basic approach is: 1) to determine if the process is benign or malignant, 2) if malignant, to characterize the origin of the malignancy (e.g., carcinoma, melanoma, lymphoma), and 3) to subclassify or identify the process. The first and second issues are clearly critical in pathology—they guide our treatment of the pathologic processes. Admittedly, the first step is not always a clear-cut decision. In several differential diagnoses in lymphoid processes, the question of benign versus malignant cannot be resolved by histomorphologic evaluation alone. The second part of the approach has become considerably easier with the advent of immunophenotypic analysis. It is important to remember that without evidence of immunophenotype, we would still be misdiagnosing anaplastic large cell lymphoma as carcinoma and some small blue cell tumors as lymphomas. The final issue, that of identification of the pathologic process, may be of greater or lesser importance, depending on the clinical situation. If an exact diagnosis can be made, it can have several benefits. In the case of neoplastic processes, it may indicate the type of treatment and the prognosis. In benign processes, there are other important benefits as well. Although some therapies may be instituted in benign conditions, especially those of infectious etiologies, often simply naming a thing can have great benefit to the patient. It is important to realize that even in the case of a purely reactive process, finding a name, a category, a classification, can provide real peace-of-mind to the patient. To have a thing named is an important part of understanding it, and this can be of great reassurance to the patient who suffers from the process.

Without doubt, great effort was put forward in completing this book. It was not only an effort of the authors but truly of the broader community of pathologists. We took the work of many others, some eminent names, others hard workers whose names will never be "recognized," and tried to find the essence and distill it in this book. One of the main reasons that this book was undertaken by these authors is that for some years there has been no single, up-to-date book that contains extensive information on benign and reactive lymphoid conditions. With respect to that issue, one eminent name that must be recognized is that of William St.Clair-Symmers.

Dr. St.Clair-Symmers edited a multi-volume pathology text, in which he wrote the chapter Systemic Pathology in volume 2, *The Lymphoreticular System* (Churchill-Livingstone, 1978). This book stands as a guide to students of benign lymphoid processes. Published in 1978, it is currently out of date and certainly out of press. The depth and breadth of coverage in this volume, however, show that Dr. St.Clair-Symmers was a man who was passionate about benign lymph nodes. Clearly, his coverage of lymphomas may not be modern enough to be practical today, but it is unlikely that even this book can better cover the descriptions of lymph node infection by *Listeria* or anthrax.

Most of these photographs were taken using an Olympus digital photomicroscope camera (DP-12) and were subsequently processed using Adobe Photoshop CS. In some cases, minimal editing was performed, but no critical information was removed or added.

To students of pathology, and hematopathology specifically, we hope that we have created a book that will serve as a useful guide to the sometimes complex world of benign and reactive lesions of the lymphoid system. It was our pleasure to create this work, and we hope that it will serve as a resource for several years.

Dennis P. O'Malley, MD
Pathologist
Clarient Diagnostics, Inc.

Tracy I. George, MD
Assistant Professor of Pathology
Stanford University

Attilio Orazi, MD, FRCPath
Professor of Pathology and Laboratory Medicine
Weill Medical College of Cornell University

Susan L. Abbondanzo, MD
Former Chairman, Department of Hematopathology
Armed Forces Institute of Pathology

ACKNOWLEDGEMENTS

A special acknowledgement is attributed to John Eble, Chairman of the Department of Pathology and Laboratory Medicine at Indiana University. Besides supplying several images for this Fascicle, he provided support and guidance throughout the production of this book.

The contributions of Peter Banks need special mention. Not only was he a mentor to one of the authors (DPO), but he also allowed us access to his massive collection of hematopathology slides. Many images in this text are from his collection and because of the sheer volume, in some cases they are not specifically acknowledged. In many ways, Peter can be considered our "fifth Beatle" in regard to the production of this book.

We received a large number of rare specimens and great technical help from the California Tumor Tissue Registry. We owe special thanks to: Donald R. Chase, MD, Executive Director; Anne E. Chism, Manager; and Linda Healy, Director of Technical Operations.

We would also like to acknowledge some last minute herculean efforts to replace some of the photos in the book. Important and excellent contributions of photos were made by Dr. Robin Cooke, as well as professors Jacque Diebold and Karl Lennert.

Other notables who contributed time, effort, photographs, and cases include the following individuals from Indiana University: Lee Ann Baldridge, Regina Bennett, Lisa Bird, Eric G. Brocken, Ryan Christy, Thomas Cibull, O.W. Cummings, Thomas Davis, Cecelia Dodson, Nick Frechette, Dean Hawley, Sylvia Hernandez, Terrance Katona, Linda Marler, Richard Neiman, Corinne Puzio, Jean Siders, Frederik Skarstedt, C.R. Stine, Attaya Suvannasankha, Saeed Vakili, and Vera Vavinski; and these indviduals from Stanford University: Daniel A. Arber, Ronald F. Dorfman, Donald P. Regula Jr., Marisela Reis, and Roger A. Warnke.

Finally, we would like to recognize the work of Mitchell Adachi, Mahul Amin, J. Bruce Beckwith, Benjaporn Chaiwun, Thomas Colby, Frank Deamant, Giovanni DePetris, Patricia Devine, Milton Drachenberg, Luis F. Fajardo, Michael E. Fitzpatrick, Christopher Fletcher, Vito Franco, Christopher Garwacki, Stephen Geller, David Grier, Anselm Hii, Peter Humphrey, Steve Kroft, Ronald Jaffe, Malisha Johnson, Young Kim, Robert Lev, Ting Li, Marie-Claire Marroum, Gary Mierau, Rodney Miles, Bharat Nathwani, Ronald Neafie, Valerie L. Ng, Stefania Pittaluga, Stefano Pileri, Valerie Purvin, Banumati Ramakrishna, Mary G. Ripple, Stanley Robboy, Janet Roepke, Victor Roggli, Jess Savala Jr., Dale Selby, Fred Silva, Bertram Schnitzer, Keith Steele, Nancy A. Twenhafel, Kurt Wegener, Mark Wick, Katrina Wood, and Craig Zuppan.

DEDICATIONS

To my wife, Karene, my parents John and Shirley, and my many teachers, colleagues, and students.

Dennis P. O'Malley

To my grandparents, Richard and Emmy Lou Levin.

Tracy I. George

To my parents and to Maria, Giulia, and Rita.

Attilio Orazi

To my mother and my husband, Jonathan, for their constant support, and to my father for teaching me when to punt in life and when to go for it on fourth down.

Susan L. Abbondanzo

Permission to use copyrighted illustrations has been granted by:

American Society for Clinical Pathology

Practical Diagnosis of Hematologic Disorders, 4th ed. Chicago: ASCP Press; 2006:281. 2006 Society for Clinical Pathology. For table 3-1.

The Pathology of the Spleen: A Functional Approach. Chicago: ASCP Press; 1976:37. For figure 15-6.

Elsevier Limited

Human Pathology 1997;28:333. For table 18-2.

Indian Council of Medical Research

Indian Journal of Medical Research 1999;109:214. For table 8-4.

Karger

The Lymphatic System and Cancer: Mechanisms and Clinical Management. Basel: Karger;1994:3. For figure 1-1.

Lippincott Williams & Wilkins

Neoplastic Hematopathology, 2nd ed. Philadelphia: Lippincott Williams & Wilkins; 2001;514, 538. For tables 3-2 and 3-3.

Masson Publishing USA

Pathology of Radiation Injury. New York: Masson Publishing; 1982:154. For figure 14-16

McGraw-Hill Companies

Infectious Diseases. Atlas Cases Text. North Ryde, NSW:McGraw-Hill Australia Pty Ltd 2008;296-422. For figures 11-4, 11-5, 11-6, 11-7, 11-8, 11-9, 11-10, 11-14, 11-15, 11-19C and D, and 11-20.

McMillan Publishers Ltd.

Modern Pathology 2004;17:921. For table 4-4.

CONTENTS

1 GENERAL IMMUNOLOGY OF LYMPH NODE AND SPLEEN

OVERVIEW OF THE IMMUNE SYSTEM AND IMMUNOLOGIC RESPONSES

Understanding the anatomy and function of lymph node and spleen allows insight into the complex mechanisms of the immune system. By studying "normal" immune responses to antigens, we have the building blocks to analyze the mechanisms by which immune dysfunction occurs, such as in congenital immunodeficiencies. In this chapter, the anatomy, morphology, and mechanisms of immunologic responses in the lymph nodes and spleen are discussed.

Whereas it is the primary lymphoid tissues of bone marrow and thymus that produce naive lymphocytes that reflect antigen-independent differentiation, it is the secondary lymphoid tissues, including lymph nodes and spleen, in which antigen-dependent reactions occur. Antigen-specific reactions include proliferation and differentiation of B and T lymphocytes in response to specific antigens. The interaction of antigen, B and T lymphocytes, macrophages, and follicular dendritic (and other accessory) cells, is responsible for effective humoral (B-cell) and cell-mediated (T-cell) responses. Uptake of antigen by the accessory cells results in presentation to the lymphocytes and subsequent expansion of both the B- and T-cell dependent areas.

LYMPH NODES

Anatomy

Lymph nodes are found in the body at specific sites designed to maximize the processing of antigens present in the lymphatic fluid draining from organs and other tissues. These locations are along major blood vessels on the proximal end of the extremities, as well as in the neck, mediastinum, mesentery, retroperitoneum, hilum of kidneys/lungs/spleen, and salivary glands. The size of the lymph nodes ranges from millimeters to centimeters depending on whether a lymph node is unstimulated or reactive or involved by a neoplasm.

Gross evaluation of an unstimulated lymph node typically shows a small bean-shaped structure enveloped by a capsule. Sectioning reveals a pale tan-gray surface with a fleshy appearance. Reactive lymph nodes are generally larger (some greater than 1 cm) and typically show a similar tan-gray appearance or may show necrosis, pigmentation, fibrosis, or prominent nodularity, findings discussed in more detail in subsequent chapters.

When dissected microscopically, lymph nodes contain functional compartments in which different cell types predominate (figs. 1-1, 1-2). Lymph enters the lymph node through multiple afferent lymphatic vessels that flow through subcapsular, intermediate, and medullary sinuses, and exits through a single efferent lymphatic vessel. The sinuses are lined by sinus endothelial cells which contain intercellular pores, especially within the medullary sinus. Fibroblastic reticular cells encase a core of type I collagen fibers, which are surrounded by a microfibrillar zone covered by a basement membrane; this forms a *conduit system,* which connects sinuses to high endothelial venules. This conduit system is richest in the paracortex and sparse throughout the cortex of the lymph node. Naive B and T cells from the blood use specific receptors to recognize ligands on the high endothelial venules in lymph nodes, and pass between these cells to enter the paracortex and then migrate to distinct B- and T-cell zones (13). Responding to cytokine secretion by follicular dendritic cells, B cells localize to follicles where they can initiate the germinal-center reaction. T cells localize to the paracortex where they interact with dendritic cells, which further drives T-cell differentiation. Local stromal cell production of cytokines and chemokines confines the T and B cells to their respective areas (31).

Primary Immune Response

The first days of a primary immune response of lymph nodes to soluble antigen can be visualized with online simulations based on static and

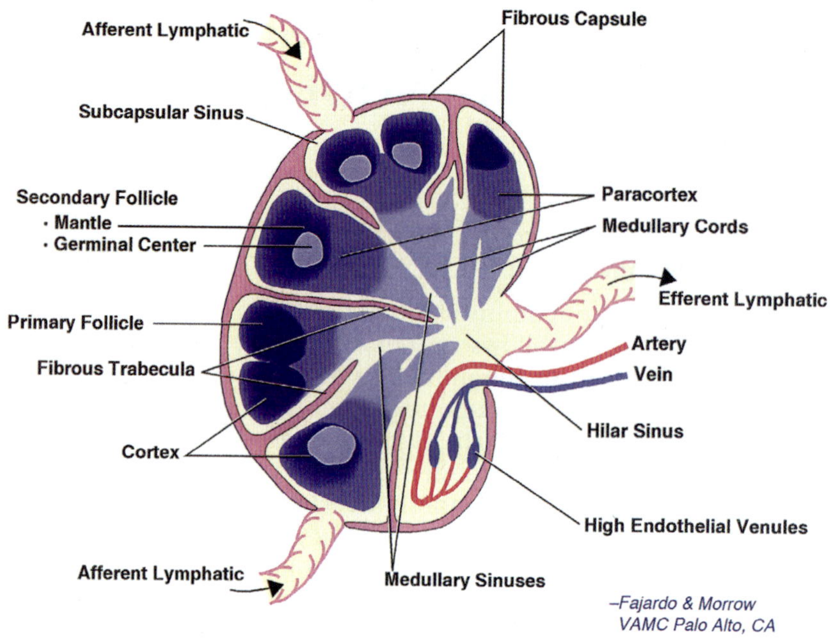

Figure 1-1

STRUCTURE OF A LYMPH NODE

Fig. 1 from Fajardo LF. Lymph nodes and cancer. A review. In: Meyer JL, ed. The lymphatic system and cancer. Basel: Karger; 1994:3. [Meyer J, ed. Frontiers of radiation therapy and oncology. Vol 28.]

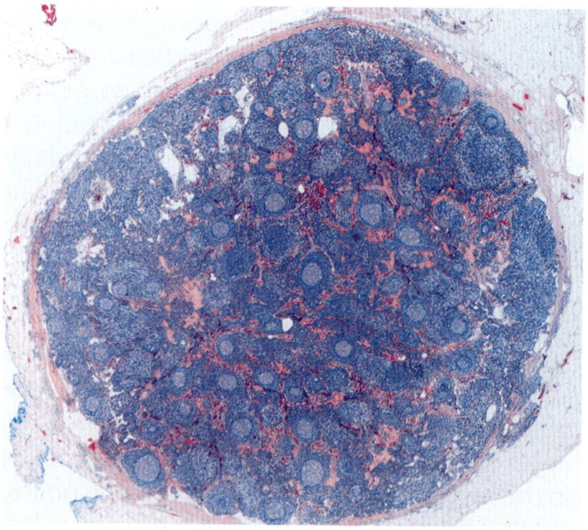

Figure 1-2

LYMPH NODE

Low-magnification image of lymph node showing normal structures including follicles, paracortex, sinuses, and capsule.

dynamic imaging methods (9). In this simulation, based on numerous experiments, soluble antigen is carried from an injection site via lymphatic vessels into afferent lymphatic vessels, draining into a lymph node within 15 to 30 minutes following injection. Dendritic cells nearest the conduits acquire antigen-producing peptide-major histocompatability complex (MHC) II complexes, which peak in number 3 hours after injection. Multiple random transient (about 5 minutes) interactions then occur between CD4-positive T cells and dendritic cells. These interactions result in induction of CD69 expression by the T cells and T-cell receptor signaling. After 18 hours, dendritic cells from the injection site bearing greater amounts of peptide-MHC I complexes appear in the lymph nodes, moving into the T-cell area. By 30 hours after injection, CD4-positive T cells have begun to divide. Continued exposure to antigen augments and sustains their cell division.

B cells require help from T-helper cells, and present peptide-MHC II ligands to these T cells in order to receive the CD40 and cytokine receptor signals necessary for proliferation, memory cell formation, and secretion of antibody. While it is not known how antigen-specific B cells acquire soluble antigen in follicles, once antigen binding occurs, the movement of the B cells to the outer follicle adjacent to the T-cell area is restricted. This location restriction is mediated via signaling through chemokine receptors: naive follicular B cells express high levels of CXCR5 and low levels of CCR7, which bind to a chemokine produced in follicles and in stromal cells, respectively (2). In contrast, after antigen binding to the B-cell receptor, the B cells express

Table 1-1

DEVELOPMENTAL STAGES OF B CELLS[a]

	Ig[b] Gene	Somatic Hyper-mutation	Ig Protein	Immunophenotype
Precursor				
Progenitor B cell	D-J/V-DJ	N	N	Pan-B[c], CD34, CD10, TdT
Precursor B cell	IgH	N	Igμ (cytoplasm)	Pan-B, CD34, CD10, TdT, CD45RB
Immature B cell	IgH/IgL	N	IgM	Pan-B, CD20, CD45RB, CD10
Naive Mature				
Recirculating, follicular B cells	IgH/IgL	N	IgM^{low},IgD^{high}	Pan-B, CD20, CD45RB, CD5, CD21, CD23
Recirculating, low affinity self-reactive (B1 cells)	IgH/IgL	N	IgM/IgD	Pan-B, CD20, CD45RB, CD5, CD11b, CD23
Sessile, marginal zone B cell	IgH/IgL	N	IgM^{high},IgD^{low}	Pan-B, CD20, CD45RB, CD5, CD21
Germinal Center				
Centroblasts	IgH/IgL	Y	Decreased/absent	Pan-B, CD20, CD45RB, CD10, bcl-6
Centrocytes	IgH/IgL	Y	Decreased/absent	Pan-B, CD20, CD45RB, CD10, bcl-6
Postgerminal Center				
Memory B cells	IgH/IgL	Y	IgM	Pan-B, CD20, CD45RB
Plasma cells	IgH/IgL	Y	IgG>IgA>IgD	CD38, CD138, VD38, MUM-1

[a]This table compares the immunoglobulin (Ig) gene configuration, presence or absence of somatic hypermutation, Ig protein, and immunophenotype of the major types of B cells. The precursor B cells are located in the bone marrow, whereas the other stages are found in lymph node or other secondary lymphoid tissues.
[b]Ig = immunoglobulin; D-J/V = diversity, joining and variable segments; IgH = immunoglobulin heavy chain; IgL = immunoglobulin light chain
[c]Pan-B immunophenotype includes expression of CD19, CD22, CD79a, and PAX5; TdT = terminal deoxynucleotidyltransferase.

increased levels of CCR7 and decreased CXCR5, resulting in the movement of the B cells toward T-cell rich areas (39). Now that the B cells are near the T cells, antigen-specific CD4-positive T cells and B cells form random interactions; this occurs 1 and 2 days following injection of antigen. These interactions result in CD40 and cytokine receptor signals from the T cell to the B cell, with the T cell receiving T-cell receptor signals from the B cell.

Two days after injection, the B cell has begun to proliferate in the follicles. B cells differentiate into plasma cells, which migrate to the bone marrow, or they become germinal center cells, which remain in the follicles and give rise to memory B cells. The antigen-specific CD4-positive T cells proliferate for several days, then die, leaving memory cells (9).

B Lymphocytes

Precursor B cells are found within the bone marrow. They arise from hematopoietic stem cells. The progenitor or pro-B cell represents the earliest stage of B-cell development and depends on multiple transcription factors including PAX5, PU.1, E2A, and early B-cell factor (6). With successful rearrangement of the immunoglobulin heavy chain gene, the pro-B cell gives rise to the precursor or pre-B cell, which while lacking surface immunoglobulin, does manufacture cytoplasmic μ heavy chain. This allows for the clonal expansion and rearrangement of immunoglobulin light chain genes. The presence of membrane immunoglobulin (Ig)M in immature B cells allows for the editing and deletion of autoreactive clones (negative selection) (19).

Precursor B cells express CD34, CD10, human leukocyte antigen (HLA)-DR, and terminal deoxynucleotidyltransferase (TdT), with sequential expression of the pan B-cell antigens CD19, CD79a, and cytoplasmic CD22, followed by expression of CD20 and the leukocyte common antigen CD45 (23,41). The precursor B cells are a result of antigen-independent B-cell differentiation and result in IgM-positive immature B cells that lack the ability to respond to antigen. These immature B cells exit the bone marrow into the peripheral blood and seed peripheral lymphoid tissues, where they acquire expression of IgD and the ability to respond to antigen (Table 1-1) (42).

In the lymph node, B lymphocytes overwhelmingly reside in the cortex of the primary and secondary follicles. *Primary B-cell follicles* are unstimulated follicles composed of naive

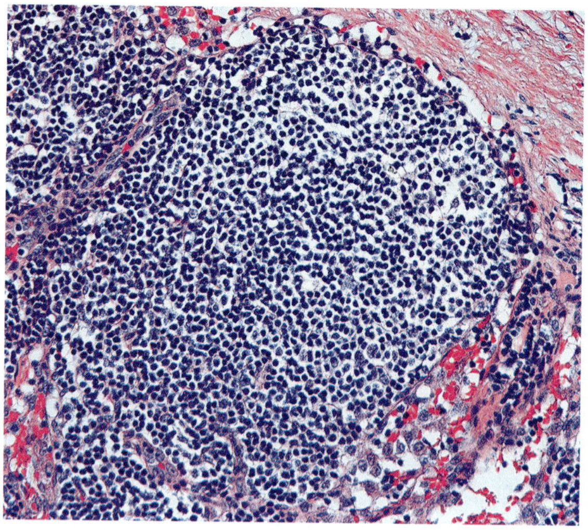

Figure 1-3

PRIMARY B-CELL FOLLICLE

Primary follicles are composed of predominantly small lymphocytes (naive B cells).

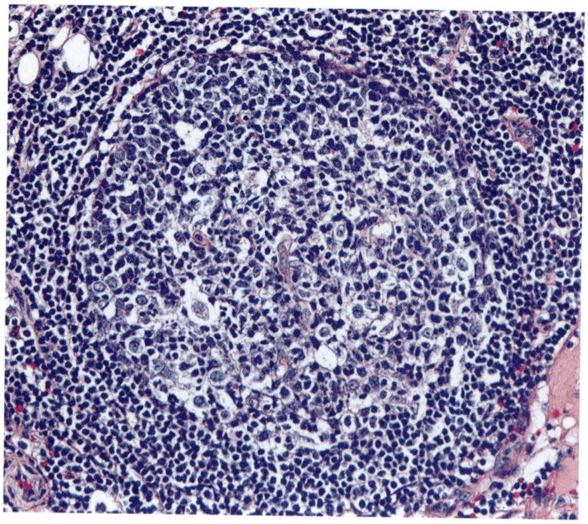

Figure 1-4

SECONDARY B-CELL FOLLICLE

Secondary follicles have a germinal center, surrounded by a mantle zone.

and memory B cells in association with follicular dendritic cells (fig. 1-3). *Naive,* or *virgin, B lymphocytes* express large amounts of immunoglobulin on their surface, with a normal ratio of kappa to lambda light chains (about 2 to 1) in combination with IgM and IgD. The naive B lymphocyte has rearranged immunoglobulin, but lacks somatic mutations in these genes (25). Naive B cells express pan-B-cell antigens (CD19, CD20, CD22, CD40, CD79a, PAX5), HLA class II molecules, surface immunoglobulin, complement receptors CD21 and CD35, and the antiapoptotic protein bcl-2, but lack markers of precursor B cells including CD10, CD34, and TdT (21,24). *Fetal B cells* in primary follicles express CD5 and CD10, but after the first year of life, CD5-positive B cells persist in a subset of cells with specificity for self antigens, and may be found in increased levels in autoimmune disease states (24). Naive B lymphocytes are present within primary follicles, circulate within the blood, and are present in mantle zones (24,26).

Secondary follicles are the sites of antigen-dependent differentiation, in which B cells are stimulated by antigens, predominantly T-cell–dependent antigens. A germinal center and surrounding mantle zone comprise each secondary follicle (figs. 1-4–1-10). Each germinal center is polarized into a pale zone and a dark zone. The dark zone is closest to the paracortex (rich in T cells) and is filled with proliferating centroblasts (large, immature-appearing lymphocytes) and tingible body macrophages. The pale zone is oriented toward the subcapsular sinus where antigens enter from afferent lymphatics. Centrocytes (small, mature lymphocytes), CD4-positive T cells, and follicular dendritic cells comprise the pale zone.

When naive B cells encounter antigen with T-cell help, they migrate toward T-cell areas and transform into extrafollicular B blasts, which produce plasma cells and primed B cells. It is these latter primed B cells that move into primary follicles and maintain the germinal center reaction, in which rounds of proliferation are accompanied by affinity maturation and class-switch recombination of immunoglobulin. The centroblasts found in the dark zone further differentiate into the centrocytes found in the pale zone. The naive B cells that have not encountered antigen in the primary follicle then form the surrounding mantle zone.

The *germinal center B cells,* centroblasts, and centrocytes show a different phenotype than the naive B cells, with an increased sensitivity to apoptosis resulting from downregulation of bcl-2 protein, upregulation of transcription factors BOB.1 and Oct2, downregulation of surface immunoglobulin, and expression of bcl-6 and CD10 (27). As part of this differentiation process

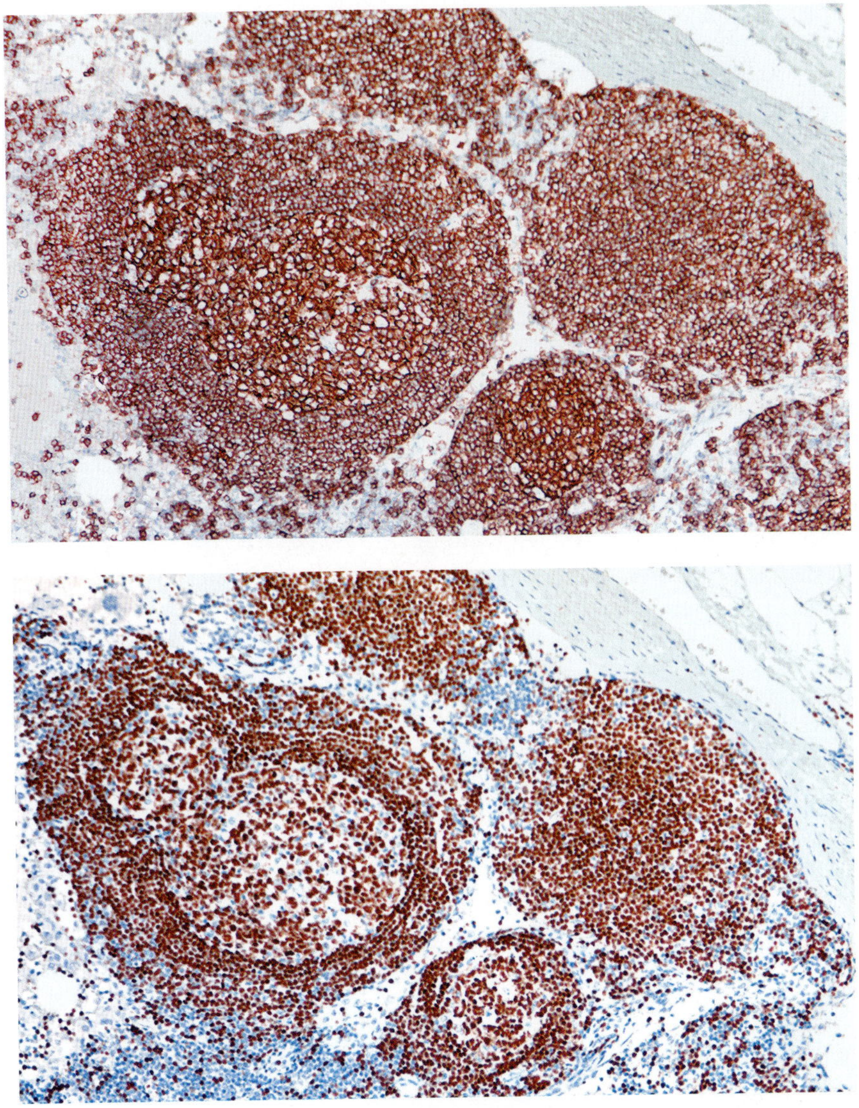

Figure 1-5

CORTEX OF LYMPH NODE

Primary and secondary follicles are labeled with CD20/PAX5.

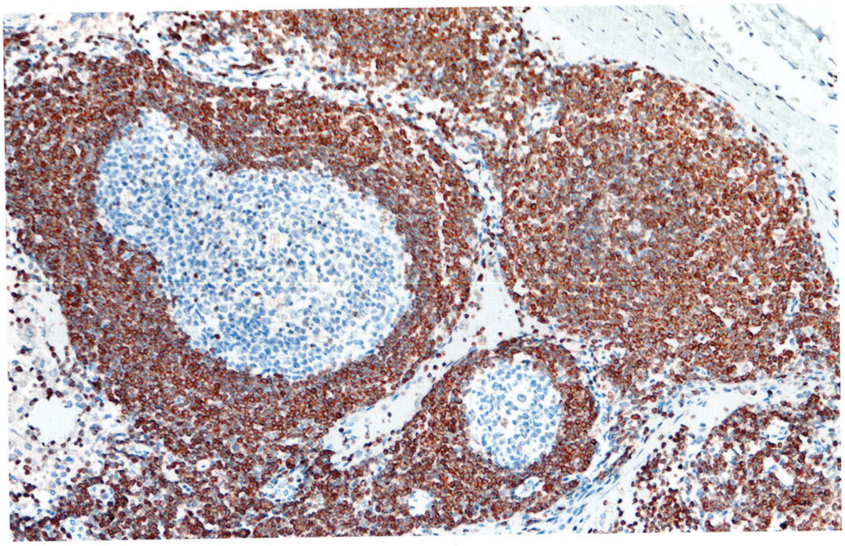

Figure 1-6

CORTEX OF LYMPH NODE

While the B cells in the primary follicles are highlighted by bcl-2 protein staining, secondary follicles lack such expression. There is strong expression, however, in the surrounding mantle lymphocytes and paracortical T cells.

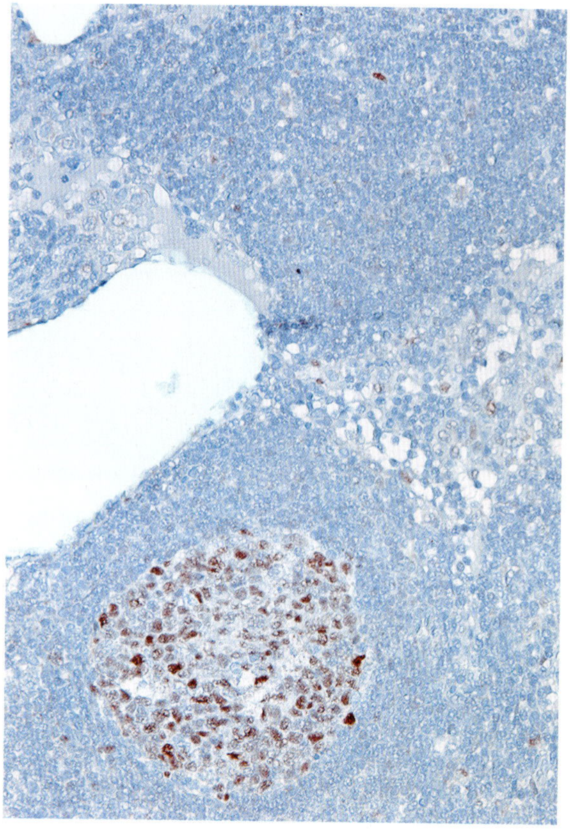

Figure 1-7

CORTEX OF LYMPH NODE

Primary and secondary follicles are labeled with bcl-6. A similar staining pattern is seen with antibody against CD10.

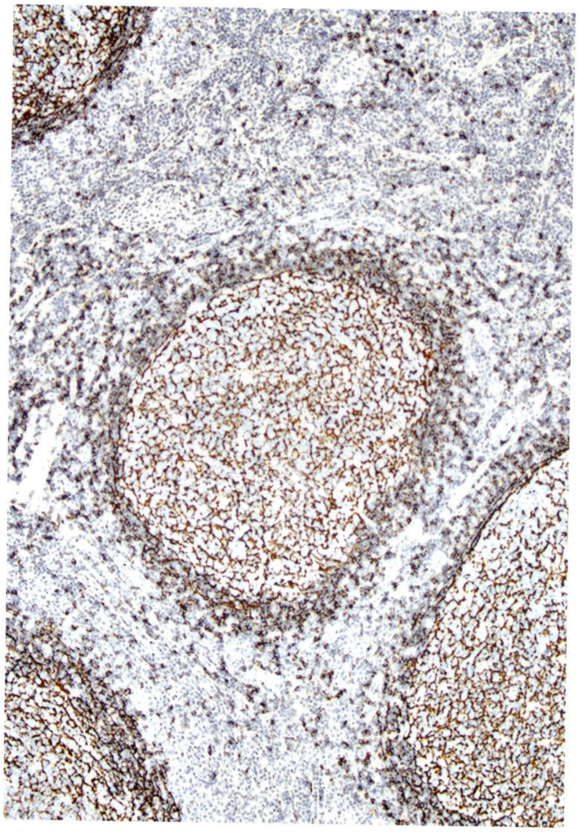

Figure 1-8

SECONDARY FOLLICLE

Follicular dendritic cells and individual mantle zone lymphocytes are positive for CD23.

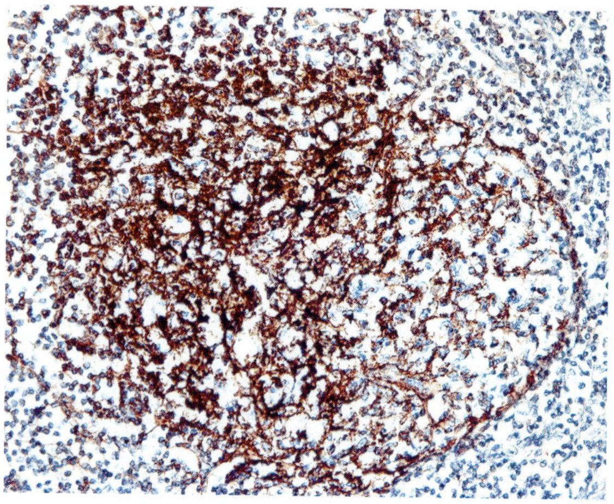

Figure 1-9

SECONDARY FOLLICLE

Follicular dendritic cells are highlighted by staining for CD21, with less prominent staining in the proliferative pole at the right.

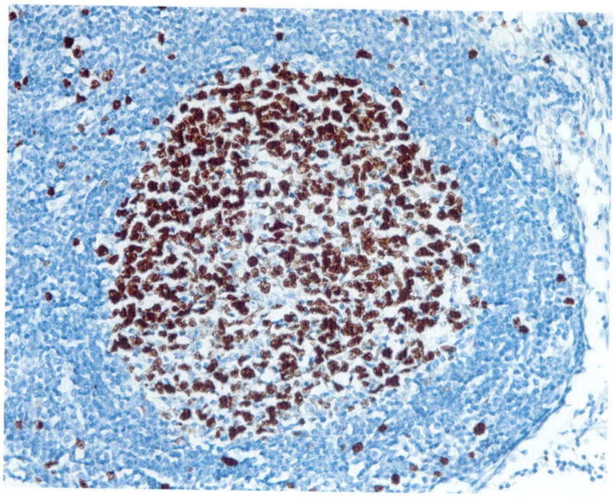

Figure 1-10

SECONDARY FOLLICLE

The dark zone, which occupies most of this germinal center, contains increased numbers of proliferating cells, as marked with MIB-1.

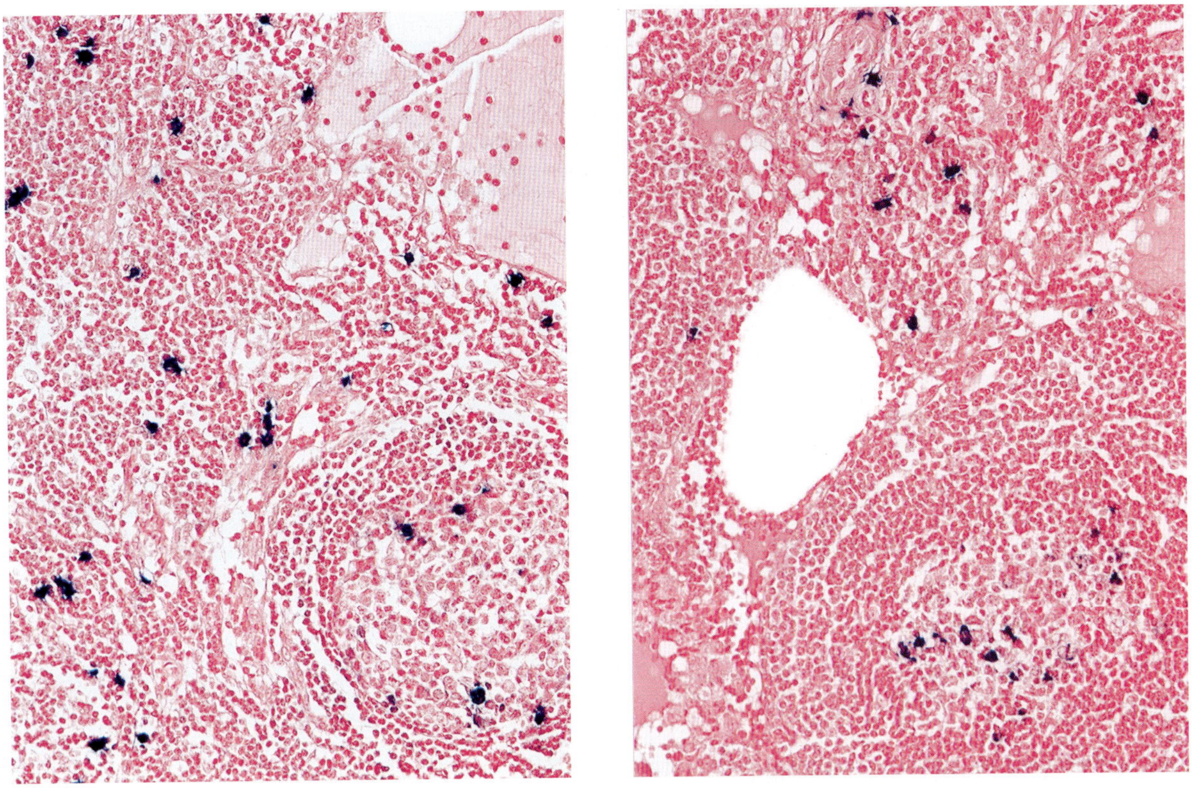

Figure 1-11

CORTEX OF LYMPH NODE

In situ hybridization for kappa (left) and lambda (right) light chains shows a polytypic pattern of plasma cells in germinal centers and interfollicular areas.

within the germinal center, the variable region of the immunoglobulin gene acquires random somatic mutations. Mutations that are favorable in the centrocyte result in an increase in the affinity of the immunoglobulin receptor (and receive survival signals from follicular dendritic cells), and the centrocyte further differentiates into a memory B cell or plasma cell (42). The intent is to refine the receptor sensitivity to the antigen and destroy cells that either have poor reactivity to antigen or reactivity to self-antigen. Thus, those centrocytes with unfavorable mutations that result in the failure of high affinity binding to antigen (the majority of centrocytes) result in apoptosis, as seen in the large number of apoptotic bodies and tingible body macrophages of the germinal center.

Postgerminal center B cells include plasma cells (fig. 1-11) and memory B cells. Beginning in the pale zone of the germinal center, plasma cell differentiation results in migration of plasma cells out of the germinal center into the bone marrow and tissues directly exposed to antigens, such as the gastrointestinal tract. Plasma cells develop after exposure to antigen and may result from naive marginal zone B cells, follicular B cells, activated germinal center B cells, or memory B cells. The location of the encounter with the antigen and the nature of the antigen determines which B-cell subset becomes terminally differentiated to plasma cells (40). Plasma cells also develop from activated B1 cells in the peritoneal and pleural cavities; after activation, the B1 cells migrate to the spleen or gut, lose CD5 expression, and become antibody-secreting plasma cells (3). Plasma cells show substantial diminishment of B-cell antigens and surface immunoglobulin, with increased cytoplasmic immunoglobulin meant for secretion. Plasma cells express transcription factor MUM-1, as well as CD38 and CD138. Memory B cells preferentially home to marginal zones, which are

Table 1-2

DEVELOPMENTAL STAGES OF T CELLS[a]

	TCR Gene	Immunophenotype	Comments
Precursor			
Prothymocyte	Germline	CD2, CD7, CD44	
Triple negative thymocyte	Rearranged	CD1, CD2, cCD3, CD7, CD25, CD44, CD45RA	Lack of sCD3, CD4, CD8
Double negative thymocyte	Rearranged	CD1, CD2, cCD3, CD7, CD45RA	Lack of CD4, CD8, expression of pre-T receptor[b]
Double positive thymocyte	Rearranged	CD1, CD2, cCD3, CD4, CD7, CD8, CD45RO	Expression of CD4, CD8
Triple positive thymocyte	Rearranged	CD1, CD2, sCD3, CD4, CD7, CD8, CD27, CD69, CD45RO	Expression of sCD3, CD4, CD8
Naive Mature T Cell	Rearranged	Pan-T[c], CD27, CD69, CD45RA	CD4 or CD8
Antigen-Dependent Interactions			
T immunoblast	Rearranged	Pan-T, HLA-DR, CD25, CD38, CD71	CD4 or CD8
Effector cell	Rearranged	Pan-T, CD45RO	CD4 or CD8
Memory cell	Rearranged	Pan-T, CD45RO	CD4 or CD8

[a]This table compares T-cell receptor (*TCR*) gene configuration and immunophenotype of the major types of T cells. While the earliest precursor T cells arise from the bone marrow, the precursor types here occupy the cortex of the thymus. Mature naive T cells circulate in the peripheral blood and in the T-cell areas of lymphoid tissues, where the latter T-cell types after antigen interaction are also found.

[b]The pre-T receptor is the β chain binding to a surrogate α chain to form a complex with CD3 at the surface of the prothymocyte, a step necessary for thymocyte maturation.

[c]Pan-T cell markers are CD2, cytoplasmic and surface CD3, CD4 or CD8, CD5 and CD7.

best developed in spleen, mucosal-associated lymphoid tissue, and mesenteric lymph nodes. Memory B cells are notable for strong IgM but little IgD expression.

T Lymphocytes

Similar to B-cell development, *precursor T cells* arise from hematopoietic stem cells; the progenitor cells travel from the bone marrow to the thymus. Within the thymus, T-cell development (Table 1-2) begins in the cortex through the interaction with soluble factors and thymic stroma. The earliest precursor T cells are pluripotent, resemble lymphoblasts, and express CD34 and CD7. Cortical thymocytes sequentially acquire antigens CD1, CD2, CD5, and cytoplasmic CD3, followed by CD4 and CD8. Rearrangement of T-cell receptor genes also occurs within the thymus (gamma [γ] and delta [δ] genes simultaneously with beta [β], followed by alpha [α] chain genes) with proteins expressed on the surface of the thymocyte. Surface CD3 and T-cell receptor beta chain appear at approximately the same time, with cortical thymocytes expressing CD45RO and lacking CD45RA and bcl-2 protein (21,41). When CD4 and CD8 expression is acquired, cortical thymocytes undergo thymic education in which T cells are selected for their ability to bind MHC (*positive selection*) and their lack of binding to self antigens (*negative selection*) (34,46). In positive selection, thymocytes interact with thymic epithelial cells expressing MHC-autologous peptides; those cells that fail to recognize autologous MHC undergo apoptosis in the medulla. In negative selection, bone marrow–derived dendritic cells expressing autologous peptides bind thymocytes; double positive thymocytes that have surface antigen receptors which bind strongly to self antigens die. Only a few T cells survive thymic education to become naive mature CD4 or CD8 cells. These cells now express increased amounts of surface CD3, lose CD1, switch from CD45RO to CD45RA, acquire CD27 and CD69, and lose either CD4 or CD8 to become virgin mature T cells (41).

Antigen *naive T cells* resemble small lymphocytes with condensed, mature chromatin and are found in the peripheral blood and paracortex of lymph nodes (figs. 1-12, 1-13). They express either CD4 or CD8, and surface CD3, CD5, CD45RA, and bcl-2. These mature cells lack the immature markers CD1 and TdT found on precursor T cells (21) and have rearranged T-cell receptor genes. Antigen-dependent T-cell differentiation requires the interaction of the CD4- or CD8-positive T cells with MHC

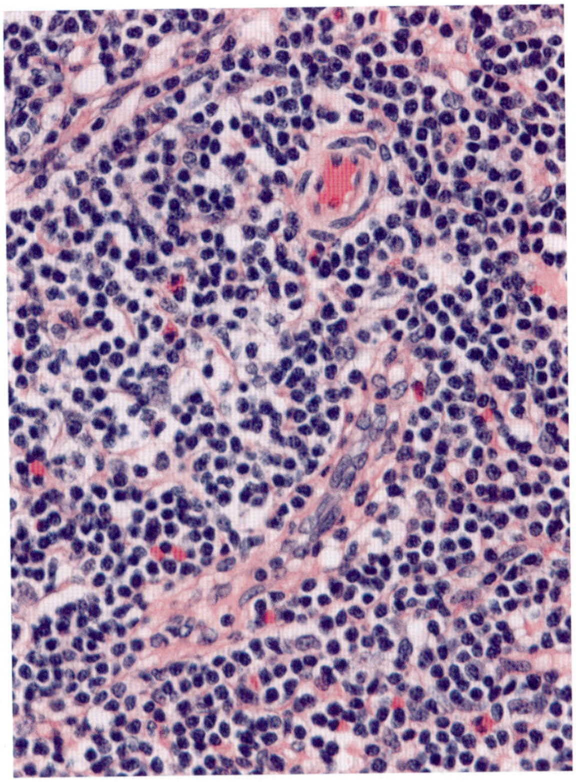

Figure 1-12

PARACORTEX OF LYMPH NODE

Numerous high endothelial venules are surrounded by small, bland lymphocytes with condensed chromatin.

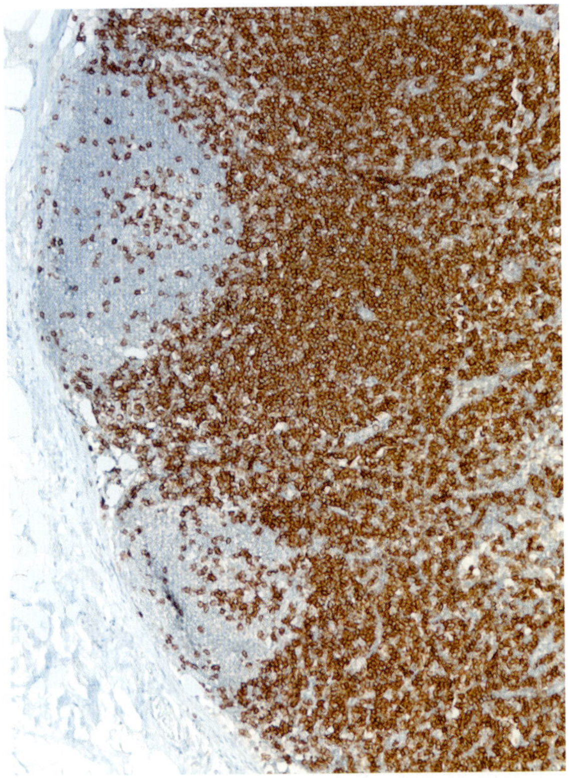

Figure 1-13

PARACORTEX OF LYMPH NODE

CD3 highlights numerous T cells within the paracortex. These T cells are a mixture of CD4- and CD8-positive T cells, and CD45RA-positive naive and CD45RO-positive memory T cells (not shown).

class II or class I molecules, respectively, on antigen-presenting cells, and occurs within the paracortex of lymph nodes and periarteriolar lymphoid sheath of the spleen.

A number of different complexes and molecules bind the T cell to the antigen presenting cell, in addition to stimulatory factors released by both cells: CD3/T-cell receptor (TCR) to antigen/MHC, adhesion molecule lymphocyte function-associated antigen (LFA)1 to intercellular adhesion molecule (ICAM)1, CD40L to CD40 (resulting in activation of both cells), CD28/CTLA4 to CD80 or CD86 (second T-cell stimulus)(15). These interactions are necessary for T-cell activation, proliferation, and differentiation.

After these interactions, naive T cells transform into T immunoblasts, large blastic cells with prominent nucleoli. These mature cells show an immunophenotype similar to that of naive T cells, with the addition of HLA-DR, CD25, CD38, and CD71. Arising from T immunoblasts are antigen-specific T-effector cells and T-memory cells. CD4-positive T-effector cells are helper cells and CD8-positive T-effector cells are suppressor cells; both act as cytotoxic T cells depending on antigen reactivity coupled with the appropriate MHC class molecule. These cells may express T-cell receptor α/β (predominantly lymphoid tissues) or γ/δ (spleen, mucosa), and also produce cytokines that modulate the immune response.

Natural Killer Cells

Natural killer (NK) *cells* are present in the paracortex of lymph nodes surrounding B-cell follicles and in close proximity to dendritic cells. These lymph node NK cells express CD56, CD94, NKG2A, and NKG2D, but lack perforin and the cytotoxic features found in circulating NK cells. The lymph node NK cells either develop into

Table 1-3

CLASSIFICATION OF DENDRITIC CELLS

B-Cell Associated	Lymphatic Tissue	T-Cell Associated Blood/Lymph	Nonlymphatic
Follicular DC[a]	Interdigitating cells Plasmacytoid DC	Veiled cells	Langerhans cells Connective tissue DC Indeterminate DC

[a]DC = dendritic cells.

cytotoxic NK cells via priming from dendritic cells or induce Th1 polarization (45).

Dendritic Cells

Dendritic cells are nonlymphoid antigen-presenting cells that lack phagocytic activity. Their complex cytoplasmic projections have the ability to activate T cells and trigger the immune response. Functionally, dendritic cells are divided into B-cell– and T-cell–associated dendritic cells (Table 1-3). Follicular dendritic cells represent the B-cell–associated dendritic cell, whereas the T-cell–associated dendritic cells include nonlymphatic tissue dendritic cells (i.e., epidermal and dermal Langerhans cells, connective tissue dendritic cells, dendritic cells of unknown origin), dendritic cells in blood and lymph (i.e., veiled cells), and interdigitating dendritic cells (22).

Follicular dendritic cells are present within the follicles (primary and secondary) of secondary lymphoid tissues (figs. 1-8, 1-9). These cells form a three-dimensional network via the interdigitation of cell processes. Follicular dendritic cells trap and retain antigen-antibody complexes, presenting them to memory B cells on their cell surface, held by Fc (CD32, CD23) or complement (CD21, CD35) receptors. Follicular dendritic cells also bind B cells via adhesion molecules (CD44, ICAM-1, vascular cell adhesion molecule [VCAM]-1), prevent apoptosis with the production of antiapoptotic molecule BAFF (B-cell–activating factor of the tumor necrosis factor family), and stimulate B-cell proliferation via 8D6 and interleukin (IL)-15 (36).

The development of the follicular dendritic cell network in the germinal center requires the proper microenvironment, including the presence of B and T cells, as suggested by mouse and in vitro human studies (36). The origin of follicular dendritic cells is either from the bone marrow or from differentiation of stromal cells. Follicular dendritic cells share numerous surface markers and ultrastructural features found in fibroblasts (35,22). Six subtypes of follicular dendritic cells have been described based on morphology, phenotype, and ability to retain immune complexes (4).

The T-cell compartment of the lymphoid tissue yields two types of dendritic cells, interdigitating and plasmacytoid dendritic cells. These dendritic cells are present in the paracortex of the lymph node where they cluster with T cells. Interdigitating dendritic cells are CD11c positive and have long cytoplasmic projections, whereas plasmacytoid dendritic cells lack CD11c and resemble plasma cells (10). Plasmacytoid dendritic cells express CD123, BDCA2, CD45RA, and Toll-like receptors 7 and 9; they produce type I interferon on exposure to viruses (45). Interdigitating dendritic cells are thought to derive from Langerhans cells, migrating from the epidermis to a draining lymph node upon acquiring antigen. Three subsets of lymph node dendritic cells were identified in one study based on the variable expression of CD1a, CD86, and CD83, and tentatively identified as immature dendritic cells migrating from epidermis, interdigitating dendritic cells, and activated interdigitating dendritic cells (43).

In the paracortex, dendritic cells take up antigen and interact with the naive T cells entering through high endothelial venules (13). There are two theories for how resident dendritic cells acquire antigen. One is that antigen is drained from the periphery into lymph, which then enters the lymphatic sinuses of the lymph node and interacts with resident dendritic cells in the lymph node (8). Or, antigen is carried by migratory dendritic cells from peripheral sites to the lymph node via lymphatic vessels, passing antigen to the resident dendritic cells of the lymph node and/or presenting antigen for T-cell stimulation directly (38). In vivo studies

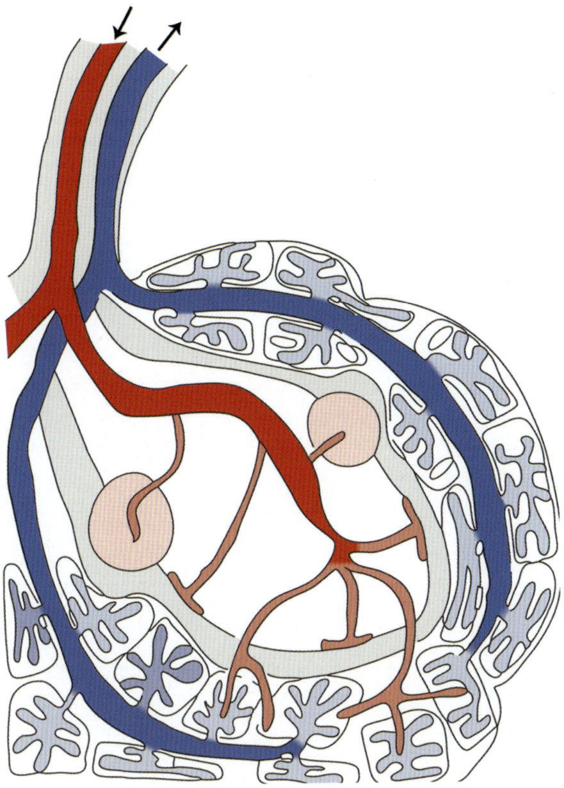

Figure 1-14

STRUCTURE OF THE SPLEEN

Arterial blood (red) travels to arterioles and passes into germinal centers, cordal macrophages (open circulation), or adjacent to sinuses (closed circulation). Blood in sinuses (pale blue) travels into trabecular veins (blue) and then into the splenic vein.

of naive T cells show that random mechanisms explain their interaction with dendritic cells (7). The dendritic cells activate these naive T cells, interacting with about 500 different T cells in 1 hour (5). Dendritic cells either induce tolerance or immunity based on the maturation or activation of the dendritic cell at the time of antigen presentation (44).

SPLEEN

The spleen as an organ is unique in its combination of functions: immunologic, hematopoietic, filtration, and storage. As an immunologic organ, the spleen has capabilities comparable to those in other secondary lymphoid tissues, with well-defined B- and T-cell zones, and is involved in both innate and adaptive immune responses. The spleen also is an important source of hematopoiesis in fetal life and a site of extramedullary hematopoiesis in certain disease states. The spleen plays an important role in the phagocytosis of blood-borne microorganisms and cellular debris. The spleen also acts in the quality control of circulating elements of the hematopoietic system, filtering out those red blood cells that lack membrane deformability. Lastly, the spleen is a site of storage of mature hematopoietic elements and may sequester cellular elements, resulting in splenomegaly.

Table 1-4

RANGE OF NORMAL SPLEEN WEIGHTS

	Male	Female
Adult[a]	168 (60-378) g	135 (46-315) g
Adult[b]	156+/-87 (30-580) g	140+/-78 (33-481) g

[a]Sprogoe-Jakobsen S, Sprogoe-Jakobsen U. The weight of the normal spleen. Forensic Sci Int 1997;88:215-223.
[b]de la Grandmaison GL, Clairand I, Durigon M. Organ weight in 684 adult autopsies: new tables for a caucasoid population. Forensic Sci Int 2001;119:149-154.

Anatomy

The spleen is encased by a fibrous capsule, penetrated at the hilus by vessels and nerves that follow an interconnected complex of fibrous trabeculae. The capsule and trabeculae form a framework on which is interposed a network of arteries and arterioles surrounded by lymphoid tissue or the white pulp of the spleen. Interspersed between the white pulp is a complex venous sinusoidal system, in which vascular sinuses collect blood, separated by a reticular network of splenic cords (red pulp). The latter drain into small pulp and trabecular veins which terminate in the splenic vein (fig. 1-14).

The normal weight of the spleen varies with age, sex, height, and body weight; normal spleen weights are given in Table 1-4. Accessory spleens occur in approximately 10 percent of people. The cut surface of the spleen is beefy red, in which small white pulp nodules (malpighian corpuscles) are scattered.

White Pulp

Microscopically, the white pulp contains T-cell and B-cell zones organized around central arterioles, similar in structure to the lymph node (figs. 1-15–1-17). The T-cell zone corresponds to

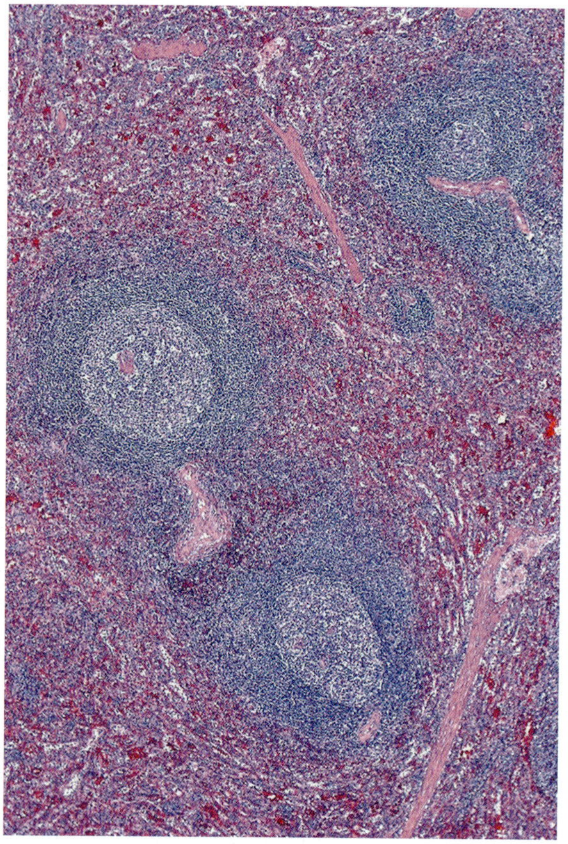

Figure 1-15

SPLENIC WHITE PULP

Low-magnification image of periarteriolar lymphoid sheath (PALS) and secondary follicles, with adjacent red pulp.

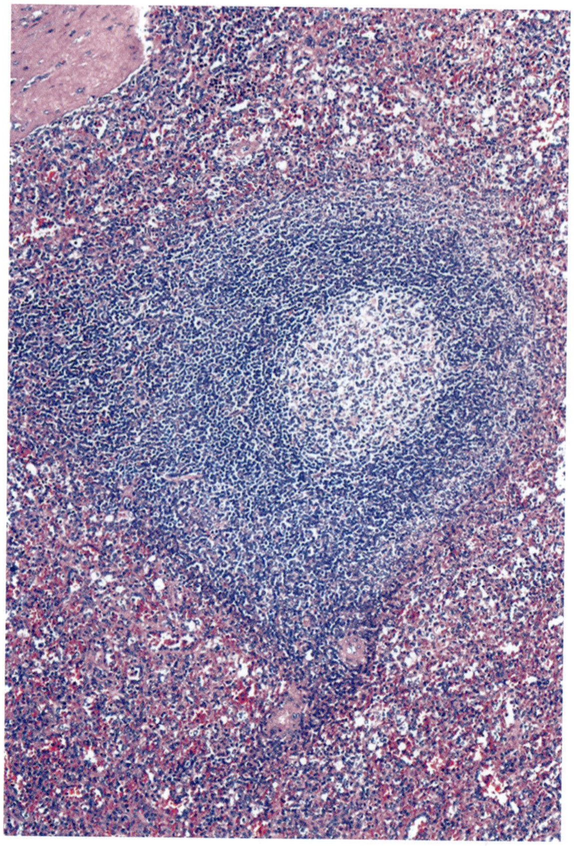

Figure 1-16

SPLENIC SECONDARY FOLLICLE WITH MARGINAL ZONE

Low-magnification image of a secondary follicle with surrounding mantle and marginal zones. A portion of the PALS is seen adjacent to the follicle.

the *periarteriolar lymphoid sheath* (PALS) while the B-cell zone is organized into follicles. T cell-dendritic cell and T cell-B cell interactions occur in the PALS and clonal expansion of activated B cells occurs in the follicles. B-cell follicles include both primary and secondary follicles. B cells are attracted to their appropriate areas by CXCL13 (produced by follicular dendritic cells and stromal cells) (2), whereas migration of T cells and dendritic cells to the T-cell zones of the white pulp is mediated by CCL19 and CCL21 (17). These chemokine ligands are controlled by stromal cells via the lymphotoxin-β and tumor-necrosis factor receptors and induce a positive-feedback loop: signaling through the B-cell receptor CXCR5 induces expression of lymphotoxin–α1β2 on the B cells, which induces differentiation of follicular dendritic cells, which then express the chemokine ligand CXCL13 (32). Similarly, the T-cell zone is regulated via other chemokine receptors, with chemokines CCL19 and CCL21 produced by stromal and dendritic cells in the T-cell area (17).

The white pulp is involved primarily in the adaptive immune response in which rare lymphocytes with appropriate antigen specificity detect foreign antigens. The initiation of this response is the entry of antigen-presenting cells to the white pulp through the marginal zone. After entry, in a manner analogous to migration of lymphocytes in lymph nodes, T cells are activated, resulting in chemokine expression and allowing them to migrate toward the edge of follicles (1). Similarly, after B cells bind antigen, upregulation of chemokine CCR7 allows B cells to migrate to the edge of follicles (39). At this location, B cells contact activated T cells,

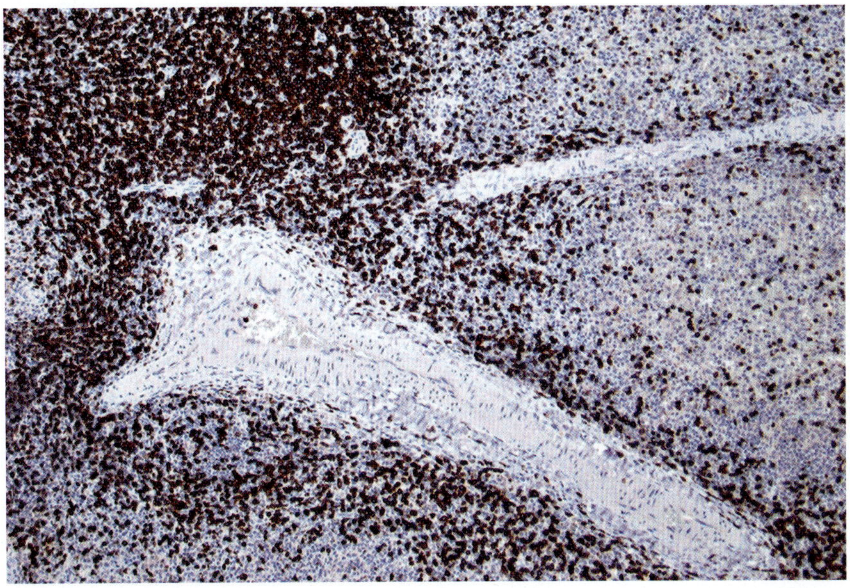

Figure 1-17

SPLENIC WHITE PULP

The PALS contains a predominance of T cells, labeled with CD3. The follicles, in contrast, are comprised of B cells.

after which they switch their isotype and either remain in the germinal center, or migrate to the marginal zone and red pulp.

Antigens and other small molecules also enter the white pulp via a conduit system similar to the conduit system described in the lymph nodes (see above) (33). Whereas in lymph nodes, this transport network carries lymph, in the spleen, this network carries small molecules in blood. Chemokines carried in the conduit system (and perhaps produced by reticular fibroblasts surrounding the transport network) are thought to direct migration and retention of cellular elements within the white pulp (33). Exit of lymphocytes from the white pulp is presumed to occur through the marginal zone into the red pulp and subsequently to the bloodstream, with the exclusion of lymphocytes from the white pulp mediated by chemokine expression (30).

Marginal Zone

The marginal zone is particularly well developed in the spleen and represents an important site in the immunologic function of the spleen when cells leave the blood and enter the white pulp; entry of lymphocytes into the white pulp depends on signaling through G-protein–coupled receptors (14). The marginal zone is composed of a framework of reticular fibroblasts, marginal zone B cells, dendritic cells, and two types of specific macrophages. The marginal zone macrophages form an outer layer of macrophages in the marginal zone, while the marginal zone metallophilic macrophages form an inner layer of macrophages within the marginal zone. Sandwiched between these layers are marginal zone B cells and dendritic cells (30). The cells of the marginal zone depend on each other for localization and maintain the structure of the marginal zone via chemokines and other molecules (30).

The marginal zone is also the site of innate immunity in which blood-borne microorganisms and antigens are trapped via specific receptors expressed by the cells of the marginal zone, as well as the site of adaptive immunity. Marginal zone macrophages express Toll-like receptors (which recognize unique structures on the surface of microorganisms), the type I scavenger receptor MARCO (recognizes *Escherichia coli* and *Staphylococcus aureus*) and the C-type lectin SIGNR1 (binds polysaccharide antigens such as in *Mycobacterium tuberculosis*). Marginal zone metallophilic macrophages are known to express SIGLEC1 and bind sialic acid–containing molecules at the cell surface of pathogens such as *Neisseria meningitidis*. Marginal zone B cells also detect blood-borne microorganisms, responding by functioning as antigen-presenting cells or differentiating into IgM-secreting plasma cells. After activation, some marginal zone B cells and dendritic cells migrate to the B-cell follicles of the white pulp (via chemokine

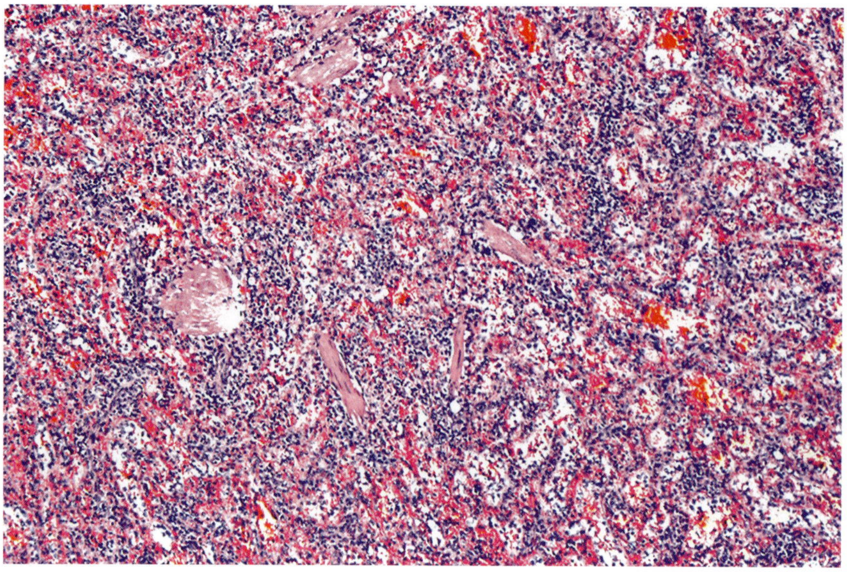

Figure 1-18

SPLENIC RED PULP

Low magnification of red pulp shows cords and sinus.

receptor signaling), becoming antigen-presenting cells and stimulating naive CD4-positive T cells. After uptake of viral pathogens, marginal zone metallophilic macrophages produce interferons alpha and beta (30).

When immature B cells leave the bone marrow, some continue to develop in the spleen where they undergo negative selection in their continued development (11). These B cells pass through two transitional stages before a small subset travels to the splenic marginal zone and remains as naive sessile marginal zone B cells (37). The decision of whether to make marginal zone B cells or follicular B cells is controlled by a complex amalgam of signals involving Notch-2 and E proteins and B-cell receptor signal strength; the exact contributions of each of these mechanisms is unclear at this time (30). For B cells to remain in the marginal zone, signaling through the lysophospholipid sphingosine 1-phosphate (S1P) receptor is necessary, which overrides the B-cell follicle chemoattractant CXCL13 (12), as well as expression of integrins LFA1 and α4β1-integrin (29). These naive marginal zone B cells express high levels of IgM, CD1d, CD9, CD21, and CD22, and low levels of IgD, CD23, and B220. Marginal zone B cells predominantly recognize T-cell–independent type 2 (TI-2) antigens and have a lower threshold for activation of antigen (35).

After these sessile cells encounter a TI-2 antigen, the marginal zone B cells migrate to the bridging channels and red pulp of the spleen. Here they proliferate and differentiate into plasmablasts (28). The majority of B cells, however, mature into naive follicular B cells, which are long-lived B cells that recirculate to follicles in the spleen, lymph nodes, and bone marrow until they encounter antigen and maturate further or die. After marginal zone B cells encounter antigen, they downregulate S1P expression and integrins LFA1 and α4β1-integrin, which allows localization to the B-cell follicle (12). Circulating mature follicular B cells may also develop into plasma cells after encountering antigen with T-cell help, forming foci of plasmablasts and plasma cells along the periphery of the periarteriolar lymphoid sheath (40).

Red Pulp

The red pulp of the spleen contains the venous sinusoidal system and is the site of blood filtration, iron recycling, removal of bacteria from the blood, and localization of plasma cells (figs. 1-18, 1-19). Arterial blood from the splenic cords (which lack an endothelial lining) passes into the venous sinuses in the red pulp. The venous sinuses are lined by discontinuous endothelial cells in a parallel arrangement. Stress fibers underpin the long axis of these endothelial cells. Perpendicular annular fibers connect the stress fibers to each other, forming a flexible tube in which blood from the cords is passed into the sinuses through endothelial cell slits.

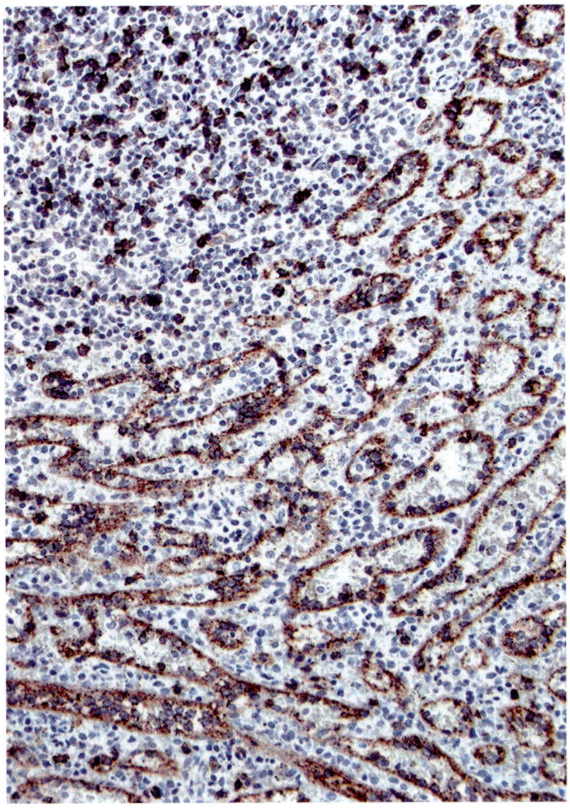

Figure 1-19

SPLENIC RED PULP

There is a predominance of CD8-positive T cells.

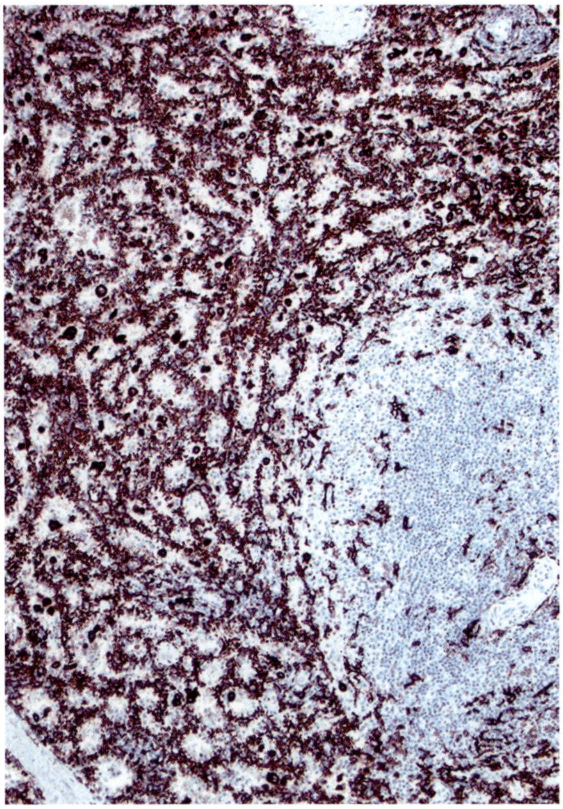

Figure 1-20

SPLENIC MACROPHAGES

CD163, the macrophage scavenger receptor, labels splenic macrophages located within the red pulp and marginal zone.

Nondeformable erythrocytes, such as older red blood cells, are unable to make this transition and are phagocytosed by macrophages within the cords (fig. 1-20) (30).

After phagocytosing erythrocytes (i.e., extravascular hemolysis), splenic macrophages recycle iron. Red blood cells are hydrolyzed in the phagolysosome of the macrophage and hemoglobin is degraded into heme. Heme is catabolized into ferrous iron, which is either stored as ferritin or released. Hemosiderin, readily seen in splenic macrophages, represents complexes of ferritin. Iron released from the macrophages is bound to plasma transferrin and is regulated by bone marrow needs. The spleen is also involved in intravascular hemolysis, in which free hemoglobin bound to haptoglobin is endocytosed by macrophages using a hemoglobin-specific receptor, CD163 (30).

The red pulp is also the site of removal of bacteria from the blood. Macrophages express Toll-like receptors, which recognize unique structures present on the surface of bacteria. Signaling through these receptors allows the macrophage to secrete lipocalin-2, which forms a complex with bacterial siderophores, successfully sequestering iron and limiting bacterial growth (16). The red pulp is also the location of plasma cells and plasmablasts, formed after antigen-specific differentiation in the white pulp (40). The plasmablasts migrate to the splenic red pulp via chemokine receptor signals. The red pulp expresses the chemokine CXCL12, which binds chemokine receptor CXCR4 present in increased levels on the plasmablasts migrating to the red pulp (20). The presence of CD11c-positive dendritic cells is also necessary for this transition (18).

REFERENCES

1. Ansel KM, McHeyzer-Williams LJ, Ngo VN, McHeyzer-Williams MG, Cyster JG. In vivo-activated CD4 T cells upregulate CXC chemokine receptor 5 and reprogram their response to lymphoid chemokines. J Exp Med 1999;190:1123-34.
2. Ansel KM, Ngo VN, Hyman PL, et al. A chemokine-driven positive feedback loop organizes lymphoid follicles. Nature 2000;406:309-14.
3. Bikah G, Carey J, Ciallella JR, Tarakhovsky A, Bondada S. CD5-mediated negative regulation of antigen receptor-induced growth signals in B-1 B cells. Science 1996;274:1906-9.
4. Bofill M, Akbar AN, Amlot PL. Follicular dendritic cells share a membrane-bound protein with fibroblasts. J Pathol 2000;191:217-26.
5. Bousso P, Robey E. Dynamics of CD8+ T cell priming by dendritic cells in intact lymph nodes. Nat Immunol 2003;4:579-85.
6. Busslinger M. Transcriptional control of early B cell development. Annu Rev Immunol 2004;22:55-79.
7. Cahalan MD, Parker I, Wei SH, Miller MJ. Real-time imaging of lymphocytes in vivo. Curr Opin Immunol 2003;15:372-7.
8. Carbone FR, Belz GT, Heath WR. Transfer of antigen between migrating and lymph node-resident DCs in peripheral T-cell tolerance and immunity. Trends Immunol 2004;25:655-8.
9. Catron DM, Itano AA, Pape KA, Mueller DL, Jenkins MK. Visualizing the first 50 hr of the primary immune response to a soluble antigen. Immunity 2004;21:341-7.
10. Cella M, Facchetti F, Lanzavecchia A, Colonna M. Plasmacytoid dendritic cells activated by influenza virus and CD40L drive a potent Th1 polarization. Nat Immunol 2000;1:305-10.
11. Chung JB, Silverman M, Monroe JG. Transitional B cells: step by step towards immune competence. Trends Immunol 2003;24:343-9.
12. Cinamon G, Matloubian M, Lesneski MJ, et al. Sphingosine 1-phosphate receptor 1 promotes B cell localization in the splenic marginal zone. Nat Immunol 2004;5:713-20.
13. Crivellato E, Vacca A, Ribatti D. Setting the stage: an anatomist's view of the immune system. Trends Immunol 2004;25:210-7.
14. Cyster JG, Goodnow CC. Pertussis toxin inhibits migration of B and T lymphocytes into splenic white pulp cords. J Exp Med 1995;182:581-6.
15. Durie FH, Foy TM, Masters SR, Laman JD, Noelle RJ. The role of CD40 in the regulation of humoral and cell-mediated immunity. Immunol Today 1994;15:406-11.
16. Flo TH, Smith KD, Sato S, et al. Lipocalin 2 mediates an innate immune response to bacterial infection by sequestrating iron. Nature 2004;432:917-21.
17. Forster R, Schubel A, Breitfeld D, et al. CCR7 coordinates the primary immune response by establishing functional microenvironments in secondary lymphoid organs. Cell 1999;99:23-33.
18. Garcia De Vinuesa C, Gulbranson-Judge A, Khan M, et al. Dendritic cells associated with plasmablast survival. Eur J Immunol 1999;29:3712-21.
19. Hardy RR, Hayakawa K. B cell development pathways. Annu Rev Immunol 2001;19:595-621.
20. Hargreaves DC, Hyman PL, Lu TT, et al. A coordinated change in chemokine responsiveness guides plasma cell movements. J Exp Med 2001;194:45-56.
21. Hockenbery D, Zutter M, Hickey W, Nahm M, Korsmeyer SJ. BCL2 protein is topographically restricted in tissues characterized by apoptotic cell death. Proc Natl Acad Sci U S A 1991;88:6961-5.
22. Imal Y, Yamakawa M. Morphology, function and pathology of follicular dendritic cells. Pathol Int 1996;46:807-33.
23. Janossy G, Bollum F, Bradstock K, Ashley J. Cellular phenotypes of normal and leukemic hematopoietic cells determined by analysis with selected antibody combinations. Blood 1980;56:430-41.
24. Kipps T. The CD5 B cell. Adv Immunol 1989; 47:117-85.
25. Klein U, Kuppers R, Rajewsky K. Human IgM+IgD+ B cells, the major B cell subset in the peripheral blood, express Vh genes with no or little somatic mutation throughout life. Eur J Immunol 1993;23:3272-7.
26. Kuppers R, Zhao M, Hansmann ML, Rajewsky K. Tracing B cell development in human germinal centres by molecular analysis of single cells picked from histological sections. EMBO J 1993;12:4955-67.
27. Lindhout E, Koopman G, Pals ST, de Groot C. Triple check for antigen specificity of B cells during germinal centre reactions. Immunol Today 1997;18:573-7.
28. Lopes-Carvalho T, Kearney JF. Development and selection of marginal zone B cells. Immunol Rev 2004;197:192-205.
29. Lu TT, Cyster JG. Integrin-mediated long-term B cell retention in the splenic marginal zone. Science 2002;297:409-12.
30. Mebius RE, Kraal G. Structure and function of the spleen. Nat Rev Immunol 2005;5:606-16.

31. Muller G, Hopken UE, Lipp M. The impact of CCR7 and CXCR5 on lymphoid organ development and systemic immunity. Immunol Rev 2003;195:117-35.
32. Ngo VN, Korner H, Gunn MD, et al. Lymphotoxin alpha/beta and tumor necrosis factor are required for stromal cell expression of homing chemokines in B and T cell areas of the spleen. J Exp Med 1999;189:403-12.
33. Nolte MA, Belien JA, Schadee-Eestermans I, et al. A conduit system distributes chemokines and small blood-borne molecules through the splenic white pulp. J Exp Med 2003;198:505-12.
34. Nossal GJ. Negative selection of lymphocytes. Cell 1994;76:229-39.
35. Oliver AM, Martin F, Gartland GL, Carter RH, Kearney JF. Marginal zone B cells exhibit unique activation, proliferative and immunoglobulin secretory responses. Eur J Immunol 1997;27:2366-74.
36. Park CS, Choi YS. How do follicular dendritic cells interact intimately with B cells in the germinal centre? Immunology 2005;114:2-10.
37. Pillai S, Cariappa A, Moran ST. Marginal zone B cells. Annu Rev Immunol 2005;23:161-96.
38. Randolph GJ, Angeli V, Swartz MA. Dendritic-cell trafficking to lymph nodes through lymphatic vessels. Nat Rev Immunol 2005;5:617-28.
39. Reif K, Ekland EH, Ohl L, et al. Balanced responsiveness to chemoattractants from adjacent zones determines B-cell position. Nature 2002;416:94-9.
40. Shapiro-Shelef M, Calame K. Regulation of plasma-cell development. Nat Rev Immunol 2005;5:230-42.
41. Spits H, Lanier L, Phillips JH. Development of human T and natural killer cells. Blood 1995;85:2654-70.
42. Stein H, Coupland SE, Hummel M. Genetic events and gene expression in B-cell differentiation: implications for lymphoma classification. Hematology (Am Soc Hematol Educ Program) 2001;194-200.
43. Takahashi K, Asagoe K, Zaishun J, et al. Heterogeneity of dendritic cells in human superficial lymph node: in vitro maturation of immature dendritic cells into mature or activated interdigitating reticulum cells. Am J Pathol 1998;153:745-55.
44. Tan JK, O'Neill HC. Maturation requirements for dendritic cells in T cell stimulation leading to tolerance versus immunity. J Leukoc Biol 2005;78:319-24.
45. Zitvogel L, Terme M, Borg C, Trinchieri G. Dendritic cell-NK cell cross-talk: regulation and physiopathology. Curr Top Microbiol Immunol 2006;298:157-74.
46. Zuniga-Pflucker JC, Jones LA, Chin LT, Kruisbeek AM. CD4 and CD8 act as co-receptors during thymic selection of the T cell repertoire. Semin Immunol 1991;3:167-75.

2 EMBRYOLOGY AND HISTOLOGY OF THE LYMPH NODE AND SPLEEN

EMBRYOLOGY OF THE SPLEEN

The tissue that will ultimately form the spleen is first identifiable in the human embryo during the 5th week of gestation. This tissue consists of condensations of mesodermal tissue between the left dorsal mesogastrium, a portion of the mesentery attaching the primitive stomach to the dorsal portion of the abdominal wall. During the 6th and 7th weeks of development, the mesenchymal nodules condense and become vascularized. These nodules, which form the splenic anlage, are the structures that underlie notches or grooves on the surface of the organ (12,57). Patterson et al. (61) illustrated that the mesodermal precursor of spleen is a symmetric bilateral structure (fig. 2-1). The left and right components seem to undergo different differentiation pathways, but not differential apoptosis, like most asymmetric organs. The development of spleen sidedness appears to be dependent on the direction of gut rotation and pancreas sidedness, suggesting a complex interplay of factors in the development of spleen location. In cases of bilateral left sidedness, two spleens would be expected to develop.

The spleen develops in three stages. The first is characterized by the proliferation of blood vessels and the differentiation of reticular or stromal cells. In the second stage, the structure of the mature spleen begins to form, including central arteries and the supporting stromal framework for both red and white pulp. The final stage is characterized by colonization of the white pulp region with lymphocytes. Although anatomically resembling the mature organ, the immature fetal spleen does not gain complete functional capacity until later into the first antenatal year.

Architecturally, the perinatal spleen consists of normal-appearing red pulp, with occasional nucleated red blood cell islands and rare megakaryocytes. The white pulp is composed of predominantly primary follicles, without reactive, secondary germinal centers. Even in septic neonates, reactive germinal centers are not seen until 2 to 4 weeks after birth. The splenic marginal zone does not develop until after birth, adding to the relative immaturity of the perinatal immune response. The periarteriolar lymphoid sheath (PALS) T-cell regions of the spleen are composed of small to intermediate-sized lymphocytes, with occasional admixed plasma cells and granulocytes.

EMBRYOLOGIC ABNORMALITIES OF THE SPLEEN

Accessory Spleen, Ectopic Spleen, and Polysplenia

Accessory spleens, or *spleniculi*, are common incidental findings that are seen in 20 to 30 percent of the population (figs. 2-2, 2-3). *Ectopic spleen* is a less desirable term for these displaced embryologic fragments, causing confusion with splenosis; *splenosis* refers to implanted fragments of splenic tissue that are usually associated with trauma. Table 2-1 describes the embryologic abnormalities associated with the spleen. Splenosis is discussed in depth in chapter 18.

Accessory spleens are most commonly single, but can be multiple. The most common locations for accessory spleens are in regions that are anatomically and embryologically related to normal spleen development. The hilum of the spleen is a common site, as is the gastrosplenic ligament as well as within the mesentery. Accessory spleen is seen in the tail of the pancreas (fig. 2-4). Rare cases of normal splenic tissue partly or entirely encapsulated by liver tissue have been reported (17).

Polysplenia is the result of incomplete fusion of splenic mesenchymal nodules in normal development. Two to nine tissue masses of approximately equal size can result. Embryologic abnormalities of splenic development may signal underlying abnormalities of asymmetry (see Asplenia, below). The most common abnormality is *situs ambiguous with polysplenia,* characterized by midline or abnormal locations

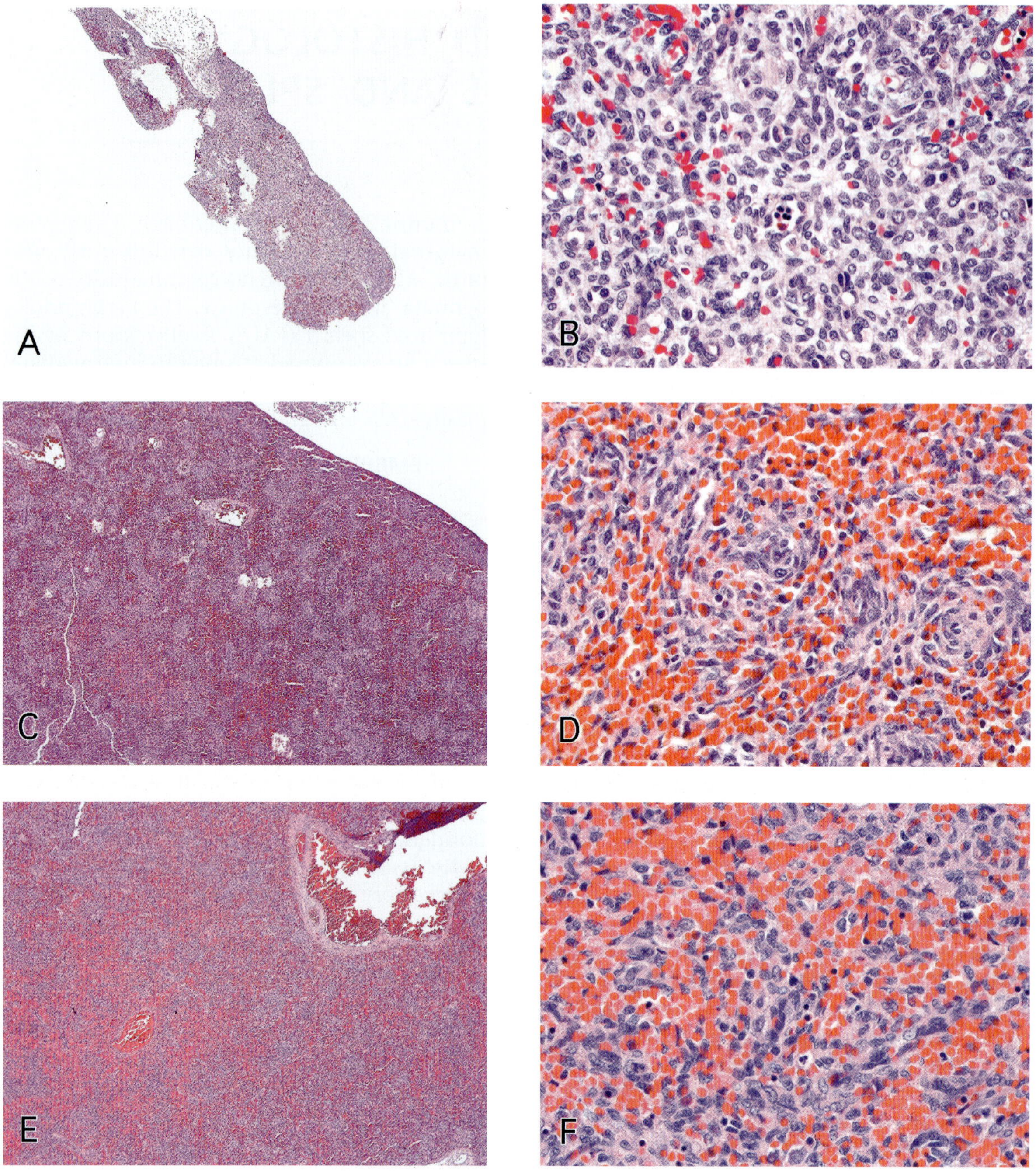

Figure 2- 1

EMBRYOLOGIC DEVELOPMENT OF SPLEEN

A,B: At the estimated gestational age (EGA) of 11 weeks, a fragment of developing spleen, composed predominantly of undifferentiated spindle-shaped stromal cells, shows the formation of some small blood vessels (A: low-power magnification; B: high-power magnification).

C,D: At EGA of 14 weeks, a vague nodular pattern is seen, suggesting division into red pulp and white pulp. Nodular elements have a storiform pattern suggesting the development of white pulp architecture. Red blood cells and nucleated erythroid precursors are present in the nascent red pulp (C: low-power magnification; D: high-power magnification).

E,F: At EGA of 17 weeks, the red pulp and white pulp divisions are more defined. Large blood vessels are apparent (E: low-power magnification; F: high-power magnification).

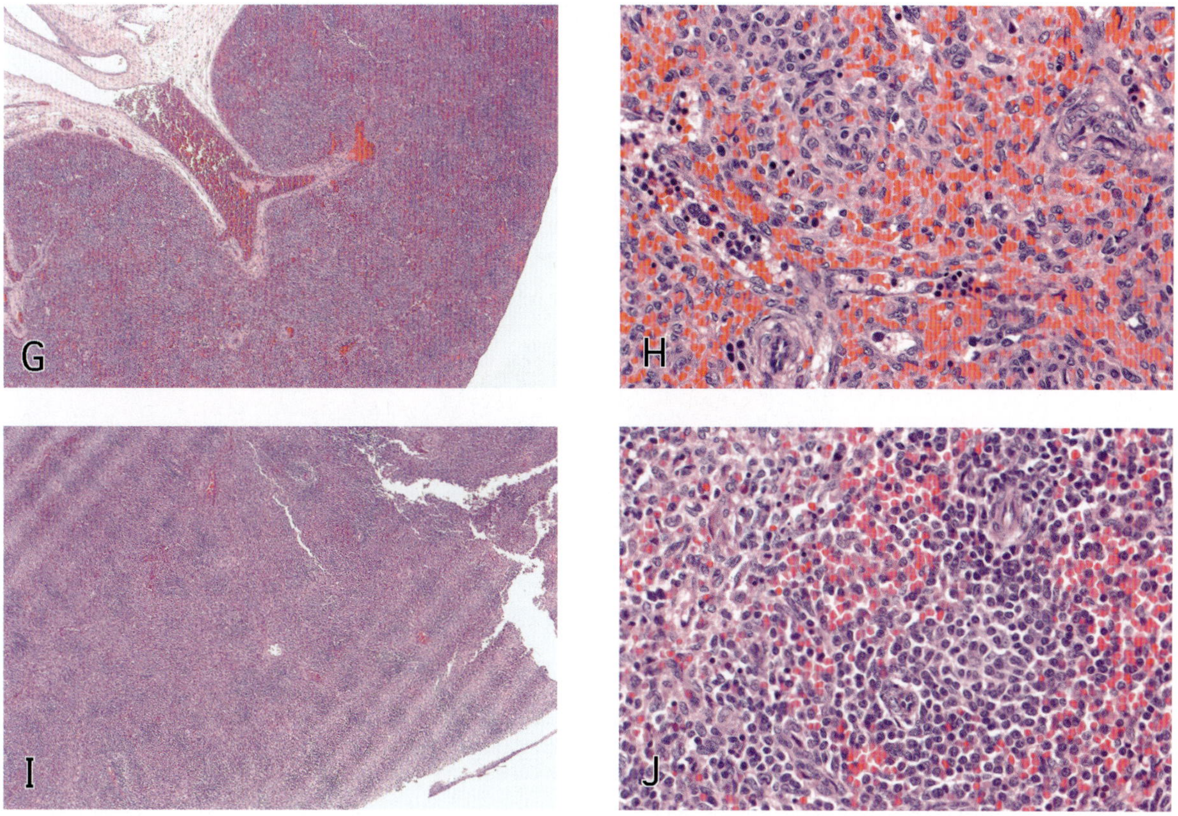

Figure 2-1 (continued)

G,H: At EGA of 19 weeks, an increase in cellularity is appreciated, and the well-formed splenic hilum is seen. Numerous nucleated erythroid precursors are present in the well-formed splenic sinuses (G: low-power magnification; H: high-power magnification).

I,J: At EGA of 24 weeks, lymphoid elements are identified in the formed white pulp (I: low-power magnification; J: high-power magnification). (Courtesy of Philip Faught, Indianapolis, IN.)

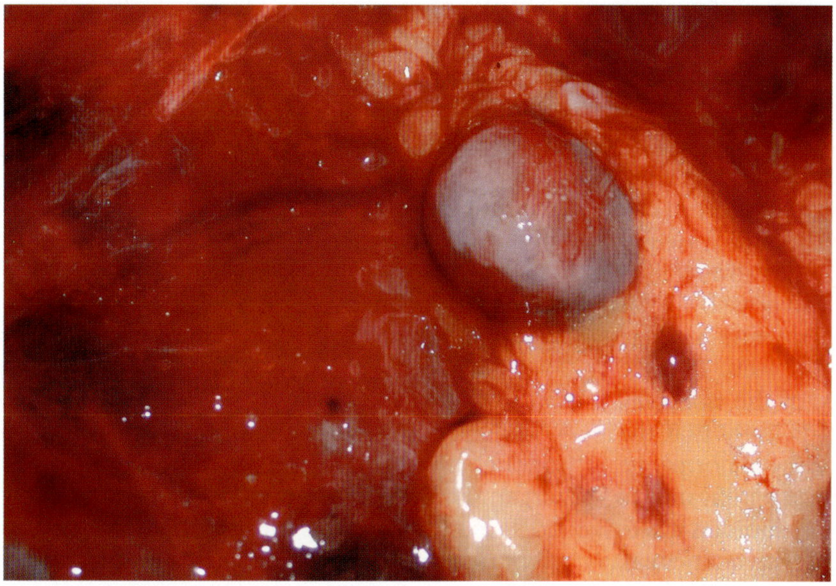

Figure 2-2

ACCESSORY SPLEEN

The accessory is present in the splenic hilum and is a red-purple, well-circumscribed nodule. (Courtesy of Michelle Elieff, Indianapolis, IN.)

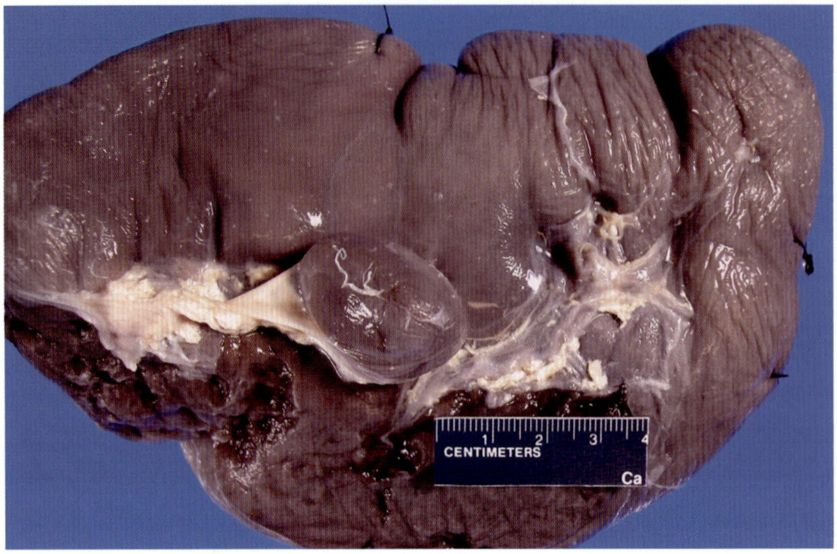

Figure 2-3

ACCESSORY SPLEEN

The accessory spleen is attached to the splenic hilum by a fibrous band. This is not present in all accessory spleens.

Table 2-1

EMBRYOLOGIC ABNORMALITIES OF THE SPLEEN

	Frequency	Features	Associated Clinical Findings
Accessory spleen	Common (10-30% of population)	Most common location in hilar area; can also be found in mesentery, pancreas, liver	
Polysplenia	Rare	Can refer to single spleen in several roughly equal nodules, or spleens on both right and left side	Can be seen in situs ambiguous with polysplenia, often associated with multiple congenital defects
Splenogonadal fusion	Rare	Continuous type has band of tissue connecting spleen with fused splenic gonadal tissue; discontinuous type has spleen tissue in region of gonad; M>>F, L>>R	Continuous type often associated with other congenital abnormalities
Splenorenal fusion	Very rare	Splenic tissue in close approximation with kidney	
Hepatolienal fusion	Very rare	Splenic tissue within parenchyma of liver	
Wandering spleen	Very rare (<0.2 % of population)	Abnormal localization of spleen in mid-abdomen or left lower quadrant	Due to laxity of splenic ligaments; may present as acute abdomen due to torsion of splenic pedicle and infarction

of abdominal organs and multiple spleens (24). This finding is associated with cardiovascular abnormalities in the majority of cases as well as abnormalities of lung, liver, and bowel.

Histologically, accessory spleens are the same as normally positioned spleen. If there is an underlying abnormality of the normally positioned spleen, however, it is likely that the accessory spleen will also share the abnormality. This concept underlies the clinical significance of accessory spleens. For example, in disorders where splenectomy is performed (i.e., hemolytic anemia), if unnoticed and not removed, an accessory spleen often will take over the function of the normal spleen. The accessory spleen will typically increase in size and contribute in a similar way to any pathologic process of the original spleen.

Wandering Spleen

Wandering spleen is an abnormal positioning of the spleen due to excessive mobility of the organ. The underlying cause is typically thought to be increased length, excessive distensibility, or abnormal formation of the splenic ligaments and

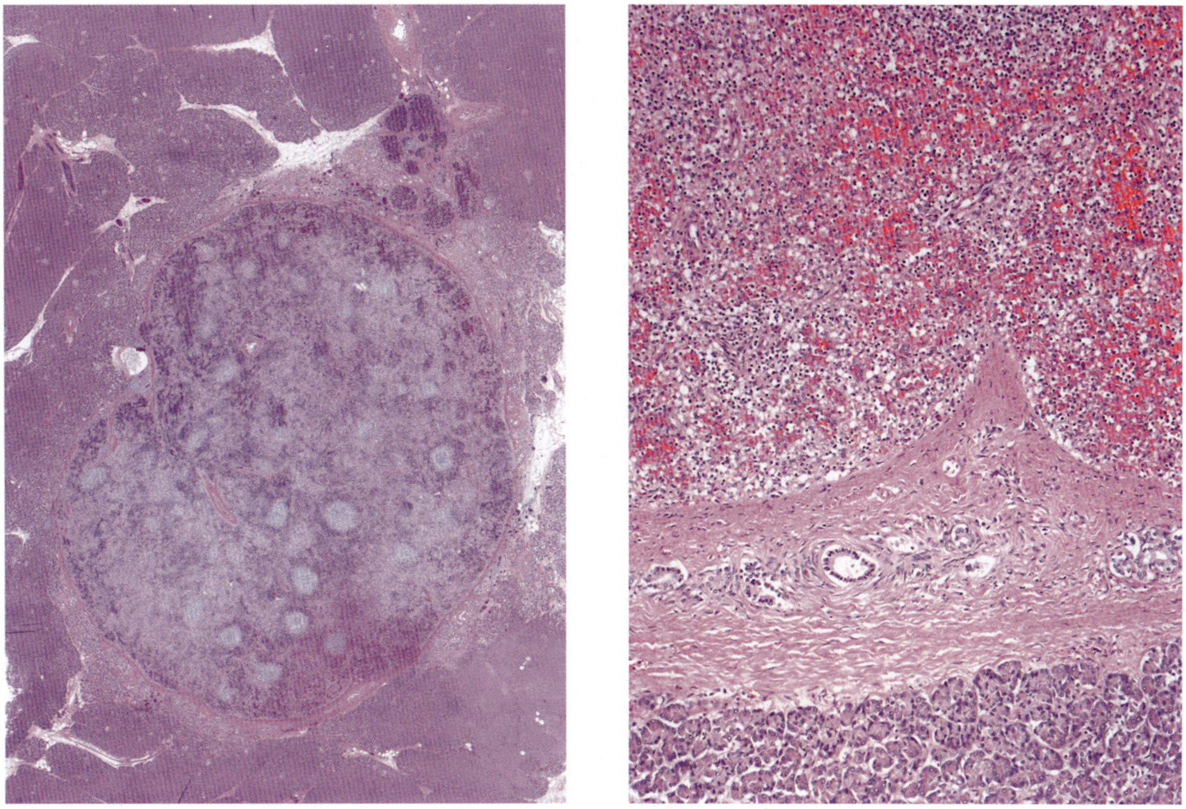

Figure 2-4

INTRAPANCREATIC SPLEEN

Left: An example of intrapancreatic splenic tissue.

Right: Higher magnification illustrates the presence of pancreatic glandular tissue in the capsule of the splenic tissue. (Courtesy of Rodney Mills, Salt Lake City, UT.)

pedicle. Typically, this occurrence is clinically silent, although occasional patients present with symptoms. Wandering spleen may present as an abdominal mass, intermittent gastrointestinal symptoms or pain, or rarely, an acute abdomen due to torsion and vascular compromise.

Abnormal Fusion: Splenogonadal, Splenorenal, Hepatolienal Fusion

The most common type of abnormal fusion of spleen is *splenogonadal fusion*. This is an abnormal anatomic fusion of gonad, epididymis, or vas deferens with a component of splenic tissue (figs. 2-5, 2-6). This condition is much more common in males than females, and left-sided occurrence is the norm, although right-sided fusions have been reported (19,42).

Clinically, this condition is often silent and may be discovered incidentally at autopsy or during inguinal hernia repair. It may also be associated with cryptorchidism, and discovered during orchiopexy. In these circumstances, intraoperative recognition of the condition may allow sparing of the gonad. Rarely, splenogonadal fusion may present as an inguinal or scrotal mass, and exceptional cases of an associated germ cell tumor have been reported (21,33). In any situation where ectopic splenic tissue is suspected, a technetium scan confirms the presence of splenic tissue.

There are two main types of splenogonadal fusion: continuous and discontinuous. The continuous type has a cord of splenic or fibrous tissue attaching the spleen proper with the gonad. This cord is composed of fibrous tissue, attenuated spleen covered by a capsule, or nodules of splenic tissue extending along a fibrous band. The gonad may descend normally,

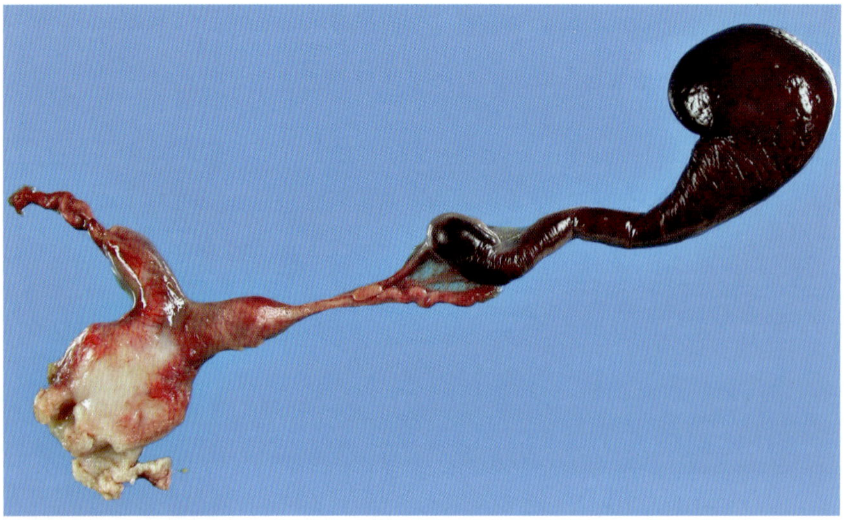

Figure 2-5

SPLENOGONADAL FUSION

The splenic tissue is attached to the ovary in this "continuous" type of fusion.

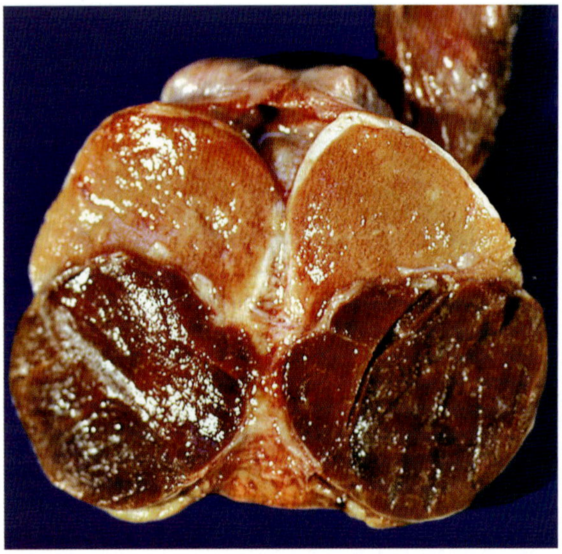

Figure 2-6

SPLENOGONADAL FUSION

The splenic tissue is dark red compared to the pale appearance of the testicular parenchyma.

but it is common for undescended testes to be a result of this process. Continuous splenic fusion is strongly associated with other congenital anomalies, especially limb defects and micrognathia (46,51).

The discontinuous type of splenogonadal fusion is probably a variant of accessory spleen. It is only rarely associated with other congenital anomalies. The spleen tissue is typically normal in architecture.

Splenorenal fusion is an exceedingly rare, but well-described, phenomenon (99). Typically, there is a distinct mass from the normally located spleen, often receiving its blood supply from the adjacent kidney. Although most commonly left sided, rare right-sided fusion has occurred (66). There are also rare reports of liver and spleen fusion, termed *hepatolienal fusion* (16).

Asplenia

Complete congenital absence of the spleen (*asplenia*) is rare, and in almost all cases, is associated with *situs ambiguous with asplenia*, also known as *right isomerism* or *bilateral right-sidedness* (24). It is characterized by the midline or abnormal location of abdominal organs, absence of the spleen, and severe congenital cardiac abnormalities in virtually all patients. There is a high mortality rate within the first year of life (95 percent), due mostly to heart abnormalities. In addition, the lack of the spleen is associated with immune deficiency, especially to encapsulated bacteria. As with other causes of asplenia, Howell-Jolly bodies are found in circulating red blood cells.

EMBRYOLOGY OF THE LYMPH NODES

Lymph node development begins during fetal life, with condensations of dendritic cells and stromal elements. Follicular dendritic cells form small nodules. Ultimately, during approximately the 16th week of gestation, primitive follicles are formed (fig. 2-7) (67). Like the spleen, lymph nodes of newborns and infants lack germinal

Table 2-2

BENIGN INCLUSIONS IN LYMPH NODES

Type of Inclusion	Common Location	Diagnostic Mimics	Comments
Nodal nevus	Axillary	Metastatic melanoma Metastatic carcinoma	S-100 protein+, –/weak staining for HMB-45; found in capsule or trabeculae of node
Hyperplastic mesothelial cells	Mediastinal (rarely abdominal, pelvic, cervical)	Dendritic cells Macrophages/histiocytes Metastatic carcinoma Metastatic melanoma	Found in patients with effusions; lack cytologic atypia; CK[a]+/vim+/calretinin+
Mullerian inclusion cysts	Femoral, inguinal	Borderline serous tumors of the ovary	Found almost exclusively in women; may represent metastases
Deciduosis	Abdominal	Metastatic carcinoma	Typically seen in pregnant women; decidualized cells typically lack pleomorphism, mitoses
Thyroid glandular inclusions	Lateral cervical and perithyroidal nodes	Thyroid carcinoma (well-differentiated)	Cytologically normal, usually found in single node; psammoma bodies not seen
Other glandular inclusions (salivary, breast, endometrial, pancreas, colonic glands)	Adjacent or draining site of organ or gland	Metastatic, well-differentiated carcinomas of glandular origin	Glandular inclusions will frequently resemble normal glands from their organ of origin

[a]CK = cytokeratin, vim = vimentin.

centers. Lymph nodes are composed of primary follicles. Secondary, or reactive, follicles develop within the first year of life (80).

Ectopia in Lymph Nodes

Benign glandular inclusions may be observed in lymph nodes in numerous anatomic sites (Table 2-2) (10,13,40,41,49,73,82,83). These inclusions are usually incidental findings with little clinical significance. Occasionally, benign inclusions result in the formation of cysts (25). Depending on the anatomic site, involved lymph nodes may contain glandular elements of mullerian, endometrial, thyroid gland, breast, salivary gland, or mesothelial origin. In these cases, it is important to distinguish the benign inclusions from micrometastases of carcinoma (55) or mesothelioma. In general, benign glandular inclusions are mature, fully differentiated structures that lack the malignant cytologic features (nuclear pleomorphism and increased mitoses) seen in carcinoma or mesothelioma. The lack of a desmoplastic response is also characteristic of a benign inclusion. Although immunohistochemical analysis helps to identify the origin of the inclusions, it usually does not help to determine the benign or malignant nature of the process. Immunoreactivity for cytokeratin and thyroglobulin, for example, suggests a thyroid process, although these markers do not differentiate heterotopic follicles from metastatic thyroid carcinoma.

One of the most vexing issues of recent years has arisen from the seemingly humble topic of ectopic tissues in lymph nodes. The presence of clusters of nevus cells in lymph nodes is, in most circumstances, simply a histologic oddity. However, with the advent of sentinel node evaluation for the presence of melanoma, these insignificant inclusions have taken on new importance. The presence of nodal nevi, including blue nevi, in nodes excised for malignancy ranges from 1 to 22 percent, with a significantly increased incidence in patients undergoing staging for melanoma (30,39,50,65). Nodal nevi are most commonly found in axillary lymph nodes, and rarely, in cervical or inguinal lymph nodes (figs. 2-8, 2-9) (9). Nodal nevi have not been reported in sites that do not drain skin. The clusters or aggregates of cells are most commonly found within the capsule of the lymph node, and occasionally, within the supporting trabeculae. They have also been rarely reported in the parenchyma or sinuses of nodes. Current studies suggest that these cells result from mechanical transport ("benign metastases"), rather than an embryologic origin (79). Their differentiation from melanoma cells can be difficult on histologic grounds alone. Immunohistochemical

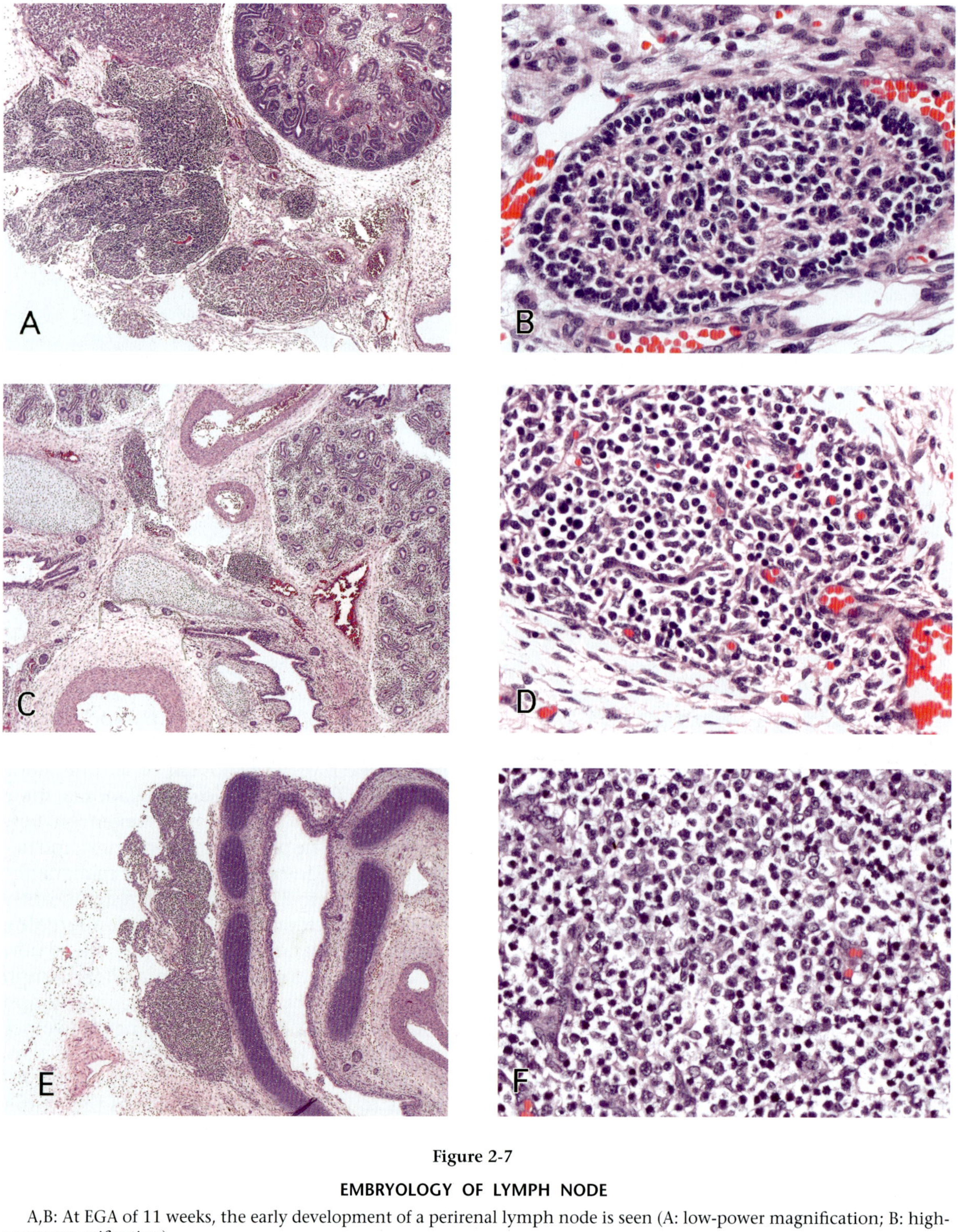

Figure 2-7

EMBRYOLOGY OF LYMPH NODE

A,B: At EGA of 11 weeks, the early development of a perirenal lymph node is seen (A: low-power magnification; B: high-power magnification).

C,D: At EGA of 14 weeks, a perihilar lymph node with relatively simple architecture is seen (C: low-power magnification; D: high-power magnification).

E,F: At EGA at 15 weeks, a hilar lymph node is seen. The vascular and sinusoidal elements are prominent (E: low-power magnification; F: high-power magnification).

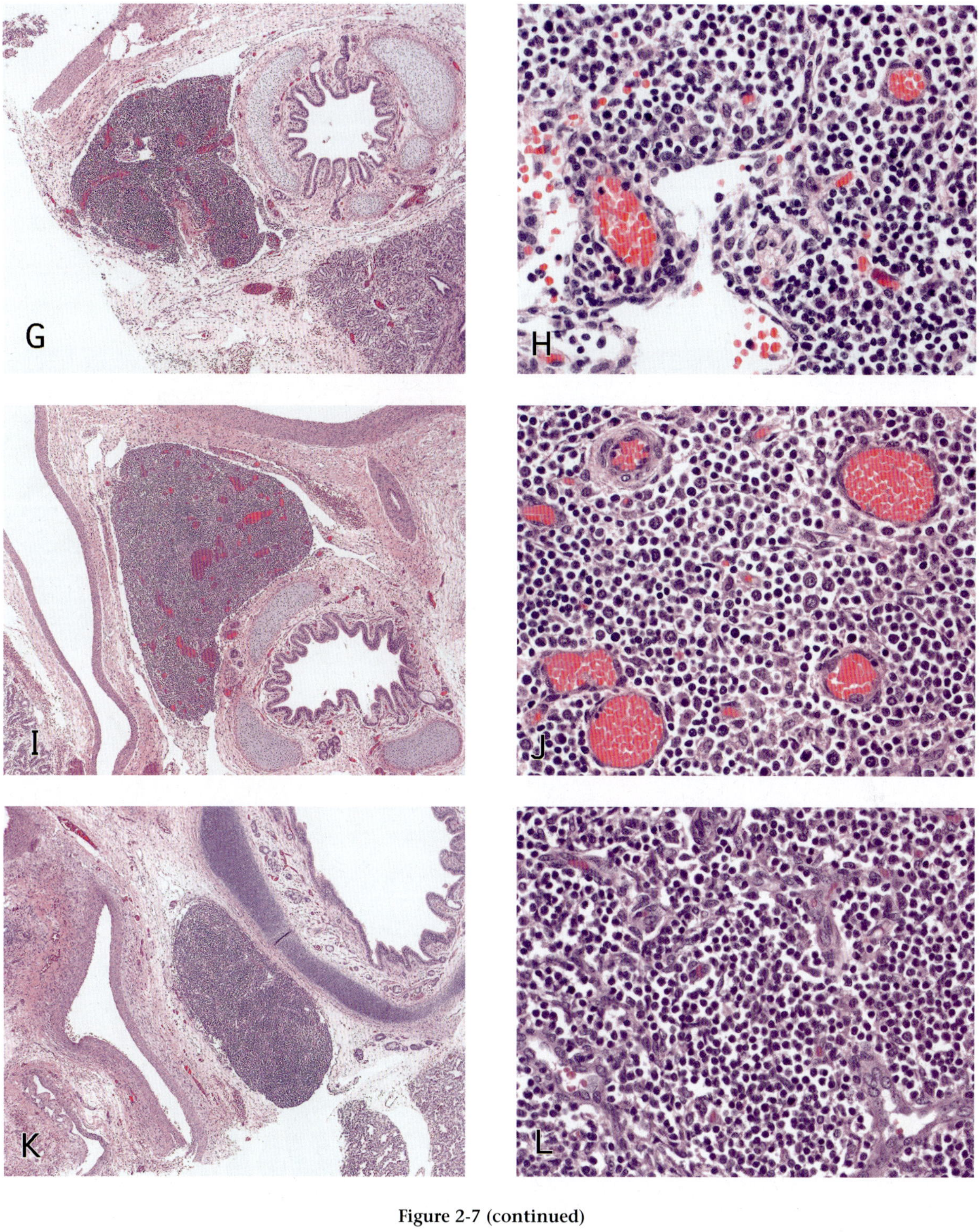

Figure 2-7 (continued)

G,H: At EGA of 17 weeks, the vascular elements have become more prominent (G: low-power magnification; H: high-power magnification).

I,J: At EGA of 19 weeks, subtle condensations of lymphoid elements surround the vascular elements, suggesting formation of separate compartments in this hilar lymph node (I: low-power magnification; J: high-power magnification).

K,L: At EGA of 24 weeks, vascular elements appear well formed in this hilar lymph node (K: low-power magnification; L: high-power magnification). (Courtesy of Philip Faught, Indianapolis, IN.)

Figure 2-8

NODAL NEVUS

A,B: Low- and high-power magnification images of nevus cells in a lymph node.

C: There is strong S-100 protein immunoreactivity.

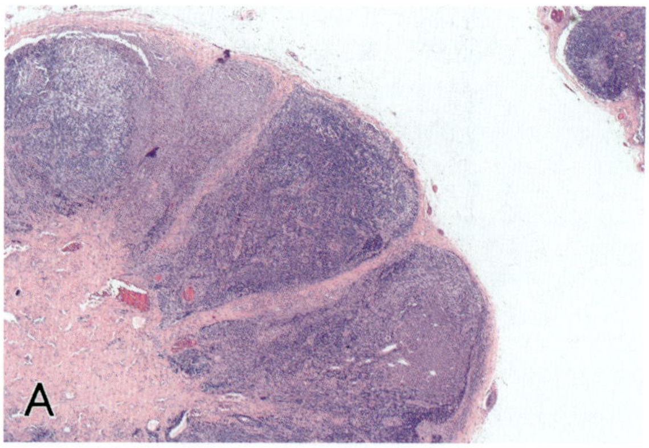

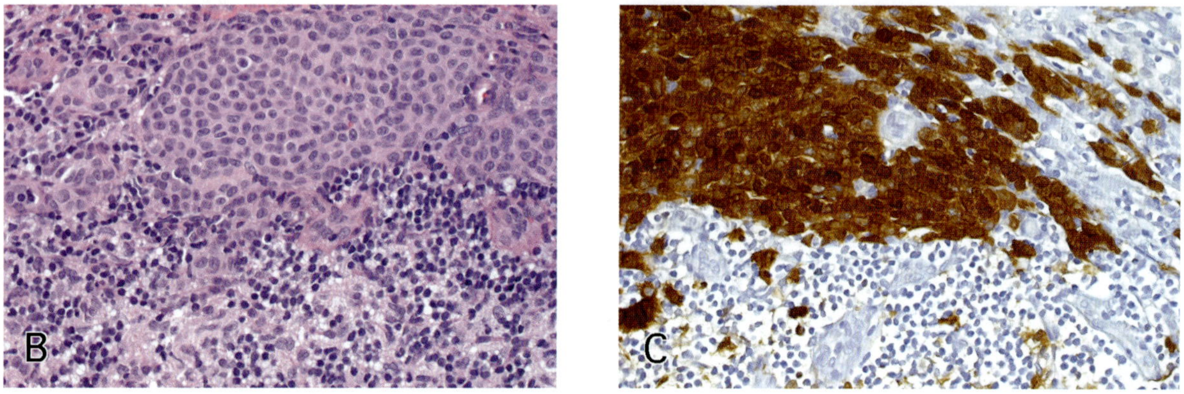

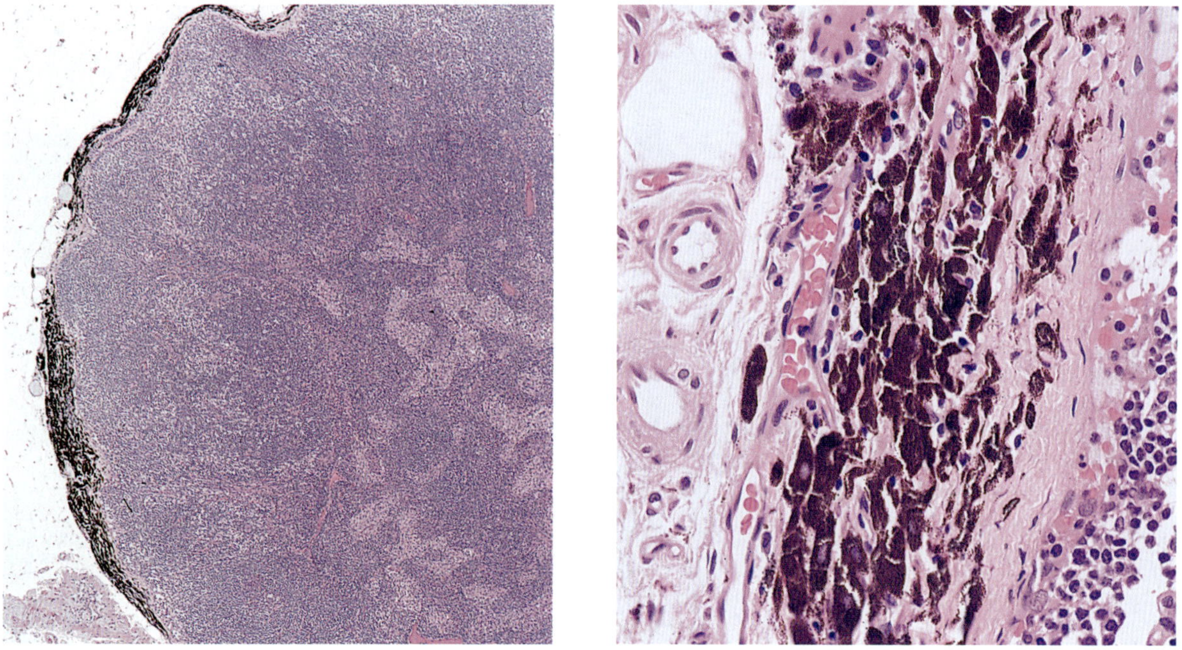

Figure 2-9

BLUE NEVUS OF LYMPH NODE

Left: A cluster of pigmented cells is present within the lymph node capsule.

Right: Higher magnification reveals the deeply pigmented blue nevus cells. (Fig. 21-66 from Fascicle 14, Third Series.)

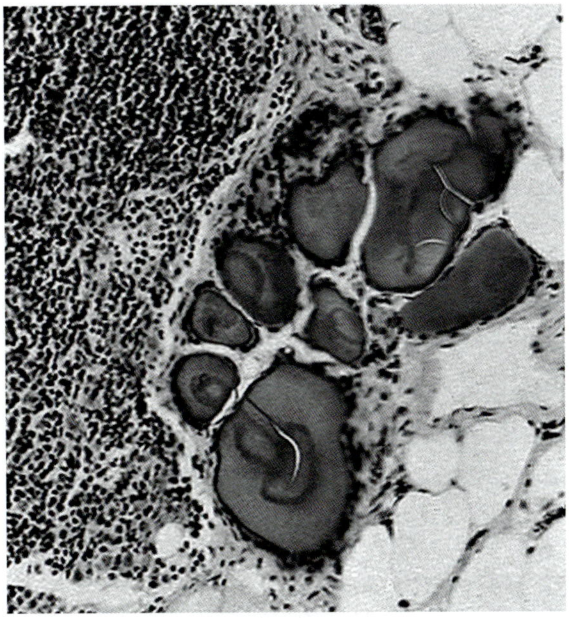

Figure 2-10

THYROID FOLLICLES IN CERVICAL LYMPH NODE

Well-developed benign-appearing thyroid follicles with colloid are seen in this lymph node. (Fig. 301 from Fascicle 5, Third Series.)

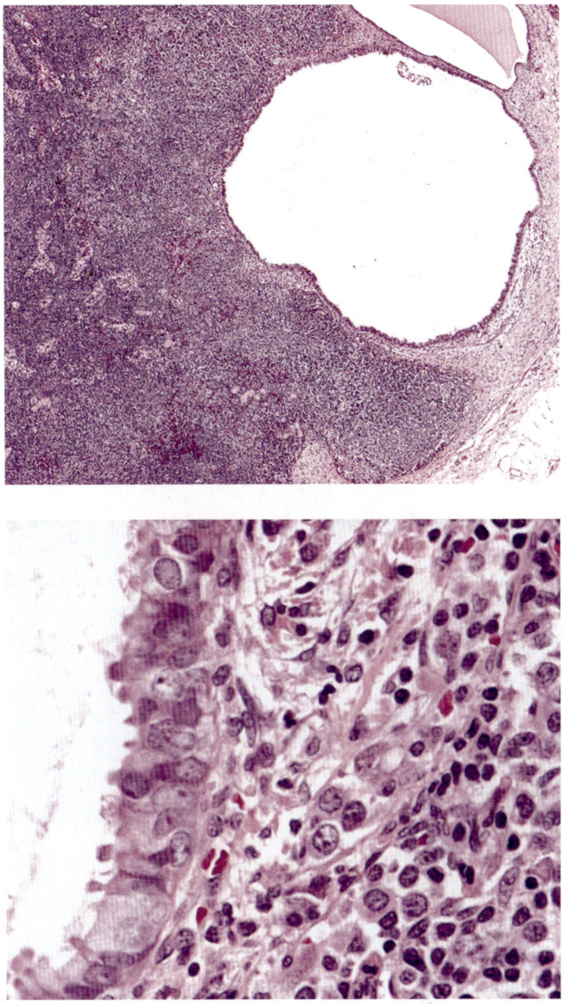

Figure 2-11

MULLERIAN INCLUSION CYST

Top: Mullerian inclusion cyst in an intraabdominal lymph node of a female.

Bottom: Ciliated columnar and secretory lining cells are seen.

staining may be helpful in the differentiation; nevus cells tend to be strongly positive for S-100 protein (similar to melanoma cells), but are typically negative or weakly positive for HMB45. In addition, nevus cells usually show no proliferation by Ki-67 staining, in contrast to most metastatic melanomas (48).

Benign thyroidal glandular elements are seen in 0.3 to 5.0 percent of lymph nodes evaluated in neck dissections (26). These glandular inclusions occur in lateral cervical or perithyroidal lymph nodes. Because of the embryologic development of the thyroid gland and neck structures, these are thought to develop from malposition or abnormal migration of thyroidal elements, rather than transport, as seen in inclusions of other types. The most important distinction is from well-differentiated thyroid carcinoma, either metastatic or developing from a previously existing inclusion. Histologic features that favor benign thyroid inclusions over metastatic carcinoma include small size, focal location, lack of desmoplasia or psammoma bodies, and bland nuclear features (52). The criteria for malignancy of thyroid glandular inclusions in lymph nodes include: cytologic atypia, more than a third of the node composed of glandular elements, more than one lymph node involved, and the presence of psammoma bodies (fig. 2-10).

Mullerian inclusion cysts are composed of small epithelial glands and are found most commonly in abdominal and pelvic lymph nodes (fig. 2-11). They rarely occur in the lymph nodes of males (32). Because of their similarity to fallopian tube epithelium, they have been referred to as endosalpingiosis; at other times, the histologic appearance is similar to endocervicosis or

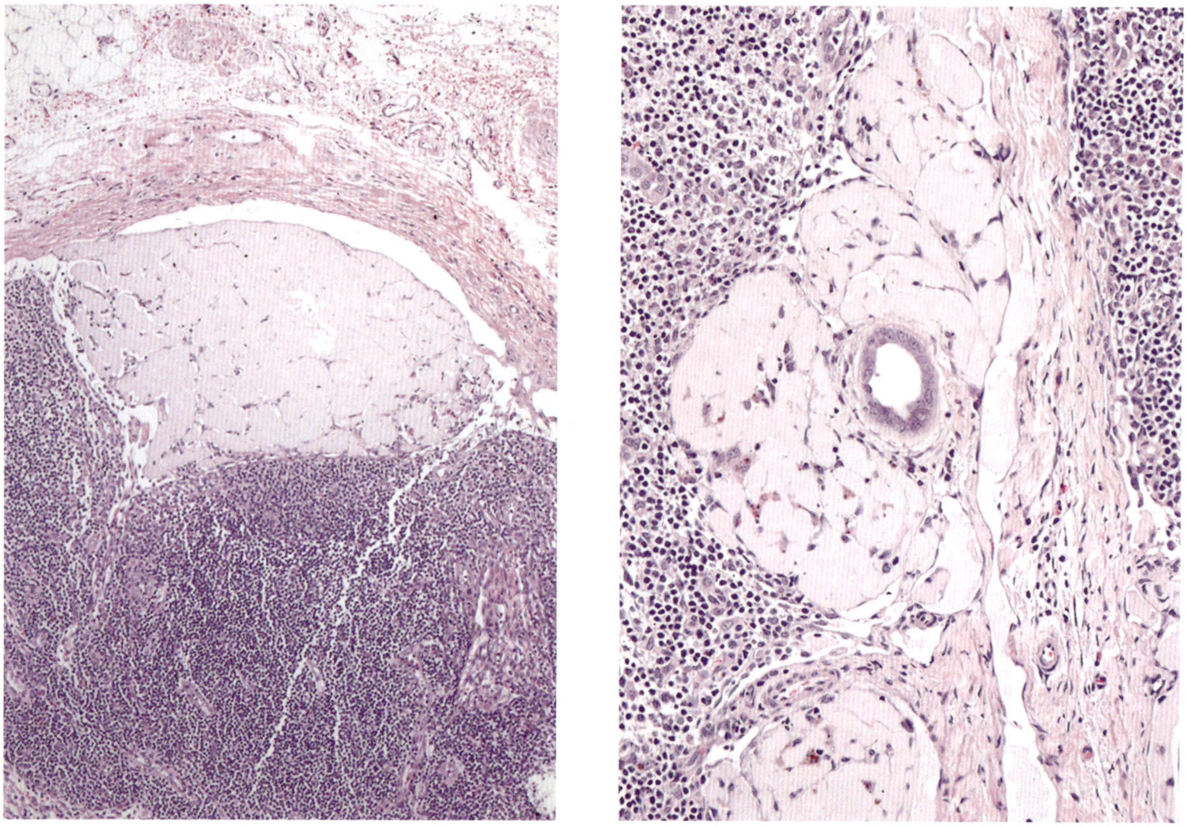

Figure 2-12

RENAL GLAND/TAMM-HORSFALL INCLUSIONS IN LYMPH NODE

Left: A benign inclusion of Tamm-Horsfall protein with entrapped epithelial cells in a perirenal lymph node from a patient with Wilms tumor.

Right: The same case with a benign entrapped renal tubule.

endometriosis. The glands usually have a round or cystic appearance and are characteristically lined by both ciliated columnar and secretory cells that do not demonstrate nuclear atypia or increased mitoses. Although typically benign, a study by Moore et al. (55) suggests that many inclusion cysts are actually metastases from serous borderline tumors of the ovary. If identified, the patient should be evaluated for the presence of ovarian or other gynecologic lesions.

When staging lymph nodes associated with pediatric renal tumors, nodal inclusions of small epithelial glands, with or without aggregates of acellular Tamm-Horsfall protein and presumably derived from damaged nephrons, may be present (fig. 2-12) (94,101). Pararenal lymph nodes may show interstitial deposition of Tamm-Horsfall protein in a variety of kidney diseases. Histologically, this appears as waxy, amorphous masses in the lymphatic vessels, peripheral sinuses, and germinal centers. These deposits are periodic acid–Schiff (PAS) positive, with or without diastase digestion, and Congo red negative. Presumably, Tamm-Horsfall protein escapes from kidney tubules, produces a localized inflammatory cell reaction in the renal interstitium, and gains access to intrarenal lymphatics and regional lymph nodes.

Rare benign epithelial inclusions or cyst-like structures are seen in the axillary lymph nodes (20). The epithelium is double-layered, usually without stroma. Apocrine- or squamous epithelium–lined cysts may also be noted. These inclusions may represent heterotopic breast tissue or sweat glands. The bland cytologic features, lack of mitoses, and absence of desmoplasia help to differentiate these benign inclusions from metastatic breast carcinoma (fig. 2-13). These

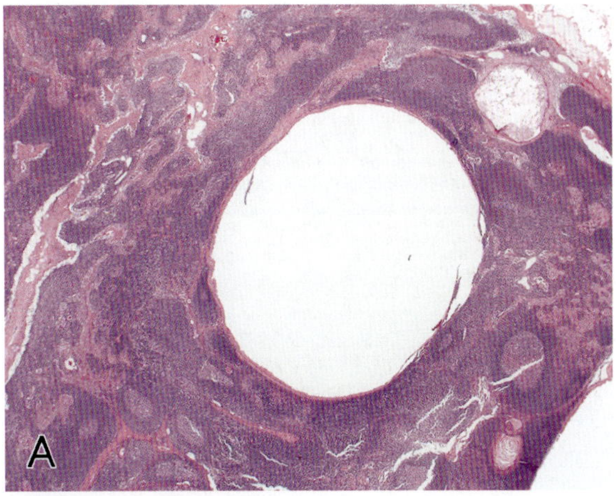

Figure 2-13

BENIGN BREAST GLAND INCLUSIONS IN LYMPH NODE

The glandular inclusions in this axillary lymph node are larger cystic inclusions (A,B) or small, benign glands (C).

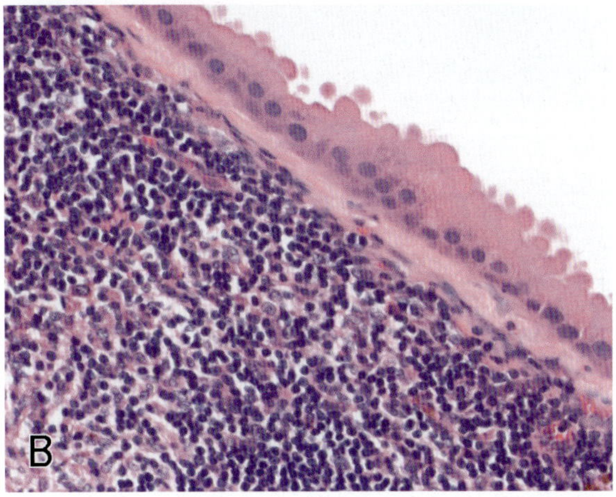

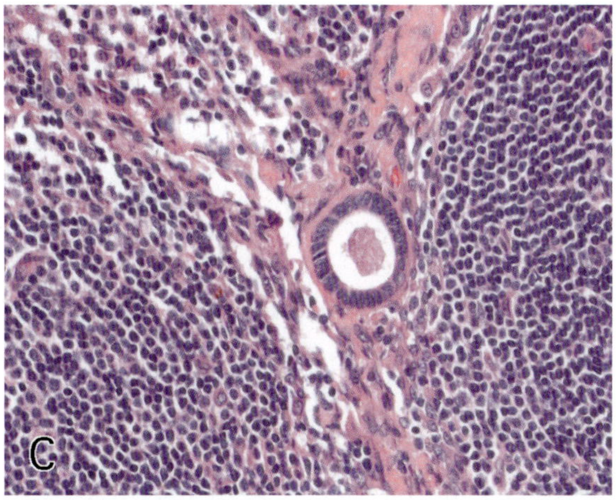

inclusions may occur in the presence of benign or malignant breast disease and result in inappropriate treatment if they are misdiagnosed as metastatic carcinoma (29). Recently, it was reported that either tumor or normal breast epithelial cells may be transported into axillary lymph nodes following a breast biopsy (6). It is believed that this finding, which reportedly occurs approximately 2 weeks after the biopsy, has little or no clinical significance. It is important, however, to distinguish these "transported" cells from a true micrometastasis. The presence of cell clusters that are identical to the main breast lesion, hemosiderin-laden macrophages, and altered red blood cells is consistent with transported cells rather than a metastasis.

Intraparotid lymph nodes may demonstrate heterotopic salivary gland inclusions (74). These inclusions are in the form of ducts that are lined by a double layer of epithelium and myoepithelium or as acini with abundant zymogen granules (fig. 2-14). In patients with acquired immunodeficiency syndrome (AIDS), the salivary gland inclusions may be the origin of benign lymphoepithelial cysts and Sjögren syndrome–like lesions (69).

Deciduosis of lymph node may be seen in the abdominal lymph nodes of pregnant women, where it may be associated with concomitant nodal endometriosis (38,58). Some cases, however, are not associated with endometriosis and originate from coelomic mesenchymal cells during pregnancy (102). The decidual cells form compact aggregates or nodules that are usually located in the subcapsular sinuses or the superficial cortex (fig. 2-15). The cells are typically polygonal and plump, with well-demarcated cell borders and amphophilic cytoplasm. Cytoplasmic vacuolization may also be noted. It is important to differentiate deciduosis of lymph node from metastatic carcinoma, especially if there is a history of abdominal cancer. Although

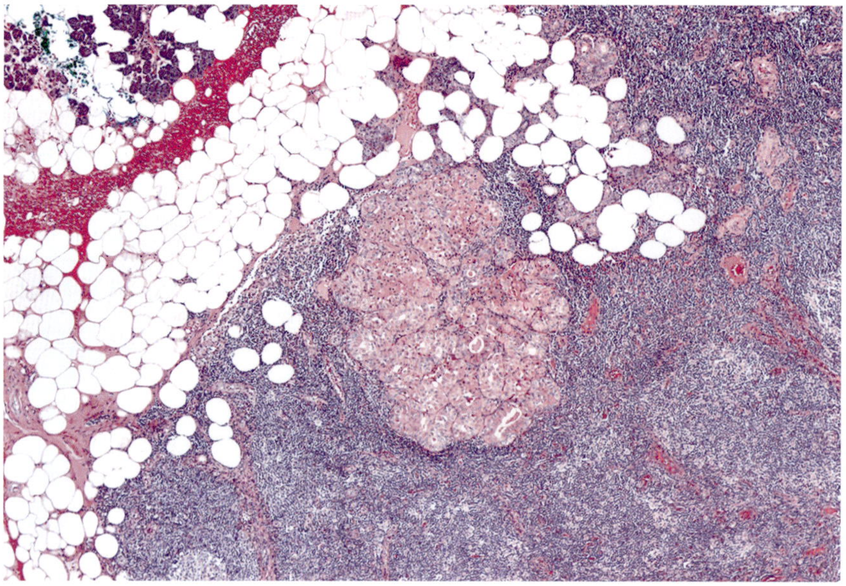

Figure 2-14

SALIVARY GLAND INCLUSIONS

Small ductular elements of salivary gland are seen in this high cervical lymph node.

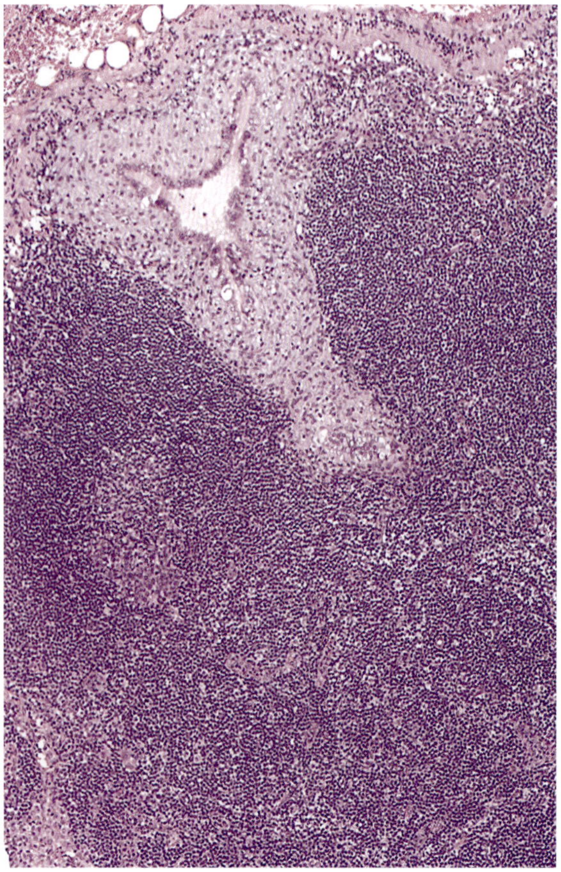

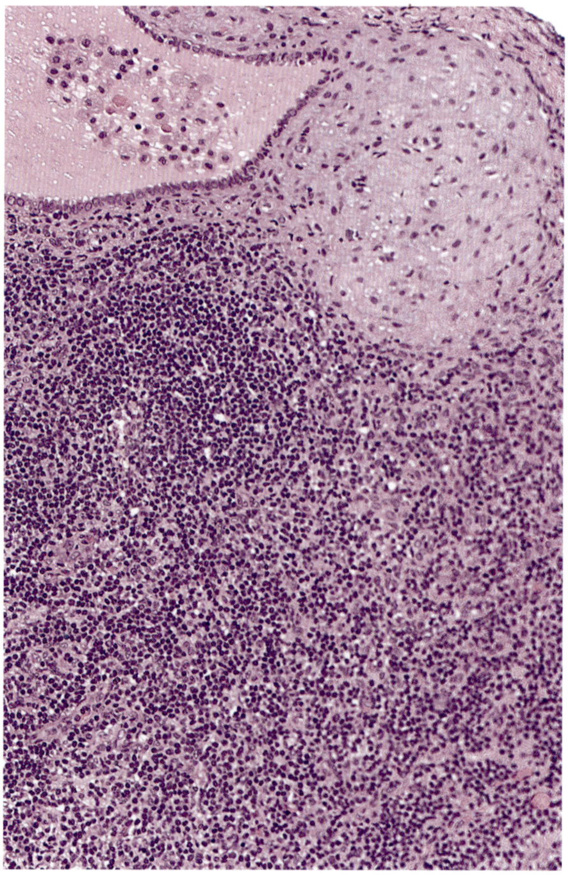

Figure 2-15

DECIDUOSIS IN LYMPH NODE

Periglandular ectopic decidua in an intraabdominal lymph node.

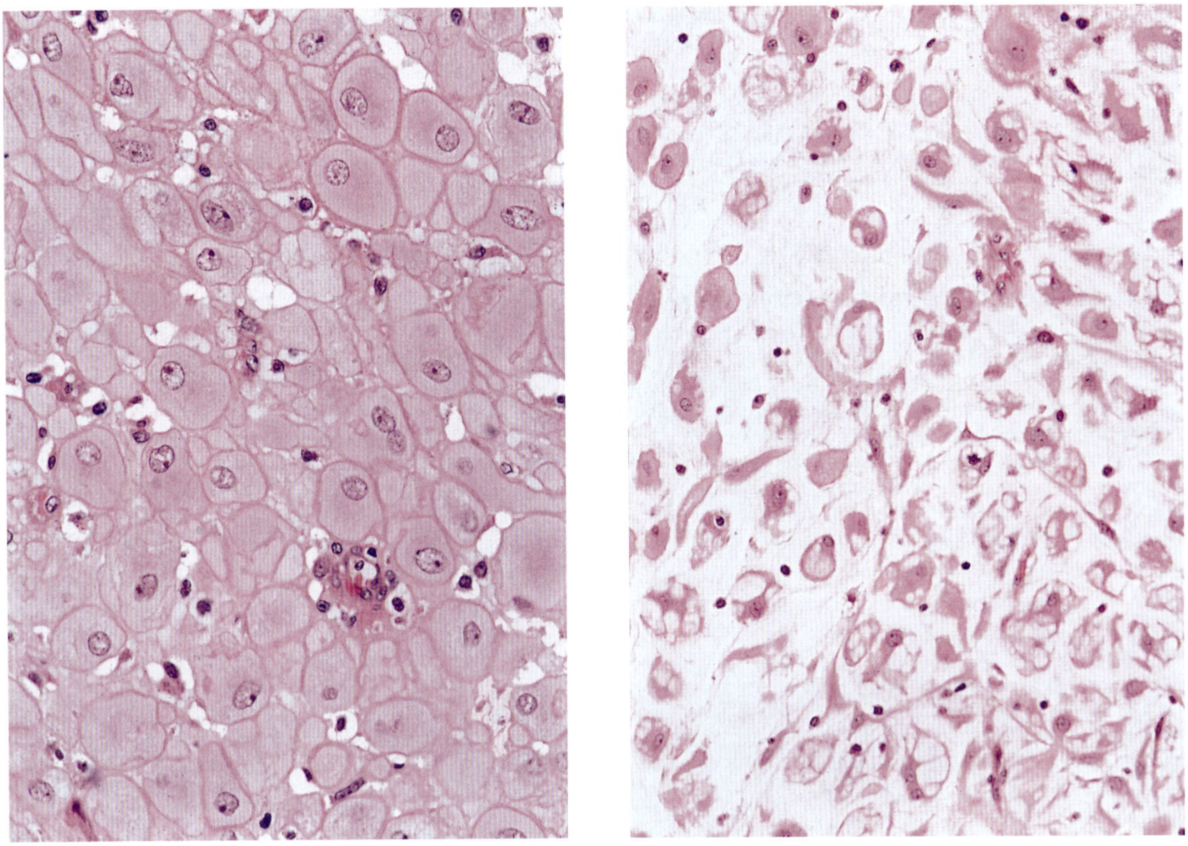

Figure 2-16

DECIDUOSIS IN LYMPH NODE

Left: The cells are polygonal and have sharp cell borders.
Right: The cells appear vacuolated. (Fig. 21-17 from Fascicle 14, Third Series.)

the decidual cells may show slight nuclear pleomorphism, they do not have an increased mitotic rate. The absence of desmoplasia and keratinization, and the lack of immunoreactivity for cytokeratin (98), help distinguish this rare, benign lesion from metastatic squamous cell carcinoma with which it may easily be confused (53). Epithelial inclusion cysts are also noted in association with ectopic decidua in intraabdominal lymph nodes (fig. 2-16).

Mediastinal, abdominal, or pelvic lymph nodes may demonstrate mesothelial inclusions, which appear as small tubular structures within the lymph node capsule or nodal sinuses (1,4, 14,15,31,32,60,68,97). Immunohistochemical reactivity with cytokeratin helps to highlight the inclusions (fig. 2-17). It is important to distinguish these benign single cells or clusters (which may be difficult to diagnose on hematoxylin and eosin (H&E)-stained slides alone) from metastatic carcinoma, melanoma, or mesothelioma. Benign mesothelial cells in lymph nodes may arise from lymphatic embolization (78) and most commonly occurs in the setting of chronic effusion, serosal inflammation, or as a reaction to adjacent lymphoma (15). In general, the same distinguishing cytologic and immunophenotypic criteria apply to benign mesothelial cell inclusions as to the previously described heterotopic lymph node inclusions. Recently, hyperplastic mesothelial cells have been reported in mediastinal lymph node sinuses in association with pericardial and pleural effusions and extranodal lymphatic involvement (36). This supports the theory that hyperplastic mesothelial cells are derived from reactive serosal mesothelium and are dislodged into draining lymphatic channels (78).

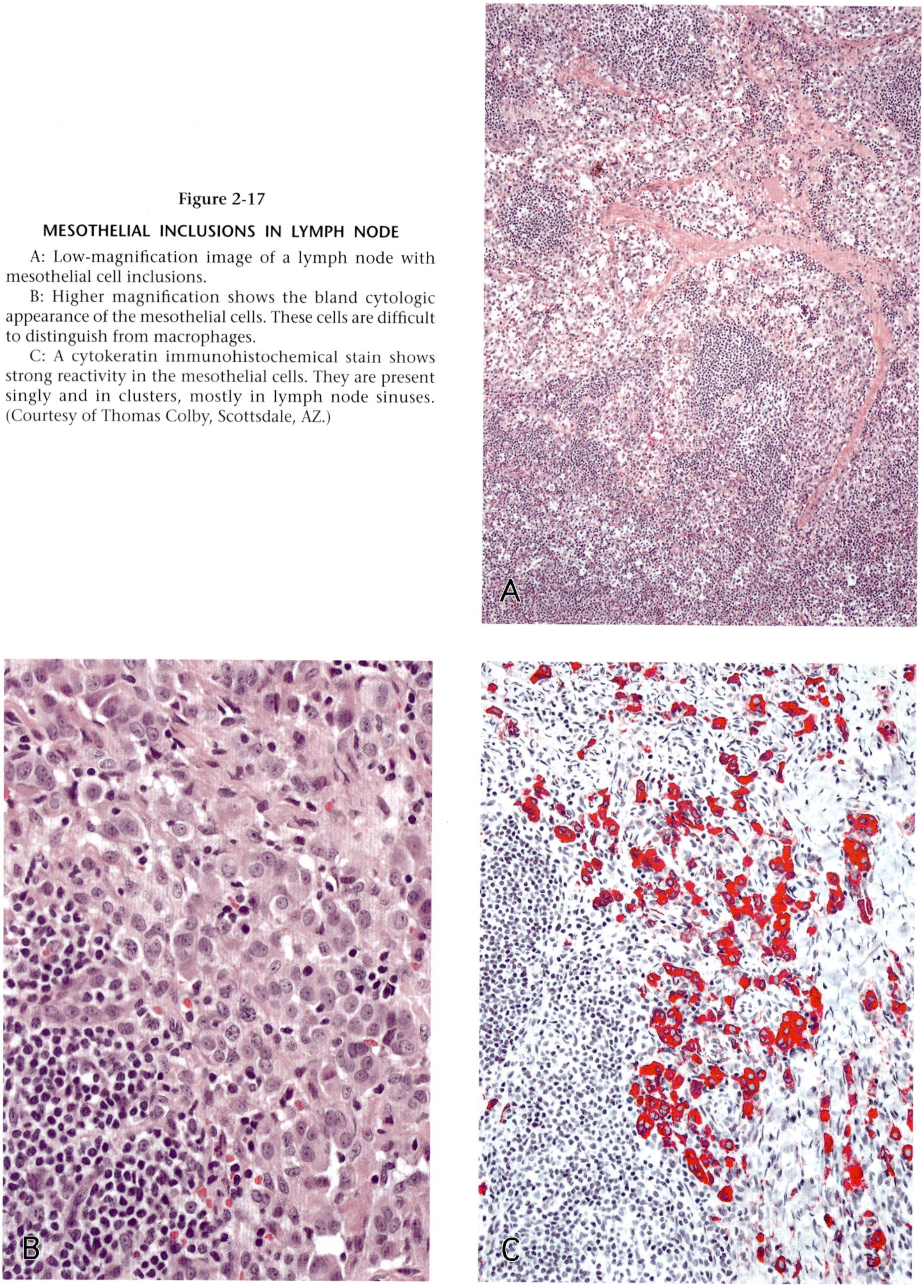

Figure 2-17

MESOTHELIAL INCLUSIONS IN LYMPH NODE

A: Low-magnification image of a lymph node with mesothelial cell inclusions.

B: Higher magnification shows the bland cytologic appearance of the mesothelial cells. These cells are difficult to distinguish from macrophages.

C: A cytokeratin immunohistochemical stain shows strong reactivity in the mesothelial cells. They are present singly and in clusters, mostly in lymph node sinuses. (Courtesy of Thomas Colby, Scottsdale, AZ.)

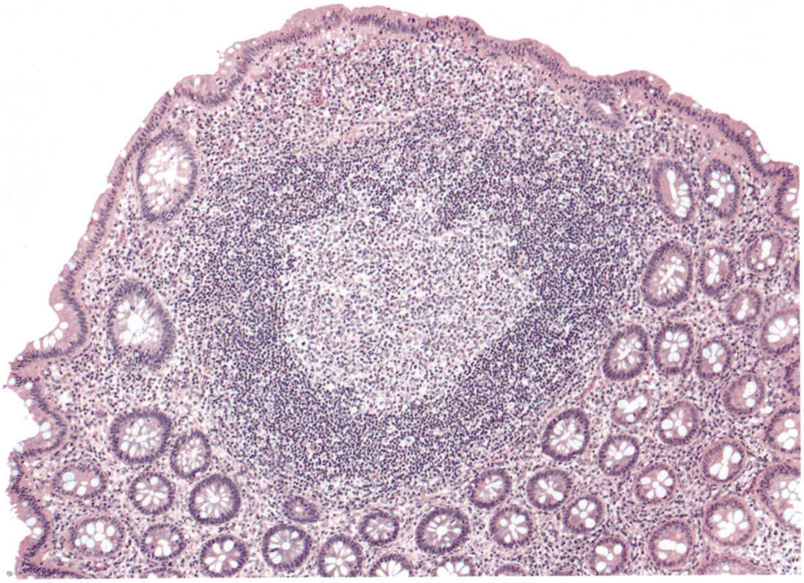

Figure 2-18

MUCOSA-ASSOCIATED LYMPHOID TISSUE (MALT) IN APPENDIX

Abundant lymphoid tissue is present in this appendix, including reactive follicles, mantle zones, and a small marginal zone.

HISTOLOGY OF LYMPH NODE (NORMAL ARCHITECTURE AND FUNCTION OF LYMPH NODES)

The primary or central lymphoid organs are the bone marrow and thymus. Here, functionally mature but naive lymphocytes develop from precursor cells. The lymph nodes comprise the body's secondary or peripheral lymphoid organs and play an extremely important role in the defense against infection. They are one of the main sites (in addition to the spleen and mucosa-associated lymphoid tissue) where antigen-specific B and T lymphocytes develop in response to exogenous antigenic stimuli.

The lymph nodes are located in several anatomic locations. They are arranged in small groups or chains and drain the lymphatic vessels of various organs. They are concentrated in the retroperitoneum, abdomen (mesentery), mediastinum, and cervical, axillary, and inguinal regions. The salivary glands, lungs, and subcutaneous tissues also contain lymph nodes. Their role in the drainage of lymphatic fluid involves not only the mechanical filtration of the foreign bodies, but also the recognition and processing of antigens. The lymph nodes exhibit a complex architecture in which many different cell populations are arranged in distinct interfacing compartments (76). This provides a favorable environment for the generation of the body's immune response.

The tertiary lymphoid tissue includes those anatomic sites that do not normally contain an abundance of lymphoid tissue, yet can be antigenically stimulated to recruit unique populations of primarily memory lymphocytes (54). These anatomic locations, including the skin and respiratory and reproductive tracts, give rise to restimulated memory and effector precursor cells that lead to clonal expansion (62).

Over the past 10 years, the concept of mucosa-associated lymphoid tissue (MALT), first described by Isaacson (35), has progressively developed (34). MALT refers to extranodal organized lymphoid tissue that does not correspond to peripheral sites of the immune system. Upon antigenic stimulation due to infection or an autoimmune process, acquired MALT is postulated to give rise to extranodal marginal zone B-cell lymphomas of MALT type (34,35). MALT is most recognizable in the appendix, Peyer patches, Waldeyer ring, and lung (fig. 2-18). It is composed of reactive germinal centers with prominent marginal zones, lymphocytes overlying the epithelium, and polyclonal plasma cells that reside beneath the surface. It has been postulated that the function of MALT involves the response to intraluminal antigens and the generation of mucosal immunity. The lymphocytes that respond to antigenic stimulation in MALT are believed to acquire homing properties that enable them to return to these tissues (3,5).

Table 2-3

NORMAL MORPHOLOGIC COMPARTMENTS OF THE LYMPH NODE

Cortex	Follicles	
	Primary	Composed of small nodules of mantle type B lymphocytes
	Secondary	Composed of a mixture of small, irregular B lymphocytes and large transformed cells, with intermixed dendritic cells and macrophages
	Mantle zone	Surrounds the germinal center; cellularity composed predominantly of small B lymphocytes with round to irregular nuclei, condensed chromatin, and scant cytoplasm
Paracortex		Adjacent to follicles and composed of a polymorphous mixture of T cells, B cells, and few granulocytes; cells may be small intermediate or large (i.e., transformed)
Medulla		Inconspicuous in most lymph nodes, this area is composed predominantly of plasma cells; located centrally within the lymph node
Supporting Stroma	Capsule and subcapsular sinus	Fibrous capsule and fibrous trabeculae are present in lymph nodes; usually thin and inconspicuous, although can become thickened in chronic inflammatory processes and neoplasms (i.e., nodular sclerosis Hodgkin lymphoma)
	Vasculature	Normally quiescent and inconspicuous; high endothelial venules can become activated with prominent endothelial cells
	Dendritic cells	Main types of dendritic cells include follicular dendritic cells and interdigitating dendritic cells located in follicles and interfollicular areas, respectively

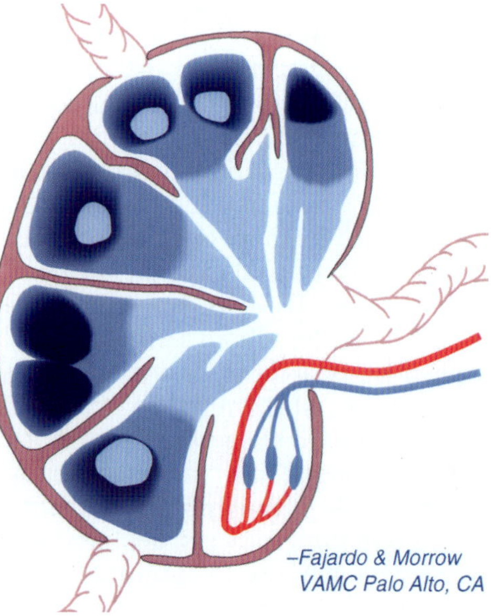

Figure 2-19

LYMPH NODE ARCHITECTURE

Diagram of the overall architecture of the lymph node. (Courtesy of Luis Fajardo, Palo Alto, CA.)

An understanding of the architecture and cellular composition of the normal lymph node (18) and the differentiation pathways of the body's immune system facilitates the correct interpretation of the histopathologic changes that characterize benign hyperplastic lymph nodes. The basic architectural structure of a lymph node includes the capsule, cortex, paracortex, medulla, sinuses (subcapsular, cortical, and medullary), and vasculature (Table 2-3) (87). These structures, in addition to the primary follicles and germinal centers, are depicted in figure 2-19.

Capsule and Subcapsular Sinus

The lymph node capsule surrounds the ovoid or round lymph node and is the site where the afferent lymphatic vessels enter into the subcapsular sinus. The capsule may become thickened or fibrotic as a result of chronic inflammation, infection, or a malignancy such as nodular sclerosing Hodgkin lymphoma. Although the subcapsular sinus is lined by endothelial cells, the branching sinuses that arise from it and drain into the efferent lymphatics in the hilum are not lined by true endothelium but by macrophages (fig. 2-20) (87).

Cortex

The cortex is located deep to the capsule and subcapsular sinus and is composed of follicular and paracortical regions, cortical sinuses, and high endothelial venules (96). The cortical region and the superficial cortex are the bone marrow–derived B-cell areas of the lymph node that are important in humoral immunity. The follicular cortex is primarily made up of B lymphocytes that reside in either primary or secondary lymphoid follicles (86). These structures have been extensively studied according to their histologic, immunophenotypic, and molecular genetic features.

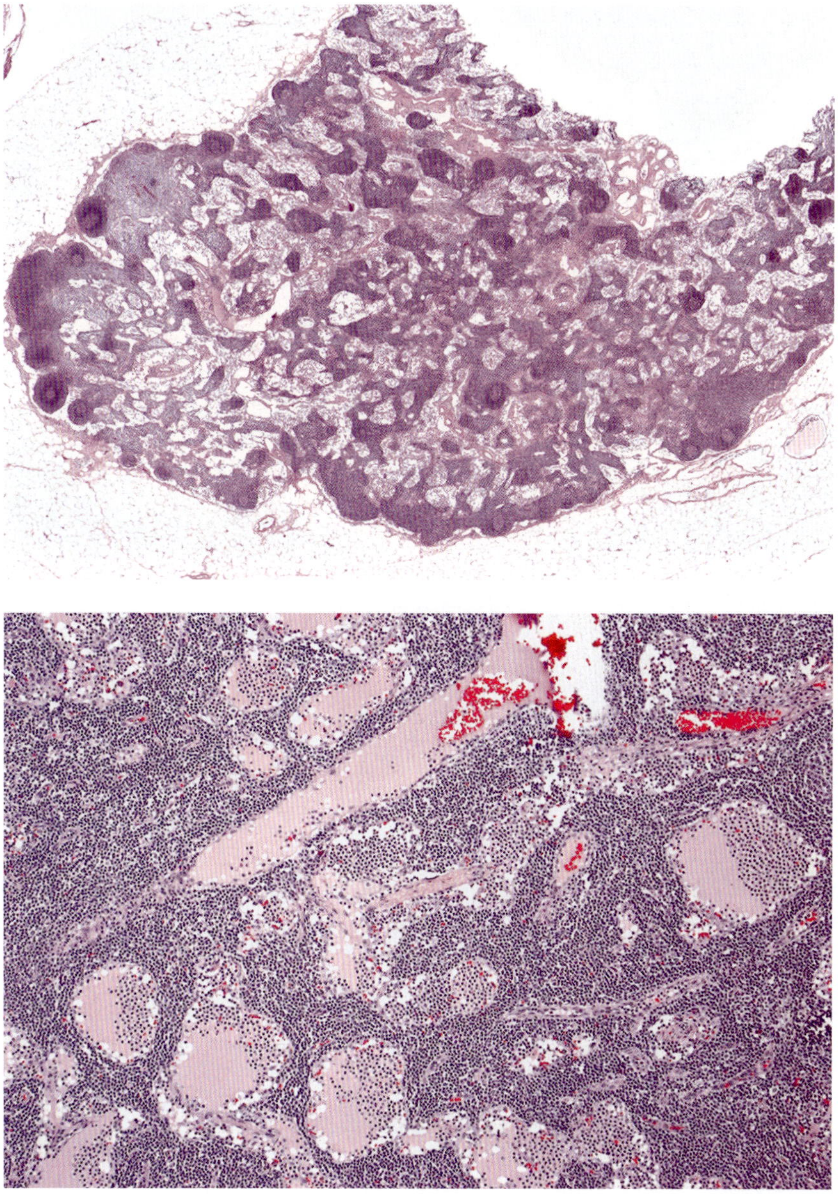

Figure 2-20

LYMPH NODE SINUS

Top: Low magnification of a lymph node shows extreme dilation of sinuses.

Bottom: At higher magnification, dilated lymphatics are filled with clear fluid, with occasional lymphocytes and other inflammatory cells.

A primary or resting follicle is composed of immunoglobulin (Ig)M-expressing B lymphocytes that are bcl-2 positive. Although they have not yet been exposed to surface receptor–specific antigen, they are able to respond to antigenic stimulation. These cells express high concentrations of surface immunoglobulin of kappa or lambda light chain type. On routine H&E-stained slides, the follicles are seen as compact nodules within the cortex (fig. 2-21) (93). There are follicular dendritic cells that express CD21 and CD35 in addition to the virgin and memory lymphocytes that comprise the primary follicles.

A secondary follicle consists of a germinal center surrounded by small B lymphocytes that form a collar or mantle zone. Germinal centers result from stimulation of B lymphocytes by primarily T-cell–dependent antigens (47,92). The cellular composition of the germinal center includes small and large cleaved cells (lymphocytes), large noncleaved cells, and a minor population of small noncleaved cells. These cells express CD10 and CD20 and low levels of immunoglobulin. Occasional small mature lymphocytes, plasma cells, follicular dendritic cells, and phagocytic (tingible body) macrophages are also normally present.

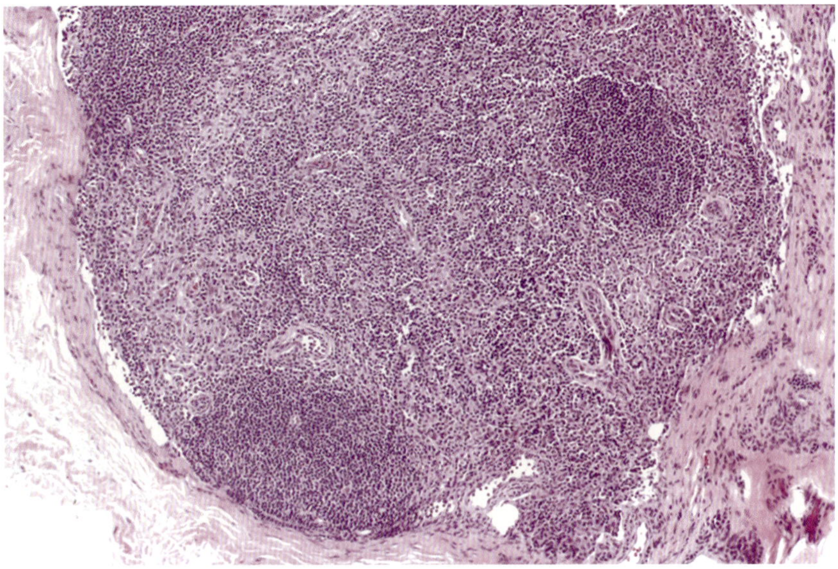

Figure 2-21

PRIMARY FOLLICLE IN LYMPH NODE

Primary follicles are formed of small, round lymphocytes with mature cytoplasm. Primary follicles are most often identified at the periphery of lymph nodes.

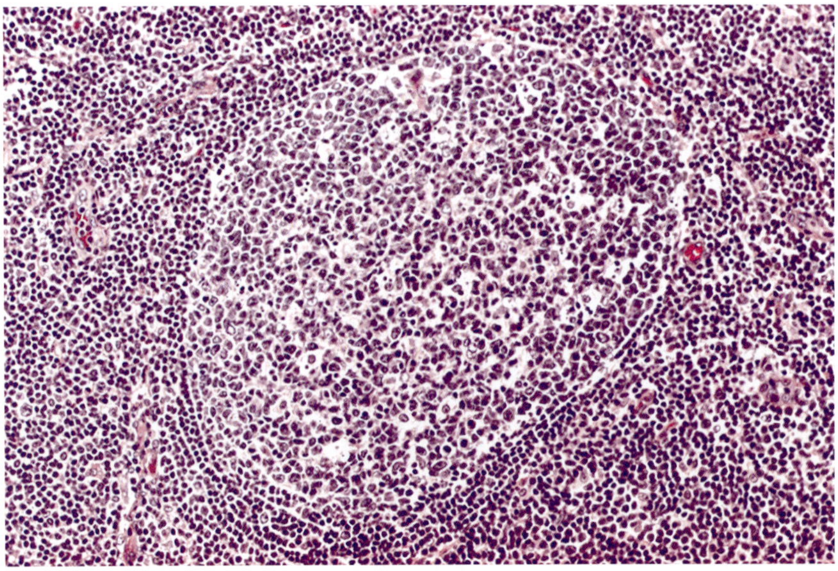

Figure 2-22

SECONDARY FOLLICLE IN LYMPH NODE

A secondary follicle, or polarized reactive germinal center, with characteristic light and dark zones.

The evolution of primary to secondary follicles begins with the accumulation of large, blast-like cells in the center of the primary follicle. Sharp demarcation from the surrounding mantle zone occurs as the reactive germinal center develops a starry sky pattern due to phagocytosis of debris by phagocytic macrophages. Large noncleaved cells are the first to appear in the germinal centers, followed by small and large cleaved follicle center cells. At this stage, the follicle becomes "polarized" toward the site of antigen presentation (fig. 2-22). Small and large cleaved B lymphocytes (centrocytes), follicular dendritic cells, and CD4-positive helper/inducer T cells comprise the light or pale-staining pole. Small and large noncleaved cells (centroblasts), in association with tingible body macrophages, form the darker-staining pole.

The majority of cells in the germinal center and those in the mantle zone show reactivity with an antibody to the B-cell–associated antigen, CD20, in paraffin-embedded tissue sections (fig. 2-23). Germinal center cells that are undergoing programmed cell death, or apoptosis, however, lack bcl-2 protein whereas mantle zone B cells express bcl-2 (fig. 2-24). Germinal center cells also express CD10 and low levels of surface immunoglobulin, with an approximate ratio of kappa to lambda light chains of 2-3 to 1.

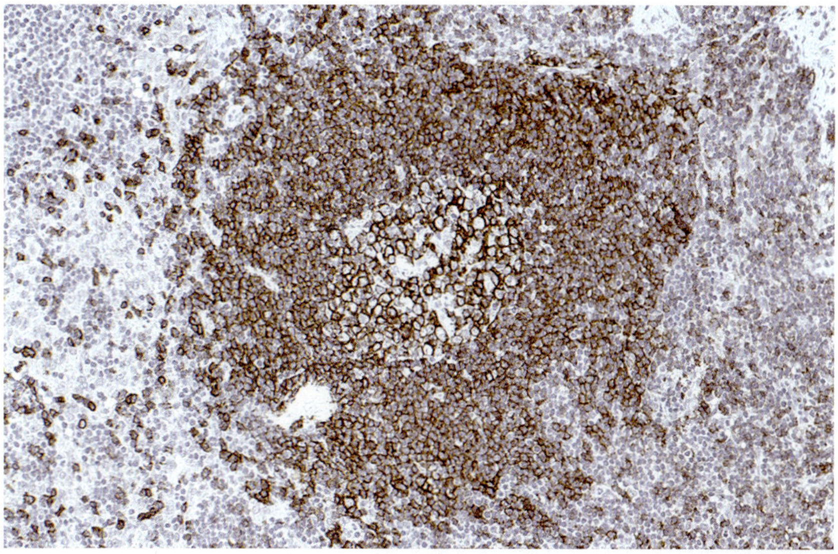

Figure 2-23

LYMPH NODE REACTIVITY FOR CD20

B lymphocytes in the germinal centers and mantle zones express the CD20 antigen in paraffin-embedded tissue sections.

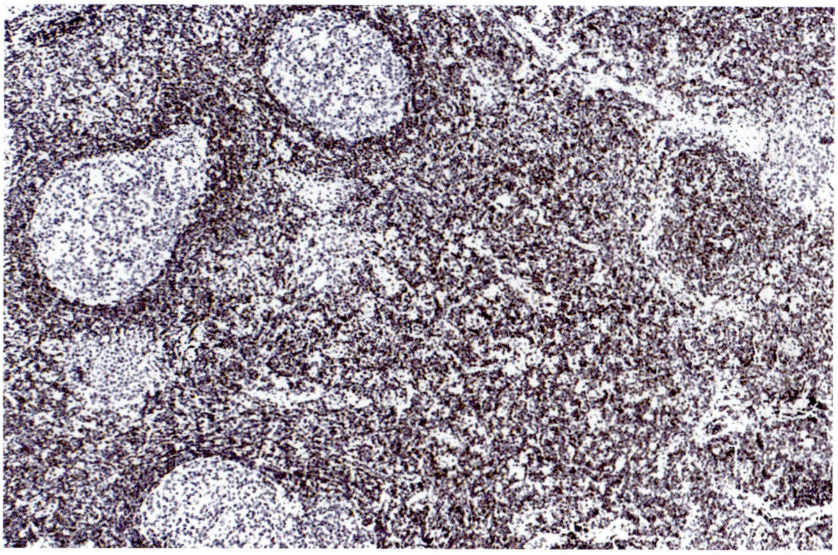

Figure 2-24

LYMPH NODE REACTIVITY FOR BCL-2

Bcl-2 reactivity is seen in the mantle zone and interfollicular T lymphocytes but not in the reactive germinal center.

Interspersed follicular dendritic cells react with antibodies to the complement receptors, CD21 (C3d) (fig. 2-25) and CD35 (C3b) (27).

B-cell development in the human lymph node has been studied on a molecular level by the analysis of single cells that have been microdissected from developing germinal centers. Sequencing and amplification of the V (variable) regions of isolated B cells, by polymerase chain reaction, show that developing germinal centers within primary follicles are dominated by a few large B-cell clones that exhibit intraclonal diversity by ongoing somatic hypermutation (44,45). Molecular analysis of different germinal centers within the same lymph node reveals a polyclonal population of activated B cells in the dark zone that continuously undergoes somatic hypermutation. These cells probably represent the initial founder cells of the germinal center reaction. Molecular studies of microdissected B cells in the light zone show that these cells have undergone a cessation of mutations, possibly indicating the late phase of the antigenic reaction.

The third, or outer, layer of the germinal center, although not as prominent as its counterpart in the spleen, represents the marginal zone component of the lymph node. The marginal zone is composed of cells that resemble parafollicular or monocytoid B cells. These cells are often noted within or adjacent to the subcapsular

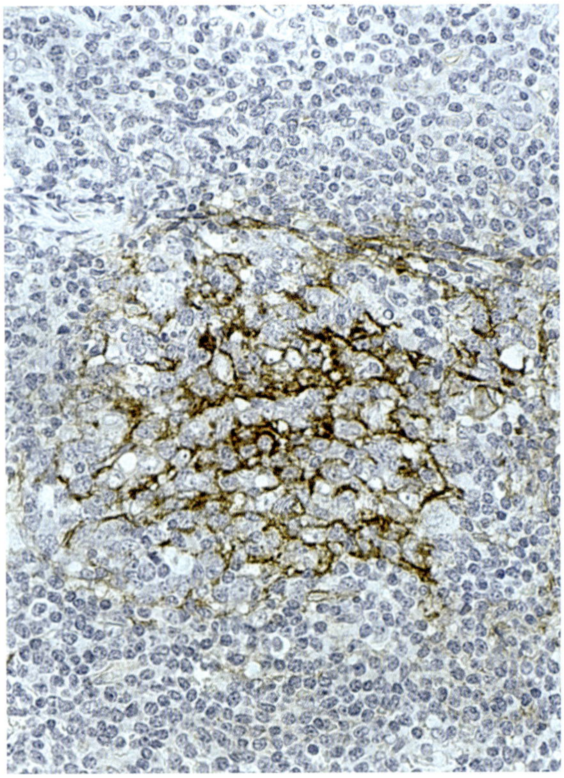

Figure 2-25

LYMPH NODE REACTIVITY FOR CD21

CD21 highlights the follicular dendritic cell network in the germinal center. A follicular dendritic cell is a specific type of mononuclear phagocyte-derived cell that captures antigen on its surface.

and cortical sinuses in some types of reactive lymphadenopathies (84). Although these distinctive mononuclear cells were previously referred to as immature sinus histiocytes, their B-cell phenotype was eventually confirmed by immunohistochemistry (8).

Monocytoid B cells, which make up the cells of the marginal zone, are intermediate to large lymphocytes with abundant clear cytoplasm and round to oval nuclei with moderately clumped chromatin and inconspicuous nucleoli. Polymorphonuclear leukocytes are invariably present in foci of marginal zone hyperplasia (fig. 2-26). This pattern is an important feature to recognize because it is characteristically seen in association with some infections such as toxoplasmosis, cat-scratch disease, and human immunodeficiency virus (HIV) and other viral-related lymphadenitides.

The exact origin of the parafollicular and marginal zone cells is still controversial. Recent molecular studies, however, have shown that some tumors composed of these cells, such as monocytoid B-cell and splenic marginal zone B-cell lymphomas, demonstrate clonal expansions of postgerminal center memory lymphocytes (54).

Paracortex

The lymph node paracortex is a specific zone containing small T lymphocytes and interdigitating reticulum cells. It is located between the B-cell follicles and the medulla. Two major subsets of T lymphocytes, CD4-positive helper/inducer and CD8-positive cytotoxic/suppressor cells, constitute the major cellular components in this location. The CD4 to CD8 ratio varies from 2-10 to1 and is characteristically reversed in viral infections such as HIV. Paracortical hyperplasia may show expansion in a nodular (fig. 2-27) or diffuse (fig. 2-28) pattern. Many of the paracortical T cells express CD45RO (fig. 2-29), which is associated with a memory function, a short lifespan, and the capacity to elaborate cytokines, or CD45RA, which has a long lifespan and an ability to elaborate interleukin-2 (IL-2) (2,37). The polyclonal antibody used in paraffin sections, CD3, is also useful for identifying these T lymphocytes (fig. 2-30). High endothelial venules are characteristically located in this region (fig. 2-31). Other regions of the paracortex often contain a mixture of both B and T lymphocytes, which are highlighted by antibodies to leukocyte common antigen, CD45RB (fig. 2-32). An increase in T immunoblasts in some reactive conditions, such as viral lymphadenitis, imparts a distinctive mottled appearance to the paracortex (81,85).

In some reactive conditions, the paracortex also contains foci of plasmacytoid dendritic cells (formerly referred to as plasmacytoid monocytes), which are medium-sized, round cells with vesicular nuclei and well-defined cytoplasmic borders (fig. 2-33). These cells are often noted in granulomatous lymphadenitis and histiocytic necrotizing lymphadenitis without neutrophils (Kikuchi-Fujimoto disease). Immunohistochemical antibodies to CD123, lysozyme, or CD68 (KP-1) may be used to highlight the clusters of plasmacytoid dendritic cells (fig. 2-34).

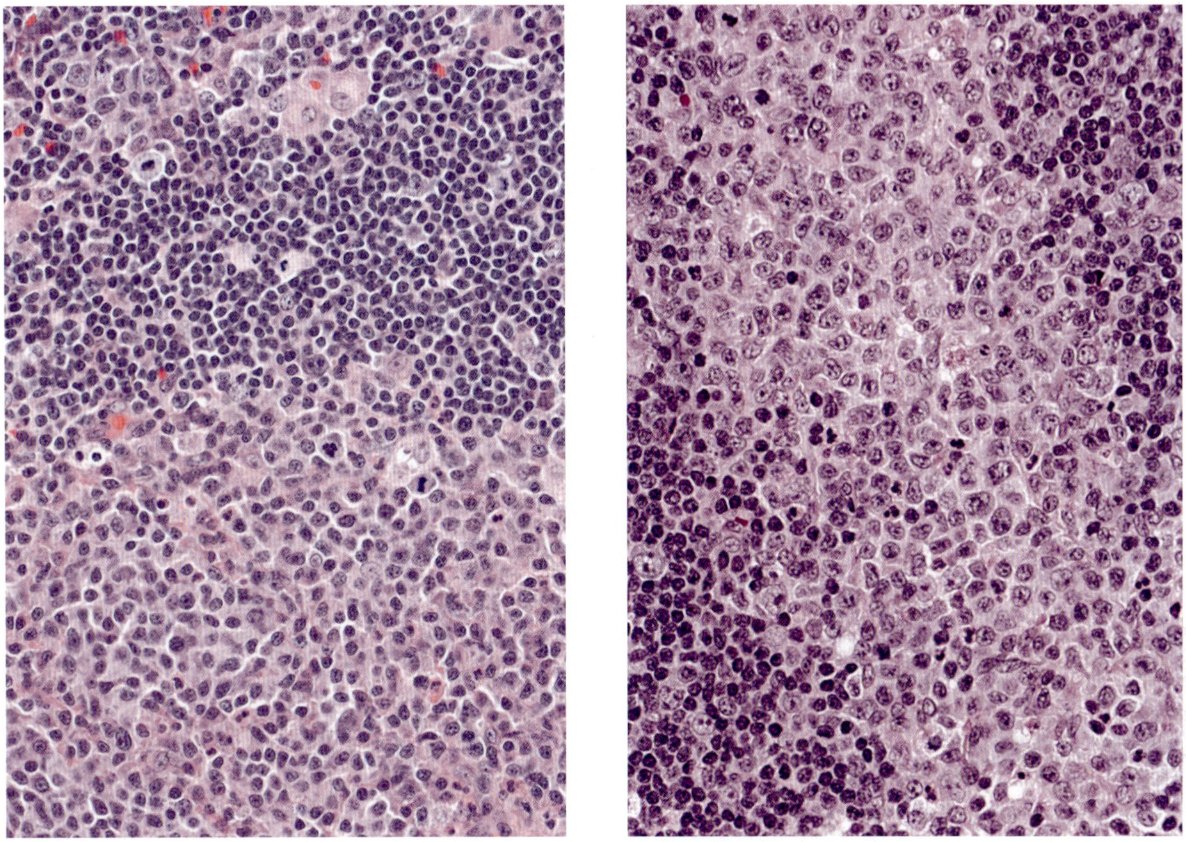

Figure 2-26

MONOCYTOID B CELLS IN MARGINAL ZONE

Two examples of marginal zone cells in lymph nodes. The cells have small to intermediated-sized nuclei, with increased amounts of pale or clear cytoplasm. Notably, there is always a small component of accompanying granulocytes in the marginal zone cell proliferations.

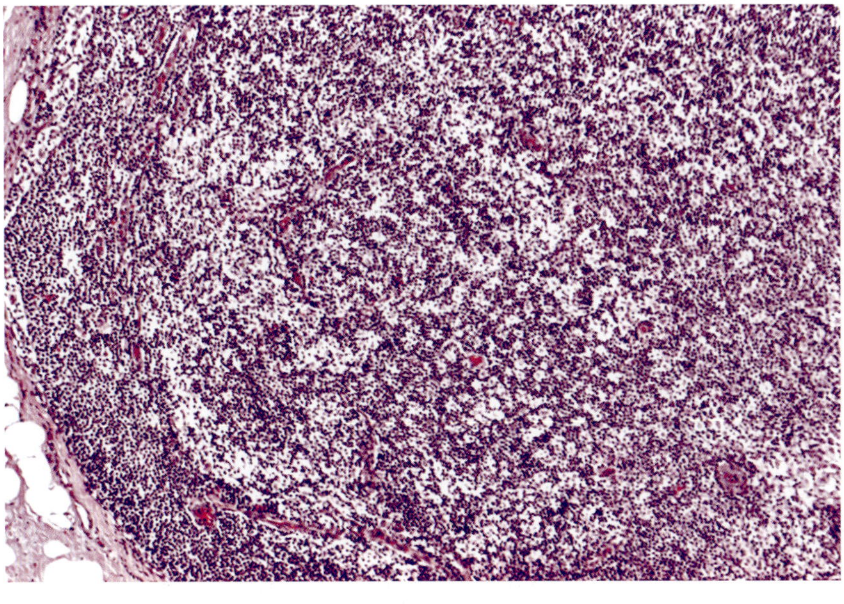

Figure 2-27

PARACORTICAL NODULAR HYPERPLASIA

Expansion of the lymph node paracortex in a nodular pattern.

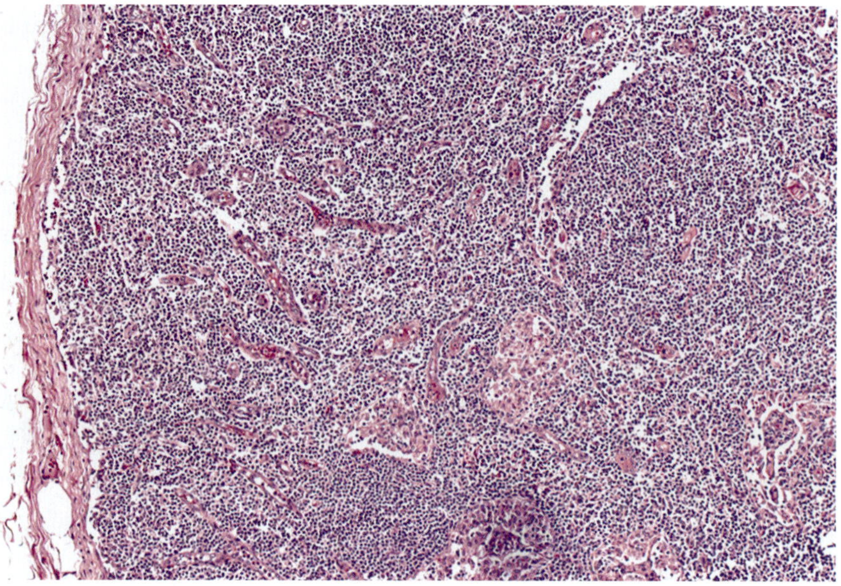

Figure 2-28

PARACORTICAL DIFFUSE HYPERPLASIA

Expansion of the paracortex in a diffuse pattern.

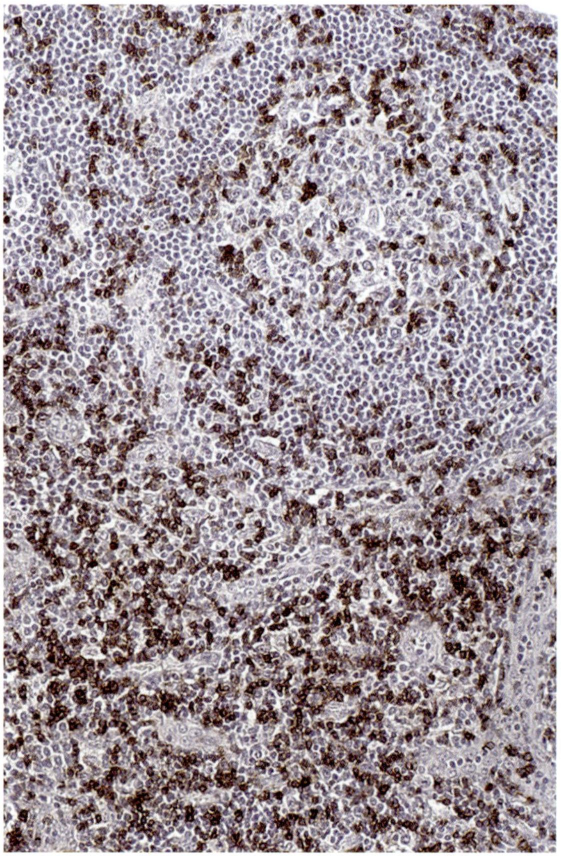

Figure 2-29

LYMPH NODE REACTIVITY FOR CD45RO IN PARACORTICAL AREAS

Scattered CD45RO-positive T cells are in the paracortex and focally within a germinal center.

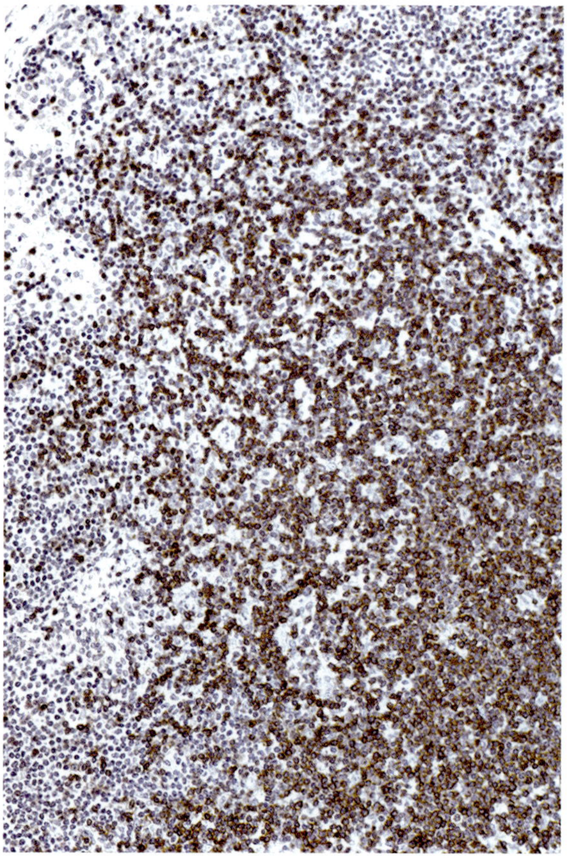

Figure 2-30

LYMPH NODE REACTIVITY FOR CD3 IN PARACORTICAL AREAS

A polyclonal antibody to CD3 reacts with T cells in the paracortex.

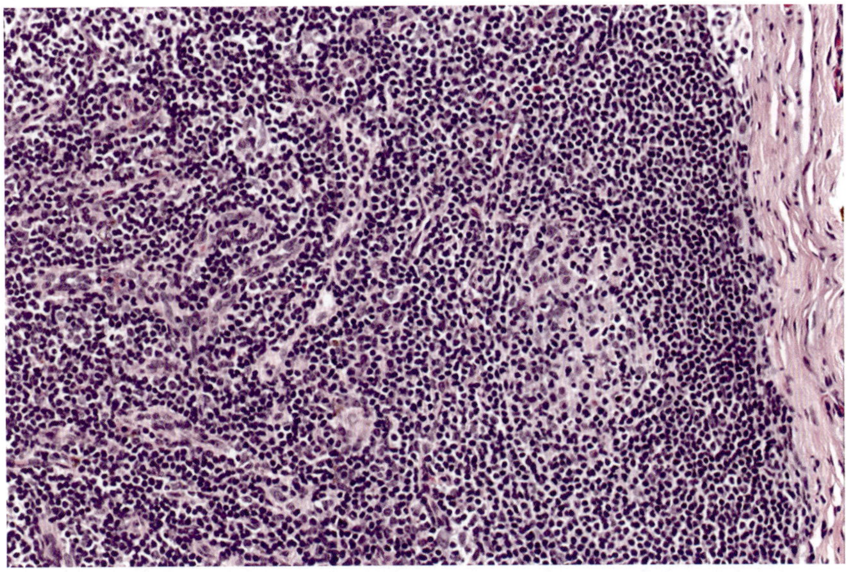

Figure 2-31

HIGH ENDOTHELIAL VENULES

Postcapillary or high endothelial venules in the lymph node paracortex.

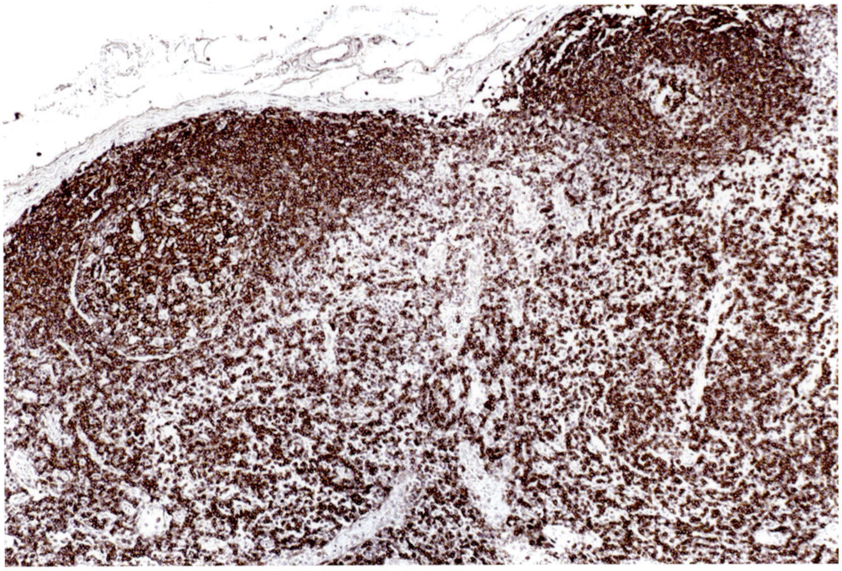

Figure 2-32

LYMPH NODE REACTIVITY FOR CD45RB

Antibody to CD45RB (leukocyte common antigen) highlights the majority of cells in the cortex and paracortex of the lymph node.

Medulla

The lymph node medulla includes both the medullary cords and the medullary sinuses that are located between the paracortex and the hilum (22). The medullary cords are primarily composed of small B and T lymphocytes, plasma cells, and occasional immunoblasts or mast cells. The medullary sinuses contain macrophages, lymphocytes, and circulating granulocytes. The sinuses are connected via the trabecular (or radial) sinuses to the afferent lymphatic vessels that penetrate the subcapsular sinus. Effector T lymphocytes and plasma cells that are generated by the body's immune reactions accumulate in the medulla and exit through the medullary sinuses. The sinuses also contain accessory cells and macrophages, which are the first cells to come in contact with exogenous antigens as they enter the lymph node. The medullary region is also the location for monocytoid B cells and plasmacytoid dendritic cells.

Vasculature

The lymph node has a complex vascular structure that consists of arteries, capillaries, postcapillary high endothelial venules, and veins, in

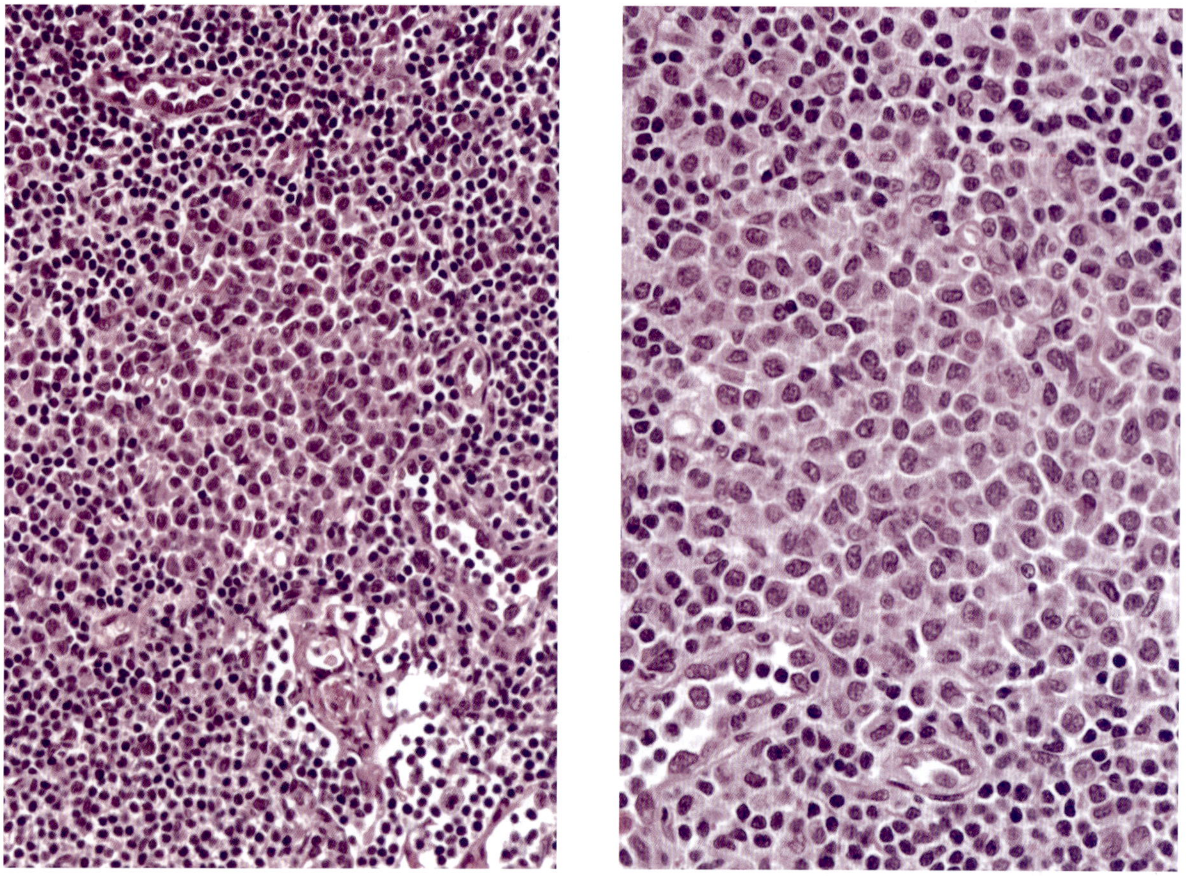

Figure 2-33

PLASMACYTOID DENDRITIC CELLS

A cluster of plasmacytoid dendritic cells in the paracortex of a reactive lymph node seen at intermediate (left) and high (right) magnification.

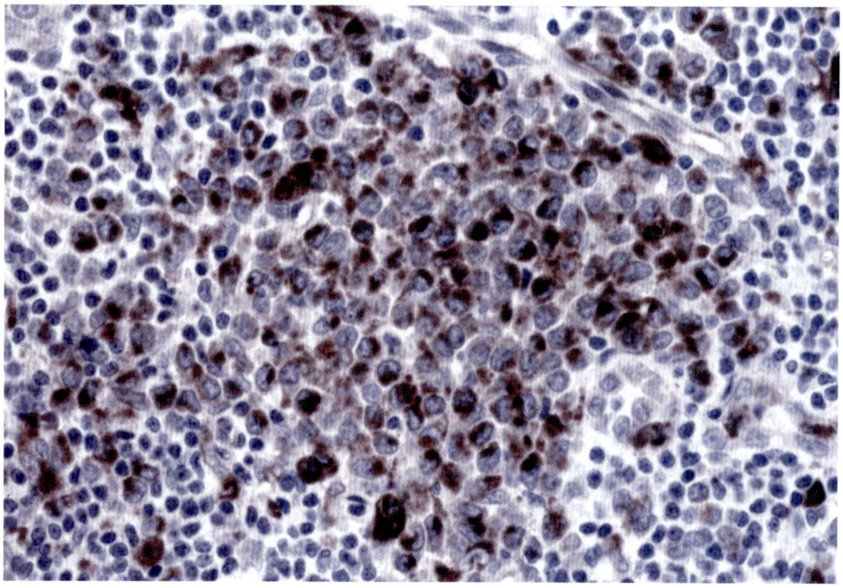

Figure 2-34

PLASMACYTOID DENDRITIC CELL REACTIVITY FOR CD68

CD68 immunoreactivity in plasmacytoid dendritic cells.

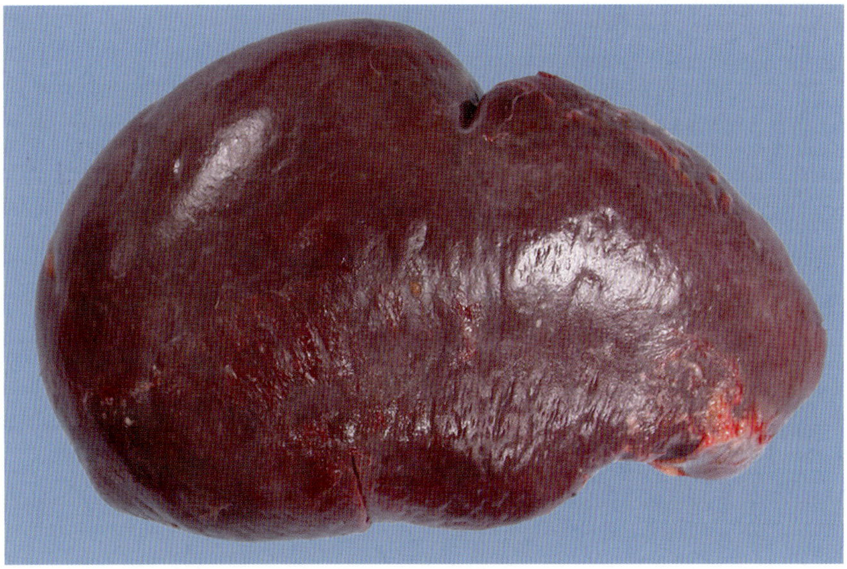

Figure 2-35

GROOVES ON SURFACE OF SPLEEN

The grooves on the spleen are remnants of the embryonic development of the spleen and are a normal variant.

addition to the afferent and efferent lymphatic vessels that drain the sinuses. The hilum is the major site of entry for the lymph node's arterial vessels. These arteries traverse the medulla and give rise to arterioles in the lymph node cortex. The arterioles subsequently lead to capillaries, which empty into the postcapillary or high endothelial venules located in the paracortex. These venules are important entry points for peripheral blood lymphocytes into the lymph node parenchyma. The high endothelial vessels lead to veins that pass through the lymph node cortex and medulla, and exit at the hilum.

HISTOLOGY OF THE SPLEEN

General Microanatomy

The human spleen is a bean-shaped organ surrounded by a fibrous capsule covered by the peritoneum. In contrast to several species, the capsule does not contain smooth muscle fibers and therefore does not have the capability of contracting in response to acute blood loss. The spleen in animals such as dogs and cats has an important red blood cell reservoir function. By undergoing rapid contraction, the spleen can squeeze out its red blood cell reservoir and, by doing so, produce a rapid increase in the amount of circulating blood.

The weight of the spleen is highly variable (56). In adults, the spleen generally weighs 150 to 250 g, but in the elderly, the spleen is often substantially smaller, even when there is no apparent hypofunction. The surface may be covered with fibrotic or even calcified plaques, the cause of which is unknown. It is common to find several grooves at the outer surface that have no clinical significance (fig. 2-35). Real, albeit short, true septa are also present in the spleen. These are connected to the capsule, lack inside vessels, and only extend for a short length into the splenic tissue. On the cut surface, the red and white pulp can be discerned, the latter consisting of small (about 2 mm) nodules (Table 2-4; fig. 2-36). Involvement of the spleen in malignant lymphoma often is observed foremost in the white pulp (91), which becomes enlarged but often not to a great extent. Therefore, the spleen should be sampled with thin sections (about 5 mm).

The spleen is innervated by nonmyelinated fibers from the major splanchnic nerves and the celiac plexus. These nerve fibers run along the splenic artery. Innervation in human spleens is less extensive than in cat and dog spleens, and this might be related to the important reservoir function of the spleen in these animals, as previously mentioned.

Vasculature

Blood reaches the spleen via the splenic artery, a large branch of the celiac artery (71,72). The splenic artery, before entering the spleen parenchyma, branches at the splenic hilum into four to six branches; their number and

Table 2-4

NORMAL MORPHOLOGIC COMPARTMENTS OF THE SPLEEN

White Pulp	Follicles	
	Primary	Composed of small nodules of mantle type B lymphocytes
	Secondary	Composed of a mixture of small, irregular B lymphocytes and large transformed cells, with intermixed dendritic cells and macrophages
	Mantle zone	Surrounds the germinal center; cellularity composed predominantly of small B lymphocytes with round to irregular nuclei, condensed chromatin, and scant cytoplasm
	Periarteriolar lymphoid sheath (PALS)	Sheaths of predominantly small T lymphocytes that surround arterioles and arteries; other cells include larger transformed lymphocytes, NK[a] cells, plasma cells, B cells
Red Pulp	Sinusoids	Lined by specialized endothelial cells with macrophage capacity (e.g., littoral cells); lack a continuous basal membrane
	Cords	Lie between the sinusoids and composed of extracellular space and cordal macrophages
Supporting Stroma	Capsule and subcapsular sinus	Composed of dense fibrous tissue and some spindle-shaped stromal cells

[a]NK = natural killer.

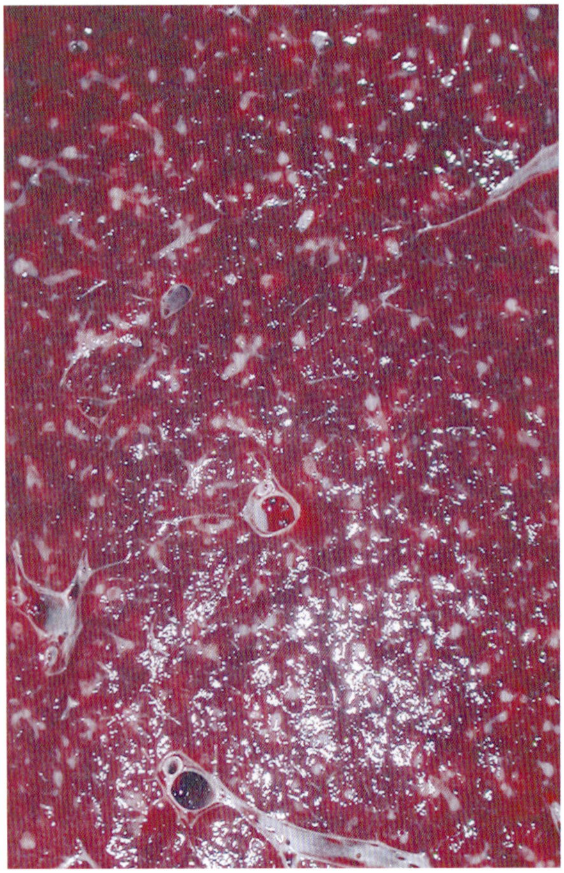

Figure 2-36

CUT SURFACE OF SPLEEN

The vascular elements and red and white pulp are distinct components. In pathologic conditions, one or more of these components may predominate.

location are, however, variable. After entering the spleen, they become surrounded by collagenous fibers. Because these perivascular collagen cuffs, which also harbor veins and lymphatics, are usually referred to as trabeculae or septa, the major intrasplenic arterial branches are termed trabecular arteries. Trabecular arteries branch to form central arteries and arterioles. These are no longer accompanied by veins and are surrounded not by a collagenous cuff but rather by lymphatic tissue predominantly composed of T lymphocytes, which is usually referred to as a periarterial or periarteriolar lymphoid sheath (PALS) (Table 2-4) (fig. 2-37). The PALS becomes smaller toward the arteriolar capillary endings. The arterioles are usually described as branching into penicilliary arterioles, which run in parallel. In humans, however, this phenomenon seems to be restricted to involuted specimens in which the disappearance of tissue between arterioles has left them lying close to each other. The branching of arterioles and capillaries often occurs at right angles, as can frequently be seen in sections.

At the arteriolar capillary endings, the endothelial lining ends abruptly and the vascular lumen is surrounded by a string of concentrically arranged macrophages forming a perivascular "sheath" of mononuclear phagocytes and rare reticulum cells. This unique splenic vascular structure (7,57,75,90) is known as sheathed capillary as well as by other names, such as ellipsoids or periarteriolar macrophage sheaths, as determined partly by the species in

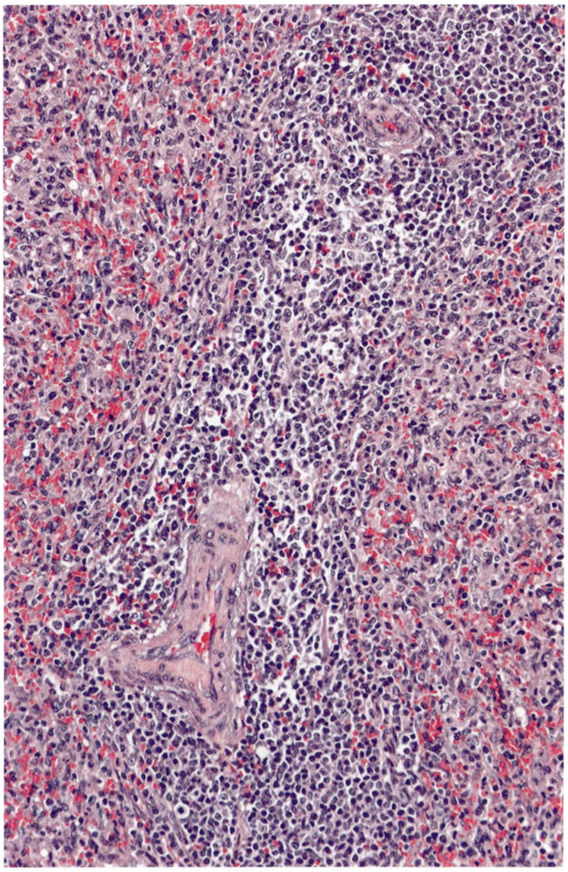

Figure 2-37

PERIARTERIOLAR LYMPHOID SHEATH (PALS) OF SPLEEN

Arterioles of the spleen are surrounded by a "cuff" of lymphocytes, termed the PALS.

which they have been originally described. The localization of the sheathed capillaries at the end of the arterial tree seems perfect for their function as a filtering unit.

Blood cells coming from an arteriole have to pass through the sheathed capillary on their way to the lumen of the venous sinus, which they reach by slowly percolating through the cord macrophages and red pulp stroma (open circulation). After that, the cells enter the splenic sinuses, the first part of the venous tree, via the slits in the basement membrane of the sinus (28,57). Although no direct anatomic connection between the arteriolar ends and the sinuses has been demonstrated, a proportion of the arteriolar branches ends close to the walls of the sinuses, allowing more rapid circulation (closed circulation) of at least a portion of the blood flow.

Venous outflow occurs via vessels that follow the trabecular arteries and exit the spleen as four to six venous branches. These combine, within the lienorenal ligament, to form the splenic vein, which drains into the portal vein.

No afferent lymphatic vessels are present in the spleen. Small efferent lymph vessels can be found in the T-lymphocyte compartment of the white pulp in about two thirds of spleens. They are not seen in the surrounding perifollicular zone. The lymph vessels form a network around arterioles and trabecular arteries, and eventually follow the arterial tree to the hilar region (23,88). The splenic lymph drainage goes to hilar lymph nodes and lymph nodes in the gastrosplenic ligament. The lymph then flows through lymphatics along the splenic artery to the celiac lymph nodes along the celiac artery.

Red Pulp

Seventy-five percent of the volume of the spleen is made up of red pulp (90). The red pulp is largely composed of cordal macrophages interconnected by their cytoplasmic processes to form a reticular meshwork which provides structural support to the venous sinuses (fig. 2-38). It is also rich in capillaries and contains the terminal ends of the penicilliary arterioles. Serial sections and ultrastructural analysis have shown, however, that the red pulp also contains a loose reticular framework. The sinus endothelial cells are surrounded by almost circular strands of discontinuous basement membrane, predominantly composed of collagen IV and laminin, known as the ring fibers (fig. 2-39). Basement type collagen and laminin constitute the vast majority of the extracellular stroma matrix of the spleen. The ring fibers are both interconnected among themselves and anchored to the dendritic processes of the cordal macrophages, the splenic adventitial reticulum cells (SARC), found predominantly in a periarteriolar location (59), and the splenic fibroblastic reticulum cells (SFRC). Stromal fibers and reticulum cells running throughout the red pulp help provide structural support to this splenic area and are collectively referred to as the reticular meshwork of the red pulp. The SARCs, which are identified by their expression of low weight nerve

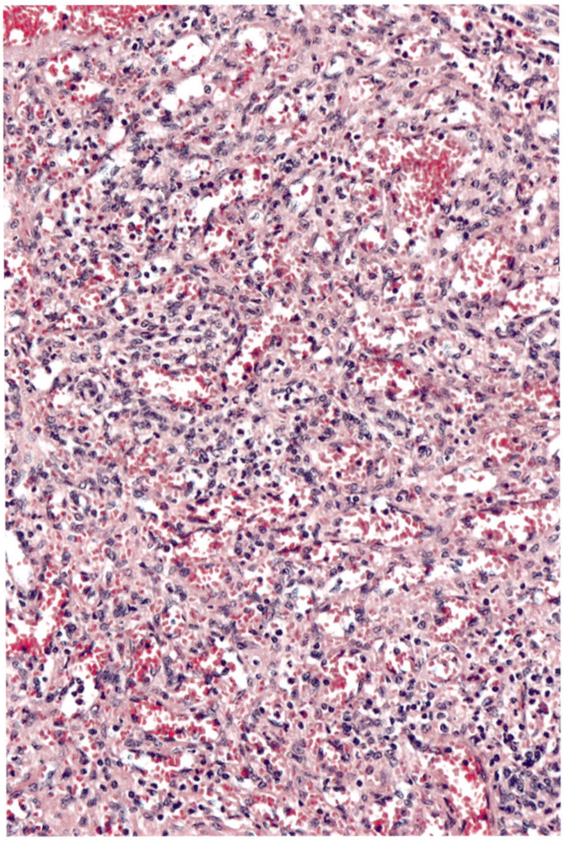

Figure 2-38

RED PULP

The red pulp is composed of splenic sinuses and splenic cords. The sinuses are lined by littoral cells, a specialized type of endothelial cell found only in the spleen.

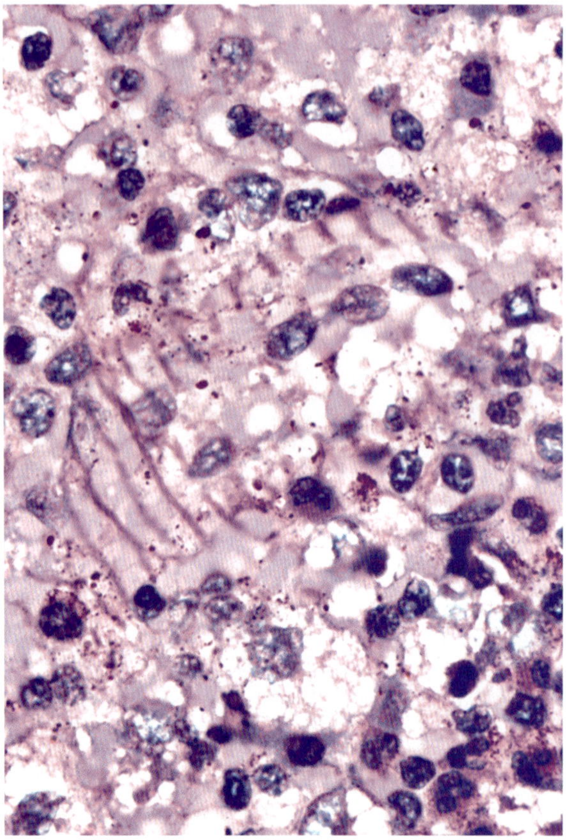

Figure 2-39

RING FIBERS, SUPPORTING EXTRACELLULAR MATRIX IN SPLEEN

Ring fibers of the spleen, seen here with a periodic acid–Schiff (PAS) stain, are analogous to metal hoops that surround the staves (i.e., endothelial cells) of a barrel.

growth factor receptor, appear similar to those present in the adventitia of blood vessels and those found in bone marrow and lymph nodes (fig. 2-40) (11,59). Splenic myoid reticulum cells (SMRC), identified by their smooth muscle actin positivity, are found scattered throughout the red pulp. These cells are, however, much more concentrated at the junction between red pulp and the marginal zone of the lymphoid follicles (perifollicular areas, see below) and in the PALS (fig. 2-41) (64,77,83). Whether these smooth actin-positive red pulp cells correspond to SFRCs which have undergone myofibroblastic differentiation, or are a truly separate population, is unclear at this time.

The red pulp sinuses, a complex vascular network with many interconnections, are lined by elongated, flat endothelial cells with typical bean-shaped nuclei having a longitudinal cleft; these cells are also known as littoral cells (95). Immunoperoxidase studies have shown their positivity for endothelial markers and, unique among other endothelial cells, to CD8 and often CD68 and CD21 (fig. 2-42). Although the predominant function of the red pulp is blood filtration, recent evidence has confirmed the presence of "nonfiltering" areas of the red pulp, which are totally devoid of capillary endings and surrounded only by sinuses. The presence in these areas of aggregates of lymphocytes and macrophages suggests that these nonfiltering areas of the splenic red pulp may represent a largely unrecognized and poorly understood lymphoid compartment, in addition to the one represented by the white pulp. Blood cells can only reach these areas by

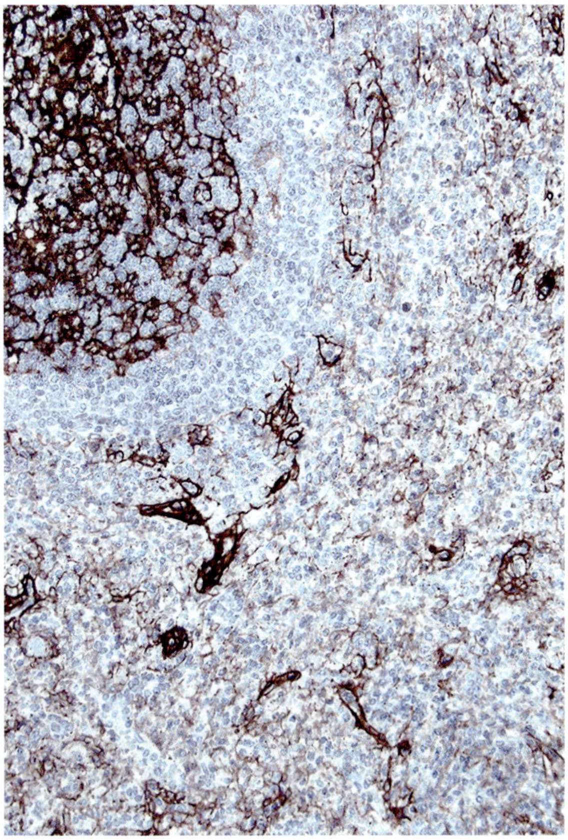

Figure 2-40

SPLEEN REACTIVITY FOR LOW AFFINITY NERVE GROWTH FACTOR RECEPTOR (LNGFR)

LNGFR highlights follicular dendritic cells in the white pulp as well as reticulum cells in the red pulp. The reticulum cells form much of the stromal framework of the red pulp.

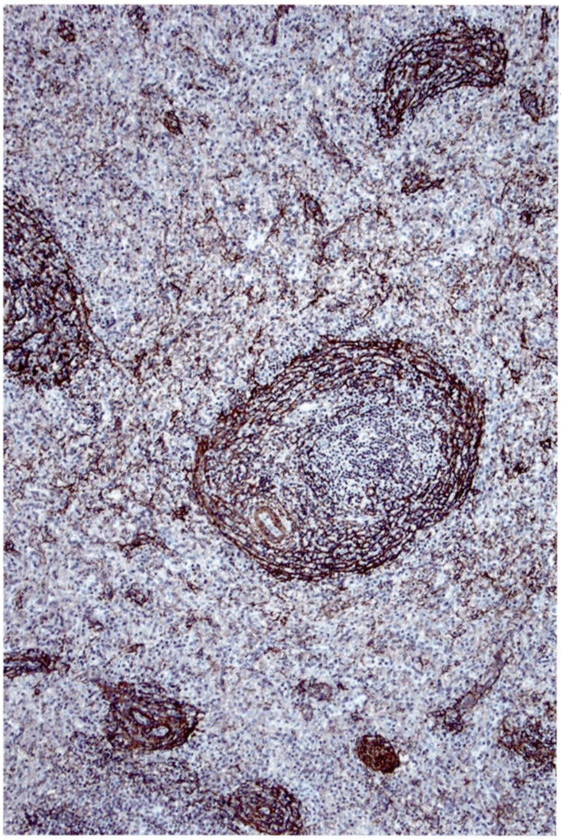

Figure 2-41

SPLEEN REACTIVITY FOR SMOOTH MUSCLE ACTIN

Smooth muscle actin highlights the distinct separation of the white pulp from the red pulp. The marginal zone of the lymphoid follicles has a discontinuous lining of these contractile cells.

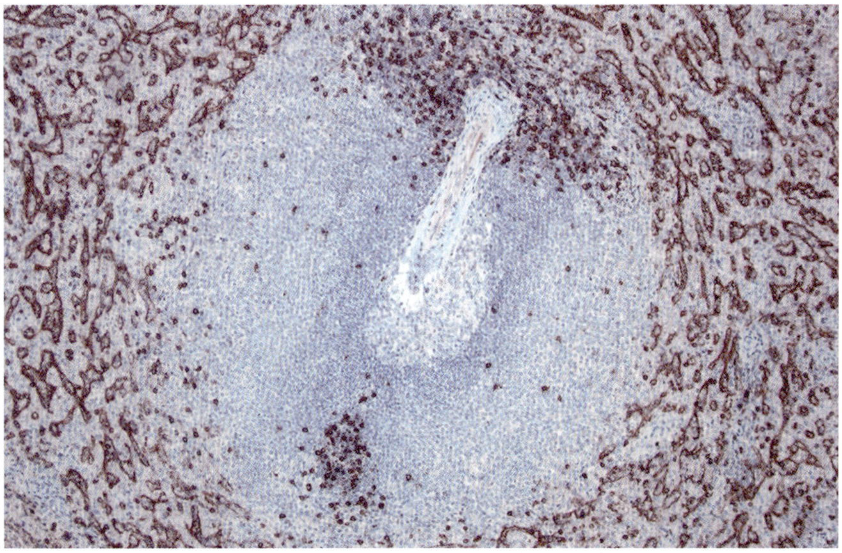

Figure 2-42

SPLENIC SINUS REACTIVITY FOR CD8

The littoral cells, which line the splenic sinuses, stain for CD8, a feature of these specialized endothelial cells of the spleen not seen at other body sites.

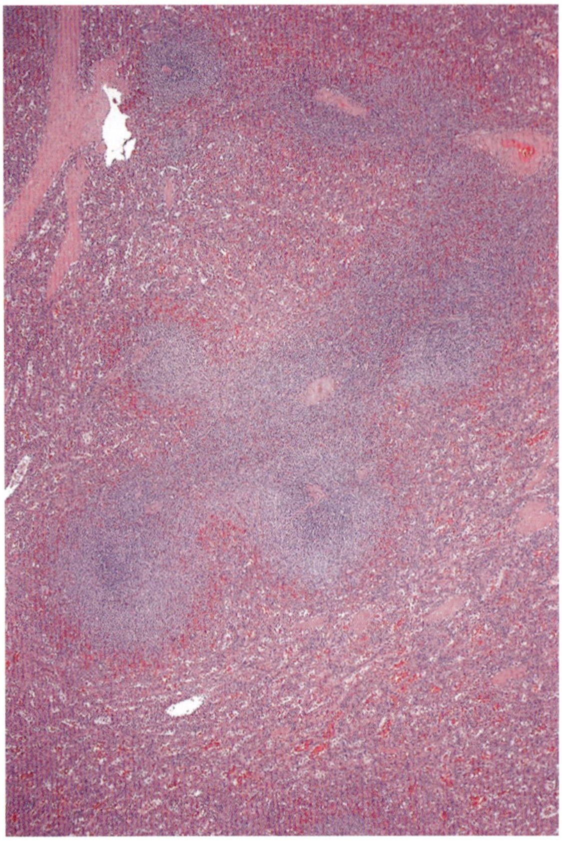

Figure 2-43

WHITE PULP OF SPLEEN

The white pulp of the spleen is arrayed along the arterioles, which are analogous to branches on a tree. The PALS surrounds the arterioles, as bark on a tree. The follicles are similar to the buds of a tree, which arise from these branches.

passing through large stretches of red pulp tissue or through their egression from the sinuses, through the sinus endothelium.

A "retrograde" return of lymphocytes from the venous sinus lumen back into the splenic tissue is known to occur in the marginal sinus of the rodent spleen, an anatomic structure that is easily seen by light microscopic examination at the interface between the marginal and mantle zones. It plays an essential role in splenic immune function as the site of entry of lymphocytes and antigens, and the site to which these cells migrate through the sinus wall into the white pulp (70). This dividing sinus is not discernible in humans, at least by light microscopy. By using electron microscopy, however, a marginal sinus-like structure has been described (71), although it seems to be, paradoxically, absent in active follicles. Neither the exact location nor functional properties of this structure are known. Since an anatomically identifiable marginal sinus is absent in the human spleen, the functional role played in rodents by the marginal sinus could be played by the perifollicular zone (PFZ), a distinct splenic compartment composed of sheathed capillaries and blood-filled vascular spaces devoid of endothelial lining, which occupies the bordering area between the red and white pulp. It has been suggested that this area is responsible for the passage of about 10 percent of the splenic blood, and is known to have a retarded flow (89). In silver-stained sections, the PFZ can be identified by its paucity of basal membrane strands and its vascular pattern of widely spaced sinuses, a pattern different from the one seen in the rest of the red pulp (77,88). The sinuses in the PFZ contain a large number of erythrocytes, which impart to those areas a deeply congested appearance evident in H&E-stained sections. Recent evidence has suggested that this zone may represent the port of entry into the white pulp for recirculating lymphocytes, since it has been shown capable of supporting influx and local proliferation of lymphoreticular cells, particularly CD4-positive T lymphocytes (77). It has also been suggested that the entry of recirculating lymphocytes may be dependent on the presence, in the perifollicular area, of specialized reticulum cells with an endothelial-like phenotype that secrete lymphokines and guide the T cells into the PALS (77).

White Pulp

The white pulp consists of PALS expanded intermittently by lymphoid follicles (fig. 2-43). Although the follicles are "within" the PALS areas, the latter appear often attenuated or even undetectable over the follicular surface.

Functionally, the white pulp consists of B- and T-cell lymphoid compartments (89). The B-cell compartment mainly consists of the splenic lymphoid follicles. The follicles have a germinal center composed of centrocytes and centroblasts (only found in secondary follicles), surrounded by a mantle zone of small lymphocytes, which in turn is surrounded by a marginal zone of mostly medium-sized lymphocytes. The germinal centers, similar to those found in other lymphoid organs, are formed by a scaffold of follicular dendritic cells, which express CD21, CD23, CD35, and the low affinity nerve growth factor receptor. The B cells of the germinal centers express CD20, CD19, CD10, bcl-6, and CD79a, but not CD5. They have a high proliferation activity with Ki-67 and do not express bcl-2. The T lymphocytes present within germinal centers are predominantly CD4 positive; CD68-positive tingible body macrophages are also present. Mantle zones consist predominantly of small lymphocytes which are IgM, IgD, CD45RA, and DBA.44 positive and alkaline phosphatase negative. The marginal zone lymphocytes are, in contrast, positive for alkaline phosphatase, and negative for IgD, CD45RA, and DBA.44 (fig. 2-44) (57,91). The marginal zone also contains macrophages functionally distinct from the cord macrophages of the red pulp, which, at least in animal models, seem to be important in maintaining the anatomic structure of the marginal zone by attracting into it newly differentiated marginal zone B lymphocytes. These cells move into the marginal zone area from the germinal center, where they are derived from a common follicular/marginal zone precursor B cell (63).

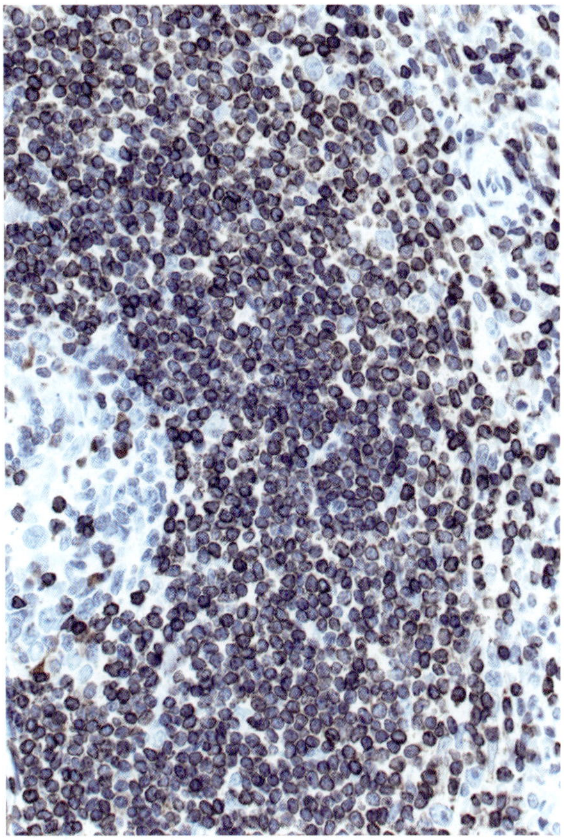

Figure 2-44

MARGINAL ZONE REACTIVITY FOR BCL-2

While the germinal center does not react for bcl-2 (lower center), the mantle cells and the marginal zone cells do.

The reticulin framework of the marginal zone is characterized by the presence of numerous smooth muscle actin (SMA)–positive reticulum cells arranged in a concentric meshwork pattern (fig. 2-45). The marginal zone SMA-positive cells continue into the T-cell zones, where reticulum cells, exhibiting the same immunophenotype, form the reticular framework of the PALS. Cells with SMA positivity are also seen, although less frequently, in the perifollicular zone and throughout the red pulp. These cells become more prominent in the presence of red pulp congestion such as seen in cases of fibrocongestive splenomegaly (43,59). Contractile capability may be important for a scaffold-like reticular structure capable of being reversibly stretched around lymphoid follicles as they expand and contract within the PALS.

The PALS region is a T-cell–rich area of the spleen (fig. 2-46). Morphologically, these areas are irregular aggregates of small polymorphic lymphocytes which lie around most of the arterioles. Contrary to what is seen in the rodent spleen, where their presence is constant, in humans the arterioles are not always covered by PALS, since they can be seen running "naked" while traversing follicles and germinal centers. Most of the lymphocytes in the PALS express CD4 reactivity (T-helper/inducer lymphocytes) (fig. 2-47). The T-cell areas are also surrounded by perifollicular-like zones similar to those previously described around follicles. Follicles and T-cell areas share a common perifollicular zone; this is clearly shown by the presence of a single continuous reticular meshwork of reticulum cells, which are clearly identifiable by their characteristic SMA positivity.

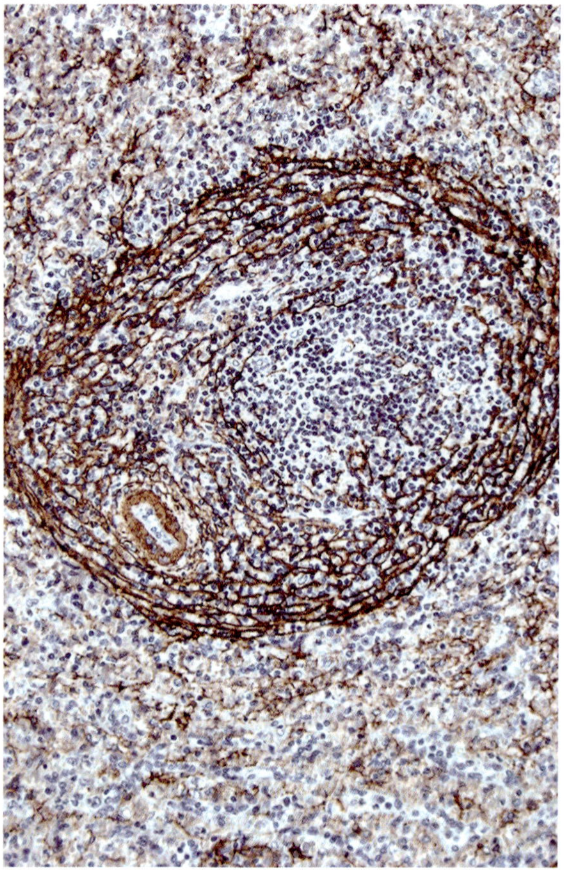

Figure 2-45

SMOOTH MUSCLE ACTIN

The reticulin framework of the splenic marginal zone is highlighted by smooth muscle actin.

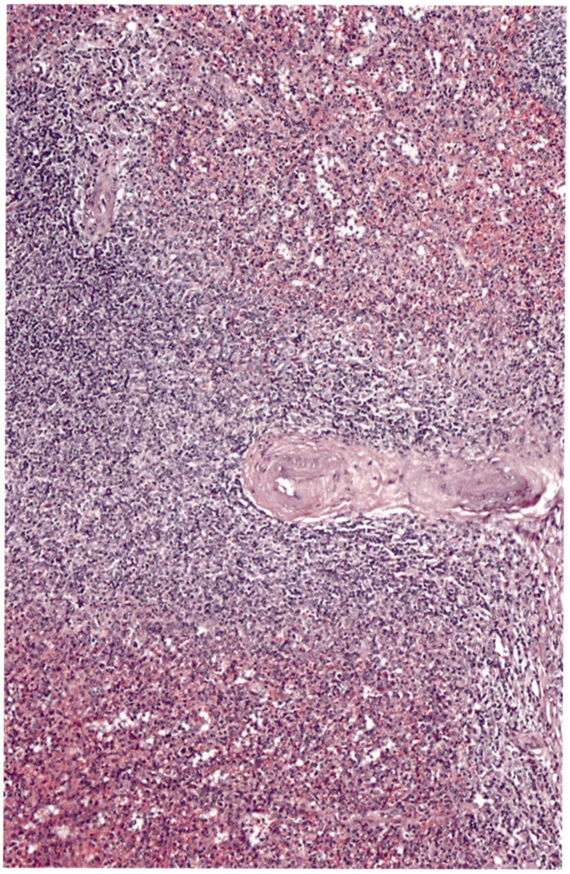

Figure 2-46

PALS OF SPLEEN

Adjacent to arterioles, the PALS is composed predominantly of T cells.

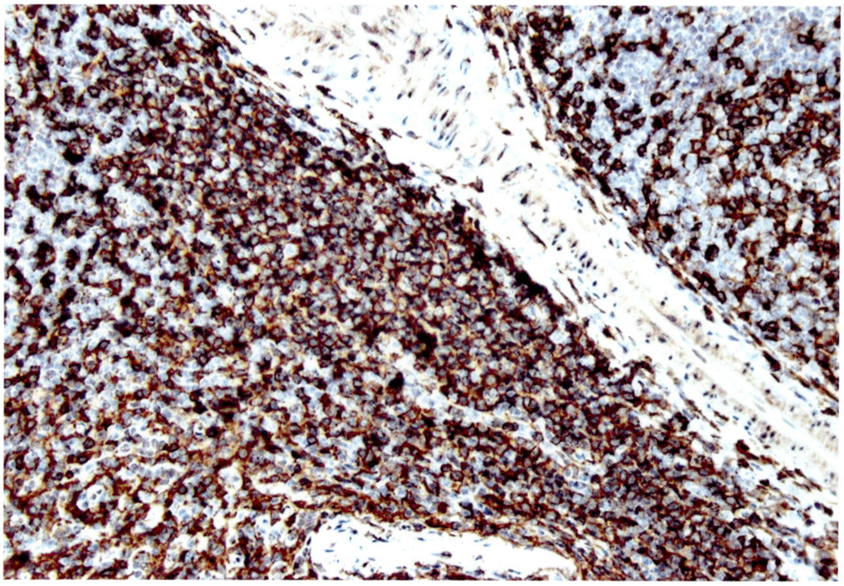

Figure 2-47

PALS REACTIVITY FOR CD4

Most T cells in the PALS express CD4.

REFERENCES

1. Argani P, Rosai J. Hyperplastic mesothelial cells in lymph nodes: report of six cases of a benign process that can simulate metastatic involvement by mesothelioma or carcinoma. Hum Pathol 1998;29:339-46.
2. Beverly PC. Functional analysis of human T cell subsets defined by CD45 isoform expression. Semin Immunol 1992;4:35-41.
3. Briskin M, Winsor-Hines D, Shyjan A, et al. Human mucosal addressin cell adhesion molecule-1 is preferentially expressed in intestinal tract and associated lymphoid tissue. Am J Pathol 1997;151:97-110.
4. Brooks JS, LiVolsi VA, Pietra GG. Mesothelial cell inclusions in mediastinal lymph nodes mimicking metastatic carcinoma. Am J Clin Pathol 1990;93:741-8.
5. Butcher EC. Warner-Lambert/Park-Davis Award Lecture. Cellular and molecular mechanisms that direct leukocyte traffic. Am J Pathol 1990;136:3-11.
6. Buxbaum JN, Chuba JV, Hellman GC, Solomon A, Gallo GR. Monoclonal immunoglobulin deposition disease: light chain and heavy chain deposition diseases and their relation to light chain amyloidosis. Clinical features, immunopathology, and molecular analysis. Ann Intern Med 1990;112:455-64.
7. Buyssens N, Paulus G, Bourgeois N. Ellipsoids in the human spleen. Virchows Arch [A] 1984; 403:27-40.
8. Cardoso De Almeida P, Harris NL, Bhan AK. Characterization of immature sinus histiocytes (monocytoid cells) in reactive lymph nodes by use of monoclonal antibodies. Hum Pathol 1984; 15:330-5.
9. Carson KF, Wen DR, Li PX, et al. Nodal nevi and cutaneous melanomas. Am J Surg Pathol 1996;20:834-40.
10. Carter BA, Jensen RA, Simpson JF, Page DL. Benign transport of breast epithelium into axillary lymph nodes after biopsy. Am J Clin Pathol 2000;113:259-65.
11. Cattoretti G, Schiro R, Orazi A, Soligo D, Colombo MP. Bone marrow stroma in humans: anti-nerve growth factor receptor antibodies selectively stain reticular cells in vivo and in vitro. Blood 1993;81:1726-38.
12. Chadburn A. The spleen: anatomy and anatomical function. Semin Hematol 2000;37(Suppl 1):13-21.
13. Chen KT. Benign glandular inclusions of the peritoneum and periaortic lymph nodes. Diagn Gynecol Obstet 1981;3:265-8.
14. Clement PB, Young RH, Oliva E, Sumner HW, Scully RE. Hyperplastic mesothelial cells within abdominal lymph nodes: mimic of metastatic ovarian carcinoma and serous borderline tumor—a report of two cases associated with ovarian neoplasms. Mod Pathol 1996;9:879-86.
15. Colby TV. Benign mesothelial cells in lymph node. Adv Anat Pathol 1999;6:41-8.
16. Cotelingam JD, Saito R. Hepatolienal fusion: case report of an unusual lesion. Hum Pathol 1978;9:234-6.
17. Davidson LA, Reid IN. Intrahepatic splenic tissue. J Clin Pathol 1997;50:532-3.
18. De Wolf-Peeters C, Delabie J. Anatomy and histophysiology of lymphoid tissue. Semin Oncol 1993;20:555-69.
19. Duncan WL Jr, Barraza MA. Splenogonadal fusion: a case report and review of literature. J Pediatr Surg 2005;40:e5-7.
20. Edlow DW, Carter D. Heterotopic epithelium in axillary lymph nodes: report of a case and review of the literature. Am J Clin Pathol 1973;59:666-73.
21. Falkowski WS, Carter MF. Splenogonadal fusion associated with an anaplastic seminoma. J Urol 1980;124:562-4.
22. Forkert PG, Thliveris JA, Bertalanffy FD. Structure of sinuses in the human lymph node. Cell Tissue Res 1977;183:115-30.
23. Fukuda T. Deep lymphatics of the spleen. Tohoku J Exp Med 1963;79:281-92.
24. Fulcher AS, Turner MA. Abdominal manifestations of situs anomalies in adults. Radiographics 2002;22:1439-56.
25. Garret R, Ada AE. Epithelial inclusion cysts in an axillary lymph node: report of a case simulating metastatic adenocarcinoma. Cancer 1957;10:173-8.
26. Gerard-Marchant R, Caillou B. Thyroid inclusions in cervical lymph nodes. Clin Endocrinol Metab 1981;10:337-49.
27. Gerdes J, Naiem M, Mason DY, Stein H. Human complement (C3b) receptors defined by a mouse monoclonal antibody. Immunology 1982;45:645-53.
28. Heusermann U, Stutte HJ. Comparative histochemical and electron microscopic studies of the sinus and venous walls of the human spleen with special reference to the sinus-venous connections. Cell Tissue Res 1975;163:519-33.

29. Holdsworth PJ, Hopkinson JM, Leveson SH. Benign axillary epithelial lymph node inclusions—a histological pitfall. Histopathology 1988;13:226-8.
30. Holt JB, Sangueza OP, Levine EA, et al. Nodal melanocytic nevi in sentinel lymph nodes. Correlation with melanoma-associated cutaneous nevi. Am J Clin Pathol 2004;121:58-63.
31. Hsu YK, Parmley TH, Rosenshein NB, Bhagavan BS, Woodruff JD. Neoplastic and non-neoplastic mesothelial proliferations in pelvic lymph nodes. Obstet Gynecol 1980;55:83-8.
32. Huntrakoon M. Benign glandular inclusions in the abdominal lymph nodes of a man. Hum Pathol 1985;16:644-6.
33. Imperial SL, Sidhu JS. Nonseminomatous germ cell tumor arising in splenogonadal fusion. Arch Pathol Lab Med 2002;126:1222-5.
34. Isaacson PG. Lymphomas of mucosa-associated lymphoid tissue (MALT). Histopathology 1990;16:617-9.
35. Isaacson P, Wright DH. Malignant lymphoma of mucosa-associated lymphoid tissue. A distinctive type of B-cell lymphoma. Cancer 1983;52:1410-6.
36. Isotalo PA, Veinot JP, Jabi M. Hyperplastic mesothelial cells in mediastinal lymph node sinuses with extranodal lymphatic involvement. Arch Pathol Lab Med 2000;124:609-13.
37. Janossy G, Bofill M, Rowe D, Muir J, Beverley PC. The tissue distribution of T lymphocytes expressing different CD45 polypeptides. Immunology 1989;66:517-25.
38. Javert CT. The spread of benign and malignant endometrium in the lymphatic system with a note on coexisting vascular involvement. Am J Obstet Gynecol 1952;64:780-806.
39. Johnson WT, Helwig EB. Benign nevus cells in the capsule of lymph nodes. Cancer 1969;23:747-53.
40. Karp LA, Czernobilsky B. Glandular inclusions in pelvic and abdominal para-aortic lymph nodes. A study of autopsy and surgical material in males and females. Am J Clin Pathol 1969;52:212-8.
41. Kempson RL. Consultation case: benign glandular inclusions in iliac lymph nodes. Am J Surg Pathol 1978;2:321-5.
42. Khairat AB, Ismail AM. Splenogonadal fusion: case presentation and literature review. J Pediatr Surg 2005;40:1357-60.
43. Kraus MD. Splenic histology and histopathology: an update. Semin Diagn Pathol 2003;20:84-93.
44. Kuppers R, Klein U, Hansmann ML, Rajewsky K. Cellular origin of human B-cell lymphomas. N Engl J Med 1999;341:1520-9.
45. Kuppers R, Zhao M, Hansmann ML, Rajewsky K. Tracing B cell development in human germinal centres by molecular analysis of single cells picked from histological sections. EMBO J 1993;12:4955-67.
46. Le Roux PJ, Heddle RM. Splenogonadal fusion: is the accepted classification system accurate? BJU Int 2000;85:114-5.
47. Liu YJ, Zhang J, Lane PJ, Chan EY, MacLennan IC. Sites of specific B cell activation in primary and secondary responses to T cell-dependent and T cell-independent antigens. Eur J Immunol 1991;21:2951-62.
48. Lohmann CM, Iversen K, Jungbluth AA, Berwick M, Busam KJ. Expression of melanocyte differentiation antigens and ki-67 in nodal nevi and comparison of ki-67 expression with metastatic melanoma. Am J Surg Pathol 2002;26:1351-7.
49. Longo S. Benign lymph node inclusions. Hum Pathol 1976;7:349-54.
50. McCarthy SW, Palmer AA, Bale PM, Hirst E. Naevus cells in lymph nodes. Pathology 1974;6:351-8.
51. McPherson F, Frias JL, Spicer D, Opitz JM, Gilbert-Barness EF. Splenogonadal fusion-limb defect "syndrome" and associated malformations. Am J Med Genet A 2003;120:518-22.
52. Meyer JS, Steinberg LS. Microscopically benign thyroid follicles in cervical lymph nodes. Serial section study of lymph node inclusions and entire thyroid gland in 5 cases. Cancer 1969;24:302-11.
53. Mills SE. Decidua and squamous metaplasia in abdominopelvic lymph nodes. Int J Gynecol Pathol 1983;2:209-15.
54. Miranda RN, Cousar JB, Hammer RD, Collins RD, Vnencak-Jones CL. Somatic mutation analysis of IgH variable regions reveals that tumor cells of most parafollicular (monocytoid) B-cell lymphoma, splenic marginal zone B-cell lymphoma, and some hairy cell leukemia are composed of memory B lymphocytes. Hum Pathol 1999;30:306-12.
55. Moore WF, Bentley RC, Berchuck A, Robboy SJ. Some mullerian inclusion cysts in lymph nodes may sometimes be metastases from serous borderline tumors of the ovary. Am J Surg Pathol 2000;24:710-8.
56. Myers J, Segal RJ. Weight of the spleen. I. Range of normal in a nonhospital population. Arch Pathol 1974;98:33-5.
57. Neiman RS, Orazi A. Disorders of the spleen, 2nd ed. Philadelphia: WB Saunders; 1999.
58. Ober WB, Black MB. Neoplasms of the subcoelomic mesenchyme. Arch Pathol 1955;59:698-705.
59. Orazi A, O'Malley DP, Thomas JL, Czader M. Stromal changes in reactive and malignant disorders of the spleen. Mod Pathol 2004;17:264A.

60. Parkash V, Vidwans M, Carter D. Benign mesothelial cells in mediastinal lymph nodes. Am J Surg Pathol 1999;23:1264-9.
61. Patterson KD, Drysdale TA, Krieg PA. Embryonic origins of spleen asymmetry. Development 2000;127:167-75.
62. Picker LJ, Butcher EC. Physiological and molecular mechanisms of lymphocyte homing. Annu Rev Immunol 1992;10:561-91.
63. Pillai S, Cariappa A, Moran ST. Marginal zone B cells. Annu Rev Immunol 2005;23:161-96.
64. Pinkus GS, Warhol MJ, O'Connor EM, Etheridge CL, Fujiwara K. Immunohistochemical localization of smooth muscle myosin in human spleen, lymph node, and other lymphoid tissues. Unique staining patterns in splenic white pulp and sinuses, lymphoid follicles, and certain vasculature, with ultrastructural correlations. Am J Pathol 1986;123:440-53.
65. Ridolfi RL, Rosen PP, Thaler H. Nevus cell aggregates associated with lymph nodes: estimated frequency and clinical significance. Cancer 1977;39:164-71.
66. Rosenthal JT, Bedetti CD, Labayen RF, Christy WC, Yakulis R. Right splenorenal fusion with associated hypersplenism. J Urol 1981;126:812-4.
67. Rudin CM, Thompson CB. B-cell development and maturation. Semin Oncol 1998;25:435-46.
68. Rutty GN, Lauder I. Mesothelial cell inclusions within mediastinal lymph nodes. Histopathology 1994;25:483-7.
69. Ryan JR, Ioachim HL, Marmer J, Loubeau JM. Acquired immune deficiency syndrome-related lymphadenopathies presenting in the salivary gland lymph nodes. Arch Otolaryngol 1985;111:554-6.
70. Sasou S, Satodate R, Katsura S. The marginal sinus in the perifollicular region of the rat spleen. Cell Tissue Res 1976;172:195-203.
71. Schmidt EE, MacDonald IC, Groom AC. Changes in splenic microcirculatory pathways in chronic idiopathioc thrombocytopenic purpura. Blood 1991;78:1485-9.
72. Schmidt EE, MacDonald IC, Groom AC. Microcirculatory pathways in normal human spleen, demonstrated by scanning electron microscopy of corrosion casts. Am J Anat 1988;181:253-66.
73. Schneider V. Benign glandular lymph node inclusions. Diagn Gynecol Obstet 1980;2:313-20.
74. Singer MI, Applebaum EL, Loy KD. Heterotopic salivary tissue in the neck. Laryngoscope 1979;89:1772-8.
75. Snook T. A comparative study of the vascular arrangements in mammalian spleens. Am J Anat 1950;87:31-77.
76. Stein H, Bonk A, Tolksdorf G, Lennert K, Rodt H, Gerdes J. Immunohistologic analysis of the organization of normal lymphoid tissue and non-Hodgkin's lymphomas. J Histochem Cytochem 1980;28:746-60.
77. Steiniger B, Barth P, Hellinger A. The perifollicular and marginal zones of the human splenic white pulp: do fibroblasts guide lymphocyte immigration? Am J Pathol 2001;159:501-12.
78. Suarez Vilela D, Izquierdo Garcia FM. Embolization of mesothelial cells in lymphatics: the route to mesothelial inclusions in lymph nodes? Histopathology 1998;33:570-5.
79. Subramony C, Lewin JR. Nevus cells within lymph nodes. Possible metastases from a benign intradermal nevus. Am J Clin Pathol 1985;84:220-3.
80. Symmers WStC. The lymphoreticular system. In: Lewis ML, Lucas RB, McMenem WH, et al eds. Systemic pathology by 38 authors, 2nd ed. Edinburgh: Churchill Livingstone; 1978:504-891.
81. Szakal AK, Kosco MH, Tew JG. Microanatomy of lymphoid tissue during humoral immune responses: structure function relationships. Annu Rev Immunol 1989;7:91-109.
82. Tazelaar HD, Vareska G. Benign glandular inclusions. Hum Pathol 1986;17:100-1.
83. Toccanier-Pelte MF, Skalli O, Kapanci Y, Gabbiani G. Characterization of stromal cells with myoid features in lymph nodes and spleen in normal and pathologic conditions. Am J Pathol 1987;129:109-18.
84. Van den Oord JJ, de Wolf-Peeters C, Desmet VJ. The marginal zone of the human reactive lymph node. Am J Clin Pathol 1986;86:475-9.
85. Van den Oord JJ, de Wolf-Peeters C, Desmet VJ, Takahashi K, Ohtsuki Y, Akagi T. Nodular alteration of the paracortical area. An in situ immunohistochemical analysis of primary, secondary, and tertiary T-nodules. Am J Pathol 1985;120:55-66.
86. Van der Valk P, Meijer CJ. The histology of reactive lymph nodes. Am J Surg Pathol 1987;11:866-82.
87. Van der Valk P, Meijer CJ. Reactive lymph nodes. In: Sternberg SS, ed. Histology for pathologists, 2nd ed. Philadelphia: Lippincott–Raven; 1997:651-73.
88. van Krieken JH, te Velde J. Normal histology of the human spleen. Am J Surg Pathol 1988;12:777-85.
89. van Krieken JH, te Velde J, Hermans J, Cornelisse CJ, Welvaart K, Ferrari M. The amount of white pulp in the spleen: a morphometrical study done in methacrylate-embedded splenectomy specimens. Histopathology 1983;7:167-82.
90. van Krieken JH, te Velde J, Hermans J, Welvaart K. The splenic red pulp: a histomorphometrical study in splenectomy specimens embedded in methylmethacrylate. Histopathology 1985;9:401-16.

91. van Krieken JH, von Schilling C, Kluin PM, Lennert K. Splenic marginal zone cells and related cells in the lymph node: a morphologic and immunohistochemical study. Hum Pathol 1989;20:320-5.
92. Wakefield JD, Thorbecke GJ. Relationship of germinal centers in lymphoid tissue to immunological memory. J Exp Med 1968;128:153-87.
93. Warnke RA, Weiss LM, Chan JK, Cleary ML, Dorfman RF. Tumors of the lymph nodes and spleen. AFIP Atlas of Tumor Pathology, 3rd Series, Fascicle 14. Washington DC: American Registry of Pathology; 1995:435-526.
94. Weeks DA, Beckwith JB, Mierau GW. Benign nodal lesions mimicking metastases from pediatric renal neoplasms: a report of the National Wilms' Tumor Study Pathology Center. Hum Pathol 1990;12:1239-44.
95. Weiss L. The spleen. In: Weiss L, ed. Cell and tissue biology: a texbook of histology, 6th ed. Baltimore: Urban & Schwarzenberg; 1988:515-38.
96. Weissman IL, Warnke R, Butcher EC, Rouse R, Levy R. The lymphoid system. Its normal architecture and the potential for understanding the system through the study of lymphoproliferative diseases. Hum Pathol 1978;9:25-45.
97. Yang XJ, Lecksell K, Epstein JI. Can immunohistochemistry enhance the detection of micrometastases in pelvic lymph nodes from patients with high-grade urothelial carcinoma of the bladder? Am J Clin Pathol 1999;112:649-53.
98. Young RH, Kurman RJ, Scully RE. Proliferations and tumors of intermediate trophoblast of the placental site. Semin Diagn Pathol 1988;5:223-37.
99. Yuan S, Vaughan M, Agoff SN. Left-sided splenorenal fusion with marked extramedullary hematopoiesis and concurrent lithium toxicity. A case report and review of the literature. Arch Pathol Lab Med 2003;127:e1-3.
100. Yunis EJ, Jaffe R. Tamm-Horsfall protein in lymph nodes. Hum Pathol 1981;12:179-83.
101. Zaytsev P, Taxy JB. Pregnancy-associated ectopic decidua. Am J Surg Pathol 1987;11:526-30.

3 TECHNICAL EVALUATION AND OVERVIEW OF LYMPH NODE AND SPLEEN

INDICATIONS FOR LYMPH NODE BIOPSY

Lymphadenopathy is a common physical sign that is associated with many benign and malignant clinicopathologic conditions. Palpable lymphadenopathy occurs as a localized or generalized process in several anatomic sites. If the lymphadenopathy persists and its cause remains undetermined, a lymph node biopsy may be necessary. It is important to be aware of the patient's past medical history, current clinical condition, and preoperative differential diagnosis at the time of the biopsy. Proper sampling and handling techniques, including adequate fixation of the tissue, should result in the correct pathologic interpretation of the adenopathy and treatment of the patient (1,5,7,11,34).

As a general rule, the largest, deepest, and most abnormal-appearing lymph node should be biopsied by the surgeon since this is likely to yield the greatest diagnostic information (4,34,37). Although overlying superficial lymph nodes are easily accessible, they often show only nonspecific reactive changes.

The differential diagnosis of lymphadenopathy varies with the patient's age. While benign reactive lymphadenopathies are more common in children and young adults, primary and secondary malignancies predominate in adults (34). Although neoplastic lesions such as Hodgkin and non-Hodgkin lymphomas are typically associated with greatly enlarged lymph nodes, pronounced lymphadenopathy is also seen in reactive conditions such as inflammatory pseudotumor of lymph node, Rosai-Dorfman disease, and infectious lymphadenitis.

The anatomic site of the lymphadenopathy may also provide a clue to the etiology and the need for an excisional biopsy (Table 3-1). Epstein-Barr virus infection and toxoplasmosis (14) are characteristically associated with enlargement of the posterior cervical lymph nodes. Enlarged occipital lymph nodes occur in the presence of scalp infections or insect bites, especially in children. The hilar lymph nodes are often involved in non-neoplastic diseases such as sarcoidosis (42), tuberculosis, histoplasmosis, and coccidioidomycosis, as well as in malignant lesions such as metastatic lung carcinoma. The mediastinal lymph nodes are a common location for Hodgkin and non-Hodgkin lymphomas. Intraabdominal and retroperitoneal lymphadenopathies often signify the presence of lymphoma or metastatic carcinoma, especially in older patients.

Table 3-1

LYMPH NODE LOCATIONS AND DISEASE ORIGINS[a]

Location	Disease
Occipital	Scalp infections, insect bites, ring worm infection
Posterior auricular	Rubella
Anterior auricular	Eye or conjunctival infections
Posterior cervical	Toxoplasmosis, scalp infections, cat-scratch disease, Epstein-Barr virus
Submental/submandibular	Dental infections, metastatic disease (oral cavity)
Anterior cervical	Infections of pharynx and oral cavity, tuberculosis, Epstein-Barr virus, nasopharyngeal carcinoma
Supraclavicular	Lymphomas, metastatic disease (lung, gastrointestinal tract)
Mediastinal	Lymphoma, sarcoidosis, histoplasmosis, coccidioidomycosis, tuberculosis, metastatic disease
Axillary	Lymphoma, cat-scratch disease, pyogenic infections of upper arms, brucellosis, dermatopathic lymphadenitis, metastatic disease (breast)
Epitrochlear	Viral diseases, sarcoidosis, tularemia, infections of hands, lymphoma
Abdominal/retroperitoneal	Lymphoma, metastatic disease, tuberculosis
Inguinal	Herpes, lymphogranuloma venereum, syphilis, gonococcal infection, HIV[b], lymphoma, metastatic disease

[a]Table 25.3 from Kjeldsberg CR, ed. Practical diagnosis of hematologic disorders, 4th ed. Chicago: ASCP Press; 2006:281.
[b]HIV = human immunodeficiency virus.

INDICATIONS FOR SPLENECTOMY

In general, spleens are removed for: "diagnostic intent," that is, identifying a cause of the splenic abnormality; "therapeutic intent," providing relief of cytopenias or rupture; and "incidental" reasons, facilitating access to left upper quadrant organs or as part of an en bloc resection (21). Diagnostic splenectomy has a yield of up to 95 percent. Approximately 1 percent of splenectomies performed for therapeutic or incidental purposes contain significant unexpected pathology. Frequent indications for splenectomy for therapeutic intent include: splenic infarcts, splenomegaly (symptomatic), hemolytic processes, sickle cell sequestration crisis, immune thrombocytopenic purpura (ITP), thrombotic thrombocytopenic purpura (TTP), and control of cytopenias in processes that cause splenic sequestration.

Despite advances in imaging techniques, the etiology of splenomegaly is unclear in 7 to 15 percent of cases (10). In cases in which the cause of splenomegaly is unclear, splenectomy is probably indicated, as 40 to 70 percent of cases have been shown to harbor occult lymphomas (10,12,32). High morbidity and complication rates (6 to 19 percent and 22 to 39 percent, respectively) have been reported (13,27); recent reports have shown no mortality and lesser morbidity (22 percent) (10).

A variety of surgical techniques are attempted in response to trauma to avoid total splenectomy. These include: splenorrhaphy, repair, and partial splenectomy. Laparoscopic splenectomy is a safe, effective alternative to open splenectomy. It is associated with a shorter hospital stay and fewer complications (2,18,35). Relative contraindications to laparoscopic removal of the spleen include known severe hematologic disease and large spleen size (2).

Staging laparotomy has been the standard for the staging of Hodgkin lymphoma and other disorders. A typical staging laparotomy includes: wedge biopsy of liver, splenectomy, periaortic mesenteric and hepatoduodenal lymph node sampling, and bone marrow biopsy. With improvement of imagining techniques, the incidence of staging laparotomy has significantly decreased, leading to a significant decrease in the number of spleen specimens evaluated in association with this procedure.

SAMPLING AND HANDLING THE FRESH LYMPH NODE

It is important to have optimal communication among the clinician, surgeon, and pathologist at the time of the lymph node biopsy. Depending on the preoperative or clinical diagnosis, portions of the fresh lymph node are allocated for routine and additional ancillary studies. Although there are several techniques available for obtaining diagnostic pathologic material, excisional biopsy of an intact lymph node is the procedure of choice for the diagnosis of hematolymphoid processes (34). In lymph node dissections for the evaluation of metastatic disease, there is no consensus on whether the nodes should be entirely submitted (26). In any study that correlates nodal status with clinical outcome, however, it is recommended that the specific method of node sampling always be stated (26).

At the time of excisional biopsy, it is important to remove the lymph node in one piece, if possible, with its capsule and adherent pericapsular fibrofatty tissue intact (fig. 3-1). Many diagnostic errors arise from improper sampling and handling of the fresh specimen. The lymph node should always be delivered as soon as possible to the pathologist in a suitable container, covered with saline-moistened gauze to prevent drying of the specimen. Placement on a dry gauze pad or dry towel may result in desiccation of the lymph node cortex and significant processing artifact, which may hinder the correct histologic and immunohistochemical interpretations (38). If an infectious disease is clinically suspected, a portion of the lymph node should be handled in a sterile manner and for the appropriate microbiologic studies. The most important consideration, however, in the procurement and processing of a lymph node biopsy, is to ensure that there is sufficient tissue for prompt fixation, paraffin embedding, and optimal diagnostic glass slides for pathologic examination (37).

Fine needle aspiration, core needle, and incisional biopsies are techniques that are also used to sample a lymph node, depending on the clinical situation (39). Fine needle aspiration biopsy (FNAB) is a procedure that is routinely performed on accessible lymph nodes, in the outpatient department or physician's office

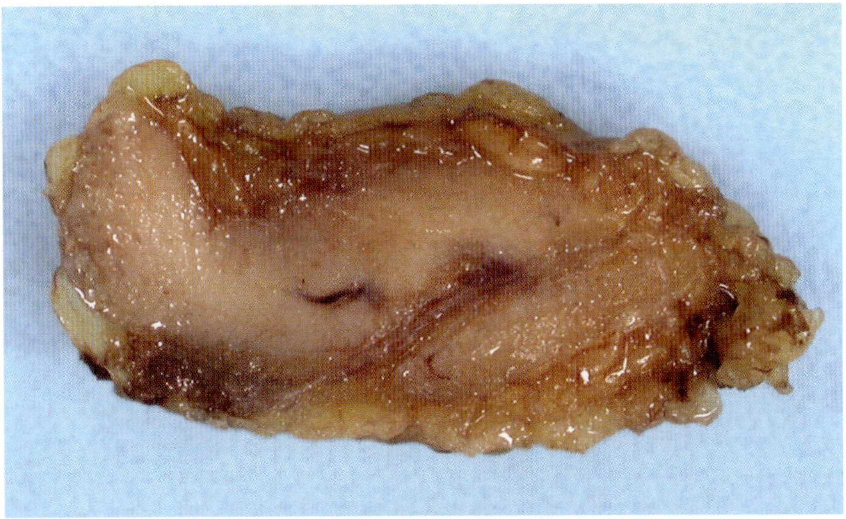

Figure 3-1

EXCISED LYMPH NODE

Excised lymph nodes are typically pink-tan and surrounded by some adherent fat. The capsule is thin and there are no apparent bands of fibrosis within the lymphoid parenchyma.

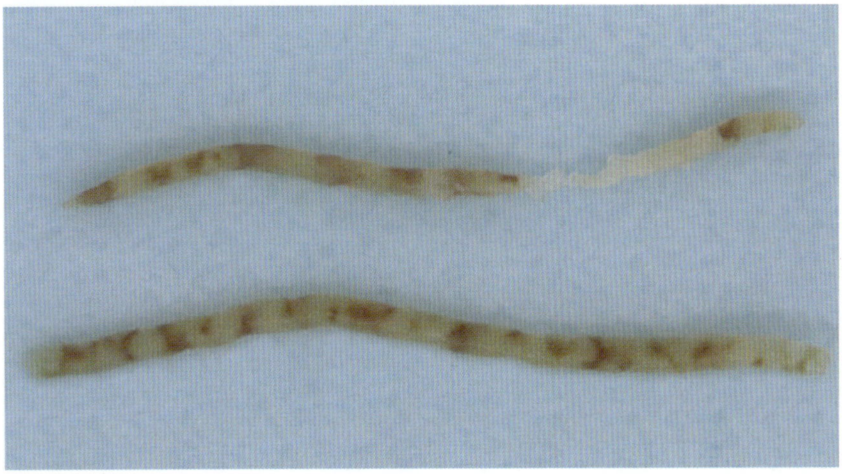

Figure 3-2

NEEDLE CORE BIOPSY

Needle core biopsy specimens may be appropriate for the evaluation of lymph node pathology, if lymph node excision is impractical.

(25,29). Radiologic or ultrasonographic guidance is required to sample inaccessible lymph nodes in intraabdominal or retroperitoneal sites (37). The procured cytologic specimens may be rapidly fixed and processed with the Papanicolaou stain or air-dried and stained with Giemsa. Specimens that are processed in cytospin preparations or paraffin-embedded tissue blocks may also be used for immunohistochemical analysis. If a malignant hematolymphoid process is suspected, fresh cell suspensions are often obtained for flow cytometric analysis. Although FNAB is reported to be very helpful in the diagnosis of metastatic malignancies, its role in the diagnosis of neoplastic and non-neoplastic hematolymphoid lesions is more limited because of the absence of architectural information (15,19,33,37). In experienced hands, however, the combination of FNAB and flow cytometry of lymph nodes can yield sufficient information to aid in the distinction between reactive and neoplastic processes (25).

Compared to a FNAB, a core needle biopsy of a lymph node provides a larger diagnostic specimen that may be used for both routine histologic and immunophenotypic analyses (fig. 3-2). Although this procedure provides more architectural details than a FNAB, the size of the specimen may still not be sufficient for a definitive diagnosis, necessitating an excisional or incisional lymph node biopsy. An incisional biopsy is used when the lymph nodes are matted, adherent, extremely large, or difficult to remove in one piece. If possible, a portion of the capsule and surrounding fibrofatty tissue should be sampled as well (34).

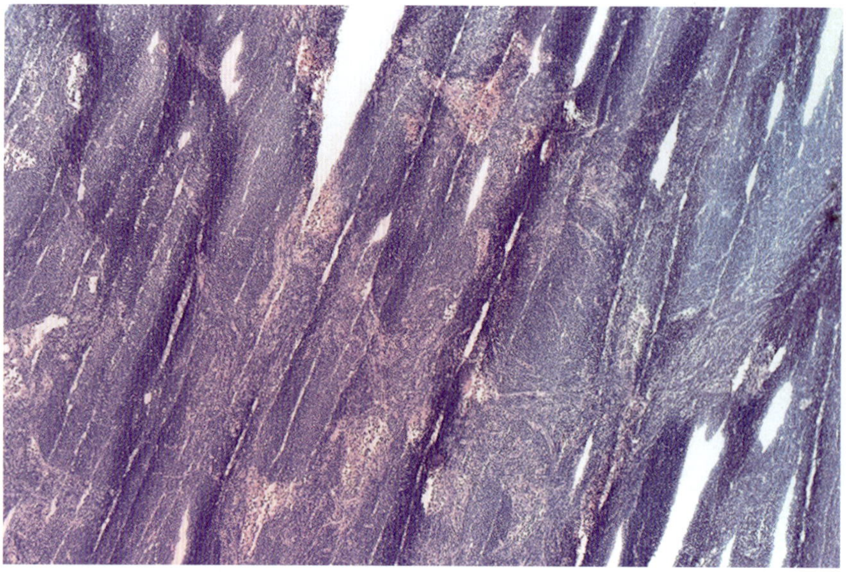

Figure 3-3

FROZEN SECTION OF LYMPH NODE

Frozen section specimens are rarely of value in evaluating lymph node pathology.

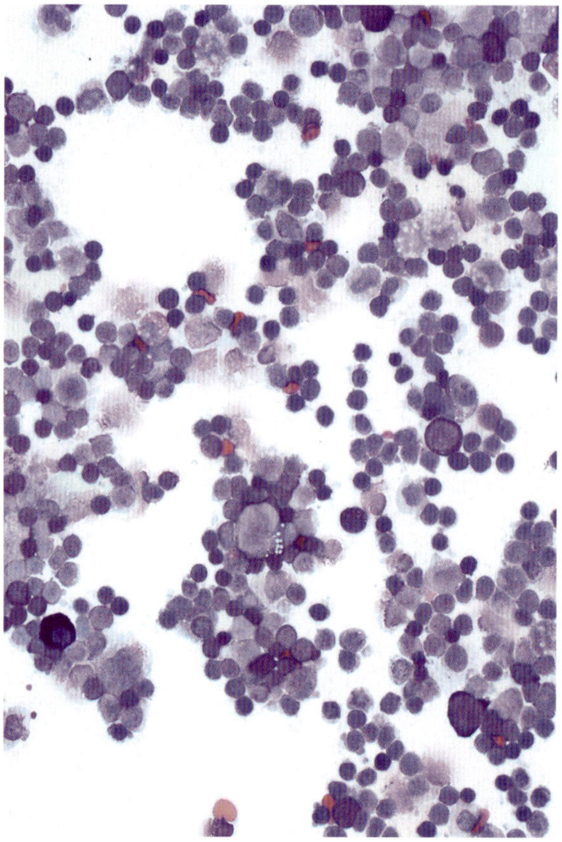

Figure 3-4

CYTOLOGIC IMPRINT OF LYMPH NODE

A well-performed and -stained cytologic imprint slide may provide valuable diagnostic information, and prevent performance of a frozen section evaluation, with the compromise of tissue for further diagnostic evaluation.

Intraoperative frozen section diagnosis on lymph nodes is generally not recommended unless the lymph node is in an inaccessible location that requires an invasive procedure such as a laparotomy or thoracotomy. In order to ensure adequate sampling of the tissue, microscopic frozen section evaluation may be used. This technique is associated with freezing artifact, which may obscure the diagnosis (fig. 3-3). Air-dried or wet-fixed smears from tissue imprints of the node may alternatively be used for this purpose (3,4). Imprint cytology has been reported to yield important diagnostic clues in the diagnosis and classification of non-Hodgkin lymphomas because of the superior nuclear and cytoplasmic details it provides (fig. 3-4) (20).

Depending on the size of the lymph node specimen and the clinical suspicion, different portions may be allocated for routine paraffin embedding and immunohistochemistry; frozen tissue immunohistochemistry; cell suspension for flow cytometric analysis; molecular genetic studies on fresh, frozen, or paraffin-embedded tissue; and, occasionally, electron microscopy. Immunophenotypic and molecular genetic studies are used in the diagnosis and classification of malignant hematolymphoid processes and the distinction from reactive processes. In reactive lymph nodes, special stains are helpful in the identification of amyloid, lipids, pigments, minerals, and microorganisms.

SAMPLING AND HANDLING THE FRESH SPLEEN

Spleens provide a unique set of problems for pathologic examination, in contrast to lymph nodes. As with lymph node examinations, appropriate communication between surgeons, clinicians, and pathologists is important in order to obtain the most appropriate material for pathologic examination and diagnosis.

If received intact, it is important to document pathologic changes in the spleen using macrophotography. In the era of digital image capture, the ease of gross photographs for pathology images is routine. If there are surface abnormalities, these should be photographed. After sectioning, documentation of abnormalities of the cut surface of the spleen may provide additional information for pathologic examination.

Gross examination of the intact spleen should include weight and dimensions, as in other pathologic specimens. Any abnormalities of the surface (capsular ruptures, residual fetal lobations, focal or diffuse fibrosis) should be recorded. Next, the splenic hilum should be carefully examined, including vascular structures and hilar lymph nodes. If hilar lymph nodes are present, these should be submitted as separate microscopic specimens, as they may add additional diagnostic information. Morcellated spleen specimens should be examined thoroughly for any focal pathology. Aggregate weight and size should be recorded.

After removal of adherent fat and dissection of splenic hilar nodes, the spleen should be bisected along its long axis. The cut surface should be examined for any characteristic pathology, and photographed if any diffuse or focal abnormalities are identified. These cuts should be continued on both halves at intervals of approximately 1 cm. Optimally, these 1-cm sections of the spleen should be allowed to fix in copious amounts of formalin-based fixative (at least 10 to 20 times the volume of tissue) overnight, before sampling for histologic examination.

Sampling for microscopic examination should include specimens of normal/unaffected spleen, any focal lesions, areas that show transitions between normal and pathologic processes, and splenic hilar lymph nodes, if present. Recent increases in laparoscopic surgeries have increased the receipt of morcellated spleen specimens. Morcellated specimens should be sampled in a similar, thorough manner.

Because of the hemorrhagic nature of the spleen, tissue samples should be made especially thin in order to assure complete fixation. Touch imprints, which may be useful for microscopic examination, and possibly for ancillary studies, should be performed on any lesional tissue. It is advisable to dab the spleen with gauze or towels before performing imprints, to minimize blood which would obscure cytologic details.

The acquisition and processing of aspiration and needle biopsies of the spleen are similar to those of lymph nodes, with the same caveats. Many difficult splenic lesions are not amenable to diagnosis by either cytologic specimens or needle biopsies, even with samples available for flow cytometry (21).

Since ample tissue is typically available from removed spleens, apportioning samples for ancillary studies is less critical than with lymph nodes. Samples for histologic examination are the most important, but tissue for flow cytometry, microbiologic studies, flow cytometry, and other studies should be obtained, as appropriate.

FIXATION AND PROCESSING

The microscopic examination of well-prepared glass slides from adequately fixed paraffin-embedded tissue sections is the gold standard for the pathologic interpretation of reactive lymphadenopathy and spleen samples. The choice of a fixative takes many factors into consideration, such as the cellular or architectural structures that are to be demonstrated and the long- or short-term storage of the tissue (33). In lymph node pathology, 10 percent neutral buffered formalin (which contains 4 percent formaldehyde) or formalin alternatives such as acetic acid-zinc formalin (AZF) are the fixatives of choice (6). Mercuric chloride fixatives, such as B5, which show excellent tissue morphology, have fallen out of favor because of antigen retrieval, possibility of overfixation, inability to perform molecular studies, safety/toxicity concerns, and disposal issues (6). Adequate fixation in a formalin-based fixative, followed by routine, balanced hematoxylin and eosin (H&E) staining (fig. 3-5), is generally sufficient to provide diagnostic slides in most cases of benign reactive lymphadenopathy (37).

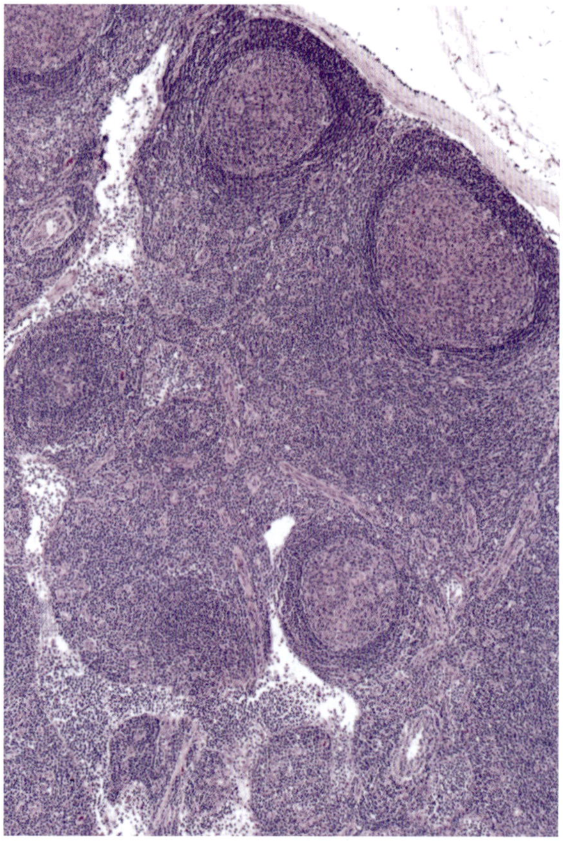

Figure 3-5

FORMALIN-FIXED LYMPH NODE

Clearly identifiable reactive germinal centers in a well-fixed lymph node with intact architecture and capsule.

Immunohistochemistry, flow cytometry, or molecular genetic analysis is sometimes necessary to confirm the benign nature of the process or to rule-out lymphoma. In the past, fresh or frozen tissue was required for molecular analysis by Southern blotting. Formalin-fixed paraffin-embedded tissue sections may now be used in the polymerase chain reaction (PCR) analysis for antigen receptor gene rearrangements (36). Properly timed adequate fixation and paraffin embedding techniques, therefore, are the two most important steps in obtaining optimal histologic sections for light microscopic interpretation and additional ancillary studies (9,16,37,40). Delayed fixation may result in weak or absent antibody staining due to increased proteolytic degradation. A short period of formalin fixation may result in adequate fixation at the periphery of the tissue but the center of the section may remain raw or unfixed (37). Prolonged formaldehyde fixation, on the other hand, may lead to excessive cross-linking of the proteins (37).

With all of the advances in diagnostic hematopathology, light microscopy remains the cornerstone of pathologic interpretation of nonneoplastic lymph nodes. The freshly excised lymph node should be sectioned at approximately 2- to 4-mm intervals before being placed in an appropriate fixative. Careful sectioning of the specimen and well-timed placement in the correct fixative result in optimal paraffin-embedded tissue sections for routine histologic and immunohistochemical analyses.

Ten percent neutral buffered formalin is generally regarded as the universal fixative. It is relatively safe to handle and inexpensive, without posing an environmental hazard. Formalin-fixed tissue sections may be stored for long periods of time. One of the disadvantages of formalin fixation is the "bubbling" artifact that occurs as a result of nuclear chromatin coalescence, obscuring cytologic detail (figs. 3-6, 3-7). The "space" that surrounds the neoplastic Reed-Sternberg cells and mononuclear cell variants ("lacunar cells") in nodular sclerosing Hodgkin lymphoma occurs as a result of formalin fixation (fig. 3-8) and is not seen in B5-fixed sections (fig. 3-9). AZF and other formalin alternatives provide sharper nuclear details (fig. 3-10). Although other fixatives, such as alcohol and Bouin and Zenker solutions also provide good nuclear detail, they may show cell shrinkage artifact and interfere with ancillary testing. Glutaraldehyde is the fixative of choice for electron microscopy. This technique, however, is rarely used in the diagnosis of reactive lymphadenopathy.

The storage of a snap-frozen portion of lymph node, prior to fixation, has traditionally been recommended for ancillary diagnostic studies such as immunohistochemistry and molecular genetic probe analysis, if necessary. In recent years, however, a large number of monoclonal and polyclonal antibodies have become available for use on paraffin tissue sections in the diagnosis of hematolymphoid lesions (28). This has broadened the applicability of immunohistochemistry, especially with regard to archival material, and has minimized the need for frozen

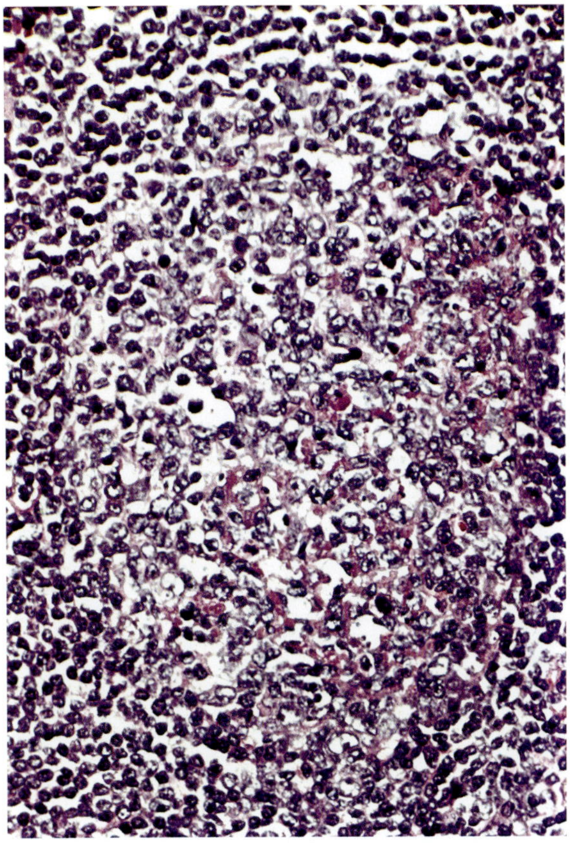

Figure 3-6

NUCLEAR ARTIFACT, POOR FIXATION

A nuclear "bubbling" artifact from chromatin coalescence secondary to formalin fixation in a reactive germinal center.

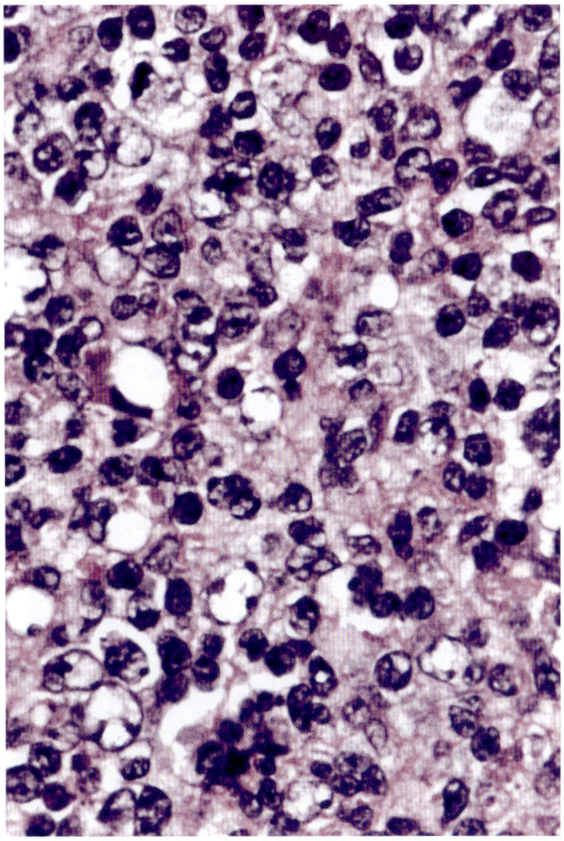

Figure 3-7

NUCLEAR ARTIFACT, POOR FIXATION

A mixed population of lymphoid cells with a nuclear bubbling artifact.

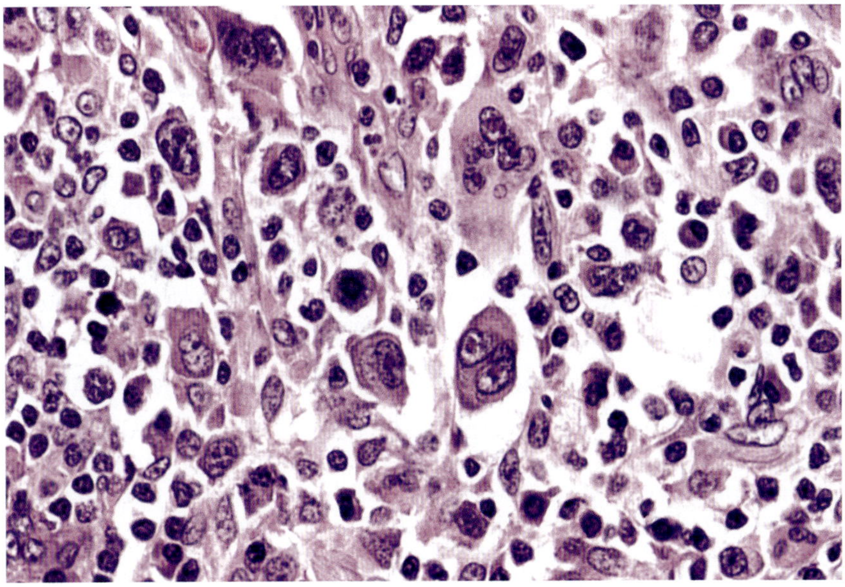

Figure 3-8

LACUNAR CELL, FORMALIN FIXATION

Lacunar cell artifact in a formalin-fixed section of nodular sclerosing Hodgkin lymphoma.

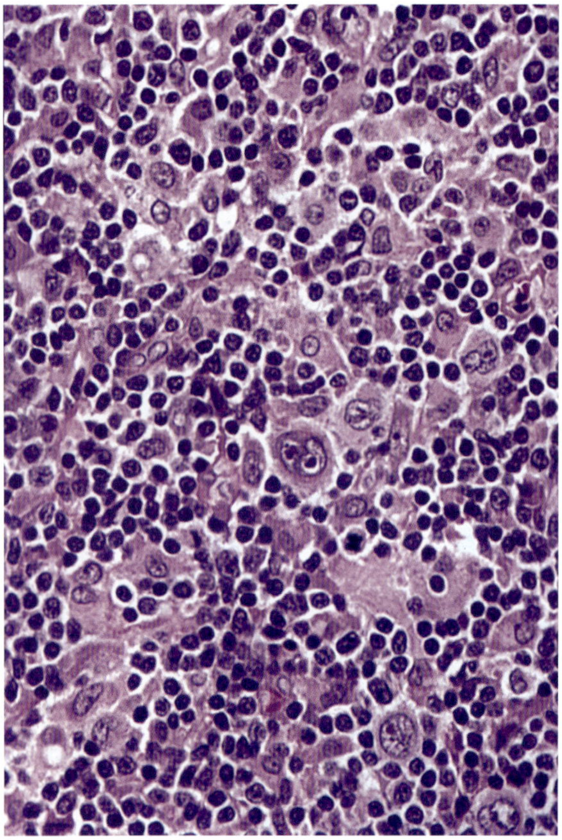

Figure 3-9

LACUNAR CELL, B5 FIXATION

Reed-Sternberg cells in a B5-fixed section of Hodgkin lymphoma do not show lacunar morphology.

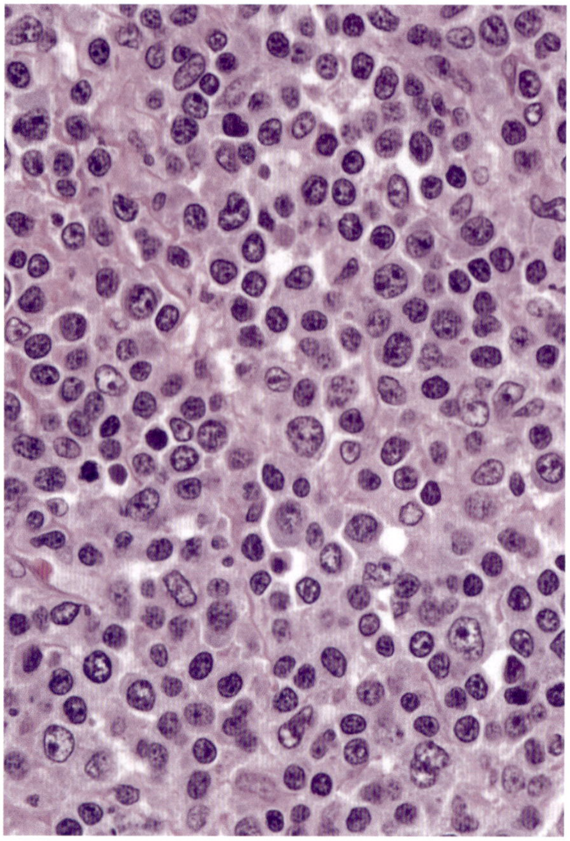

Figure 3-10

ACIDIFIED ZINC FORMALIN (AZF)–FIXED LYMPH NODE

Sharp nuclear details are seen in an AZF-fixed lymph node.

section immunohistochemistry. Antigen retrieval techniques have enhanced the antigenicity of formalin-fixed paraffin-embedded tissue sections and subsequent immunohistochemical antibody reactivity (31). Most cases of benign reactive lymphadenopathy can be correctly interpreted with adequate H&E-stained slides and paraffin immunohistochemistry.

Although flow cytometric and cytogenetic analyses are extremely valuable in the diagnosis and classification of leukemias and lymphomas (17,43), they are generally less helpful in making specific diagnoses of non-neoplastic lymph node lesions. Flow cytometry can, however, play an important role in confirming the non-neoplastic nature of a lesion. Molecular genetic analysis for B-and T-cell antigen receptor gene rearrangements, which has revolutionized the field of hematopathology, has traditionally been performed on fresh or frozen tissue. In recent years, however, it has become possible to amplify small segments of DNA and perform molecular genetic probe analysis on current or archival paraffin-embedded sections (22). Molecular genetic studies to detect clonal populations of B or T cells are usually not necessary for the diagnosis of reactive lymphadenopathy. In some cases, however, it may be difficult to distinguish a benign lymph node that has atypical features from a malignant lymphoma, thereby necessitating molecular genetic analysis.

ROUTINE AND HISTOCHEMICAL STAINS

Lymph nodes that have been fixed in formalin are processed in an automated processor that follows a standard sequence of dehydration, clearing, and paraffin embedding. Sections from the paraffin block are routinely cut by a histotechnologist on a microtome at approximately 4-µm sections, a thickness that helps to reduce nuclear overlap. The importance of a well-maintained microtome and careful sectioning of the paraffin block cannot be over emphasized. Lines or tears in the tissue section may occur as a result of incorrect placement or positioning of the paraffin block or a microtome knife that is not well sharpened (fig. 3-11). The cut sections or ribbons are placed onto the surface of a flotation bath and then positioned on glass slides. The slides are dried and cooled before an appropriately balanced H&E counterstain is applied. Attention to these important details will ensure optimal glass slides for histologic interpretation. Other histochemical stains can be used, if necessary.

Most benign reactive lymphadenopathies are diagnosed by conventional processing methods and H&E-stained slides alone. In some cases, however, special histochemical stains, such as Giemsa, provide useful diagnostic clues. A Giemsa stain, when applied to air-dried or wet-fixed imprint slides, is helpful in distinguishing the heterogeneity of a reactive hematolymphoid process from the monotony of a neoplastic process. Giemsa- or Wright-stained imprints also provide excellent nuclear details. A Giemsa stain may be used to highlight vascularity and pigments such as iron, lipofuscin, or melanin, and to identify infectious organisms.

A periodic acid–Schiff (PAS) stain also helps identify organisms in infectious lymphadenitis. Depending on the histologic features and the clinical suspicion, other special stains for infectious organisms (e.g., Warthin-Starry or Gomori methenamine silver) may also be used. The utility of these stains will be discussed in greater detail in regard to individual diagnoses. Chapter 4 discusses ancillary studies, including immunohistochemistry, which is one of the most important techniques in hematopathology.

EVALUATION OF THE LYMPH NODE

A systematic approach to the diagnosis of lymphoid pathology is based on a thorough understanding of the normal cellular components and compartments of the lymph nodes as well as the spleen. It is important to remember that in the diagnosis of splenic and lymphoid processes, one primary aim is to distinguish a benign from a malignant process. It has long been assumed that lymphoid neoplasms arise from the benign counterparts of specific cells or compartments, for example, mantle cell lymphoma or follicular (e.g., follicular center) lymphoma.

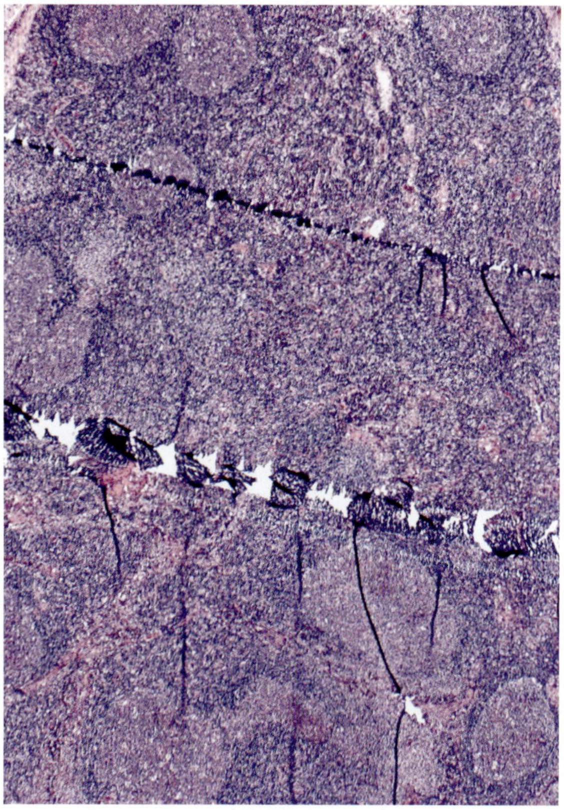

Figure 3-11

POOR SECTIONING, LYMPH NODE

Knife marks from irregularities in the edge of the blade and folds in the tissue from improper handling of the paraffin ribbon in the water bath.

In almost all circumstances, microscopic examination of a specimen generates a differential diagnosis rather than a single definitive answer. Diagnostic surety rests on the character of the morphologic findings and the clinical context, and in many cases, results in ancillary studies. As stated by Nathwani et al. (23), morphologic evaluation becomes magnified in importance in benign disorders because of the frequent nonspecific immunohistochemical or flow cytometric findings.

The ultimate step in diagnosis is weighing varying sources of information and drawing a conclusion. In almost all circumstances, there is

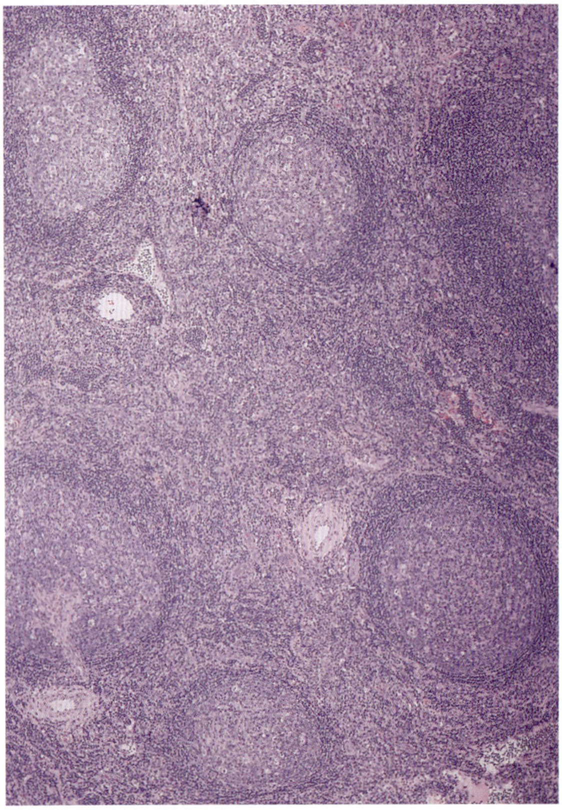

Figure 3-12

NORMAL LYMPH NODE COMPARTMENTS

Low-magnification examination of a lymph node gives an overview of the functional compartments.

no one "gold standard." Discordant or uninformative results may cloud appropriate evaluation but finally, the sources must be combined to discern a final diagnosis. This is the fundamental role of the pathologist.

One approach to the evaluation of lymphoid tissues, both nodal and extranodal, is to evaluate them in terms of functional compartments. Using the lymph node as the archetype, this prototypical lymphoid tissue can be divided into several components (fig. 3-12). The first of these is the germinal center, which is predominantly composed of B cells. Additionally, there is the interfollicular compartment, composed of a mixture of both B and T cells. Another component is the sinus compartment. Although there are other distinctive components of the lymph node, such as medullary cords, stromal elements, and other functional areas, these can be easily considered in the context of this other, simpler system.

The combination of histologic patterns with cytologic features typically allows identification of specific cell types. Identifying cell types then allows for a better understanding of proliferative or abnormal populations of cells, leading to more information for diagnosis. Although ancillary testing, such as flow cytometry or immunohistochemistry, can be used, recognizing the combined histologic and cytologic features of cells often makes the use of additional studies unnecessary.

In the sections below, an approach to lymphoid tissue evaluation is described using normal histologic features, including the cytologic features of individual components. For ease of discussion, features of the lymph nodes are described although the discussion is also applicable to non-nodal lymphoid tissue and splenic white pulp.

The earliest point of histologic diagnosis is to examine the slide with the unaided eye (fig. 3-13). Questions to be asked are: Is the tissue (i.e., lymph node) enlarged? Is it of uniform appearance or varied? Is there a mixture of colors or a predominant single color? All of these findings help guide microscopic examination and establish the differential diagnosis.

Using a low-power objective (preferably 2X or 2.5X), the entire structure is scanned. Is there tissue surrounding the node? Is it fat, as expected; or is there extension of lymphoid or other processes outside the capsule of the node? The capsule should be thin and uniform outside the lymph node. If it is thickened, varies in thickness, or has cellular infiltrates, this should be noted. The capsule should be composed of sparsely cellular fibrous tissue. Spindle-shaped fibroblasts and collagen are the most prominent components of the capsule, as well as rare inconspicuous capillaries. Fibrous trabeculae may extend from the capsule for a short distance into the parenchyma of the lymph node. Conditions associated with capsular thickening include chronic inflammatory, autoimmune, or infectious processes; slow-growing neoplasms; and nodular sclerosing Hodgkin lymphoma.

Perhaps the most notable compartment of the lymph node is *the follicle*. This round (spherical in three dimensions) structure is the basic unit of the B-cell/antigen immunologic response (see chapter 1). As such, the state of

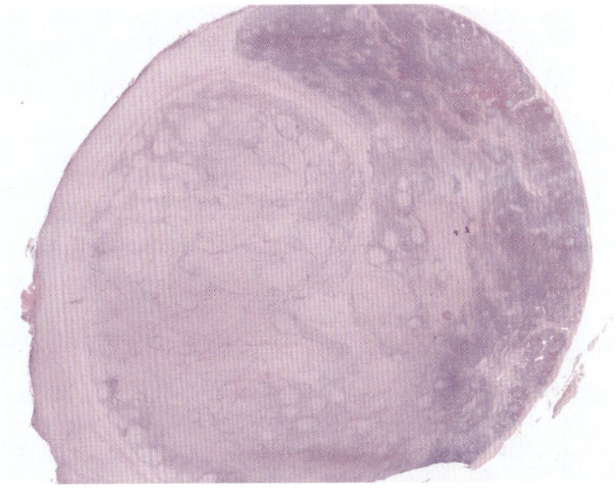

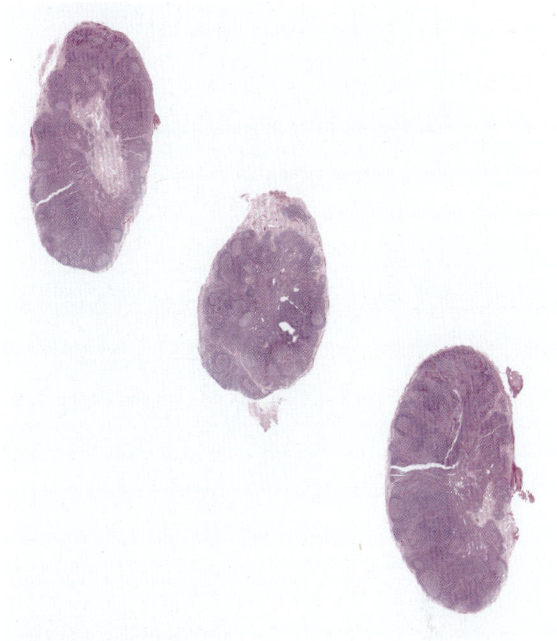

Figure 3-13

NORMAL AND ABNORMAL LYMPH NODES

Whole slide scans of an abnormal (above) and normal (right) lymph node at the same magnification. Examination with the unaided eye may give important clues to the type of pathology present.

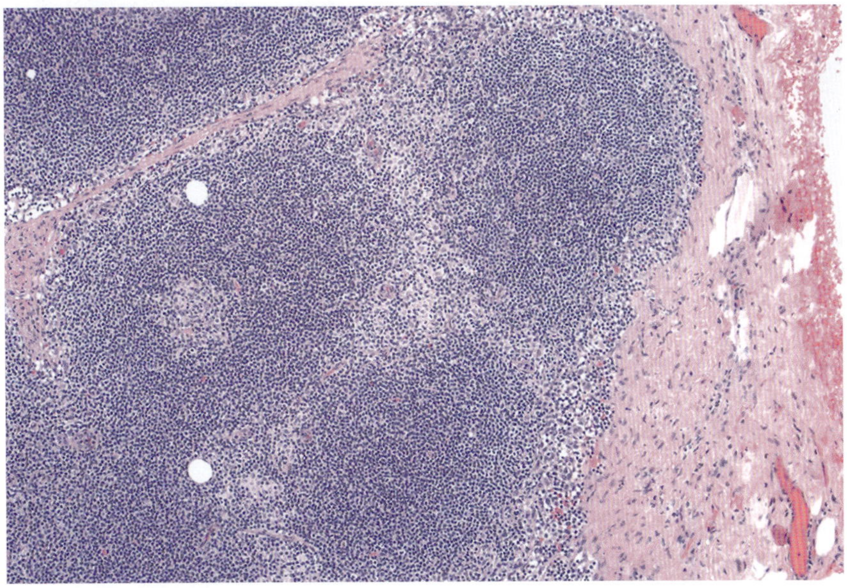

Figure 3-14

PRIMARY FOLLICLES

This image highlights two primary follicles (right) and early formation of a secondary follicle (left). Primary follicles are composed of lymphocytes that make up the mantle zone.

the follicle depends greatly on the immunologic status of the node. *Primary follicles* are composed of small lymphocytes (7 to 10 mm) with mature condensed chromatin, round to irregular nuclei, and scant inconspicuous cytoplasm (fig. 3-14). At low magnification, these small lymphocytes appear dark blue and can be densely packed due to their paucity of cytoplasm. These cells, and the primary follicle itself, are the basic component of the mantle zone (see below).

The *secondary follicle,* or *germinal center*, is the most recognizable component of the lymph node (fig. 3-15). This is a round structure, typically with a well-defined margin. In pathologic states, the germinal center may be increased in size (e.g., hyperplastic) or regressed/atretic. The germinal center is composed of a mixture of centrocytes (small, cleaved, irregular lymphocytes), centroblasts (large, transformed lymphocytes) with large round or irregular nuclei

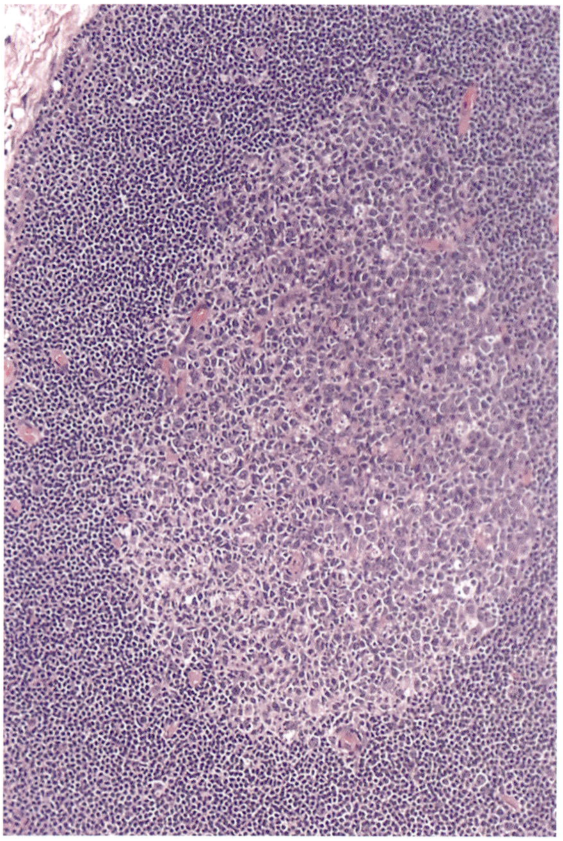

Figure 3-15

REACTIVE FOLLICLES

A follicle undergoing an immunologic response shows a mixture of cell types.

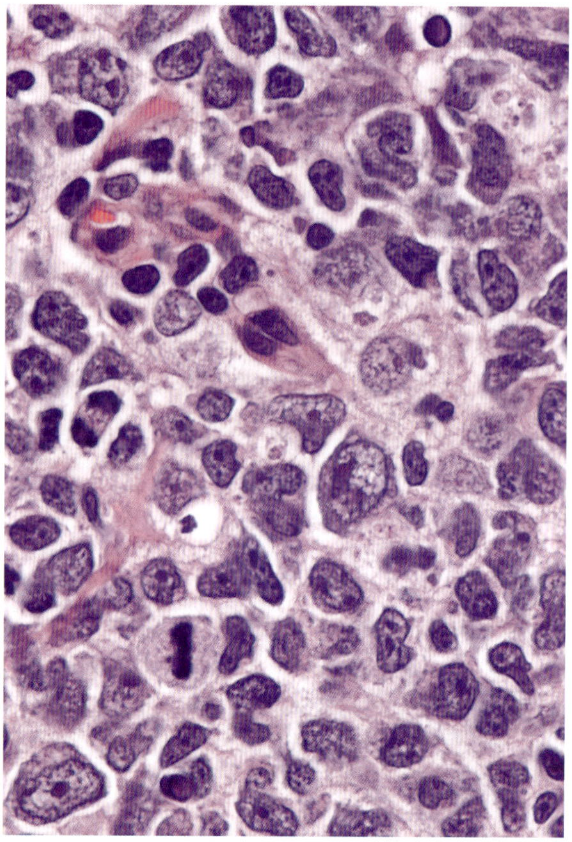

Figure 3-16

CENTROBLASTS

Centroblasts are mostly found in the "dark zone" of the germinal center and are large cells with multiple nucleoli, relatively open chromatin, and scant cytoplasm.

and moderate amounts of cytoplasm, and some intermediate forms. Centroblasts have open chromatin and usually multiple small nucleoli (fig. 3-16). Other cells found within the germinal center include small round lymphocytes (T cells), macrophage/histiocytic cells, and dendritic cells. Macrophages may have broken down fragments of cellular material, and such macrophages are called tingible body macrophages (fig. 3-17). Follicular dendritic cells are large, with round to ovoid nuclei, delicate marginated chromatin, and little cytoplasm (fig. 3-18). They have an overall pale appearance and may occasionally present as closely approximated pairs ("kissing cells"). Rarely, plasma cells are also found within the germinal center, usually associated with pathologic states.

Surrounding the germinal center is the *mantle zone*. This mantle is composed of small, round mature lymphocytes (fig. 3-14). These cells make up the dominant component of the primary follicle. The marginal zone is normally a third outermost layer of the follicle of the spleen and mesenteric lymph nodes. When present in pathologic states, it may be uniform or appear as irregular, parafollicular clusters or nodules. Cytologically, marginal zone cells, also known as monocytoid B cells, are small to intermediate sized with round nuclei and mature nuclear chromatin. They differ from typical small lymphocytes by an increased amount of pale or clear cytoplasm.

The *interfollicular*, or *paracortical, zone* is typically heterogeneous in its cellular composition (fig. 3-19). It is typically composed of a mixture of small lymphocytes, larger transformed lymphocytes, plasma cells, occasional granulocytes,

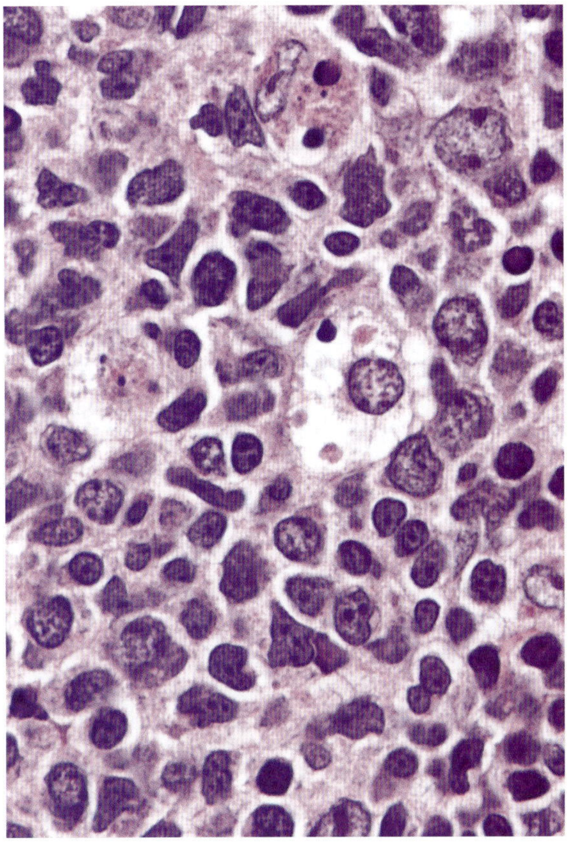

Figure 3-17

TINGIBLE BODY MACROPHAGES

Tingible body macrophages are apparent in germinal centers and have round, bland-appearing nuclei with fragments of cellular debris in their cytoplasm.

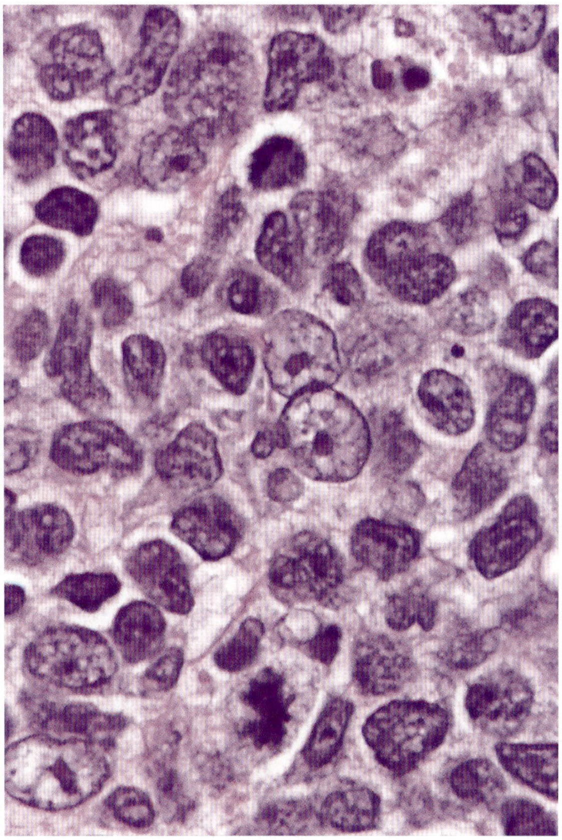

Figure 3-18

FOLLICULAR DENDRITIC CELLS

Follicular dendritic cells have very open, delicate chromatin, often with a single prominent nucleolus. They are often seen in pairs, as in this image, and are sometimes referred to as "kissing cells."

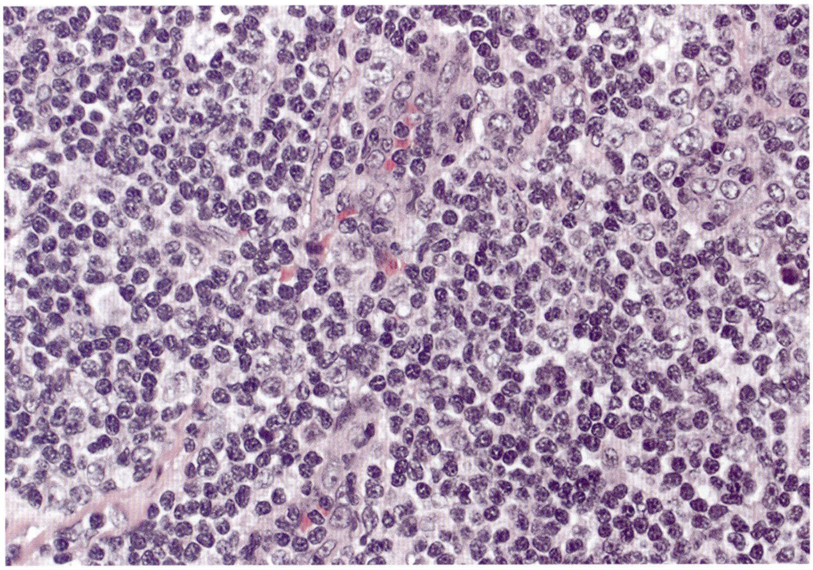

Figure 3-19

PARACORTICAL ZONE

The cells that are typically found in the paracortical zone include numerous small lymphocytes, occasional larger transformed lymphocytes, occasional macrophages, vascular elements, and rare elements such as plasma cells and granulocytes.

and scattered stromal elements. These stromal elements include macrophages, dendritic cells, and vascular elements. This area becomes more prominent in states of immunoblastic hyperplasia, where there is an increase of large transformed lymphocytes (see Table 3-2; also chapter 5). This portion of the lymph node can also be preferentially involved in several specific types of lymphoma, notably many of T-cell type.

Table 3-2

ETIOLOGIES ASSOCIATED WITH INTERFOLLICULAR EXPANSIONS[a]

Focal
Kikuchi-Fujimoto disease
Necrotizing lymphadenitis
Cat-scratch disease
Dermatopathic lymphadenitis
Nodular paracortical T-cell hyperplasia
Multifocal
Necrotizing lymphadenitis
Kikuchi-Fujimoto disease
Cat-scratch disease
HIV/AIDS[b] lymphadenitis
Lymphogranuloma venereum
Syphilis
Dermatopathic lymphadenitis
Nodular paracortical T-cell hyperplasia
Viral lymphadenitis
Castleman disease
Diffuse
Interfollicular hyperplasia
HIV/AIDS lymphadenitis
Lymphogranuloma venereum
Dermatopathic lymphadenitis
Nodular paracortical T-cell hyperplasia
Viral lymphadenitis
Castleman disease

[a]Table 14.6 from Nathwani BN, Hernandez AM, Drachenberg MR. In: Knowles DM, ed. Neoplastic hematopathology, 2nd ed. Philadelphia: Lippincott Williams & Wilkins; 2001:514.
[b]HIV = human immunodeficiency virus; AIDS = acquired immunodeficiency syndrome.

Another component of the lymph node that deserves special attention is the *lymph node sinuses*. Just beneath the lymph node capsule is the aptly named subcapsular sinus (fig. 3-20). In addition, there are sinuses that course from the periphery to the central portion of the node. Often, these sinuses are inapparent in inactive lymph nodes, and only become apparent when they are distended by either cells or other pathologic processes. Several pathologic processes preferentially involve the lymph node sinuses, including benign and malignant histiocytic/macrophage processes, leukemic involvement of lymph nodes, metastatic carcinomas, and anaplastic large cell lymphoma.

A deviation from the normal architecture can present in several forms. An expansion of a compartment or component of lymphoid tissue is often simply referred to as hyperplasia (e.g., follicular hyperplasia) (Table 3-3). The loss of a compartment or structure can be due to regression or replacement by another structure or pathologic process. An example of this is the apparent "loss" of sinuses in lymphomas, caused by compression of the sinuses by the expansion of the neoplastic lymphoid components. Replacement of the normal architecture of the lymph node is often referred to as effacement. Many pathologic processes cause complete effacement in a diffuse pattern. This should be

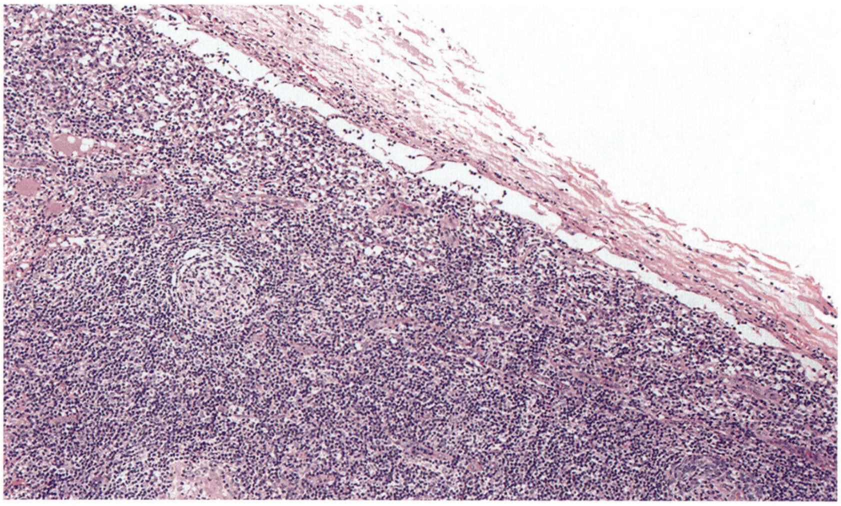

Figure 3-20

SUBCAPSULAR SINUS

Often inapparent, the subcapsular sinus of the lymph node is a potential space that exists beneath the capsule. This sinus connects to lymphatic sinuses that run into the cortical and medullary regions of the lymph node.

distinguished from focal or partial involvement of a lymph node (or nodal compartment) by a pathologic process.

EVALUATION OF THE SPLEEN

The initial pathologic evaluation of the spleen should be based on gross examination of the organ (fig. 3-21) (24,41). The two general patterns of splenic involvement are diffuse and focal processes. Among the diffuse processes, one type is caused by abnormal expansion of preexisting nodular lymphoid structures (i.e., splenic lymphoid follicles, periarteriolar lymphoid sheaths). Grossly, this appears as multiple small, whitish nodules on the cut surface, and is referred to as a miliary pattern because of its resemblance to millet seeds (fig. 3-22). This pattern is a caricature of the normal appearance of tiny whitish flecks seen on the cut surface, which represent the normal lymphoid follicles of the spleen (8). These nodules may coalesce and present as larger, dominant masses.

Expansion of the red pulp gives the spleen a more homogeneous red or "beefy" appearance (fig. 3-23). The normal nodularity of the white pulp is typically diminished and the white pulp is often atrophic or compressed by the expanded red pulp. Disorders of circulation, such as congestion, or disorders of the macrophages system, such as red blood cell disorders, parasites, and storage diseases present with red pulp expansion. Focal pathology of the spleen, including cysts and masses, can be caused by a variety of disorders, both benign and malignant.

Table 3-3

PATTERNS OF LYMPHOID HYPERPLASIA[a]

Follicular
Benign follicular hyperplasia
HIV/AIDS[b]
Rheumatoid arthritis
Syphilis
Castleman disease
Progressive transformation of germinal centers
Sinus Pattern
Sinus histiocytosis
Rosai-Dorfman disease
Monocytoid B-cell hyperplasia (marginal zone hyperplasia)
Hemophagocytic syndrome
Whipple disease
Lymphangiogram effect
Langerhans cell histiocytosis
Vascular transformation of sinuses
Kaposi sarcoma
Diffuse Pattern
Infectious mononucleosis
Herpes zoster and herpes simplex lymphadenitis
Postvaccinial lymphadenitis
Drug-induced hypersensitivity reaction
Angioimmunoblastic lymphadenopathy
Mixed Pattern
Toxoplasma lymphadenitis
Dermatopathic lymphadenitis
Granulomatous lymphadenitis
Non-necrotizing (e.g., sarcoid)
Necrotizing (e.g., cat-scratch disease, lymphogranuloma venereum, *Yersinia* lymphadenitis)
Kikuchi-Fujimoto lymphadenitis
Systemic lupus lymphadenitis
Kawasaki disease

[a]Table 15.1 from Schnitzer B. In: Knowles DM, ed. Neoplastic hematopathology, 2nd ed. Philadelphia: Lippincott Williams & Wilkins; 2001:538.
[b]HIV = human immunodeficiency virus; AIDS = acquired immunodeficiency syndrome.

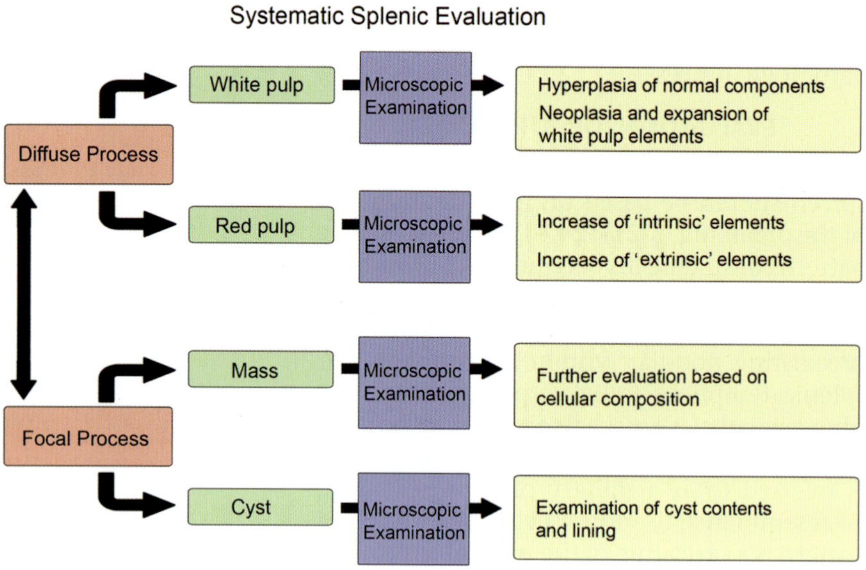

Figure 3-21

SYNOPSIS OF SYSTEMATIC SPLENIC EVALUATION

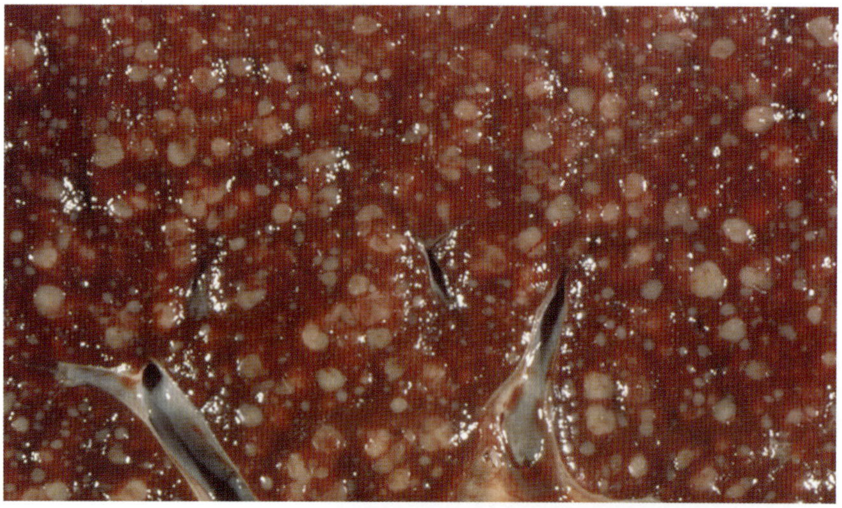

Figure 3-22

CUT SURFACE OF SPLEEN WITH WHITE PULP DISEASE

The cut surface of a spleen with a white pulp disease, such as splenic marginal zone lymphoma, shows accentuation of the white pulp portion, with increased numbers of small white nodules.

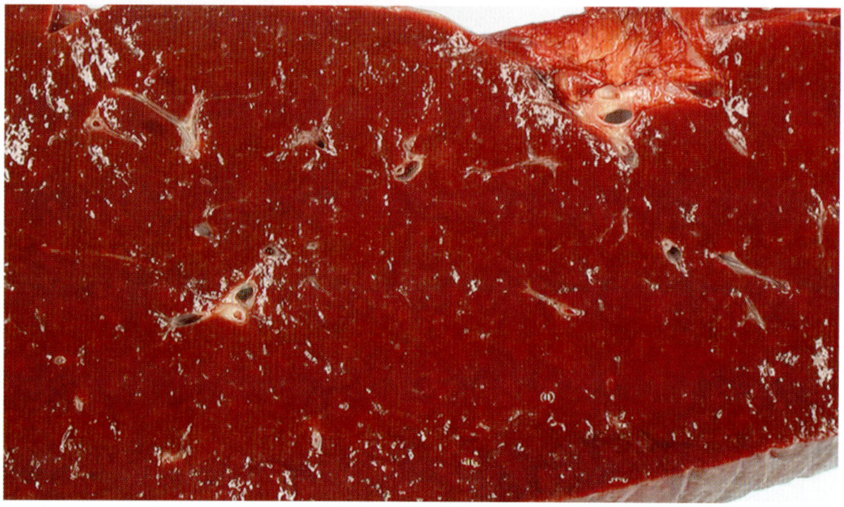

Figure 3-23

CUT SURFACE OF SPLEEN WITH RED PULP DISEASE

Red pulp diseases often impart a red, "beefy" appearance to the spleen.

REFERENCES

1. Association of Directors of Anatomic and Surgical Pathology. Recommendations for the reporting of lymphoid neoplasms: a report from the Association of Directors of Anatomic and Surgical Pathology. Virchows Arch 2002;441:314-9.
2. Balague C, Targarona EM, Cerdan G, et al. Long-term outcome after laparoscopic splenectomy related to hematologic diagnosis. Surg Endosc 2004;18:1283-7.
3. Banks PM. Technical aspects of specimen preparation and introduction to special studies. In: Jaffe ES, ed. Surgical pathology of the lymph nodes and related organs. Philadelphia: W.B. Saunders; 1995:1-21.
4. Banks PM. Technical factors in the preparation and evaluation of lymph node biopsies. In: Knowles DM, ed. Neoplastic hematopathology, 2nd ed. Philadelphia: Lippincott Williams & Wilkins; 2001:467-82.
5. Beard C, Nabers K, Bowling MC, Berard CW. Achieving technical excellence in lymph node specimens: an update. Lab Med 1985;16:468-75.
6. Bonds LA, Barnes P, Foucar K, Sever CE. Acetic acid-zinc-formalin: a safe alternative to B-5 fixative. Am J Clin Pathol 2005;124:205-11.
7. Bowling MC. Lymph node specimens: achieving technical excellence. Lab Med 1979;10:467-76.
8. Burke JS. Diagnosis of lymphoma and lymphoid proliferations in the spleen. In: Jaffe ES, ed. Surgical pathology of the lymph nodes and related organs, 2nd ed. Philadelphia: WB Saunders; 1995:448-475.
9. Butler JJ. Non-neoplastic lesions of lymph nodes of man to be differentiated from lymphomas. Natl Cancer Inst Monogr 1969;32:233-55.
10. Carr JA, Shurafa M, Velanovich V. Surgical indications in idiopathic splenomegaly. Arch Surg 2002;137:64-8.
11. Cousar JB. Surgical pathology examination of lymph nodes. Practice survey by American Society of Clinical Pathologists. Am J Clin Pathol 1995;104:126-32.
12. Cronin CC, Brady MP, Murphy C, Kenny E, Whelton MJ, Hardiman C. Splenectomy in patients with undiagnosed splenomegaly. Postgrad Med J 1994;70:288-91.
13. Danforth DN Jr, Fraker DL. Splenectomy for the massively enlarged spleen. Am Surg 1991;57:108-13.
14. Gray GF Jr, Kimball AC, Kean BH. The posterior cervical lymph node in toxoplasmosis. Am J Pathol 1972;69:349-58.
15. Hehn ST, Grogan TM, Miller TP. Utility of fine-needle aspiration as a diagnostic technique in lymphoma. J Clin Oncol 2004;22:3046-52.
16. Hsi ED, Yegappan S. Lymphoma immunophenotyping: a new era in paraffin-section immunohistochemistry. Adv Anat Pathol 2001;8:218-39.
17. Jennings CD, Foon KA. Recent advances in flow cytometry: application to the diagnosis of hematologic malignancy. Blood 1997;90:2863-92.
18. Katkhouda N, Hurwitz MB, Rivera RT, et al. Laparoscopic splenectomy: outcome and efficacy in 103 consecutive patients. Ann Surg 1998;228:568-78.
19. Kline TS, Kannan V, Kline IK. Lymphadenopathy and aspiration biopsy cytology: review of 376 superficial nodes. Cancer 1984;54:1076-81.
20. Koo CH, Rappaport H, Sheibani K, Pangalis GA, Nathwani BN, Winberg CD. Imprint cytology of non-Hodgkin's lymphomas based on a study of 212 immunologically characterized cases: correlation of touch imprints with tissue sections. Hum Pathol 1989;20(Suppl 1):1-137.
21. Kraus MD, Fleming MD, Vonderheide RH. The spleen as a diagnostic specimen: a review of 10 years' experience at two tertiary care institutions. Cancer 2001;91:2001-9.
22. Mies C, Houldsworth J, Chaganti RS. Extraction of DNA from paraffin blocks for Southern blot analysis. Am J Surg Pathol 1991;15:169-74.
23. Nathwani BN, Hernandez AM, Drachenberg MR. Diagnostic significance of morphologic patterns of lymphoid proliferations in lymph nodes. In: Neoplastic hematopathology, 2nd ed. Knowles DM, ed. Philadelphia: Lippincott Williams & Wilkins; 2001;507-36.
24. Neiman, RS and Orazi A. Disorders of the spleen. 2nd ed. Philadelphia: WB Saunders; 1999.
25. Nicol TL, Silberman M, Rosenthal DL, Borowitz MJ. The accuracy of combined cytopathologic and flow cytometric analysis of fine-needle aspirates of lymph nodes. Am J Clin Pathol 2000;114:18-28.
26. Niemann TH, Yilmaz AG, Marsh WL Jr, Lucas JG. A half a node or a whole node: a comparison of methods for submitting lymph nodes. Am J Clin Pathol 1998;109:571-6.
27. Patel AG, Parker JE, Wallwork B, et al. Massive splenomegaly is associated with significant morbidity after laparoscopic splenectomy. Ann Surg 2003;238:235-40.
28. Perkins SL, Kjeldsberg CR. Immunophenotyping of lymphomas and leukemias in paraffin-embedded tissues. Am J Clin Pathol 1993;99:362-73.

29. Pitts DB, Hilsinger RL Jr, Karandy E, Ross JC, Caro JE. Fine-needle aspiration in the diagnosis of salivary gland disorders in the community hospital setting. Arch Otolaryngol Head Neck Surg 1992;118:479-82.
30. Prophet EB. Fixation. In: Prophet EB, Mills B, Arrington JB, Sobin LH, eds. In: Laboratory methods in histotechnology. Washington, DC: Armed Forces Institute of Pathology & American Registry of Pathology; 1994;25-8.
31. Shi SR, Cote RJ, Taylor CR. Antigen retrieval immunohistochemistry: past, present, and future. J Histochem Cytochem 1997;45:327-43.
32. Simu G, Bancu VE, Macavei I, Fazekas A, Tohati MT. Microscopic patterns in surgically removed spleens. Rom J Morphol Embryol 1991;37:81-6.
33. Steel BL, Schwartz MR, Ramzy I. Fine needle aspiration biopsy in the diagnosis of lymphadenopathy in 1,103 patients. Role, limitations and analysis of diagnostic pitfalls. Acta Cytol 1995;39:76-81.
34. Strauchen JA. The lymph node biopsy. In: Strauchen JA, ed. Diagnostic histopathology of the lymph node. New York: Oxford University Press; 1998:3-9.
35. Targarona EM, Balague C, Trias M. Is the laparoscopic approach reasonable in cases of splenomegaly? Semin Laparosc Surg 2004;11:185-90.
36. Tbakhi A, Totos G, Pettay JD, Myles J, Tubbs RR. The effect of fixation on detection of B-cell clonality by polymerase chain reaction. Mod Pathol 1999;12:272-78.
37. Warnke RA, Weiss LM, Chan JK, Cleary ML, Dorfman RF. Tumors of the lymph nodes and spleen. AFIP Atlas of Tumor Pathology, 3rd Series, Fascicle 14. Washington, DC: American Registry of Pathology; 1994;15-42.
38. Weiss LM, Dorfman RF, Warnke RA. Lymph node work-up. In: Fenoglio-Preiser C, Weinstein RS, Anderson E, Benson ES, Cotran R, Vogel FS, eds. Advances in pathology. Chicago: Year Book Medical Pub; 1988;1:111-30.
39. Weiss LM, Pitts WC. The role of fine needle aspiration biopsy in diagnosis and management of hematopoietic neoplasms. In: Knowles DM, ed. Neoplastic hematopathology, 2nd ed. Philadelphia: Lippincott Williams & Wilkins; 2001:483-506.
40. Werner M, Chott A, Fabiano A, Battifora H. Effect of formalin tissue fixation and processing on immunohistochemistry. Am J Surg Pathol 2000;24:1016-9.
41. Wilkins BS, Wright DH. Illustrated pathology of the spleen. Cambridge: Cambridge University Press; 2000.
42. Winterbauer RH, Belic N, Moores KD. Clinical interpretation of bilateral hilar adenopathy. Ann Intern Med 1973;78:65-71.
43. Witzig TE, Banks PM, Stenson MJ, et al. Rapid immunotyping of B-cell non-Hodgkin's lymphomas by flow cytometry. A comparison with the standard frozen-section method. Am J Clin Pathol 1990;94:280-6.

4 ANCILLARY STUDIES FOR EVALUATION OF LYMPH NODE AND SPLEEN

BASIC CONCEPTS

In the past two decades, there have been many advances in the use of immunologic techniques in diagnostic pathology, with a substantial impact on all areas of laboratory medicine, especially surgical pathology and hematopathology. Immunohistochemistry is now accepted as the most important ancillary technique for the analysis of fresh frozen and paraffin-embedded histologic material (66). Immunophenotypic analysis has been universally accepted as an adjunct technique that aids in the diagnosis and classification of lymphomas and leukemias (32,51,52). This methodology has proven to be essential in assessing the histogenesis or pathogenesis of these neoplasms. The recognition of lineage-associated and lineage-restricted antigen/antibody combinations has provided great insight into these malignancies.

Immunohistochemical analysis primarily uses high-affinity monoclonal (and occasionally polyclonal) antibodies to identify proteins and leukocyte cell surface antigens. In an attempt to standardize the nomenclature and unify the terminology, many antigens have been grouped into so-called clusters of differentiation (CD). The CD number may be used to refer to either the antigen or the corresponding antibody. Immunohistochemical antibodies are most often used in the identification and classification of lymphomas and other neoplasms, such as melanoma and carcinoma. They are also helpful in the diagnosis of reactive lymphoid processes and in their distinction from malignant processes.

Many hospital laboratories use immunohistochemical marker studies routinely. Hematopathology, in particular, has become increasingly reliant on immunohistochemistry since this ancillary technique greatly aids in the identification of the lineage-associated or lineage-restricted antigens present in hematolymphoid processes.

Increasing numbers of antibodies have become available for use in routinely processed paraffin-embedded histologic material. This greatly facilitates the collection, processing, shipping, and storage of tissue specimens for immunohistochemical analysis (41). Frozen section immunohistochemistry is rarely needed today. Paraffin tissue sections preserve cytologic and architectural features better than frozen sections, and provide better assessment of antigen cellular localization.

This chapter discusses the basic concepts of immunohistochemistry and its applicability to the diagnosis of reactive lymphoid hyperplasia, especially in paraffin-embedded tissue sections. It also describes the most relevant antibodies that are routinely used in panels for the diagnosis and classification of hematolymphoid lesions.

Immunohistochemistry Techniques

Different techniques are used to detect the presence of antigen in frozen and fixed tissue sections. The *direct method* refers to the labeling of an antibody with a fluorescent dye or enzyme for subsequent reaction and visualization with either a fluorescent or light microscope. The *indirect method* is much more important in immunohistochemistry. With this technique, a bridge or "sandwich" consisting of primary and secondary antibodies linked to enzyme substrates and detection reagents is used to identify tissue antigens on glass slides. Some of the most widely used indirect antibody techniques are the peroxidase-antiperoxidase (PAP), biotin-streptavidin, alkaline phosphatase-antialkaline phosphatase, and avidin-biotin complex (ABC) methods, of which the latter is probably the most commonly applied. The ABC indirect antibody technique basically uses an unlabeled primary antibody, which binds to its corresponding antigen, followed by the use of a biotinylated secondary antibody to which ABC (1 avidin molecule, 3 biotin-labeled peroxidase molecules) attaches. If the sought-after antigen is present in the section, this procedure results in an antibody-antigen interaction and an enzymatic

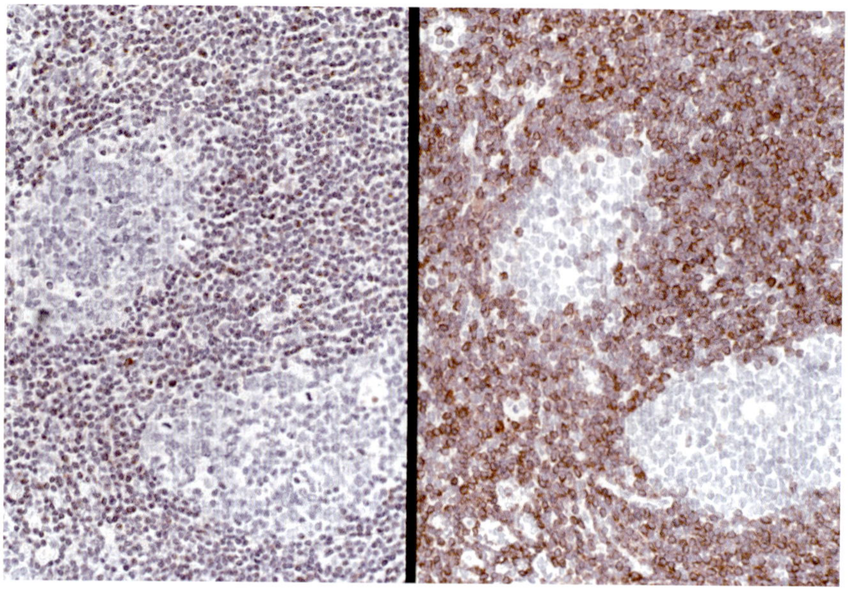

Figure 4-1

EFFECT OF ANTIGEN RETRIEVAL

Without (left) and with (right) antigen retrieval in bcl-2 reactivity in a lymph node

reaction which can be detected by a chromogen, most often diaminobenzidine (DAB), and visualized by light microscopy (26). There are few areas in surgical pathology where immunohistochemistry has had a more important role than in the area of hematopathology.

Highly sensitive frozen tissue immunohistochemical assays, using both the ABC and alkaline phosphatase-antialkaline phosphatase systems, have led to the detection and characterization of a wide spectrum of cell surface antigens. Most of these antigens are now routinely detected on paraffin-embedded tissue sections, which are easier to process, store, and transport than frozen sections (10). Paraffin immunohistochemistry lacks the sensitivity and specificity of frozen tissue or cell suspensions. Nevertheless, it still provides sufficient diagnostic immunophenotypic information from routinely processed tissue to arrive at a definitive diagnosis in most cases (58).

Antigen Retrieval

The cross-linking of molecules in formalin-fixed paraffin-embedded tissue sections can result in a decrease in antigenicity and antibody reactivity. Over the years, different techniques, including refixation in zinc-sulfate formalin (1) and, most important, heat-induced epitope retrieval (HIER) (22,67), have been used in an attempt to enhance the immunoreactivity of antigens that have been altered by fixation and paraffin embedding (fig. 4-1). Currently, the most common procedure relies on the immersion of the glass slide in a microwave oven or a steamer for "antigen retrieval" and enhancement of immunoreactivity in paraffin-embedded tissue sections (56,57). This technique alters the cross-linking of proteins caused by formaldehyde fixation, thereby exposing hidden antigenic sites (22). This procedure has been shown to reduce artifacts or "changes" in immunophenotype that are most likely related to inconsistent fixation and processing of the tissue (62).

Antibodies: Clusters of Differentiation (CD) Groups

Over the years, large numbers of different monoclonal antibodies reactive to leukocyte cell surface antigens have been produced. The continuous classification of human leukocyte antigens (HLA) has been accomplished during numerous international workshops held between 1982 and 2004. Cell surface antigens have been grouped as clusters of differentiation (CD) based on the recognition of the antigen by more than one antibody (29–31). Reference to the CD number provides uniformity in the discussion of immunohistochemical analysis of hematolymphoid lesions and eliminates the variability in antibody designation by different manufacturers. Increasing numbers of cell origin markers are being discovered and added to the list of useful antibodies.

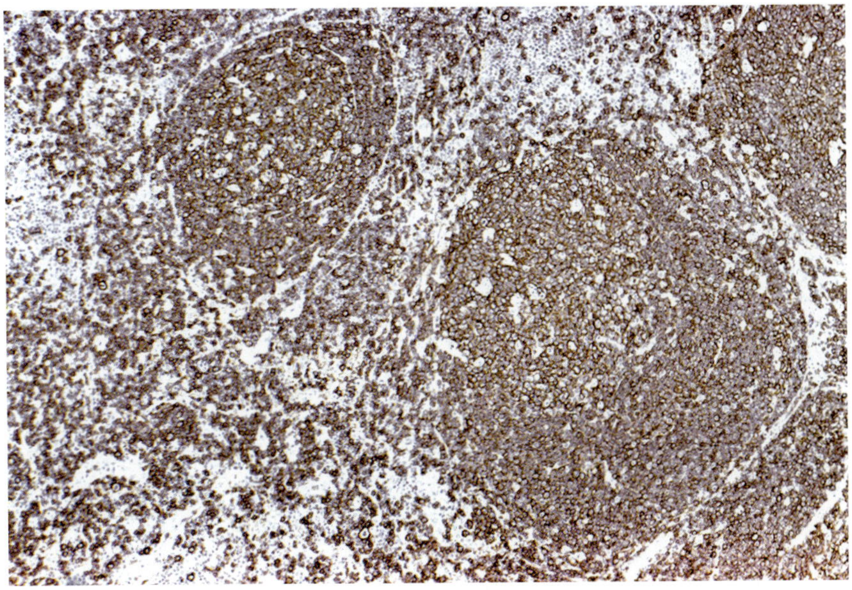

Figure 4-2

CD20 REACTIVITY, LYMPH NODE

CD20 stains B cells, with reactivity in the lymphoid follicles.

A panel of immunohistochemical antibodies, rather than one or two, is routinely used in the workup of benign and malignant lesions, since no single antibody reactivity is diagnostic of a particular disease. In the workup of a histiocytic lesion, for example, immunoreactivity for S-100 protein, CD68, and CD1a supports a diagnosis of Langerhans cell histiocytosis. Although the subject of this Fascicle is nontumor pathology, it is important to discuss the most important monoclonal and polyclonal antibodies used in paraffin sections in the diagnosis of benign and neoplastic hematolymphoid lesions. Many cases of reactive lymphoid hyperplasia can be diagnosed solely by light microscopic features. There are some benign lesions, however, that simulate neoplasms and are difficult or impossible to distinguish without immunohistochemical studies.

IMMUNOHISTOCHEMISTRY OF LYMPHOID TISSUES

One useful approach to the evaluation of lymphoid tissue is to examine it in terms of functional compartments. Using a benign lymph node as the archetype, the lymphoid tissue can be divided into several components. The first of these is the lymphoid follicle, which is predominantly composed of B cells. Additionally, there is the interfollicular compartment, composed of a mixture of both B and T cells, with predominance of the latter. Other distinctive components of the lymph node include the lymphoid sinuses, medullary cords, stromal framework, and other functional areas.

B Cells

The evaluation of B cells is facilitated by a wide variety of antibodies (9,12). The most commonly used antibody is CD20, an antibody directed at the surface molecule involved in activation, proliferation, and differentiation of B cells (fig. 4-2). This antibody is robust in its technical performance and in its sensitivity and specificity for identification of B cells. CD20 expression is limited in B-cell development; it is not expressed on the earliest B-lymphoid precursors (e.g., as in precursor B-cell acute lymphocytic leukemia [ALL]), and is also not expressed in plasma cells.

There are other B-cell antibodies that are also useful. CD79a is a molecule which has a functional role in supporting and maintaining the surface immunoglobulin receptors of B cells (fig. 4-3). It is expressed throughout the lifespan of B cells, from the stage of early, committed B-cell lymphoblasts, through immature and mature B cells, as well as in plasma cells. PAX-5, CD22, CD74, CD45RA, MUM-1 are other antibodies that are preferentially expressed on B cells, both benign and malignant (39,55,60). Plasma cell neoplasms are identified with great specificity and sensitivity by using CD138 (47).

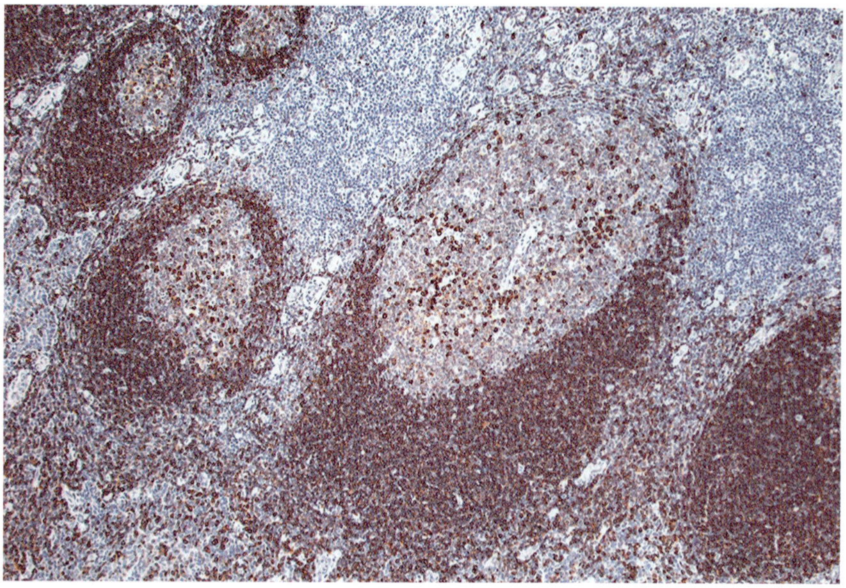

Figure 4-3

CD79A REACTIVITY, LYMPH NODE

Another pan-B-cell antigen, CD79a, parallels the reactivity of CD20, but in addition, stains plasma cells.

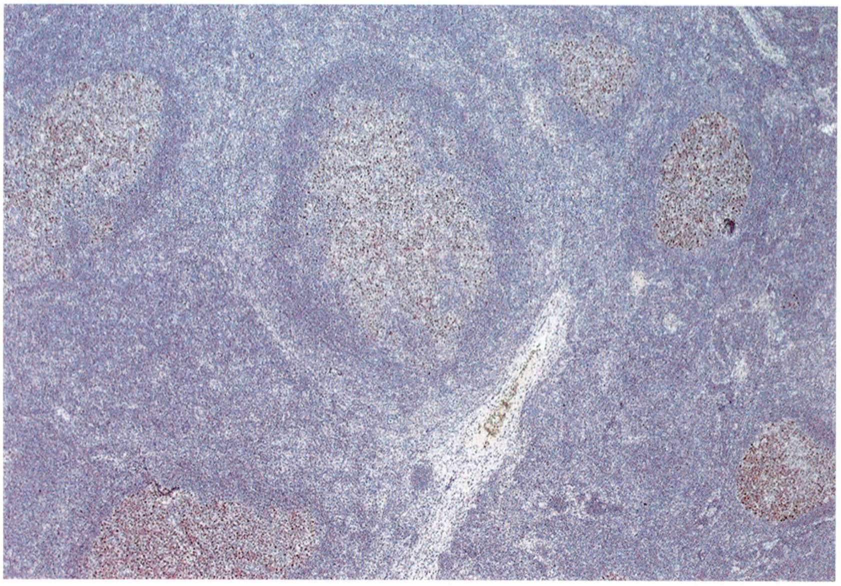

Figure 4-4

BCL-6 REACTIVITY, LYMPH NODE

Follicle center cells show nuclear reactivity for bcl-6.

The follicles of the lymph node are home to the B-cell component of the immune response. Follicle composition, morphology, and cellular composition are affected by the state of the immune response.

Several antibodies are selectively expressed on germinal center B cells (16,28,36,48). Bcl-6 is preferentially expressed in B cells of follicle center derivation (fig. 4-4). Besides normal secondary follicles/germinal centers, bcl-6 is also expressed in neoplasms of follicle center cell derivation including follicular lymphoma, subsets of diffuse large B-cell lymphoma (DLBCL), and Burkitt lymphoma. Bcl-6 expression is not seen in other B-cell lymphomas, such as mantle cell lymphoma or marginal zone lymphoma. Bcl-6 is a nuclear protein, and the pattern of immunohistochemical expression is that of distinct nuclear positivity. CD10 is also expressed on cells of follicle center derivation (fig. 4-5). Besides follicle center cells, it is also expressed on a subset of ALL/lymphomas, DLBCL, and Burkitt lymphoma. Some of the malignant cells in angioimmunoblastic T-cell lymphoma co-express CD10 and T-cell antigens.

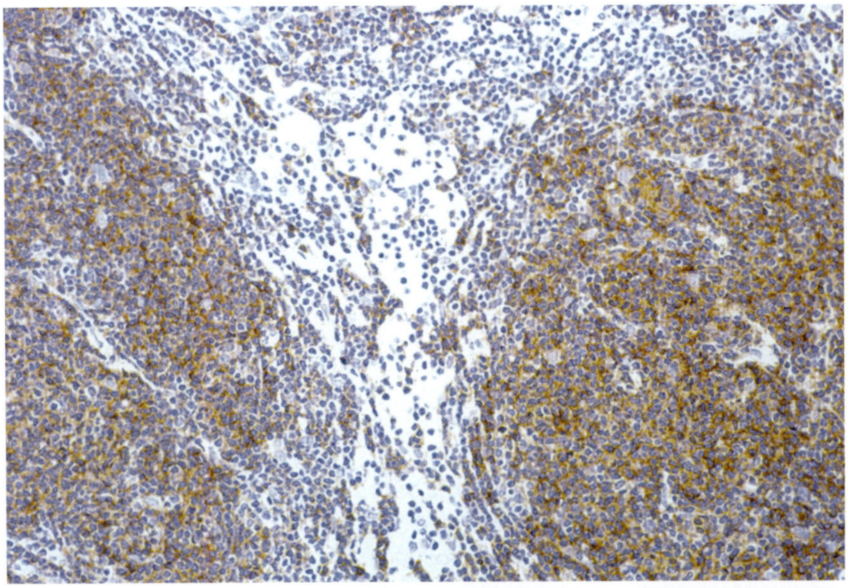

Figure 4-5

CD10 REACTIVITY, LYMPH NODE

Expression of CD10 in the neoplastic cells of follicular lymphoma. Benign cells of follicle center origin are also CD10 positive.

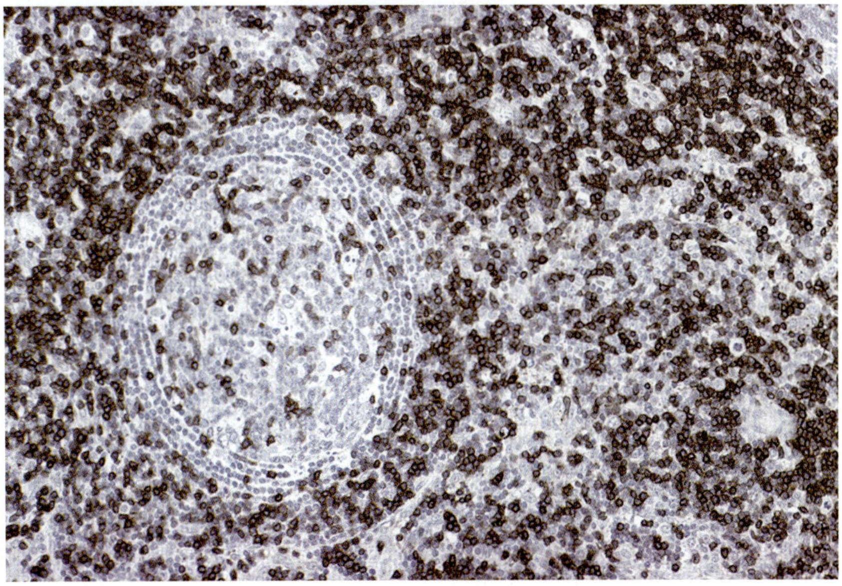

Figure 4-6

CD3 REACTIVITY, LYMPH NODE

Only rare T cells are seen in follicles, but the interfollicular compartment of the lymph node has many CD3-positive T cells.

T Cells

Numerous antibodies reactive with T cells have become available during the last decade. Among these, CD3 and CD2 are widely used as pan-T-cell markers since they are expressed throughout the entire lifespan of the T cell, from the stage of early T-cell precursor lymphoblasts, through immature and mature CD4- or CD8-positive T cells (fig. 4-6). CD45RO and CD43 antibodies, which were previously used extensively as pan-T-cell markers, lack specificity and should not be considered as "first line" T-cell markers. Other paraffin-reactive antibodies frequently used to characterize T cells and T-cell malignancies include: TdT, CD1a, CD5, CD4, CD8, CD7, CD30, Alk-1, CD56, and TIA-1.

Occasionally, the distinction needs to be drawn between reactive hyperplasia and focal infiltration with precursor T-cell lymphoma/ALL. Precursor T cells are normally absent or extremely rare in lymph nodes. They are, however, normally found in the normal and hyperplastic thymus, thymoma, spleen, and appendix as well as in the interfollicular areas of reactive tonsil (fig. 4-7) (49). Precursor T-cell lymphoblastic

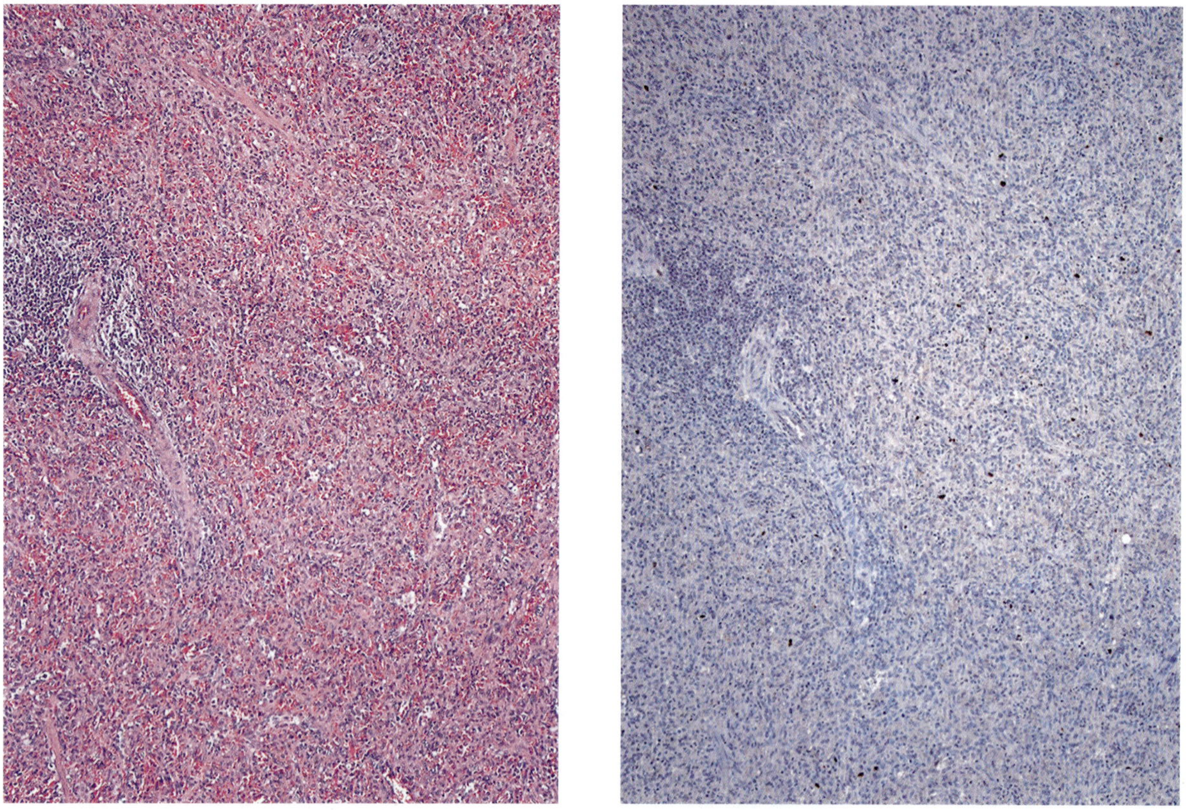

Figure 4-7

TERMINAL DEOXYNUCLEOTIDYLTRANSFERASE (TDT) REACTIVITY, SPLEEN

Rare TdT-positive cells are seen in the spleen. This degree of reactivity should not be mistaken for involvement with a lymphoblastic neoplasm.

lymphoma often expresses an immature T-cell immunophenotype (50). This includes expression of TdT and often CD1a. The lack of CD4 and CD8 expression (as seen in hepatosplenic T-cell lymphoma) or coexpression of CD4 and CD8 (as in T-cell prolymphocytic leukemia) is occasionally helpful in the differential diagnosis of T-cell lymphomas.

Reactive Conditions Versus Malignancies

Lymph nodes may be the site of a primary or secondary malignancy, especially a lymphoma, carcinoma, or melanoma. Occasionally, the malignant cells are difficult to distinguish from the reactive cellular background. Cytokeratin, vimentin, S-100 protein, and CD45RB (leukocyte common antigen) are often used in an initial screening panel in an attempt to identify and categorize metastatic lesions involving the lymph node (Table 4-1).

Cytokeratin is an intermediate filament in epithelial tissues. Antibodies are used to identify approximately 95 percent of epithelial tumors. There are rare, anecdotal reports of immunoreactivity in malignant lymphomas (19), usually with a dot-like paranuclear pattern of reactivity. Cytokeratin is often used to highlight the lymphoepithelial lesions in extranodal marginal zone lymphomas (fig. 4-8).

Vimentin is a ubiquitous cytoplasmic protein that is expressed in mesenchymal cells. Reactivity may also be seen in malignant melanoma and lymphoma (6,53).

S-100 protein is a highly soluble, acidic, nervous tissue-specific protein that is present in glial cells. Antibodies are very sensitive (but not specific) for malignant melanoma. This antigen is expressed in the macrophages (histiocytes) of Rosai-Dorfman disease and Langerhans cell histiocytosis, as well as in interdigitating

Table 4-1

IMMUNOHISTOCHEMISTRY OF LARGE CELL UNDIFFERENTIATED MALIGNANCIES[a]

	Cytokeratin	Vimentin	S-100 Protein	CD45RB
Carcinoma	Positive	Negative	Negative	Negative
Melanoma	Negative	Positive	Positive	Negative
Lymphoma	Negative	Pos[b]/Neg	Negative	Positive

[a]Confirmatory markers include epithelial membrane antigen (EMA) for carcinomas and HMB45 for melanomas.
[b]Diffuse large cell type.

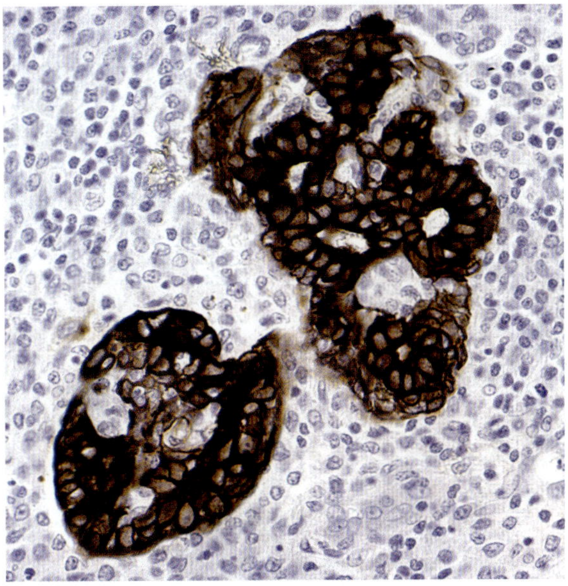

Figure 4-8

CYTOKERATIN REACTIVITY, MARGINAL ZONE LYMPHOMA

The cytokeratin stain highlights lymphoepithelial lesions in extranodal marginal zone lymphomas.

dendritic cells and their corresponding tumors (fig. 4-9).

CD45RB, leukocyte common antigen, is a member of the CD45 cluster of antibodies, which is present on pre-B and B cells, most T cells, macrophages, and myeloid cells (fig. 4-10). This antibody is considered to be a pan-leukocyte antibody that reacts with approximately 95 percent of non-Hodgkin lymphomas (97 percent B-cell, 90 percent T-cell types) and most cases of nodular lymphocyte-predominant Hodgkin lymphoma. Depending on the CD45RB result in the initial screening panel, additional supportive or confirmatory markers such as epithelial membrane antigen or HMB45 may be necessary.

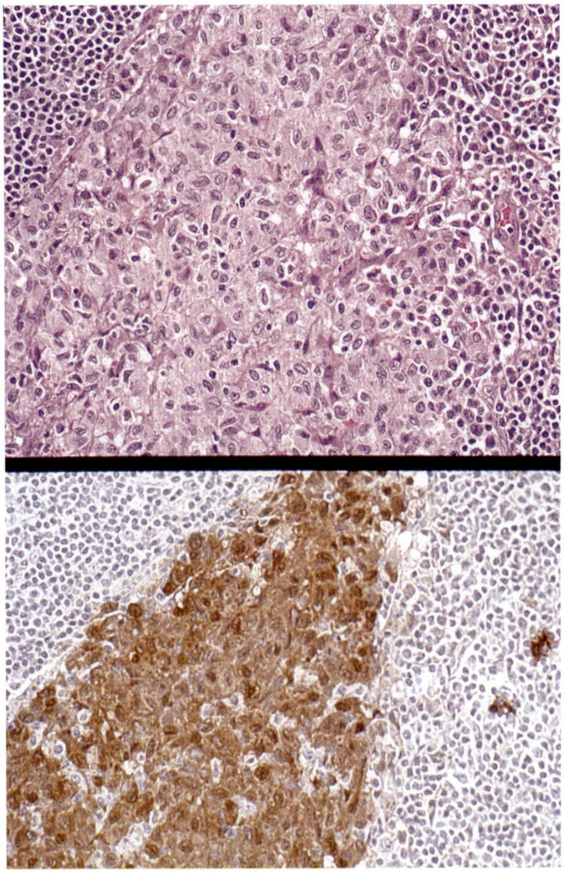

Figure 4-9

S-100 PROTEIN REACTIVITY, LANGERHANS CELL HISTIOCYTOSIS, LYMPH NODE

Langerhans cell histiocytes (top) are strongly reactive for S-100 protein (bottom).

Epithelial membrane antigen (EMA) is a sensitive marker of epithelial cells, which is often used as a confirmatory marker for carcinoma. Immunoreactivity for EMA is seen in benign and neoplastic plasma cells, anaplastic large cell lymphoma, and nodular lymphocyte-predominant Hodgkin lymphoma (fig. 4-11) (13).

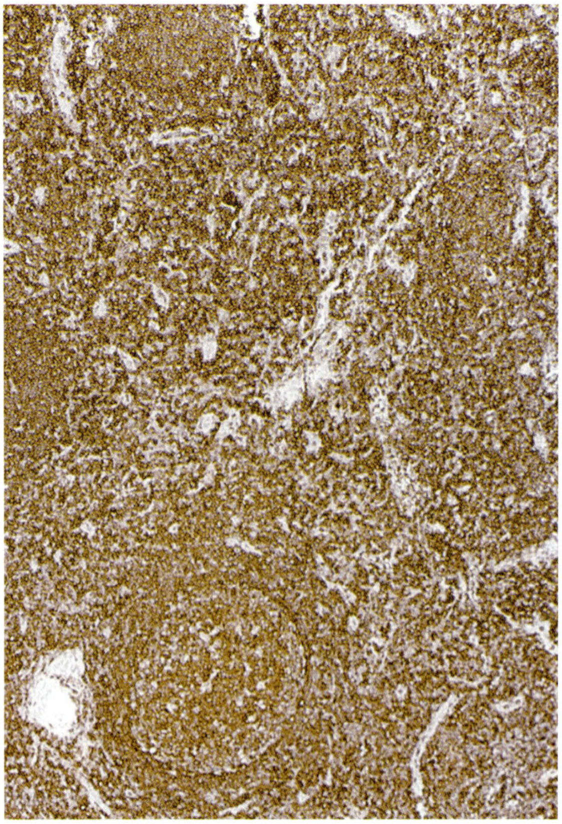

Figure 4-10

CD45RB REACTIVITY, LYMPH NODE

An antigen that stains most of the cells that express leukocyte common antigen (LCA), CD45RB is expected to stain most cells in a normal lymph node.

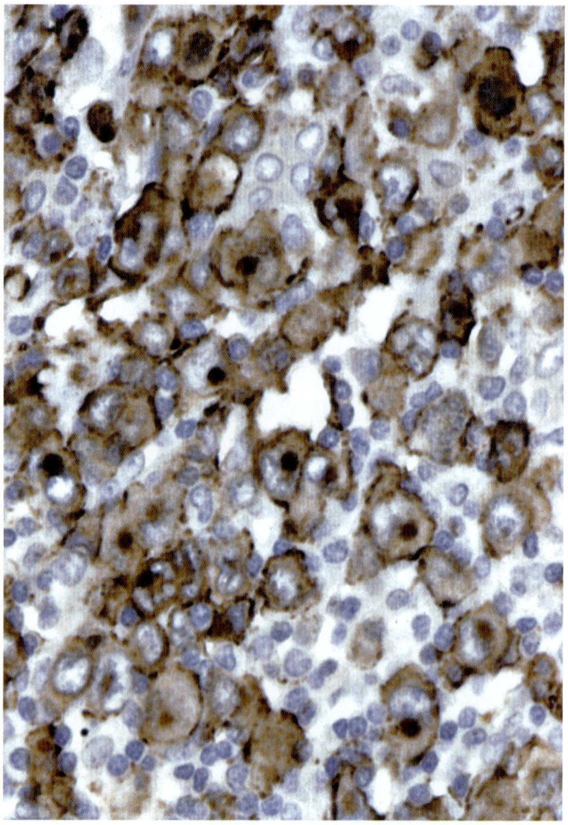

Figure 4-11

EPITHELIAL MEMBRANE ANTIGEN (EMA) REACTIVITY, ANAPLASTIC LARGE CELL LYMPHOMA, LYMPH NODE

EMA positivity is seen in the majority of cases of anaplastic large cell lymphoma, and is often associated with ALK positivity.

HMB45 is a highly sensitive and specific marker for malignant melanoma. It is used as a confirmatory marker in the presence of S-100 protein positivity (23).

Reactive Conditions Versus Lymphomas

There are several commonly used antigens (listed in Table 4-2) that are used to separate reactive conditions from lymphomas (in addition to CD45RB).

CD20 is a cluster of antibodies that recognizes a restricted B-cell antigen. CD20 reacts with approximately 98 percent of B-cell lymphomas and most cases of nodular lymphocyte-predominant Hodgkin lymphomas (8).

CD45RO is a T-cell antigen that is also present on some macrophages and granulocytes (fig. 4-12). Antibodies identify approximately 77 percent of T-cell lymphomas and may show coexpression in approximately 5 percent of B-cell lymphomas (24,40).

CD3 is a T-cell antigen associated with the T-cell receptor. A polyclonal antibody is used in paraffin sections to identify the majority of T-cell lymphomas but essentially no cases of B-cell lymphoma.

CD5 is an antigen that is present in 95 percent of thymocytes, almost all immature and mature peripheral T cells, more than 95 percent of chronic lymphocytic leukemias/small lymphocytic lymphomas, and 93 percent of mantle cell lymphomas (3,17,59).

CD43 antigen is expressed by normal T cells, granulocytes, and a subset of plasma cells (but not normal B cells). Reactivity is seen in almost all cases of T-cell lymphoma. CD43 is coexpressed with CD20 on a subset of B-cell lymphomas (37,45).

Table 4-2

IMMUNOHISTOCHEMISTRY OF NON-HODGKIN LYMPHOMA (NHL) VERSUS HODGKIN LYMPHOMA (HL)

	CD45RB	CD20	CD45RO	CD3	CD5	CD43	CD15	CD30	ALK
B-cell NHL	+	+	-/+	-	-/+[c]	-/+[d]	-	-	-[e]
T-cell NHL	+	-	+	+	+	+	-	-	-
ALCL-T[a]	+/-	-	+	+	+	+	-	+	+
Classic HL[b]	-	-	-	-	-	-	+	+	-
NLPHL	+	+	-	-	-	-	-	-	-

[a]ALCL-T = anaplastic large cell lymphoma, T cell; NLPHL = nodular lymphocyte-predominant Hodgkin lymphoma.
[b]Results refer to the immunoreactivity of the neoplastic Reed-Sternberg cells and variants.
[c]Coexpression of CD5 and CD20 in a subset of B cell lymphomas.
[d]Coexpression of CD43 and CD20 in a subset of B cell lymphomas.
[e]B-cell neoplasms may express ALK protein but lack the t(2;5) translocation (14).

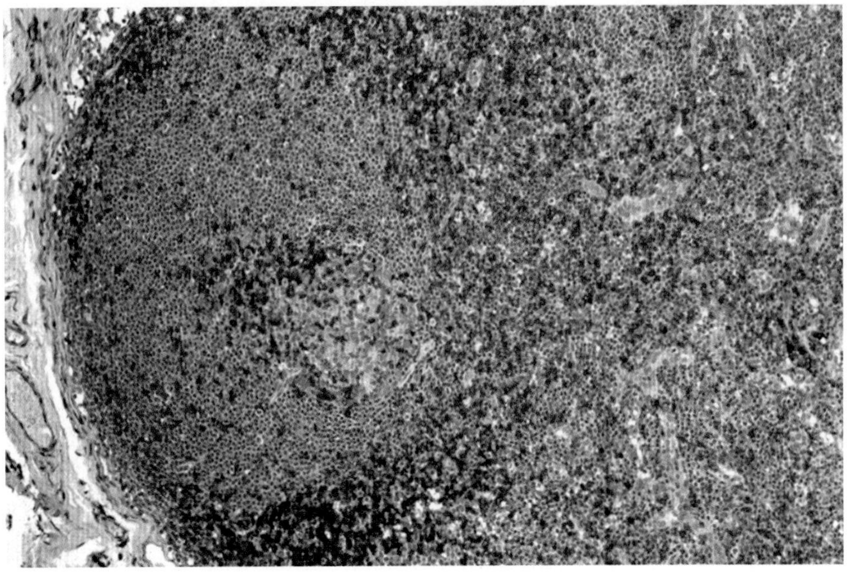

Figure 4-12

CD45RO REACTIVITY, LYMPH NODE

CD45RO stains the majority of T cells as well as granulocytes and macrophages.

CD15 protein is present in granulocytes and some macrophages. Antibodies are used to identify the Reed-Sternberg cells in classic Hodgkin lymphoma as well as granulocytic sarcoma and some myeloid leukemias (fig. 4-13). It is also coexpressed in some large cells in cases of cytomegalovirus lymphadenitis.

CD30 activation antigen is present on a subset B and T cells (fig. 4-14). Reactivity is seen in most cases of classic Hodgkin lymphoma and anaplastic large cell lymphoma. Antibodies also react with the immunoblasts in Epstein-Barr virus–related lymphadenitis and other benign proliferations of immunoblasts (2).

ALK-1 protein is the product of the t(2;5) translocation and is associated with approximately 85 percent of cases of anaplastic large cell lymphoma (4,14,38,54). Rare cases of B-cell lymphoma express the ALK protein but lack t(2;5) (14).

CD56 is a natural killer (NK) cell antigen expressed by resting and activated NK cells. It is present in a subset of cytotoxic T cells.

CD57 antigen is present on a subset of germinal center T cells and NK cells (27). This antibody reacts with NK cells and a subset of T cells. It is also important in the diagnosis of large granular lymphocytosis, T-cell lymphoma/leukemia, and some NK-cell neoplasms.

Reactive Conditions Versus B-Cell Neoplasms

Immunohistochemistry in paraffin sections can help to distinguish a B-cell malignancy from reactive lymphoid hyperplasia. The demonstration of one or more of the following features

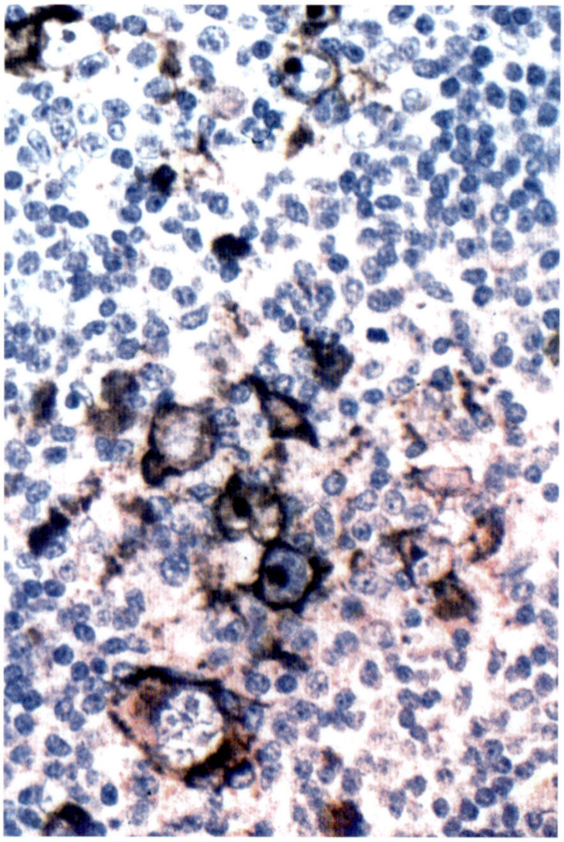

Figure 4-13

CD15 REACTIVITY, HODGKIN LYMPHOMA, LYMPH NODE

CD15 reactivity in Hodgkin lymphoma is often accentuated in the Golgi apparatus, giving the cytoplasm a strongly staining paranuclear dot.

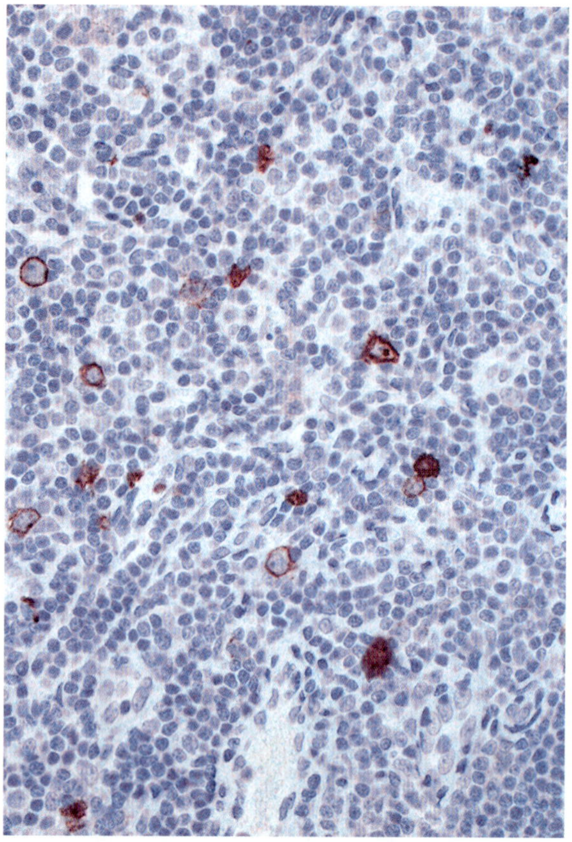

Figure 4-14

CD30 REACTIVITY, LYMPH NODE

Activated lymphocytes, both T and B cells, stain for CD30, as do Hodgkin cells.

supports a neoplastic rather than a reactive B-cell process: immunoglobulin light chain restriction, bcl-2 immunoreactivity in germinal centers, cyclin D1 overexpression, coexpression of CD5 or CD43 with CD20, and rearrangement of immunoglobulin heavy/light chain gene by Southern blotting or polymerase chain reaction (PCR) technique.

Antibodies to CD20 are extremely valuable for identifying most B-cell lymphomas, although plasma cell neoplasms are usually negative. Alternative B-cell markers, such as PAX-5, CD79a, or CD22, are used to document the presence of residual lymphoma cells in cases treated with anti-CD20 monoclonal antibodies (e.g., rituximab). Although the immunoglobulin light chain antibodies work more reliably in frozen tissue sections or flow cytometric cell suspensions, they are available for use in paraffin-embedded tissue sections by both immunohistochemical and in situ hybridization techniques (fig. 4-15). Polyclonal reactivity for kappa and lambda light chains in a 3-5 to 1 ratio supports the diagnosis of reactive hyperplasia rather than a B-cell neoplasm in most cases.

CD23 is an antigen expressed by mature B cells and follicular dendritic cells (fig. 4-16). It is reactive in chronic lymphocytic leukemia/small lymphocytic lymphoma but not in mantle cell lymphoma.

Cyclin D1 is a cell cycle protein that is not normally expressed in lymphocytes. The characteristic translocation, t(11;14), which is seen in mantle cell lymphoma, results in overexpression of the *PRAD1* gene that encodes for cyclin D1. Nuclear reactivity in a small B-cell

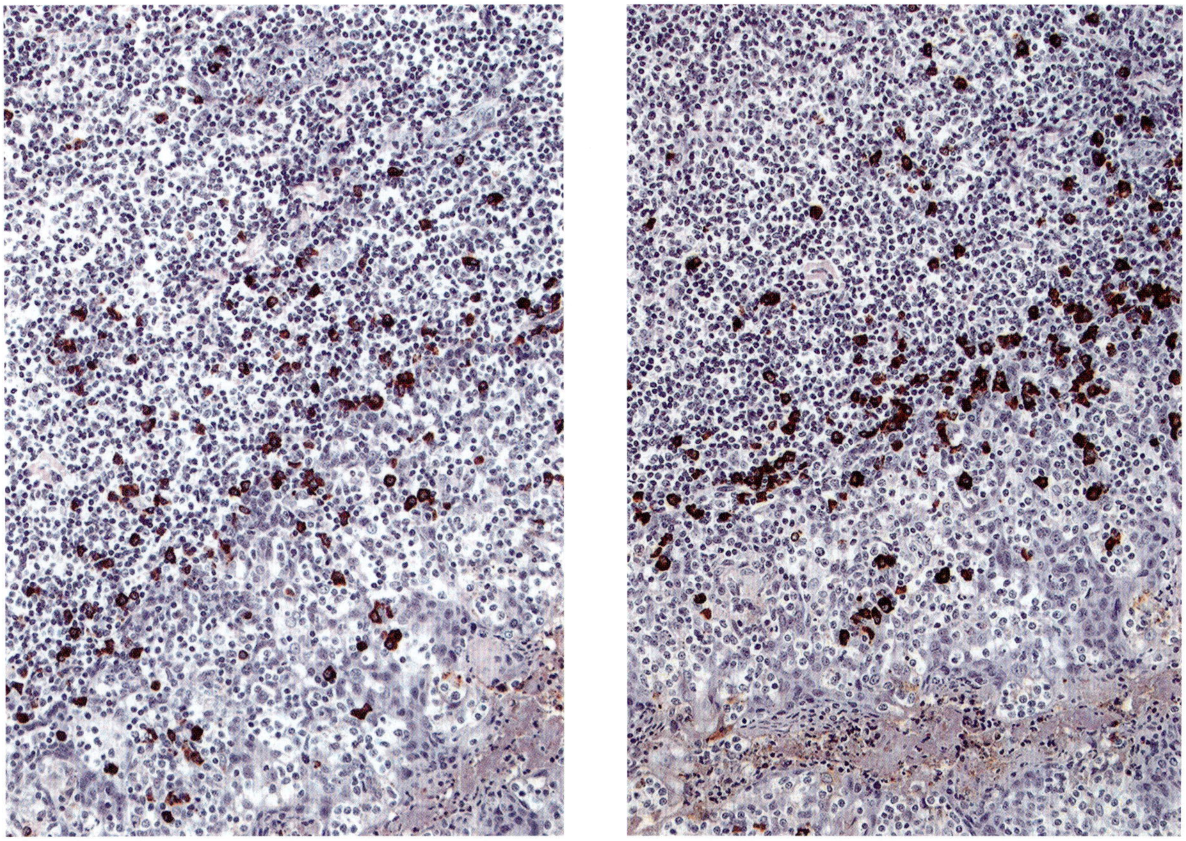

Figure 4-15

KAPPA AND LAMBDA LIGHT CHAIN REACTIVITY, LYMPH NODE

Immunohistochemical staining for light chains shows a polyclonal pattern in the plasma cells in this lymph node (left, kappa; right, lambda).

lymphoma supports a diagnosis of mantle cell lymphoma (63,69).

Bcl-2 antibody recognizes an oncogene that prevents apoptosis and decreases the rate of cell death. Bcl-2 protein is normally present on mantle zone cells, rare T cells in the germinal centers, normal T cells, and plasma cells (fig. 4-17). Overexpression of the bcl-2 protein caused by the t(14;18) translocation is seen in the majority of follicular lymphomas, but is overexpressed in many other B-cell lymphomas (36). Reactivity for antibodies to the bcl-2 protein (44) is used to support a diagnosis of follicular lymphoma, especially of grades 1 and 2 (36), or to distinguish follicular lymphoma from follicular hyperplasia. Follicular lymphoma, grade 3, shows less frequent immunoreactivity for bcl-2 than grades 1 and 2 lymphomas (36).

Reactive Conditions Versus T-Cell Neoplasms

Viral infections, other infectious conditions, and inflammatory conditions often show a preponderance of T cells. Occasionally, these conditions may suggest a peripheral T-cell malignancy. Histologically, peripheral T-cell lymphomas are heterogeneous. They may display a high content of epithelioid macrophages or granulomas and therefore simulate granulomatous inflammatory conditions.

An immunohistochemical test to evaluate T-cell clonality that is analogous to immunoglobulin light chain evaluation is not available for distinguishing T-cell neoplasms from reactive lesions. An aberrant phenotype with the loss of pan-T-cell antigens in more than 50 percent of the total T cells supports a diagnosis of peripheral T-cell lymphoma (65). Antibodies

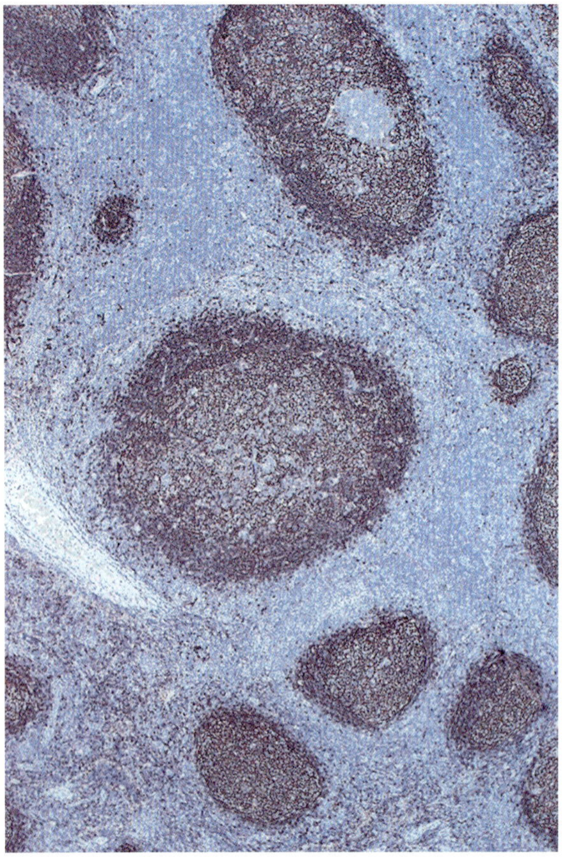

Figure 4-16

CD23 REACTIVITY, LYMPH NODE

CD23 is useful for highlighting the follicular dendritic cells, but often with a slightly different pattern of reactivity than CD21 or CD35.

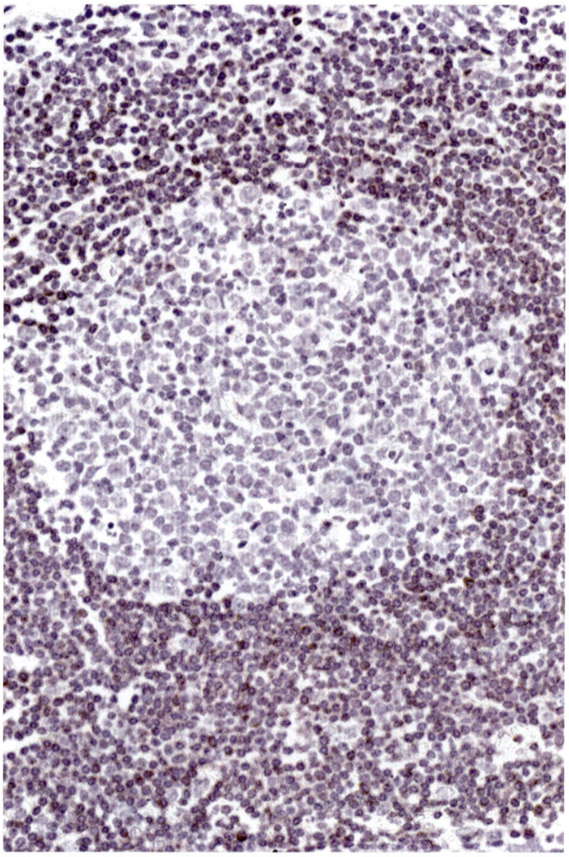

Figure 4-17

BCL-2 REACTIVITY, LYMPH NODE

Normal follicle center cells do not express bcl-2.

to CD4 identify helper/inducer T cells whereas antibodies to CD8 label the cytotoxic/suppressor subset. Mature T cells usually express either CD4 or CD8. The ratio of CD4 to CD8 cells varies in reactive T-cell processes and cannot be used in an analogous fashion to the immunoglobulin light chains. In general, however, coexpression of CD4 and CD8 or the absence of both CD4 and CD8 in a mature T-cell population suggests a diagnosis of T-cell lymphoma (10,65). Besides CD3, other pan-T-cell markers such as CD2, CD5, and CD7 are expressed early in T-cell differentiation and throughout the life of T cells; loss of expression supports a diagnosis of lymphoma over T-cell hyperplasia. TdT and CD1a identify immature T cells which are absent or rare in reactive conditions. The presence of immature T cells in significant numbers suggests a diagnosis of a precursor cell lymphoid neoplasm, most commonly T-cell lymphoblastic lymphoma. To evaluate cytotoxic differentiation in T cells and NK cells both in reactive and neoplastic proliferations, CD56, TIA-1, perforin, and granzyme-B are helpful.

Reactive Conditions Versus Hodgkin Lymphoma

The immunophenotyping of Hodgkin lymphoma is characteristic (CD15/CD30 positive, CD45 negative) and allows its distinction both from reactive lymphoid proliferations and from most cases of non-Hodgkin lymphoma. The distinction between Hodgkin lymphoma and an immunoblast-rich paracortical hyperplasia, such as infectious mononucleosis, is particularly important in cases of Hodgkin lymphoma characterized by minimal (interfollicular) nodal involvement.

Histiocytic and Myelomonocytic Antibodies

Immunoreactivity with S-100 protein is useful in making the diagnosis of malignant melanoma. It is also characteristically seen, however, in important histiocytic disorders, Langerhans cell histiocytosis and Rosai-Dorfman disease. It can also be expressed in cases of histiocytic sarcoma and in interdigitating dendritic cells and their corresponding neoplasms. CD1a is particularly useful to confirm a diagnosis of Langerhans cell histiocytosis in paraffin sections (18). Other macrophages, such as those seen in Rosai-Dorfman disease and juvenile xanthogranuloma, are negative with antibodies to CD1a.

Other useful antibodies for identifying macrophages and monocytic cells in paraffin sections include CD68R, CD163, and lysozyme. Plasmacytoid dendritic cells, which are seen in Kikuchi-Fujimoto disease and other reactive lymph nodal conditions, are positive for CD68, lysozyme, and myeloperoxidase, but the most specific for these cells is CD123.

Several antibodies are important in the diagnosis of histiocytic lesions. *CD1a* is a formalin-resistant epitope recognized by a mouse monoclonal antibody originally reported to be specific for Langerhans cell macrophages (18). *CD68R (PG-M1)* and *CD163* antigens are present on cells of the histiocytic lineage; these antibodies are mainly used to identify histiocytic processes and myeloid leukemias with monocytic differentiation (fig. 4-18). *CD68 (KP-1)* reacts with macrophages, mast cells, and myeloid cells. A potential pitfall is the staining of nonhematopoietic malignancies (fig. 4-19). *Lysozyme* is present on macrophages and myeloid cells and is useful in the diagnosis of histiocytic processes and myeloid sarcoma. *CD123* is the most specific marker for highlighting plasmacytoid dendritic cells in paraffin sections (fig. 4-20).

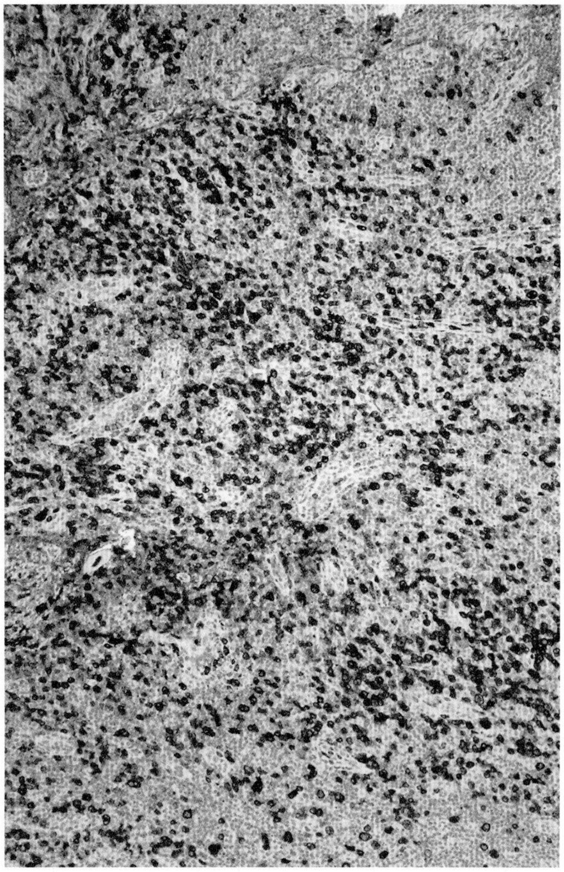

Figure 4-18

CD163 REACTIVITY, KIKUCHI-FUJIMOTO DISEASE, LYMPH NODE

In addition to other stains that are positive in the plasmacytoid dendritic cells of Kikuchi-Fujimoto disease, CD163 also shows reactivity.

Myeloid Cell Antibodies

Occasionally, myeloid cells are encountered in lymph nodes and (more commonly) spleen. Immunohistology can be used to confirm the nature of myeloid infiltrates in these cases. Myeloid sarcoma may have to be distinguished from benign myeloid proliferations or from proliferations of large, undifferentiated cells. Important antibodies that aid in this differential diagnosis include: myeloperoxidase, lysozyme, CD34, CD117, CD68, and CD163 (Table 4-3).

CD34 is an antigen present on hematopoietic progenitor/precursor cells and endothelial cells. CD34 immunostaining is used to identify leukemias and vascular lesions in lymph nodes and in spleen.

CD117 antigen is present on early myeloid precursor cells and mast cells. Antibodies are used to identify extramedullary acute myeloid leukemia and mastocytosis (fig. 4-21). CD117 also stains several nonhematopoietic malignancies.

Myeloperoxidase is normally present in the primary granules of neutrophilic myeloid cells. It is useful in the diagnosis of acute myeloid leukemia and myeloid sarcoma (fig. 4-22) (53).

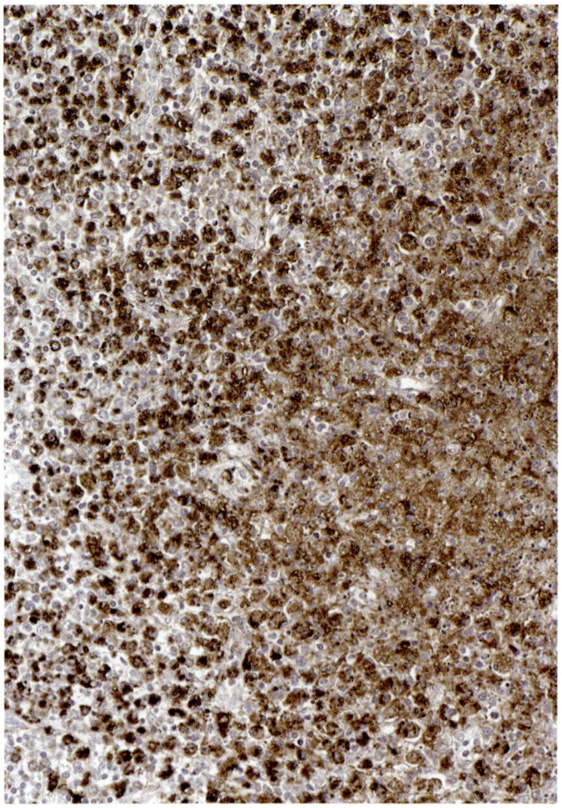

Figure 4-19

CD68 REACTIVITY, KIKUCHI-FUJIMOTO DISEASE, LYMPH NODE

CD68 (KP-1) is a very sensitive, but nonspecific, stain for cells of myeloid and related lineages. In this case of Kikuchi-Fujimoto disease, the plasmacytoid dendritic cells and other myeloid elements (e.g., macrophages) are strongly positive for CD68.

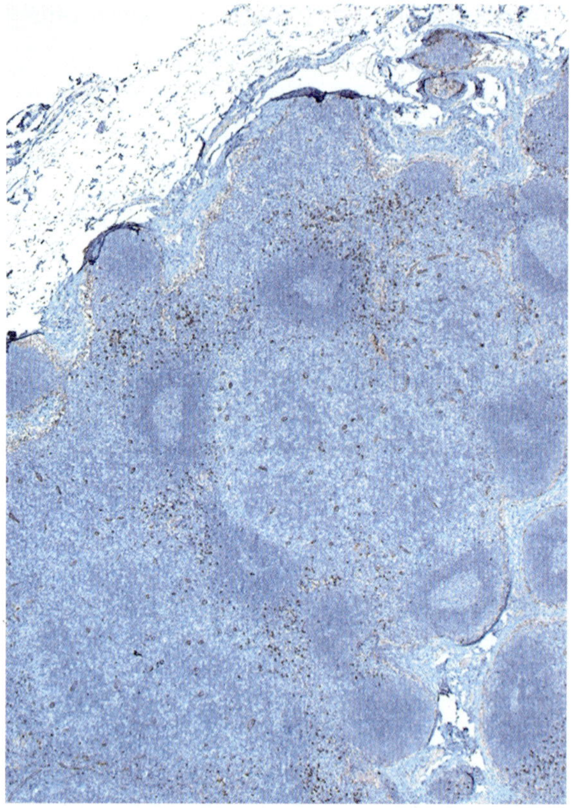

Figure 4-20

CD123 REACTIVITY, LYMPH NODE

Immature dendritic cells are highlighted in this lymph node with dermatopathic lymphadenitis by CD123 reactivity.

TdT, terminal deoxynucleotidyltransferase, is an important antibody. It demonstrates reactivity in lymphoblastic lymphoma and precursor cells of the bone marrow and thymus.

Dendritic Cell Antibodies

Follicular dendritic cells (FDCs) are accessory cells that help make up the skeleton of normal follicles. Because of their antigen-presenting capability, they play an important role in the ongoing immune response and B-cell maturation. CD21 is useful for staining FDCs, although CD35 has similar reactivity (fig. 4-23). CD23 also stains FDCs, but has a slightly different staining pattern than the other two markers. The differences observed depend on the activity level of the germinal centers.

Staining for FDCs facilitates the identification of lymphoid follicles in cases characterized by expanded paracortical areas and in benign lymph nodes where those structures are inapparent (e.g., mesenteric lymph nodes). Staining demonstrates follicular germinal center colonization such as is seen in cases of nodal involvement by marginal zone lymphoma or other parafollicular hematologic malignancies. Expanded FDC networks are seen in reactive lymphadenopathies. Spindle cell proliferations of FDCs may be encountered in lymph node and spleen. In these cases, the main distinction is between reactive conditions (e.g., inflammatory pseudotumor) and neoplastic proliferations (see chapter 18).

Smooth muscle actin (SMA) is useful in identifying myofibroblastic proliferations seen in reactive and pseudoneoplastic conditions such as inflammatory pseudotumor.

Table 4-3

IMMUNOHISTOCHEMISTRY OF LYMPHOMA VERSUS MYELOID SARCOMA

	CD45RB	CD20	CD3	CD68	CD34	MPO[a]	CD15
Lymphoma	Positive	Pos/Neg	Pos/Neg	Negative	Negative	Negative	Negative
Myeloid sarcoma	Pos/Neg	Negative	Negative	Positive[b]	Positive	Positive[c]	Positive

[a]MPO = myeloperoxidase.
[b]Monocytic differentiation.
[c]Myeloid differentiation.

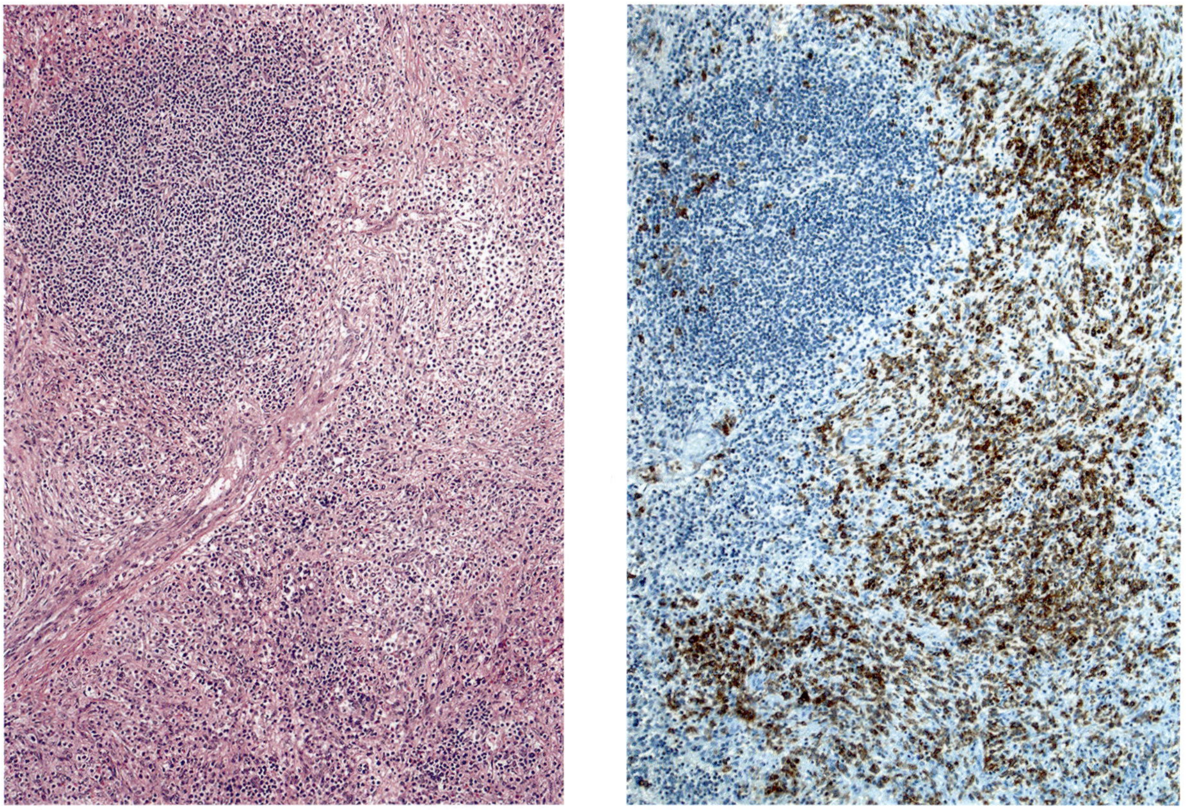

Figure 4-21

CD117 REACTIVITY, MASTOCYTOSIS, SPLEEN

In this case of splenic mastocytosis (left), the (neoplastic) mast cells are strongly positive for CD117 (right). The mast cells, both benign and malignant, would also be positive for tryptase.

POTENTIAL PITFALLS IN IMMUNOHISTOCHEMISTRY

Immunohistochemistry is a powerful adjunct technique in the diagnosis of hematolymphoid lesions. There are potential problems and pitfalls, however, which may occur from procedural errors (i.e., technician error, machine failure), poor tissue fixation, loss of antigenicity, suboptimal processing (62,64), and incorrect interpretation of results. Inconsistent or different phenotypes in sequential biopsy specimens of the same diagnosis may be the result of variation in tissue processing techniques (62,66). The lack of antigenic specificity may result in an incorrect diagnosis (such as CD15 reactivity in cytomegalovirus-infected cells that simulate the neoplastic cells of Hodgkin lymphoma) (fig. 4-24). A problem with the immunohistochemical detection method or

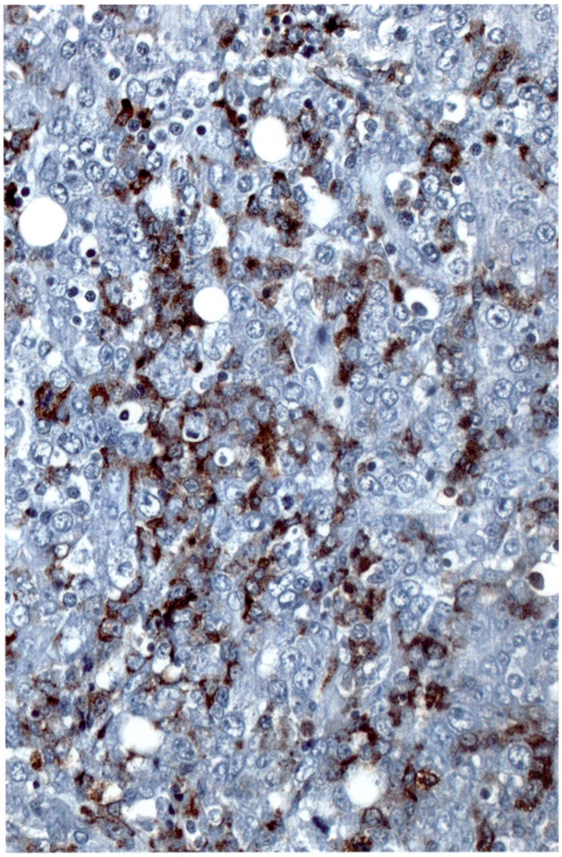

Figure 4-22

MYELOPEROXIDASE REACTIVITY, MYELOID SARCOMA, LYMPH NODE

Myeloperoxidase is positive in the large pleomorphic cells of myeloid sarcoma of lymph node.

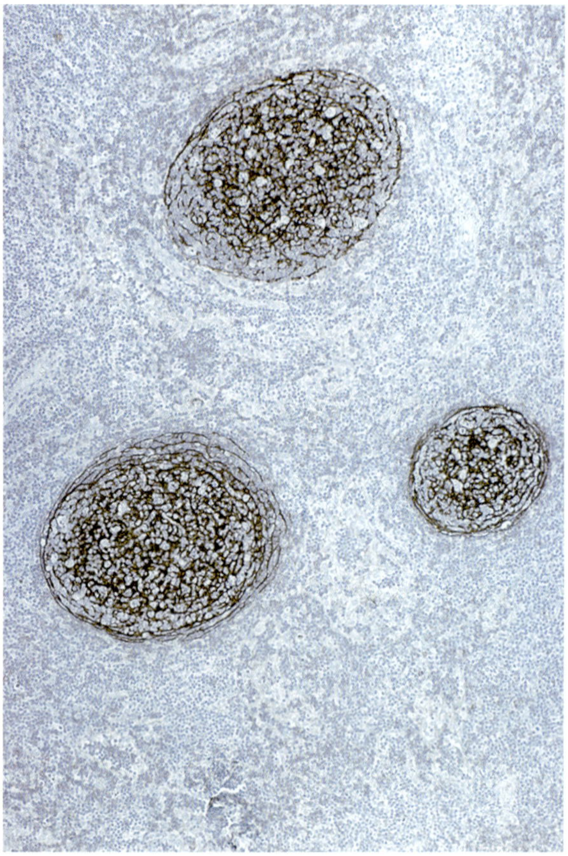

Figure 4-23

CD21 REACTIVITY, LYMPH NODE

CD21 highlights the follicular dendritic cells.

Figure 4-24

CD15 REACTIVITY, CYTOMEGALOVIRUS (CMV) LYMPHADENITIS

A potential pitfall, CD15 reactivity in the large cells of CMV lymphadenitis can cause some confusion with Hodgkin lymphoma.

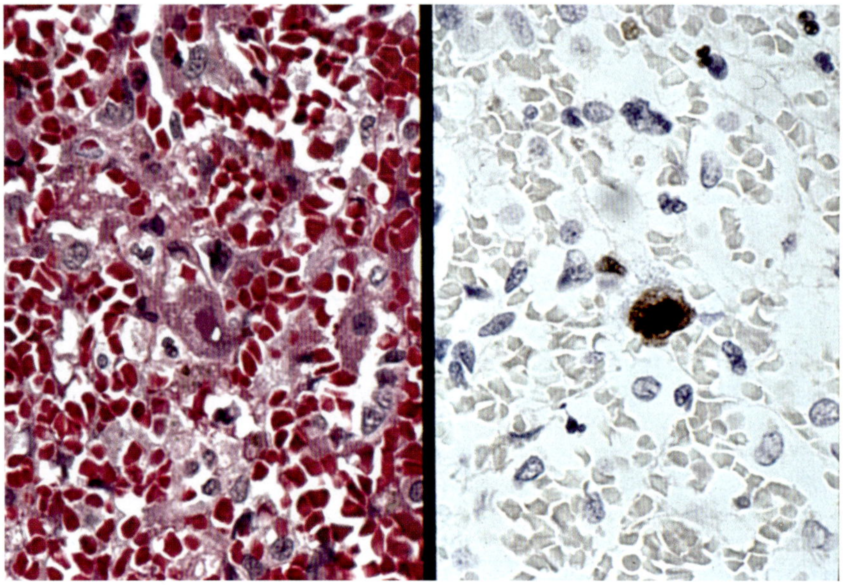

endogenous peroxidase activity may result in high background staining, which can give false positive results; to avoid high background staining, endogenous peroxide should be blocked and the highest possible dilution of primary antibody used (10).

Misinterpretation of the immunoreactivity pattern (i.e., whether the benign or neoplastic cell population is reactive) can result in a serious misdiagnosis. Familiarity with pertinent leukocyte cell surface antigens and antibodies, anticipated patterns of reactivity, and potential pitfalls optimizes the use of this important ancillary technique.

IMMUNOHISTOCHEMISTRY OF THE SPLEEN

Immunohistochemistry is a valuable tool in the evaluation of splenic disorders. It provides unique challenges, however, because of the functional complexity of the spleen and the variety of its histologic components. The purpose of this section is to provide general guidelines on evaluating the complex splenic microanatomy, stressing in particular the morphologic and the immunohistologic characteristics of the white pulp and red pulp compartments (61).

As a functional compartment, the stroma of the spleen is often overlooked. It does, however, give rise to both neoplastic and non-neoplastic proliferations that may be complex and difficult to evaluate. The splenic stroma is divided into three components: the vascular component, the reticuloendothelial or monocyte/macrophage component, and the remainder (43). This remaining portion consists of various mesenchymal cells and extracellular matrix, which forms the structural framework of the spleen.

The large arteries, arterioles, and veins of the spleen are similar to those of other sites in the body, and can be evaluated with the battery of immunostains used to stain endothelial cells as well as vascular tumors at other sites: CD34, CD31, factor VIII (von Willebrand factor), and, more recently, FLi-1 (fig. 4-25). A specialized endothelial cell unique to the spleen is the littoral cell, which lines the vascular sinuses. The littoral cells share features of both endothelial cells and monocyte/macrophages. They are usually flat, inconspicuous cells along the edges of sinuses. When activated, they become plump and appear larger. These cells are strongly and uniformly positive for CD8, a marker that is more commonly associated with cytotoxic or suppressor T cells. Therefore, CD8 is a useful stain for delineating the sinusoidal architecture in the spleen; however, the strong vascular reactivity with CD8 can make the evaluation of CD8-positive T cells difficult (fig. 4-26).

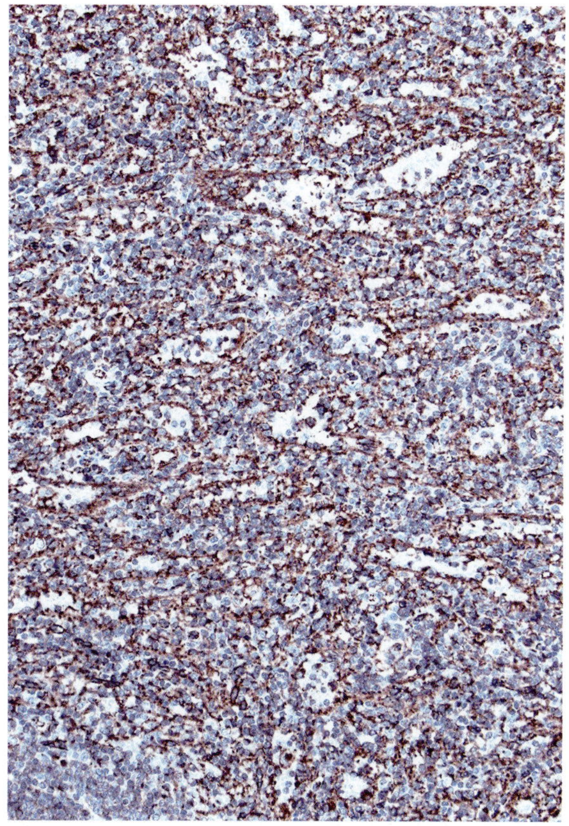

Figure 4-25

CD31 REACTIVITY, SPLEEN

A variety of vascular markers can be used to evaluate the vascular architecture of the spleen. In this case, CD31 is reactive in both the sinuses (littoral cells) as well as arterioles.

The monocyte/macrophage system is one of the more important anatomic and functional components of the spleen; it forms the bulk of the red pulp (cordal macrophages), but often receives little specific attention. Only when there is a significant derangement of the monocyte/macrophage system is it even noticed. Evaluation of this system using immunohistochemistry is accomplished by a number of antibodies, which include CD68, CD163, lysozyme, antichymotrypsin, and others. When there is accumulation of

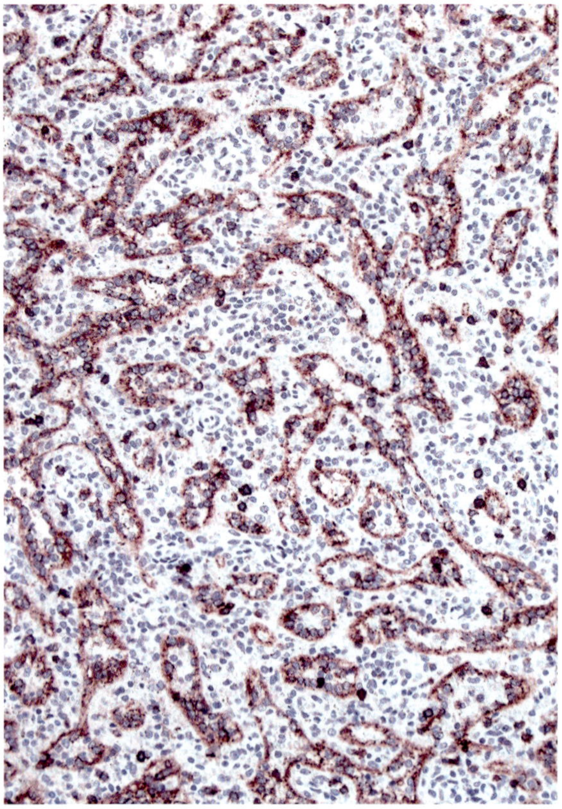

Figure 4-26

CD8 REACTIVITY, SPLEEN

Splenic cytotoxic T cells are positive for CD8, but must be interpreted in the background of staining in the littoral cells.

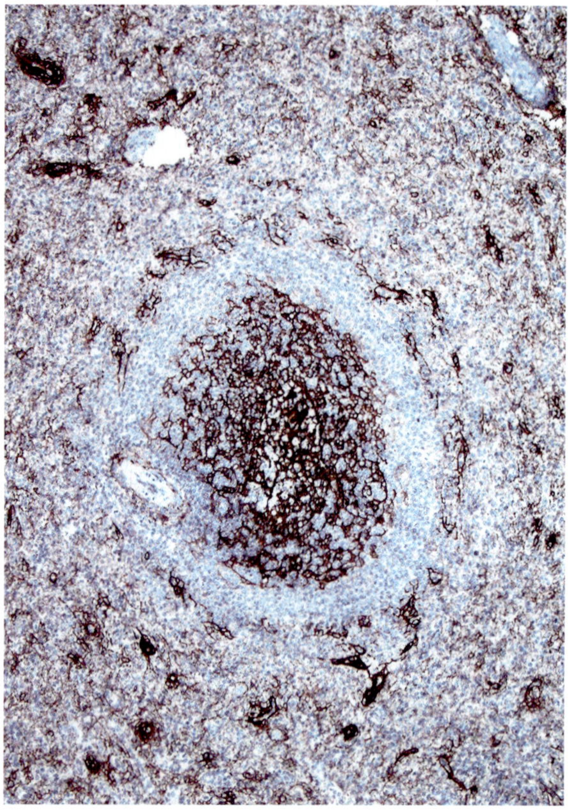

Figure 4-27

LOW-AFFINIITY NERVE GROWTH FACTOR RECEPTOR (LNGFR) REACTIVITY, SPLEEN

LNGFR stains both stromal elements of the red pulp as well as the follicular dendritic cells of the white pulp.

intracellular material in macrophages, histologic stains may be of considerable value, depending on the accumulated product. Most abnormal storage proteins are periodic acid–Schiff (PAS) positive. Infectious organisms can be evaluated by the judicious use of acid-fast bacillus (AFB), Gomori methenamine silver (GMS), tissue Gram, and PAS stains. In the case of immunoglobulin accumulation, immunohistochemistry for kappa and lambda light chains may be of benefit.

A considerable portion of the spleen (white pulp) is devoted to its function as a lymphoid organ. A notable component of the white pulp are the dendritic cells (FDCs and interdigitating dendritic cells [IDCs]). Dendritic cells are distinguished by immunohistochemistry: depending on the type, dendritic cells are varyingly positive for monocyte/macrophage-associated markers such as CD21, CD23, CD35, CD68, S-100 protein, CD1a, lysozyme, and alpha-1-antitrypsin (as previously described).

Various antibodies are used to evaluate structural mesenchymal cells and extracellular matrix. Low-affinity nerve growth factor receptor (LNGFR) identifies reticulum cells in the splenic cords, periarteriolar and pericapillary adventitial cells, and FDCs (fig. 4-27). The LNGFR-positive cell subsets typically share a fibroblastic or spindle cell morphology and perform mainly structural functions. SMA identifies pericytes and cells with myofibroblastic differentiation (myoid cells). A concentric reticular meshwork of SMA-positive cells is present at the interface between the red pulp and the marginal zones (35,68). SMA staining of perivascular cells within the red pulp is also observed. Extracellular matrix is evaluated by immunohistochemistry for collagen IV and by reticulin staining. Collagen

IV highlights the "ring fibers" which incompletely surround the littoral cells of the splenic sinusoids (61). Various patterns of stromal cell hyperplasia or alterations in the architectural distribution of extracellular matrix proteins are observed in a variety of splenic disorders.

FLOW CYTOMETRY

Flow cytometry has the advantage of allowing the evaluation of several thousand cells in a rapid manner, and it has the ability to assess the expression of multiple antigens on a single cell. Also, the use of CD45 versus side scatter gating strategies allows cells with specific characteristics (such as blast cells or abnormal lymphoid cells) to be evaluated. This method greatly increases the ability to detect a population of abnormal hematolymphoid cells which may be "diluted" by the presence of a reactive cellular background. Flow cytometry is also the best technique for the assessment of clonality in B-cell lymphoid neoplasms (using surface immunoglobulin light chain analysis) and, as such, helps in establishing a diagnosis of lymphoid malignancy. Several consensuses reports and reviews regarding the use of flow cytometric immunophenotyping in hematologic malignant neoplasms offer guidelines to the use of this methodology (5,15,20,21,33,42).

Flow Cytometry of the Spleen

The spleen has been only rarely investigated by flow cytometry. Relatively recently, the immunophenotypic characteristics of the lymphocytes of the human spleen were investigated and reference values established for normal and reactive spleens (11). Although the results obtained showed T-cell antigen patterns of expression comparable to those seen in other lymphoid organs, a few differences were noted (Table 4-4). In contrast to the thymus and bone marrow, the spleen contains only rare TdT-positive lymphoid precursors (7). Within the B-cell subsets, the spleen shows a frequency of CD19-positive/CD20-negative B cells that is higher than in the peripheral blood or lymph node. This corresponds to the presence, in the spleen, of a sizable proportion of early plasma cells (CD138 negative) as well as more mature plasma cells. Other differences include a significant population of CD20/CD5-positive B cells,

Table 4-4

EXPRESSION OF SURFACE AND INTRACELLULAR ANTIGENS IN HUMAN SPLEEN LYMPHOCYTES[a]

Cell Marker	Normal (Cadaveric) Spleen Mean ± s.d. (%)	Reactive (Non-malignant) Spleen Mean ± s.d. (%)	P Value
CD2	38 ± 10	50 ± 14	0.015
CD3	31 ± 9	43 ± 14	0.009
CD4	17 ± 8	23 ± 7	NS[b]
CD5	32 ± 8	42 ± 13	0.028
CD7	37 ± 11	44 ± 12	NS
CD8	14 ± 5	19 ± 7	0.028
CD4/CD8 ratio	1.2 ± 3	1.2 ± 0.2	NS
CD10	1 ± 1	1 ± 1	NS
CD11c	28 ± 10	25 ± 10	NS
CD13	1 ± 1	1 ± 1	NS
CD16/56+CD3-	15 ± 7	12 ± 5	NS
CD16/56+CD3+	5 ± 2	5 ± 4	NS
CD19	55 ± 11	45 ± 14	0.04
CD20	49 ± 9	42 ± 12	NS
CD20+CD5+	8 ± 6	11 ± 7	NS
CD23	34 ± 13	35 ± 12	NS
CD30	1 ± 1	1 ± 1	NS
CD34	2 ± 2	2 ± 1	NS
CD38	79 ± 13	83 ± 12	NS
CD103	2 ± 1	2 ± 1	NS
cy CD79[b]	52 ± 12	44 ± 10	NS
HLA-DR	71 ± 11	71 ± 12	NS
IgM	42 ± 14	40 ± 17	NS
IgG	5 ± 5	3 ± 2	NS
IgA	9 ± 7	6 ± 2	NS
IgD	36 ± 12	35 ± 12	NS
FMC7	38 ± 13	30 ± 10	NS
Kappa (κ)	28 ± 5	25 ± 8	NS
Lambda (λ)	21 ± 5	17 ± 6	NS
Kappa/Lambda (κ/λ)	1.3 ± 0.2	1.4 ± 0.2	NS
cy Kappa (cy κ)	31 ± 6	29 ± 8	NS
cy Lambda (cy λ)	22 ± 5	16 ± 6	NS
cy TdT	<1	<1	NS
TCR alpha/beta (TCR α/β)	29 ± 9	37 ± 12	NS
TCR gamma/delta (TCR γ/δ)	2 ± 2	5 ± 1	NS

[a]Table 2 from Colovai AI, Giatzikis C, Ho EK, et al. Flow cytometric analysis of normal and reactive spleen. Mod Pathol 2004;17:921.

[b]NS = not significant (P>0.05); cy = cytoplasmic; TdT = terminal deoxynucleotidyltransferase; Ig = immunoglobulin; TCR = T-cell receptor.

accounting for approximately 10 percent of the B lymphocytes; a CD4/CD8 ratio of 1.2 to 1.0 (lower than in the blood but similar to that seen in lymph nodes; and a mean number of gamma/delta-positive T cells (of all CD3-positive cells) of 6 percent in normal and 10 percent in reactive spleens. While in the peripheral blood, NK/T cells account for less than 6 percent of the CD3-positive circulating lymphocytes, Colovai et al. (11) showed a high frequency of these cells in the spleen. Similar results have been observed in the liver by others and support the concept that spleen and liver lymphocytes have specific, although yet unknown, immunoregulatory functions (46).

ULTRASTRUCTURAL EXAMINATION OF THE LYMPH NODE AND SPLEEN

Ultrastructural examination of the lymph node is a useful technique in research but it is rarely, if at all, applied to diagnostic problems. Electron microscopy (especially scanning electron microscopy) has been used mainly to study the functional microanatomy of the spleen (25, 34). These studies have shown the routes that blood cells take through the spleen and have clearly illustrated the pitting function (removal of inclusions in erythrocytes) exerted by the sinusoids (34). In spleens examined in a diagnostic-oriented setting, however, there is hardly, if ever, the necessity of using ultrastructural studies.

REFERENCES

1. Abbondanzo SL, Allred DC, Lampkin S, Banks PM. Enhancement of immunoreactivity among lymphoid malignancies in paraffin-embedded tissues by refixation in zinc sulfate-formalin. Arch Pathol Lab Med 1991;115:31-3.
2. Abbondanzo SL, Sato N, Straus SE, Jaffe ES. Acute infectious mononucleosis. CD30 (Ki-1) antigen expression and histologic correlations. Am J Clin Pathol 1990;93:698-702.
3. Arber DA, Weiss LM. CD5: a review. Applied Immunohistochemistry: official publication of the Society for Applied Immunohistochemistry 1995;3:1-22.
4. Benharroch D, Meguerian-Bedoyan Z, Lamant L, et al. ALK-positive lymphoma: a single disease with a broad spectrum of morphology. Blood 1998;91:2076-84.
5. Bryan CF, Eastman PJ, Conner JB, Baier KA, Durham JB. Clinical utility of a lymph node normal range obtained by flow cytometry. Ann N Y Acad Sci 1993;677:404-6.
6. Caselitz J, Janner M, Breitbart E, Weber K, Osborn M. Malignant melanomas contain only the vimentin type of intermediate fibers. Virchows Arch A 1983;400:43-51.
7. Cattoretti G, Parravicini C, Bonati A, et al. Terminal deoxynucleotidyl transferase-positive B cell precursors in fetal lymph nodes and extrahemopoietic tissues. Eur J Immunol 1989;19:493-500.
8. Chang KL, Arber DA, Weiss LM. CD20: a review. Applied Immunohistochemistry: official publication of the Society for Applied Immunohistochemistry 1996;4:1-15.
9. Chen CC, Raikow RB, Sonmez-Alpan E, Swerdlow SH. Classification of small B-cell lymphoid neoplasms using a paraffin section immunohistochemical panel. Appl Immunohistochem Mol Morphol 2000;8:1-11.
10. Chu PG, Chang KL, Arber DA, Weiss LM. Practical applications of immunohistochemistry in hematolymphoid neoplasms. Ann Diagn Pathol 1999;3:104-33.
11. Colovai AI, Giatzikis C, Ho EK, et al. Flow cytometric analysis of normal and reactive spleen. Mod Pathol 2004;17:918-27.
12. Contos MJ, Kornstein MJ, Innes DJ, Ben-Ezra J. The utility of CD20 and CD43 in subclassification of low-grade B-cell lymphoma on paraffin sections. Mod Pathol 1992;5:631-3.
13. Delsol G, Al Saati T, Gatter KC, et al. Coexpression of epithelial membrane antigen (EMA), Ki-1, and interleukin-2 receptor by anaplastic large-cell lymphomas. Diagnostic value in so-called malignant histiocytosis. Am J Pathol 1988;130:59-70.
14. Delsol G, Lamant L, Mariame B, et al. A new subtype of large B-cell lymphoma expressing the ALK kinase and lacking the 2; 5 translocation. Blood 1997;89:1483-90.
15. Deneys V, Mazzon AM, Marques JL, Benoit H, De Bruyere M. Reference values for peripheral blood B-lymphocyte subpopulations: a basis for multiparametric immunophenotyping of abnormal lymphocytes. J Immunol Methods 2001;253:23-36.
16. Dogan A, Bagdi E, Munson P, Isaacson PG. CD10 and BCL-6 expression in paraffin sections of normal lymphoid tissue and B-cell lymphomas. Am J Surg Pathol 2000;24:846-52.

17. Dorfman DM, Shahsafaei A. Usefulness of a new CD5 antibody for the diagnosis of T-cell and B-cell lymphoproliferative disorders in paraffin sections. Mod Pathol 1997;10:859-63.
18. Emile JF, Wechsler J, Brousse N, et al. Langerhans' cell histiocytosis: definitive diagnosis with the use of monoclonal antibody O10 on routinely processed paraffin-embedded samples. Am J Surg Pathol 1995;19:636-41.
19. Frierson HF Jr, Bellafiore FJ, Gaffey MJ, McCary WS, Innes DJ Jr, Williams ME. Cytokeratin in anaplastic large cell lymphoma. Mod Pathol 1994;7:317-21.
20. Fukushima PI, Nguyen PK, O'Grady P, Stetler-Stevenson M. Flow cytometric analysis of kappa and lambda light chain expression in evaluation of specimens for B-cell neoplasia. Cytometry 1996;26:243-52.
21. Ginaldi L, De Martinis M, D'Ostilio A, et al. Changes in the expression of surface receptors on lymphocyte subsets in the elderly: quantitative flow cytometric analysis. Am J Hematol 2001;67:63-72.
22. Gown AM, de Wever N, Battifora H. Microwave-based antigenic unmasking: a revolutionary new technique for routine immunohistochemistry. Applied Immunohistochemistry: official publication of the Society for Applied Immunohistochemistry 1993;1:256-66.
23. Gown AM, Vogel AM, Hoak D, Gough F, McNutt MA. Monoclonal antibodies specific for melanocytic tumors distinguish subpopulations of melanocytes. Am J Pathol 1986;123:195-203.
24. Hall PA, d'Ardenne AJ, Stansfeld AG. Paraffin section immunohistochemistry I. Non-Hodgkin's lymphoma. Histopathology 1988;13:149-60.
25. Heusermann U, Stutte HJ. Comparative histochemical and electron microscopic studies of the sinus and venous walls of the human spleen with special reference to the sinus–venous connections. Cell Tissue Res 1975;163:519-33.
26. Hsu SM, Raine L, Fanger H. The use of avidin-biotin-peroxidase complex (ABC) in immunoperoxidase techniques: a comparison between ABC and unlabeled antibody (PAP) procedures. J Histochem Cytochem 1981;29:577-80.
27. Kamel OW, Gelb AB, Shibuya RB, Warnke RA. Leu 7 (CD57) reactivity distinguishes nodular lymphocyte predominance Hodgkin's disease from nodular sclerosing Hodgkin's disease, T-cell-rich B-cell lymphoma and follicular lymphoma. Am J Pathol 1993;142:541-6.
28. King BE, Chen C, Locker J, et al. Immunophenotypic and genotypic markers of follicular center cell neoplasia in diffuse large B-cell lymphomas. Mod Pathol 2000;13:1219-31.
29. Kishimoto T, Goyert S, Kikutani H, et al. CD antigens 1996. Blood 1997;89:3502.
30. Kishimoto T, Kikutani H, von dem Borne AE, et al. eds. In: Leukocyte typing VI: white cell differentiation antigens. New York, NY: Garland Publishing; 1997.
31. Knapp W, Dorken B, Rieber P, Schmidt RE, Stein H, von dem Borne AE. CD antigens 1989. Blood 1989;74:1448-50.
32. Knowles DM, Chadburn A, Inghirami G. Immunophenotypic markers useful in the diagnosis and classification of hematopoietic neoplasms. In Knowles DM, ed. Neoplastic hematopathology. Baltimore: Williams & Wilkins; 1992:73-167.
33. Kotylo P, Fineberg NS, Freeman KS, Redmond NL, Charland C. Reference ranges for lymphocyte subsets in pediatric patients. Am J Clin Pathol 1993;100:111-5.
34. Koyama S, Aoki S, Deguchi D. Electron microscopic observations of the splenic red pulp with special reference to the pitting function. Mie Med J 1964;14:143-88.
35. Kraus MD. Splenic histology and histopathology: an update. Semin Diagn Pathol 2003;20:84-93.
36. Lai R, Arber DA, Chang KL, Wilson CS, Weiss LM. Frequency of bcl-2 expression in non-Hodgkin's lymphoma: a study of 778 cases with comparison of marginal zone lymphoma and monocytoid B-cell hyperplasia. Mod Pathol 1998;11:864-9.
37. Lai R, Weiss LM, Chang KL, Arber DA. Frequency of CD43 expression in non-Hodgkin's lymphoma. A survey of 742 cases and further characterization of rare CD43+ follicular lymphomas. Am J Clin Pathol 1999;111:488-94.
38. Lamant L, Meggetto F, al Saati T, et al. High incidence of the t (2; 5) (p23; q35) translocation in anaplastic large cell lymphoma and its lack of detection in Hodgkin's disease. Comparison of cytogenetic analysis, reverse transcriptase-polymerase chain reaction, and P-80 immunostaining. Blood 1996;87:284-91.
39. Loddenkemper C, Anagnostopoulos I, Hummel M, et al. Differential Emu enhancer activity and expression of BOB.1/OBF.1, Oct2, PU.1, and immunoglobulin in reactive B-cell populations, B-cell non-Hodgkin lymphomas, and Hodgkin lymphomas. J Pathol 2004;202:60-9.
40. Macon WR, Casey TT, Kinney MC, Collins RD, Cousar JB. Leu-22 (L60): a more sensitive marker than UCHL1 for peripheral T-cell lymphomas, particularly large-cell types. Am J Clin Pathol 1991;95:696-701.
41. Mason DY, Biberfeld P. Technical aspects of lymphoma immunohistology. J Histochem Cytochem 1980;28:731-45.
42. McCoy JP Jr, Overton WR. Quality control in flow cytometry for diagnostic pathology: II. A conspectus of reference ranges for lymphocyte immunophenotyping. Cytometry 1994;18:129-39.
43. Neiman RS, Orazi A. Histopathologic manifestation of lymphoproliferative and myeloproliferative disorders involving the spleen. In: Knowles DM, ed. Neoplastic hematopathology, 2nd ed. Baltimore: Lippincott Williams & Wilkins; 2000:1881-1914.

44. Ngan BY, Chen-Levy Z, Weiss LM, Warnke RA, Cleary ML. Expression in non-Hodgkin lymphoma of the bcl-2 protein associated with the t (14;18) chromosomal translocation. N Engl J Med 1988;318:1638-44.
45. Ngan BY, Picker LJ, Medeiros LJ, Warnke RA. Immunophenotypic diagnosis of non-Hodgkin's lymphoma in paraffin sections. Co-expression of L60 (Leu-22) and L26 antigens correlates with malignant histologic findings. Am J Clin Pathol 1989;91:579-83.
46. Norris S, Doherty DG, Collins C, et al. Natural T cells in the human liver: cytotoxic lymphocytes with dual T cell and natural killer cell phenotype and function are phenotypically heterogeneous and include Valpha24-JalphaQ and gamma delta T cell receptor bearing cells. Hum Immunol 1999;60:20-31.
47. O'Connell, FP, Pinkus JL, Pinkus GS. CD138 (syndecan-1), a plasma cell marker immunohistochemical profile in hematopoietic and nonhematopoietic neoplasms. Am J Clin Pathol 2004;121:254-63.
48. Ohshima K, Kawasaki C, Muta H, et al. CD10 and Bcl10 expression in diffuse large B-cell lymphoma: CD10 is a marker of improved prognosis. Histopathology 2001;39:156-62.
49. O'Malley DP, Orazi A. Terminal deoxynucleotidyl transferase-positive precursor cells in spleen, appendix, and branchial cleft cysts in pediatric patients. Haematologica 2006;91:1139-40.
50. Orazi A, Cattoretti G, John K, Neiman RS. Terminal deoxynucleotidyl transferase staining of malignant lymphomas in paraffin sections. Mod Pathol 1994;7:582-6.
51. Perkins SL, Kjeldsberg CR. Immunophenotyping of lymphomas and leukemias in paraffin-embedded tissues. Am J Clin Pathol 1993;99:362-73.
52. Picker LJ, Weiss LM, Medeiros LJ, Wood GS, Warnke RA. Immunophenotypic criteria for the diagnosis of non-Hodgkin's lymphoma. Am J Pathol 1987;128:181-201.
53. Pinkus GS, Pinkus JL. Myeloperoxidase: a specific marker for myeloid cells in paraffin sections. Mod Pathol 1991;4:733-41.
54. Pulford K, Lamant L, Morris SW, et al. Detection of anaplastic lymphoma kinase (ALK) and nucleolar protein nucleophosmin (NPM)-ALK proteins in normal and neoplastic cells with the monoclonal antibody ALK1. Blood 1997;89:1394-404.
55. Saez AI, Artiga MJ, Sanchez-Beato M, et al. Analysis of octamer-binding transcription factors Oct2 and Oct1 and their coactivator BOB.1/OBF.1 in lymphomas. Mod Pathol 2002;15:211-20.
56. Shi SR, Cote RJ, Taylor CR. Antigen retrieval immunohistochemistry: past, present, and future. J Histochem Cytochem 1997;45:327-43.
57. Shi SR, Key ME, Kalra KL. Antigen retrieval in formalin-fixed, paraffin-embedded tissues: an enhancement method for immunohistochemical staining based on microwave heating of tissue sections. J Histochem Cytochem 1991;39:741-8.
58. Strauchen JA. Immunologic and molecular techniques. In: Strauchen JA, ed. Diagnostic histopathology of the lymph node. New York: Oxford University Press; 1998:10-28.
59. Sundeen JT, Longo DL, Jaffe ES. CD5 expression in B-cell small lymphocytic malignancies. Correlations with clinical presentation and sites of disease. Am J Surg Pathol 1992;16:130-7.
60. Torlakovic E, Torlakovic G, Nguyen PL, Brunning RD, Delabie J. The value of anti-pax-5 immunostaining in routinely fixed and paraffin-embedded sections: a novel pan pre-B and B-cell marker. Am J Surg Pathol 2002;26:1343-50.
61. van Krieken JM, te Velde J. "Spleen." In: Sternberg SS, Alsabeh R, Medeiros LJ, Weiss LM, eds. Histology for pathologists, 2nd ed. Philadelphia: Lippincott-Raven; 1997:675-686.
62. Vasef MA, Alsabeh R, Medeiros LJ, Weiss LM. Immunophenotype of Reed-Sternberg and Hodgkin's cells in sequential biopsy specimens of Hodgkin's disease: a paraffin-section immunohistochemical study using the heat-induced epitope retrieval method. Am J Clin Pathol 1997;108:54-9.
63. Vasef MA, Medeiros LJ, Koo C, McCourty A, Brynes RK. Cyclin D1 immunohistochemical staining is useful in distinguishing mantle cell lymphoma from other low-grade B-cell neoplasms in bone marrow. Am J Clin Pathol 1997;108:302-7.
64. Warnke RA, Rouse RV. Limitations encountered in the application of tissue section immunodiagnosis to the study of lymphomas and related disorders. Hum Pathol 1985;16:326-31.
65. Weiss LM, Crabtree GS, Rouse RV, Warnke RA. Morphologic and immunologic characterization of 50 peripheral T-cell lymphomas. Am J Pathol 1985;118:316-24.
66. Werner M, Chott A, Fabiano A, Battifora H. Effect of formalin tissue fixation and processing on immunohistochemistry. Am J Surg Pathol 2000;24:1016-9.
67. Werner M, Von Wasielewski R, Komminoth P. Antigen retrieval, signal amplification and intensification in immunohistochemistry. Histochem Cell Biol 1996;105:253-60.
68. Wilkins BS, Wright DH. Illustrated pathology of the spleen. Cambridge: Cambridge University Press; 2000.
69. Zukerberg LR, Yang WI, Arnold A, Harris NL. Cyclin D1 expression in non-Hodgkin's lymphomas. Detection by immunohistochemistry. Am J Clin Pathol 1995;103:756-60.

5 GENERAL REACTIVE CONDITIONS IN LYMPH NODE AND SPLEEN

In addition to making the correct pathologic diagnosis, it is important to understand the personal perspective of a patient who has clinical lymphadenopathy necessitating a lymph node biopsy. In this situation, there is usually serious concern that the cause of the lymph node enlargement is a primary or metastatic malignancy. When the pathologic examination reveals a benign reactive process, it is important that the patient and clinician understand the most likely etiology for the nodal enlargement so that the appropriate treatment is given. Furthermore, some types of reactive lymphadenopathy, such as those related to infection, are curable.

Histologic examination of benign lymph nodes often shows architectural as well as cytologic changes that are important to recognize. Familiarity with the normal components of a reactive lymph node is important in order to distinguish reactive from malignant processes (77,85,89). There are nonspecific and specific causes of benign reactive lymphoid hyperplasia, such as autoimmune, infectious, and immunodeficient conditions. Some pathologic entities are associated with consistent, characteristic changes while others show nonspecific or inconsistent patterns of reactivity.

The aim of this chapter is to review many of the nonspecific morphologic findings that are encountered in reactive lymph nodes and spleens. While these findings may be characteristic or strongly associated with specific pathologic states, they may also be seen as isolated, idiopathic findings. Some miscellaneous conditions or morphologic findings that fit best in a general overview are also included.

FOLLICULAR HYPERPLASIA

Definition. *Follicular hyperplasia* is defined as an increase, per unit area, of secondary (reactive) follicles, or germinal centers. In addition to hyperplasia, the follicles are often hypertrophic as well, with an increase in size and the presence of irregular shapes. A variety of etiologies are associated with follicular hyperplasia, but most often, the specific causative agent is unknown.

General Features. The underlying biology of follicular hyperplasia is outlined in detail in chapter 1. Briefly, follicular hyperplasia is a result of the activation of the immune system by an antigen (most often nonself antigens, although self antigens are also occasionally responsible). The ultimate effect of the process of antigen processing, somatic mutation, affinity maturation, and clonal selection is the production of plasma cells, which may produce antibody (e.g., humoral immunity) to a specific antigen. This process is the raison d'etre of the germinal center: to produce a specific antibody to an antigen.

This physiologic process is played out in exquisite histologic detail in reactive lymph nodes. The individual processes cannot all be seen, but some are apparent from microscopic examination. The presence of numerous apoptotic bodies and tingible body macrophages is evidence of clonal selection, the presence of mitotic figures highlights the proliferative nature of the process, and the cytologic changes from small lymphocyte (naive or mantle cell) to proliferative blastic cell (centroblast) to the mature lymphocyte with completed antigen selection (centrocyte) are the histologic evidence of the active immune system.

Clinical Features. The exact incidence of follicular hyperplasia is difficult to calculate. It is a common enough occurrence that it typically goes unnoticed in lymph nodes removed for other purposes, such as cancer staging. As an isolated clinical finding, however, it is of more concern. An important consideration is the age of the patient. Adenopathy in children is relatively common and is associated with exposure to antigens. Anxious parents often find lumps and bumps in their children that lead to evaluation by a healthcare provider. Clinical clues for distinguishing between benign and malignant lymph nodes are frequently used in the

Table 5-1

CLINICAL SIGNS AND SYMPTOMS OF LYMPHADENOPATHY

Sign/Symptom	Benign	Malignant
Age	Younger	Older
Associated pain	Painful	Painless
Palpation	Freely moveable; tender	Fixed to adjacent structure; nontender
Onset	Rapid	Slowly progressive
History	Recent illness (e.g., viral infection) or inflammatory state	No history or generalized symptoms such as fever, weight loss, weakness
Location	Localized	Generalized

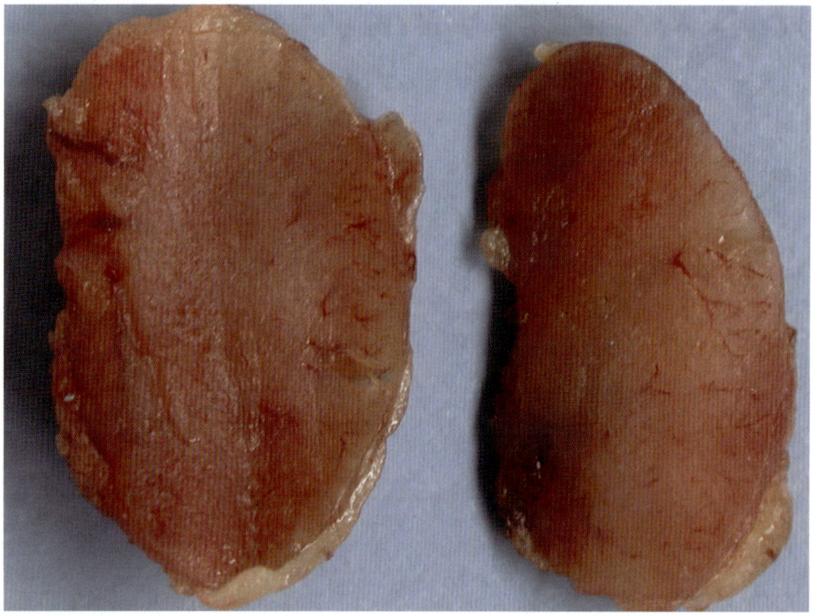

Figure 5-1

FOLLICULAR HYPERPLASIA, LYMPH NODE

The cut surface shows a subtle nodular architecture.

evaluation of patients. These are summarized in Table 5-1.

Lymph nodes of older patients, as compared to those of children and adolescents, often show less florid germinal center hyperplasia, which may be attributable to a subdued immune response in this age group. Enlarged lymph nodes with follicular hyperplasia in elderly patients have reportedly been associated with concomitant or subsequent development of non-Hodgkin lymphoma (42, 43,63). Other associated causes of follicular hyperplasia in elderly patients include autoimmune disorders, nonlymphoid cancer-related adenopathy, and Epstein-Barr virus (EBV) infections (42). Since follicular hyperplasia in older patients may be a harbinger of lymphoma, it is advisable to alert the clinician of the need for a thorough clinical evaluation and adequate follow-up.

Some cases of reactive follicular hyperplasia show so-called follicular lysis, which is a peculiar "dissolution" of the germinal center by clusters of small lymphocytes (11,69,92). This finding is especially important to recognize because it is characteristically associated with human immunodeficiency virus (HIV)-related lymphadenopathy. The following specific etiologies of lymphadenopathy are usually characterized by follicular hyperplasia: rheumatoid arthritis, HIV-related lymphadenopathy, syphilis, and angiofollicular lymph node hyperplasia (Castleman disease).

Gross Findings. Lymph nodes with follicular hyperplasia show a slightly mottled, shiny, granular cut surface (fig. 5-1). Close examination reveals tiny, raised nodules, which represent the follicles. Unfortunately, a similar gross appearance can be seen in follicular lymphoma.

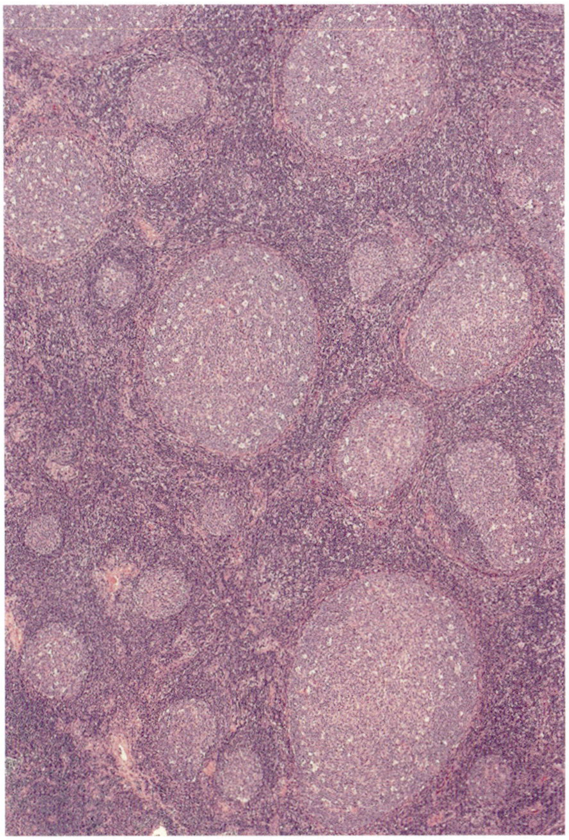

Figure 5-2

FOLLICULAR HYPERPLASIA, LYMPH NODE

Increased numbers of reactive follicles have a variety of sizes.

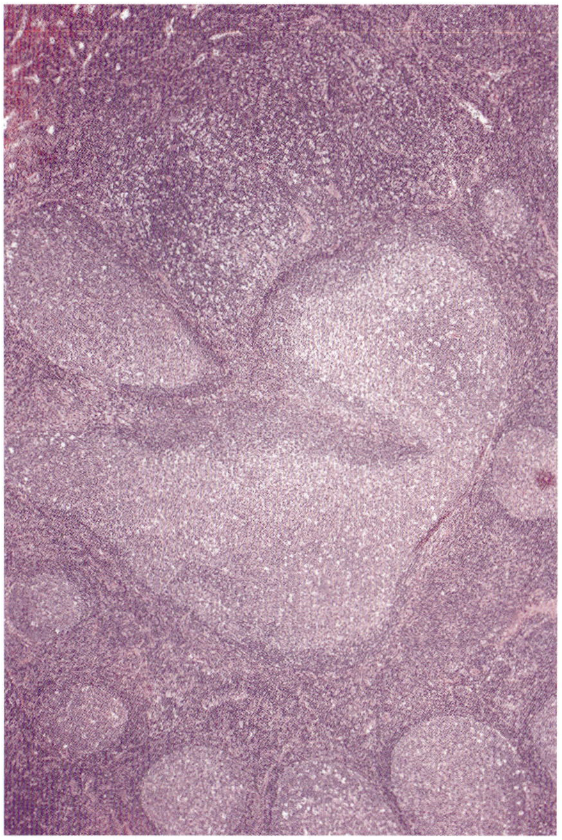

Figure 5-3

FOLLICULAR HYPERPLASIA, LYMPH NODE

The shape of the follicles varies, as is often seen in follicular hyperplasia.

Microscopic Findings. Variably sized and shaped follicles that are located primarily in the cortex (fig. 5-2) characterize reactive follicular hyperplasia. Some of these may assume a "dumb-bell" appearance. Close examination reveals a polymorphic rather than a monotypic population of follicle center cells. The presence of tingible body macrophages, the polarization of the follicle, and the retention of the mantle zones suggest a reactive rather than neoplastic follicular process (fig. 5-3; Table 5-2) (70).

In contrast, follicular lymphoma usually shows a back-to-back arrangement of similarly sized and shaped neoplastic follicles that are present throughout the lymph node. These neoplastic follicles are composed of a monotonous rather than polymorphous population of atypical lymphocytes. Tingible body macrophages are generally absent. The mantle zones,

Table 5-2

MORPHOLOGIC CRITERIA OF FOLLICULAR LYMPHOMA VERSUS FOLLICULAR HYPERPLASIA

Criteria	Follicular Lymphoma	Follicular Hyperplasia
Increase in follicle density	Yes	Yes
Back-to-back follicles	Yes	No
Lack of tingible body macrophages	Yes	No
Mantle zone	Poorly formed or absent	Present
Follicle polarization	Not present	Often present
Expansion beyond LN[a] capsule	Common	Rare
Dysplastic/abnormal cytology	Yes	No

[a]LN = lymph node.

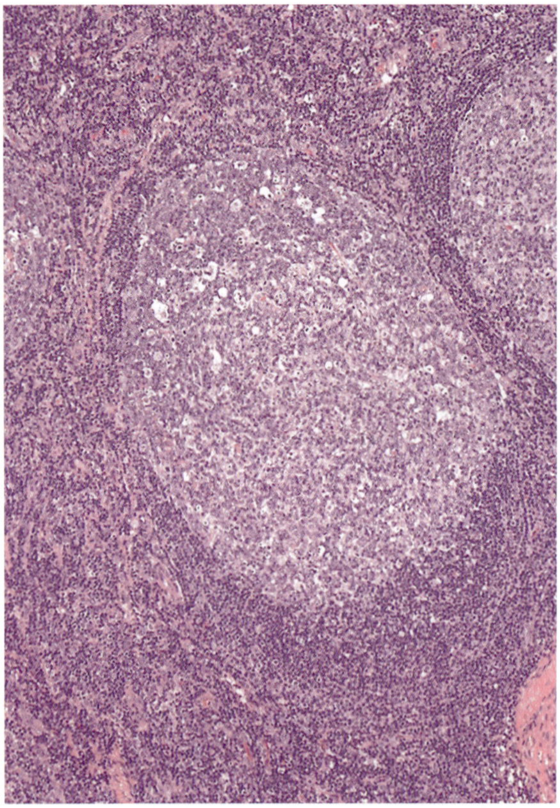

Figure 5-4

FOLLICULAR HYPERPLASIA, LYMPH NODE

Follicular polarization is a feature of hyperplastic follicles.

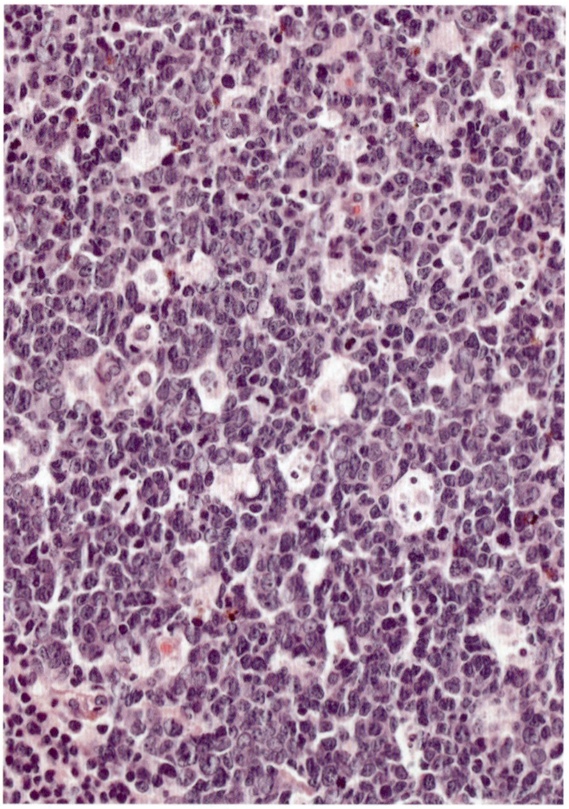

Figure 5-5

FOLLICULAR HYPERPLASIA, LYMPH NODE

Tingible body macrophages, a feature of benign hyperplastic follicles, are present.

which surround the germinal centers, are usually attenuated or absent whereas they are well preserved in most reactive follicles (fig. 5-4). Germinal center polarization is another important finding in reactive follicles that is typically not seen in lymphoma (fig. 5-5).

An important architectural characteristic of lymphoid hyperplasia in general is the overall preservation of the normal nodal architecture. Follicular hyperplasia, in contrast to follicular lymphoma, does not show extension of the reactive germinal centers beyond the capsule of the lymph node. In the presence of the above features, it is usually not difficult to distinguish between typical reactive follicular hyperplasia and a malignant lymphoma. In some cases, however, the histologic features overlap, resulting in a diagnosis of atypical follicular hyperplasia.

Benign germinal centers do not normally express bcl-2 protein because the transforming, proliferating B cells are programmed for apoptosis or cell death (fig. 5-6; Table 5-3). Interspersed, reactive T cells, however, do express this protein. Bcl-2 stains that distinguish between follicular hyperplasia and follicular lymphoma should not be interpreted without review of a CD3 stain to evaluate the number of T cells in the follicles. In a well-performed bcl-2 stain, the T cells will have strong cytoplasmic staining, while the neoplastic B cells of follicular lymphoma will tend to have weaker staining. Another useful distinguishing stain is Ki-67/MIB-1 (6): the highly proliferative follicles of follicular hyperplasia have a distinctive pattern of proliferation, while grade 1 or 2 follicular lymphoma shows a lower proliferative rate (fig. 5-7); grade 3 follicular lymphoma may show a somewhat similar proliferation rate to follicular hyperplasia, but is typically distinctive enough to be distinguished with Ki-67 in combination with other immunohistochemical

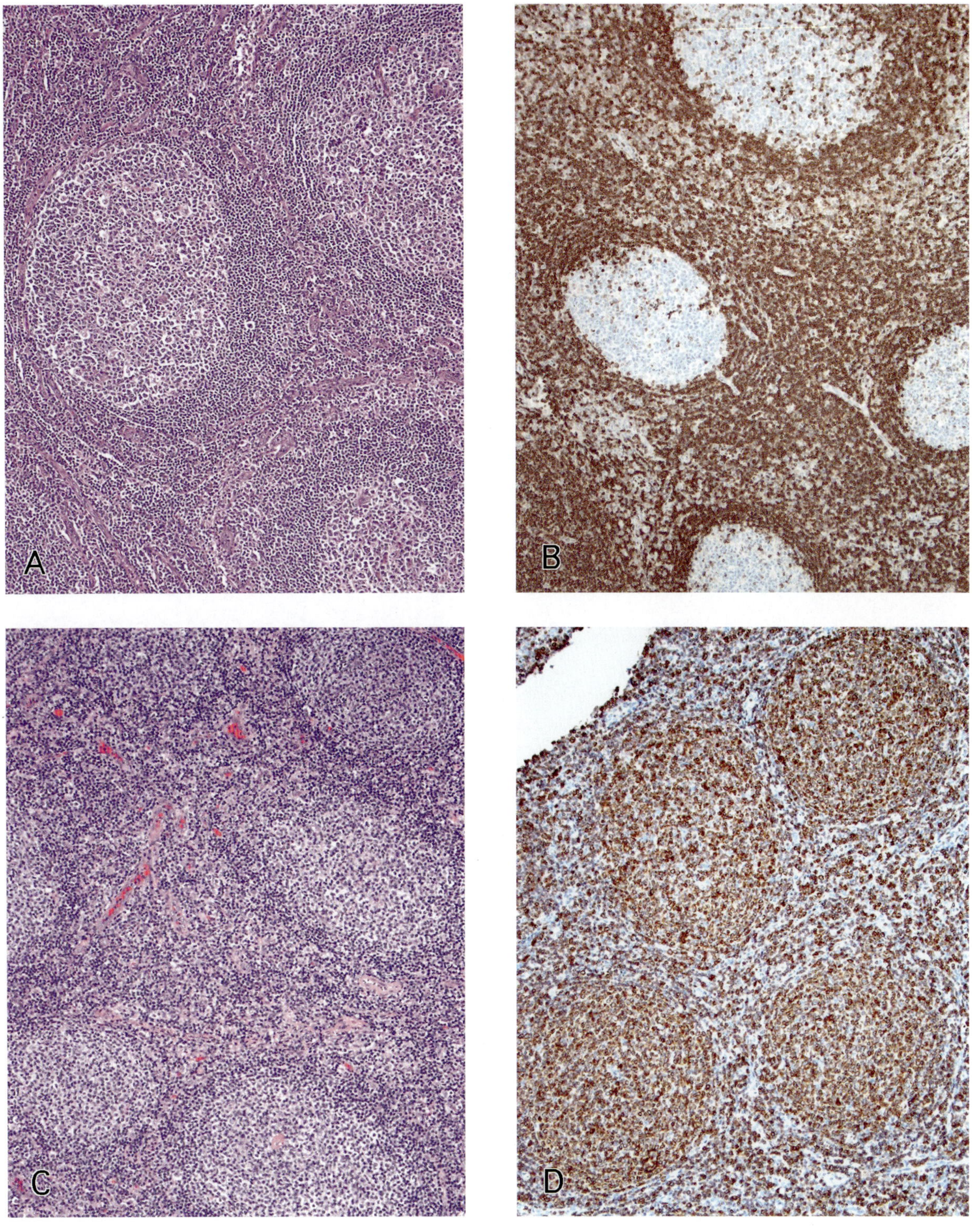

Figure 5-6

BCL-2 REACTIVITY IN FOLLICULAR HYPERPLASIA AND FOLLICULAR LYMPHOMA

A,B: Follicular hyperplasia with lack of bcl-2 staining in the follicles.
C,D: Low-grade follicular lymphoma with bcl-2 expression in the neoplastic follicles.

Table 5-3

IMMUNOHISTOCHEMICAL FEATURES OF FOLLICULAR HYPERPLASIA VERSUS FOLLICULAR LYMPHOMA

Immuno-histochemical	Follicular Hyperplasia	Follicular Lymphoma
Bcl-2	Negative	Positive (~75%)
Bcl-6	Positive	Positive
CD10	Positive	Positive
Ki-67	High proliferation	Low proliferation
CD21/CD23 (in follicular dendritic cell networks)	Positive	Positive

and histologic stains. Expression of bcl-6 and CD10 can be seen in both follicular lymphoma and benign follicles. However, these stains may have some indirect value; if there are significant numbers of CD10/bcl-6-positive cells outside the follicles, this is suspicious for follicular lymphoma, as this phenotype is restricted to follicles in normal lymphocytes.

In some cases, additional studies may become necessary when morphologic or immunohistochemical evaluation proves inadequate. Flow cytometric analysis may be of great benefit in proving light chain restriction, especially in small samples. The presence of a polyclonal

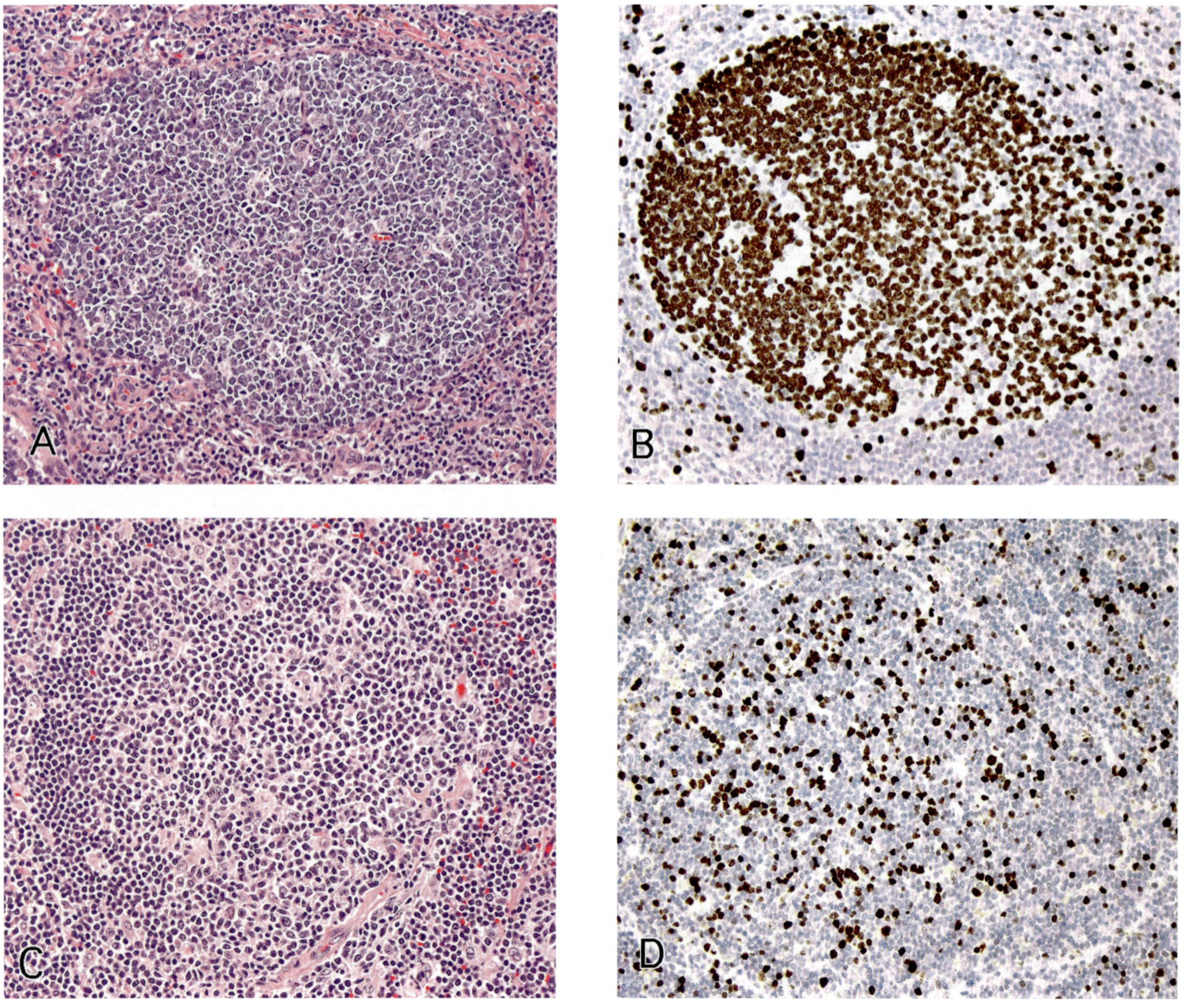

Figure 5-7

KI-67 REACTIVITY IN FOLLICULAR HYPERPLASIA AND FOLLICULAR LYMPHOMA

A,B: Follicular hyperplasia shows a high Ki-67 proliferation rate.
C,D: Low-grade follicular lymphoma shows an abnormal, low Ki-67 proliferation rate.

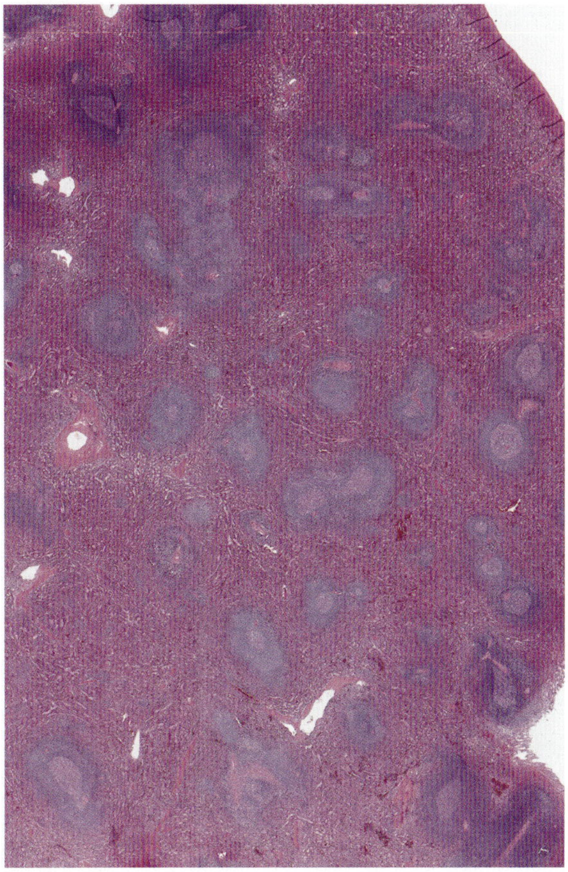

Figure 5-8

FOLLICULAR HYPERPLASIA IN SPLEEN

Follicular hyperplasia may mimic involvement of the spleen by follicular lymphoma or other B-cell lymphomas.

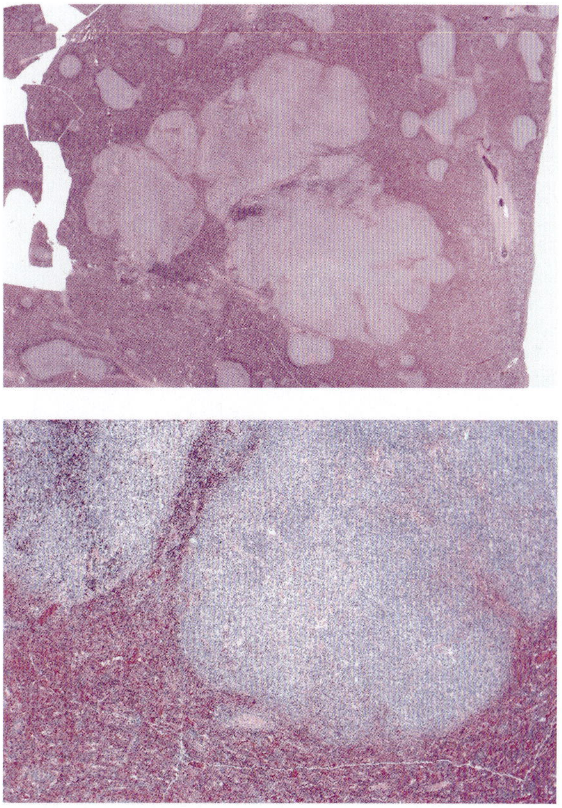

Figure 5-9

LOCALIZED REACTIVE LYMPHOID HYPERPLASIA, SPLEEN

Localized (nodular) lymphoid hyperplasia of the spleen occasionally mimics a neoplasm when it presents as a distinct mass (top). Upon examination, however, the white pulp mass is composed of a dense focus of hyperplastic, benign follicular elements (bottom).

population of B lymphocytes cannot entirely rule out the presence of a B-cell neoplasm, but can certainly support the morphologic findings. Evaluation of tissues for the presence of the characteristic chromosomal translocation, t(14;18), by fluorescence in situ hybridization (FISH), Southern blot, or polymerase chain reaction (PCR) studies is supportive evidence of a follicular lymphoma rather than reactive follicular hyperplasia. The lack of t(14;18), however, does not exclude the possibility of follicular lymphoma, as a percentage of cases do not have this translocation.

In the spleen, reactive follicular hyperplasia with the formation of germinal centers, seen in evolving immune responses, is usually easily recognized as benign (59,61). Follicular hyperplasia with prominent germinal centers, however, occasionally needs to be distinguished from follicular lymphoma (fig. 5-8) (8). As in lymph node, there are several criteria which help distinguish between benign and malignant splenic follicular processes.

A rare entity seen in spleen that may grossly simulate lymphoma is *localized (nodular) reactive lymphoid hyperplasia*. The area of nodular hyperplasia appears distinct from adjacent normal spleen and may raise the suspicion of lymphoma. Microscopic examination typically resolves the issue; the nodules are formed by focal aggregation of hyperplastic follicles, which have typical benign features (fig. 5-9) (8). If necessary, immunohistochemistry or molecular studies can be undertaken.

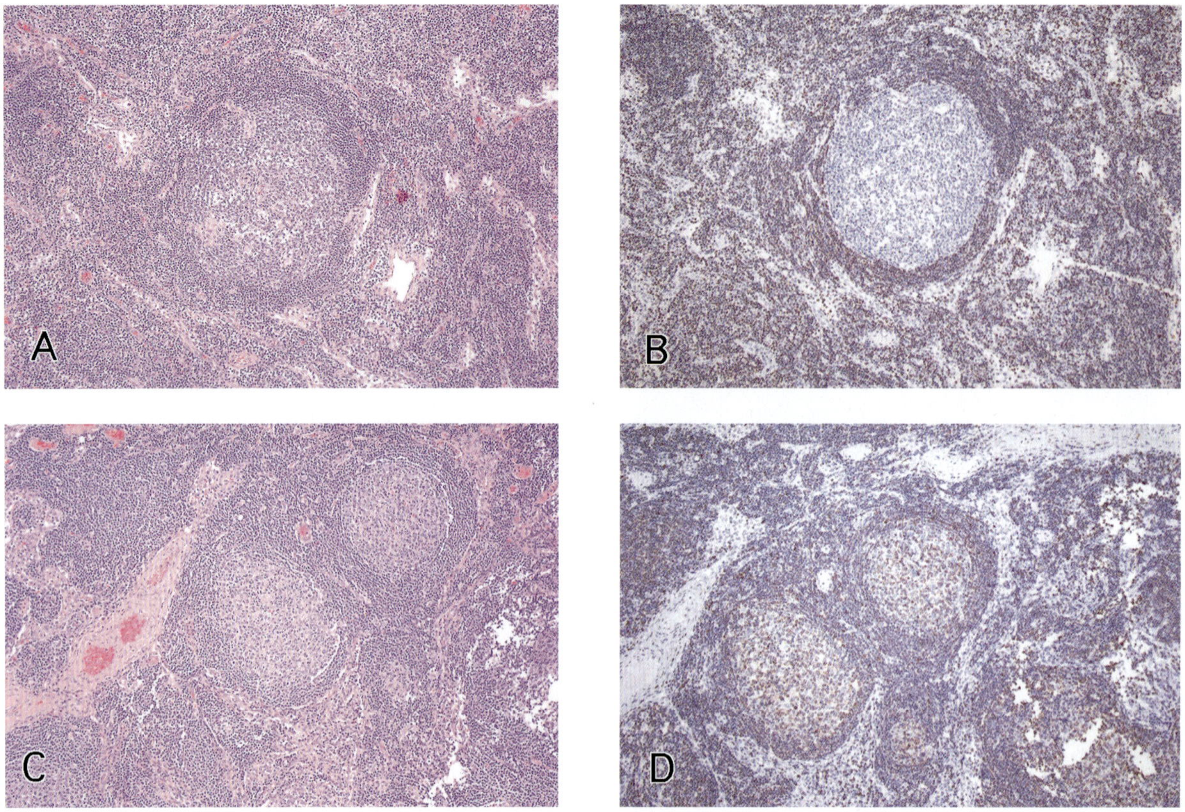

Figure 5-10

IN SITU FOLLICULAR LYMPHOMA

In a lymph node resected for carcinoma, the follicles in A, B, C, and D were adjacent to one another.
A,B: Follicular hyperplasia with no expression of bcl-2 in benign follicles.
C,D: Low-grade follicular lymphoma with expression of bcl-2 in neoplastic follicles.

Differential Diagnosis. As discussed above, the primary entity in the differential diagnosis is follicular lymphoma. Other lymphomas may also mimic follicular hyperplasia, especially those with a predominantly nodular pattern, such as marginal zone lymphoma, small lymphocytic lymphoma, and mantle cell lymphoma. In these circumstances, careful histologic examination and appropriate use of ancillary studies usually resolve the problem.

In situ follicular lymphoma refers to focal or minimal involvement of a lymph node by follicular lymphoma (15). Only a minority of follicles have evidence of follicular lymphoma, which is usually identified by aberrant bcl-2 staining in the abnormal follicles (fig. 5-10). The individual follicles have similar morphologic features to those of more extensive follicular lymphoma. The value of bcl-2 immunohistochemical staining in cases in which follicles appear atypical and vary from the classic appearance of hyperplasia is clear here.

As mentioned previously, evaluation of ancillary studies can be of great benefit in distinguishing benign processes (such as follicular hyperplasia) from neoplasms. As with all studies, however, it is important to be aware of caveats. Clonal populations of lymphocytes have been identified in cases of follicular hyperplasia by flow cytometry (49). Cytogenetic aberrations that can be seen in lymphoma, can also be seen in reactive lymph nodes, but are nonclonal (4). Both false negative and false positive results are seen with Southern blot and PCR assays of immunoglobulin gene rearrangements. Results can be affected by the amount and quality of the DNA obtained (35,81).

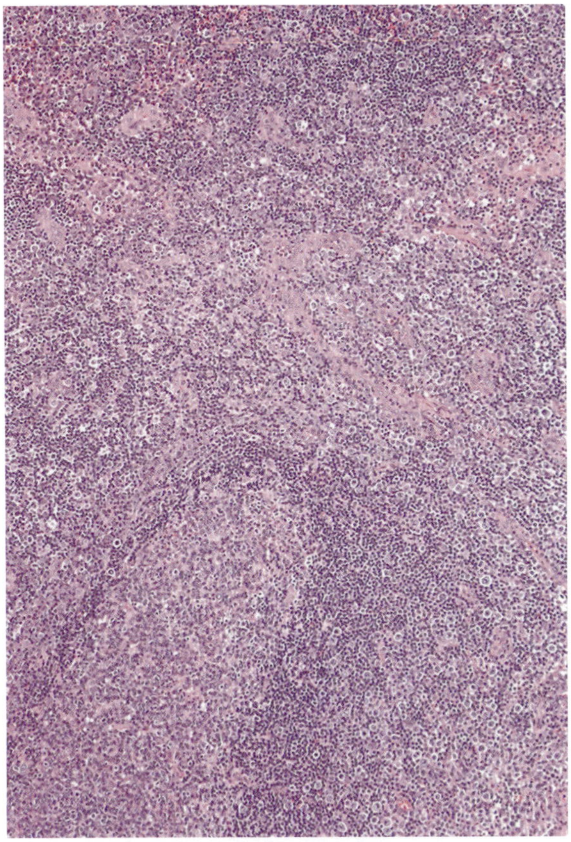

Figure 5-11

IMMUNOBLASTIC HYPERPLASIA

Proliferations of immunoblasts typically occur in the interfollicular region of the lymph node.

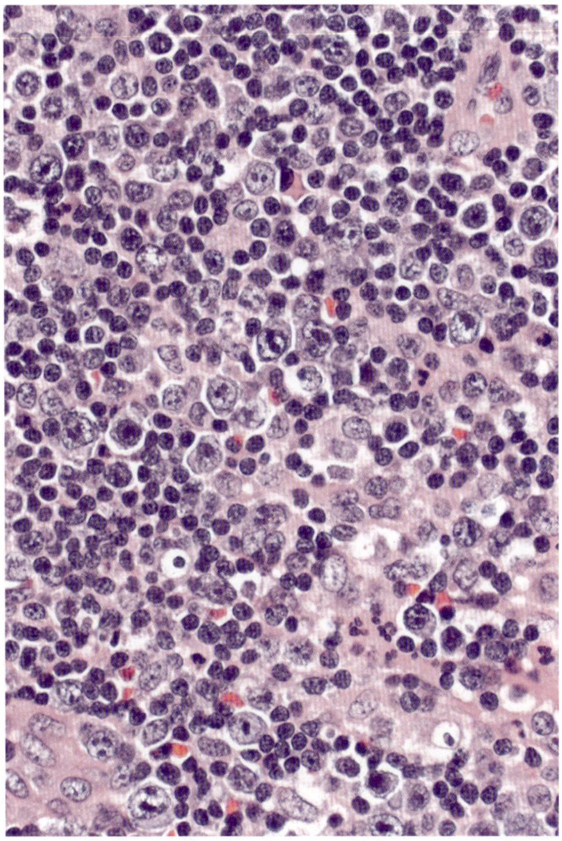

Figure 5-12

IMMUNOBLASTIC HYPERPLASIA

Immunoblasts are large, transformed lymphocytes, with open chromatin, a single prominent nucleolus, and a small amount of cytoplasm, which may stain deep blue.

INTERFOLLICULAR/IMMUNOBLASTIC HYPERPLASIA

Definition. *Interfollicular/immunoblastic hyperplasia* is characterized by the proliferation and expansion of the interfollicular areas in lymph nodes, or alternatively, the periarteriolar regions in spleens, with increased numbers of large transformed lymphocytes (immunoblasts).

General Features. Interfollicular/immunoblastic hyperplasia is usually not difficult to recognize. This pattern may be observed in viral (especially EBV) (12,22,27,70), postvaccinial (32), and drug (Dilantin)-related lymphadenopathies (1). These same clinicopathologic conditions, however, may result in atypical hyperplastic lymphoid changes that simulate malignant lymphoma (see later in this chapter).

Microscopic Findings. In its typical form, interfollicular/immunoblastic hyperplasia preserves the normal lymph node architecture (fig. 5-11). Cytologically, there is a diffuse population of mixed inflammatory cells, including small reactive lymphocytes, eosinophils, neutrophils, macrophages (histiocytes), and immunoblasts, in the interfollicular or paracortical areas (fig. 5-12). Scattered immunoblasts and interdigitating reticulum cells may impart a mottled appearance.

In many circumstances, the use of immunohistochemical stains complicates the interpretation of interfollicular/immunoblastic hyperplasia. Most of the immunoblasts are B cells and express CD20, although some are T cells. In some circumstances, B-cell activation causes the large transformed cells to downregulate the expression of CD20. Many of these cells express CD30, which is particularly troublesome

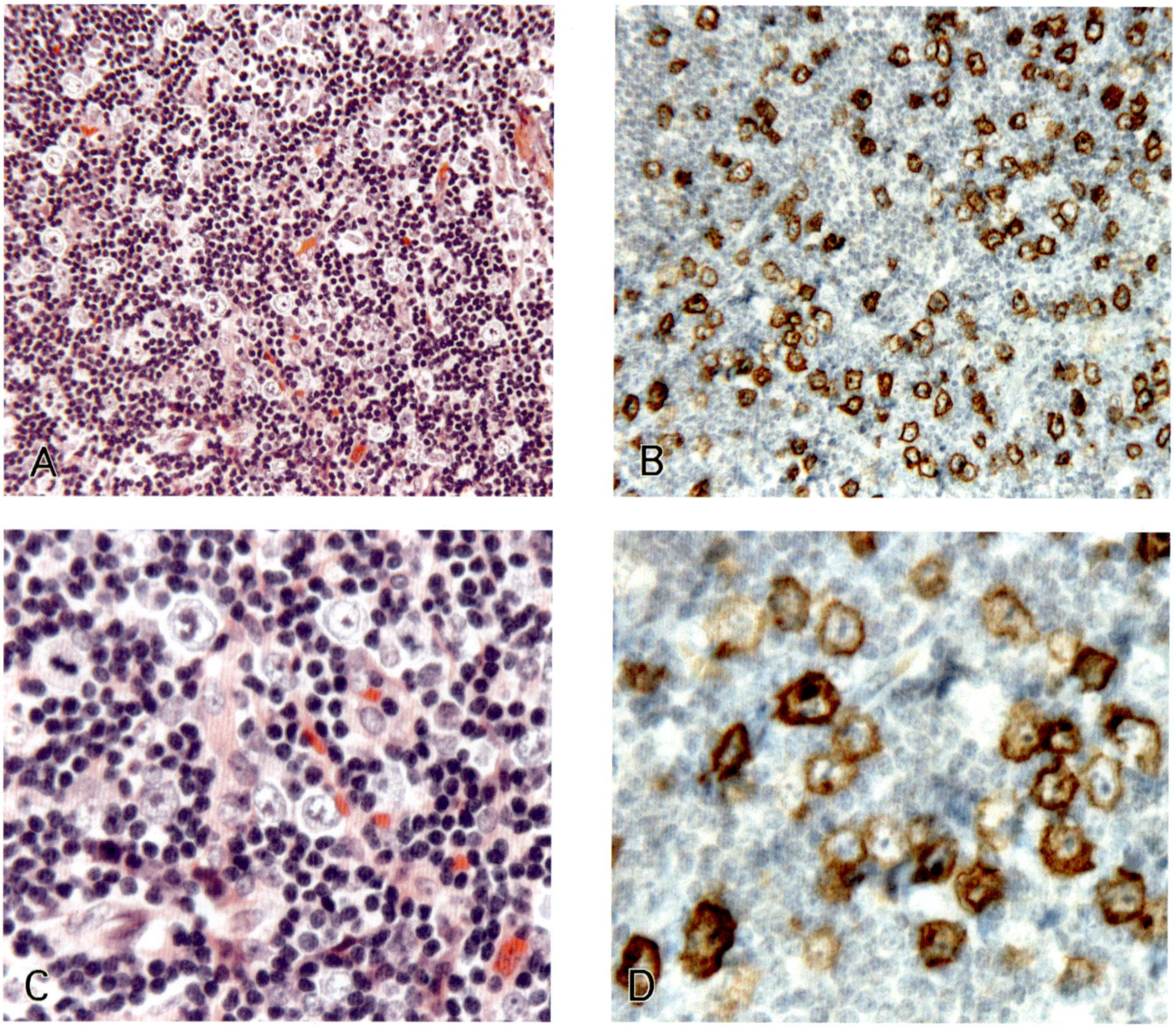

Figure 5-13

CD30 REACTIVITY IN IMMUNOBLASTIC HYPERPLASIA

The histologic appearance of immunoblasts (A,B) and the corresponding immunohistochemical reactivity for CD30 (C, D) are shown. CD30 expression by immunoblasts often suggests Hodgkin lymphoma.

if classic Hodgkin lymphoma is a differential consideration (fig. 5-13). Immunoblasts do not express CD15, however, and this stain is useful in distinguishing partial or interfollicular involvement by Hodgkin lymphoma.

Differential Diagnosis. Other specific causes of interfollicular/immunoblastic proliferations should be considered in the differential diagnosis. As mentioned above, viral, postvaccinial, and medication-related adenopathies should be considered, and correlation with clinical findings and patient history attempted.

One consideration in the differential diagnosis is the presence of early nodal involvement by Hodgkin lymphoma. Early/partial nodal involvement by Hodgkin lymphoma may be quite subtle and the features of Hodgkin/Reed-Sternberg cells may overlap those of transformed lymphocytes/immunoblasts. In these circumstances, the clinical information and immunohistochemical results are useful. In classic Hodgkin lymphoma, the Hodgkin/Reed-Sternberg cells have the typical immunophenotype (CD15+, CD30+, CD45-). In contrast, immunoblasts are

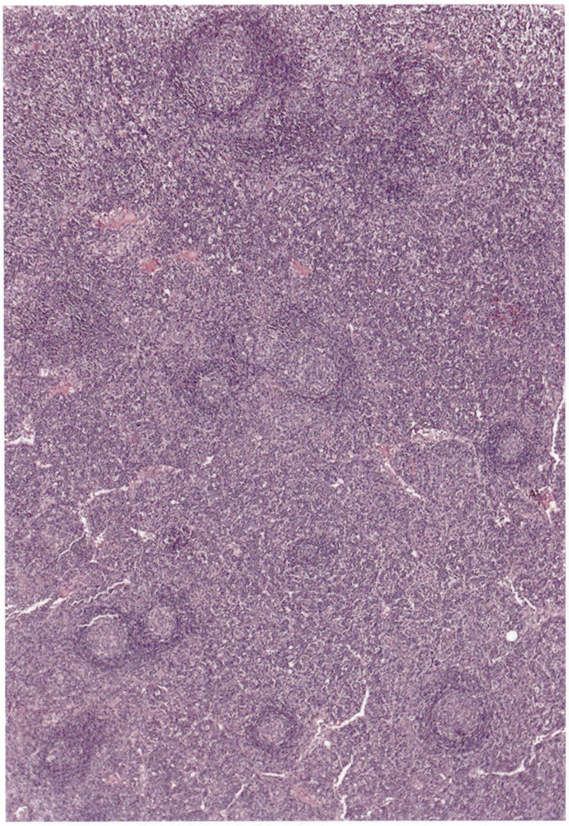

Figure 5-14

INTERFOLLICULAR LYMPH NODE INVOLVEMENT BY LYMPHOMA

In this lymphoplasmacytic lymphoma, there is extensive interfollicular replacement by the neoplastic lymphocytes, but sparing of the follicles.

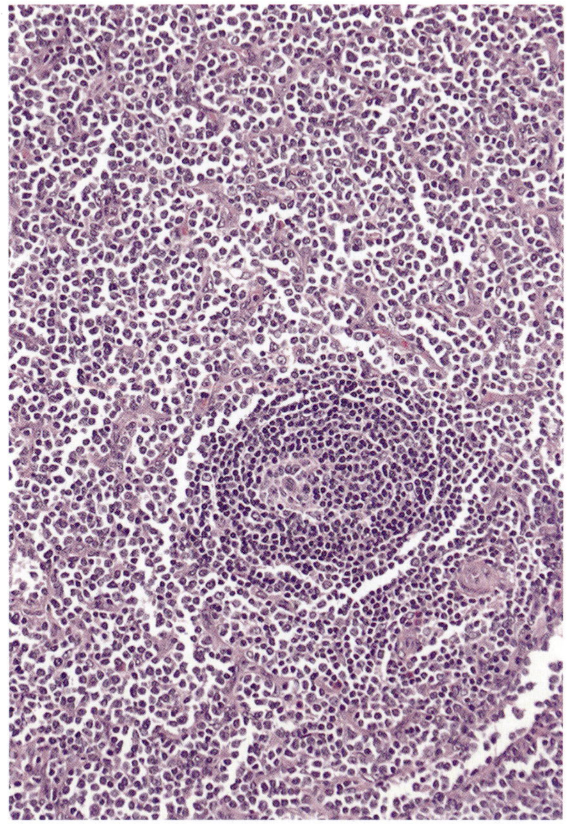

Figure 5-15

INTERFOLLICULAR LYMPH NODE INVOLVEMENT BY LEUKEMIA

Myeloid sarcoma (lymph node involvement by myeloid leukemia) is illustrated by the infiltration of medium-sized, atypical cells in the interfollicular area, adjacent to the relatively normal follicle.

only occasionally positive for CD30, lack CD15 expression, express CD45, and may express either CD20 or CD3 depending on whether they are derived from B or T cells, respectively.

Some lymphomas and other neoplasms preferentially involve the interfollicular zones of lymph nodes and may cause interfollicular expansion simulating hyperplasia. Nodal marginal zone lymphoma, lymphoplasmacytic lymphoma, interfollicular small lymphocytic lymphoma, anaplastic large cell lymphoma, peripheral T-cell lymphoma, and plasmacytoma have preferential distribution in the interfollicular zones (fig. 5-14). Langerhans cell histiocytosis, carcinomas, and leukemic processes preferentially involve the interfollicular zones (fig. 5-15). In most of these circumstances, careful application of morphology resolves the diagnosis. In select cases, ancillary studies are necessary.

MANTLE ZONE (PRIMARY FOLLICLE) HYPERPLASIA

Definition. The expansion of mantle zones, or a proliferation of unreacted primary follicles, is a rare form of hyperplasia. *Mantle zone (primary follicle) hyperplasia* is seen in a variety of conditions, and may precede more typical follicular hyperplasia.

General Features. Since the components of the mantle zones or primary follicles are predominantly naive B cells, the expansion of the mantle zones may represent an immunologic stimulus for expansion of the mantle zone. This may be the earliest part of the antigen

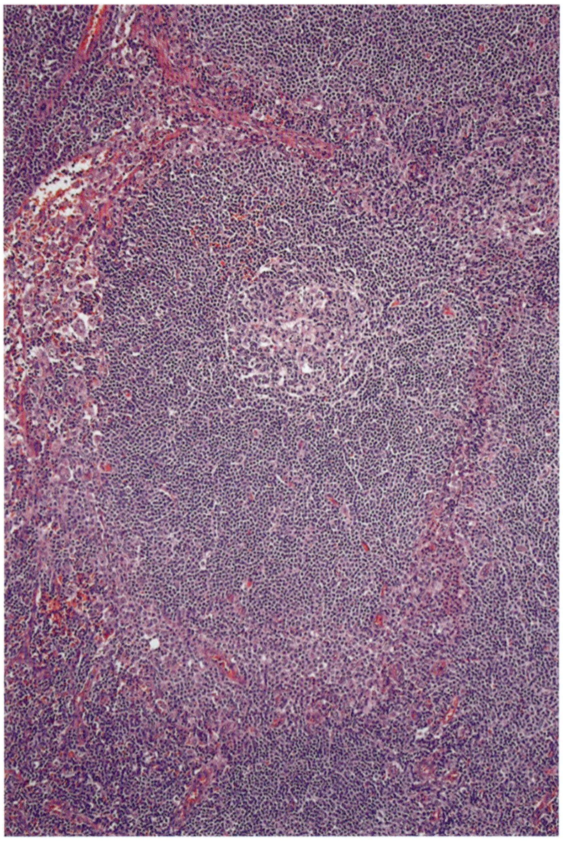

Figure 5-16

MANTLE ZONE HYPERPLASIA, LYMPH NODE

The mantle zone is expanded around follicles.

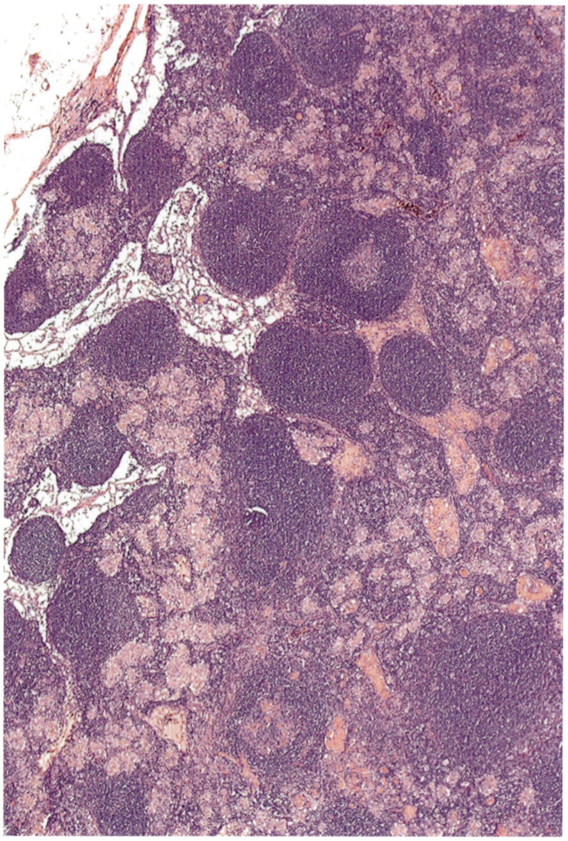

Figure 5-17

PRIMARY FOLLICLE HYPERPLASIA, LYMPH NODE

The number of unreacted follicles (primary follicles) is increased. The primary follicles are composed of mantle cells.

response, with mobilization of the naive B cells in preparation for the germinal center reaction (see chapter 1). Specific etiologies causing hyperplastic mantle zones or increased primary follicles in lymph nodes include progressive transformation of germinal centers (see later in this chapter) and hyaline-vascular Castleman disease (see chapter 6).

Reactive lymphoid hyperplasia without germinal center formation is a frequent finding in the spleen. The white pulp resembles the immunologically unstimulated spleen. The hyperplasia may simulate Hodgkin and non-Hodgkin lymphomas (59,61).

Microscopic Findings. Mantle cell hyperplasia is characterized by either the expansion of the normal mantle zone to an excessive thickness, or an increase in the number of primary follicles beyond that which is expected in a usual lymph node (figs. 5-16, 5-17). Mantle cells are small lymphocytes, with round to slightly irregular nuclear contours, dense mature chromatin, and scant cytoplasm (fig. 5-18). Occasionally, mantle cells have moderate amounts of cytoplasm, thus resembling cells of the marginal zone (36).

In the spleen, the white pulp may lack germinal centers and on low-power magnification, resembles the immunologically unstimulated spleen (59, 61,70). Higher magnification, however, reveals reactive changes including the presence of lymphocytes in varying stages of transformation (small and large lymphocytes and immunoblasts). Transformed lymphocytes/immunoblasts also proliferate around the splenic arterioles and may infiltrate the subendothelial zone of the trabecular veins and the connective tissue framework, resulting in splenic rupture in rare cases (88).

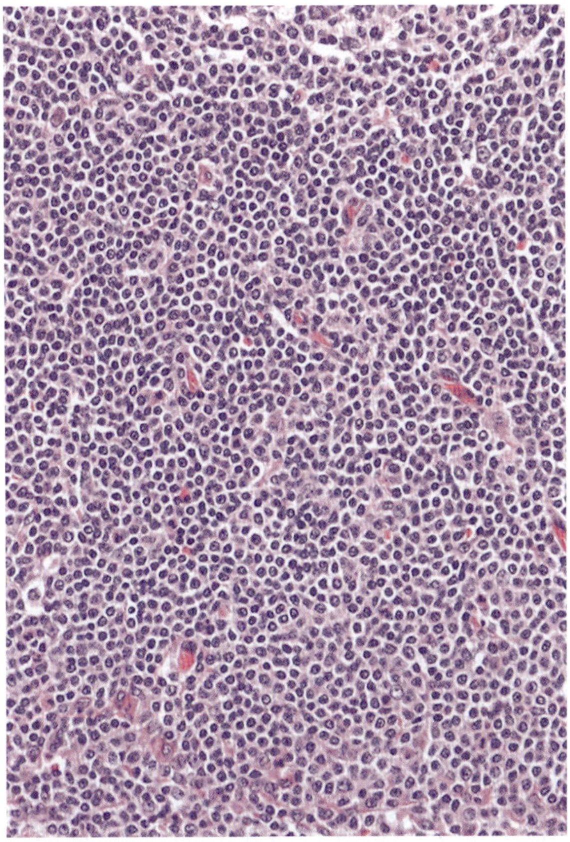

Figure 5-18

MANTLE ZONE

Small, mature lymphocytes, with a generally round nuclear contour and condensed chromatin, are characteristic of mantle zone cells.

This is characteristic of infectious mononucleosis, herpes simplex, and other viral infections. Steroid-treated immune thrombocytopenic purpura and autoimmune hemolytic anemia may show predominantly primary follicles due to the atrophy of follicular germinal centers (33).

Differential Diagnosis. Because of the nature of mantle cell proliferations, they may be confused with lymph node involvement by small B-cell lymphomas, especially mantle cell lymphoma (Table 5-4). Normal mantle cells do not express cyclin D1 and, in contrast to most cases of mantle cell lymphoma and small lymphocytic lymphoma, do not express CD43. Nodular proliferations of lymphocytes which coexpress CD20 and bcl-2 may cause diagnostic difficulty, as this staining pattern can be seen in both normal mantle cells and mantle cell lymphoma.

Table 5-4

IMMUNOREACTIVITY OF NORMAL MANTLE CELLS VERSUS SMALL B-CELL LYMPHOMA

	Normal Mantle Cells	MCL[a]	CLL/SLL	FL	MZL
CD20	+	+	+	+	+
Bcl-2	+	+	+	+	+
CD43	–	+	+	–	–/+
Cyclin D1	–	+	–	–	–
Bcl-6	–	–	–	+	–

[a]MCL = mantle cell lymphoma; CLL/SLL = chronic lymphocytic leukemia/small lymphocytic lymphoma; FL = follicular lymphoma; MZL = marginal zone lymphoma.

Such staining patterns may also cause confusion with a follicular lymphoma, and emphasize the point that there are many benign cells in lymph nodes (T cells, mantle cells, marginal zone cells) that may be bcl-2 positive and care should be taken in interpretation.

MARGINAL ZONE (MONOCYTOID B-CELL) HYPERPLASIA

Definition. *Marginal zone*, or *monocytoid B-cell, hyperplasia* is characterized by a proliferation of clusters or aggregates of small to intermediate-sized lymphocytes with increased pale cytoplasm in paracortical or interfollicular areas. This pattern may be seen in several specific benign etiologies, but is also an isolated finding without a specific identifiable etiology. It is a frequent finding in immunologically active spleens.

General Features. The exact pathogenesis and origin of marginal zone lymphocytes (such as seen in the spleen) and those seen in hyperplastic proliferations and in neoplasms of marginal zone cells have been debated. Marginal zone cells of the spleen have been shown to be different from the cells of monocytoid B-cell hyperplasia (78,82). Much of this debate is based on the derivation of different types of marginal zone lymphoma: nodal marginal zone lymphoma, splenic marginal zone lymphoma, and extranodal marginal zone lymphoma (5,83). Undoubtedly, these debates will continue, but for practical purposes, this section defines marginal zone hyperplasia as increased numbers of lymphocytes with pale or clear cytoplasm.

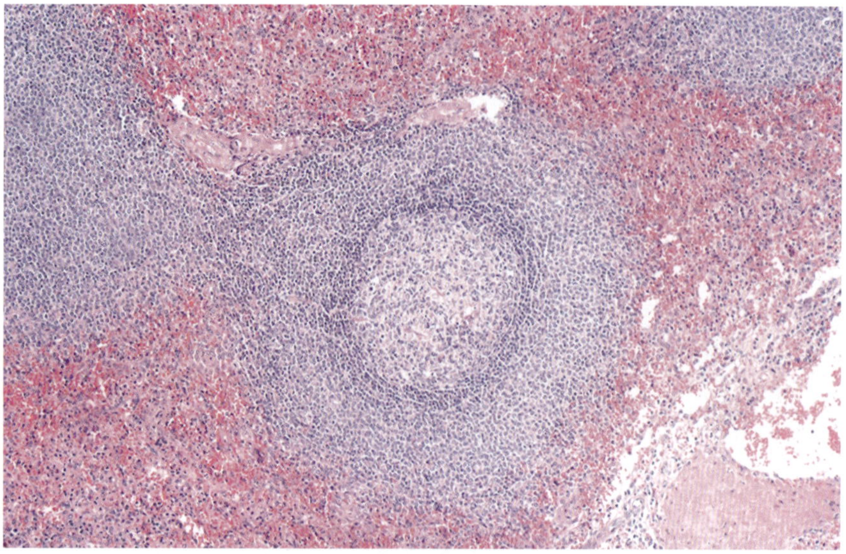

Figure 5-19

MARGINAL ZONE HYPERPLASIA, SPLEEN

Expansion of the marginal zone to greater than 12 cells is considered marginal zone hyperplasia. In this case, this pale third layer of the follicle is expanded.

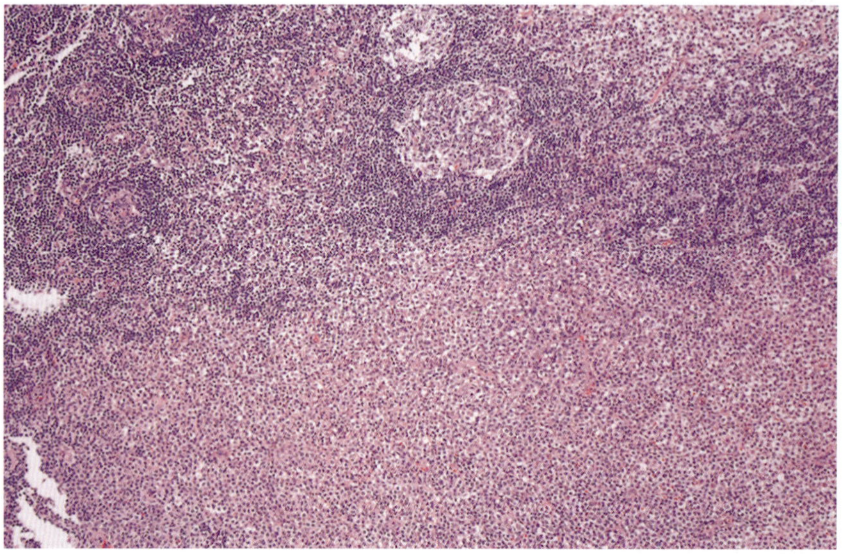

Figure 5-20

MARGINAL ZONE HYPERPLASIA, LYMPH NODE

In the lymph nodes, marginal zone hyperplasia is usually seen adjacent to the follicles, and is not necessarily concentrically arranged around follicles, as in splenic marginal zones.

Microscopic Findings. Under normal circumstances, distinct marginal zones are present in the spleen and mesenteric lymph nodes, but are rare in peripheral lymph nodes (fig. 5-19) (36,44). The marginal zone is a pale, third layer around the otherwise familiar two-layer follicle, with the light-colored germinal center and dark mantle zone. Hyperplasia of marginal zone cells takes several forms. The most common is the expansion of the preexisting marginal zone beyond a usual degree (23,26,31,47). Other forms include formation of a distinct third layer of clear cells surrounding follicular mantles in nodes where this is not an expected finding (e.g., nonmesenteric lymph nodes) (fig. 5-20). Another form of hyperplasia is the presence of sheets or clusters of pale-appearing lymphocytes in parafollicular or interfollicular areas that are distinct from surrounding cell populations (fig. 5-21). This form is appropriately described as *monocytoid B-cell hyperplasia* when the cells are not in a typical distribution for marginal zone cells.

Reactive marginal zone cells do not show nuclear atypia or a high mitotic rate, and are only rarely transformed or nucleolated (fig. 5-22). Interspersed polymorphonuclear leukocytes are consistently seen in marginal zone hyperplasia but are also commonly present in marginal zone lymphoma. Cytologically, these lymphocytes are small to intermediate sized, with rounded

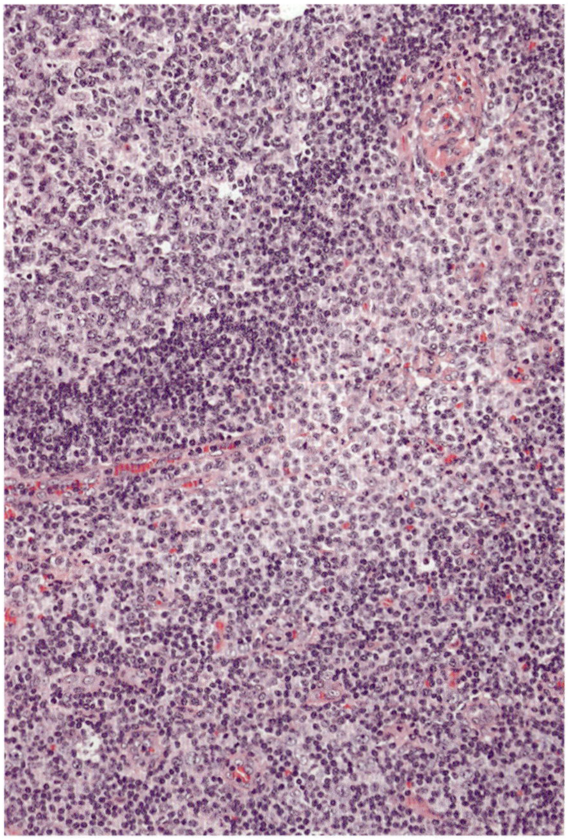

Figure 5-21

MARGINAL ZONE CELL NODULE, LYMPH NODE

Although nonspecific, marginal cell nodules are seen in a variety of benign pathologic conditions.

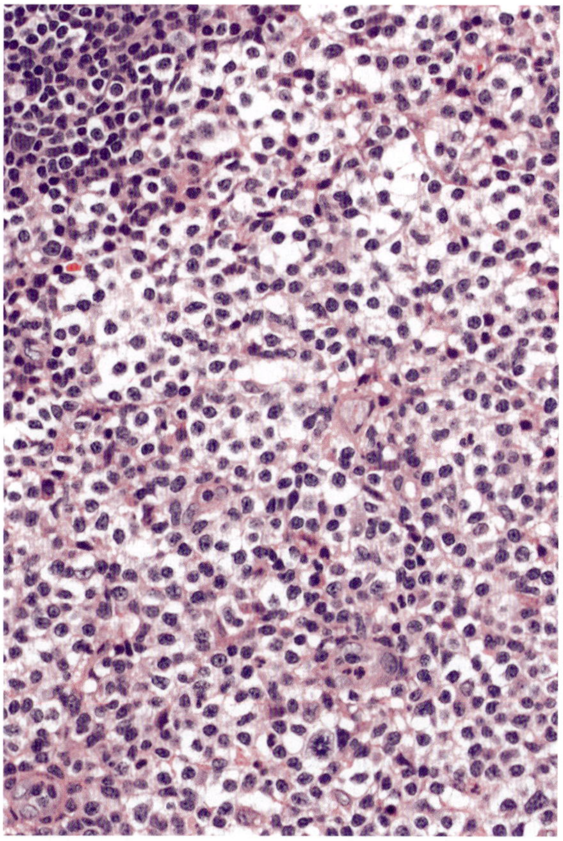

Figure 5-22

MARGINAL ZONE

The classic monocytoid appearance of marginal zone cells is seen. These B cells have increased amounts of pale or clear cytoplasm, giving them an appearance similar to peripheral blood monocytes.

or indented nuclei. The chromatin is mature and nucleoli may be inconspicuous. They often have a moderate to abundant amount of pale to clear cytoplasm.

An unusual type of marginal zone hyperplasia has been described in tonsils and appendices (3). In children, this expansion of marginal zones shows lambda-light chain restriction, but is polyclonal when immunoglobulin genes are examined. These cases are benign, but raise the diagnostic consideration of pediatric marginal zone lymphoma.

In the spleen, marginal zone hyperplasia is a common finding. It usually occurs in association with follicular hyperplasia and may, occasionally, be impossible to distinguish from indolent marginal zone lymphoma on morphologic grounds alone. The marginal zones become expanded; a marginal zone layer wider than 12 cells has been arbitrarily defined as "hyperplasia" (fig. 5-23) (23,26,47). Features that help distinguish the two conditions are listed in Table 5-5. It is important to be fully aware of any underlying condition that may be associated with the presence of hyperplastic splenic marginal zones, such as immune thrombocytopenic purpura, systemic lupus erythematosus, and other chronic autoimmune disorders.

Differential Diagnosis. Distinguishing marginal zone hyperplasia from marginal zone lymphoma may be extremely difficult although certain criteria have been well described (57). In hyperplasia, the monocytoid B-cell component does not predominate but, rather, occurs in focal areas; in lymphoma, the monocytoid B cells are confluent or totally efface the lymph node.

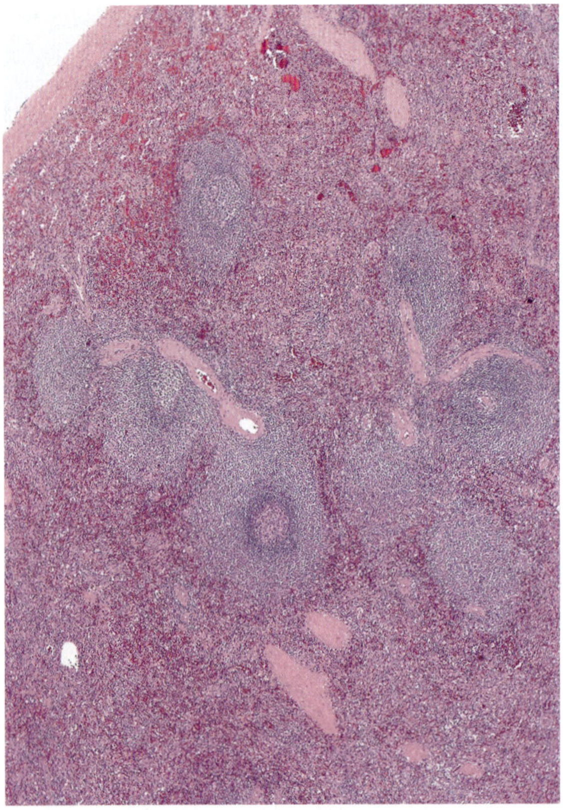

Figure 5-23

MARGINAL ZONE HYPERPLASIA, SPLEEN

The expanded marginal zones in the spleen may be difficult to differentiate from involvement by splenic marginal zone lymphoma, or less commonly, mantle cell lymphoma or small lymphocytic lymphoma.

Lymphocytes with pale cytoplasm and a perifollicular distribution (monocytoid cells) in lymph node suggest the following diagnoses: hairy cell leukemia, T-cell lymphoma, and mastocytosis. Marginal zone hyperplasia is a distinctive pattern that is seen in several specific infectious etiologies of lymphadenitis including toxoplasmosis (21,73), acquired immunodeficiency syndrome (AIDS) (76), cat-scratch disease (56), and EBV-related lymphadenopathy (57) and other viral adenopathies (Table 5-6).

T-CELL HYPERPLASIAS INCLUDING NODULAR PARACORTICAL T-CELL HYPERPLASIA AND OTHER T-CELL NODULES

Definition. T cells are an integral component of the lymph nodes and spleen. In their most typical arrangement, T cells form nodules, which upon stimulation, enlarge and have a characteristic structure, *nodular paracortical T-cell hyperplasia* (NPTCH). This nonspecific reaction can be seen in a variety of reactive conditions. Splenic T cells are distributed throughout the red pulp and in the periarteriolar lymphoid sheath. Hyperplasia of splenic T cells can be seen in many situations comparable to those of the lymph nodes, but with a different morphologic appearance.

Table 5-5

COMPARISON OF MARGINAL ZONE HYPERPLASIA AND MARGINAL ZONE LYMPHOMA OF SPLEEN

Features	Marginal Zone Hyperplasia	Marginal Zone Lymphoma
Expanded marginal zone (>12 cell layers)	Yes	Yes
Numerous B cells in periarteriolar lymphoid sheath	No	Yes
Follicles	3 layers	Loss of layers; often uniform single layer
Red pulp	No increase in red pulp B cells	Often has clusters of red pulp B cells
Clonality	No	Yes
Kappa/lambda	Polyclonal	Monoclonal
Ki-67	Normal secondary follicles with high proliferation	Colonized follicles have low proliferation in neoplastic cells

Clinical Features. There are three general types of T-cell nodule encountered in the lymph node (20). Primary T-cell nodules are small, circumscribed collections of T cells, with a central core of CD4-positive T cells and a meshwork of interdigitating dendritic cells (IDCs). Secondary nodules are less well demarcated, with increased IDCs and a more scattered distribution of CD8/CD4-positive lymphocytes. The most characteristic of the nodules is the tertiary nodule, also known as NPTCH. This is most often seen in dermatopathic lymphadenitis (16,37,50) (see chapter 6), but may also be seen in a variety of reactive conditions.

T-cell hyperplasia is occasionally encountered in the spleen and may be a cause of white pulp expansion. There are varied etiologies that can cause selective expansion of the white pulp T-cell compartment including congenital or acquired immunodeficiencies (see chapter 7) and autoimmune conditions (see chapter 12). Morphologically, these conditions may simulate white pulp involvement by lymphoma.

Table 5-6

SPECIFIC CAUSES OF LYMPHADENOPATHY ASSOCIATED WITH MARGINAL ZONE OR MONOCYTOID B-CELL HYPERPLASIA

Viral infections
Cytomegalovirus
Epstein-Barr virus
HIV/AIDS[a]
Toxoplasmosis
Cat-scratch disease
Lymphogranuloma venereum

[a]HIV = human immunodeficiency virus; AIDS = acquired immunodeficiency syndrome.

Microscopic Features. Isolated or confluent nodules that are composed primarily of small lymphocytes, interdigitating reticulum cells that impart a "mottled" appearance, occasional macrophages, and high endothelial venules characterize NPTCH (fig. 5-24) (84). In addition, nodular expansion of the paracortex by confluent areas of pale-staining macrophages, interspersed Langerhans cells and IDCs, and small reactive lymphocytes (figs. 5-25–5-27) is seen. Immunoreactivity for S-100 protein may be demonstrated in the IDCs and Langerhans cells and CD1a in the Langerhans cells (fig. 5-28). Follicular hyperplasia and/or sinus histiocytosis is commonly associated with the nodular paracortical expansion of dermatopathic lymphadenopathy.

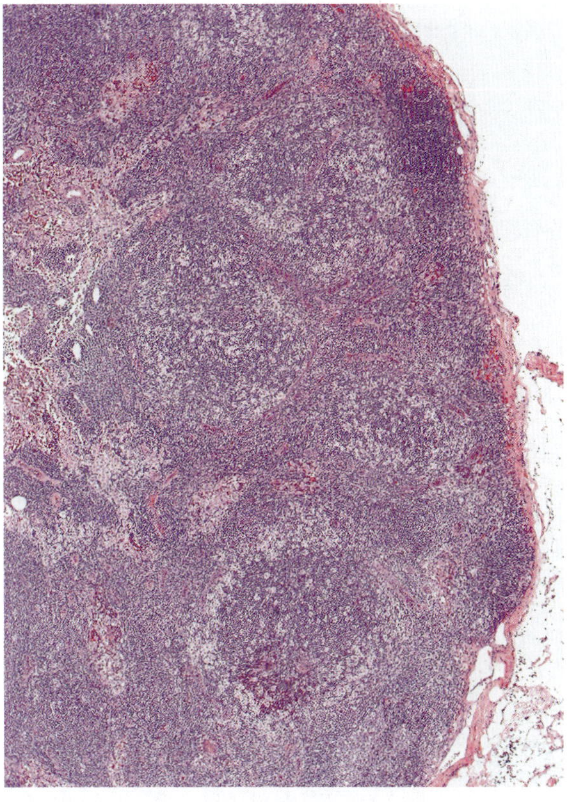

Figure 5-24

NODULAR PARACORTICAL T-CELL HYPERPLASIA, LYMPH NODE

At low magnification, nodular paracortical T-cell hyperplasia has a classic mottled appearance.

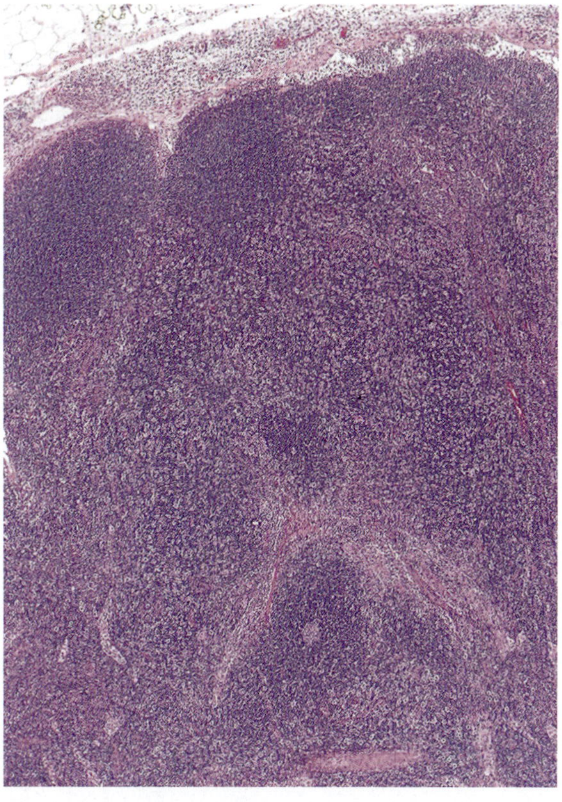

Figure 5-25

NODULAR PARACORTICAL T-CELL HYPERPLASIA, LYMPH NODE

This example of nodular paracortical T-cell hyperplasia is more extensive than that seen in figure 5-24, but still has an apparent mottled appearance and spares the subcapsular primary follicles (right).

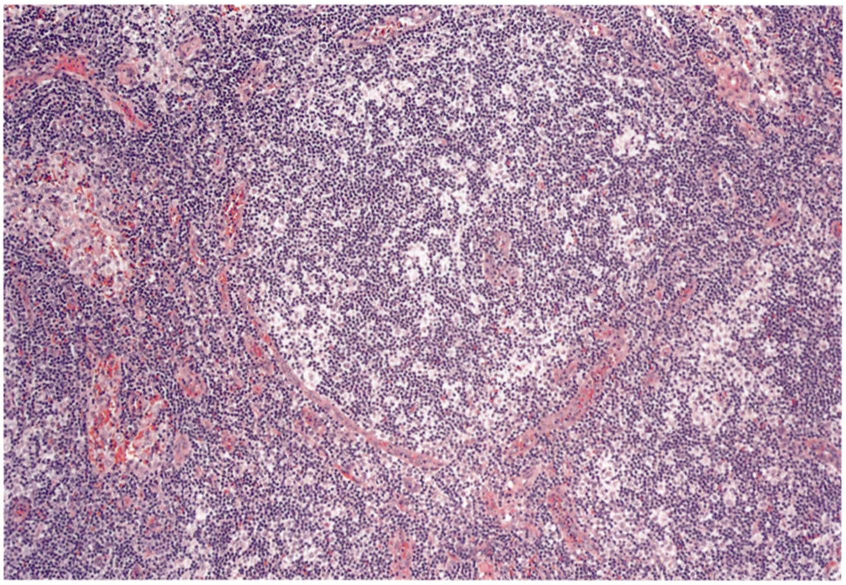

Figure 5-26

NODULAR PARACORTICAL T-CELL HYPERPLASIA, LYMPH NODE

Higher magnification highlights the macrophages and small lymphocytes.

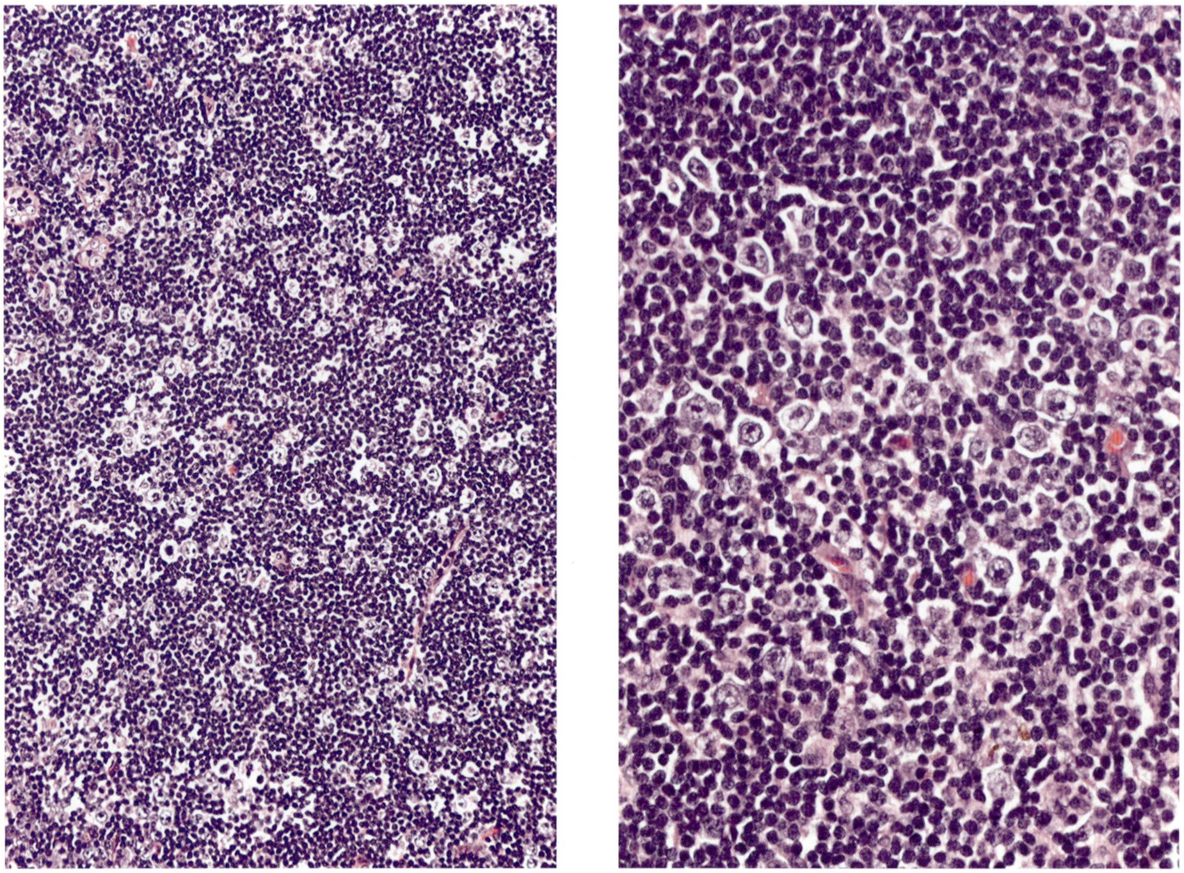

Figure 5-27

NODULAR PARACORTICAL T-CELL HYPERPLASIA, LYMPH NODE

The cytologic appearance is a mixture of small mature lymphocytes, large lymphocytes, macrophages, and dendritic cells.

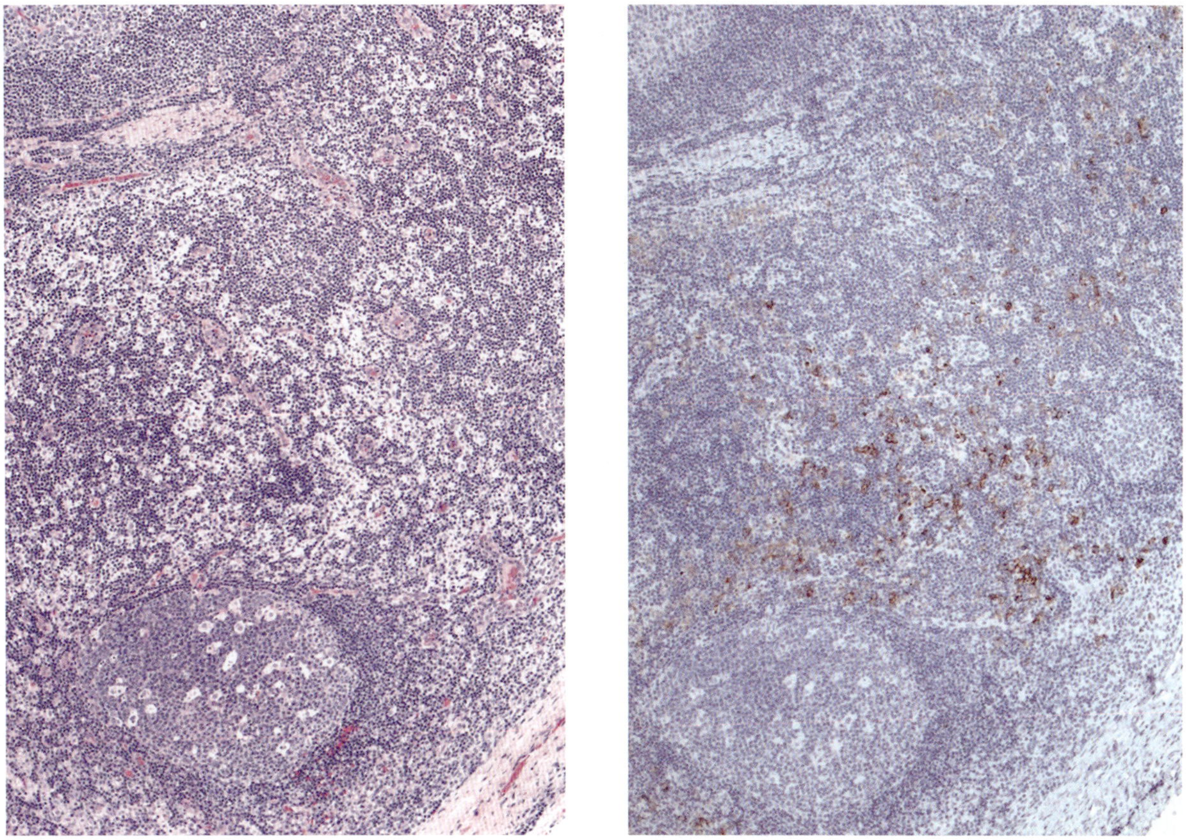

Figure 5-28

CD1A REACTIVITY IN NODULAR PARACORTICAL T-CELL HYPERPLASIA, LYMPH NODE

Nodular paracortical T-cell hyperplasia (left) involves antigen presenting cells/macrophages, as evidenced by the CD1a stain (right).

An expansion of the T-cell compartment in the spleen is usually appreciated after basic immunohistochemical staining (CD3, CD20) is performed. The periarteriolar lymphoid sheaths may be thickened to a degree that is similar to the size of germinal centers. There is typically a mixture of small T cells and larger, transformed T cells (immunoblasts). Extensive panels of T-cell reactive antibodies may be necessary for evaluation to rule out the possibility of an unusual population of T cells or an aberrant immunophenotype. In addition, PCR for T-cell gene rearrangements may provide important diagnostic help. Rarely, in patients treated with phenytoin, NPTCH simulates a peripheral T-cell lymphoma (67).

Differential Diagnosis. In most cases, the histologic features of NPTCH are not difficult to recognize. Distinction from lymph node involvement by mycosis fungoides, however, may pose a diagnostic challenge unless there is significant architectural effacement of the lymph node that is easily recognizable and consistent with a neoplastic process (fig. 5-29) (7,9). A complete clinical history is particularly important in such cases. In general, overall preservation of the normal lymph node architecture, in the absence of atypical T cells or increased mitoses, supports a diagnosis of NPTCH rather than involvement of the lymph node by peripheral T-cell lymphoma. Involvement of lymph node by mycosis fungoides presents a more atypical morphology. Early involvement by mycosis fungoides, however, may pose a significant diagnostic dilemma, and thus immunophenotypic studies are appropriate; they reveal a predominance of CD4-positive T cells that often lack expression of CD7.

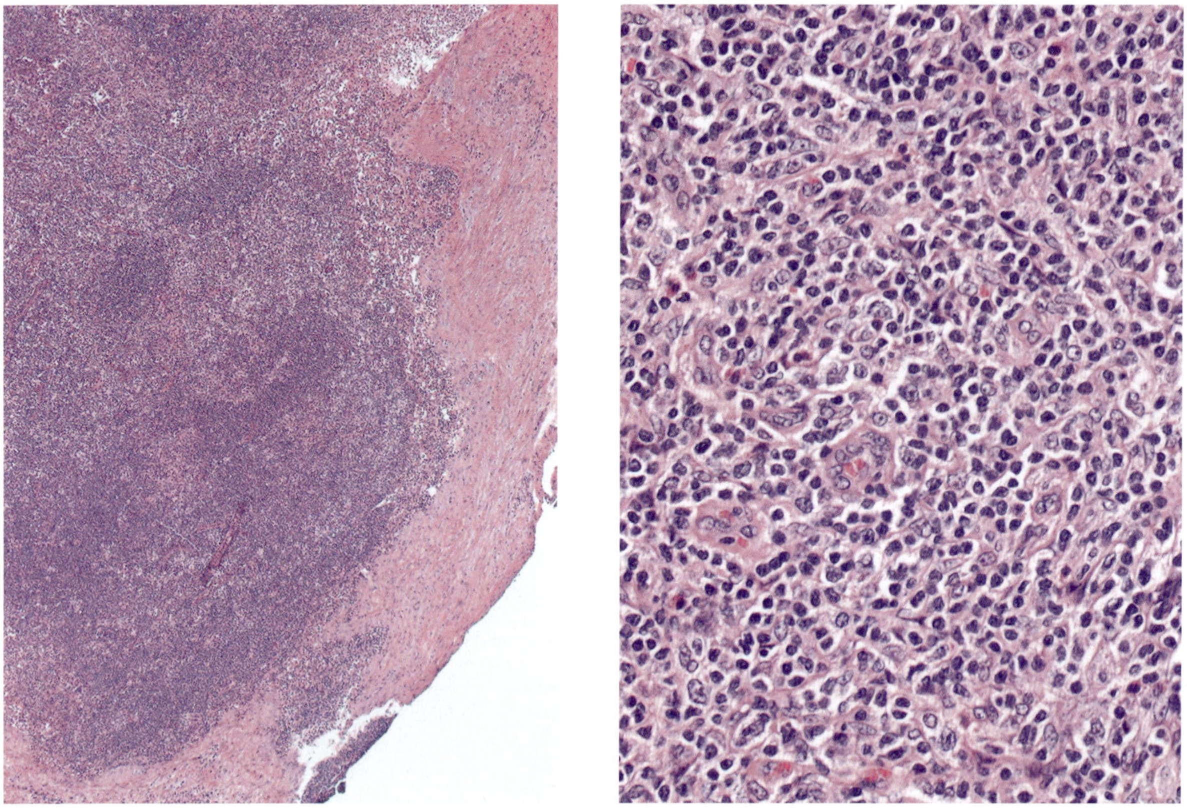

Figure 5-29

MYCOSIS FUNGOIDES IN LYMPH NODE

Left: Although subtle, this lymph node is involved by mycosis fungoides.

Right: Higher magnification of the paracortical areas reveals an increase in larger, atypical lymphocytes. Immunohistochemical staining (not shown) would highlight the abnormal lymphocyte population.

MIXED PATTERN HYPERPLASIA

Definition. *Mixed pattern hyperplasia* is lymphoid hyperplasia with a combination of histopathologic features of other types of hyperplasia (i.e., follicular, marginal zone), and lacking a specific etiology.

Clinical Features. Mixed pattern hyperplasia is a descriptive term, suggesting a combination of histologic features of more than one type of well-characterized lymphoid hyperplasia. These combinations are undoubtedly expressions of activation of different response mechanisms within the immune system. If given the opportunity to observe the immune responses in lymph nodes and spleen over time, they would show different evolving combinations of features (11).

Microscopic Findings. Individual microscopic features of hyperplasias (follicular, marginal zone, interfollicular/immunoblastic, mantle cell, T cell) are covered in their respective sections in this chapter (figs. 5-30, 5-31).

Differential Diagnosis. Each individual type of hyperplasia in a lymph node carries its own differential diagnoses. However, complex mixtures of patterns in a lymph node may raise other, less common differential diagnoses which should be considered. Included in these are early or partial involvement of a lymph node by lymphoma, including typical small B-cell lymphomas, in situ follicular lymphoma, interfollicular Hodgkin lymphoma, and T-cell lymphoma. Rare composite lymphomas (such as a combination of diffuse large B-cell lymphoma and angioimmunoblastic T-cell lymphoma) may present complex architectural features, which may mimic benign processes. In many circumstances, ancillary studies, such as immunohistochemistry and

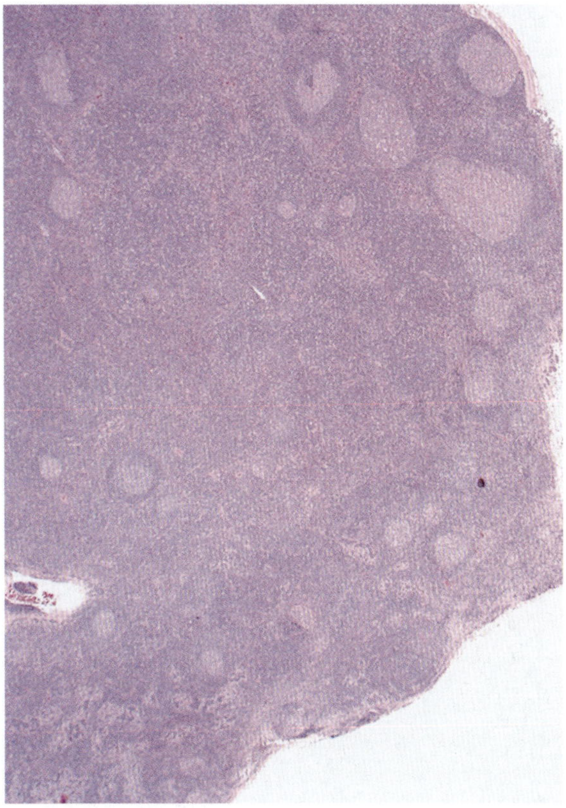

Figure 5-30

MIXED PATTERN HYPERPLASIA, LYMPH NODE

The common combination of hyperplastic features, follicular hyperplasia, and nodular paracortical T-cell hyperplasia is seen in this lymph node.

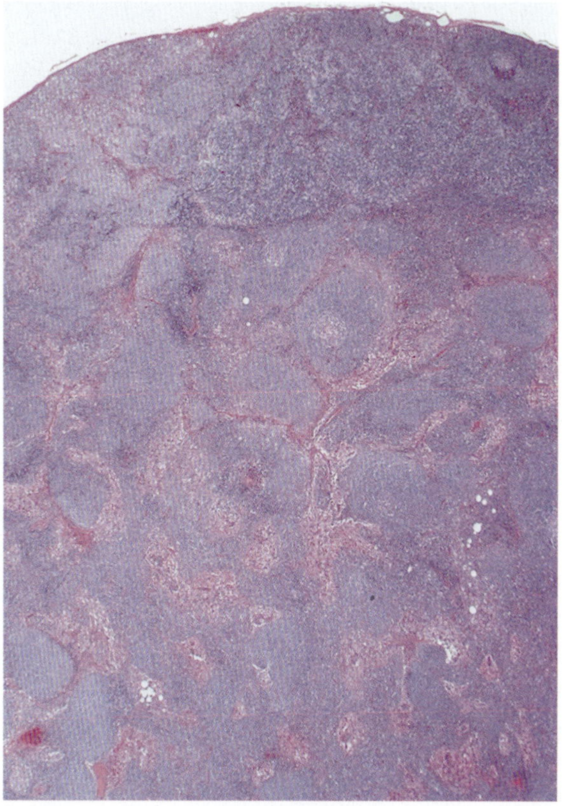

Figure 5-31

MIXED PATTERN HYPERPLASIA, LYMPH NODE

In another combination of hyperplastic features, this lymph node has mantle cell/zone hyperplasia, nodular paracortical T-cell hyperplasia, and sinus histiocytosis.

flow cytometry, provide reassuring evidence of complex patterns of hyperplasia, or reveal the presence of lymphoma.

ATYPICAL LYMPHOID HYPERPLASIA

Definition. *Atypical lymphoid hyperplasia* (ALH) is not a specific pattern of histologic or clinical findings, but rather a hyperplastic lymph node with sufficient deviation from normal patterns of hyperplasia to raise suspicion of a lymphoproliferative disorder, but without achieving a degree of abnormality to warrant a diagnosis of lymphoma.

Clinical Features. ALH is not a specific diagnosis, but occupies the borderline between a benign reactive hyperplastic process and a neoplastic lymphomatous process. In older studies, ALH was used as a strictly morphologic description (17,62,68,71,91). When evaluated by ancillary studies, a significant portion of these cases progressed to lymphoma; many had unequivocal evidence of lymphoma.

Microscopic Findings. Although the ALH designation can refer to any combination of "not-quite-lymphoma-but-not-quite-benign" features, there are generally three circumstances that usually warrant the ALH designation. The first is the presence of individual or a few follicles with features of follicular lymphoma in a background of normal follicles. As discussed above, consideration of the individual features of follicular hyperplasia, in situ follicular lymphoma, and outright follicular lymphoma need to be considered (fig. 5-32). The second circumstance is the presence of interfollicular proliferations of atypical mixtures of polymorphous cells, including immunoblasts. In this circumstance, there may be associated vascular proliferation

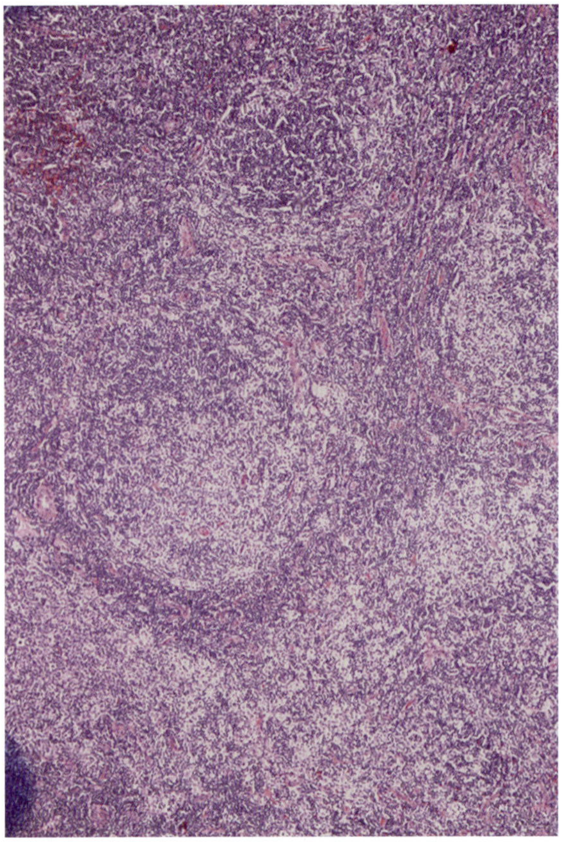

Figure 5-32

ATYPICAL LYMPHOID HYPERPLASIA

Atypical lymphoid follicles often have some of the features of follicular lymphoma, but not enough to be entirely sure that the are benign or malignant.

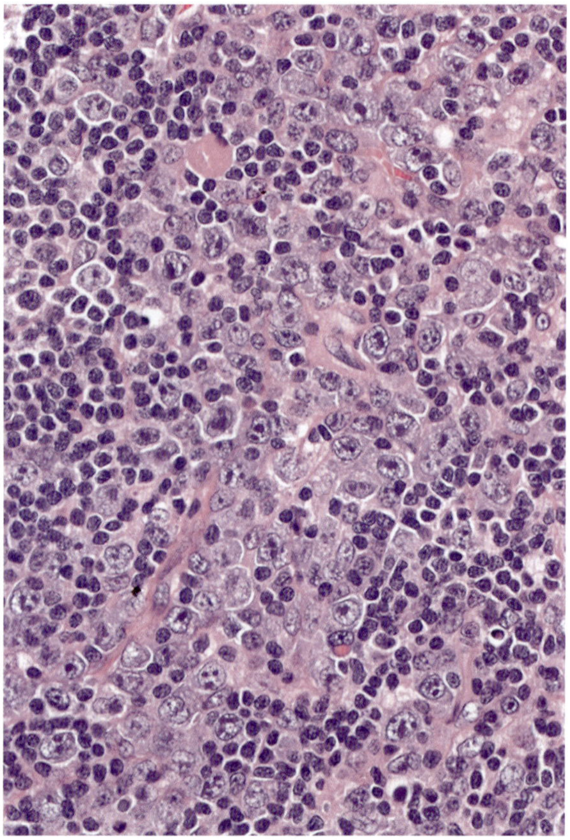

Figure 5-33

ATYPICAL LYMPHOID HYPERPLASIA

Immunoblastic proliferations are often difficult to distinguish from large cell lymphomas, without the benefit of clinical information and evaluation of the entire lymph node.

and increases in granulocytes, eosinophils, and plasma cells (fig. 5-33). Peripheral T-cell lymphomas (especially angioimmunoblastic T-cell lymphoma), partial nodal involvement by a lymphoplasmacytic lymphoma, diffuse large B-cell lymphoma, and other lymphomas with a polymorphous cellular composition need to be considered. The final common circumstance is the presence of large atypical lymphoid cells in a variety of cellular backgrounds (fig. 5-34). The differential diagnosis is broad, but the most common implication is the possibility of Hodgkin lymphoma or a T-cell–rich/histiocyte-rich large B-cell lymphoma.

In cases of ALH, it is prudent to perform additional ancillary studies, as necessary, in an attempt to clarify the diagnosis. Careful consideration of all appropriate laboratory studies and the clinical history cannot be overemphasized. Batteries of immunohistochemical stains are appropriate, but may not lead to a conclusive diagnosis. Performance of either immunoglobulin heavy chain or T-cell receptor gene rearrangement studies is prudent, but negative results are not necessarily indicative of the lack of a lymphomatous process. If available, the results of cytogenetic studies should be correlated with morphologic findings. If a specific genetic abnormality can be tested, such as t(14;18) for follicular lymphoma, then FISH or PCR studies should be attempted to clarify a diagnosis of ALH.

Even after all ancillary studies have been attempted, some cases may retain the ALH designation. In these circumstances, it is important to communicate with clinicians to allow for appropriate follow-up studies. If adenopathy persists or if new

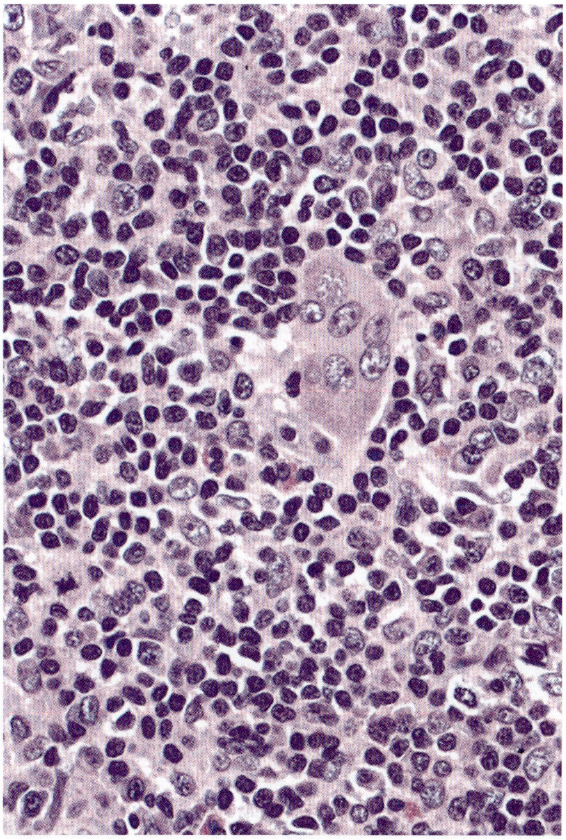

Figure 5-34

ATYPICAL LYMPHOID HYPERPLASIA

Individual large, atypical cells often raise the possibility of Hodgkin lymphoma. Although this lymph node is benign, the large cell in the center is worrisome, and would elicit a flurry of immunohistochemical stains.

adenopathy arises, it may be appropriate to perform an additional biopsy at another site or after an appropriate interval. Follow-up biopsies may yield a more definitive diagnosis.

SINUS HISTIOCYTOSIS

Definition. *Sinus histiocytosis* refers to the filling and expansion of lymph node sinuses by benign macrophages (histiocytes). This process occurs as a result of a variety of situations, such as a node draining cancer or infection, but frequently there is no identifiable cause.

Clinical Features. Sinus histiocytosis is a type of hyperplasia that is seen in specific or nonspecific clinicopathologic conditions. It is a common finding in reactive lymph nodes that drain infectious sites or tumors (20,74). Sinus histiocytosis should be distinguished from metastatic carcinoma or melanoma and anaplastic large cell lymphoma (79), all of which are commonly identified in the lymph node sinuses.

Microscopic Findings. Sinuses are always present in lymph nodes, but are often not apparent unless they are distended by a cellular component, which highlights their presence. Sinus histiocytosis is characterized by sinusoidal infiltration by bland-appearing macrophages that lack nuclear atypia or increased mitoses and may exhibit phagocytosis (fig. 5-35). The macrophages are uniform in size, with round to oval nuclei and abundant cytoplasm. Rarely, they exhibit erythrophagocytosis or the presence of pigment. Although rare, the macrophages may have a signet ring appearance, which can be suggestive of metastatic signet ring type carcinoma (fig. 5-36) (2,29). Immunohistochemical studies prove the histiocytic nature of the cells, depending on the clinical situation.

Another rare finding is the presence of muciphages in lymph nodes (figs. 5-37, 5-38) (19). These cells, which closely mimic the cells of signet ring cell carcinoma, have been reported in nodes draining mucin-producing carcinomas. The muciphages have ingested mucin and are mucin and Alcian blue positive. They are distinguished from carcinoma cells by their immunohistochemical profile (CD68+, CD163+, keratin-).

Differential Diagnosis. A sinus pattern of reactive lymph node hyperplasia includes sinus histiocytosis, marginal zone/monocytoid B-cell hyperplasia, infection-associated hemophagocytic syndrome, histiocytic disorders, vascular transformation of lymph node sinuses, and lymphangiectasis. In addition, metastatic carcinomas can occasionally be deceptively bland on low-magnification examination (fig. 5-39). Careful examination of the cells that expand the sinuses usually reveals their nature. In some circumstances, immunohistochemistry is necessary to highlight the histiocytic nature of the cells. Stains for macrophages include CD68, CD163, HAM56, lysozyme, CD31, CD43, CD45, antitrypsin, and antichymotrypsin.

GRANULOMATOUS INFLAMMATION

Definition. *Granulomas* are the result of an organized immune response with activation and organization of mononuclear phagocytic cells.

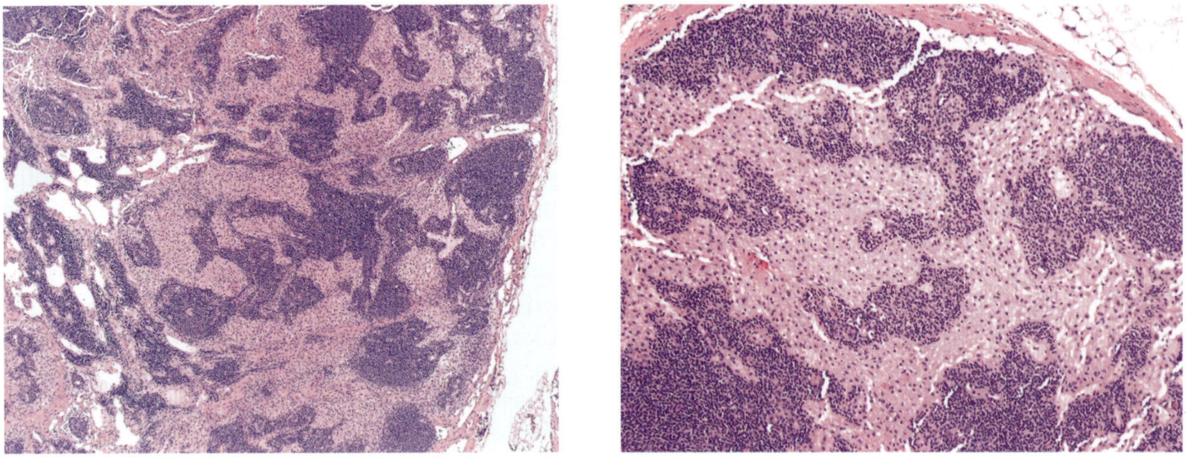

Figure 5-35

SINUS HISTIOCYTOSIS, LYMPH NODE

Two examples of florid sinus histiocytosis expanding the lymphoid sinuses with histiocytes/macrophages.

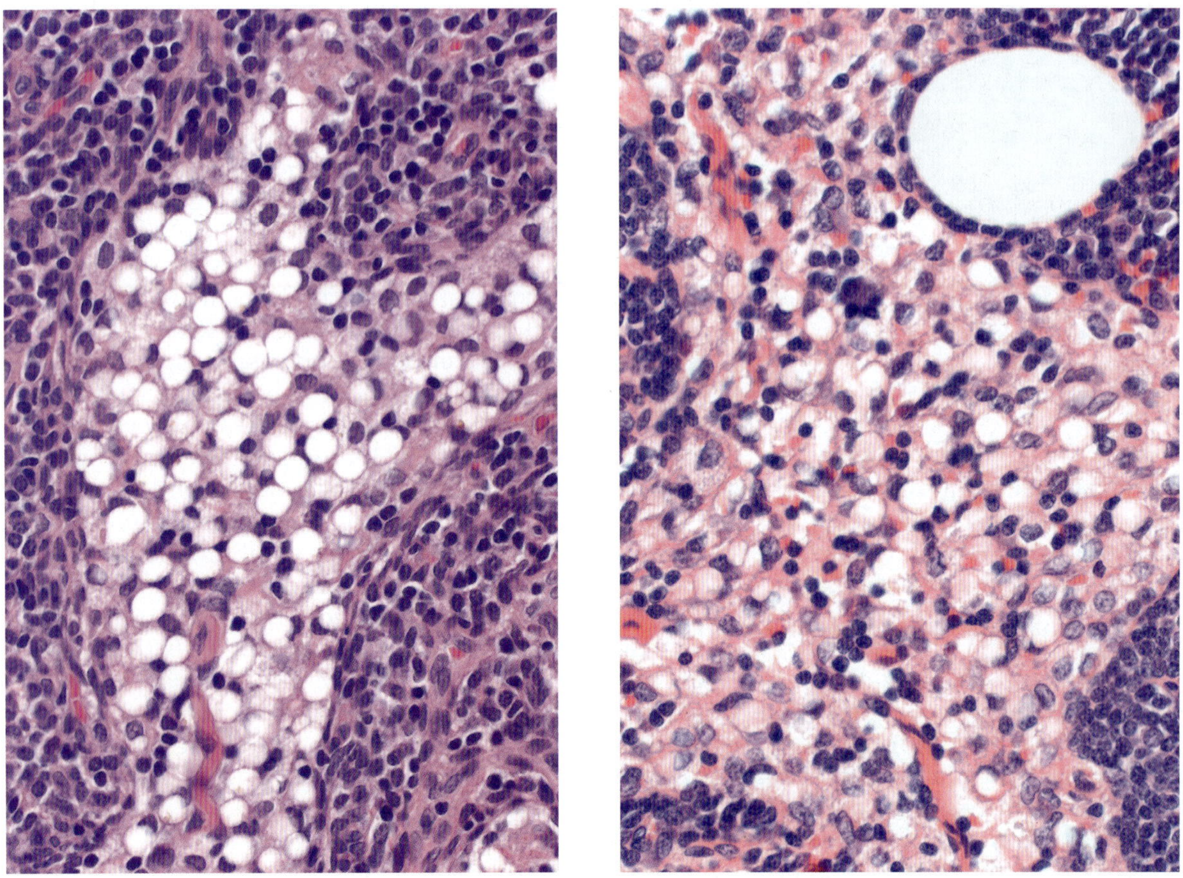

Figure 5-36

SIGNET RING MACROPHAGES, SINUS HISTIOCYTOSIS, LYMPH NODE

These macrophages have a clear vacuole in the cytoplasm. This appearance could raise suspicion of a signet ring cell carcinoma in some circumstances. (Right courtesy of Peter Humphreys, St. Louis, MO.)

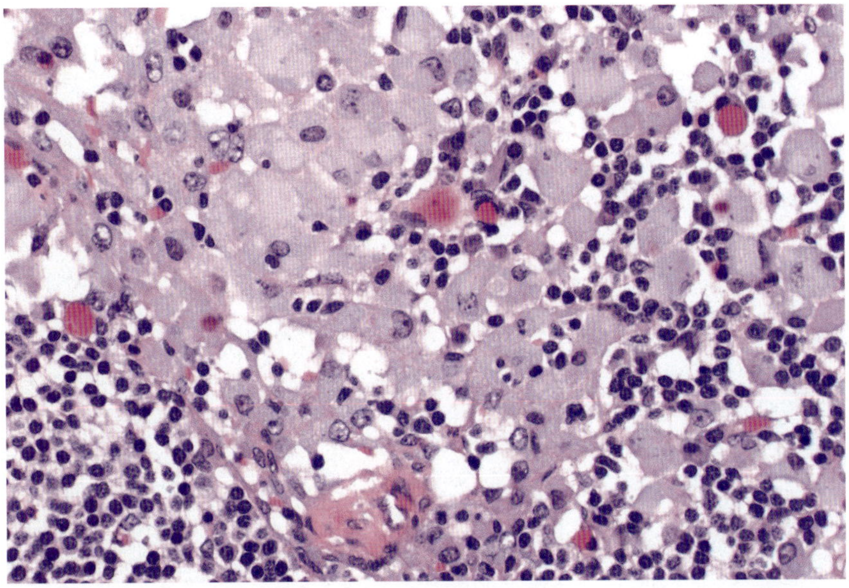

Figure 5-37

NODAL MUCIPHAGES, LYMPH NODE

A rare finding, muciphages are seen in lymph nodes draining sites of mucin production, as in this lymph node draining a mucin-producing carcinoma. (Courtesy of Robert Lev, Providence, RI.)

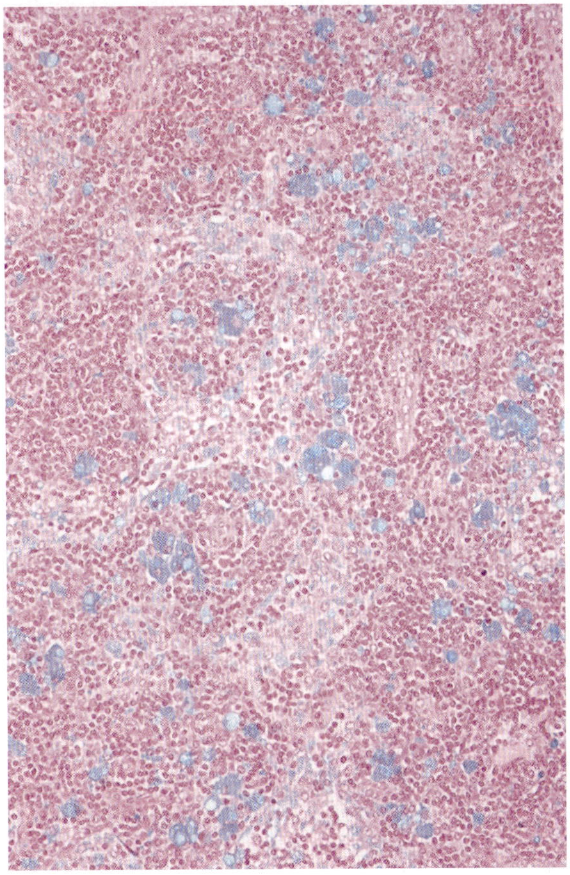

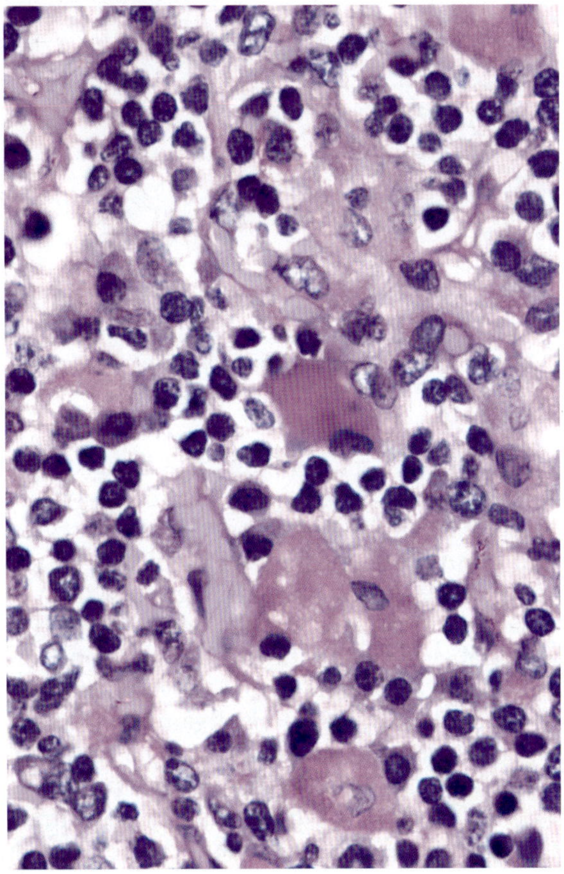

Figure 5-38

NODAL MUCIPHAGES, LYMPH NODE

Sulfated Alcian blue (left) and periodic acid–Schiff (PAS) (right) stain nodal muciphages. (Same case as in fig. 5-37; courtesy of Robert Lev, Providence, RI.)

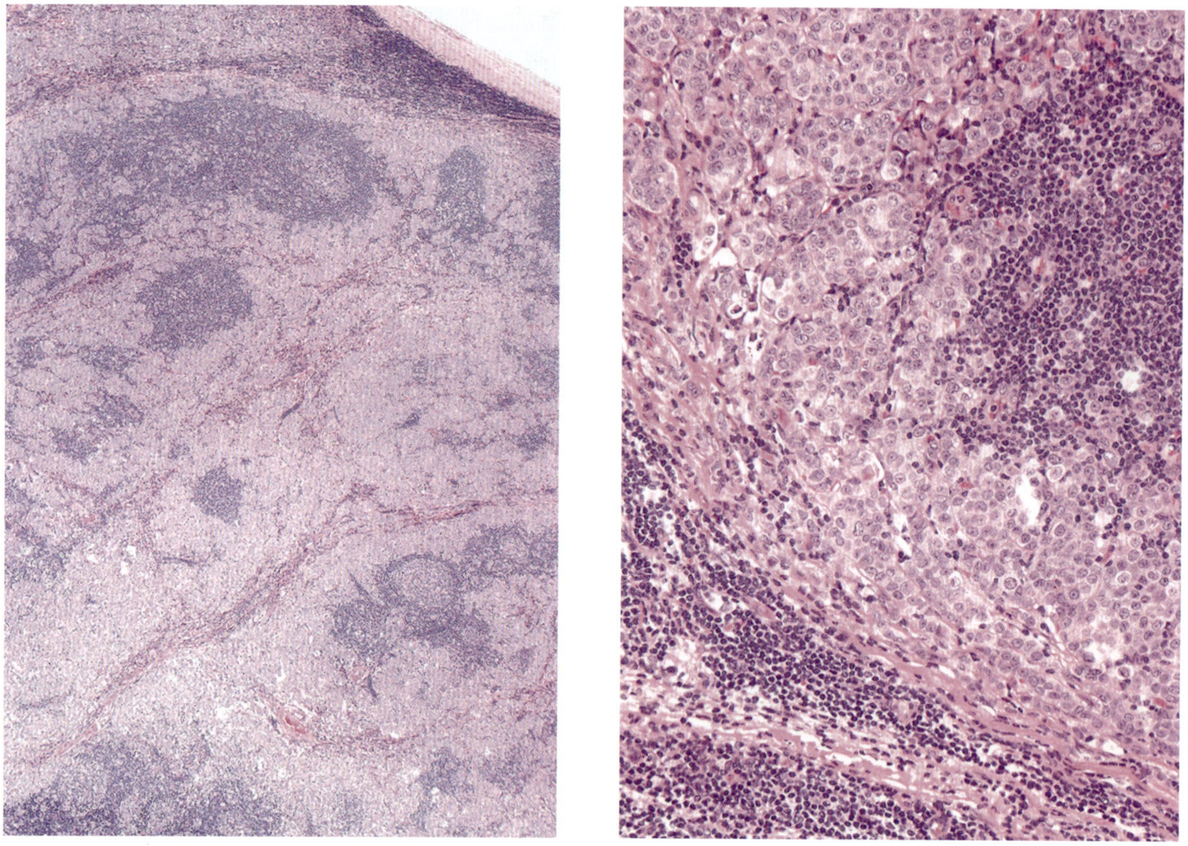

Figure 5-39

METASTATIC CARCINOMA INVOLVING LYMPH NODE SINUS

Left: Low magnification image of a carcinoma involving the lymph node sinus.

Right: Higher magnification highlights the large size of the cells in comparison to the background lymphocytes. The cells show moderate nuclear pleomorphism and ample amounts of granular, pink cytoplasm.

These activated macrophages may be accompanied by various numbers of other inflammatory elements including granulocytes, lymphocytes, and plasma cells, and a variable degree of necrosis, depending on the etiology.

General Features. Granuloma formation is a specialized immune function. Inciting agents are varied, and many studies have focused on those caused by infectious organisms, such as *Mycobacterium tuberculosis*. Additional causes include foreign materials, autoimmune processes, cancers (including lymphomas), and primary diseases of granuloma formation, such as sarcoidosis. Granuloma formation is a process to contain a pathogen (or other antigenic stimulus), in order to prevent dissemination to the organism. It is a primary example of a delayed type hypersensitivity reaction.

Granuloma formation is divided into four phases: initiation, accumulation, effector stage, and resolution (14). Macrophages probably are primary in the initiation of granuloma formation. Undoubtedly, a complex interplay of cytokines and adhesion molecules plays a role in initiation and subsequent phases. "Frustrated phagocytosis" is believed to be the key cause of foreign body granuloma formation, while chronic immune stimulation underlies other types. In the accumulation phase, CD4-positive T cells play the primary role. Their production of cytokines, including CCL2, CCL4, CCL6, CCL7, CCL8, and CCL12, serves to recruit appropriate effector cells to the site. The effector stage is characterized by CD4-positive T cells, CD8-positive cytotoxic T cells, natural killer (NK) cells, and occasionally, granulocytes and additional macrophages. The resolution phase involves the successful destruction of the antigenic stimulus, with reduction of the inflammatory cells and the formation of a fibrous scar.

Clinical Features. Granulomas or generalized granulomatous inflammation can be seen in a variety of disorders (Table 5-7). Granulomas are probably most frequently due to infectious etiologies or sarcoidosis, particularly in young patients (41,48,72).

Splenic granulomas are often associated with systemic disease (48). If granulomas are identified or suspected in a spleen specimen, material for microbiologic cultures should be obtained.

Gross Findings. When granulomas are of an appropriate size, they can be seen on gross examination. They appear as pale or tan, well-circumscribed nodules (fig. 5-40). Compared to the surrounding tissue, they are firm and fibrous. Central portions of the granuloma may be necrotic, having a crumbly, cheese-like quality (caseous). Some granulomas are only seen microscopically.

Microscopic Findings. Although a granuloma can be as simple as a loose collection of macrophages, it is perhaps best recognized by the presence of epithelioid macrophages (fig. 5-41) (38). These are activated macrophages, with increased amounts of pink granular cytoplasm and indistinct cell borders. The nucleus is delicate and oval or elongated, with an irregular nuclear contour. Clusters of the macrophages may be surrounded by a rim of inflammatory cells including lymphocytes (both small and transformed), plasma cells, and acute inflammatory cells. Multinucleated giant cells and fused macrophages, with multiple nuclei and large amounts of cytoplasm, may also be seen (fig. 5-42)

The form of, or the inclusions in, a granuloma may give clues to its etiology. Structures within the central portions of a granuloma or within the macrophages should be carefully sought. Polarizable material may highlight foreign body inclusions. Infectious organisms, such as fungi,

Table 5-7

FREQUENT CAUSES OF LYMPH NODE OR SPLENIC GRANULOMA

Cause
Infectious
Viral (chapter 9)
Fungal (chapter 10)
Mycobacterial (chapter 8)
Bacterial (chapter 8)
Parasitic/protozoal (chapter 11)
Systemic
Sarcoidosis (chapter 12)
Vasculitis (chapter 12)
Crohn disease
Rheumatoid arthritis (chapter 9)
Malignancy Associated
Carcinoma
Melanoma
Lymphoma
Hodgkin lymphoma
B-cell lymphoma
T-cell lymphoma
Immunodeficiency (chapter 7)
Foreign Body (chapter 15)
Idiopathic

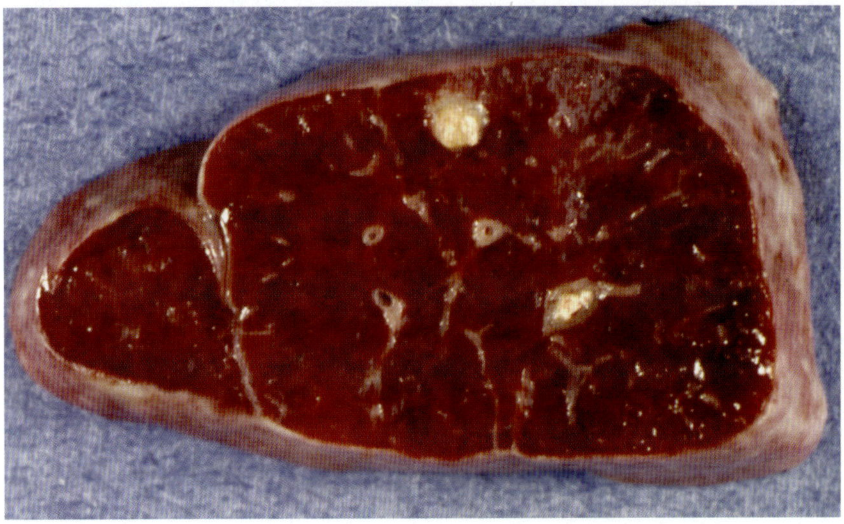

Figure 5-40

GRANULOMA, SPLEEN

Granulomas in spleen are often nodular and well circumscribed. Their appearance is distinct from the adjacent normal spleen. (Courtesy of John Eble, Indianapolis, IN.)

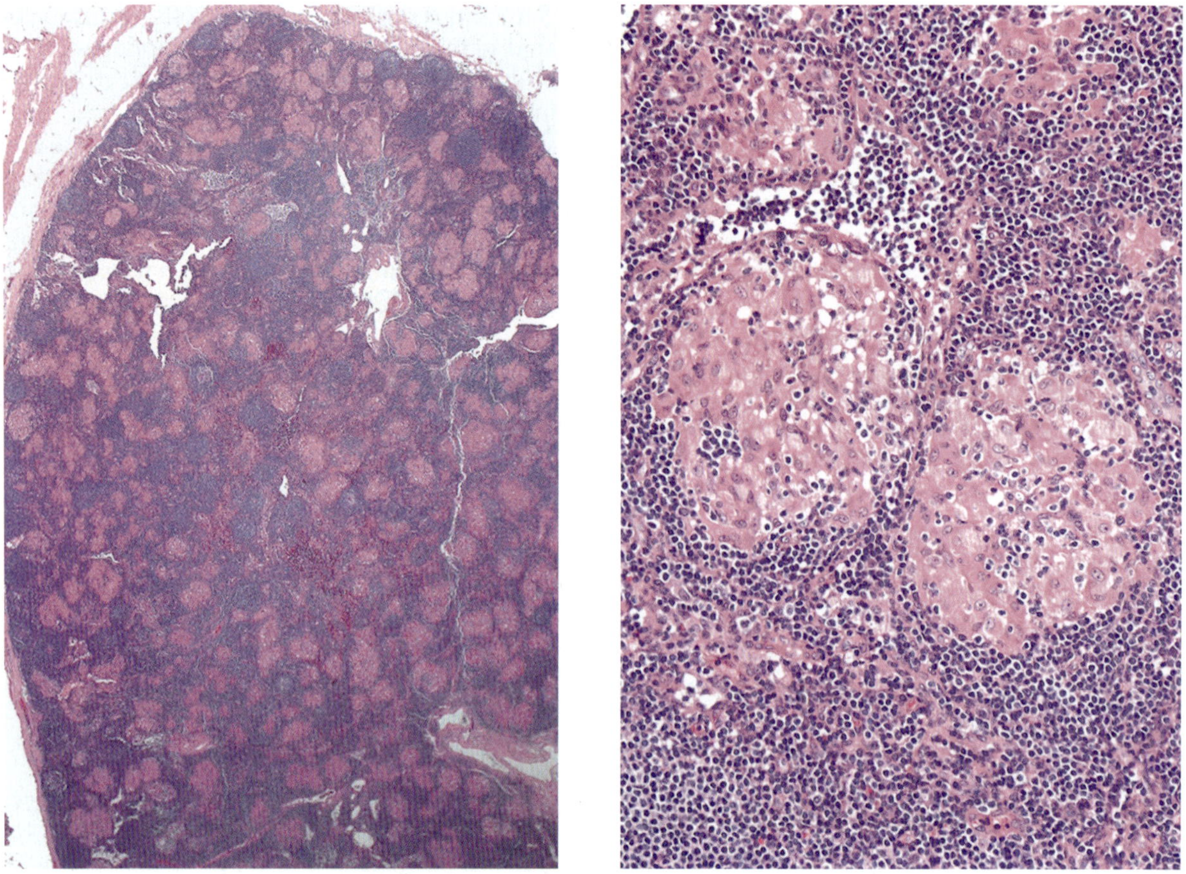

Figure 5-41

EPITHELIOID MACROPHAGES IN GRANULOMA

The lymph nodes are adjacent to carcinoma, but there was no histologic evidence of carcinoma in the lymph nodes. A striking granulomatous reaction, however, was present in the lymph nodes.

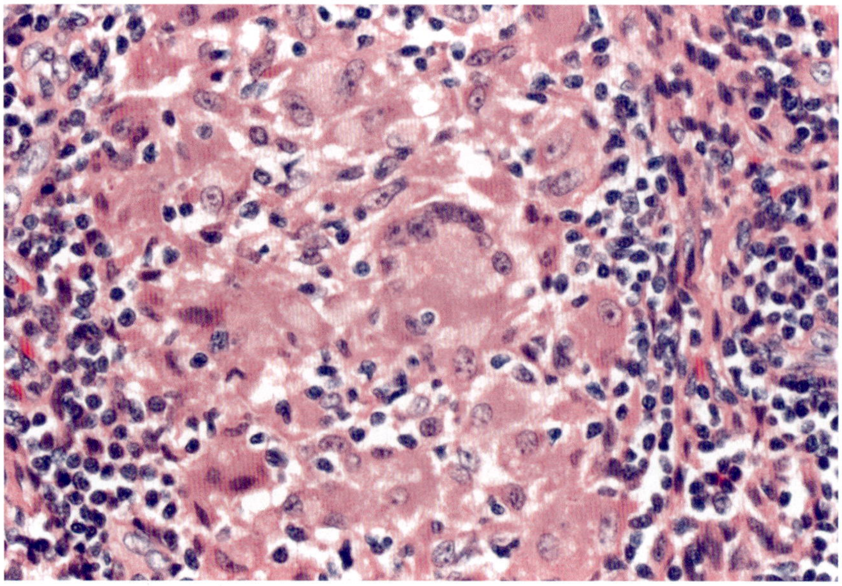

Figure 5-42

GIANT CELLS IN GRANULOMA

Multinucleated giant cells are formed from the epithelioid macrophages (histiocytes) that make up this sarcoidal granuloma.

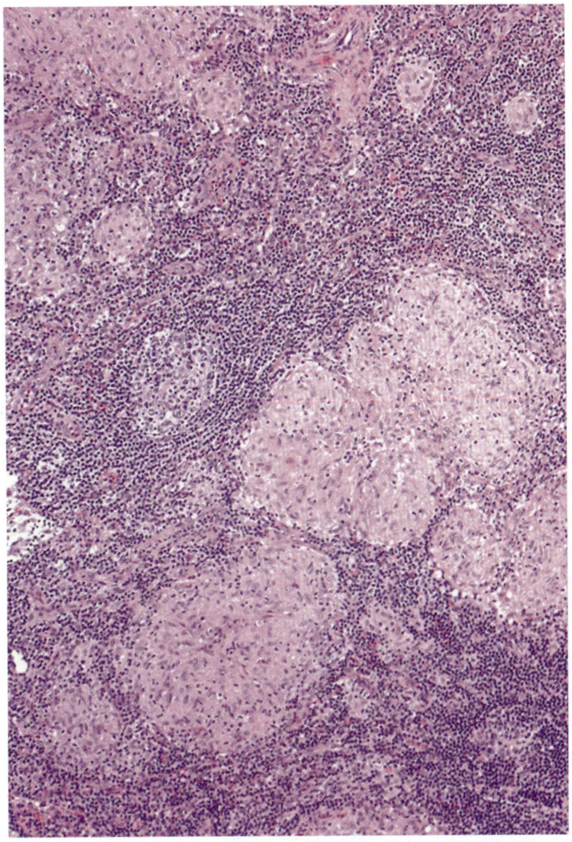

Figure 5-43

SARCOID TYPE GRANULOMAS

Sarcoidal type granulomas are composed of macrophages with abundant cytoplasm (epithelioid macrophages), and have well-circumscribed borders.

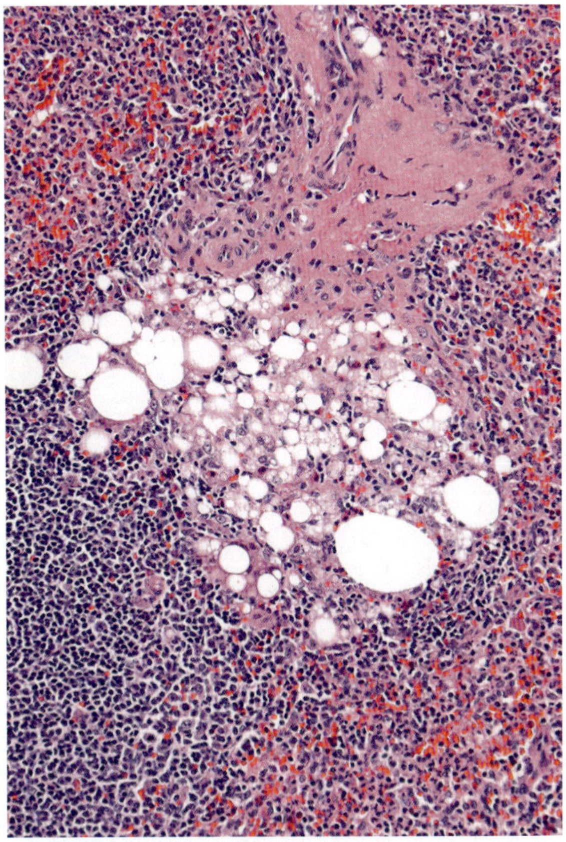

Figure 5-44

LIPOGRANULOMAS, SPLEEN

Usually located in perivascular areas, lipogranulomas are common findings in spleen. They consist of foci of fat, with associated macrophages and lymphocytes.

may be seen microscopically (for additional details, see following chapters).

Sarcoidal granulomas are characterized by well-defined borders and a cohesive, solid appearance (fig. 5-43). Sarcoidosis is discussed in detail in chapter 12. *Lipogranuloma* is a frequent finding in the spleen, and occasionally, in lymph nodes. A lipogranuloma is a focus of macrophages (with small clusters of 5 to 10), with ingested fat in the vacuoles, surrounded by various inflammatory cells, usually lymphocytes and plasma cells (fig. 5-44). Lipogranulomas can be numerous, especially in perivascular areas. Their etiology is unknown, but they may represent either focal disruption of adipocytes, with subsequent cellular reaction, or trapped circulating lipids, with a subsequent immune response.

In any circumstance, it is prudent to evaluate a granuloma for the presence of organisms. Even in cases of known systemic or neoplastic disorders, the possibility of concurrent infection is not excluded. In most circumstances, a stain for mycobacteria (acid-fast bacillus [AFB]) and a silver stain for organisms, such as Gomori methenamine silver (GMS), are appropriate. Other special stains should be performed if the individual circumstance warrants.

Differential Diagnosis. Multiple granulomas in lymph nodes and spleen can be seen in a wide variety of circumstances, as mentioned. Important general categories that should be considered include epithelial malignancies and lymphomas, infections (fungal, mycobacterial, others), and systemic disorders.

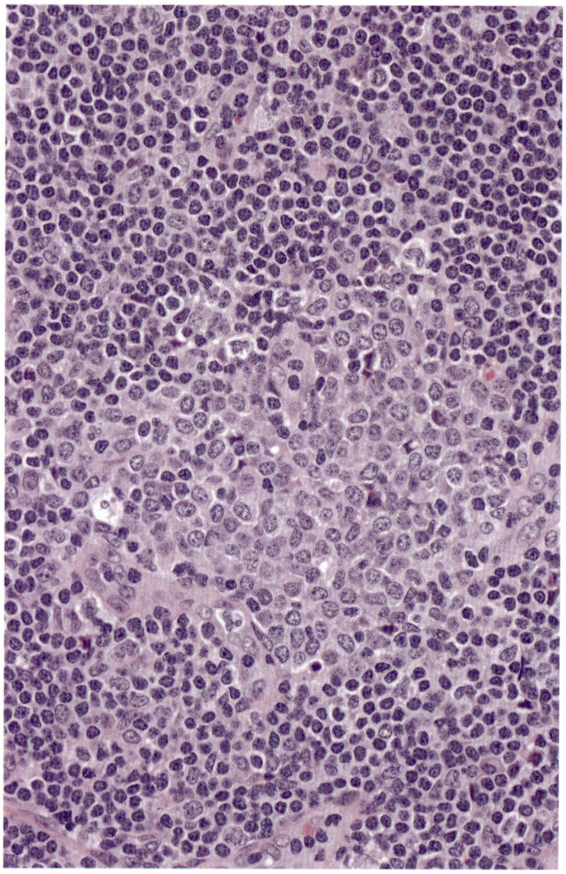

Figure 5-45

PLASMACYTOID DENDRITIC CELLS

Plasmacytoid dendritic cells are intermediate in size (compared to small lymphocytes), and have eccentrically placed nuclei. They are more apparent in nodules.

PLASMACYTOID DENDRITIC CELLS

Definition. Proliferations of *plasmacytoid dendritic cells* (pDCs), formerly known as plasmacytoid monocytes, are an uncommon reactive finding in lymph nodes. Although seen more frequently with some specific etiologies (e.g., Kikuchi-Fujimoto lymphadenitis), they may be seen in a variety of circumstances.

General Features. Originally described by Lennert and Remmele (54), these cells came to be identified as T-cell–associated plasma cells, with the terminology subsequently clarified as plasmacytoid T cells, based on ultrastructural studies (52,53). Later studies with immunohistochemistry identified the enigmatic cell type to be derived from the monocyte/macrophage lineage, and they were subsequently renamed plasmacytoid monocytes (24,34,46). More recently, these cells have been identified as dendritic cell precursors (28), and so termed plasmacytoid dendritic cells (pDCs).

pDCs mature into interferon-producing cells, which are derived from bone marrow hematopoietic progenitor cells (55). They migrate to the T-cell zones of lymph nodes, mucosal-associated lymphoid tissue, and the marginal zone regions of spleens. They appear to play a role in T-cell activation as well as production of large amounts of interferon-α during viral infections (10,25,55).

Clinical Features. pDCs increase in a variety of reactive conditions including those due to specific as well as nonspecific etiologies. Some of the benign adenopathies associated with proliferations of pDCs include tuberculosis, sarcoidosis, Kikuchi-Fujimoto disease, and hyaline-vascular Castleman disease (25). In addition, a variety of dermatologic conditions are associated with accumulations of pDCs, including lymphocytic infiltrate of Jessner, lupus erythematosus, psoriasis, and contact dermatitis (25). An important consideration is the proliferation of pDCs in association with myeloproliferative disorders, especially chronic myelomonocytic leukemia. A tumor thought to be of pDC derivation has been identified; termed *CD4/CD56-positive hematodermic neoplasm*, or alternatively, *CD4/CD56-positive blastic neoplasm*, this entity is an aggressive malignancy with leukemic, bone marrow, and skin involvement. The tumor cells share immunophenotypic features with benign pDCs, with the addition of CD56 expression and occasional terminal deoxynucleotidyltransferase (TdT) expression.

Microscopic Findings. pDCs are slightly larger than lymphocytes, and have a round, oval, or indented nucleus; fine chromatin; and inconspicuous nucleoli (fig. 5-45). They have moderate amounts of pink cytoplasm and well-defined cytoplasmic borders. They are most easily observed as clusters of cells. Tingible body macrophages are often associated with clusters of pDCs. These clusters are frequently in the parafollicular areas, often near high endothelial venules. Individual pDCs are distributed throughout tonsils, lymph nodes, and thymus. In spleens, they are located in the periarteriolar regions or at the border of the marginal zones.

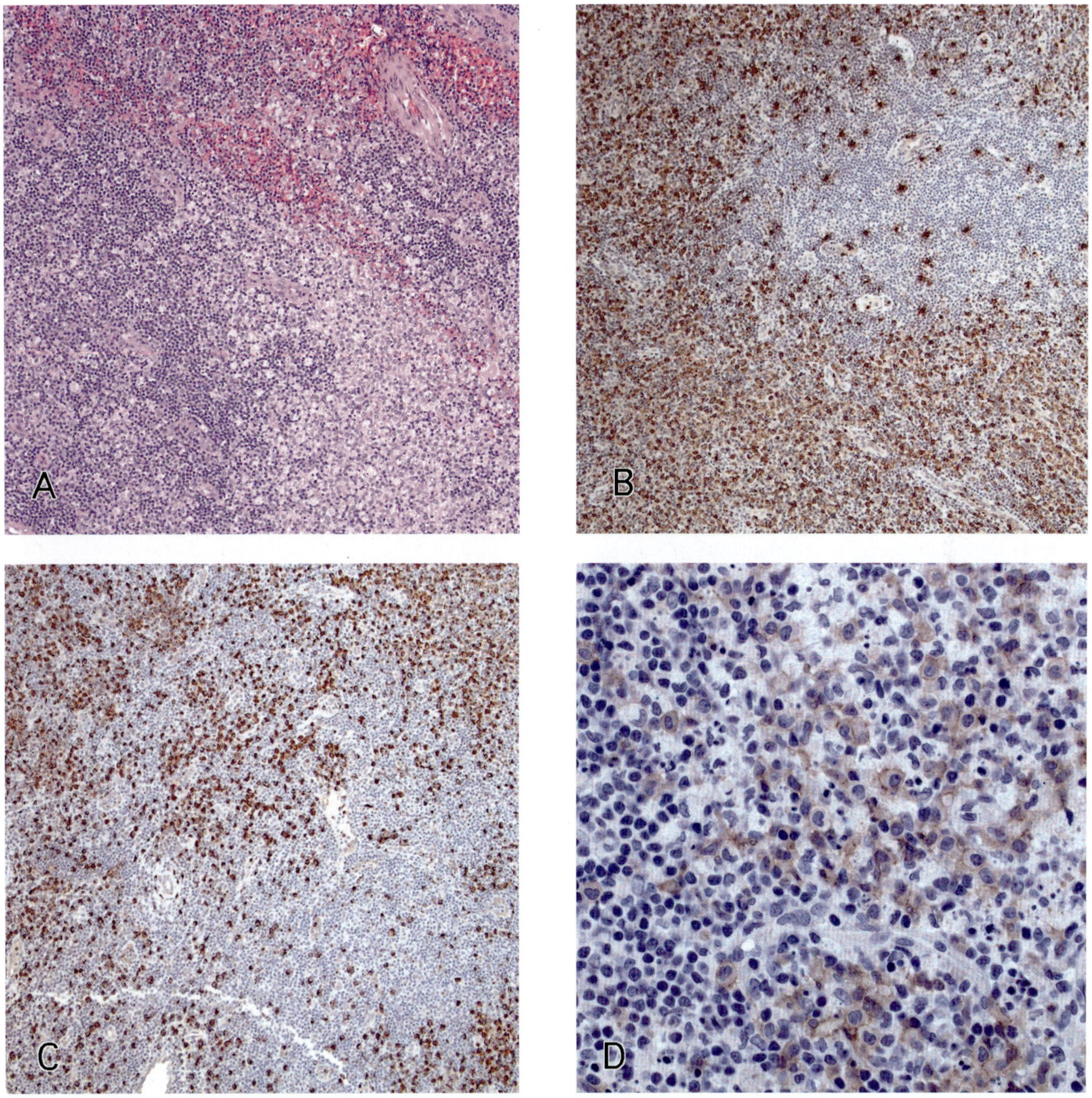

Figure 5-46

IMMUNOHISTOCHEMICAL REACTIVITY OF PLASMACYTOID DENDRITIC CELLS

Plasmacytoid dendritic cells in this case of Kikuchi-Fujimoto disease (A) are positive for lysozyme (B), CD68 (C), and CD123 (D).

The immunophenotype is distinctive, but only taken in a broader context. Individual stains that are positive underlie the previous misclassification of the unusual cell type (fig. 5-46). Perhaps most helpful in identifying pDCs is the following phenotype: CD3-, CD4+, CD68+, and CD123+. Other stains that help confirm the identity of pDC (but could equally likely cause confusion under less than optimal circumstances) include: CD1-, CD31+, CD43+, CD45RA+, CD45RB+, CD45RO-, cutaneous lymphocyte antigen (CLA)+, granzyme B+, lysozyme-, myeloperoxidase-, perforin-, TCL-1+, TIA-1-, T cell receptor α/β-, and T-cell receptor γ/δ- (25). pDCs do not have evidence of T-cell or immunoglobulin heavy chain gene rearrangements.

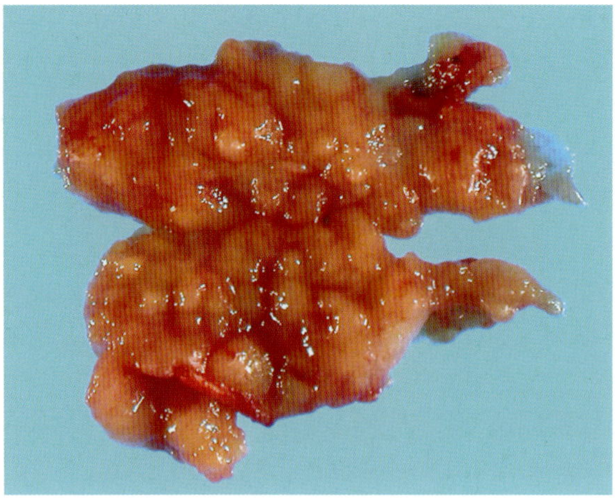

Figure 5-47

NECROTIZING LYMPHADENITIS

Small foci of chalky, yellow necrosis are seen in this case of necrotizing granulomatous lymphadenitis. (Courtesy of Peter Banks, Charlotte, NC.)

NECROTIZING LYMPHADENITIS

Definition. *Necrotizing lymphadenitis* is defined as focal or geographic areas of necrosis in a lymph node, with an organized cellular response to the reaction. This is in contrast to infarctive necrosis of lymph nodes, which is discussed later in this chapter.

General Features. Necrotizing lymphadenitis is a rare finding associated with several specific etiologies that should be evaluated when possible (Table 5-8). In some cases, however, it is not possible to render a specific diagnosis based on morphologic findings alone, and a diagnosis of necrotizing lymphadenitis may be used.

The cellular reaction to necrosis varies, depending on the underlying etiology. *Necrotizing granulomatous lymphadenitis* can be differentiated from *suppurative lymphadenitis*. In the former, an organized granulomatous response is seen in the lymph node, surrounding the areas of necrosis. This type of response occurs with cat-scratch disease and tuberculous lymphadenitis. In contrast, suppurative lymphadenitis is seen in lymph nodes with bacterial infections.

Microscopic Findings. Areas of necrosis are easily recognizable at low magnification by their eosinophilic character and lack of distinct nuclei (fig. 5-47). In some cases, closer examination reveals the composition of the necrotic areas.

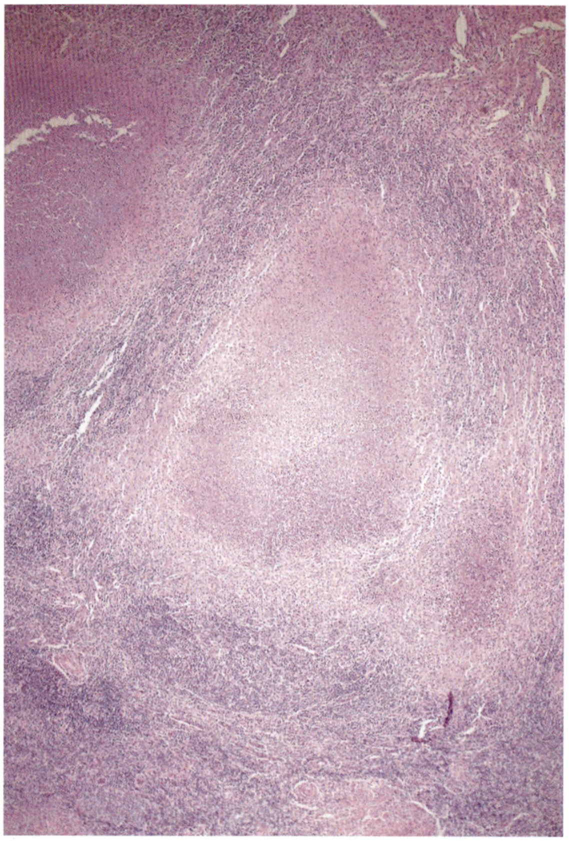

Figure 5-48

NECROTIZING GRANULOMATOUS LYMPHADENITIS

As the name implies, there is a combination of necrosis with a surrounding rim of granulomatous inflammation, as in this case of cat-scratch disease.

Masses of neutrophils and cellular debris are more characteristic of suppurative lesions. An organized epithelioid macrophage reaction, surrounding an area of necrosis, is more characteristic of a granulomatous reaction (fig. 5-48). Sometimes, these findings overlap.

Because several of the specific etiologies associated with necrosis are infectious, it may be appropriate to perform histochemical stains in such cases. A Warthin-Starry or other silver stain is useful to evaluate for cat-scratch disease, although the immunohistochemical stain for the causative organism, *Bartonella henselae,* is more sensitive and specific. AFB stains are appropriate for mycobacterial infections. A GMS stain may be used to evaluate for fungal infections. Immunohistochemical stains for other organisms or viruses (EBV, herpes) may be appropriate.

Table 5-8

SPECIFIC ETIOLOGIES ASSOCIATED WITH NECROTIZING LYMPHADENITIS

Cat-scratch disease
Tularemia
Lymphogranuloma venereum
Other bacterial infections

Viral infections
  Epstein-Barr virus
  Herpes lymphadenitis
  Other viruses

Kikuchi-Fujimoto disease

Differential Diagnosis. Necrotizing lymphadenitis must always be considered as a descriptive diagnosis, which excludes other, more specific diagnoses associated with known etiologies (Table 5-8). It is distinct from lymph node infarction, which is discussed in a later section. The features of cat-scratch disease, Kikuchi-Fujimoto disease, and lymphogranuloma venereum are discussed in the following chapters.

PROGRESSIVE TRANSFORMATION OF GERMINAL CENTERS

Definition. *Progressive transformation of germinal centers* (PTGCs) refers to a morphologic appearance consisting of large lymphoid nodules, typically in a background of hyperplastic follicles. These large nodules are composed of numerous small B cells, with clusters or islands of larger, germinal center type lymphocytes in the more central portions. PTGC is thought to arise from an aberrant or unusual expression of the immune response.

Clinical Features. PTGC is a self-limited phenomenon involving less than 5 percent of hyperplastic follicles (39). *Generalized PTGC,* also known as *florid PTGC,* is a rare condition that usually occurs in young men. The process is characterized by the expansion of the follicle and subsequent migration of mantle cells into the central portion of the germinal center, causing its fragmentation. This eventually results in islands of germinal center cells, separated into small nodules and divided by populations of mantle cells. Disruption and dissolution of the follicular dendritic cell network ultimately lead to fragmentation and dissolution of the germinal center structure. This process may ultimately be due to an abnormal proliferation of germinal center T cells.

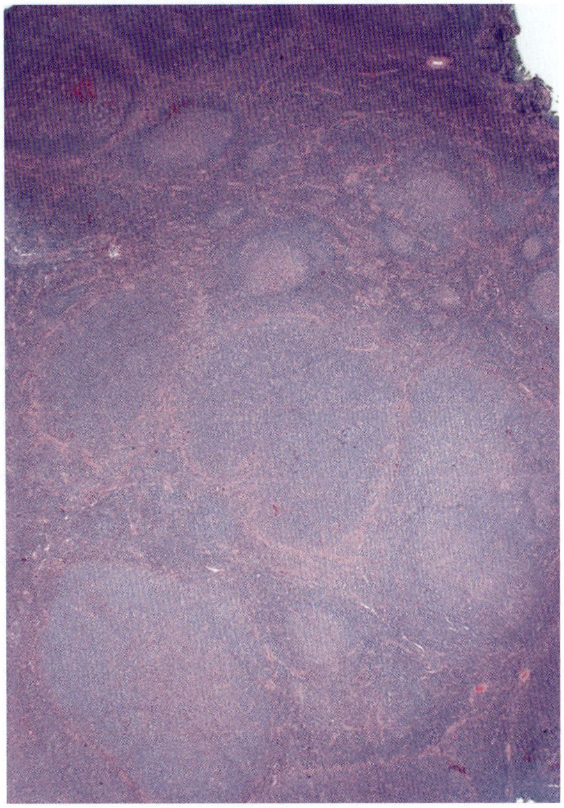

Figure 5-49

PROGRESSIVE TRANSFORMATION OF GERMINAL CENTER

Progressively transformed germinal centers have numerous small lymphocytes, sparse residual follicle center cells, and typical reactive germinal centers.

Microscopic Findings. PTGCs are made up of enlarged, ill-defined germinal centers that are composed primarily of small lymphocytes that are predominantly mantle zone cells (fig. 5-49) (11,65,66). The B-cell nature may be demonstrated by immunoreactivity with antibodies to CD20 (figs. 5-50, 5-51). Occasional follicle center and dendritic reticulum cells are also present.

PTGC may be a nonspecific finding in reactive lymph nodes. It is also described in association with Hodgkin lymphoma, especially the nodular lymphocyte-predominant type (NLPHL) (11,65,66). In this setting, PTGC occurs before, with, or after the diagnosis of the lymphoma.

Differential Diagnosis. The most significant entities in the differential diagnosis are NLPHL

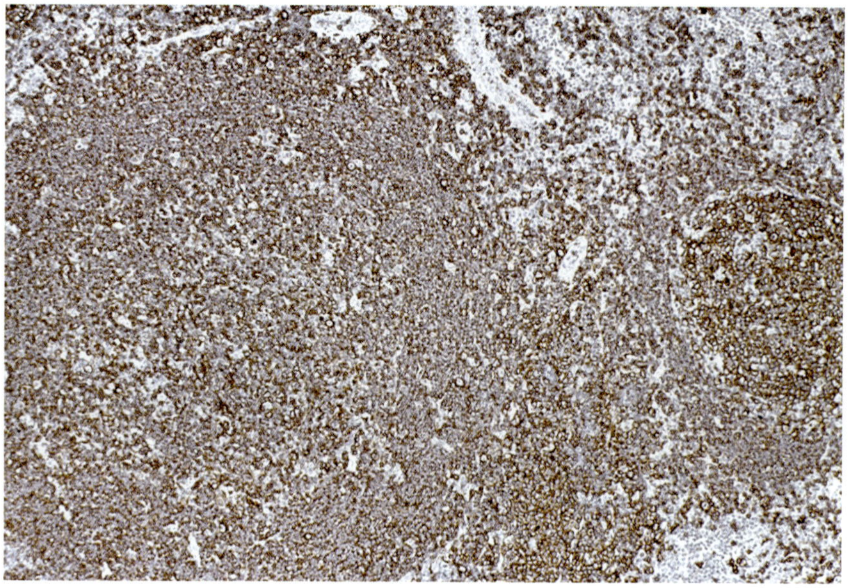

Figure 5-50

PROGRESSIVE TRANSFORMATION OF GERMINAL CENTER

CD20 is reactive in this example of a progressively transformed germinal center.

and lymphocyte-rich classic Hodgkin lymphoma (LRCHL). The morphologic similarities between PTGC, NLPHL, and LRCHL are significant (figs. 5-51, 5-52). Each is composed of large nodules, composed of predominantly small, blue, mature lymphocytes, with larger lymphocytes within the central portion. An important initial consideration is the degree of involvement in the lymph node and the composition of the background. It is relatively rare to have only single or rare scattered nodules in Hodgkin lymphoma, while this is typical in PTGC; however, partial involvement can occur, although rarely, in Hodgkin lymphoma. Furthermore, PTCG almost always occurs in a background of classic follicular hyperplasia, with many hyperplastic follicles and occasional follicles showing regressive features. This may also be seen in cases of Hodgkin lymphoma, but is rare.

Cytologically, the hallmark of NLPHL is the lymphocytic and histiocytic (L&H) cells, or "popcorn" cells. These individual malignant cells appear, under the best conditions, quite distinctive from other surrounding cells. They are extremely large, and have open, vesicular nuclei, frequently with multiple lobations, and moderate amounts of pale cytoplasm. Other forms are similar to classic Reed-Sternberg cells. Unfortunately, ideal conditions are rarely obtained, and the neoplastic cells often have features that overlap with those of large dendritic cells or centroblasts.

Immunohistochemistry is used to distinguish between PTGC, NLPHL and LRCHL in difficult cases. Typical stains to evaluate Hodgkin lymphoma (CD3, CD20, CD15, CD30, and CD45) should be used (Table 5-9). Other stains may be necessary or useful depending on individual circumstances. Perhaps the most critical stain for interpretation is CD20. In NLPHL, the individual L&H cells are strikingly positive, but are surrounded by a collar of nonstaining small lymphocytes. These cells are specialized germinal center T cells, and can be highlighted by CD3 and often CD57, giving a target or ring appearance of staining around the large, nonstaining neoplastic cells. LRCHL is often mistaken for NLPHL by histologic examination alone, but the large cells have the typical staining pattern of classic Hodgkin lymphoma (CD15+, CD30+, CD45-). The large cells in PTGC are negative for most stains, in the case of dendritic cells, or stain as B cells (CD20+). In contrast to NLPHL, these cells are surrounded by small B cells, without the nonstaining collar of T cells.

Another possible neoplastic mimic of PTGC is the floral variant of follicular lymphoma (fig. 5-53). This variant has large numbers of small, mature mantle type B cells, which invade and invaginate the neoplastic follicles. In contrast to the cells of PTGC, the floral variant of follicular lymphoma has neoplastic features that include monotony of the follicle center cells, lack of tingible body macrophages, and other

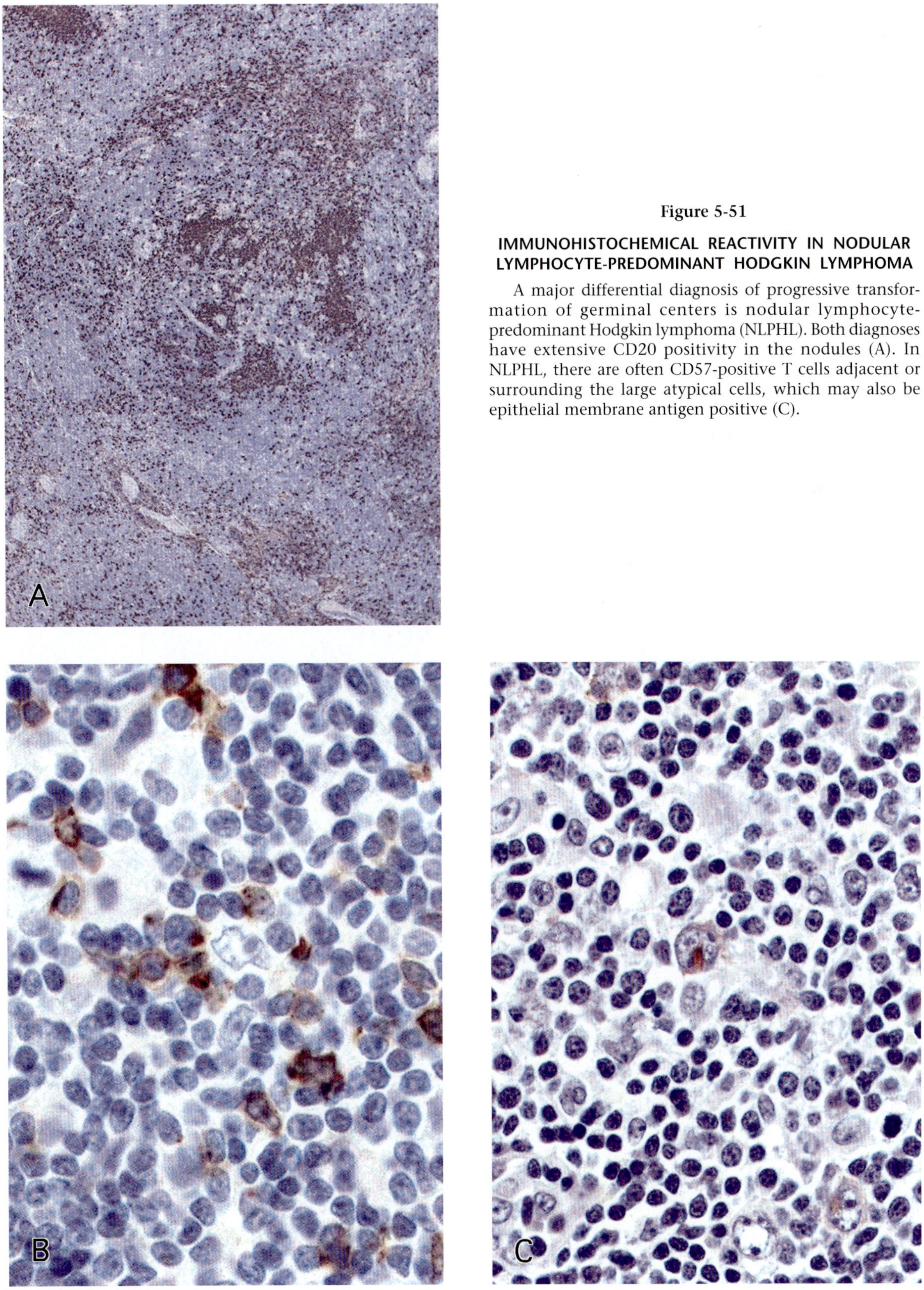

Figure 5-51

IMMUNOHISTOCHEMICAL REACTIVITY IN NODULAR LYMPHOCYTE-PREDOMINANT HODGKIN LYMPHOMA

A major differential diagnosis of progressive transformation of germinal centers is nodular lymphocyte-predominant Hodgkin lymphoma (NLPHL). Both diagnoses have extensive CD20 positivity in the nodules (A). In NLPHL, there are often CD57-positive T cells adjacent or surrounding the large atypical cells, which may also be epithelial membrane antigen positive (C).

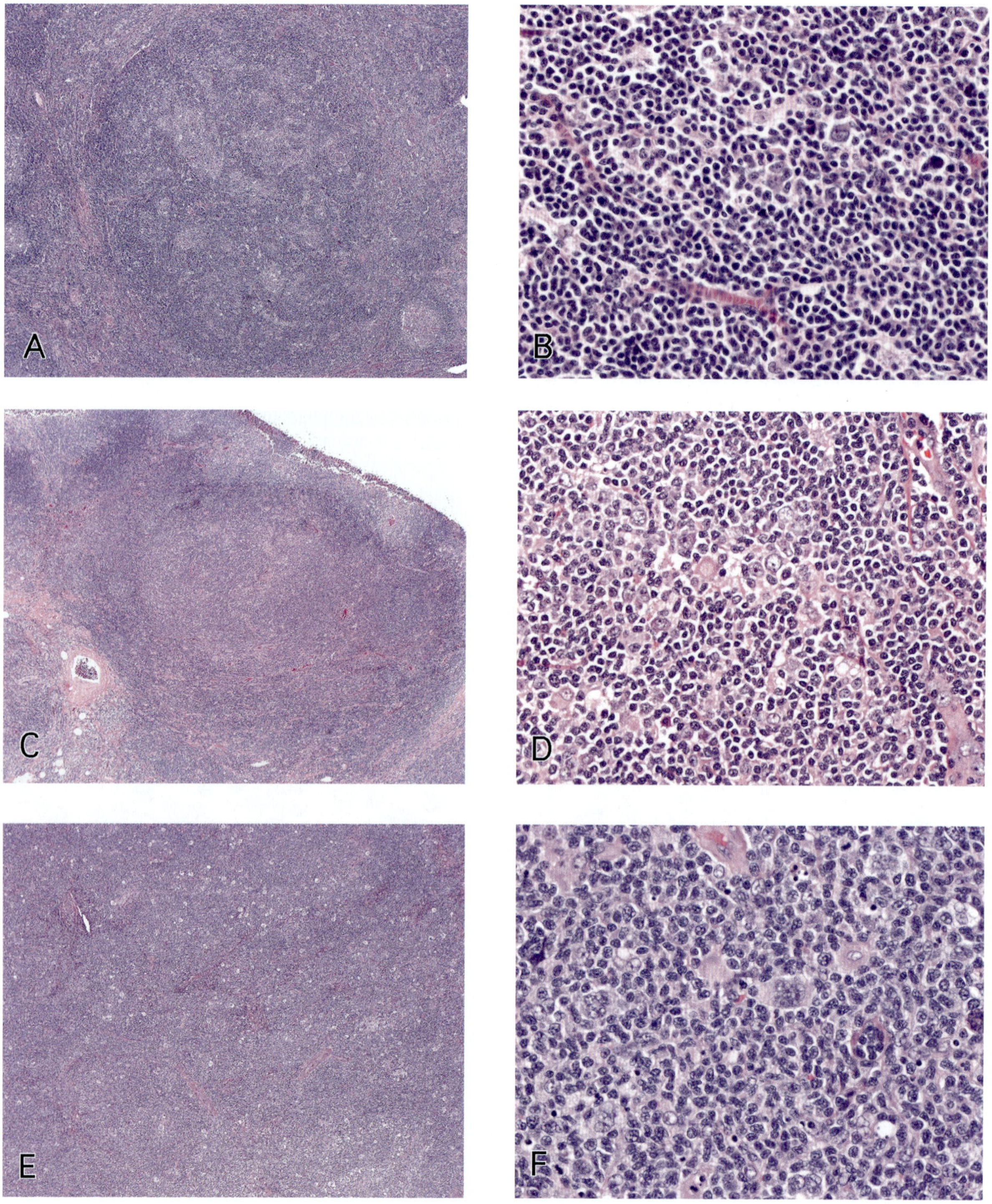

Figure 5-52

COMPARISON OF PROGRESSIVE TRANSFORMATION OF GERMINAL CENTERS, NODULAR LYMPHOCYTE-PREDOMINANT HODGKIN LYMPHOMA, AND LYMPHOCYTE-RICH CLASSIC HODGKIN LYMPHOMA

Low and high magnification images of progressively transformed germinal centers (A,B), NLPHL (C,D), and lymphocyte-rich classic Hodgkin lymphoma (E,F). Although there are some apparent histologic differences, immunohistochemical staining differentiates these processes.

Table 5-9

STAINING PATTERNS IN CELLS OF PROGRESSIVE TRANSFORMATION OF GERMINAL CENTERS (PTGC), NODULAR LYMPHOCYTE-PREDOMINANT HODGKIN LYMPHOMA (NLPHL), AND LYMPHOCYTE-RICH CLASSIC HODGKIN LYMPHOMA (LRCHL)

	PTGC	NLPHL	LRCHL
CD20	Diffuse positive	Positive in L&H[a] cells	Negative in RS cells
CD3	Scattered small cells	Positive in cells surrounding L&H cells ("collar")	Scattered positive cells
CD15	Negative	Negative in L&H cells	Positive in RS cells
CD45	Positive	Positive in L&H cells	Negative in RS cells
CD57	Rare cells positive	Often positive in cells surrounding L&H cells	Negative in RS cells

[a]L&H = lymphocytic/histiocytic; RS = Reed-Sternberg.

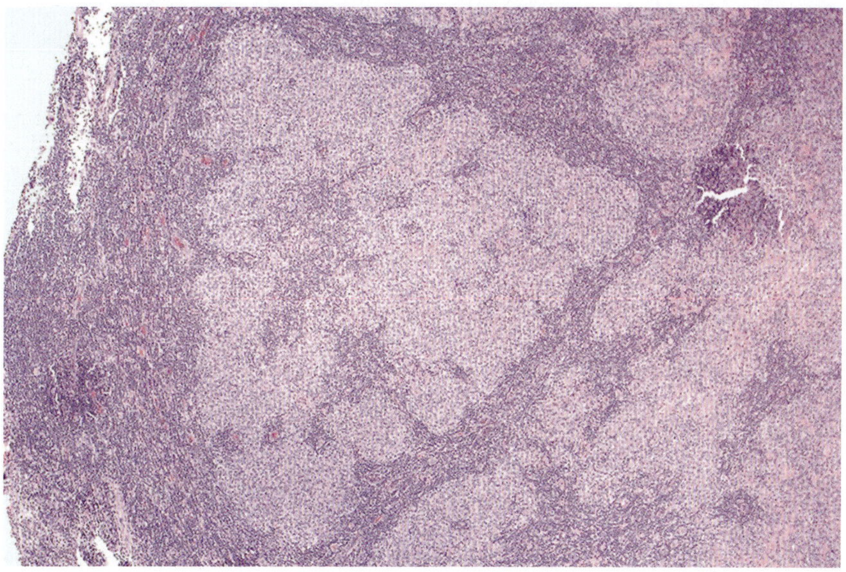

Figure 5-53

FOLLICULAR LYMPHOMA, FLORAL VARIANT

The neoplastic follicle is irregular in shape; the outer border is indented by small, non-neoplastic lymphocytes.

characteristic features (see discussion of follicular hyperplasia versus follicular lymphoma earlier in this chapter).

Treatment and Prognosis. In most circumstances, PTCG is a self-limited condition which regresses spontaneously; however, it may rarely persist or recur. Because of the associations with subsequent lymphoma development, patients with PTGC should be followed closely. If there is recurrent adenopathy, or significant changes in the size of persistent adenopathy, additional biopsies should be evaluated.

REGRESSIVE CHANGES IN GERMINAL CENTERS

Definition. *Regressive changes in germinal centers* are characterized by small, compact, well-circumscribed B-cell nodules that retain their stromal architecture, but have lost most, or all, of their germinal center lymphocytes. Although these findings are commonly associated with hyaline-vascular Castleman disease, they can be seen in other conditions.

General Features. Regressed follicles are presumed to be evidence of the completion or termination of the immune response of a follicle. The depletion of germinal center cells may be due to persistent exposure to potent antigenic stimuli, EBV infection, longstanding connective tissue disease, nodal irradiation, systemic immunosuppression or chemotherapy, syphilis, HIV/AIDS adenopathy, and of course, hyaline-vascular Castleman disease (39,93).

Microscopic Findings. Regressive transformation of germinal centers refers to atretic or small follicles. The follicles often have concentric layers of small, mature mantle cells (fig. 5-54). The central portion of the follicle may have

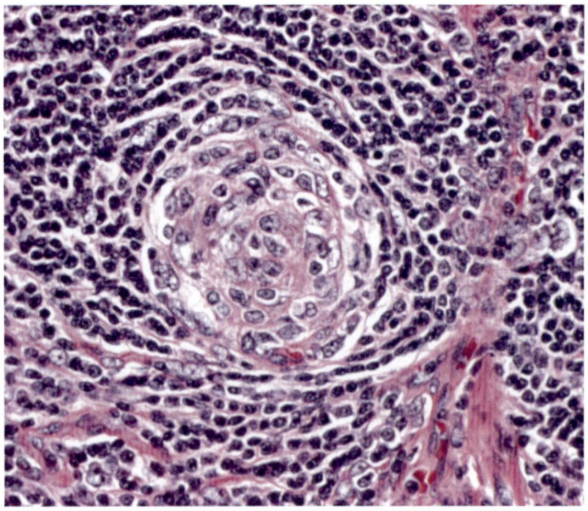

Figure 5-54

REGRESSIVE CHANGES IN GERMINAL CENTER, LYMPH NODE

High magnification of a regressed follicle shows depletion of the lymphocytes and prominence of stromal components, including follicular dendritic cells.

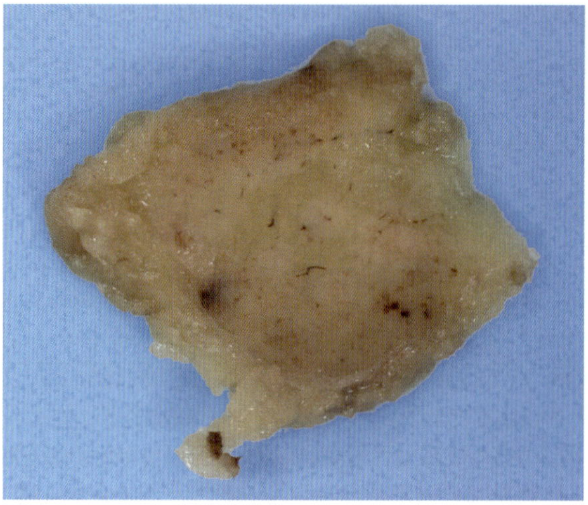

Figure 5-55

FATTY TRANSFORMATION OF LYMPH NODE

Gross appearance of a lymph node with fatty replacement shows the shiny yellow appearance of fat, but the vague outline of the residual lymph node can be appreciated by the slight pink-tan coloration.

a few residual lymphocytes, plasma cells, and larger cells with more open, delicate cytoplasm. Follicular dendritic cells are often the most prominent residual component of regressed follicles, and are revealed by staining for CD21. Frequently, small, penetrating hyalinized vessels are seen in the regressed follicles.

FATTY TRANSFORMATION OF LYMPH NODES

Definition. The partial or complete replacement of the structure of a lymph node by benign, mature fat is referred to as *fatty transformation of lymph node*.

General Features. The perinodal adipose tissue has different properties than non-nodal fat, including the composition of the fatty acids and the response to cytokines and endocrine stimulation (64). These differences in lipid are probably due to an ability to make polyunsaturated fatty acids available to immune cells almost instantly without disrupting the metabolism of the entire body. The fatty changes in the lymph nodes are probably related to these underlying differences in lipid metabolism and the state of immune function in an individual.

Clinical Features. Fatty transformation of lymph nodes appears to be an age- and location-related phenomenon. By far, the most frequent locations of fatty transformation are the femoral/inguinal region and axillary lymph nodes. By radiologic examination, fatty lymph nodes are easily identified by their difference in density from normal lymph nodes. Rarely, fatty lymph nodes can clinically mimic lymphomas (75).

Gross Findings. Fatty lymph nodes appear as well-circumscribed nodules with a yellow, greasy, lobulated cut surface (fig. 5-55). A thin rim of tan residual lymphoid tissue or remnants of a thin fibrous capsule may be seen.

Microscopic Findings. Microscopic examination of lymph nodes with fatty transformation reveals replacement of the lymph node structure by unremarkable adipocytes (fig. 5-56) (90). The residual stromal architecture may be present to varying degrees. A thin rim of lymphocytes or lymphoid structures may be present at the periphery of the node. The fibrous capsule or preservation of the pericapsular sinus may be the only way to recognize that the nodular structure is, in fact, the remnant of a lymph node.

Differential Diagnosis. Fatty changes in lymph nodes are usually easily identified. Of academic interest is the differential diagnosis of a benign process of transformation to fat in a lymph node versus the development of a

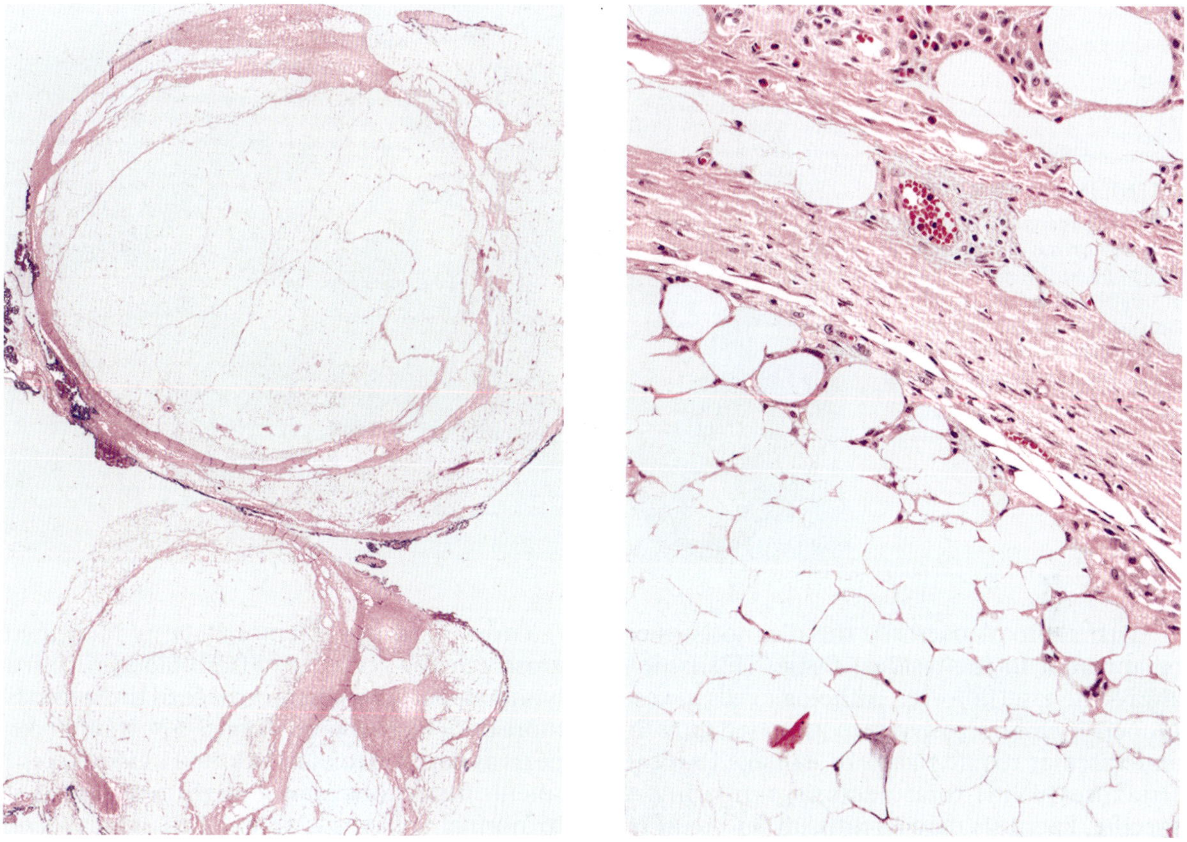

Figure 5-56

FATTY TRANSFORMATION OF LYMPH NODE

The architecture of the lymph node is maintained, including the capsule, but the parenchymal portion is replaced by mature adipocytes.

benign, neoplastic proliferation of fat, such as lipoma (see chapter 18).

HEMORRHAGE AND INFARCTION

Definition. *Hemorrhage* is a common finding in lymph nodes or spleen, and is most often related to iatrogenic issues associated with lymph node biopsy or splenectomy. *Infarction* refers to partial or complete, spontaneous, coagulative necrosis of lymphoid tissues.

Clinical Features. Hemorrhage is a common finding in sampled lymph nodes. In most circumstances, this finding is incidental, and usually is due to issues of handling or sampling. Splenic hemorrhage is also common, and is seen in many removed spleens, especially those removed because of associated trauma. On occasion, hemorrhage in lymph nodes or spleen is due to the underlying pathology, as in some vascular lesions, or as a result of a pathologic process that damages vessels, as seen in metastases in the spleen. Hemorrhage in lymph nodes and spleen is nonspecific, and although seen in association with some specific pathologies, should not be used as a strong diagnostic criterion.

Complete lymph node infarction is rare. Many etiologies are associated with lymph node infarction. It can occur in association with a variety of benign conditions including infections, autoimmune disorders, systemic/vascular diseases, trauma, and medical procedures (e.g., fine needle aspiration biopsy). However, the importance of recognizing lymph node infarction lies in its other, more ominous, associations, such as lymphomas and other epithelial and nonepithelial malignancies. Lymph node infarction has proven to be a clinical presentation of lymphoma in 27 to 89 percent of cases (13,60,80).

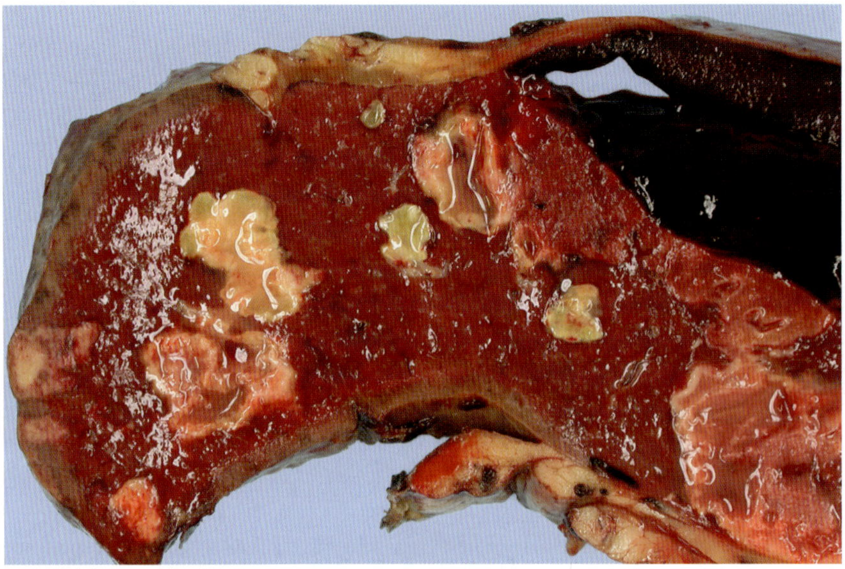

Figure 5-57

RECENT INFARCTION, SPLEEN

Splenic infarction has a bright red, hemorrhagic appearance, compared to the dark red color of unaffected spleen (right). In addition to recent infarction, there are several abscesses in this spleen, characterized by irregular yellow-gray foci.

With subtotal necrosis, the diagnosis may be apparent in the residual tissue. This is not always the case, however; pathologic cells have a propensity for necrosis due to increased growth and vascular requirements or damage to local structures. With total necrosis, rendering a specific diagnosis may be difficult and require a careful, systematic approach.

When dealing with necrotic tissue, evaluating any residual viable tissue for evidence of disease is important. The lack of pathology in viable tissue, however, does not rule out the presence of a pathologic process, as outlined above. Careful evaluation of the clinical history and laboratory studies, and communication with clinicians may yield a likely cause, or at least minimize an expensive, but potentially fruitless work-up. Finally, performance of immunohistochemical stains on the necrotic tissue may yield important information in guiding further biopsies or treatment. Several studies have been performed on necrotic tissues, and some antigenic reactivity is retained, depending on the antibody used and the qualities of the sampled tissues. In any circumstance, immunohistochemical stains performed on necrotic tissue must be interpreted carefully. Nonspecific staining may occur, nonreactivity is common, and only the most basic interpretations can be made, with limited reliability. In all cases, attempts should be made to procure additional, viable tissue for more complete evaluation.

Gross Findings. Hemorrhage is identified grossly by the presence of fresh blood within a lymph node. Recent hemorrhage in the spleen is more difficult to identify (fig. 5-57). It often appears as dark red to black, clotted blood. Recent splenic infarctions appear bright red compared to normal spleen. As splenic infarcts resolve, they become firm and tan, and are often wedged shaped, belying their frequent traumatic origins (fig. 5-58).

Grossly, areas of necrosis are visible as uniform, yellow or gray areas. They are more apparent if there is adjacent viable tissue. Necrotic tissue may have a discohesive, crumbly quality (grumous).

Microscopic Features. Hemorrhage is easily identified in tissues. Intact red blood cells are seen on hematoxylin and eosin (H&E)-stained sections as ovoid or round, bright pink structures. In lymph nodes, red blood cells are seen only in small numbers, and large areas of red blood cells usually indicate hemorrhage. Areas of resolved hemorrhage appear as pale, hypocellular areas of bland spindle cells with interstitial fibrosis. In the spleen, areas of remote hemorrhage are identified by the deposition of hemosiderin pigment, usually in perivascular areas. These areas are termed Gamna-Gandy bodies (fig. 5-59).

The histopathologic appearance of necrosis is familiar to most pathologists. Areas of necrosis are pale pink. There may be focal fragments of

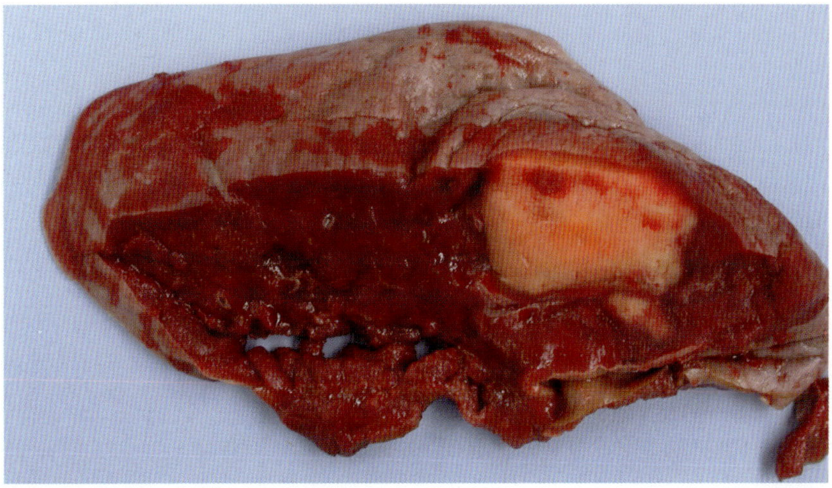

Figure 5-58

REMOTE INFARCTION, SPLEEN

The remote infarction in the spleen is firm, yellow-tan, and wedge shaped.

purple nuclear debris, but these are present only in cases of recent infarction (fig. 5-60). Depending on the remoteness of the infarction and the strength of the associated inflammatory/macrophage response, the cell outlines are variably intact ("ghost cells"). More remote infarcts show only uniform fields of amorphous eosinophilic material without visible cell outlines. In some cases, residual viable cells are present. These may be stromal cells, such as fibroblasts or endothelial cells, which are relatively more resistant to hypoxic effects than the lymphoid elements, or they may be inflammatory agents or regenerative cells that have arrived after the infarctive event. Typically, if viable lymphoid cells are present, they are in areas that are adjacent to blood vessels (in cases of tissue hypoxia) or distant from the site of damage (as in infarction after needle biopsy).

Ancillary Studies. Several studies have addressed the usefulness of antibody combinations and antigen preservation in infarcted lymph nodes (44,45,60,80,86). The conclusions drawn from these studies include: CD79a staining is better preserved than CD20 staining; the T cell stains CD3, CD45RO, and CD43 are all relatively well preserved; and cytokeratins and epithelial membrane antigen are all variably preserved (80). Other B-cell markers, such as bcl-6 and bcl-2, are poorly preserved (45). Although these are useful guidelines, any results, whether positive or negative, should be evaluated with care and with the understanding that they may not be valid in a particular case.

Gene rearrangement studies have also been successfully applied to infarcted tissues (51,86). The same caveats to interpretation as those in immunohistochemistry should be considered.

PERISPLENITIS ("SUGAR-COATED" SPLEEN)

Definition. Fibrotic, hyaline thickening of the splenic capsule is referred to as *perisplenitis* or *sugar-coated spleen*. It occurs more frequently in patients with portal hypertension. A variety of names have been historically used for this process including zuckergussmilz, splenic capsular sclerosis, and perisplenitis chronica cartilaginea (in response to the cartilaginous appearance of the plaques) (58).

Clinical Features. Perisplenitis is a paucicellular plaque formed on the surface of the spleen. It is most commonly seen in patients with portal hypertension due to a liver disease such as cirrhosis. Other causes of fibrocongestive splenomegaly are also associated with perisplenitis. Perisplenitis is also associated with pulmonary tuberculosis, pleural plaques, and asbestosis (58).

Gross Findings. Perisplenitis appears as a focal or diffuse lesion on the surface of the spleen. The lesion is pearly white to yellow, and of varying thickness (fig. 5-61). Moderate to severe thickening is considered to be greater than 0.33 mm (87).

Microscopic Findings. Perisplenitis consists of plaques of dense collagen on the outer surface of the true capsule of the spleen. Hemosiderin deposition and small vessels may be seen within the body of the plaques.

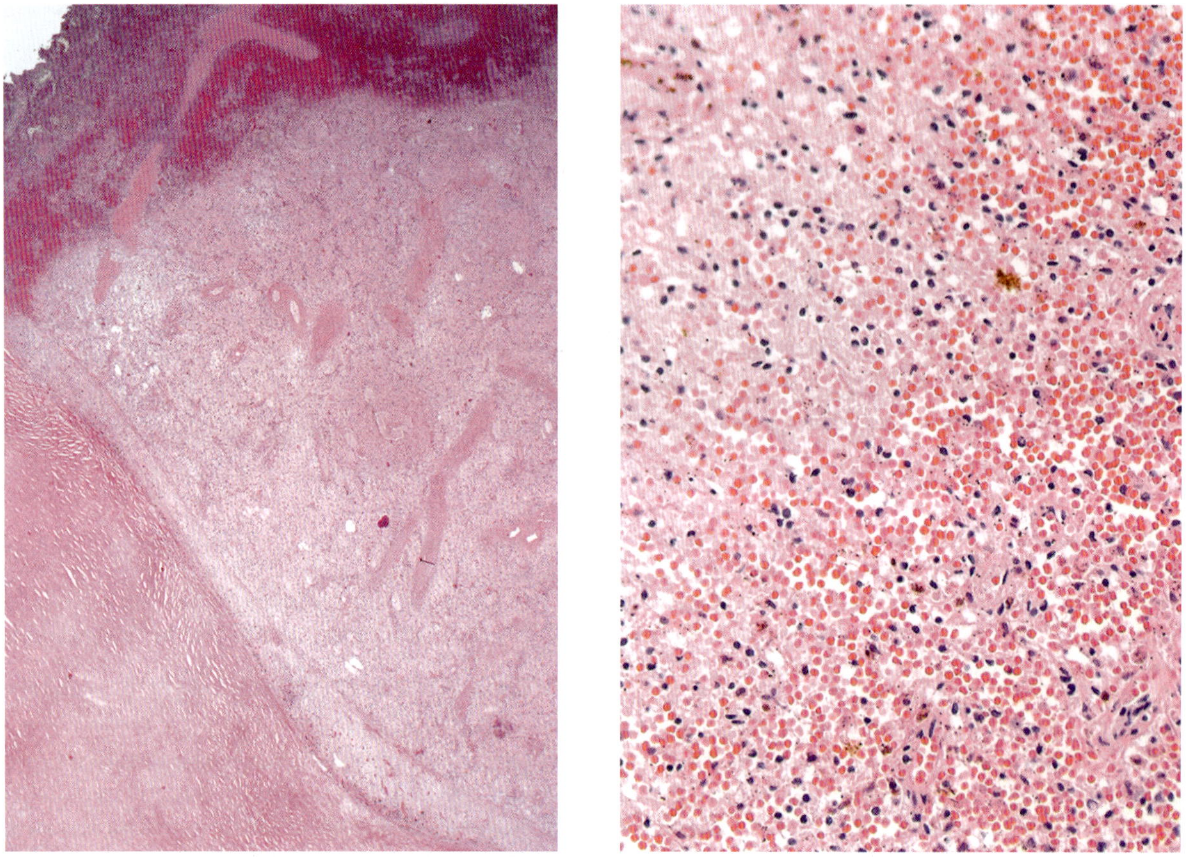

Figure 5-59

HEMORRHAGE AND INFARCTION, SPLEEN

Hemorrhage surrounds an infarcted spleen (left). Coagulative necrosis, with hemorrhage, is seen in this higher magnification image (right). Ghosts of the splenic sinuses are barely visible.

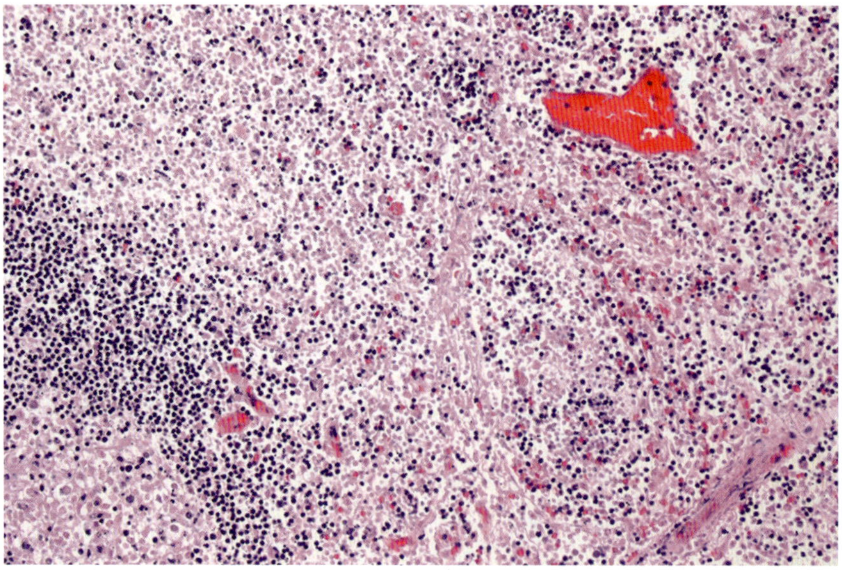

Figure 5-60

INFARCT, LYMPH NODE

The remnants of a partially viable germinal center are seen in the lower left corner, while most of the lymph node is necrotic. Note the prominence of vascular elements.

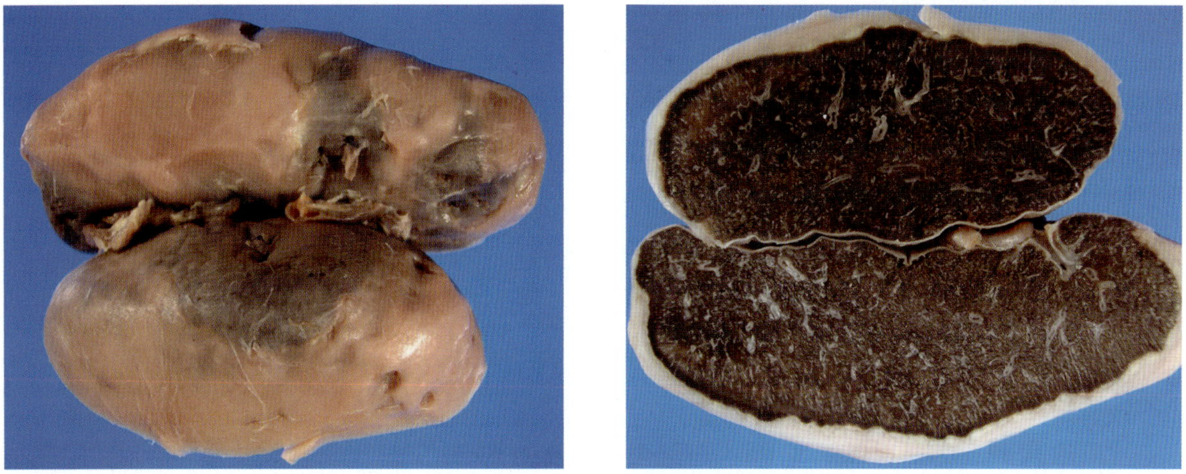

Figure 5-61

PERISPLENITIS ("SUGAR-COATED" SPLEEN)

The outer surface of spleen with extensive perisplenitis (left) shows the shiny, firm appearance, while the cut surface (right) shows the thick "sugar-coating" on the surface.

REFERENCES

1. Abbondanzo SL, Irey NS, Frizzera G. Dilantin-associated lymphadenopathy. Spectrum of histopathologic patterns. Am J Surg Pathol 1995;19:675-86.
2. Arista-Nasr J, Nuncio J, Martinez B. Atypical histiocytic infiltration simulating diffuse-type carcinoma in a gastric ulcer due to non-steroidal anti-inflammatory drugs. Pathol Oncol Res 2002;8:272-4.
3. Attygalle AD, Liu H, Shirali S, et al. A typical marginal zone hyperplasia of mucosa-associated lymphoid tissue: a reactive condition of childhood showing immunoglobulin lambda light-chain restriction. Blood 2004;104:3343-8.
4. Au WY, Horsman DE, Connors JM, Klasa RJ, Gascoyne RD. Cytogenetic findings in reactive lymphoid hyperplasia: significance of non-clonal t(3;14) and t(3;22). Am J Hematol 2002;70:133-8.
5. Bahler DW, Pindzola JA, Swerdlow SH. Splenic marginal zone lymphomas appear to originate from different B cell types. Am J Pathol 2002;161:81-8.
6. Bryant RJ, Banks PM, O'Malley DP. Ki67 staining pattern as a diagnostic tool in the evaluation of lymphoproliferative disorders. Histopathology 2006;48:505-15.
7. Burke JS, Colby TV. Dermatopathic lymphadenopathy. Comparison of cases associated and unassociated with mycosis fungoides. Am J Surg Pathol 1981;5:343-52.
8. Burke JS, Osborne BM. Localized reactive lymphoid hyperplasia of the spleen simulating malignant lymphoma. A report of seven cases. Am J Surg Pathol 1983;7:373-80.
9. Burke JS, Sheibani K, Rappaport H. Dermatopathic lymphadenopathy: an immunophenotypic comparison of cases associated and unassociated with mycosis fungoides. Am J Pathol 1986;123:256-63.
10. Cella M, Jarrossay D, Facchetti F, et al. Plasmacytoid monocytes migrate to inflamed lymph nodes and produce large amounts of type I interferon. Nat Med 1999;5:919-23.
11. Chang CC, Osipov V, Wheaton S, Tripp S, Perkins SL. Follicular hyperplasia, follicular lysis, and progressive transformation of germinal centers. A sequential spectrum of morphologic evolution in lymphoid hyperplasia. Am J Clin Pathol 2003;120:322-6.
12. Childs CC, Parham DM, Berard CW. Infectious mononucleosis. The spectrum of morphologic changes simulating lymphoma in lymph nodes and tonsils. Am J Surg Pathol 1987;11:122-32.

13. Cleary KR, Osborne BM, Butler JJ. Lymph node infarction foreshadowing malignant lymphoma. Am J Surg Pathol 1982;6:435-42.
14. Co DO, Hogan LH, Il-Kim S, Sandor M. T cell contributions to the different phases of granuloma formation. Immunol Lett 2004;92:135-42.
15. Cong P, Raffeld M, Teruya-Feldstein J, Sorbara L, Pittaluga S, Jaffe ES. In situ localization of follicular lymphoma: description and analysis by laser capture microdissection. Blood 2002;99:3376-82.
16. Cooper RA, Dawson PJ, Rambo ON. Dermatopathic lymphadenopathy: a clinicopathologic analysis of lymph node biopsy over a fifteen-year period. Calif Med 1967;106:170-5.
17. Davis RE, Warnke RA, Dorfman RF, Cleary ML. Utility of molecular genetic analysis for the diagnosis of neoplasia in morphologically and immunophenotypically equivocal hematolymphoid lesions. Cancer 1991;67:2890-9.
18. Delsol G, Gatter KC, Stein H, et al. Human lymphoid cells express epithelial membrane antigen. Implications for diagnosis of human neoplasms. Lancet 1984;2:1124-9.
19. De Petris G, Lev R, Siew S. Peritumoral and nodal muciphages. Am J Surg Pathol 1998;22:545-9.
20. De Wolf-Peeters C, Tierens A, Achten R. Normal histology and immunoarchitecture of the lymphohematopoietic system. In: Knowles DM, ed. Neoplastic hematopathology, 2nd ed. Philadelphia: Lippincott, William & Wilkins; 2001;271-305.
21. Dorfman RF, Remington JS. Value of lymph node biopsy in the diagnosis of acute acquired toxoplasmosis. N Engl J Med 1973;289:878-81.
22. Dorfman RF, Warnke R. Lymphadenopathy simulating the malignant lymphomas. Hum Pathol 1974;5:519-50.
23. Dunphy CH, Bee C, McDonald JW, Grosso LE. Incidental early detection of a splenic marginal zone lymphoma by polymerase chain reaction analysis of paraffin-embedded tissue. Arch Pathol Lab Med 1998;122:84-6.
24. Facchetti F, de Wolf-Peeters C, Mason DY, Pulford K, van den Oord JJ, Desmet VJ. Plasmacytoid T cells. Immunohistochemical evidence for their monocyte/macrophage origin. Am J Pathol 1988;133:15-21.
25. Facchetti F, Vermi W, Mason D, Colonna M. The plasmacytoid monocyte/interferon producing cells. Virchows Arch 2003;443:703-17.
26. Farhi DC, Ashfaq R. Splenic pathology after traumatic injury. Am J Clin Pathol 1996;105:474-8.
27. Frizzera G. The clinico-pathological expressions of Epstein-Barr virus infection in lymphoid tissues. Virchows Arch B Cell Pathol Incl Mol Pathol 1987;53:1-12.
28. Galibert L, Maliszewski CR, Vandenabeele S. Plasmacytoid monocytes/T cells: a dendritic cell lineage? Semin Immunol 2001;13:283-9.
29. Gould E, Perez J, Albores-Saavedra J, Legaspi A. Signet ring cell sinus histiocytosis. A previously unrecognized histologic condition mimicking metastatic adenocarcinoma in lymph nodes. Am J Clin Pathol 1989;92:509-12.
30. Gould E, Porto R, Albores-Saavedra J, Ibe MJ. Dermatopathic lymphadenitis. The spectrum and significance of its morphologic features. Arch Pathol Lab Med 1988;112:1145-50.
31. Harris S, Wilkins BS, Jones DB. Splenic marginal zone expansion in B-cell lymphomas of gastrointestinal mucosa-associated lymphoid tissue (MALT) is reactive and does not represent homing of neoplastic lymphocytes. J Pathol 1996;179:49-53.
32. Hartsock RJ. Postvaccinial lymphadenitis. Hyperplasia of lymphoid tissue that simulates malignant lymphomas. Cancer 1968;21:632-49.
33. Hassan NM, Neiman RS. The pathology of the spleen in steroid-treated immune thrombocytopenic purpura. Am J Clin Pathol 1985;84:433-8.
34. Horny HP, Feller AC, Horst HA, Lennert K. Immunocytology of plasmacytoid T cells: marker analysis indicates a unique phenotype of this enigmatic cell. Hum Pathol 1987;18:28-32.
35. Horsman DE, Gascoyne RD, Coupland RW, Coldman AJ, Adomat SA. Comparison of cytogenetic analysis, southern analysis, and polymerase chain reaction for the detection of t(14; 18) in follicular lymphoma. Am J Clin Pathol 1995;103:472-8.
36. Hunt JP, Chan JA, Samoszuk M, et al. Hyperplasia of mantle/marginal zone B cells with clear cytoplasm in peripheral lymph nodes. A clinicopathologic study of 35 cases. Am J Clin Pathol 2001;116:550-9.
37. Hurwitt E. Dermatopathic lymphadenitis: focal granulomatous lymphadenitis associated with chronic generalized skin disorders. J Invest Dermatol 1942;5:197-204.
38. Jaffe ES. Histiocytoses of lymph nodes: biology and differential diagnosis. Semin Diagn Pathol 1988;5:376-90.
39. Jones D. Dismantling the germinal center: comparing the processes of transformation, regression, and fragmentation of the lymphoid follicle. Adv Anat Pathol 2002;9:129-38.
40. Kamel OW, Gelb AB, Shibuya RB, Warnke RA. Leu 7 (CD57) reactivity distinguishes nodular lymphocyte predominance Hodgkin's disease from nodular sclerosing Hodgkin's disease, T-cell-rich B-cell lymphoma and follicular lymphoma. Am J Pathol 1993;142:541-6.

41. Karadeniz C, Oguz A, Ezer U, Ozturk G, Dursun A. The etiology of peripheral lymphadenopathy in children. Pediatr Hematol Oncol 1999;16:525-31.
42. Kojima M, Nakamura S, Itoh H, et al. Clinical implication of florid reactive follicular hyperplasia in Japanese patients 60 years or older: a study of 46 cases. J Surg Pathol 2005;13:175-80.
43. Kojima M, Nakamura S, Shimizu K, et al. Florid reactive follicular hyperplasia in elderly patients. A clinicopathological study of 23 cases. Pathol Res Pract 1998;194:391-7.
44. Kojima M, Nakamura S, Shimizu K, Yamane Y, Itoh H, Masawa N. Granulocytic sarcoma presenting with lymph node infarction at disease onset. APMIS 2003;111:1133-6.
45. Kojima M, Nakamura S, Yamane Y, et al. Antigen preservation in infarcted nodal B-cell lymphoma, with special reference to follicular center cell markers. Int J Surg Pathol 2004;12:251-5.
46. Koo CH, Mason DY, Miller R, Ben-Ezra J, Sheibani K, Rappaport H. Additional evidence that "plasmacytoid T-cell lymphoma" associated with chronic myeloproliferative disorders is of macrophage/monocyte origin. Am J Clin Pathol 1990;93:822-7.
47. Kroft SH, Singleton TP, Dahiya M, Ross CW, Schnitzer B, Hsi ED. Ruptured spleens with expanded marginal zones do not reveal occult B-cell clones. Mod Pathol 1997;10:1214-20.
48. Kuo T, Rosai J. Granulomatous inflammation in splenectomy specimens. Clinicopathologic study of 20 cases. Arch Pathol 1974;98:261-8.
49. Kussick SJ, Kalnoski M, Braziel RM, Wood BL. Prominent clonal B-cell populations identified by flow cytometry in histologically reactive lymphoid proliferations. Am J Clin Pathol 2004;121:464-72.
50. Laipply TC. Lipomelanotic reticular hyperplasia of lymph nodes: report of 6 cases. Arch Intern Med 1948;81:19-36.
51. Laszewski MJ, Belding PJ, Feddersen RM, et al. Clonal immunoglobulin gene rearrangement in the infarcted lymph node syndrome. Am J Clin Pathol 1991;96:116-20.
52. Lennert K, Mohri N. Malignant lymphomas other than Hodgkin's disease: histology, cytology, ultrastructure, immunology. New York: Springer-Verlag; 1977.
53. Lennert K, Kaiserling E, Muller-Hermelink HK. Letter: T-associated plasma-cells. Lancet 1975;1:1031-2.
54. Lennert K, Remmele W. [Karyometric research on lymph node cells in man. I. Germinoblasts, lymphoblasts and lymphocytes]. Acta Haematol 1958;19:99-113. [German]
55. Liu YJ. IPC: professional type 1 interferon-producing cells and plasmacytoid dendritic cell precursors. Annu Rev Immunol 2005;23:275-306.
56. Miller-Catchpole R, Variakojis D, Vardiman JW, Loew JM, Carter J. Cat scratch disease. Identification of bacteria in seven cases of lymphadenitis. Am J Surg Pathol 1986;10:276-81.
57. Mohrmann RL, Nathwani BN, Brynes RK, Taylor C, Hansmann M, Sheibani K. Morphologic criteria to distinguish malignant from reactive monocytoid B cell (MBC) proliferations. Mod Pathol 1991;4:79A.
58. Mollo F, Bellis D, Magnani C, Delsedime L, Andrion A. Hyaline splenic and hepatic plaques. Correlation with cirrhosis, pulmonary tuberculosis, and asbestos exposure. Arch Pathol Lab Med 1993;117:1017-21.
59. Neiman RS, Orazi A. Disorders of the spleen, 2nd ed. Philadelphia: WB Saunders; 1999.
60. Norton AJ, Ramsay AD, Isaacson PG. Antigen preservation in infarcted lymphoid tissue. A novel approach to the infarcted lymph node using monoclonal antibodies effective in routinely processed tissues. Am J Surg Pathol 1988;12:759-67.
61. Orazi A, O'Malley DP. Pathology of the spleen. In: Jaffe ES, Vardiman J, Harris NL, eds. Disorders of lymph nodes and spleen. Philadelphia: W.B. Saunders; 2006.
62. Orphanos V, Anagnostou D, Papadaki T, Maniatis GM, Athanassiadou A. Detection of gene rearrangements in reactive lymphoid processes. Leuk Lymphoma 1993;9:103-6.
63. Osborne BM, Butler JJ. Clinical implications of nodal reactive follicular hyperplasia in the elderly patient with enlarged lymph nodes. Mod Pathol 1991;4:24-30.
64. Pond CM. Long-term changes in adipose tissue in human disease. Proc Nutr Soc 2001;60:365-74.
65. Poppema S, Kaiserling E, Lennert K. Hodgkin's disease with lymphocytic predominance, nodular type (nodular paragranuloma) and progressively transformed germinal centres—a cytohistological study. Histopathology 1979;3:295-308.
66. Poppema S, Kaiserling E, Lennert K. Nodular paragranuloma and progressively transformed germinal centers. Ultrastructural and immunohistologic findings. Virchows Arch B Cell Pathol Incl Mol Pathol 1979;31:211-25.
67. Rodriguez-Garcia JL, Sanchez-Corral J, Martinez J, Bellas C, Aguado M, Serrano M. Phenytoin-induced benign lymphadenopathy with solid spleen lesions mimicking a malignant lymphoma. Ann Oncol 1991;2:443-5.
68. Sadek I, Greer W, Foyle A. Diagnosis of lymphoproliferative disorders: experience of a single institution in the long-term follow-up of discordant cases. Clin Invest Med 2000;23:366-75.

69. Said JW. AIDS-related lymphadenopathies. Semin Diagn Pathol 1988;5:365-75.
70. Schnitzer B. Reactive lymphoid hyperplasias. In: Jaffe ES, ed. Surgical pathology of the lymph nodes and related organs, 2nd ed. Philadelphia: W.B. Saunders; 1995:98-132.
71. Schroer KR, Franssila KO. Atypical hyperplasia of lymph nodes: a follow-up study. Cancer 1979;44:1155-63.
72. Segal GH, Perkins SL, Kjeldsberg CR. Benign lymphadenopathies in children and adolescents. Semin Diagn Pathol 1995;12:288-302.
73. Sheibani K, Fritz RM, Winberg CD, Burke JS, Rappaport H. "Monocytoid" cells in reactive follicular hyperplasia with and without multifocal histiocytic reactions: an immunohistochemical study of 21 cases including suspected cases of toxoplasmic lymphadenitis. Am J Clin Pathol 1984;81:453-8.
74. Silverberg SG, Frable WJ, Brooks JW. Sinus histiocytosis in non-diagnostic scalene lymph node biopsies. Cancer 1973;32:177-80.
75. Smith T. Fatty replacement of lymph nodes mimicking lymphoma relapse. Cancer 1986;58:2686-8.
76. Sohn CC, Sheibani K, Winberg CD, Rappaport H. Monocytoid B lymphocytes: their relation to the patterns of the acquired immunodeficiency syndrome (AIDS) and AIDS-related lymphadenopathy. Hum Pathol 1985;16:979-85.
77. Stein H, Bonk A, Tolksdorf G, Lennert K, Rodt H, Gerdes J. Immunohistologic analysis of the organization of normal lymphoid tissue and non-Hodgkin's lymphomas. J Histochem Cytochem 1980;28:746-60.
78. Stein K, Hummel M, Korbjuhn P, et al. Monocytoid B cells are distinct from splenic marginal zone cells and commonly derive from unmutated naive B cells and less frequently from postgerminal center B cells by polyclonal transformation. Blood 1999;94:2800-8.
79. Stein H, Mason DY, Gerdes J, et al. The expression of the Hodgkin's disease associated antigen Ki-1 in reactive and neoplastic lymphoid tissue: evidence that Reed-Sternberg cells and histiocytic malignancies are derived from activated lymphoid cells. Blood 1985;66:848-58.
80. Strauchen JA, Miller LK. Lymph node infarction. An immunohistochemical study of 11 cases. Arch Pathol Lab Med 2003;127:60-3.
81. Taylor JM, Spagnolo DV, Kay PH. B-cell target DNA quantity is a critical factor in the interpretation of B-cell clonality by PCR. Pathology 1997;29:309-12.
82. Tierens A, Delabie J, Michiels L, Vandenberghe P, De Wolf-Peeters C. Marginal-zone B cells in the human lymph node and spleen show somatic hypermutations and display clonal expansion. Blood 1999;93:226-34.
83. Tierens A, Delabie J, Pittaluga S, Driessen A, DeWolf-Peeters C. Mutation analysis of the rearranged immunoglobulin heavy chain genes of marginal zone cell lymphomas indicates an origin from different marginal zone B lymphocyte subsets. Blood 1998;91:2381-6.
84. Van den Oord JJ, De Wolf-Peeters C, Desmet VJ, Takahashi K, Ohtsuki Y, Akagi T. Nodular alteration of the paracortical area. An in situ immunohistochemical analysis of primary, secondary, and tertiary T-nodules. Am J Pathol 1985;120:55-66.
85. Van der Valk P, Meijer CJ. The histology of reactive lymph nodes. Am J Surg Pathol 1987;11:866-82.
86. Vega F, Lozano MD, Alcalde J, Pardo-Mindan FJ. Utility of immunophenotypic and immunogenotypic analysis in the study of necrotic lymph nodes. Virchows Arch 1999;434:245-8.
87. Wanless IR, Bernier V. Fibrous thickening of the splenic capsule. A response to chronic splenic congestion. Arch Pathol Lab Med 1983;107:595-9.
88. Weisenburger DD. Multicentric angiofollicular lymph node hyperplasia. Pathology of the spleen. Am J Surg Pathol 1988;12:176-81.
89. Weissman IL, Warnke R, Butcher EC, Rouse R, Levy R. The lymphoid system. Its normal architecture and the potential for understanding the system through the study of lymphoproliferative diseases. Hum Pathol 1978;9:25-45.
90. Werbin N. Fatty changes and metastases in axillary lymph nodes. J Surg Oncol 1984;25:145-7.
91. Williams ME, Lee JT, Innes DJ, et al. Immunoglobulin gene rearrangement in abnormal lymph node hyperplasia. Am J Clin Pathol 1991;96:746-54.
92. Wood GS, Garcia CF, Dorfman RF, Warnke RA. The immunohistology of follicle lysis in lymph node biopsies from homosexual men. Blood 1985;66:1092-7.
93. Yamakawa M, Ikeda I, Masuda A, Enomoto H, Ando A, Kasajima T. An unusual regressive germinal center, the 'FDC-only lymphoid follicle,' in lymph nodes of organ transplant recipients. Am J Surg Pathol 1999;23:536-45.

6 SPECIFIC CLINICAL ENTITIES

The entities discussed in this chapter are heterogeneous in terms of etiology and histologic appearance. The unifying theme is that each entity is a distinct clinical syndrome and has characteristic lymph node or splenic findings as a cornerstone of the diagnosis. Although not necessarily the most common benign disorders seen in hematopathology practice, many of the entries in this chapter have been thoroughly studied and described because of their distinctive histologic findings.

DERMATOPATHIC LYMPHADENITIS

Definition. *Dermatopathic lymphadenitis* is a predominantly T-cell hyperplasia associated with lymph nodes draining sites of skin irritation, inflammation, or infection.

General Features. Langerhans cells are an immature form of dendritic cell of the skin, which are exposed to antigen, and then migrate to the lymph nodes to mature (49). They interact with other mature dendritic cells to present antigen to T cells to initiate an immune response. This migration and maturation process can be induced by disruption of the epidermis, inflammatory cytokines, necrotic cells, and other agents including bacterial components (49).

Clinical Features. Dermatopathic lymphadenitis (65), which historically has been referred to as *lipomelanotic reticular hyperplasia* (85), consists of changes in the lymph node paracortex that may be associated with a variety of chronic generalized skin disorders (25,65). In some cases, these changes occur in the absence of dermatitis, and with the exception of pigment deposition, are identical to the findings seen in nodular paracortical T-cell hyperplasia (see chapter 5) (52). Since follicular hyperplasia and sinus histiocytosis are commonly associated with the nodular paracortical expansion of dermatopathic lymphadenopathy, this entity is also classified as *mixed pattern of lymphoid hyperplasia*.

Microscopic Findings. Dermatopathic lymphadenitis is characterized by a nodular expansion of the paracortex by confluent areas of pale-staining macrophages (histiocytes) that usually contain brown pigment, interspersed Langerhans and interdigitating dendritic cells, and small reactive lymphocytes (fig. 6-1). Interdigitating dendritic cells cannot be reliably distinguished from Langerhans cells by morphology alone, although the latter are more numerous (128). The pigment within the macrophages is typically melanin (fig. 6-2). In rare cases, the dendritic cells and macrophages become numerous, leaving only rare lymphocytes. These cases may be more difficult to distinguish from other conditions. However, even in cases with a predominance of these large pale cell proliferations, the overall nodular architecture is still maintained.

Immunoreactivity for S-100 protein is demonstrated in the interdigitating and Langerhans cells (fig. 6-3). CD1a highlights the Langerhans cells, and CD123 marks the DC2 type dendritic cells, which play a role in this type of immune response. The DC2 cells are increased within the nodular T-cell areas and in lymph node sinuses.

Differential Diagnosis. In most circumstances, isolated enlarged lymph nodes are removed to rule out the possibility of localized lymphoma. The histologic features of dermatopathic lymphadenitis are usually not difficult to recognize and distinguish from lymphoma. Distinction from lymph node involvement by mycosis fungoides, however, may pose a diagnostic challenge unless there is the significant architectural effacement of the lymph node that is easily recognizable and consistent with a neoplastic process (7,8). A complete clinical history is essential in such cases. In general, overall preservation of the normal lymph node architecture, in the absence of atypical T cells or increased mitoses, supports a diagnosis of dermatopathic lymphadenitis rather than involvement of the lymph node by peripheral T-cell lymphoma.

Less commonly, dermatopathic lymphadenitis is confused with nodal involvement by Hodgkin lymphoma, Langerhans cell histiocytosis, and

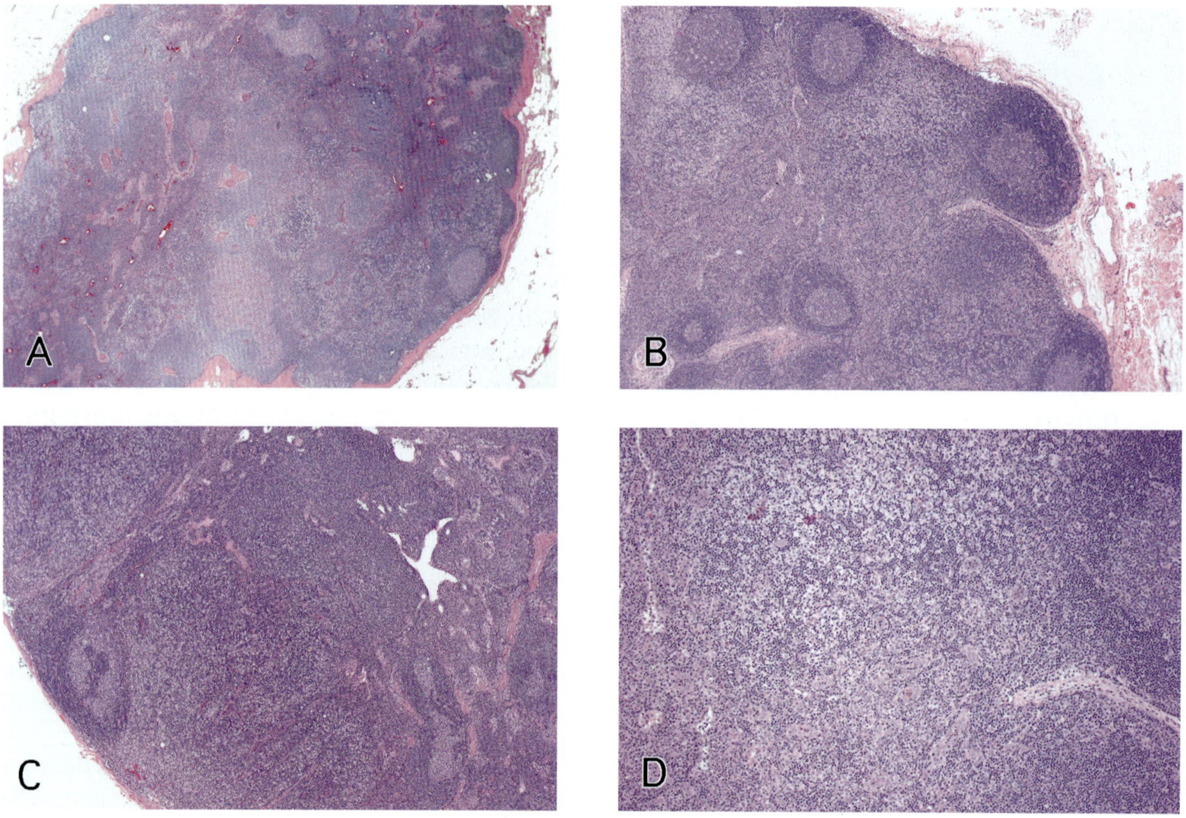

Figure 6-1

DERMATOPATHIC LYMPHADENITIS, LYMPH NODE

Low magnification (A-C) and intermediate magnification (D) of dermatopathic lymphadenitis. This morphologic appearance is essentially identical to that of paracortical T-cell hyperplasia.

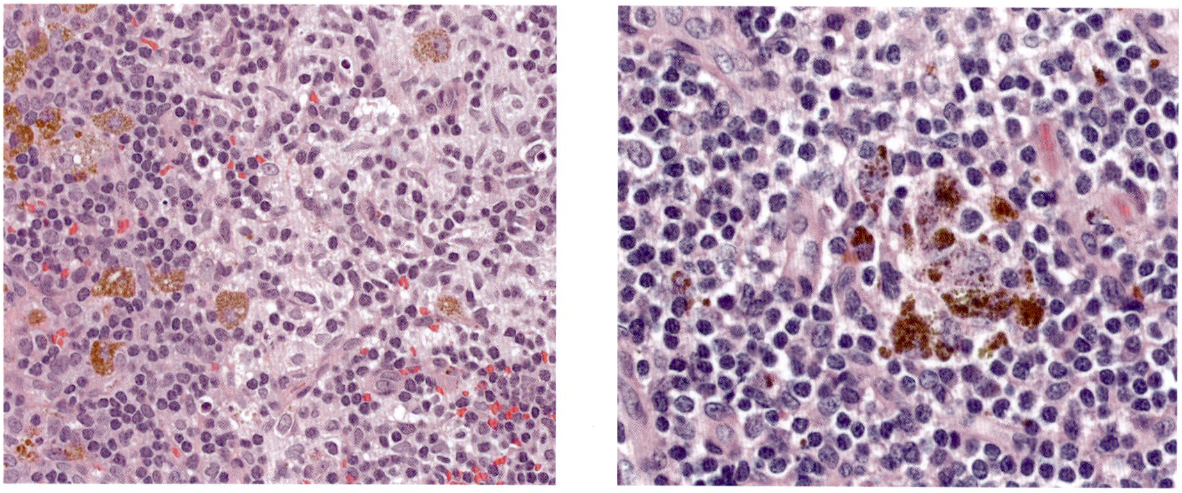

Figure 6-2

MELANIN PIGMENT IN DERMATOPATHIC LYMPHADENITIS, LYMPH NODE

Pigmented macrophages are seen.

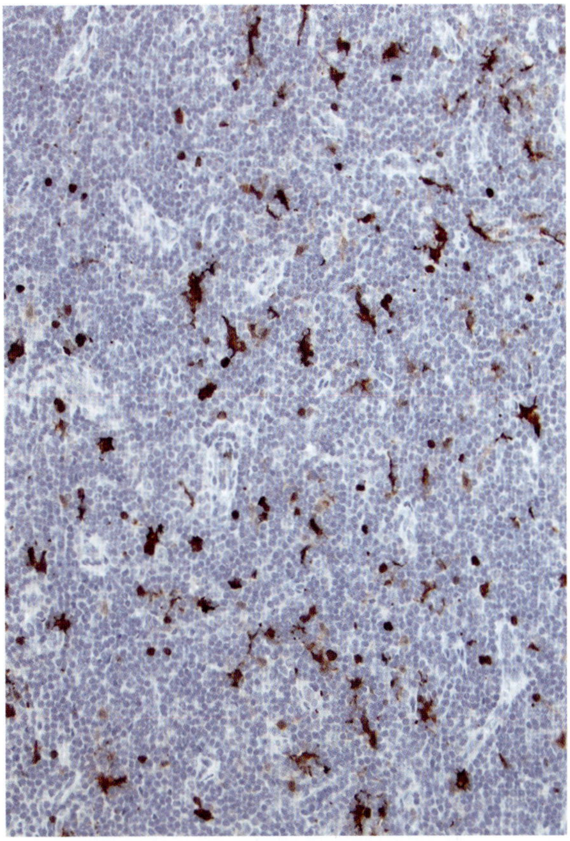

Figure 6-3

S-100 PROTEIN IMMUNOHISTOCHEMICAL REACTIVITY IN DERMATOPATHIC LYMPHADENITIS, LYMPH NODE

S-100 protein highlights the Langerhans and dendritic cells in this area of dermatopathic lymphadenitis.

monocytic leukemia. In each of these circumstances, the clinical history, a careful histologic examination, and in some cases, evaluation of immunohistochemical stains generally make the distinction.

Treatment and Prognosis. Typically, no specific treatment is required. Treatment of the underlying skin condition prevents recurrence.

KIMURA DISEASE

Definition. A distinctive clinical syndrome causing lymphadenopathy, *Kimura disease* is a rare disorder of unknown etiology associated with eosinophilia.

General Features. Allergic reactions to a variety of potential causative agents, including parasites, viruses, fungi, and toxins, have been postulated as a cause of Kimura disease (18). The finding of multinucleated giant cells has been one feature suggesting a viral etiology of this mysterious disorder, and reports have found evidence of Epstein-Barr virus (EBV) and human herpesvirus (HHV)-8 in some cases, but these results have not been validated in larger studies (68,102). To date, no specific etiology has been definitively elucidated.

Table 6-1

HISTOLOGIC FINDINGS IN KIMURA DISEASE

Follicular hyperplasia
Eosinophilia
Eosinophilic microabscesses
Eosinophils within germinal centers
Polykaryotic cells
Vascular proliferation
Fibrosis

Clinical Features. Kimura disease occurs predominantly in young to middle-aged adults and shows a slight male predominance. It is a chronic inflammatory disorder that is prevalent in Asia but rare in Western countries. This intriguing clinicopathologic syndrome was first described by Kimura et al. 1948 (77). Sporadic cases have been subsequently reported in Western countries.

Clinically, the disease manifests as subcutaneous nodules in the head and neck, including salivary glands, and regional lymphadenopathy (18,64). Nephrotic syndrome may develop as a result of immunoglobulin (Ig)E- immune complex deposition.

Laboratory Findings. Peripheral blood eosinophilia and increased levels of serum IgE are associated with this disorder.

Microscopic Findings. The histologic features in Kimura lymphadenopathy primarily include reactive follicular hyperplasia and prominent eosinophilia (Table 6-1). The architecture of the lymph nodes is generally preserved, but the capsule may be thickened (18,64). Eosinophils may be increased in the interfollicular areas, as well as within follicles. Eosinophilic abscesses and microabscesses may be seen in the paracortex, and, less commonly, within or replacing follicles (fig. 6-4). Occasionally, germinal center necrosis is present. Polykaryotic cells (multinucleated giant cells) are seen, both in paracortical areas and in germinal centers. Hyperplastic postcapillary

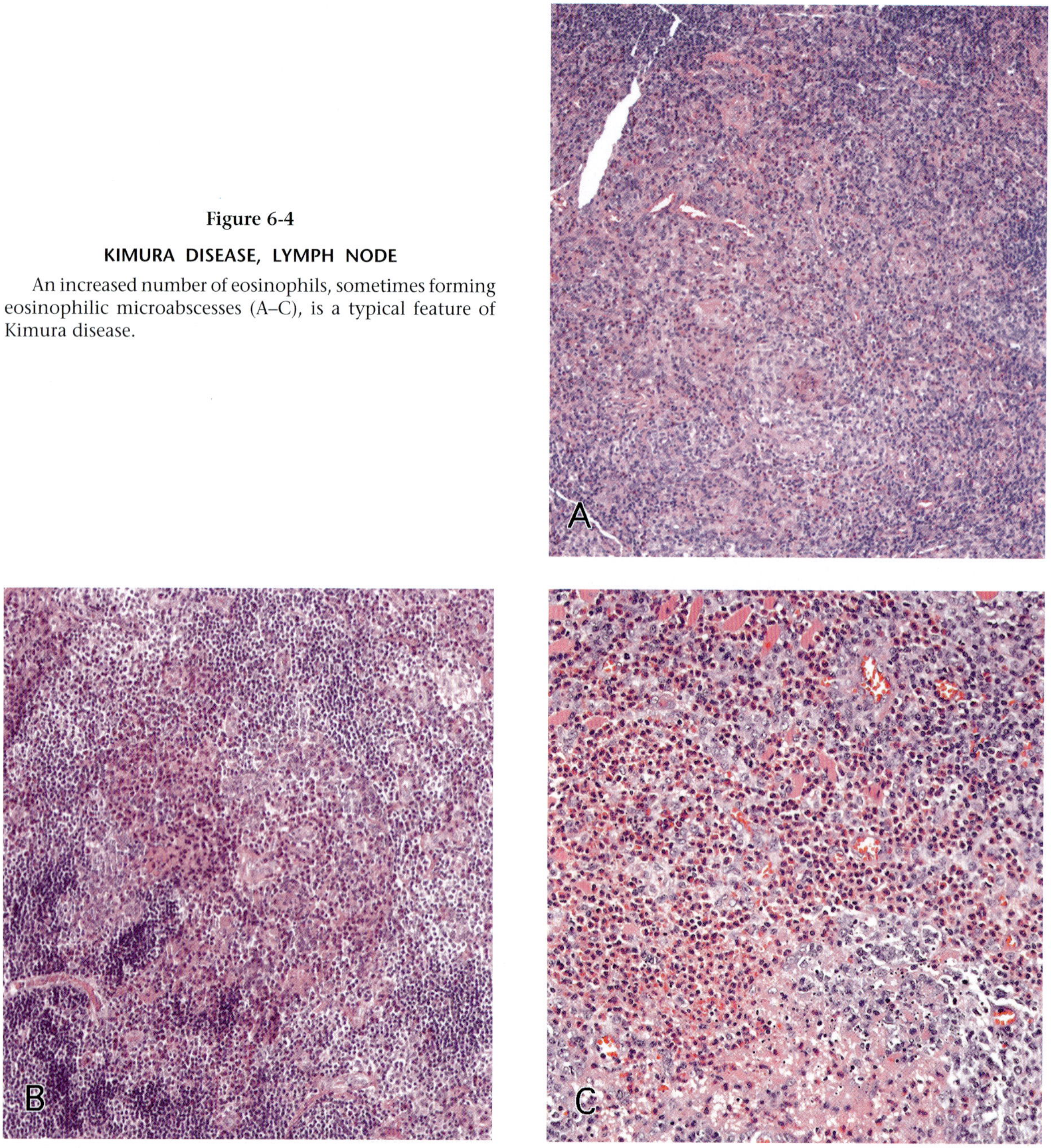

Figure 6-4

KIMURA DISEASE, LYMPH NODE

An increased number of eosinophils, sometimes forming eosinophilic microabscesses (A–C), is a typical feature of Kimura disease.

venules are frequent and may be sclerotic (fig. 6-5). Deposits of IgE within the germinal centers are demonstrated by immunofluorescent or immunohistochemical antibody studies (fig. 6-6). Mast cells and T cells are increased in lymph nodes; these cells produce increased amounts of cytokines such as interleukin (IL)-4, IL-5, eotaxin, and RANTES (regulated on activation normal T expressed and secreted) which may regulate IgE synthesis and recruit eosinophils (78).

A single case of Kimura disease was reported with the presence of clonal T-cell receptor gene rearrangements (21,22). This is unlikely to be present in most cases.

Differential Diagnosis. The differential diagnosis of Kimura disease includes angiolymphoid hyperplasia with eosinophilia (fig. 6-7) (14,83), drug- or parasitic-related eosinophilia with lymphadenopathy, Langerhans cell histiocytosis, peripheral T-cell lymphoma, Hodgkin

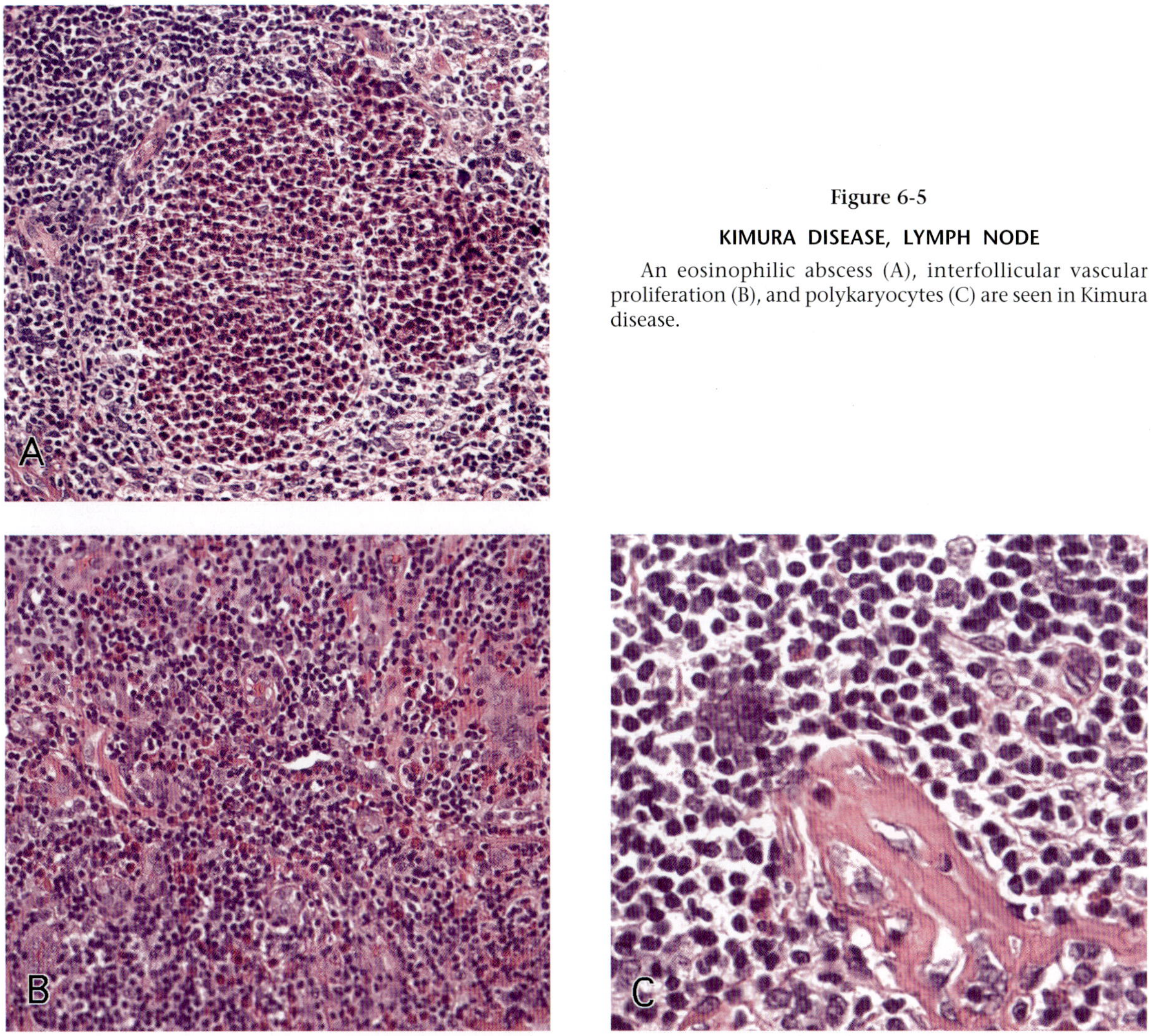

Figure 6-5

KIMURA DISEASE, LYMPH NODE

An eosinophilic abscess (A), interfollicular vascular proliferation (B), and polykaryocytes (C) are seen in Kimura disease.

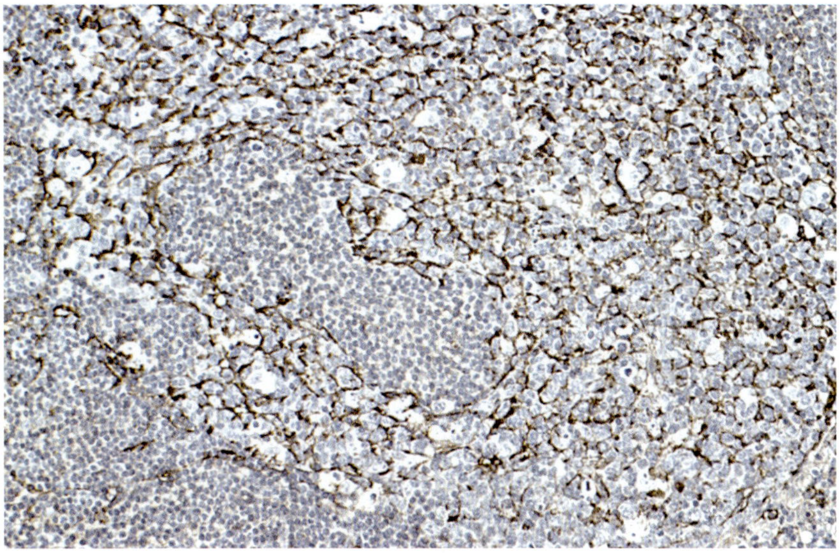

Figure 6-6

KIMURA DISEASE, LYMPH NODE

Immunohistochemical staining for immunoglobulin (Ig)E.

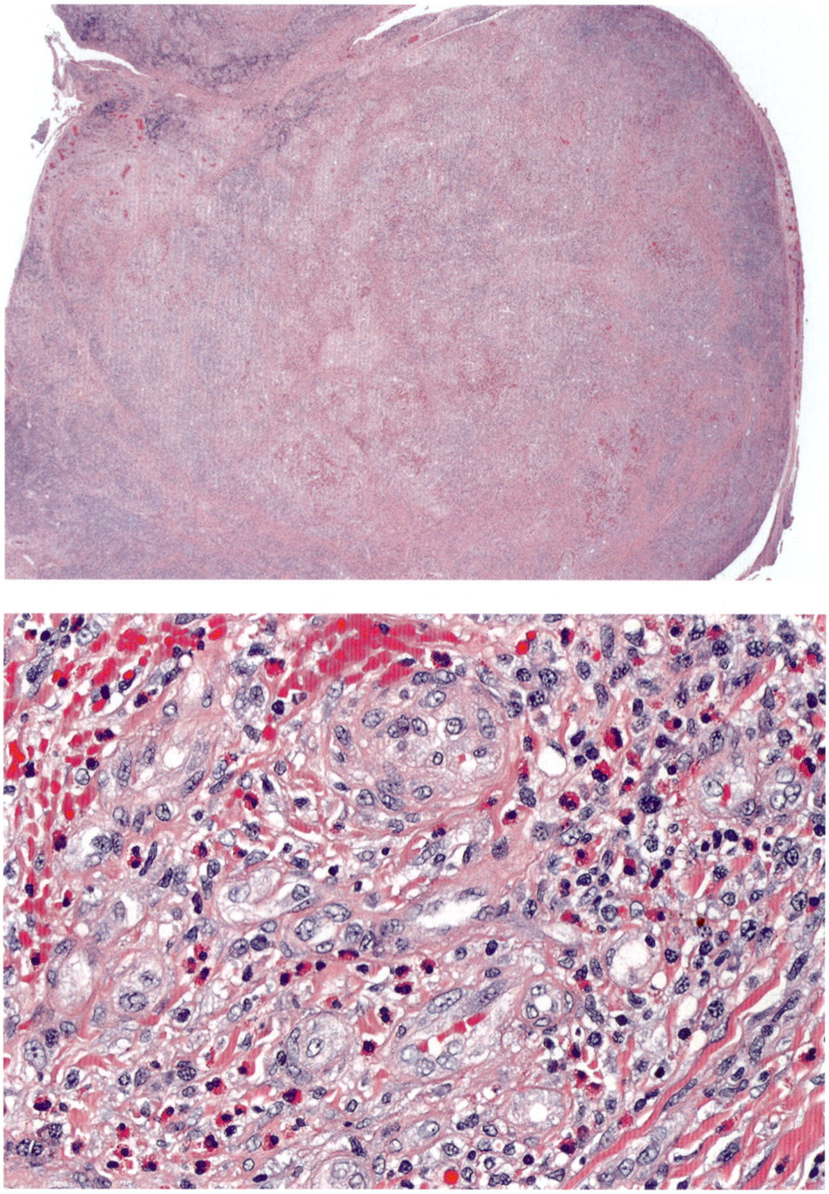

Figure 6-7

EPITHELIOID HEMANGIOMA WITH EOSINOPHILIA (ANGIOLYMPHOID HYPERPLASIA WITH EOSINOPHILIA)

Low magnification (top) and high magnification (bottom) show a primarily vascular proliferation.

lymphoma, and rarely, nodal involvement by hypereosinophilic syndrome.

Angiolymphoid hyperplasia with eosinophilia has been definitively proven to be a variant of epithelioid hemangioma with eosinophilia. It is distinct from Kimura disease in many ways: it is a disease seen primarily in Western countries, lymph node involvement is lacking, and endothelial cell markers are positive (83).

Distinction from classic Hodgkin lymphoma or T-cell lymphoma is not difficult when Hodgkin/Reed-Sternberg cells or atypical T lymphocytes are present. Langerhans cell histiocytosis can usually be differentiated by the constellation of histologic features described later in this chapter. Other causes of systemic eosinophilia with lymphadenopathy should be distinct from Kimura disease based on the clinical history.

Treatment and Prognosis. Kimura disease has a benign clinical course following surgical excision of the subcutaneous masses and lymph nodes and treatment of any associated inflammatory conditions. Occasional cases, however, persist and treatment includes steroids, other antiinflammatory agents, and, in some cases, chemotherapy.

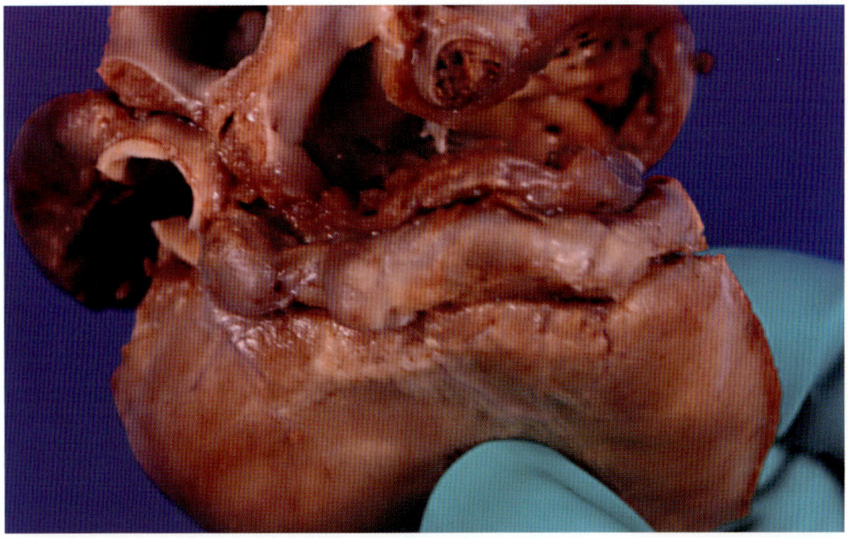

Figure 6-8

CORONARY ARTERY ANEURYSM, KAWASAKI DISEASE

There is massive dilation of the circumflex coronary artery.

KAWASAKI DISEASE

Definition. *Kawasaki disease*, also known as *mucocutaneous lymph node syndrome*, is a rare acute, self-limited vasculitic disorder associated with lymphadenopathy and other systemic symptoms.

General Features. Although an infectious etiology has been proposed for Kawasaki syndrome, including viral (9), rickettsial (10), and *Proprionibacterium* (which has been cultured from involved lymph nodes) (61), definitive evidence of an infectious etiology remains inconclusive (98) and continued epidemiologic investigations are necessary. Exposure to drugs, toxins, pesticides, chemicals, or heavy metals does not appear to be responsible (106). An infectious agent does seem to be a likely possibility in Kawasaki disease because of its self-limited course, clinical manifestations, which include fever and rash, and the documentation of epidemic outbreaks (61). It is possible that a ubiquitous infectious agent, combined with specific genetic susceptibility, particularly in Japan, may underlie the disorder (106). Patients with Kawasaki disease also have numerous immunoregulatory problems such as circulating immune complexes and T-cell and polyclonal B-cell activation (61). The presence of lytic autoantibodies to cytokine-activated endothelial cells that disappear in the convalescent stage may be responsible for the vasculitis (88).

Clinical Features. Although Kawasaki disease was first reported by Kawasaki in Japan in 1967 (72), it has also been described in the United States and other Western countries, but is markedly more prevalent in Japan and in those of Japanese ancestry (96,106). The clinicopathologic syndrome affects infants and children, and most patients are younger than 10 years of age (6). There is a modest male prevalence of 1.5-2.0 to 1.0.

Diagnostic symptoms include five or more of the following not due to some other known etiology: 1) fever of 5 or more days; 2) bilateral congestion of conjunctiva; 3) oral mucous membrane lesions including fissuring of lips, diffuse erythema, and prominence of tongue papillae; 4) distal extremity lesions including erythema, indurative edema of hands and feet, and periungual desquamation of fingertips; 5) polymorphous exanthem; and 6) acute nonsuppurative cervical adenopathy. Later stages of the disorder may include arthritis, diarrhea, vomiting, and abdominal pain. Important clinical complications include the development of vasculitis and aneurysms. Particularly affected are the vessels of the heart, which may lead to myocarditis, congestive heart failure, pericarditis with pericardial effusion, mitral or aortic insufficiency, arrhythmias, and coronary artery aneurysms (fig. 6-8). Outcomes may include myocardial infarction, sudden death, or ischemic heart disease.

Laboratory Findings. Up to 50 percent of affected patients have leukocytosis and elevation of acute phase reactants (such as erythrocyte sedimentation rate [ESR] and C-reactive

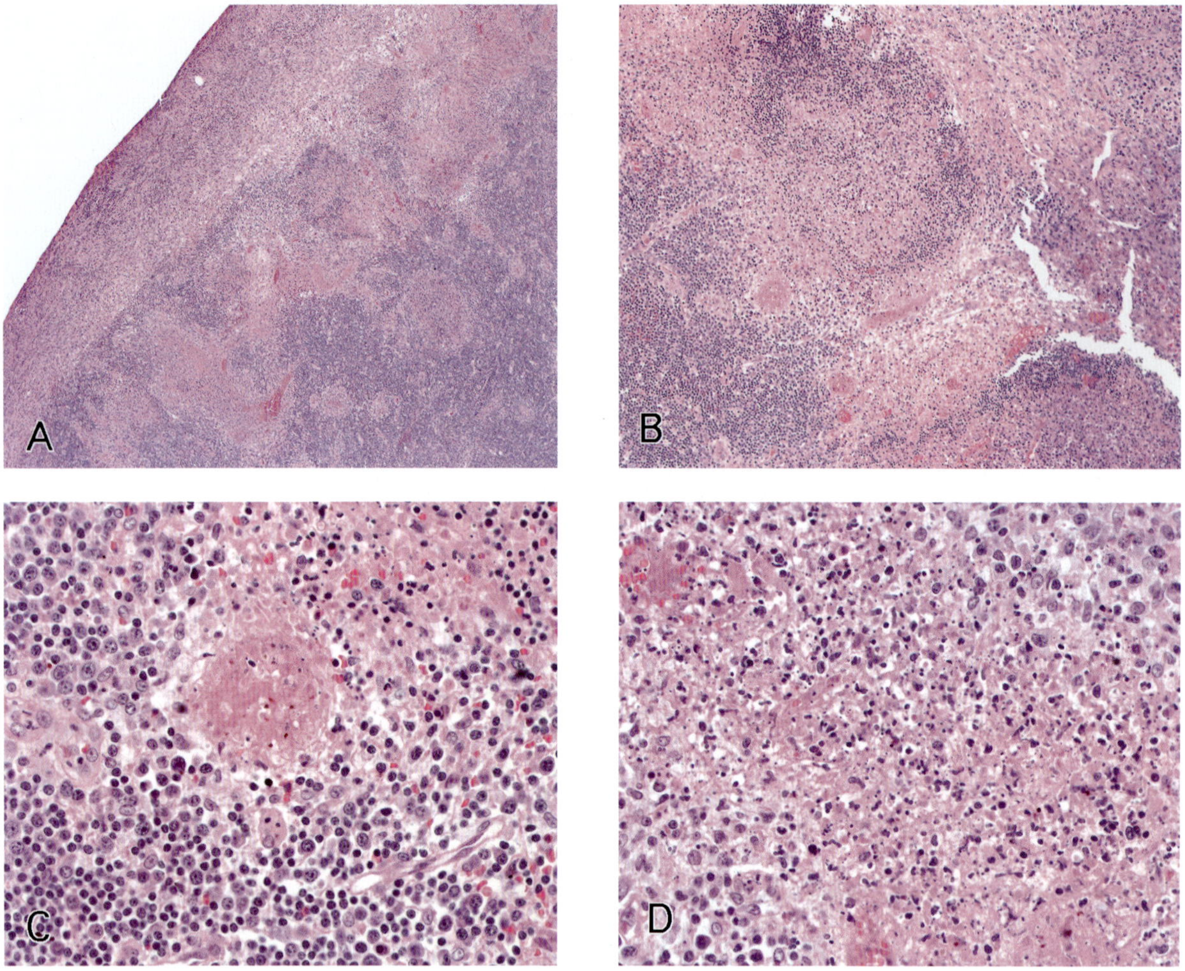

Figure 6-9

KAWASAKI DISEASE, LYMPH NODE

Kawasaki lymphadenitis in a child shows patchy necrosis in the paracortex and depletion of lymphocytes and germinal centers. (Courtesy of Randy Gascoyne, Vancouver, BC.)

protein). Thrombocytosis of 500-700 x 10^9/L is frequently seen (126).

Microscopic Findings. The histopathologic changes in the lymph nodes include effacement of the architecture and expansion of interfollicular areas (50). There are multiple foci of necrosis, which may be small or large and may become confluent (figs. 6-9, 6-10). Within the areas of necrosis are scattered neutrophils and nuclear debris. Microthrombosis of small blood vessels is also seen (50). Adjacent to areas of necrosis, the endothelial cells swell. Vascular proliferation may be seen, but granulomas are not present.

Differential Diagnosis. The presence of thrombi and neutrophils helps distinguish Kawasaki disease from Kikuchi disease by histomorphologic criteria alone.

Treatment and Prognosis. Treatment includes the use of intravenous immunoglobulin, antiinflammatory agents, steroids, and anticoagulants (106). Plasma exchange and monoclonal antibodies to inflammatory agents have been used with success as well.

KIKUCHI-FUJIMOTO DISEASE (HISTIOCYTIC NECROTIZING LYMPHADENITIS)

Definition. *Kikuchi-Fujimoto disease,* also known as *histiocytic necrotizing lymphadenitis*, is a benign, self-limited disorder with localized lymphadenopathy and systemic symptoms.

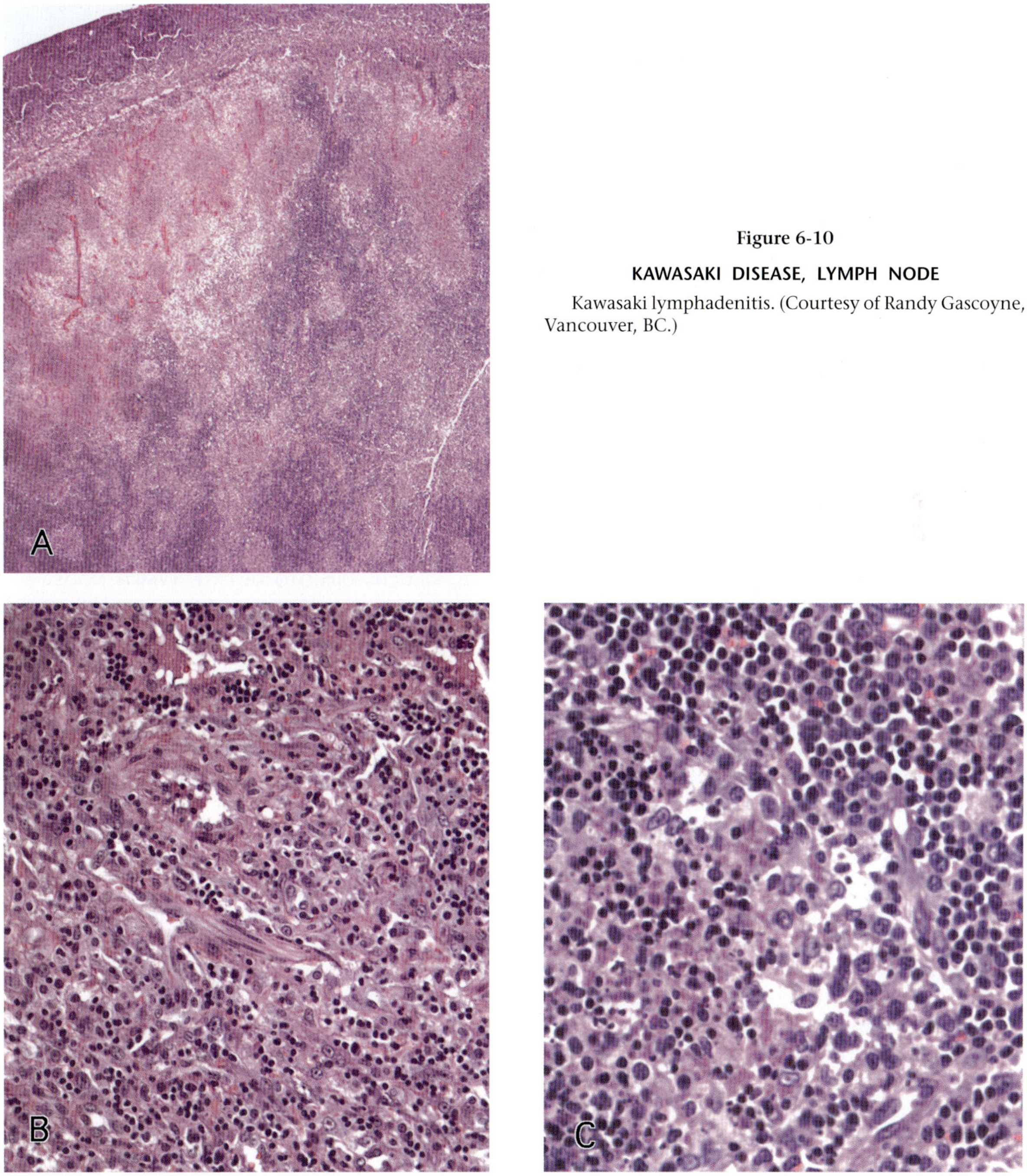

Figure 6-10

KAWASAKI DISEASE, LYMPH NODE

Kawasaki lymphadenitis. (Courtesy of Randy Gascoyne, Vancouver, BC.)

General Features. The exact etiology of Kikuchi-Fujimoto disease remains unknown although infection has been suggested. Several potential organisms have been proposed over the years including *Yersinia enterocolitica* (36,124), *Toxoplasma gondii* (36,76), and a variety of viruses (66,81, 124,138), especially EBV (23,124,133) and HHV-6 (81). Follow-up studies, however, have shown a lack of definitive evidence for either EBV or HHV-6 in this disease (62). Although human immunodeficiency virus (HIV) type 1 has been associated with cases showing similar histologic features (30), investigation continues as to the exact cause of this disease. Recent polymerase chain reaction (PCR) studies have shown the presence of HHV-8 in

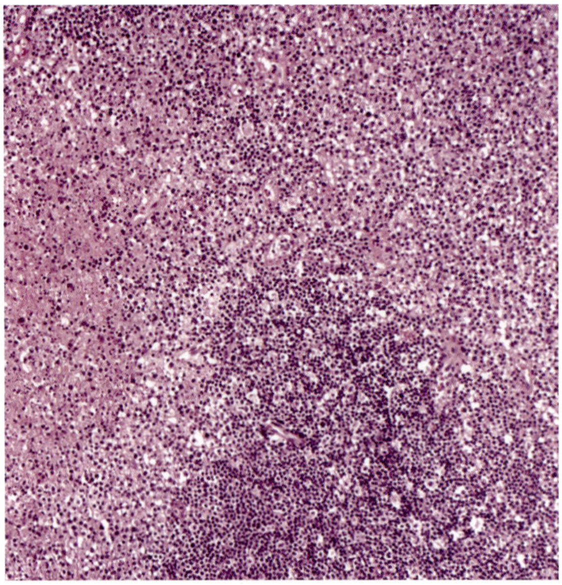

Figure 6-11

KIKUCHI-FUJIMOTO DISEASE, LYMPH NODE

Discreet areas of necrosis and adjacent mottled paracortex.

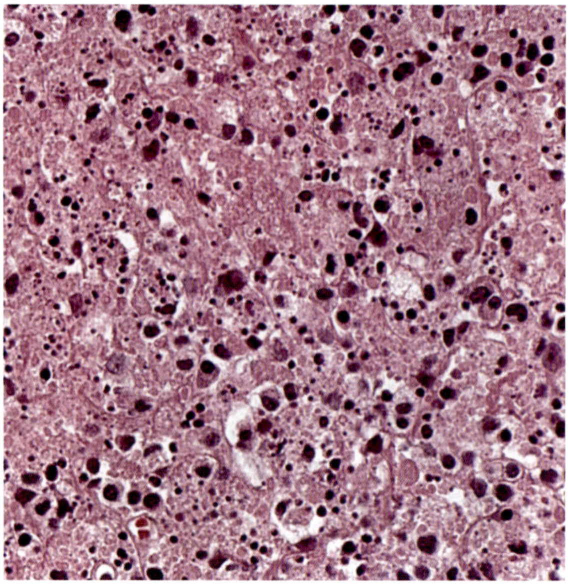

Figure 6-12

KIKUCHI-FUJIMOTO DISEASE, LYMPH NODE

Karyorrhexis and the absence of neutrophils in Kikuchi-Fujimoto disease.

lymph nodes involved by Kikuchi-Fujimoto disease, suggesting this virus as a possible etiologic agent in a subset of cases (63).

The relationship of EBV, type 1 human T-cell lymphotropic virus (HTLV-1), and parvovirus B19 to Kikuchi-Fujimoto disease in Taiwan has recently been investigated (23). EBV was detected by in situ hybridization for EBV-encoded RNA expression in all 10 cases whereas HTLV-1 and parvovirus B19 were not detected in any cases. Future studies are necessary to elucidate the possible association of viral infection with the apoptosis and histiocytic interaction that are characteristic of this disorder.

Clinical Features. Kikuchi-Fujimoto disease was first reported in Japan in 1972 by Kikuchi and independently by Fujimoto et al. (47,75). Shortly thereafter, other cases with similar clinicopathologic features were reported in Europe (120) and later in the United States (30,137).

The classic clinical presentation of Kikuchi-Fujimoto disease was first described as solitary, painless cervical lymphadenopathy in a predominantly young adult or adolescent Oriental female with a mean age of 30 years. Following excisional lymph node biopsy, these patients had a benign clinical course with no progression to malignant lymphoma. Since the initial reports, this disease has been described in both males and females with a wide age range, presenting as either localized or generalized lymphadenopathy (114). Patients complain of migratory large joint arthralgias, variable fever, malaise, and regional (most commonly cervical) or widespread lymphadenopathy.

Laboratory Findings. Neutropenia, mild lymphocytosis and granulocytopenia, and an elevated ESR are often associated with Kikuchi-Fujimoto disease (114). Laboratory studies for evaluation of autoimmune diseases, such as lupus erythematosus, should be performed (114).

Microscopic Findings. Histologically, the lymph nodes involved by Kikuchi-Fujimoto disease usually show a well-circumscribed paracortical focus of necrosis with a variable mixture of karyorrhectic nuclear debris, single cell necrosis, transformed lymphocytes, and foamy macrophages (figs. 6-11, 6-12). The conspicuous absence of polymorphonuclear leukocytes contrasts with the histologic findings of an acute bacterial infection such as cat-scratch disease. In the early stages of Kikuchi-Fujimoto disease, plasmacytoid dendritic cells (formerly called plasmacytoid T cells or plasmacytoid monocytes) predominate,

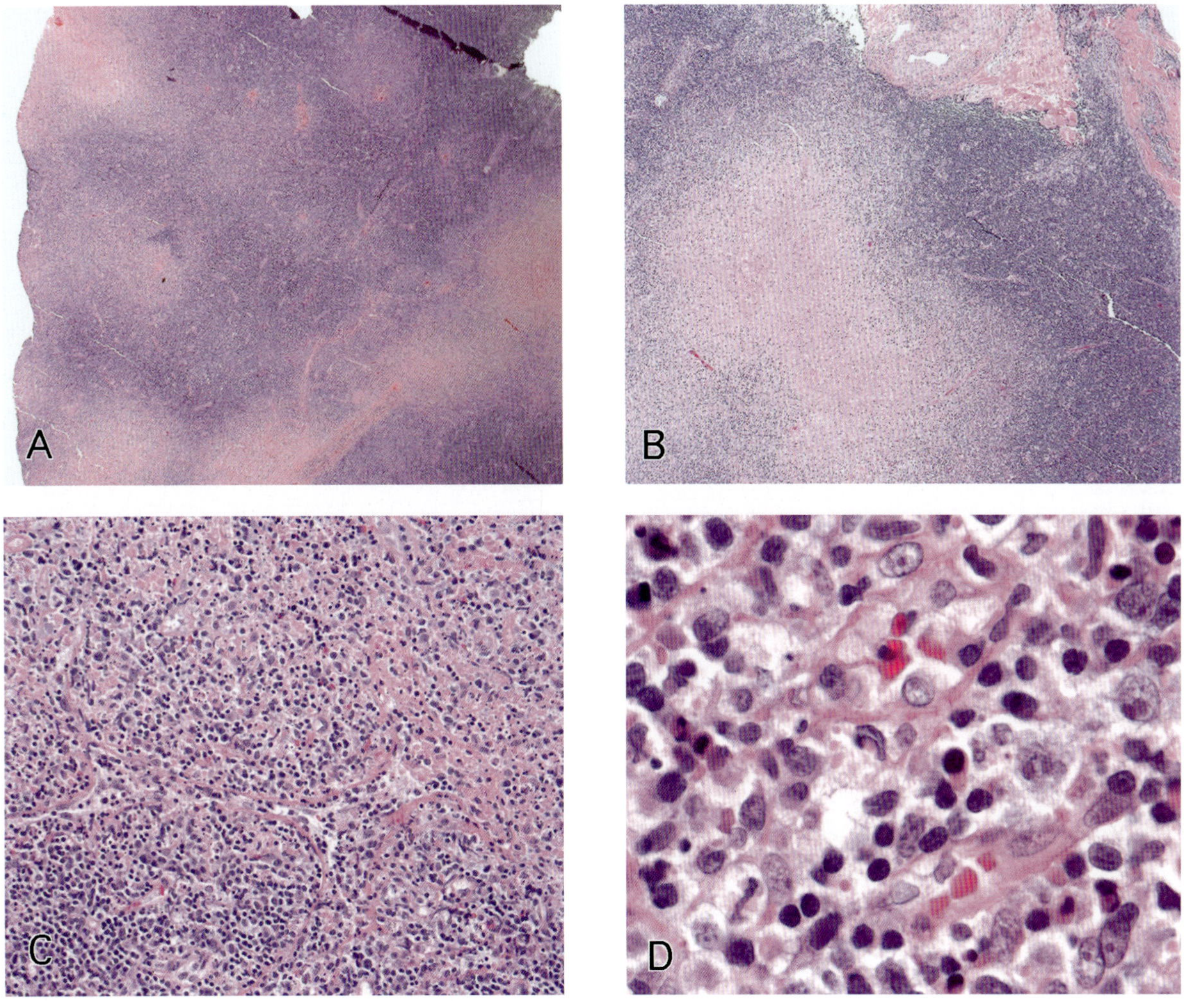

Figure 6-13

KIKUCHI-FUJIMOTO DISEASE, LYMPH NODE

Areas of neutrophil-poor necrosis, which often have surrounding areas of activated, large lymphocytes, are seen. (Courtesy of Patricia Devine, Lowell, MA.)

in association with activated lymphocytes with a CD8 (cytotoxic-suppressor) phenotype (34,124). Subsequent areas of necrosis due to an abnormal granulomatous response result. Transformed lymphocytes and macrophages impart a mottled appearance to the residual paracortex (fig. 6-13). Focal clusters of plasmacytoid dendritic cells may be demonstrated in this region.

The histopathologic changes have been classified into three types: proliferative (early phase), necrotizing (intermediate phase), and xanthomatous (late phase) depending on the histologic features (82). The late phase contains zones of amorphous cellular debris surrounded by palisading epithelioid macrophages. In all stages, the predominant cells are various types of macrophages, including plasmacytoid dendritic cells. Occasionally, more than one histologic pattern is observed in the same patient (32).

Although not necessary for diagnosis, the plasmacytoid dendritic cells are highlighted with immunohistochemical stains including CD123 (very specific), CD68, CD163, lysozyme (sensitive, but less specific), or myeloperoxidase (fig. 6-14).

Recent molecular probe studies have demonstrated clonal, or oligoclonal, patterns with PCR methods using primers for the T-gamma gene, suggesting a clonal expansion of T cells in

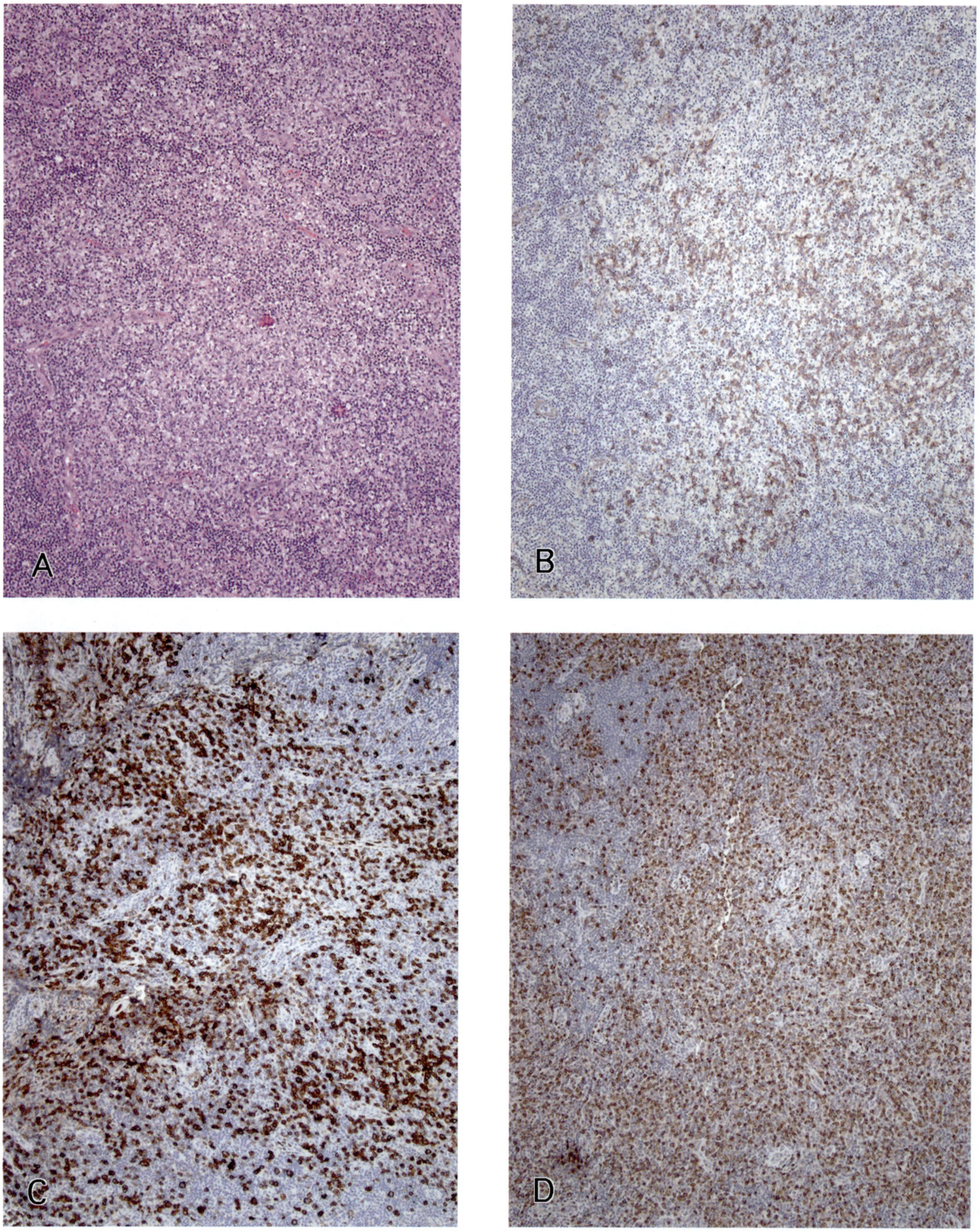

Figure 6-14

KIKUCHI-FUJIMOTO DISEASE, LYMPH NODE

Plasmacytoid dendritic cells are difficult to distinguish by hematoxylin and eosin (H&E) alone (A), but can be recognized by staining with CD123 (B), CD163 (C), and lysozyme (D).

this clinically self-limited disorder (114). This is an example of a situation in which this highly sensitive test should not be used as a criterion for malignancy.

Differential Diagnosis. The histologic appearance of Kikuchi-Fujimoto disease, especially the large transformed cells and occasional mitoses, can simulate a malignant lymphoma (12,30). Important histologic features that help in this distinction are the overall preservation of the lymph node architecture, with residual lymphoid tissue, and the absence of nuclear atypia or significant numbers of mitoses in Kikuchi-Fujimoto disease. Immunohistochemical studies show CD68 and CD123 reactivity in the plasmacytoid monocytes and other macrophages, which helps to differentiate this lesion from a large B-cell lymphoma.

Treatment and Prognosis. This self-limited disease has been shown to resolve spontaneously in weeks (31). Most cases of Kikuchi-Fujimoto disease have resolved following excisional lymph node biopsy although the anecdotal use of antibiotics has also been reported. Although local recurrences can occur, transformation to malignant lymphoma has never been described and fatalities are exceptional (111,136). Of interest, however, is one reported case in which a disease with the same pathologic features of histiocytic necrotizing lymphadenitis without granulocytic infiltration presented in a 19-month-old child and had a fulminant, progressive course that resulted in the child's death (111).

CASTLEMAN DISEASE (ANGIOFOLLICULAR LYMPH NODE HYPERPLASIA), HYALINE-VASCULAR TYPE, PLASMA CELL TYPE, AND MULTICENTRIC TYPE

Definition. *Castleman disease* (CD) has come to represent a spectrum of disorders, with at least two types of localized disease (*hyaline-vascular type* [HV], and *plasma cell type* [PC]) and a systemic or multicentric form of the disease. Each of the localized types has a distinct histologic appearance and suggested etiology. *Multicentric CD* (M) has a distinctive clinical presentation, but shares histologic features of one or both of the localized types.

General Features. The exact pathogenesis of CD is still unknown. The spontaneous production of high levels of B-cell differentiation factor in cultured lymph nodes from patients with M-CD has been reported, supporting the possibility of an unregulated B-cell proliferation (146). In other studies, the germinal centers in systemic CD have been immunohistochemically shown to produce excess IL-6, a cytokine associated with B-cell proliferation and differentiation to plasma cells and encoded by HHV-8 (109,147). Recent studies show an association between CD and IL-6 expression (115,132). This suggests that CD may be a syndrome encompassing multiple etiologies that involve aberrant IL-6 activity from either endogenous or viral sources. In some cases of systemic CD, EBV has been demonstrated, suggesting a possible role of this virus in the disorder (57).

Recently, it has been recognized that HV-CD may actually represent a neoplasm of dendritic or angiomyoid cells. Clonal cytogenetic abnormalities of these cell types have been reported (19,24,117). This intriguing evidence suggests that the dysplastic dendritic cells seen in HV-CD may represent a neoplasm, and that the other histologic and clinical findings may be a generalized response to a localized tumor. Cytogenetic abnormalities reported in these cells include: t(1;22)(qter;q13); t(7;8)(q37.3;q12); t(1;16)(p11;p11),del(7)(q21q22),del(8)(q12q22); and a dd(1)(q21),der(6)t(6;12) (q23;q15),add(7)(p22), -9,inv(9)(p11q13),del(12)(q15),+mar.

Clinical Features. HV-CD is more common and more frequently localized than PC-CD, which occurs either as a localized form or as M-CD. Sites of involvement are remarkably varied (Table 6-2). In general, the most common sites for HV-CD are mediastinal and abdominal or peripheral lymph nodes. PC-CD occurs more commonly in lymph nodes. As is suggested by Table 6-3, CD is associated with a wide array of disorders and malignancies. It is a diagnosis of exclusion that should only be made in the appropriate clinical setting (127).

HV-CD was first described in mediastinal lymph nodes by Castleman et al. in 1956 (11). Over the years, this intriguing disorder has been extensively studied and referred to as *angiofollicular lymph node hyperplasia, angiomatous lymphoid hamartoma* (37), *follicular lymphoreticuloma*, and *giant lymph node hyperplasia* (74). HV-CD has a wide age range and no gender predilection. The lymphadenopathy associated with HV-CD

Table 6-2

REPORTED LOCATIONS OF CASTLEMAN DISEASE

Epidural	Parotid gland	Paravertebral	Liver	Vaginal wall
Dura	Submandibular gland	Mediastinum	Porta hepatis	Broad ligament
Leptomeninges	Nasopharynx	Thymus	Spleen	Urachus
Intracranial	Retropharyngeal	Pleura	Mesentery	Pelvis
Cerebral spinal fluid	Neck	Pericardium	Omentum	Arm
Eye (globe)	Thyroid gland	Breast	Kidney	Leg
Orbit	Skin	Stomach	Adrenal gland	Bone marrow
Lacrimal gland	Skeletal muscle	Pancreas	Retroperitoneum	

Table 6-3

DISEASES REPORTED IN ASSOCIATION WITH CASTLEMAN DISEASE

Cutaneous	**Other Conditions**
Paraneoplastic pemphigus	Acute adrenal insufficiency
Bullous pemphigoid	Bronchiolitis obliterans
Epidermolysis bullosa	Cardiomyopathy
Vitiligo	Chronic inflammatory demyelinating polyradiculoneuropathy
Lichen planus	Cytomegalovirus colitis
	Klinefelter syndrome
Hematologic	Neurofibromatosis
Evan syndrome	Neuropathy
Pure red cell aplasia	Peliosis hepatis
Autoimmune hemolytic anemia	POEMS syndrome
Immune thrombocytopenic purpura	Pregnancy
Hyperviscosity syndrome	Primary pulmonary hypertension
Cold agglutinin disease	Schizophrenia
	Secondary amyloidosis
Autoimmune	Superior vena cava thrombi
Systemic lupus erythematosus	Tumor lysis syndrome
Rheumatoid arthritis	Ulcerative colitis
Sjögren syndrome	
Sicca syndrome	**Neoplasms**
Scleroderma	Hematologic
Myasthenia gravis	Classic Hodgkin lymphoma
Behcet syndrome	Diffuse large B-cell lymphoma
	Primary body cavity lymphoma
Renal	Peripheral T-cell lymphoma
Nephrotic syndrome	Follicular dendritic cell tumor (sarcoma)
Acute renal failure	Nonhematologic
Glomerulonephritis	Carcinoma
Membranoproliferative glomerulonephritis	Thyroid carcinoma
Rapidly progressive glomerulonephritis	Renal carcinoma
Linear IgA disease	Pheochromocytoma
Hydronephrosis	Glomeruloid hemangioma
	Kaposi sarcoma
	Leiomyosarcoma

usually occurs as a solitary, asymptomatic lesion, unaccompanied by constitutional symptoms in 90 percent of cases (94). Common sites of involvement are mediastinal, cervical, axillary, and pulmonary lymphoid tissues. Rare cases of HV-CD have been reported in the spleen. The clinical manifestations usually regress after excision of the lymph node.

In contrast, PC-CD is often associated with clinical signs and symptoms, such as fever, anemia, and hypergammaglobulinemia, and is often disseminated. It is also associated with HIV/acquired immunodeficiency syndrome (AIDS), possibly in association with HHV-8 infection (see above). In cases of localized disease, systemic manifestations may be reversed by the

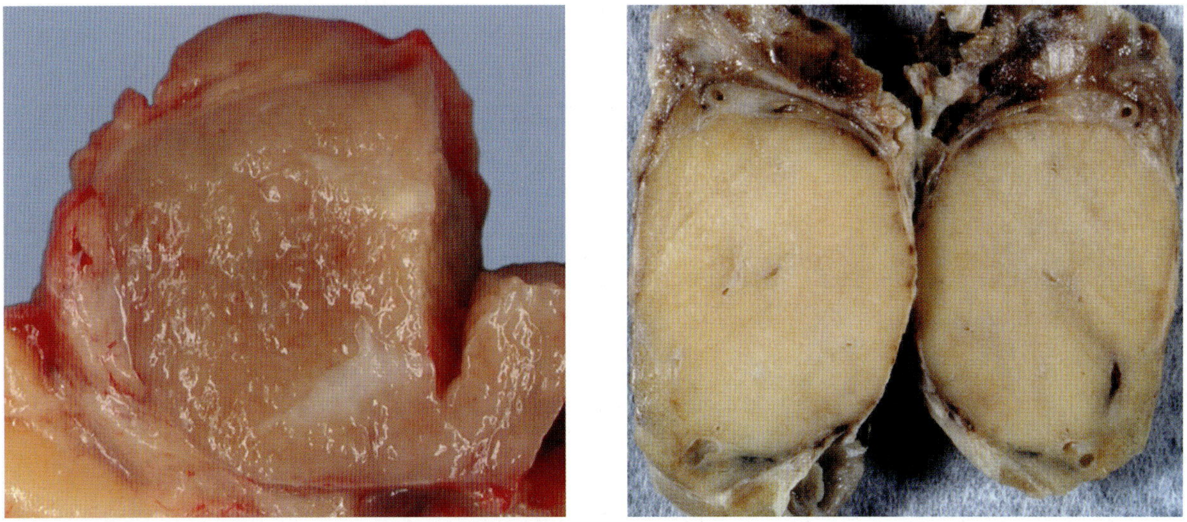

Figure 6-15

CASTLEMAN DISEASE, LYMPH NODE

Left: Plasma cell Castleman disease.
Right: Hyaline-vascular Castleman disease. (Courtesy of Stefano Pileri, Bologna, Italy.)

removal of the affected lymph node. Often, however, the symptoms continue. PC-CD has been reported more frequently in the spleen than HV-CD.

Leibetseder and Thurner (86) originally reported the disorder known as multicentric CD (M-CD) in 1973. In 1978, Gaba et al. (48) described a similar condition as "multicentric giant lymph node hyperplasia." Over the years, M-CD has been described in the literature as *multicentric angiofollicular lymph node hyperplasia* (140), *angiofollicular and plasmacytic polyadenopathy* (28), *systemic lymphoproliferative disorder with morphologic features of CD* (43), and *idiopathic plasmacytic lymphadenopathy with polyclonal hypergammaglobulinemia* (100). Other investigators described it as a *plasma cell dyscrasia with polyneuropathy* (99), *endocrine disturbances*, and *lymphadenopathy with abnormal germinal centers* (79).

M-CD is an idiopathic multisystem disorder that predominantly involves multiple peripheral lymph nodes (40,46). Patients with M-CD tend to be older than those with the localized form. There is a male predominance (42). Abnormal laboratory findings are similar to those of PC-CD and include anemia, thrombocytopenia, leukopenia, proteinuria, hypoalbuminemia, and an elevated ESR (54). Physical findings include peripheral lymphadenopathy (100 percent), abdominal lymphadenopathy (53 percent), mediastinal lymphadenopathy (47 percent), splenomegaly (79 percent), and hepatomegaly (63 percent) (54). Edema or pleural effusions are seen in 48 percent of patients, rash in 37 percent, and neurologic findings in 24 percent (54). M-CD is associated with neuropathies, endocrinopathies, osteoblastic bone lesions (5,79), and rheumatoid arthritis (4).

M-CD differs from localized CD in several ways. Although both may show similar histopathologic changes in lymph nodes, the clinical presentations differ. In general, the patients with M-CD have a more aggressive disease, often associated with the development of malignancies. They present with peripheral lymphadenopathy rather than central nodal disease. They require systemic therapy whereas patients with localized CD are usually cured by excisional lymph node biopsy (41).

Gross Findings. Lymph nodes can be enlarged, but retain normal architectural landmarks. Areas of hemorrhage or necrosis are not typically seen (fig. 6-15).

Microscopic Findings. The histopathologic features of HV-CD are distinctive (Table 6-4; fig. 6-16) and include germinal centers that vary in size (usually small) and shape, and are located throughout the lymph node parenchyma.

Table 6-4

COMPARISON OF FEATURES OF HYALINE-VASCULAR AND PLASMA CELL CASTLEMAN DISEASE

Feature	Hyaline-Vascular Type	Plasma Cell Type
Regressed follicles	+	-/+
Onion skinning of mantle zones	+	+/-
Follicular hyperplasia	+[a]	+
Dysplastic dendritic cells	+	-
Vascular proliferation	+	-/+
Plasmacytosis	-	+
Human herpesvirus-8	-	+

[a]Although the follicles are small (atretic), they are typically increased in number per unit area of the lymph node in comparison to normal.

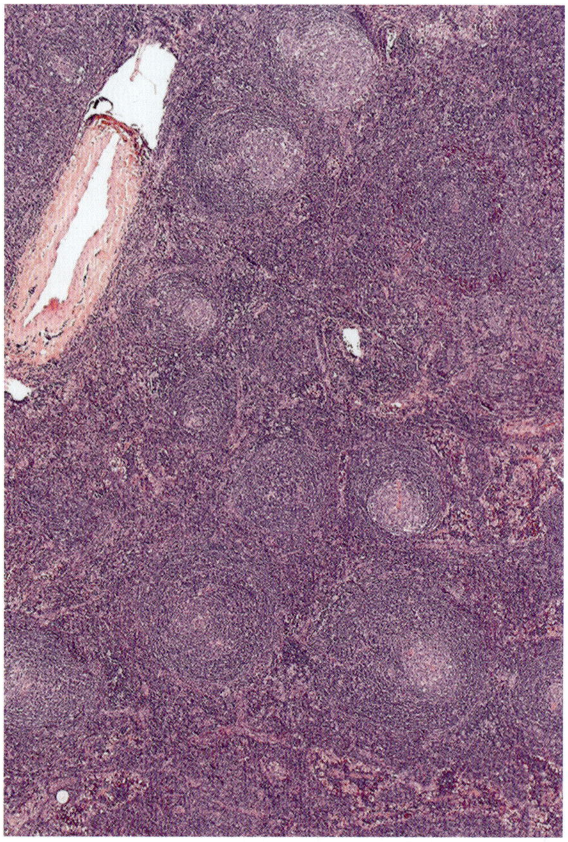

Figure 6-16

HYALINE-VASCULAR CASTLEMAN DISEASE, LYMPH NODE

Low magnification of hyaline-vascular Castleman disease shows small regressed follicles with prominent mantle zones.

Although the germinal centers are small, it is important to recognize that there is actually follicular hyperplasia (i.e., an increase of follicles per unit area) even though they are reduced in size. Some of the germinal centers are atrophic and depleted of lymphocytes (regressively transformed) and have radially penetrating hyalinized capillaries, resulting in "lollipop" follicles (fig. 6-17) (73). The lymphocytes in the surrounding mantle zones are expanded and arranged in multiple concentric layers, imparting an "onion-skin" appearance (fig. 6-18). In the localized form of CD, the sinuses are usually inapparent.

Hyalinization or increased eosinophilic material around blood vessels is often seen. There is a vascular proliferation in the interfollicular space, often with hyalinization of the vessels in the interfollicular space. Importantly, there are dysplastic and degenerating dendritic cells, both in the follicles and in the interfollicular spaces (fig. 6-19). As mentioned previously, it has been shown that clonal translocations are present in these dendritic cells. In rare cases of splenic HV-CD, there are grossly visible masses composed of hyperplastic nodules of white pulp surrounded by dense fibrous tissue.

The most characteristic finding in PC-CD is the interfollicular expansion of plasma cells (Table 6-4; figs. 6-20, 6-21). These are typically a mixture of mature kappa- and lambda-expressing plasma cells; monotypic plasma cells should raise the suspicion of a plasma cell neoplasm. There is often follicular hyperplasia, and follicles may vary in size from large and hyperplastic to small and regressed. Vascular proliferation is not seen. The features of splenic involvement by PC-CD are similar to those of the lymph node. Some cases may show expansion of the marginal zones by plasma cells.

The histologic findings in M-CD are similar to those seen in the PC-CD (41,112), including overall preservation of the normal nodal architecture with prominent interfollicular plasmacytosis and numerous abnormal germinal centers (figs. 6-22–6-24) (40). The sinuses are characteristically open and dilated. The germinal centers are either hyperplastic or atrophic; the latter resemble the regressively transformed germinal centers of HV-CD.

Some investigators believe that the lymph nodes in M-CD progress from a proliferative to

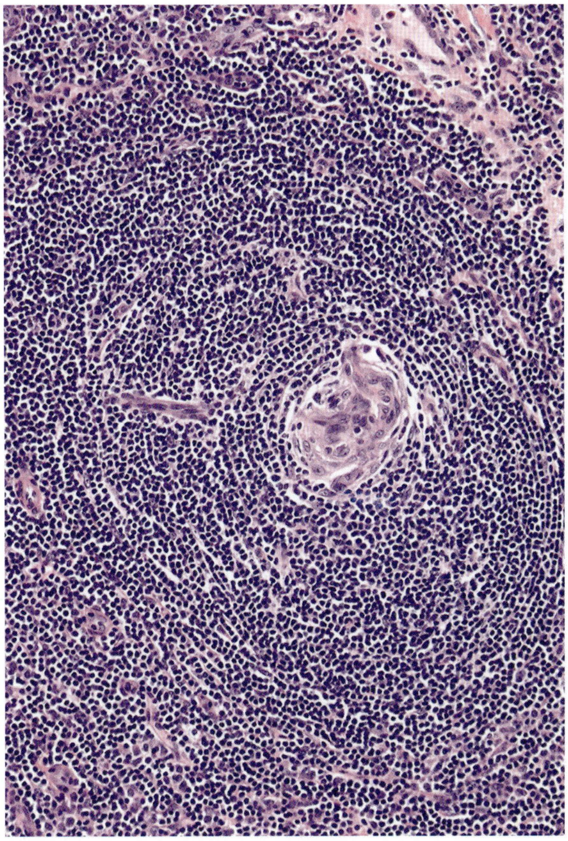

Figure 6-17

HYALINE-VASCULAR CASTLEMAN DISEASE, LYMPH NODE

An atretic follicle with a prominent, hyalinized penetrating blood vessel gives the appearance of a lollipop.

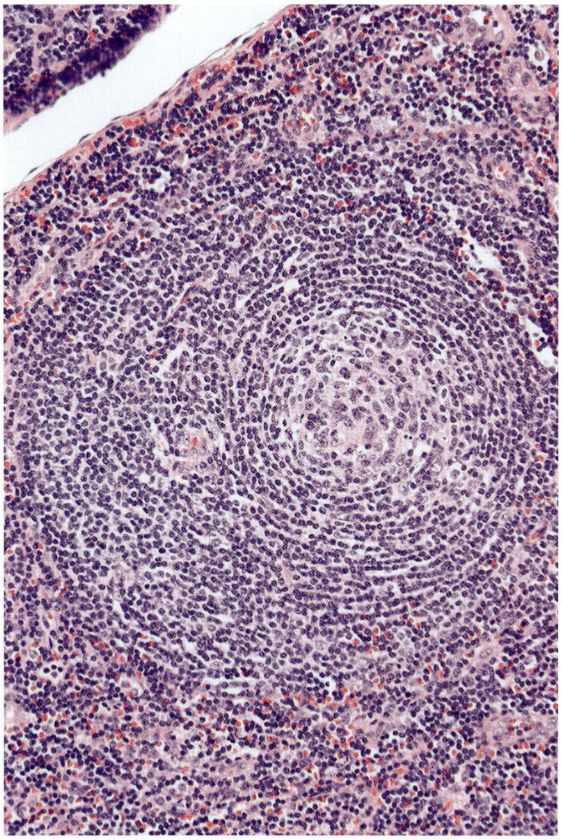

Figure 6-18

HYALINE-VASCULAR CASTLEMAN DISEASE, LYMPH NODE

Lamination of the mantle cell layers leads to the characteristic "onion-skin" appearance of the follicles.

an accumulative phase (40). In the proliferative phase, there is an increase in the number of high endothelial venules and a spectrum of plasma cells, including immature forms. Numerous immunoblasts and mitotic figures may be present, giving a worrisome histologic appearance. Other involved lymph nodes, however, even from the same patient, do not show an increase in vascularity, immature plasma cells, immunoblasts, or mitoses and may represent the accumulative phase (43). Although the plasma cells usually demonstrate polyclonal light-chain expression, some cases of M-CD reportedly have a monoclonal population of plasma cells in a polytypic background (121). Other cases have shown clonal rearrangements of the immunoglobulin gene (57).

Ancillary Studies. Although a specialized technique, cytogenetic analysis of the dendritic cells in HV-CD may be of benefit. The presence of clonal abnormalities in the dendritic cells supports the diagnosis of HV-CD, although does not suggest a different clinical course.

An abnormal immunophenotype of the mantle cells in HV-CD has been reported (97,118). In situ or immunohistochemical staining of PC-CD by HHV-8 is usually positive (fig. 6-25). Staining for immunoglobulin light chains (kappa and gamma) by either immunohistochemistry or in situ hybridization typically reveals a polyclonal pattern in most cases. However, lambda light chain restriction and IgA heavy chain have been reported in some cases (56). Clonal gene rearrangements are also seen occasionally in PC-CD (112).

Differential Diagnosis. The histologic changes of HV-CD are not pathognomonic, and as mentioned previously, CD is a diagnosis of exclusion. Similar changes are seen in lymph

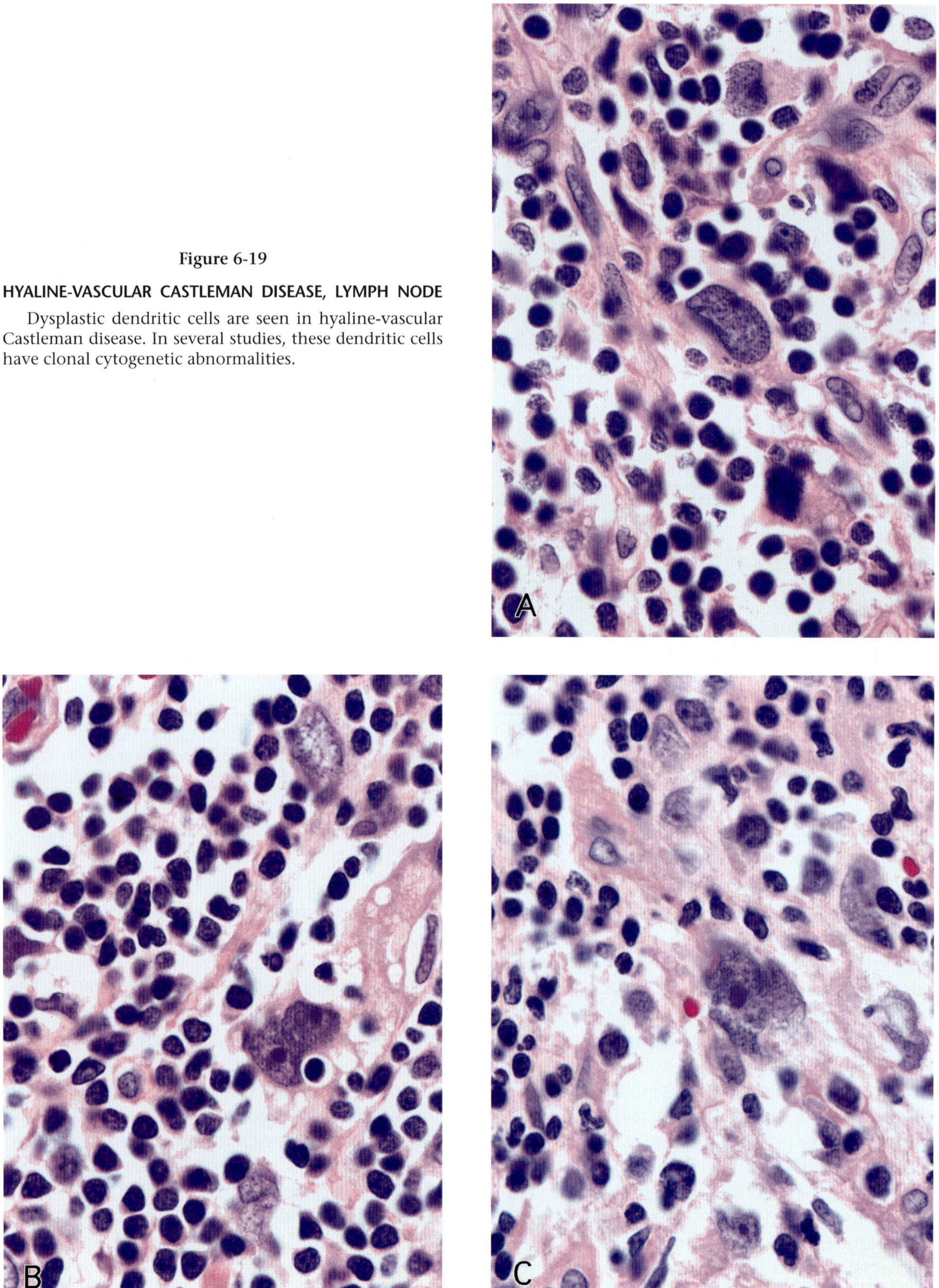

Figure 6-19

HYALINE-VASCULAR CASTLEMAN DISEASE, LYMPH NODE

Dysplastic dendritic cells are seen in hyaline-vascular Castleman disease. In several studies, these dendritic cells have clonal cytogenetic abnormalities.

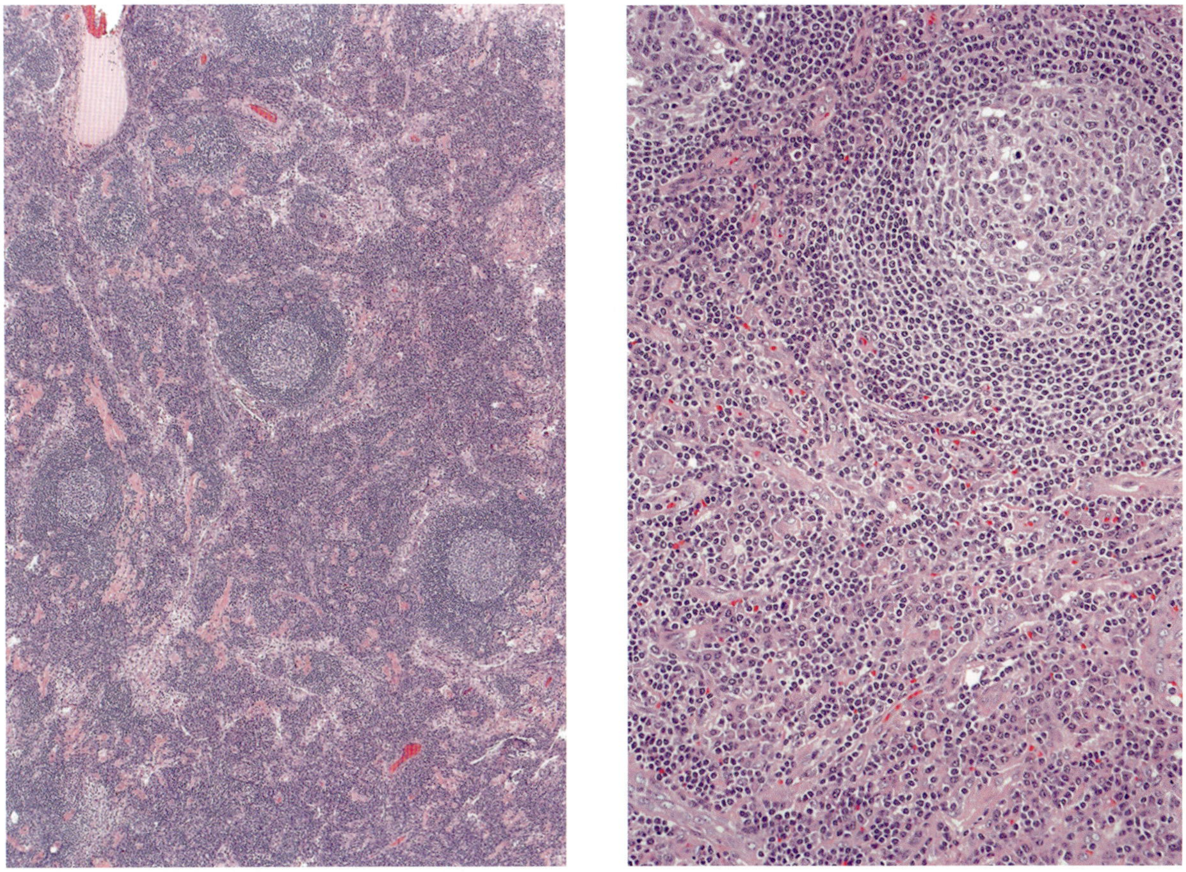

Figure 6-20

PLASMA CELL CASTLEMAN DISEASE, LYMPH NODE

Interfollicular expansion of a lymph node (left), composed predominantly of plasma cells (right).

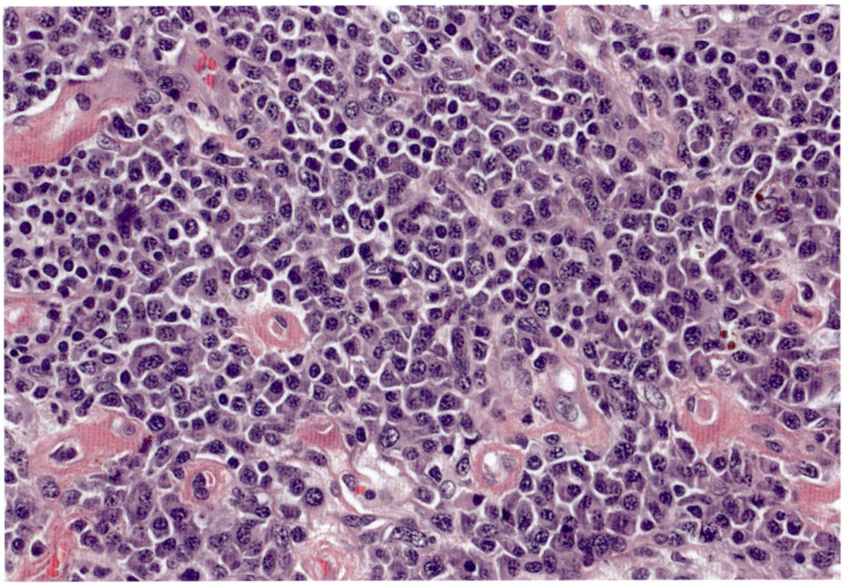

Figure 6-21

PLASMA CELL CASTLEMAN DISEASE, LYMPH NODE

Some cytologic atypia in the plasma cells of Castleman disease is not unusual.

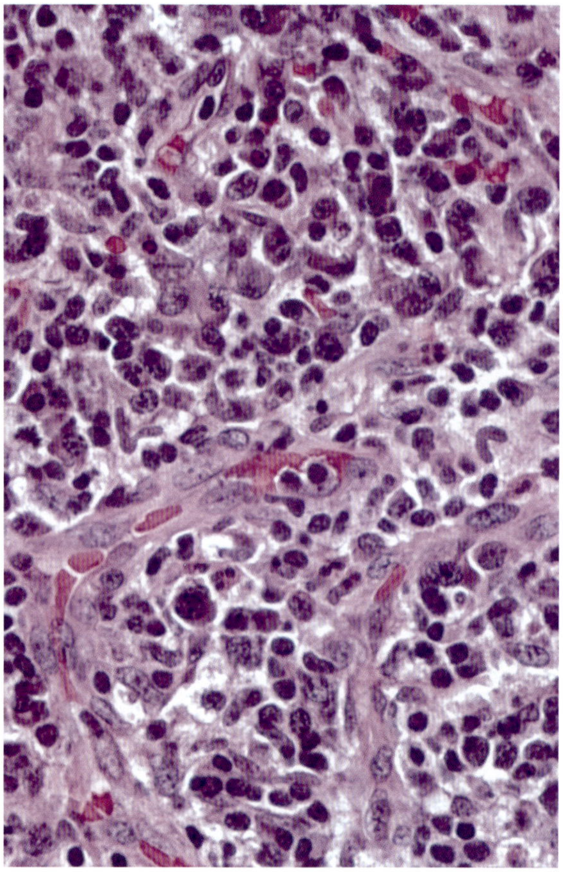

Figure 6-22

MULTICENTRIC CASTLEMAN DISEASE, LYMPH NODE

There is often vascular proliferation as well as plasma cell proliferation in multicentric Castleman disease.

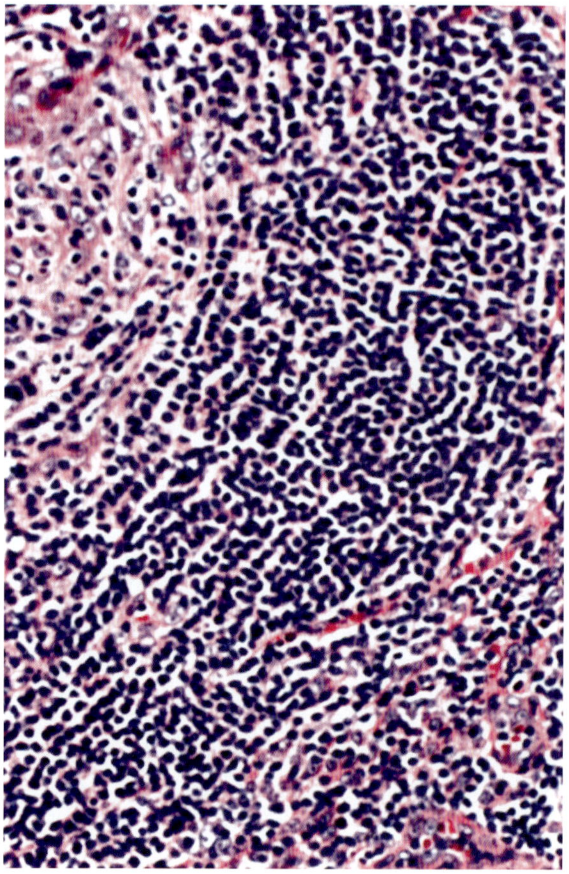

Figure 6-23

MULTICENTRIC CASTLEMAN DISEASE, LYMPH NODE

Small, hyalinized follicles, with some suggestion of onion skinning.

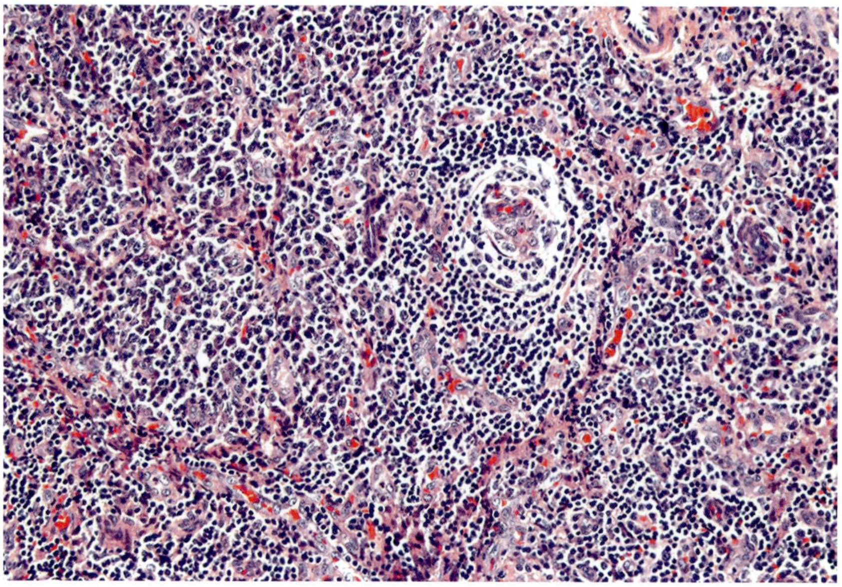

Figure 6-24

MULTICENTRIC CASTLEMAN DISEASE, LYMPH NODE

Small atretic follicles, interfollicular vascular proliferation, and numerous polyclonal plasma cells are seen.

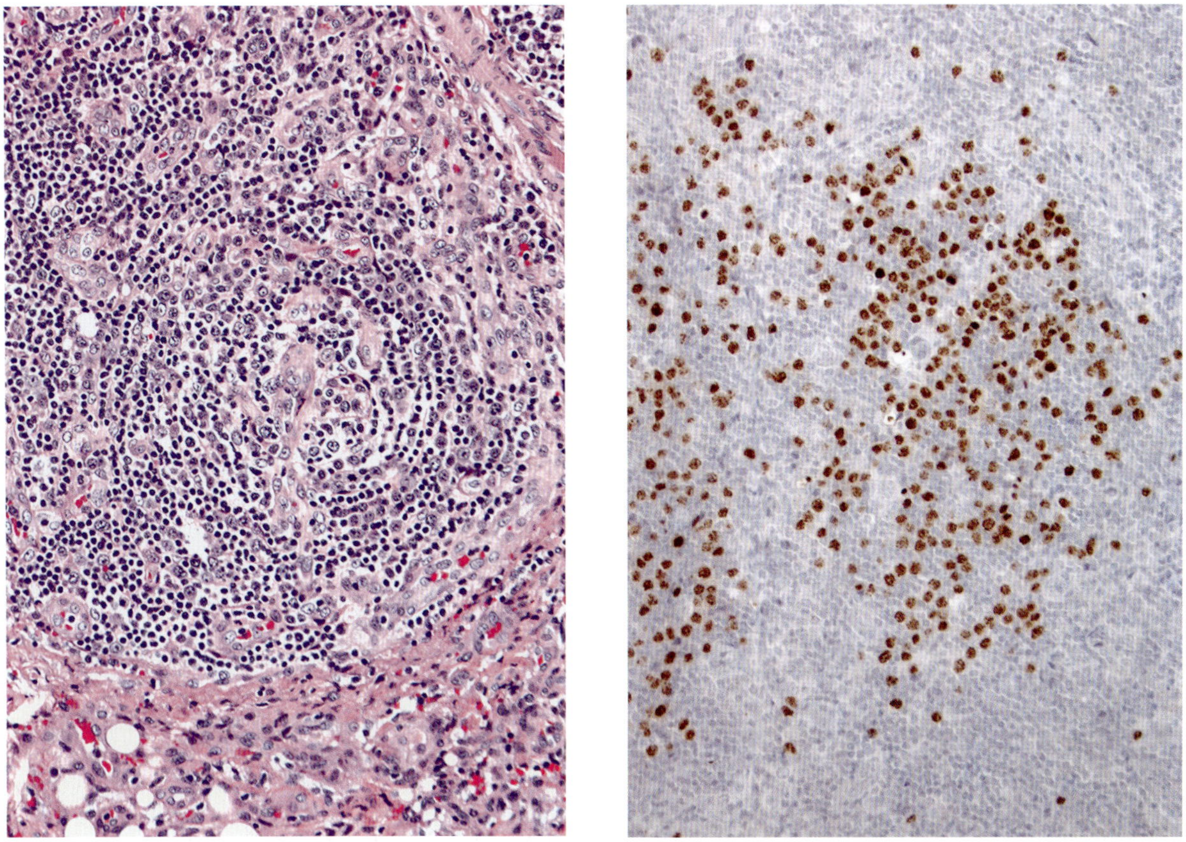

Figure 6-25

HUMAN HERPESVIRUS (HHV)-8 REACTIVITY IN PLASMA CELL CASTLEMAN DISEASE, LYMPH NODE

Lymph node with plasma cell Castleman disease (left) and extensive immunoreactivity for HHV-8 (right). (Courtesy of Anselm Hii, Irvine, CA.)

nodes adjacent to malignancies, both hematopoietic and nonhematopoietic. The individual histologic features of CD, including regressed follicles, onion-skinning of mantle zones, sclerosis/hyalinization, and interfollicular vascular proliferation, can be seen in a variety of conditions. The combination of all these features, however, is not typically seen in other conditions. Also, the presence of dysplastic dendritic cells, in association with the aforementioned features, likely represents HV-CD.

Lymph node changes similar to those seen in PC-CD and M-CD have been reported in AIDS patients, both with and without Kaposi sarcoma (1,58,84,113). HIV infection causes a variety of B-cell abnormalities that result in abnormal immunoregulation and polyclonal B-cell activation. A higher incidence of non-Hodgkin lymphoma and Kaposi sarcoma is also associated with HIV infection. It has been suggested that both the CD-like changes and the presence of Kaposi sarcoma reflect the underlying abnormality of immunoregulation that is the hallmark of AIDS (41).

PC-CD needs to be distinguished from syphilitic lymphadenitis and neoplastic proliferations with an excess of plasma cells such as lymphoplasmacytic lymphoma, marginal zone lymphoma, and plasma cell dyscrasias. In neoplastic conditions, the plasma cells demonstrate light chain restriction, which is not the case in PC-CD.

Treatment and Prognosis. A wide variety of modalities have been used in the treatment of CD; a partial list is presented in Table 6-5. Complete surgical resection is the primary treatment of HV-CD, which is usually a benign and self-limited disease (73). HV-CD may rarely develop into sarcomas

Table 6-5

VARIOUS THERAPIES USED FOR TREATMENT OF CASTLEMAN DISEASE

2-chlorodeoxyadenosine (2-CDA)
Antiinterleukin (anti-IL)-6 (infusional)
Cimetidine
Combination chemotherapy
Cyclophosphamide/cyclosporine A
Danazol
Etoposide (oral)
Ganciclovir
HAART (highly active antiretroviral therapy)
Interferon-alpha
Melphalan
Rituximab
Steroids
Thalidomide
Retinoic acid
Vincristine
Radiotherapy
Autologous bone marrow transplant
Splenectomy

(13,71). These are usually of follicular dendritic cell type, but may have the features of other mesenchymal elements (e.g., vascular) (17).

ANGIOIMMUNOBLASTIC LYMPHADENOPATHY

Definition. *Angioimmunoblastic lymphadenopathy with dysproteinemia* (AILD) is a controversial clinicopathologic entity that shares clinical and morphologic features with angioimmunoblastic T-cell lymphoma (AITL). Some consider it to represent the most indolent end of a spectrum of disorders. If it exists as an entity separate from AITL, it is exceedingly rare.

General Features. Histologic findings identical to those of AILD have been reported in association with a variety of medications. EBV genomes have been detected in both AILD and AITL by PCR and in situ hybridization, suggesting a possible etiologic role for the virus (141).

Clinical Features. AILD was first reported in 1974 by Frizzera et al. (44) as a clinicopathologic syndrome of fever, generalized lymphadenopathy, rash, hepatosplenomegaly, and increased susceptibility to infections. Abnormal laboratory values are seen in most patients (see below).

Over time, similar disorders were described using a variety of terms including immunoblastic lymphadenopathy (93) and lymphogranulomatosis X (87). Because of the similarity in the histopathologic and clinical features, it appears that AILD, *immunoblastic lymphadenopathy*, and *lymphogranulomatosis X* all represent the same entity (40).

Studies suggest that the vast majority of cases of AILD are part of a spectrum of T-cell lymphomas (105,129,139), with clonal T-cell populations in most cases (110,142) and immunoglobulin gene rearrangements in some cases (55,91). Frizzera (40) suggests that there is a spectrum of related disorders, possibly with similar etiologies, that are represented by AILD as a non-neoplastic, and possibly precursor, lesion to AITL as a neoplastic, malignant T-cell proliferation. It is possible that AILD may progress to AITL under some circumstances.

The above disorders can be morphologically grouped into three categories: AILD, AITL, and *atypical lymphoid hyperplasia* (ALH) (see chapter 5) (104). ALH resembles AILD or AITL but does not exactly fit the criteria for either of these disorders. It is possible that ALH represents an abnormal immune response that may be associated with autoimmune diseases (80).

Laboratory Findings. Laboratory abnormalities include Coombs-positive hemolytic anemia with an attendant drop in hemoglobin, low haptoglobin levels, and elevated lactate dehydrogenase (LDH) levels (41,54). Polyclonal hypergammaglobulinemia and protein electrophoresis occasionally reveal small monoclonal proteins.

Microscopic Findings. The histologic findings in lymph nodes involved by AILD are essentially identical to those seen in AITL and include effacement and disarray of the normal architecture (40). In contrast to many neoplastic processes in the lymph nodes, the peripheral and central lymph node sinuses are often patent in both AILD and AITL. The nodes are populated by a polymorphic cellular infiltrate that consists of prominent immunoblasts, small lymphocytes, macrophages, and plasma cells. Eosinophils are frequently increased. There is a prominent increase in vascularity, mostly of high endothelial vessels, with thickened, activated endothelial cells. Other inconsistent features include eosinophilic amorphous periodic acid–Schiff (PAS)-

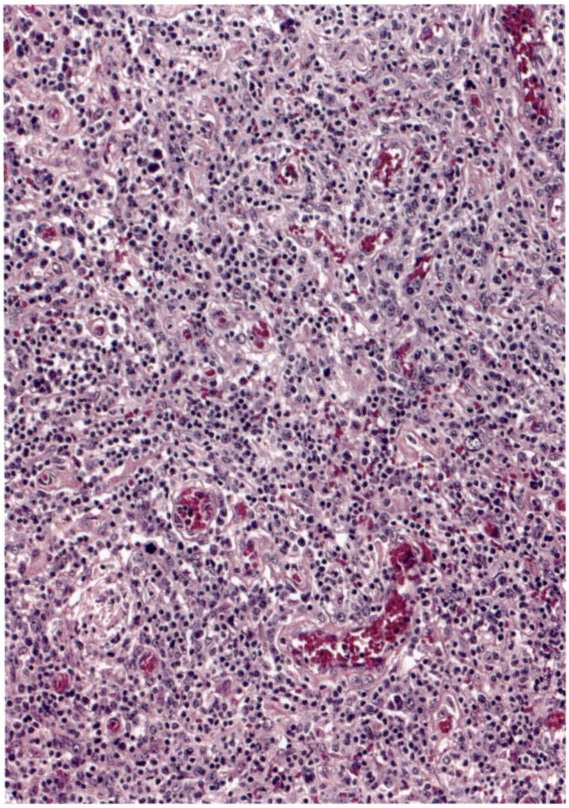

Figure 6-26

ANGIOIMMUNOBLASTIC LYMPHADENOPATHY WITH DYSPROTEINEMIA

A depleted lymphoid pattern with accentuated vascularity is seen.

Table 6-6

COMPARISON OF ANGIOIMMUNOBLASTIC LYMPHADENOPATHY WITH DYSPROTEINEMIA (AILD) AND ANGIOIMMUNOBLASTIC T-CELL LYMPHOMA (AITL)

		AILD	AITL
Histology	Effaced nodal architecture	+	+
	Increased immunoblasts	+	+
	Polymorphous cellularity	+	+
	Vascular proliferation	+	+
	Burned-out germinal centers	+	+
	Plasmacytosis	+/-	+/-
	Increased eosinophils	+/-	+/-
Immuno-histo-chemistry	Predominantly T cells (CD3)	+	+
	Abnormal T-cell immuno-phenotype[a]	-	+/-
	CD30 expression by numerous cells	-	-/+
	Increased follicular dendritic cell networks (CD21, CD35)	+	+
Molecular	Clonal TCR[b]	-	+/-
	Clonal IgH	-	-/+

[a]Loss of pan-T-cell antigens or coexpression of CD10 in T cells.
[b]TCR = T-cell receptor; IgH = immunoglobulin H.

positive intercellular material and burned-out or regressively transformed germinal centers in a lymphoid depleted background (fig. 6-26). An additional feature of AITL is the presence of clusters, islands, or sheets of atypical T cells that may have clear cytoplasm.

Immunohistochemical evaluation of lymph nodes is of great value when assessing AILD and AILD-like processes. The predominant cell type is the T cell, with an excess of the cytotoxic type (positive for CD8, TIA-1, perforin, and granzyme B) (40,103). In spite of this excess of cytotoxic T cells, the neoplastic population of lymphocytes are CD4 positive. Expression of CD30 or loss of pan-T-cell antigens (such as CD2, CD3, CD5, or CD7) should not be seen, and would suggest a diagnosis of AITL. The proliferation of dendritic cell networks, as highlighted by CD21, CD35, or other markers, occurs in both AILD and AITL.

Ancillary Studies. Analysis of both T-cell receptor and B-cell immunoglobulin receptor, either by Southern blot or PCR, should be undertaken in undetermined cases. The presence of clonal populations of either T or B cells is contrary to a diagnosis of AILD, and suggests a lymphomatous process. The presence of oligoclonal bands (especially strong, distinct oligoclonal bands), is considered supportive of a diagnosis of AILD, if other features of lymphoma are lacking. The presence of any clonal cytogenetic abnormalities supports a diagnosis of lymphoma, rather than AILD.

Differential Diagnosis. The most important considerations in the differential diagnosis of AILD are the exclusion of AITL and an immunoblastic large B-cell lymphoma, which are discussed above (Table 6-6). As mentioned, AILD is a controversial diagnosis. Some authorities believe that all cases are in fact AITL, or represent reactive lymph nodes (29); with this in mind, the validity of a diagnosis of AILD should be given serious consideration. Other benign conditions that can mimic AILD are PC-CD/M-CD and other general changes that would be categorized as atypical lymphoid hyperplasia (see chapter 5).

Treatment and Prognosis. When considering the spectrum of diseases that include AILD and AITL, the heterogeneity of clinical outcomes should be considered. In many cases, AILD has an aggressive clinical course and requires treatment that is comparable to that of T-cell lymphoma. In spite of aggressive therapy, patients with AILD have mortality rates of up to 60 percent (45,54). It is important to consider that either or both T-cell lymphoma (e.g., AITL) and B-cell lymphoma (e.g., immunoblastic diffuse large B-cell lymphoma) can develop as a progression of AILD.

ROSAI-DORFMAN DISEASE (SINUS HISTIOCYTOSIS WITH MASSIVE LYMPHADENOPATHY)

Definition. *Rosai-Dorfman disease,* also known as *sinus histiocytosis with massive lymphadenopathy,* is a pathologic process involving a nonclonal proliferation of distinctive cells of macrophage/histiocytic lineage. These cells may cause local enlargement of lymph nodes, or present in extranodal sites. Emperipolesis is a characteristic finding of the cells of Rosai-Dorfman disease.

General Features. No specific etiology for Rosai-Dorfman disease is known at present. The macrophages are distinctive from the remainder of the histiocytic "family." They are definitely not derived from follicular dendritic cells, interdigitating dendritic cells, or Langerhans cells, and are thought to represent an unusual type of activated macrophage (92). They have been shown to be polyclonal by human androgen receptor assay (HUMARA) (116). Rare cases are associated with EBV, *Klebsiella*, and HHV-6 infections (16,89). Some patients have underlying immune dysfunction, which may play a role in the development of Rosai-Dorfman disease.

Clinical Features. Rosai-Dorfman disease was first reported by Rosai and Dorfman in 1969 (125). The disease characteristically presents as bilateral, often bulky, painless cervical lymphadenopathy. Other lymph nodes, most commonly axillary, mediastinal, and paraaortic, can be involved. Fever and other systemic symptoms are present in approximately 25 percent of patients. Rosai-Dorfman disease is a benign, self-limited disorder that usually spontaneously resolves. The lymphadenopathy may persist or recur. This disorder is most commonly seen in children in the first two decades of life although it may be seen at any age. There is a slight male predominance.

Extranodal Rosai-Dorfman disease, with or without lymph node involvement, represents about 40 percent of cases and is a well-described clinicopathologic condition that has been reported in many sites. These sites include the sinonasal region (16 percent), skin and soft tissues (16 percent), orbit (11 percent), bone (11 percent), salivary gland (7 percent), central nervous system (7 percent), kidney (3 percent), and respiratory tract (3 percent) (16,38,53,94, 135,143). In extranodal sites, this lesion can be challenging to diagnose since it usually presents with increased fibrosis and less obvious emperipolesis than in a lymph node.

Some patients with Rosai-Dorfman disease develop lymphoma (both Hodgkin and non-Hodgkin types); rarely, the disease and lymphoma are concurrent (39,92,130). In these cases, lymphoma-associated hemophagocytic syndromes should be considered in the differential diagnosis.

Laboratory Findings. Laboratory abnormalities include low albumin levels, leukocytosis, polyclonal hypergammaglobulinemia, and an elevated ESR. A reversed CD4 to CD8 ratio and mild anemia may also be seen (16).

Microscopic Findings. Histologically, involved lymph nodes show a sinusoidal pattern of dilatation by large macrophages with round vesicular nuclei, distinct nucleoli, and foamy cytoplasm (figs. 6-27–6-29). The hallmark of this disease is emperipolesis, which is the presence of viable inflammatory and hematopoietic cells (plasma cells, lymphocytes, neutrophils, and erythrocytes) within the cytoplasm of the macrophages (fig. 6-30). In contrast to Langerhans cell histiocytosis, eosinophils are not prominent.

Other histologic features include a variable amount of fibrosis, residual germinal centers, and scattered lymphocytes. Prominent polyclonal plasmacytosis within the medullary cords is also characteristically noted. The lymph node capsule is often thickened.

The macrophages are typically reactive with S-100 protein (fig. 6-31) and with histiocyte/macrophage markers such as lysozyme, CD163, and CD68. They are also positive for CD31, although this will not distinguish Rosai-Dorfman disease

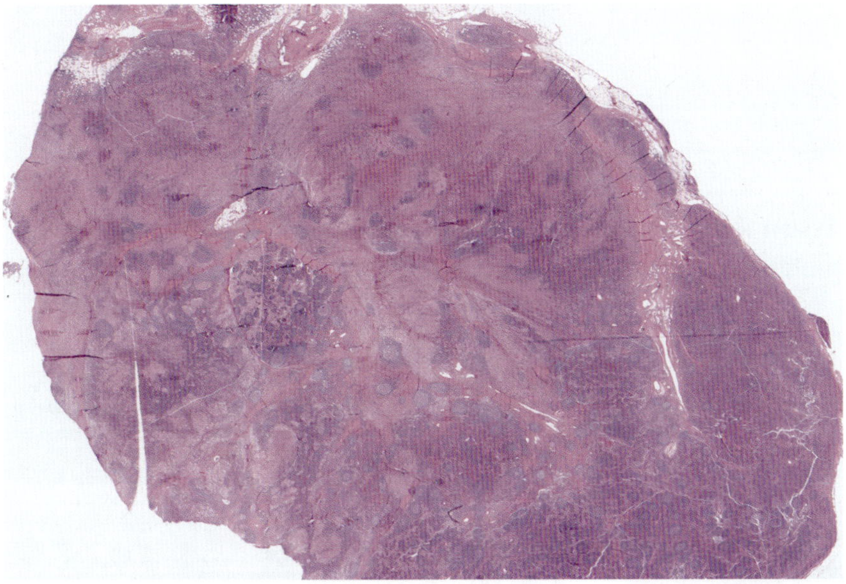

Figure 6-27

ROSAI-DORFMAN DISEASE, LYMPH NODE

The lymphoid sinuses are expanded by pale-staining cells in a portion of this lymph node (top and left).

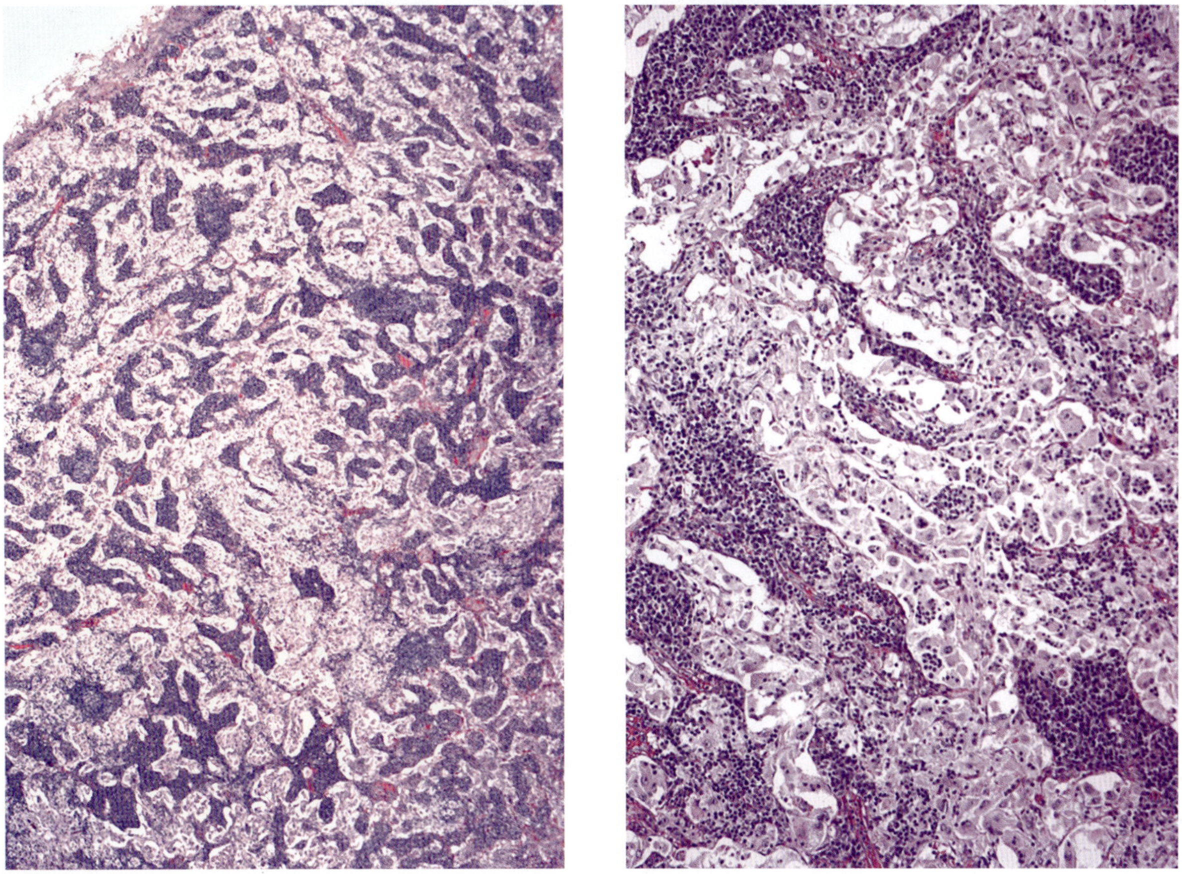

Figure 6-28

ROSAI-DORFMAN DISEASE, LYMPH NODE

The lymph node sinuses are filled with pale-staining macrophages.

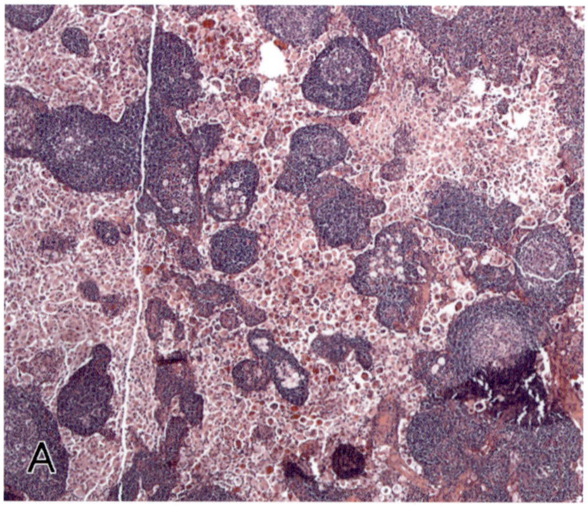

Figure 6-29

ROSAI-DORFMAN DISEASE, LYMPH NODE

In some cases of Rosai-Dorfman disease, the sinus macrophages are more "epithelioid" appearing.

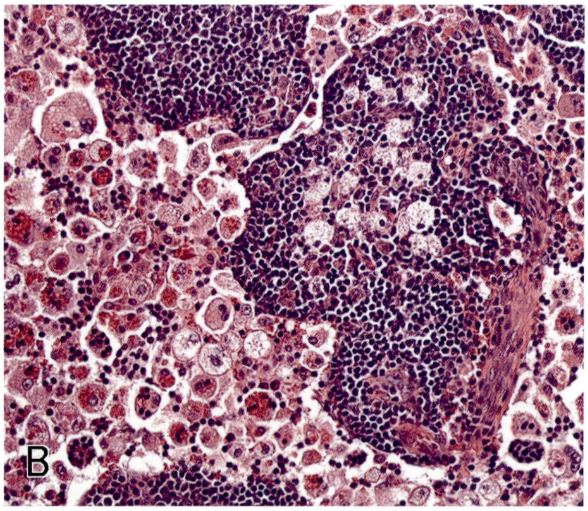

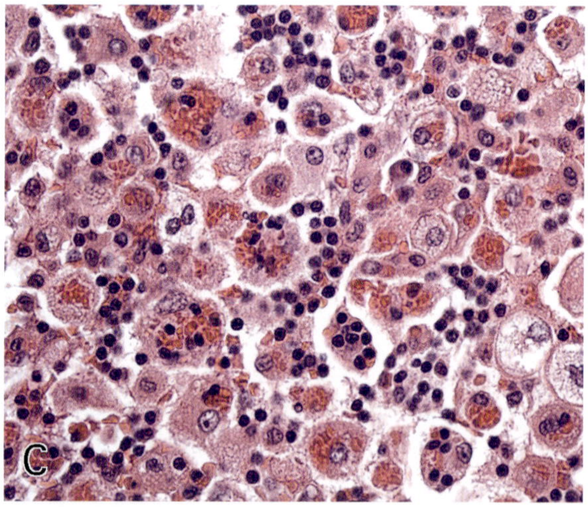

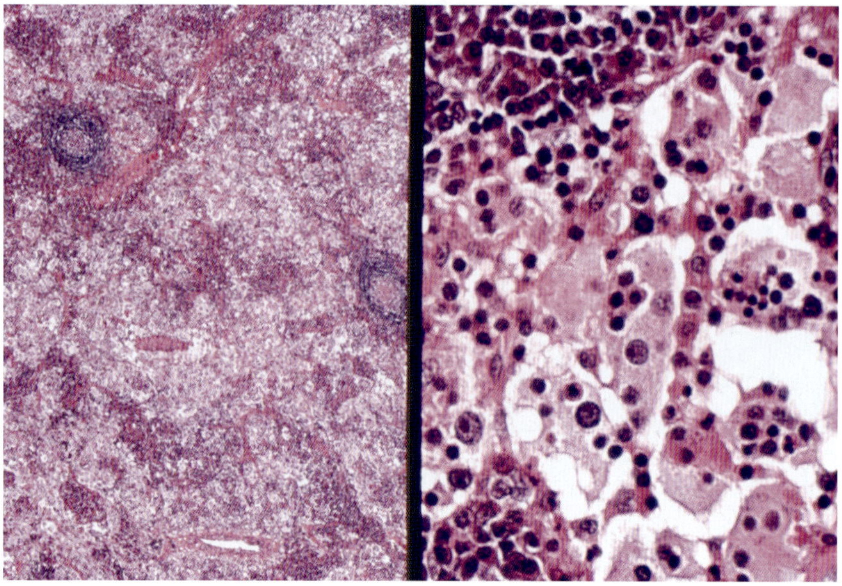

Figure 6-30

ROSAI-DORFMAN DISEASE, LYMPH NODE

The sinuses are infiltrated by large macrophages (left). Emperipolesis is present (right).

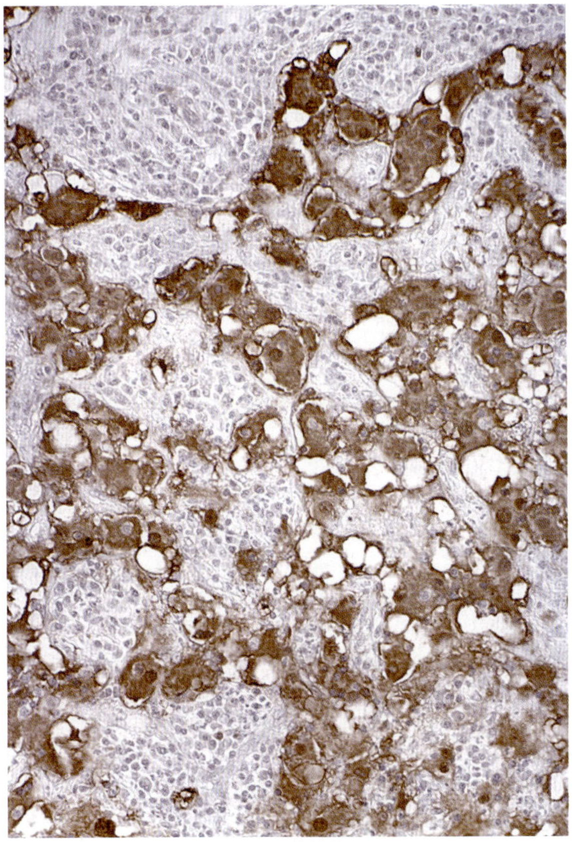

Figure 6-31

S-100 REACTIVITY IN ROSAI-DORFMAN DISEASE, LYMPH NODE

The cells are positive for S-100 protein.

Table 6-7

COMPARISON OF ROSAI-DORFMAN DISEASE AND OTHER HISTIOCYTIC DISORDERS

	Rosai-Dorfman Disease	Langerhans Cell Histiocytosis	Sinus Histiocytosis	Histiocytic Sarcoma
Predominant sinus distribution	+	+	+	+/-
Eosinophils	-	+	-	-
Emperipolesis	+	-	-	-/+
CD68 positive	+	+	+	+/-
S-100 positive	+	+	-	-/+
CD1a positive	-	+	-	-

Table 6-8

DISORDERS ASSOCIATED WITH HEMOPHAGOCYTOSIS IN THE SPLEEN AND LYMPH NODES

Benign
- Virus associated (Epstein-Barr virus, other viruses)
- Associated with other infections (bacterial, fungal, rickettsial, parasitic)
- Congenital hemophagocytic syndromes
- Drug induced (e.g., fludarabine)
- Autoimmune hemolytic anemias
- Storage diseases

Malignant
- Histiocytic sarcoma (e.g., malignant histiocytosis)
- T-cell lymphoma including hepatosplenic T-cell lymphoma
- B-cell lymphomas
- Rare nonhematopoietic malignancies

from Langerhans cell histiocytosis (131); however, nonreactivity with antibodies to CD1a helps to distinguish the former from the latter (33).

Differential Diagnosis. Table 6-7 compares Rosai-Dorfman disease to other histiocytic disorders. Often because of the sinus distribution of Rosai-Dorfman disease, it is mistaken for metastatic carcinoma, melanoma, or even lymphoma. Careful histologic examination typically eliminates these as diagnoses, although occasionally, immunohistochemical stains are necessary.

Treatment and Prognosis. As mentioned above, most cases of Rosai-Dorfman disease regress spontaneously. Rare patients, however, have local relapses or persistent, nonprogressive disease. A mortality rate of approximately 7 percent is primarily due to the massive involvement of vital organs or sites (16).

HEMOPHAGOCYTIC SYNDROMES

Definition. The *hemophagocytic syndromes* are a group of systemic disorders characterized by systemic symptoms, pancytopenia, and phagocytosis of hematopoietic elements. They occur in a variety of tissues and organs, including lymph nodes and spleen.

General Features. The hemophagocytic syndromes are associated with various infectious agents, hematologic malignancies, and nonhematologic familial disorders (Table 6-8) (35,51,59,69,107). Whether all cases of hemophagocytic syndrome represent the same underlying mechanism(s) is unclear. The common denominator appears to be an immunodeficiency state with a superimposed condition, most often, but not always, of an infectious nature. Some investigators have proposed that hyperproduction

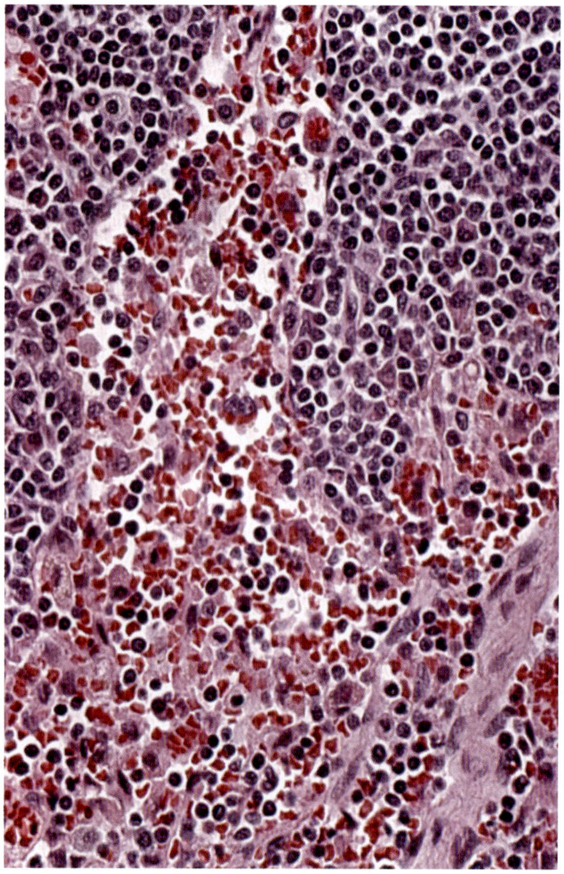

Figure 6-32

HEMOPHAGOCYTIC SYNDROME, LYMPH NODE

Sinuses contain abnormally large macrophages with red blood cells in their cytoplasm.

of cytokines, resulting from a deficient immune stimulus, may result in the hyperplasia and hyperactivity of the macrophages characteristically seen in this disorder (15,60).

Familial hemophagocytic lymphohistiocytosis (FHLH), a congenital hemophagocytic syndrome, has an autosomal recessive manner of inheritance and is caused by the overwhelming activation of T lymphocytes and macrophages associated with defective triggering of apoptosis and reduced cytotoxic activity. FHLH exhibits genetic heterogeneity; cases are linked to chromosome 9q, mutations at 10q22 (*PRF1* gene), mutations at 17q25.1 (*UNC13D* gene), and mutation in the *syntaxin-11* gene (149).

Clinical Features. The hemophagocytic syndromes are characterized by the acute onset pancytopenia. This is caused by the proliferation of macrophages in lymphoreticular organs and is associated with prominent phagocytosis of hematopoietic elements. Manifestations include fever, cytopenias, liver dysfunction, coagulopathies, abnormal lipid metabolism, and hepatosplenomegaly (67).

Because the acute clinical course culminates in death in many cases, an immediately obvious etiology is lacking, and the systemic distribution and striking proliferation of cells are present in all lymphoreticular organs, these cases were previously considered to represent malignant histiocytosis. Risdall et al. (123) were the first to identify their reactive nature. They described a distinct clinical syndrome characterized by a proliferation of benign macrophages demonstrating prominent hemophagocytosis, fever, and varying cytopenias in a clinical context of underlying viral infection. They termed the disorder viral-associated and, later, *infection-associated hemophagocytic syndrome* (IAHS) (122). Since that time, it has been associated with a variety of viral (95), bacterial (122), and other infectious processes (134) including HIV/AIDS. Hemophagocytic syndrome also has been reported in association with several autoimmune disorders including systemic lupus erythematosus, rheumatoid arthritis, juvenile rheumatoid arthritis (Still disease), polyarteritis nodosa, and others (27). In some cases, no definitive etiology is established.

Many cases have been reported in conjunction with hematologic and nonhematologic malignancies. T-cell lymphomas, especially subcutaneous panniculitis-like T-cell lymphoma and hepatosplenic T-cell lymphoma, are associated with hemophagocytic syndrome. Prominent hemophagocytosis, however, may also be seen in all subtypes of T-cell as well as B-cell lymphomas.

Microscopic Findings. Histologically, involved lymph nodes show lymphoid depletion and prominent dilatation of the sinuses by bland-appearing hemophagocytic macrophages (figs. 6-32, 6-33). The process may extend beyond the capsule into the perinodal tissues. Focal hemorrhage may be seen. Although phagocytosis of red blood cells is most prominent, other hematopoietic components (granulocytes, lymphocytes, platelets) are found within the cytoplasm of the macrophages.

Spleens with IAHS are usually moderately enlarged, although significant enlargement may occur. The red pulp shows a proliferation of macrophages, which display prominent hemophagocytosis (figs. 6-34, 6-35). The red pulp is frequently congested. The macrophages vary from normal size to massive, with cytoplasm distended by cells and debris. Fibrosis, focal infarctions, and lymphoid depletion of the white pulp may occur (67,70). Besides lymph nodes and spleen, phagocytic macrophages are also prominent in the bone marrow and liver.

Differential Diagnosis. The differential diagnosis of hemophagocytic syndrome includes malignant neoplasms of true histiocytic origin (e.g., histiocytic sarcoma), hairy cell leukemia, monocytoid B-cell lymphoma, anaplastic large cell lymphoma, and nonhematopoietic metastatic malignancies that involve the lymph node sinuses, such as carcinoma or melanoma (figs. 6-36, 6-37). In most circumstances, careful morphologic examination and the use of ancillary studies, such as immunohistochemistry, flow cytometry, and molecular/cytogenetic testing, distinguish these processes.

Hemophagocytic syndromes associated with malignancies of the hematopoietic system

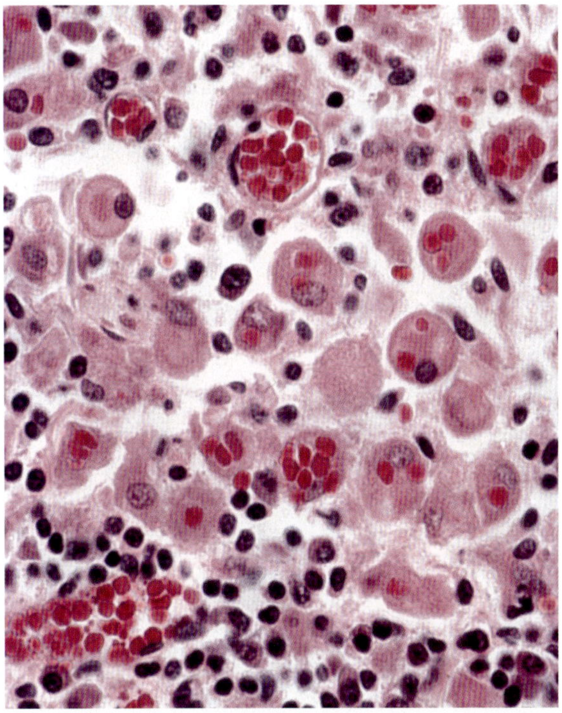

Figure 6-33

HEMOPHAGOCYTIC SYNDROME, LYMPH NODE

Bland-appearing macrophages are filled with red blood cells in infection-associated hemophagocytic syndrome.

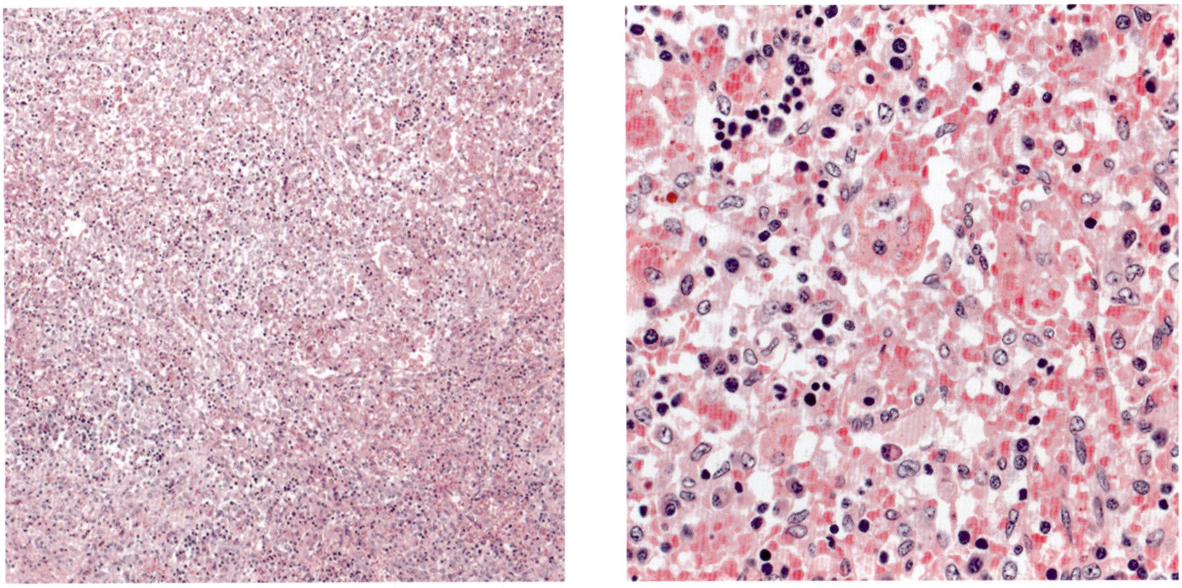

Figure 6-34

HEMOPHAGOCYTIC SYNDROME, SPLEEN

In this example of viral-associated hemophagocytic syndrome, the red pulp is expanded (left) and hemophagocytic macrophages are present in the cords and sinuses (right).

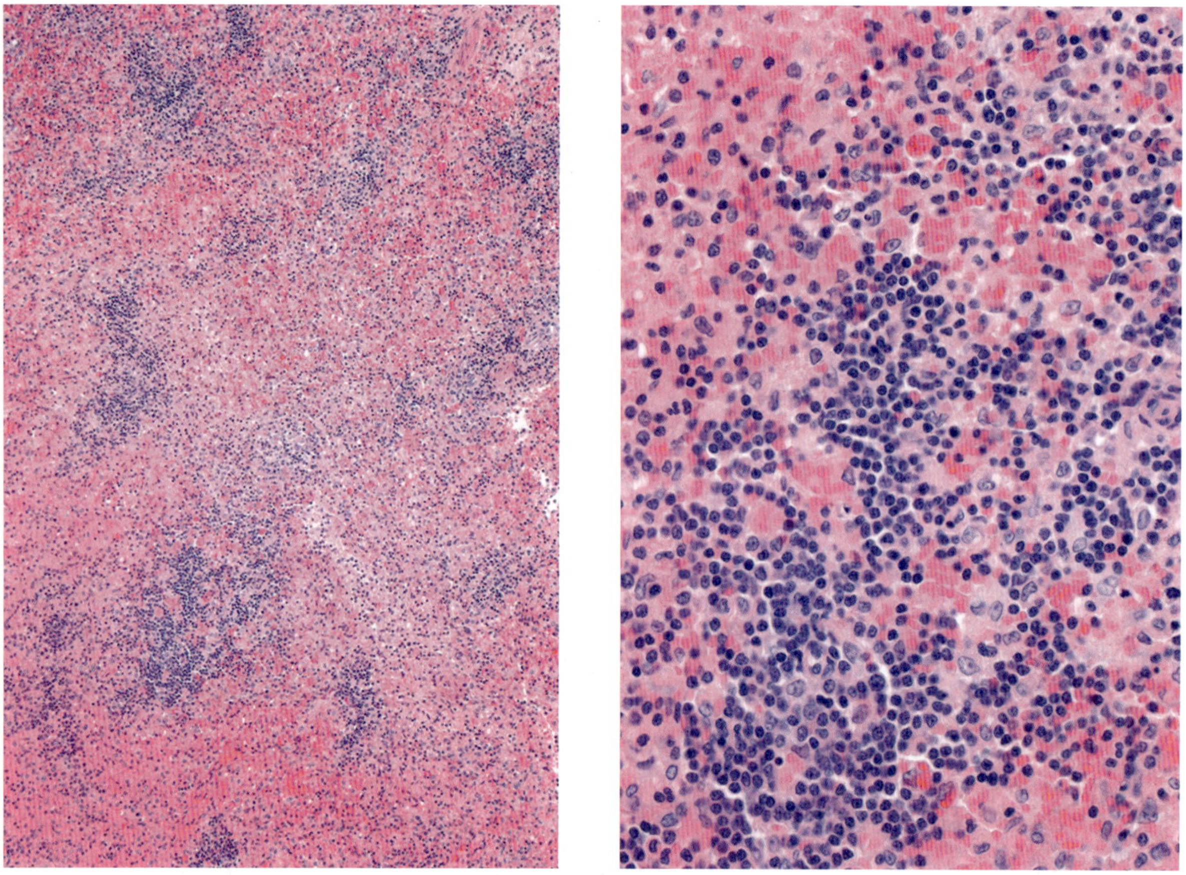

Figure 6-35

HEMOPHAGOCYTIC SYNDROME, SPLEEN

Phagocytosis predominantly involves red blood cells.

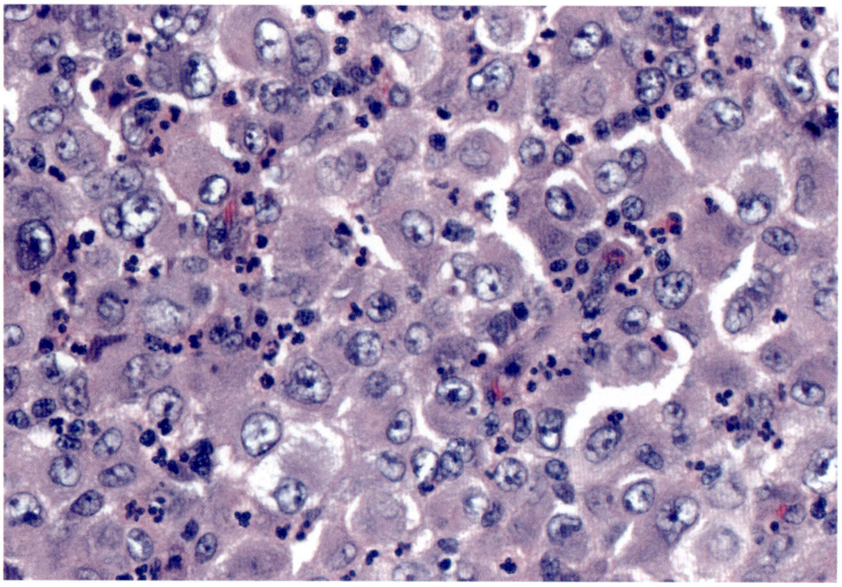

Figure 6-36

HISTIOCYTIC SARCOMA

Large, atypical macrophages are seen. (Courtesy of Dale Selby, San Antonio, TX.)

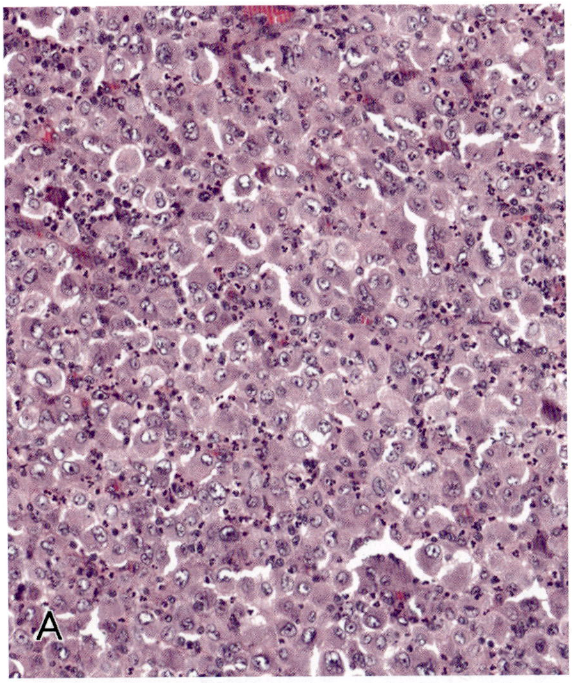

Figure 6-37

HISTIOCYTIC SARCOMA

This histiocytic sarcoma (A) is immunoreactive for CD163 (B) and S-100 protein (C). (Courtesy of Dale Selby, San Antonio, TX.)

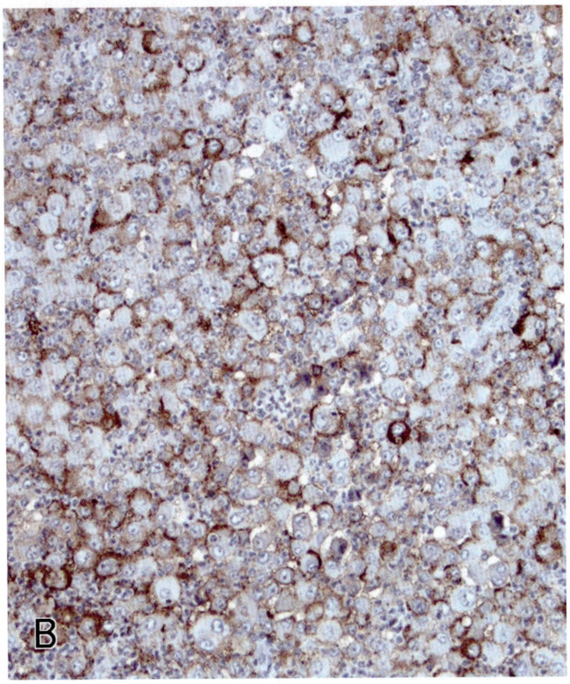

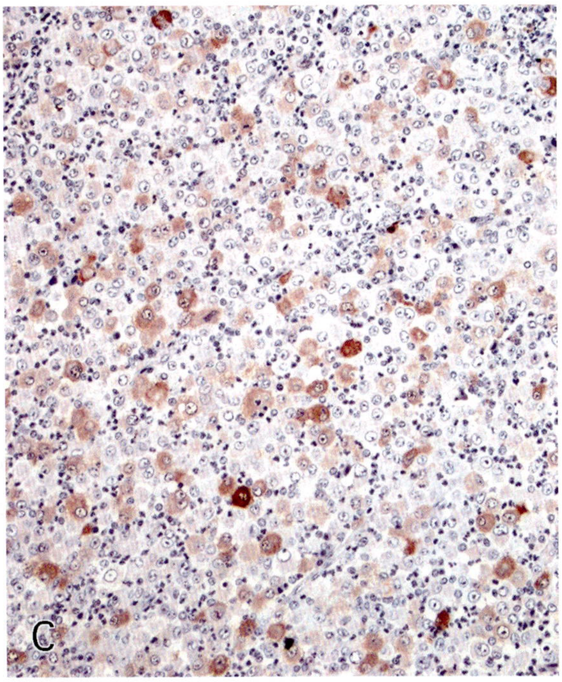

include a component of malignant cells. Lymphomas associated with hemophagocytic syndrome are most often of peripheral T-cell type (fig. 6-38). When only rare neoplastic T cells are found admixed with the numerous macrophages, the resemblance to malignant histiocytosis may be considerable. The diagnosis of T-cell lymphoma in these cases usually requires molecular confirmation.

Treatment and Prognosis. The treatment of hemophagocytic syndrome is usually directed at the associated infection, if known, in addition to supportive measures for the underlying immunosuppressive condition. Bone marrow

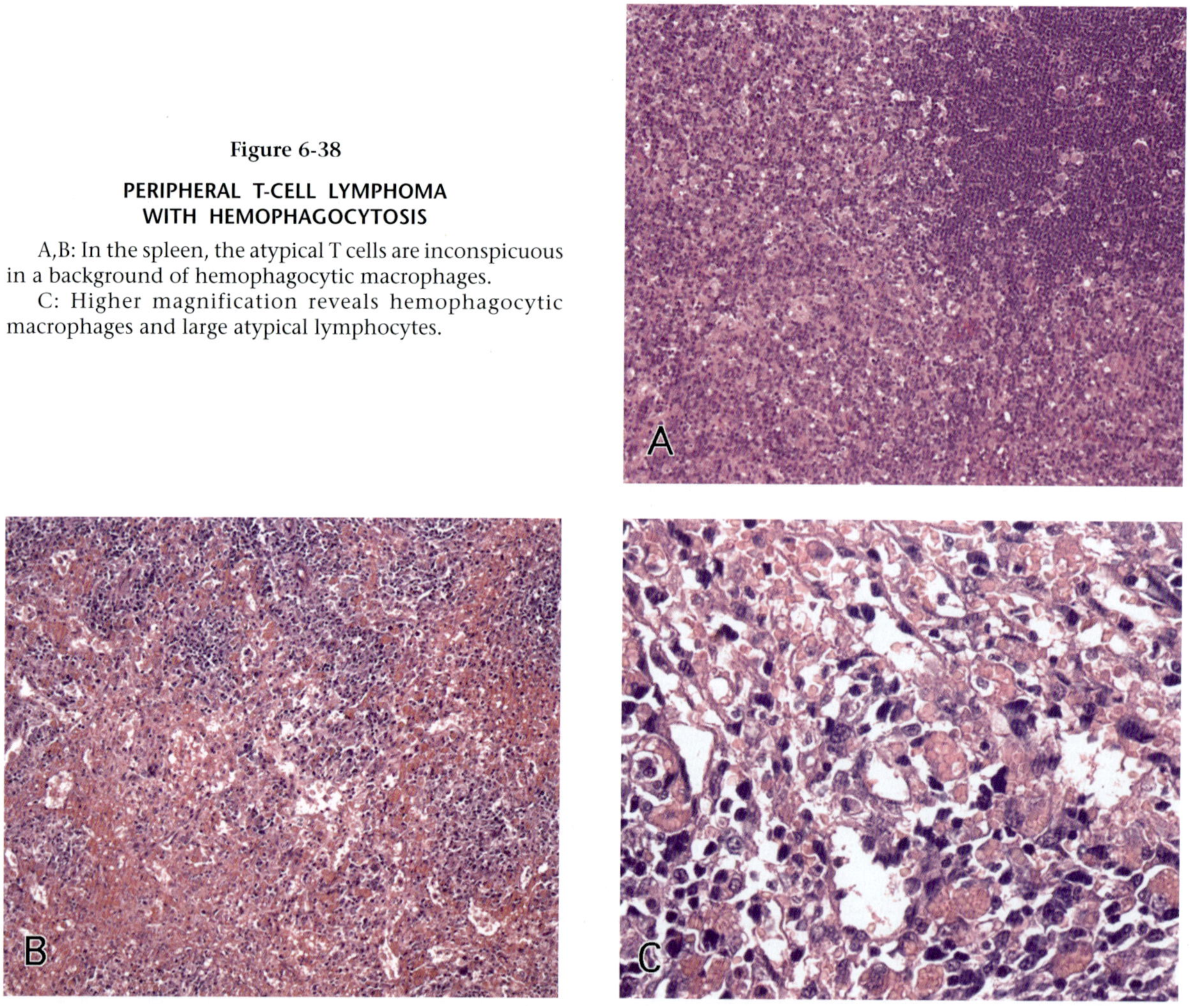

Figure 6-38

PERIPHERAL T-CELL LYMPHOMA WITH HEMOPHAGOCYTOSIS

A,B: In the spleen, the atypical T cells are inconspicuous in a background of hemophagocytic macrophages.

C: Higher magnification reveals hemophagocytic macrophages and large atypical lymphocytes.

transplantation has proven effective as a treatment for FHLH.

LANGERHANS CELL HISTIOCYTOSIS

Definition. *Langerhans cell histiocytosis* (LCH) is a family of disorders that is derived from an immature immune accessory cell, the Langerhans cell. Lymph node and spleen are sites of primary disease or secondary involvement.

General Features. The exact etiology of LCH remains unknown. In the past, most cases were felt to represent benign reactive processes rather than true neoplasms. Some studies, however, have used X-linked polymorphic DNA probes to detect histiocytic clonality in lesions from female patients (145). Studies using loss of heterozygosity and comparative genomic hybridization have also shown frequent abnormalities involving chromosome 1p, chromosome 7, chromosome 9, and chromosome 22q (26,101). These abnormalities suggest that in many cases LCH is probably a clonal neoplastic disorder with a variable clinical course. Other studies using HUMARA DNA, however, have shown that some cases of adult LCH (e.g., pulmonary) are not clonal (148). Recent studies have suggested that the proliferation of Langerhans cells may be due to autocrine and paracrine cytokine signaling between T cells, Langerhans cells, and eosinophils (2,94). Under these conditions, the microenvironment may be responsible for the proliferation of Langerhans cells.

Clinical Features. LCH has multiple clinical presentations, ranging from unifocal lesions, usually of bone, to disseminated systemic disease. The historic eponyms of *eosinophilic granuloma* (usually unifocal LCH), *Hand-Schüller-Christian disease* (skull lesions, exophthalmos,

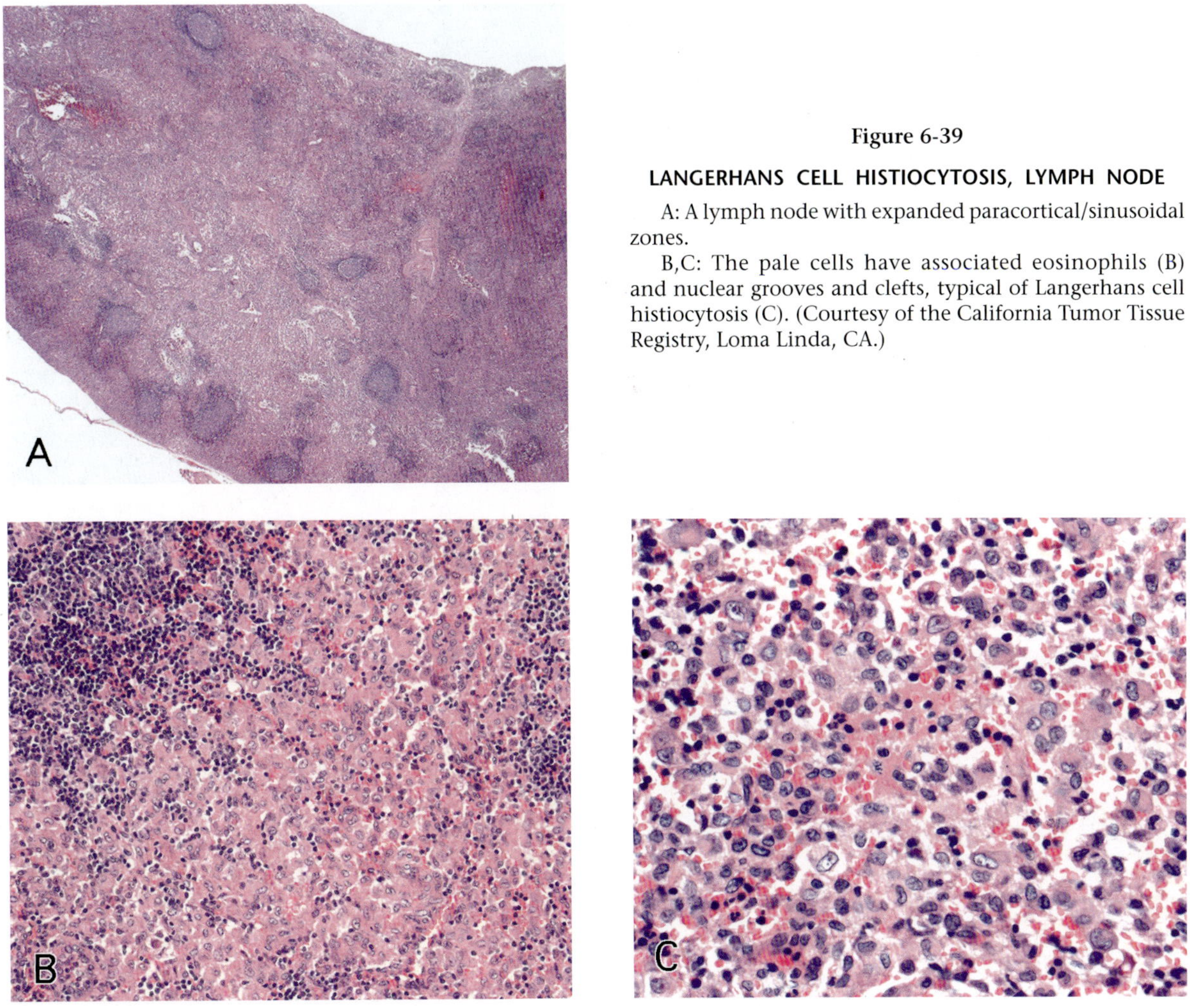

Figure 6-39

LANGERHANS CELL HISTIOCYTOSIS, LYMPH NODE

A: A lymph node with expanded paracortical/sinusoidal zones.

B,C: The pale cells have associated eosinophils (B) and nuclear grooves and clefts, typical of Langerhans cell histiocytosis (C). (Courtesy of the California Tumor Tissue Registry, Loma Linda, CA.)

and diabetes insipidus, or, more commonly, multifocal LCH), and *Letterer-Siwe disease* (systemic LCH) are all examples of the clinical spectrum of LCH but not specific disease entities (2). The lymph node or spleen may represent a primary or secondary site of disease, but is usually involved in the systemic form of the disease (2,90,144). It is not possible to distinguish localized from systemic disease by light microscopic features alone.

Males are more frequently affected than females and most cases occur in children, although the disease can occur at any age (2). Several malignancies have been reported at increased frequency in association with LCH: acute lymphoblastic leukemia, acute myeloid leukemia, myelodysplastic syndrome, Hodgkin lymphoma, non-Hodgkin lymphoma, and a variety of solid tumors (2). Rare familial cases also occur.

Laboratory Findings. Patients with LCH may have leukocytosis and an elevated ESR. A urinalysis should be performed in all LCH patients to evaluate for diabetes insipidus.

Microscopic Findings. The histologic features of the involved lymph nodes include an intact architecture and expansive sinusoidal dilatation by Langerhans cells (fig. 6-39). These cells typically have elongated irregular nuclei with a linear groove, inconspicuous nucleoli, and eosinophilic cytoplasm (fig. 6-40). Multinucleated giant cells and eosinophils are often associated with LCH. In addition to the classic variant of LCH, there is an epithelioid variant that may be mistaken for a metastatic melanoma or anaplastic large cell lymphoma (figs. 6-41, 6-42).

The abnormalities observed in the spleen include hemorrhages and areas of necrosis and infarction. The red pulp is predominantly

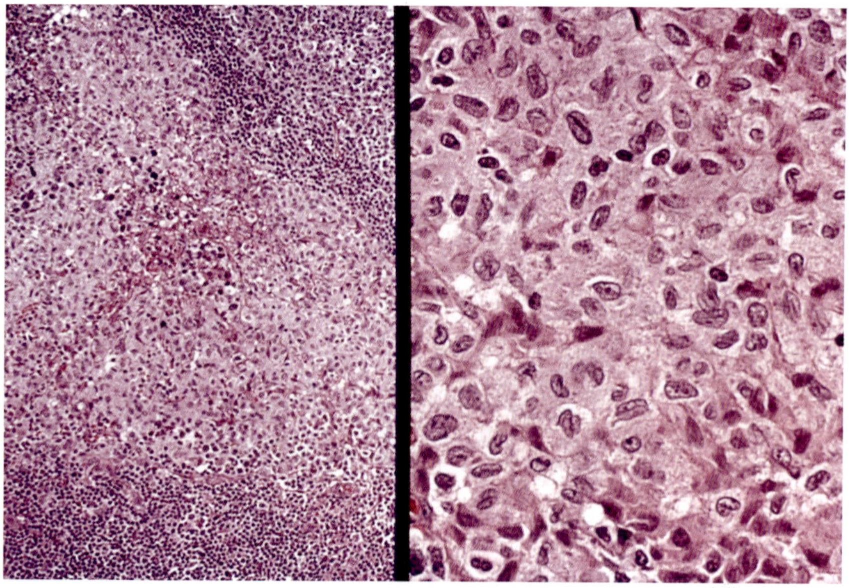

Figure 6-40

LANGERHANS CELL HISTIOCYTOSIS, LYMPH NODE

Dilatation of the sinuses (left) by cells with characteristic elongated nuclei and nuclear grooves (right) is seen in the classic variant of Langerhans cell histiocytosis.

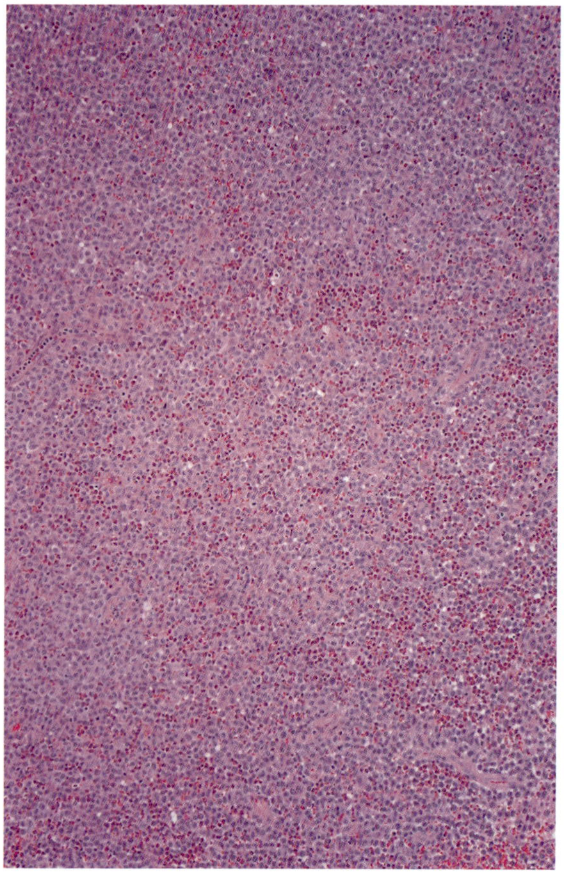

Figure 6-41

LANGERHANS CELL HISTIOCYTOSIS, LYMPH NODE

The sinuses are infiltrated by epithelioid Langerhans cells.

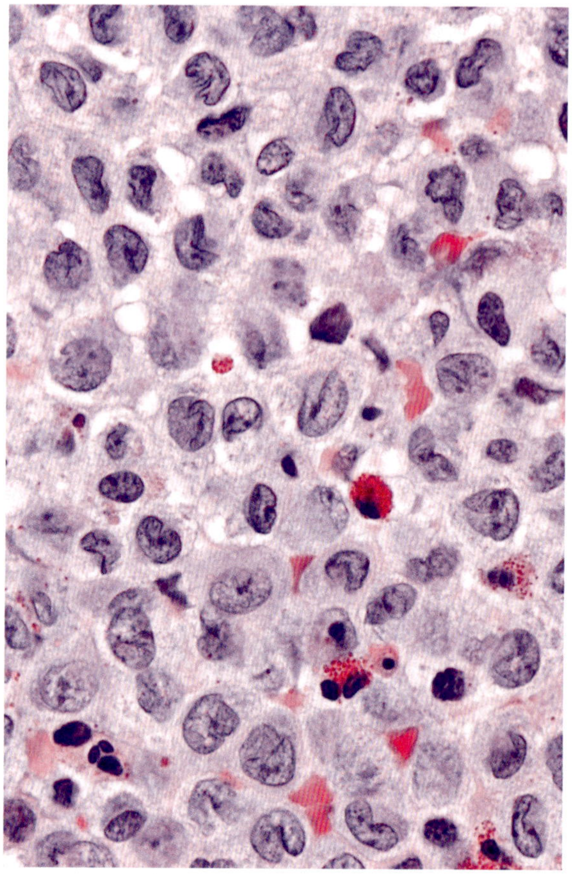

Figure 6-42

LANGERHANS CELL HISTIOCYTOSIS, LYMPH NODE

Langerhans cell histiocytosis, epithelioid cell variant.

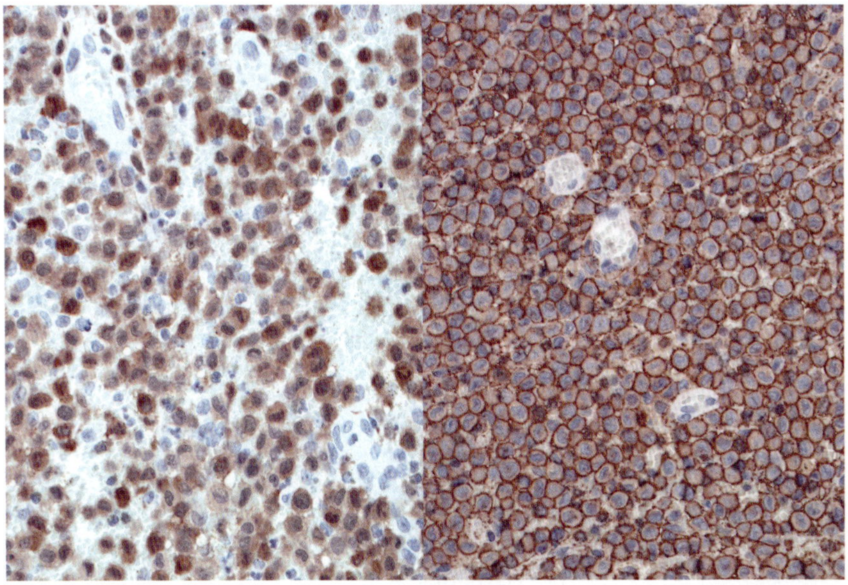

Figure 6-43

LANGERHANS CELL HISTIOCYTOSIS, LYMPH NODE

The Langerhans cells are reactive with S-100 protein (left) and CD1a (right).

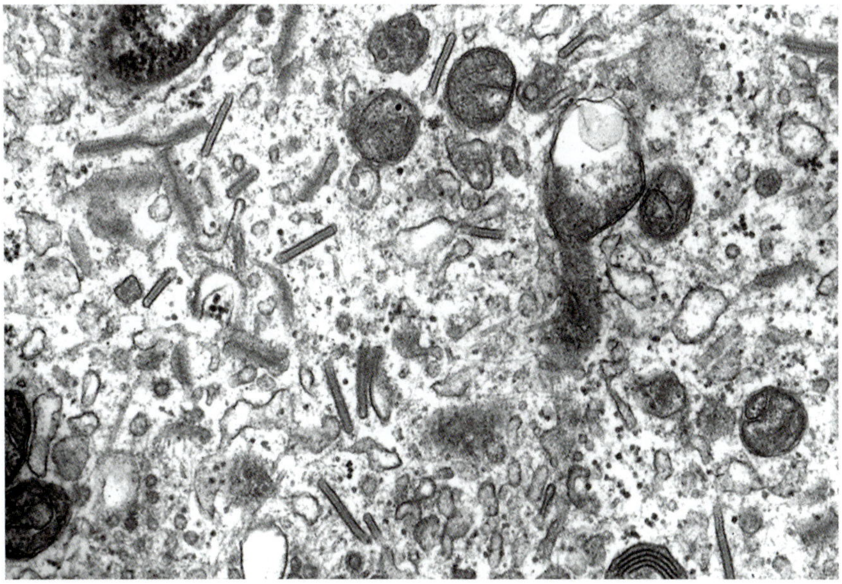

Figure 6-44

BIRBECK GRANULE, LANGERHANS CELL HISTIOCYTOSIS

Electron microscopy shows the Birbeck granules as multilaminated tubular and round structures. In the most fortuitous sections, they have a "tennis racquet" shape.

affected, often by a diffuse infiltrate, or by ill-defined tumor aggregates resembling loosely formed granulomas.

The cells of LCH are typically both S-100 protein and CD1a positive (fig. 6-43) (33). They are also positive for other markers of macrophages including CD68, CD163, and CD31 (108). CD31 does not stain normal Langerhans cells seen in skin (131). Cell cycle and other cellular mechanisms are abnormal in LCH, with the lesional cells staining for transforming growth factor-beta (TGF-β), MDM2, p53, p21, p16, Rb, and bcl-2 (3). An additional antibody, langerin (CD207), is also available, with staining that is as sensitive and specific as CD1a (20). Electron microscopy helps demonstrate the characteristic cytoplasmic organelle, the Birbeck granule (fig. 6-44).

Differential Diagnosis. The differential diagnosis of LCH includes both benign and malignant lesions that have a sinusoidal pattern of infiltration in the lymph node. The benign entities primarily include Rosai-Dorfman disease and IAHS while the malignant neoplasms include metastatic melanoma and carcinoma, anaplastic large cell lymphoma, and malignant histiocytosis. Although reactivity with S-100 protein is also seen in Rosai-Dorfman disease and melanoma, CD1a positivity supports a diagnosis of LCH. The absence of emperipolesis in LCH also aids in the distinction from Rosai-Dorfman disease.

Rare cases of Langerhans cell sarcoma, the malignant counterpart of LCH, have been reported (119). Features include a male predominance, older patient age, and disseminated involvement frequently including the spleen. In these cases, the Langerhans cells appear cytologically malignant with marked atypia.

Treatment and Prognosis. The clinical course of LCH is often unpredictable. Usually, localized disease is treated with local therapy (e.g., radiation), with excellent outcome. Systemic disease is treated with combination chemotherapy and the outcome is dependent on the extent of the disease.

REFERENCES

1. Aboulafia DM, Picozzi VJ, Patterson S. Castleman's disease, Kaposi's sarcoma, and immunoblastic lymphoma in a patient with AIDS. AIDS Reader 1998;8:107-13.
2. Arceci RJ, Longley BJ, Emanuel PD. Atypical cellular disorders. Hematology Am Soc Hematol Educ Program 2002;297-314.
3. Arico M. Langerhans cell histiocytosis in adults: more questions than answers? Eur J Cancer 2004;40:1467-73.
4. Ben-Chetrit E, Flusser D, Okon E, Ackerman Z, Rubinow A. Multicentric Castleman's disease associated with rheumatoid arthritis: a possible role of hepatitis B antigen. Ann Rheum Dis 1989;48:326-30.
5. Bitter MA, Komaiko W, Franklin WA. Giant lymph node hyperplasia with osteoblastic bone lesions and the POEMS (Takatsuki's) syndrome. Cancer 1985;56:188-94.
6. Bradley DJ, Glode MP. Kawasaki disease. The mystery continues. West J Med 1998;168:23-9.
7. Burke JS, Colby TV. Dermatopathic lymphadenopathy. Comparison of cases associated and unassociated with mycosis fungoides. Am J Surg Pathol 1981;5:343-52.
8. Burke JS, Sheibani K, Rappaport H. Dermatopathic lymphadenopathy. An immunophenotypic comparison of cases associated and unassociated with mycosis fungoides. Am J Pathol 1986;123:256-63.
9. Burns JC, Geha RS, Schneeberger EE, et al. Polymerase activity in lymphocyte culture supernatants from patients with Kawasaki disease. Nature 1986;323:814-6.
10. Carter R, Haynes ME, Morton J. Rickettsia-like bodies and splenitis in Kawasaki disease. Lancet 1976;2:1254-5.
11. Castleman B, Iverson L, Menendez VP. Localized mediastinal lymph-node hyperplasia resembling thymoma. Cancer 1956;9:822-30.
12. Chamulak GA, Brynes RK, Nathwani BN. Kikuchi-Fujimoto disease mimicking malignant lymphoma. Am J Surg Pathol 1990;14:514-23.
13. Chan AC, Chan KW, Chan JK, Au WY, Ho WK, NG WM. Development of follicular dendritic cell sarcoma in hyaline-vascular Castleman's disease of the nasopharynx: tracing its evolution by sequential biopsies. Histopathology 2001;38:510-8.
14. Chan JK, Hui PK, Ng CS, Yuen NW, Kung IT, Gwi E. Epithelioid haemangioma (angiolymphoid hyperplasia with eosinophilia) and Kimura's disease in Chinese. Histopathology 1989;15:557-74.
15. Chan JK, Ng CS, Law CK, Ng WF, Wong KF. Reactive hemophagocytic syndrome: a study of 7 fatal cases. Pathology 1987;19:43-50.
16. Chan JK, Tsang WY. Uncommon syndromes of reactive lymphadenopathy. Semin Oncol 1993;20:648-57.
16. Chan JK, Tsang WY, Ng CS. Follicular dendritic cell tumor and vascular neoplasm complicating hyaline-vascular Castleman's disease. Am J Surg Pathol 1994;18:517-25.
18. Chen H, Thompson LD, Aguilera NS, Abbondanzo SL. Kimura disease: a clinicopathologic study of 21 cases. Am J Surg Pathol 2004;28:505-13.
19. Chen WC, Jones D, Ho CL, et al. Cytogenetic anomalies in hyaline vascular Castleman disease: report of two cases with reappraisal of histogenesis. Cancer Genet Cytogenet 2006;164:110-7.
20. Chikwava K, Jaffe R. Langerin (CD207) staining in normal pediatric tissues, reactive lymph nodes, and childhood histiocytic disorders. Pediatr Dev Pathol 2004;7:607-14.

21. Chim CS, Fung A, Shek TW, Liang R, Ho WK, Kwong YL. Analysis of clonality in Kimura's disease. Am J Surg Pathol 2002;26:1083-6.
22. Chim CS, Liang R, Fung A, Kwong YL, Shek TW. Further analysis of clonality in Kimura's disease. Am J Surg Pathol 2003;27:703-4.
23. Chiu CF, Chow KC, Lin TY, Tsai MH, Shih CM, Chen LM. Virus infection in patients with histiocytic necrotizing lymphadenitis in Taiwan. Detection of Epstein-Barr virus, type 1 human T-cell lymphotropic virus, and parvovirus B19. Am J Clin Pathol 2000;113:774-81.
24. Cokelaere K, Debiec-Rychter M, De Wolf-Peeters C, Hagemeijer A, Sciot R. Hyaline vascular Castleman's disease with HMGIC rearrangement in follicular dendritic cells: molecular evidence of mesenchymal tumorigenesis. Am J Surg Pathol 2002;26:662-9.
25. Cooper RA, Dawson PJ, Rambo ON. Dermatopathic lymphadenopathy: a clinicopathologic analysis of lymph node biopsy over a fifteen-year period. Calif Med 1967;106:170-5.
26. Dacic S, Trusky C, Bakker A, Finkelstein SD, Yousem SA. Genotypic analysis of pulmonary Langerhans cell histiocytosis. Hum Pathol 2003;34:1345-9.
27. Dhote R, Simon J, Papo T, et al. Reactive hemophagocytic syndrome in adult systemic disease: report of twenty-six cases and literature review. Arthritis Rheum 2003;49:633-9.
28. Diebold J, Tulliez M, Bernadou A, et al. Angiofollicular and plasmacytic polyadenopathy: a pseudotumourous syndrome with dysimmunity. J Clin Pathol 1980;33:1068-76.
29. Dogan A, Attygalle AD, Kyriakou C. Angioimmunoblastic T-cell lymphoma. Br J Haematol 2003;121:681-91.
30. Dorfman RF. Histiocytic necrotizing lymphadenitis of Kikuchi and Fujimoto. Arch Pathol Lab Med 1987;111:1026-9.
31. Dorfman RF, Berry GJ. Kikuchi's histiocytic necrotizing lymphadenitis: an analysis of 108 cases with emphasis on differential diagnosis. Semin Diagn Pathol 1988;5:329-45.
32. El Menzi F, Mrad K, el Menzi-Benzarti A, Zermani R, Ben Abdeladhim A, Ben Jilani S. [Kikuchi-Fujimoto subacute necrotizing lymphadenitis: two histologic forms observed in the same patient.] Ann Pathol 1998;18:422-44. [French]
33. Emile JF, Wechsler J, Brousse N, et al. Langerhans' cell histiocytosis. Definitive diagnosis with the use of monoclonal antibody O10 on routinely paraffin-embedded samples. Am J Surg Pathol 1995;19:636-41.
34. Facchetti F, de Wolf-Peeters C, van den Oord JJ, de Vos R, Desmet VJ. Plasmacytoid monocytes (so-called plasmacytoid T cells) in Kikuchi's lymphadenitis. An immunohistologic study. Am J Clin Pathol 1989;92:42-50.
35. Falini B, Pileri S, De Solas I, et al. Peripheral T-cell lymphoma associated with hemophagocytic syndrome. Blood 1990;75:434-44.
36. Feller AC, Lennert K, Stein H, Bruhn HD, Wuthe HH. Immunohistology and aetiology of histiocytic necrotizing lymphadenitis. Report of three instructive cases. Histopathology 1983;7:825-39.
37. Fisher ER, Sieracki JC, Goldenberg DM. Identity and nature of isolated lymphoid tumors (so-called nodal hyperplasia, hamartoma, and angiomatous hamartoma) as revealed by histologic, electron microscopic, and heterotransplantation studies. Cancer 1970;25:1286-300.
38. Foucar E, Rosai J, Dorfman RF. Sinus histiocytosis with massive lymphadenopathy: current status and future directions. Arch Dermatol 1988;124:1211-4.
39. Foucar E, Rosai J, Dorfman R. Sinus histiocytosis with massive lymphadenopathy (Rosai-Dorfman disease): review of the entity. Semin Diagn Pathol 1990;7:19-73.
40. Frizzera G. Atypical lymphoproliferative disorders. In: Knowles DM, ed. Neoplastic hematopathology, 2nd ed. Baltimore: Lippincott Williams & Wilkins; 2001:569-622.
41. Frizzera G. Castleman's disease: more questions than answers. Hum Pathol 1985;16:202-5.
42. Frizzera G. Castleman's disease and related disorders. Semin Diagn Pathol 1988;5:346-64.
43. Frizzera G, Banks PM, Massarelli G, Rosai J. A systemic lymphoproliferative disorder with morphologic features of Castleman's disease. Pathological findings in 15 patients. Am J Surg Pathol 1983;7:211-31.
44. Frizzera G, Moran EM, Rappaport H. Angioimmunoblastic lymphadenopathy with dysproteinemia. Lancet 1974;1:1070-3.
45. Frizzera G, Moran EM, Rappaport H. Angioimmunoblastic lymphadenopathy: diagnosis and clinical course. Am J Med 1975;59:803-17.
46. Frizzera G, Peterson BA, Bayrd ED, Goldman A. A systemic lymphoproliferative disorder with morphologic features of Castleman's disease: clinical findings and clinicopathologic correlation in 15 patients. J Clin Oncol 1985;3:1202-16.
47. Fujimoto Y, Kuzima Y, Yamaguchi K. [Cervical subacute necrotizing lymphadenitis: a new clinicopathologic entity.] Naika 1972;20:920-7. [Japanese]
48. Gaba AR, Stein RS, Sweet DL, Variakojis D. Multicentric giant lymph node hyperplasia. Am J Clin Pathol 1978;69:86-90.

49. Geissmann F, Dieu-Nosjean MC, Dezutter C, et al. Accumulation of immature Langerhans cells in human lymph nodes draining chronically inflamed skin. J Exp Med 2002;196:417-30.
50. Giesker DW, Pastuszak WT, Forouhar FA, Krause PJ, Hine P. Lymph node biopsy for early diagnosis in Kawasaki disease. Am J Surg Pathol 1982;6:493-501.
51. Gonzalez CL, Medeiros LJ, Braziel RM, Jaffe ES. T-cell lymphoma involving subcutaneous tissue. A clinicopathologic entity commonly associated with hemophagocytic syndrome. Am J Surg Pathol 1991;15:17-27.
52. Gould E, Porto R, Albores-Saavedra J, Ibe MJ. Dermatopathic lymphadenitis. The spectrum and significance of its morphologic features. Arch Pathol Lab Med 1988;112:1145-50.
53. Green I, Dorfman RF, Rosai J. Breast involvement by extranodal Rosai-Dorfman disease: report of seven cases. Am J Surg Pathol 1997;21:664-8.
54. Greiner T, Armitage JO, Gross TG. Atypical Lymphoproliferative diseases. Hematology (Am Soc Hematol Educ Program) 2000:133-46.
55. Griesser H, Feller A, Lennert K, Minden M, Mak TW. Rearrangement of the beta chain of the T cell antigen receptor and immunoglobulin genes in lymphoproliferative disorders. J Clin Invest 1986;78:1179-84.
56. Hall PA, Donaghy M, Cotter FE, Stansfeld AG, Levison DA. An immunohistological and genotypic study of the plasma cell form of Castleman's disease. Histopathology 1989;14:333-46; discussion 429-32.
57. Hanson CA, Frizzera G, Patton DF, et al. Clonal rearrangement for immunoglobulin and T- cell receptor genes in systemic Castleman's disease: association with Epstein-Barr virus. Am J Pathol 1988;131:84-91.
58. Harris NL. Hypervascular follicular hyperplasia and Kaposi's sarcoma in patients at risk for AIDS. N Engl J Med 1984;310:462-3.
59. Henter JI, Arico M, Elinder G, Imashuku S, Janka G. Familial hemophagocytic lymphohistiocytosis. Primary hemophagocytic lymphohistiocytosis. Hematol Oncol Clin North Am 1998;12:417-33.
60. Henter JI, Elinder G, S`der O, Hansson M, Andersson B, Andersson U. Hypercytokinemia in familial hemophagocytic lymphohistiocytosis. Blood 1991;78:2918-22.
61. Hicks RV, Melish ME. Kawasaki syndrome. Pediatr Clin North Am 1986;33:1151-75.
62. Hollingsworth HC, Peiper SC, Weiss LM, Raffeld M, Jaffe ES. An investigation of the viral pathogenesis of Kikuchi-Fujimoto disease. Lack of evidence for Epstein-Barr virus or human herpesvirus type 6 as the causative agents. Arch Pathol Lab Med 1994;118:134-40.
63. Huh J, Kang GH, Gong G, Kim SS, Ro JY, Kim CW. Kaposi's sarcoma-associated herpesvirus in Kikuchi's disease. Hum Pathol 1998;29:1091-6.
64. Hui PK, Chan JK, Ng CS, Kung IT, Gwi E. Lymphadenopathy of Kimura's disease. Am J Surg Pathol 1989;13:177-86.
65. Hurwitt E. Dermatopathic lymphadenitis: focal granulomatous lymphadenitis associated with chronic generalized skin disorders. J Invest Dermatol 1942;5:197-204.
66. Imamura M, Ueno H, Matsuura A, et al. An ultrastructural study of subacute necrotizing lymphadenitis. Am J Pathol 1982;107:292-9.
67. Imashuku S, Obayashi M, Hosoi G, et al. Splenectomy in haemophagocytic lymphohistiocytosis: report of histopathological changes with CD19+ B-cell depletion and therapeutic results. Br J Haematol 2000;108:505-10.
68. Jang KA, Ahn SJ, Choi JH, et al. Polymerase chain reaction (PCR) for human herpesvirus 8 and heteroduplex PCR for clonality assessment in angiolymphoid hyperplasia with eosinophilia and Kimura's disease. J Cutan Pathol 2001;28:363-7.
69. Janka G, Imashuku S, Elinder G, Schneider M, Henter JI. Infection- and malignancy- associated hemophagocytic syndromes: secondary hemophagocytic lymphohistiocytosis. Hematol Oncol Clin North Am 1998;12:435-44.
70. Kakkar N, Vasishta RK, Banerjee AK, Marwaha RK, Thapa BR. Familial hemophagocytic lymphohistiocytosis: an autopsy study. Pediatr Pathol Mol Med 2003;22:229-42.
71. Katano H, Kaneko K, Shimizu S, Saito T, Irie T, Mori S. Follicular dendritic cell sarcoma complicated by hyaline-vascular type Castleman's disease in a schizophrenic patient. Pathol Int 1997;47:703-6.
72. Kawasaki T. [Acute febrile mucocutaneous syndrome with lymphoid involvement with specific desquamation of the fingers and toes in children: clinical observation of 50 cases.] Jpn J Allergy 1967;16:178-222. [Japanese]
73. Keller AR, Hochholzer L, Castleman B. Hyaline-vascular and plasma-cell types of giant lymph node hyperplasia of the mediastinum and other locations. Cancer 1972;29:670-83.
74. Kessler E. Multicentric giant lymph node hyperplasia: a report of 7 cases. Cancer 1985;56:2446-51.
75. Kikuchi M. [Lymphadenitis showing focal reticulum cell hyperplasia with nuclear debris and phagocytosis.] Nippon Ketsueki Gakkai Zasshi 1972;35:379-80. [Japanese]
76. Kikuchi M, Yoshizumi T, Nakamura H. Necrotizing lymphadenitis: possible acute toxoplasmic infection. Virchows Arch A Pathol Anat 1977;376:247-53.

77. Kimura T, Yoshimura S, Ishikawa E. On the unusual granulation combined with hyperplastic changes of lymphatic tissue. Trans Soc Pathol Jpn 1948;37:179-80.
78. Kimura Y, Pawankar R, Aoki M, Niimi Y, Kawana S. Mast cells and T cells in Kimura's disease express increased levels of interleukin-4, interleukin-5, eotaxin and RANTES. Clin Exp Allergy 2002;32:1787-93.
79. Kojima M, Sakuma H, Mori N. Histopathological features of plasma cell dyscrasia with polyneuropathy and endocrine disturbances, with special reference to germinal center lesions. Jpn J Clin Oncol 1983;13:557-75.
80. Koo CH, Nathwani BN, Winberg CD, Hill LR, Rappaport H. Atypical lymphoplasmacytic and immunoblastic proliferation in lymph nodes of patients with autoimmune disease (autoimmune-disease-associated lymphadenopathy). Medicine 1984;63:274-90.
81. Krueger GR, Sander C. What's new in human herpesvirus-6? Clinical immunopathology of the HHV-6 infection. Pathol Res Pract 1989;185:915-29.
82. Kuo TT. Kikuchi's disease (histiocytic necrotizing lymphadenitis). A clinicopathologic study of 79 cases with an analysis of histologic subtypes, immunohistology, and DNA ploidy. Am J Surg Pathol 1995;19:798-809.
83. Kuo TT, Shih LY, Chan HL. Kimura's disease: involvement of regional lymph nodes and distinction from angiolymphoid hyperplasia with eosinophilia. Am J Surg Pathol 1988;12:843-54.
84. Lachant NA, Sun NC, Leong LA, Oseas RS, Prince HE. Multicentric angiofollicular lymph node hyperplasia (Castleman's disease) followed by Kaposi's sarcoma in two homosexual males with the acquired immunodeficiency syndrome (AIDS). Am J Clin Pathol 1985;83:27-33.
85. Laipply TC. Lipomelanotic reticular hyperplasia of lymph nodes: report of 6 cases. Arch Intern Med 1948;81:19-36.
86. Leibetseder F, Thurner J. [Angiofollicular lymph node hyperplasia (onion-skin lymphoma).] Med Klin 1973;68:817-20. [German]
87. Lennert K. Pathologisch-histologische Klassifizierung der malignen Lymphome. In: Stacher A, ed. Leukaemien und maligne Lymphome, Pathophysiologie, Klinik, Chemo-und Immunotherapie. Munich: Urban & Schwarzenberg; 1973:181-94.
88. Leung DY, Geha RS, Newburger JW, et al. Two monokines, interleukin 1 and tumor necrosis factor, render cultured vascular endothelial cells susceptible to lysis by antibodies circulating during Kawasaki syndrome. J Exp Med 1986;164:1958-72.
89. Levine PH, Jahan N, Murari P, Manak M, Jaffe ES. Detection of human herpesvirus 6 in tissues involved by sinus histiocytosis with massive lymphadenopathy (Rosai-Dorfman disease). J Infect Dis 1992;166:291-5.
90. Lieberman PH, Jones CR, Steinman RM, et al. Langerhans cell (eosinophilic) granulomatosis. A clinicopathologic study encompassing 50 years. Am J Surg Pathol 1996;20:519-52.
91. Lipford EH, Smith HR, Pittaluga S, Jaffe ES, Steinberg AD, Cossman J. Clonality of angioimmunoblastic lymphadenopathy and implications for its evolution to malignant lymphoma. J Clin Invest 1987;79:637-42.
92. Lu D, Estalilla OC, Manning JT Jr, Medeiros LJ. Sinus histiocytosis with massive lymphadenopathy and malignant lymphoma involving the same lymph node: a report of four cases and review of the literature. Mod Pathol 2000;13:414-9.
93. Lukes RJ, Tindle BH. Immunoblastic lymphadenopathy: a hyperimmune entity resembling Hodgkin's disease. N Engl J Med 1975;292:1-8.
94. McClain KL, Natkunam Y, Swerdlow SH. Atypical cellular disorders. Hematology (Am Soc Hematol Educ Program) 2004:283-96.
95. McKenna RW, Risdall RJ, Brunning RD. Virus associated hemophagocytic syndrome. Hum Pathol 1981;12:395-8.
96. Melish ME, Hicks RV. Kawasaki syndrome: clinical features. Pathophysiology, etiology and therapy. J Rheumatol Supp 1990;24:2-10.
97. Menke DM, Tiemann M, Camoriano JK, et al. Diagnosis of Castleman's disease by identification of an immunophenotypically aberrant population of mantle zone B lymphocytes in paraffin-embedded lymph node biopsies. Am J Clin Pathol 1996;105:268-76.
98. Morens DM, O'Brien RJ. Kawasaki disease in the United States. J Infect Dis 1978;137:91-3.
99. Mori N, Tsunoda R, Kojima K. Multicentric lymphadenopathy histologically simulating Castleman's disease. J Jpn Soc RES 1981;20:55-66.
100. Mori S, Mohri N, Uchida T, Shimamine T. Idiopathic plasmacytic lymphadenopathy with polyclonal hyperimmunoglobulinemia: a syndrome related to giant lymph node hyperplasia of plasma cell type. J Jpn Soc RES 1981;56:85-94.
101. Murakami I, Gogusev J, Fournet JC, Glorion C, Jaubert F. Detection of molecular cytogenetic aberrations in langerhans cell histiocytosis of bone. Hum Pathol 2002;33:555-60.
102. Nagore E, Llorca J, Sanchez-Motilla JM, Ledesma E, Fortea JM, Aliaga A. Detection of Epstein-Barr virus DNA in a patient with Kimura's disease. Int J Dermatol 2000;39:618-20.

103. Namikawa R, Suchi T, Ueda R, et al. Phenotyping of proliferating lymphocytes in angioimmunoblastic lymphadenopathy and related lesions by the double immunoenzymatic staining technique. Am J Pathol 1987;127:279-87.
104. Nathwani BN, Jaffe ES. Angioimmunoblastic lymphadenopathy (AILD) and AILD-like T-cell lymphomas. In: Jaffe ES, ed. Surgical pathology of the lymph nodes and related organs, 2nd ed, vol. 16. Philadelphia: W.B. Saunders; 1995:390-412.
105. Nathwani BN, Rappaport H, Moran EM, Pangalis GA, Kim H. Malignant lymphoma arising in angioimmunoblastic lymphadenopathy. Cancer 1978;41:578-606.
106. Newburger JW, Takahashi M, Gerber MA, et al. Committee on Rheumatic Fever, Endocarditis and Kawasaki Disease; Council on Cardiovascular Disease in the Young; American Heart Association; American Academy of Pediatrics. Diagnosis, treatment, and long-term management of Kawasaki disease: a statement for health professionals from the Committee on Rheumatic Fever, Endocarditis and Kawasaki Disease, Council on Cardiovascular Disease in the Young, American Heart Association. Circulation 2004;110:2747-71.
107. Nezelof C. Hemophagocytic lymphohistiocytosis as a syndrome: correlation of clinicopathological data. Pediatr Hematol Oncol 1989;6:207-11.
108. Nguyen TT, Schwartz EJ, West RB, Warnke RA, Arber DA, Natkunam Y. Expression of CD163 (hemoglobin scavenger receptor) in normal tissues, lymphomas, carcinomas, and sarcomas is largely restricted to the monocyte/macrophage lineage. Am J Surg Pathol 2005;29:617-24.
109. Nishimoto N, Sasai M, Shima Y, et al. Improvement in Castleman's disease by humanized anti-interleukin-6 receptor antibody therapy. Blood 2000;95:56-61.
110. O'Connor NT, Crick JA, Wainscoat JS, et al. Evidence for monoclonal T-lymphocyte proliferation in angioimmunoblastic lymphadenopathy. J Clin Pathol 1986;39:1229-32.
111. O'Neill D, O'Grady J, Variend S. Child fatality associated with pathological features of histiocytic necrotizing lymphadenitis (Kikuchi-Fujimoto disease). Pediatr Pathol Lab Med 1998;18:79-88.
112. Ohyashiki JH, Ohyashiki K, Kawakubo K, et al. Molecular genetic, cytogenetic, and immunophenotypic analyses in Castleman's disease of the plasma cell type. Am J Clin Pathol 1994;101:290-5.
113. Oksenhendler E, Duarte M, Soulier J, et al. Multicentric Castleman's disease in HIV infection: a clinical and pathological study of 20 patients. AIDS 1996;10:61-7.
114. Onciu M, Medeiros LJ. Kikuchi-Fujimoto lymphadenitis. Adv Anat Pathol 2003;10:204-11.
115. Parravicini C, Corbellino M, Paulli M, et al. Expression of a virus-derived cytokine, KSHV vIL-6, in HIV-seronegative Castleman's disease. Am J Pathol 1997;151:1517-22.
116. Paulli M, Bergamaschi G, Tonon L, et al. Evidence for a polyclonal nature of the cell infiltrate in sinus histiocytosis with massive lymphadenopathy (Rosai-Dorfman disease). Br J Haematol 1995;91:415-8.
117. Pauwels P, Dal Cin P, Vlasveld LT, Aleva RM, van Erp WF, Jones D. A chromosomal abnormality in hyaline vascular Castleman's disease: evidence for clonal proliferation of dysplastic stromal cells. Am J Surg Pathol 2000;24:882-8.
118. Peh SC, Shaminie J, Poppema S, Kim LH. The immunophenotypic patterns of follicle centre and mantle zone in Castleman's disease. Singapore Med J 2003;44:185-91.
119. Pileri SA, Grogan TM, Harris NL, et al. Tumours of histiocytes and accessory dendritic cells: an immunohistochemical approach to classification from the International Lymphoma Study Group based on 61 cases. Histopathology 2002;41:1-29.
120. Pileri S, Kikuchi M, Helbron D, Lennert K. Histiocytic necrotizing lymphadenitis without granulocytic infiltration. Virchows Arch A Pathol Anat 1982;395:257-71.
121. Radaszkiewicz T, Hansmann ML, Lennert K. Monoclonality and polyclonality of plasma cells in Castleman's disease of the plasma cell variant. Histopathology 1989;14:11-24.
122. Risdall RJ, Brunning RD, Hernandez JI, Gordon DH. Bacteria-associated hemophagocytic syndrome. Cancer 1984;54:2968-72.
123. Risdall RJ, McKenna RW, Nesbit ME, et al. Virus-associated hemophagocytic syndrome: a benign histiocytic proliferation distinct from malignant histiocytosis. Cancer 1979;44:993-1002.
124. Rivano MT, Falini B, Stein H, et al. Histiocytic necrotizing lymphadenitis without granulocytic infiltration (Kikuchi's lymphadenitis). Morphological and immunohistochemical study of eight cases. Histopathology 1987;11:1013-27.
125. Rosai J, Dorfman RF. Sinus histiocytosis with massive lymphadenopathy. A newly recognized benign clinicopathological entity. Arch Pathol 1969;87:63-70.
126. Royle J, Burgner D, Curtis N. The diagnosis and management of Kawasaki disease. J Paediatr Child Health 2005;41:87-93.
127. Shahidi H, Myers JL, Kvale PA. Castleman's disease. Mayo Clin Proc 1995;70:969-77.

128. Shamoto M, Osada A, Shinzato M, Kaneko C, Yoshida A. Do epidermal Langerhans cells, migrating from skin lesions, induce the paracortical hyperplasia of dermatopathic lymphadenopathy? Pathol Int 1996;46:348-54.
129. Shimoyama M, Minato K, Saito H, et al. Immunoblastic lymphadenopathy (IBL)-like T-cell lymphoma. Jpn J Clin Oncol 1979;9(Suppl 1):347-56.
130. Shoda H, Oka T, Inoue M, et al. Sinus histiocytosis with massive lymphadenopathy associated with malignant lymphoma. Intern Med 2004;43:741-5.
131. Slone SP, Fleming DR, Buchino JJ. Sinus histiocytosis with massive lymphadenopathy and Langerhans cell histiocytosis express the cellular adhesion molecule CD31. Arch Pathol Lab Med 2003;127:341-4.
132. Soulier J, Grollet L, Oksenhendler E, et al. Kaposi's sarcoma-associated Herpesvirus-like DNA sequences in multicentric Castleman's disease. Blood 1995;86:1276-80.
133. Sumiyoshi Y, Kikuchi M, Minematu T, Ohshima K, Takeshita M, Minamishima Y. Analysis of herpesvirus genomes in Kikuchi's disease. Virchows Arch 1994;424:437-40.
134. Suster S, Hilsenbeck S, Rywlin AM. Reactive histiocytic hyperplasia with hemophagocytosis in hematopoietic organs: a reevaluation of the benign histiocytic proliferations. Hum Pathol 1988;19:705-12.
135. Thawerani H, Sanchez RL, Rosai J, Dorfman RF. The cutaneous manifestations of sinus histiocytosis with massive lymphadenopathy. Arch Dermatol 1978;114:191-7.
136. Tsai MK, Huang HF, Hu RH, et al. Fatal Kikuchi-Fujimoto disease in transplant recipients: a case report. Transplant Proc 1998;30:3137-8.
137. Turner RR, Martin J, Dorfman RF. Necrotizing lymphadenitis. A study of 30 cases. Am J Surg Pathol 1983;7:115-23.
138. Unger PD, Rappaport KM, Strauchen JA. Necrotizing lymphadenitis (Kikuchi's disease). Report of four cases of an unusual pseudolymphomatous lesion and immunologic marker studies. Arch Pathol Lab Med 1987;111:1031-4.
139. Watanabe S, Sato Y, Shimoyama M, Minato K, Shimosato Y. Immunoblastic lymphadenopathy, angioimmunoblastic lymphadenopathy, and IBL-like T-cell lymphoma: a spectrum of T-cell neoplasia. Cancer 1986;58:2224-32.
140. Weisenberger DD, Nathwani BN, Winberg CD, Rappaport H. Multicentric angiofollicular lymph node hyperplasia: a clinicopathologic study of 16 cases. Hum Pathol 1985;16:162-72.
141. Weiss LM, Jaffe ES, Liu XF, Chen YY, Shibata D, Medeiros LJ. Detection and localization of Epstein-Barr viral genomes in angioimmunoblastic lymphadenopathy and angioimmunoblastic lymphadenopathy-like lymphoma. Blood 1992;79:1789-95.
142. Weiss LM, Strickler JG, Dorfman RF, Horning SJ, Warnke RA, Sklar J. Clonal T-cell populations in angioimmunoblastic lymphadenopathy and angioimmunoblastic lymphadenopathy-like lymphoma. Am J Pathol 1986;122:392-7.
143. Wenig BM, Abbondanzo SL, Childers EL, Kapadia SB, Heffner DR. Extranodal sinus histiocytosis with massive lymphadenopathy (Rosai-Dorfman disease) of the head and neck. Hum Pathol 1993;24:483-92.
144. Williams JW, Dorfman RF. Lymphadenopathy as the initial manifestation of histiocytosis X. Am J Surg Pathol 1979;3:405-21.
145. Willman CL, Busque L, Griffith BB, et al. Langerhans'-cell histiocytosis (histiocytosis X)—a clonal proliferative disease. N Engl J Med 1994;331:154-60.
146. Yabuhara A, Yanagisawa M, Murata T et al. Giant lymph node hyperplasia (Castleman's disease) with spontaneous production of high levels of B-cell diferentiation factor activity. Cancer 1989;63:260-5.
147. Yoshizaki K, Matsuda T, Nishimoto N, et al. Pathogenic significance of interleukin- 6 (IL-6/BSF-2) in Castleman's disease Blood 1989;74:1360-7.
148. Yousem SA, Colby TV, Chen YY, Chen WG, Weiss LM. Pulmonary Langerhans' cell histiocytosis: molecular analysis of clonality. Am J Surg Pathol 2001;25:630-6.
149. zur Stadt U, Schmidt S, Kasper B, et al. Linkage of familial hemophagocytic lymphohistiocytosis (FHL) type-4 to chromosome 6q24 and identification of mutations in syntaxin 11. Hum Mol Genet 2005;14:827-34.

7 CONGENITAL IMMUNODEFICIENCY DISEASES

Congenital immunodeficiency diseases have a wide range of clinical severity, from asymptomatic to fatal (Table 7-1). These disorders usually present early in life, and although signs and symptoms are variable, recurrent infections and other manifestations may provide diagnostic clues (Table 7-2). Our knowledge of the underlying cytogenetic and molecular defects of these diseases is growing (Table 7-3).

Often, the characteristic findings of the congenital immunodeficiency diseases are in the hematolymphoid organs, which, while typically not completely specific, show significant morphologic abnormalities. The recognition of these findings as benign and associated with an immunodeficiency is of great clinical importance. In many cases, the recognition of an immunodeficiency disorder leads to appropriate treatment.

There is an association between primary immunodeficiencies and the subsequent development of malignant neoplasms (47,52,124). The malignancies primarily involve the lymphoid system (Table 7-4) (47). An association between congenital immunodeficiency and so-called pseudolymphomas or atypical lymphoid proliferations associated with Epstein-Barr virus (EBV) has been reported (9,105,135). It seems likely that there is a pathologic spectrum of changes in congenital immunodeficiency–associated lesions that ranges from nonspecific reactive lymphoid hyperplasia, to atypical lymphoproliferative disease, to malignant lymphoma (44).

Lymphadenopathy that shows changes consistent with atypical lymphoid hyperplasia commonly occurs in immunodeficiency-related conditions. The abnormalities seen with such hyperplasia occur in both the cytologic and architectural components of the lymph node (figs. 7-1, 7-2). Many cases consist of diffuse paracortical immunoblastic hyperplasia with ill-defined or unrecognized germinal centers. A lymphoid-depleted background may be present, as well as prominent high endothelial venules, increased mitoses, and focal necrosis (45,105). Prominent plasmacytic hyperplasia is another pattern associated with immunodeficiency diseases (Tables 7-5, 7-6) (44).

Table 7-1

1995 WORLD HEALTH ORGANIZATION (WHO) CLASSIFICATION OF PRIMARY AND SECONDARY IMMUNODEFICIENCY DISORDERS[a]

Combined immunodeficiencies
Predominantly antibody defects
Predominantly T-cell defects
Immunodeficiencies associated with other major defects
Defects of phagocytic function
Complement deficiencies
Immunodeficiencies associated with or secondary to other diseases
Chromosomal instability or defective repair
Chromosomal defects
Skeletal abnormalities
Immunodeficiency with generalized growth retardation
Immunodeficiency with dermatologic defects
Hereditary metabolic defects
Hypercatabolism of immunoglobulin
Other

[a]Adapted from Tables 1–3 from Rosen FS. Primary immunodeficiency diseases: Report of a WHO scientific group. Clin Exp Immunol 1995;99(Suppl 1):11-13.

Table 7-2

COMMON CLINICAL AND LABORATORY FINDINGS IN IMMUNODEFICIENT PATIENTS

Frequent/severe bacterial infections
Sinus
Otitis
Pneumonia
Frequent opportunistic infections
Pneumocystis
Giardia
Absent/hypoplastic thymus (on radiographic examination)
Absent/hypoplastic tonsils and adenoids
No palpable lymph nodes, especially cervical (in spite of infection)
Autoimmune phenomena (including hematologic)
Lymphopenia
Decreased serum immunoglobulin level(s)
Abnormal response to vaccination
Disseminated infection after live-virus vaccines
Graft versus host disease (maternal origin or non-irradiated transfusions)

Table 7-3

GENE AND CHROMOSOME LOCATIONS IN CONGENITAL IMMUNODEFICIENCIES

Disorder	Gene(s) Involved	Chromosome Location
Severe combined immunodeficiency (SCID)	*Artemis* *IL2RG* *JAK3*	10q Xq13.1-q13.3 19p13
Omenn syndrome	*RAG1, RAG2*	11p13
Adenosine deaminase deficiency SCID	*ADA*	20q13.11
Purine nucleoside phosphorylase deficiency SCID	*PNP*	14q13.1
DiGeorge syndrome	*TUPLE1, TBX1*	22q11.2
Major histocompatibility complex (MHC) deficiency	*CIITA* *RFXAN P* *RFX5* *RFXAP*	16p13 19p12 1q21.1-q21.3 13q14
Autoimmune lymphoproliferative syndrome (ALPS)	*fas* *caspase 10, caspase 8*	10q24.1 2q33-q34
Selective IgA deficiency	*IGAD1*	6p21.3
Hyper-IgM syndrome	*CD40L*	Xq26
Hyper-IgE syndrome	unknown	4q21
X-linked agammaglobulinemia	*BTK*	Xq21.3-q22
X-linked lymphoproliferative disorder	*SH2D1A, SLAM-associated protein*	Xq26
Griscelli syndrome	*RAB27A, MYO5A*	15q21
Chediak-Higashi syndrome	*CHS1, LYST*	1q42.1-q42.2
Wiskott-Aldrich syndrome	*WAS, WASP*	Xp11.23-p11.22
Ataxia-telangiectasia	*ATM*	11q23.1
Nijmegen breakage syndrome/Berlin breakage syndrome	*NBS1, LIG4, nibrin/p95*	8q21
Chronic granulomatous disease	*NADPH oxidase* *NCF1* *NCF2* *CYBA* *CYBB*	22q12.3-q13.2 7q11.23 1q21-q32 16q24 Xp21.1

Table 7-4

CONGENITAL IMMUNODEFICIENCIES COMMONLY ASSOCIATED WITH INCREASED INCIDENCE OF LYMPHOPROLIFERATIVE DISORDERS

Ataxia-telangectasia
Wiskott-Aldrich syndrome
Common variable immunodeficiency
Severe combined immunodeficiency
X-linked lymphoproliferative disorder
Nijmegen breakage syndrome
Hyper-IgM syndrome
Autoimmune lymphoproliferative syndrome
DiGeorge syndrome
X-linked agammaglobulinemia
Chediak-Higashi syndrome

Table 7-5

HISTOPATHOLOGIC FEATURES COMMON IN LYMPH NODES WITH CONGENITAL IMMUNODEFICIENCY

Hypocellularity
Absent or atrophic germinal centers
Stromal proliferation Vascular prominence Increased dendritic cells
+/– Hemophagocytosis/erythrophagocytosis
+/– Plasmacytosis
+/– Eosinophilia
+/– Fibrosis

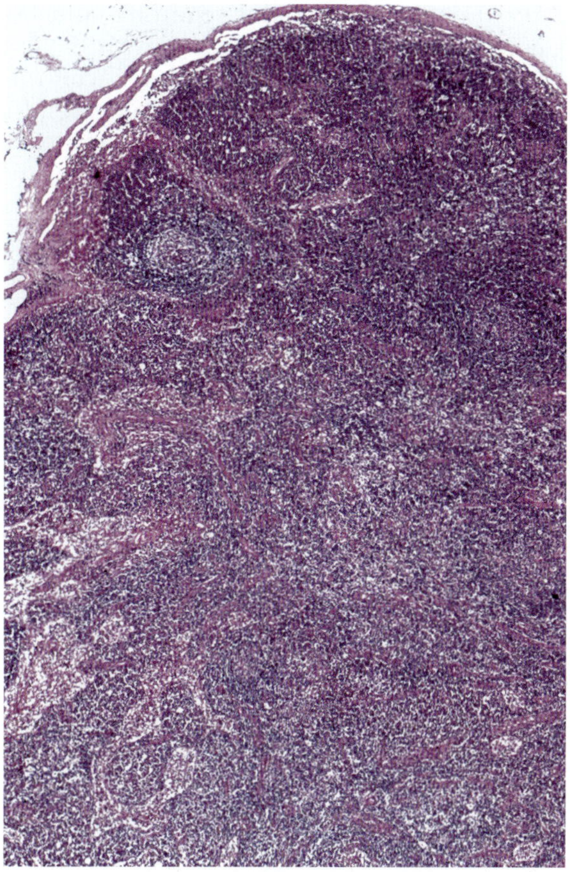

Figure 7-1

ATYPICAL LYMPHOID HYPERPLASIA

Disruption of the normal nodal architecture, with only small, barely recognizable germinal centers, in diffuse atypical paracortical hyperplasia.

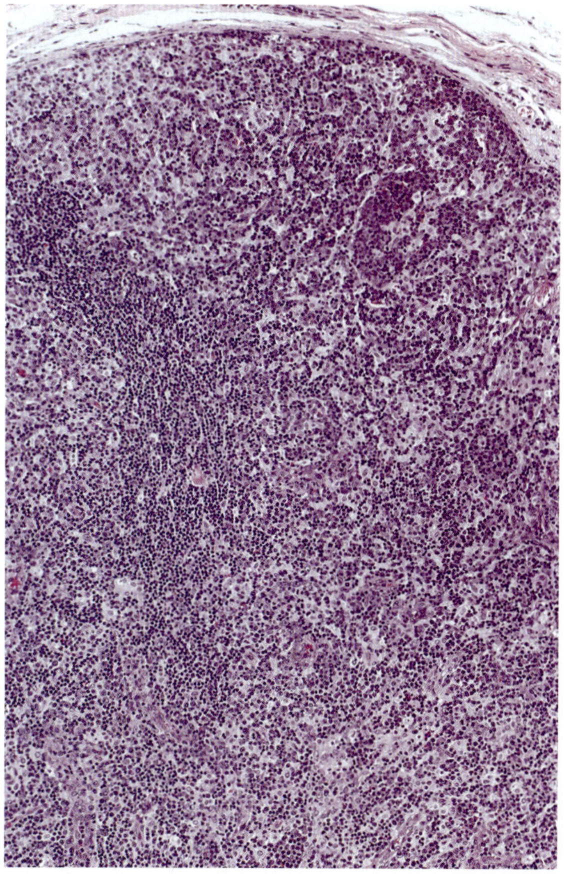

Figure 7-2

ATYPICAL LYMPHOID HYPERPLASIA

There are no clearly recognizable germinal centers.

Table 7-6

SUMMARY OF LYMPH NODE AND SPLENIC PATHOLOGY IN CONGENITAL IMMUNODEFICIENCY DISORDERS[a]

	T-cell Areas (Paracortex or PALS)[b]	Germinal Centers	Plasma Cells	Comments
Wiskott-Aldrich syndrome	↓ - A[c]	N - ↓	N - ↑	Atypical plasma cells; EMH
Ataxia-telangectasia	↓ - A	N - ↓	N - ↓	Sinus histiocytosis
Common variable immunodeficiency (CVID)	N - ↓	↓ - A	↓ - A	
Severe combined immunodeficiency (SCID)				
Autosomal recessive	A	A	A	
X-linked	↓ - A	↓ - A	↓ - A	
DiGeorge syndrome	A	N	N	
X-linked agammaglobulinemia	N	A	A	
Selective IgA deficiency	N	N	N	Absence of IgA+ plasma cells

[a]Data taken from reference 135.
[b]PALS = periarteriolar lymphoid sheath, EMH = extramedullary hematopoiesis.
[c]A = absent; N = normal; ↑ = increased; ↓ = decreased.

Excisional lymph node biopsy is not necessary to establish the diagnosis of an immunodeficiency disorder, but it may help in the classification (108). Under optimal circumstances, lymph node biopsies should be performed 5 to 7 days after antigenic stimulation by the application of diphtheria or tetanus toxoids. Since ideal conditions are rarely realized, if performed, the biopsies should be evaluated carefully. When lymph nodes are diffusely enlarged or rapidly enlarge, a biopsy may provide significant diagnostic information.

Lymphomas develop at an increased frequency in patients with congenital immunodeficiency, as much as 100 times the frequency of the general population. They occur most commonly in extranodal sites such as the gastrointestinal tract or the central nervous system. Lung and kidney are common sites for the appearance of lymphomatoid granulomatosis. EBV is associated with the development of many lymphoproliferative disorders found in patients with congenital immunodeficiencies. The postulated pathogenetic mechanism is defective immune surveillance.

SEVERE COMBINED IMMUNODEFICIENCY

Definition. *Severe combined immunodeficiency* (SCID) is a spectrum of disorders characterized by severe combined deficits of cellular and humoral immunity. Diseases in this spectrum are *Omenn syndrome, adenosine deaminase deficiency, purine nucleoside phosphorylase deficiency, Nezelof syndrome, reticular dysgenesis, DiGeorge syndrome*, and *defects in major histocompatibility complex expression.*

General Features. There are five general categories of etiology for the various types of SCID: 1) abnormal cytokine receptors or signaling; 2) defects in antigen receptor genes of B or T cells; 3) defects in purine pathway enzymes; 4) specific gene disorders of lymphocytes; and 5) SCID as a component of other genetic syndromes. X-linked SCID, which accounts for 50 to 60 percent of cases, is caused by a mutation in the interleukin (IL)-2 receptor (Xq13). Another cause is the deficiency of purine degradation enzymes, adenosine deaminase (ADA-SCID) and purine nucleoside phosphorylase (PNP-SCID). Omenn syndrome is due to mutations of the recombinase activating genes (*RAG1, RAG2*). Other causes of SCID include: *Artemis* deficiency, *JAK3* deficiency, defects of IL-7 receptor, CD3 deficiency, and ZAP-70 deficiency. Nezelof syndrome and DiGeorge syndrome are associated with defects of thymus formation, which cause T-cell immunodeficiency. DiGeorge syndrome results from deletions of 22q11 region, which leads to abnormalities in the formation of the third and fourth branchial arch derivatives. Although apparently a stem cell defect, the underlying etiology has not been completely described. Reticular dysgenesis is a very severe form of SCID. Finally, defects in the expression of major histocompatibility complex (MHC) molecules, which play a primary role in identifying cells as self or nonself, result in immunodeficiency.

Clinical Features. SCID is estimated to occur in 1/50,000 to 100,000 births. The inheritance pattern may be autosomal recessive, X-linked, or sporadic. SCID, therefore, is not a single disorder, but rather a spectrum of underlying pathologic and biochemical defects that leads to similar phenotypic expressions.

As is implied in the name, cases of SCID are accompanied by the manifestations of severe immunodeficiency. Infections are not only frequent but are particularly severe, despite appropriate treatment. Fatal perinatal infections from varicella virus, herpesvirus, adenovirus, and cytomegalovirus occur (108). Recurrent pyogenic sinopulmonary infections are common. Opportunistic infections, including with *Pneumocystis*, mycobacteria, and fungi also occur. Recurrent bouts of herpes simplex are seen, as well as frequent infection with *Giardia*. Thymic defects are common and types of SCID may be characterized by the type of thymic abnormalities present (50).

ADA-SCID and PNP-SCID are both autosomal recessive in inheritance. The clinical course of Nezelof syndrome is mild compared to other types of combined immunodeficiencies. Patients with Nezelof syndrome and ADA-SCID may appear immunologically normal at birth and early infancy, with the severe immunologic deficits occurring in a delayed fashion.

Reticular dysgenesis is one of the rarest and most severe forms of SCID. It is characterized by congenital agranulocytosis, lymphopenia, and lymphoid and thymic hypoplasia resulting in absent cellular and humoral immunity functions. Without almost immediate intervention, reticular dysgenesis results in death in the first few weeks of life.

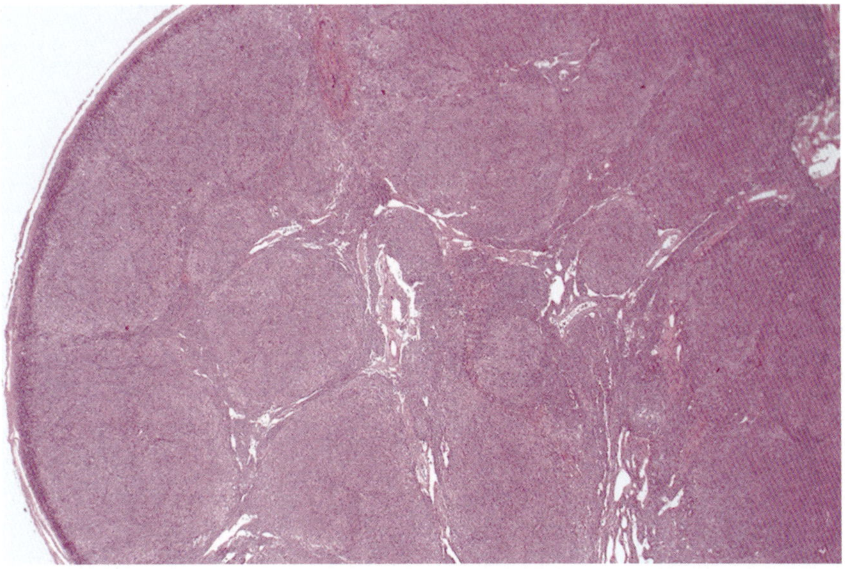

Figure 7-3

OMENN SYNDROME, LYMPH NODE

On low magnification, the nodular appearance of Omenn syndrome is highlighted. The nodules are relatively hypocellular.

DiGeorge syndrome is a disorder of thymic hypoplasia or aplasia resulting in severe T-cell defects. It is due to the abnormal formation of the third and fourth pharyngeal pouches, leading to abnormalities of the organs that develop from these regions. These include the thymus, parathyroid glands, and aortic arch. Many patients with DiGeorge syndrome have severe cardiac abnormalities. Severe hypocalcemia due to the abnormal formation of the parathyroid gland is common. Numerous infections are seen in these patients, including bacterial, viral, and fungal.

Defects in MHC expression are sometimes referred to as the *bare lymphocyte syndrome*. It is an autosomal recessive syndrome of immune deficits associated with abnormal expression of MHC antigens (type I or type II).

Laboratory Findings. Severe lymphopenia (less than 1.0 x 10^9/L) is present in most patients with SCID and other combined immunodeficiency diseases. Evaluation of lymphocyte subsets may reveal decreases in B cells as well as natural killer (NK) cells. Hypogammaglobulinemia is a common finding, although elevated immunoglobulin (Ig)E may be seen in Omenn syndrome. Lymphocytes typically have a poor cellular response to lymphocytic mitogens. In DiGeorge syndrome, CD4-positive lymphocytes are often severely decreased (less than 0.4 x 10^9/L); cytogenetic studies show the characteristic 22q11 deletion.

Lymphopenia is not present in MHC deficits, although CD4-positive cells are reduced in MHC type II. Marked decreases in all classes of immunoglobulins are seen, despite a normal number of B cells.

Microscopic Findings. In some cases of SCID, the lymph nodal tissue is completely absent; in other cases, the lymph nodes are either lacking or markedly depleted of lymphoid cells (26). The "empty" nodes are predominantly composed of dendritic cells, endothelial cells, macrophages, and granulocytes. Germinal centers are not seen. Empty nodes are often associated with significant graft versus host disease after transplantation. Erythrophagocytosis may be prominent. In occasional cases, there are small primary follicles, and rarely, small germinal centers with few centroblasts. Plasma cells are moderate in number in SCID lymph nodes. All of the histologic findings may be complicated by the presence of coexisting opportunistic bacterial, fungal, or viral infection.

The lymph nodes of Omenn syndrome are hypocellular and empty appearing (figs. 7-3, 7-4). There is significant lymphoid depletion and the architecture is effaced; no follicles or cortical regions are seen. The most prominent cellular components are interdigitating dendritic cells (S-100 protein–positive cells) with prominent eosinophils. There are clusters of macrophages and rare plasma cells. The lymph node sinuses

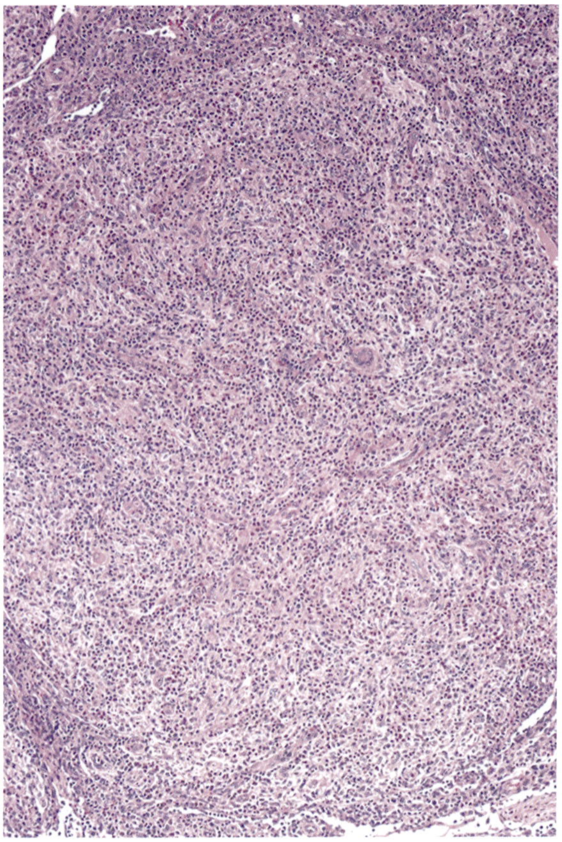

Figure 7-4

OMENN SYNDROME, LYMPH NODE

Intermediate magnification of the nodules in Omenn syndrome shows increased eosinophils and stromal elements. Lymphocytes are decreased while macrophages are increased.

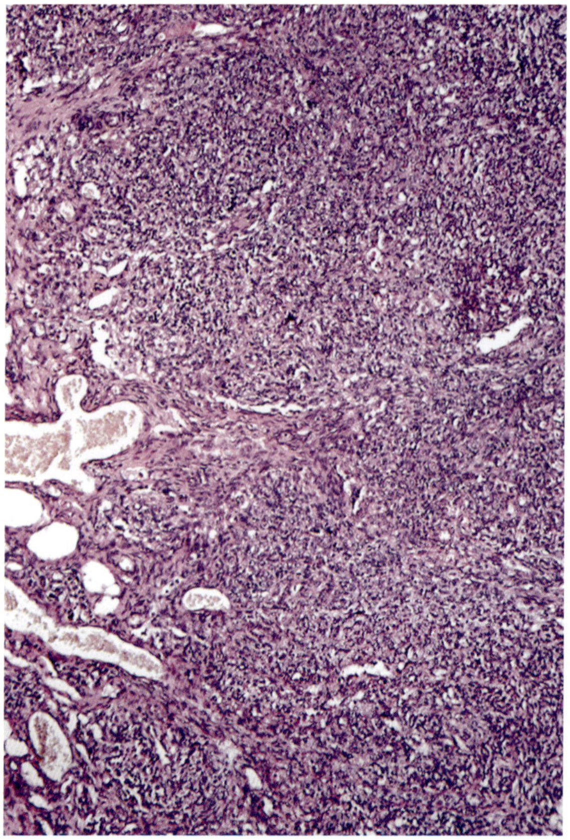

Figure 7-5

ADENOSINE DEAMINASE (ADA) DEFICIENCY, LYMPH NODE

Lymph node biopsy of 3-month-old male after local antigenic stimulation. The cortex and medulla are present, with only minimal follicle formation. (Courtesy of Ronald Jaffe, Pittsburgh, PA.)

are intact and there is no vascular proliferation, fibrosis, granulomas, or necrosis.

The lymph nodes in ADA-SCID have residual, normal-appearing architecture but reduced numbers of lymphocytes (fig. 7-5). In some cases, erythrophagocytosis is seen. Follicles are typically poorly formed and only rarely have reactive germinal centers. Paracortical areas are often hypocellular. The cellularity consists of plasma cells and variable numbers of lymphocytes. Granulocytes or eosinophils may be prominent (116). PNP-SCID has reduced T-cell–associated areas (paracortical) and a lack of CD8-positive T cells (26).

Nezelof syndrome is similar to other types of SCID. Although B cells are present, germinal centers are still not formed (figs. 7-6–7-8). The lymph nodes in reticular dysgenesis are small, have virtually no lymphocytes, and consist almost entirely of dendritic cells (fig. 7-9) (26).

The lymph nodes of DiGeorge syndrome show changes in the paracortical regions; they are small and depleted of lymphocytes (fig. 7-10). There are no significant abnormalities of germinal center formation. In MHC class deficits, B-cell areas (follicles) are small and poorly formed or absent (79).

In general, spleens affected by SCID show findings similar to those of lymph nodes. Follicles and germinal centers are poorly developed. The periarteriolar lymphoid sheath (PALS) areas are often atrophic, and distinguishing follicles from PALS regions is difficult. In some cases, the spleens lack lymphoid cells, and consist of

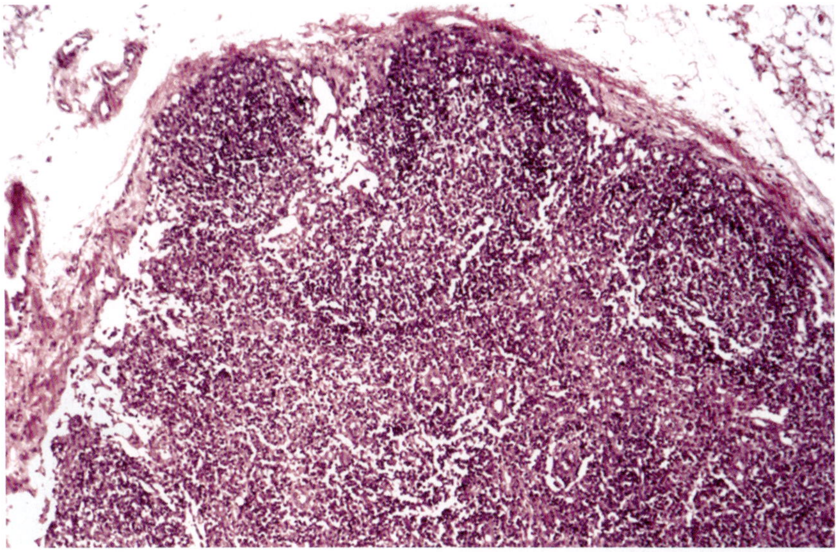

Figure 7-6

NEZELOF SYNDROME, LYMPH NODE

Lymph node biopsy of 7.5-month-old male after local antigenic stimulation. Although small in size, germinal centers are present. (Courtesy of Ronald Jaffe, Pittsburgh, PA.)

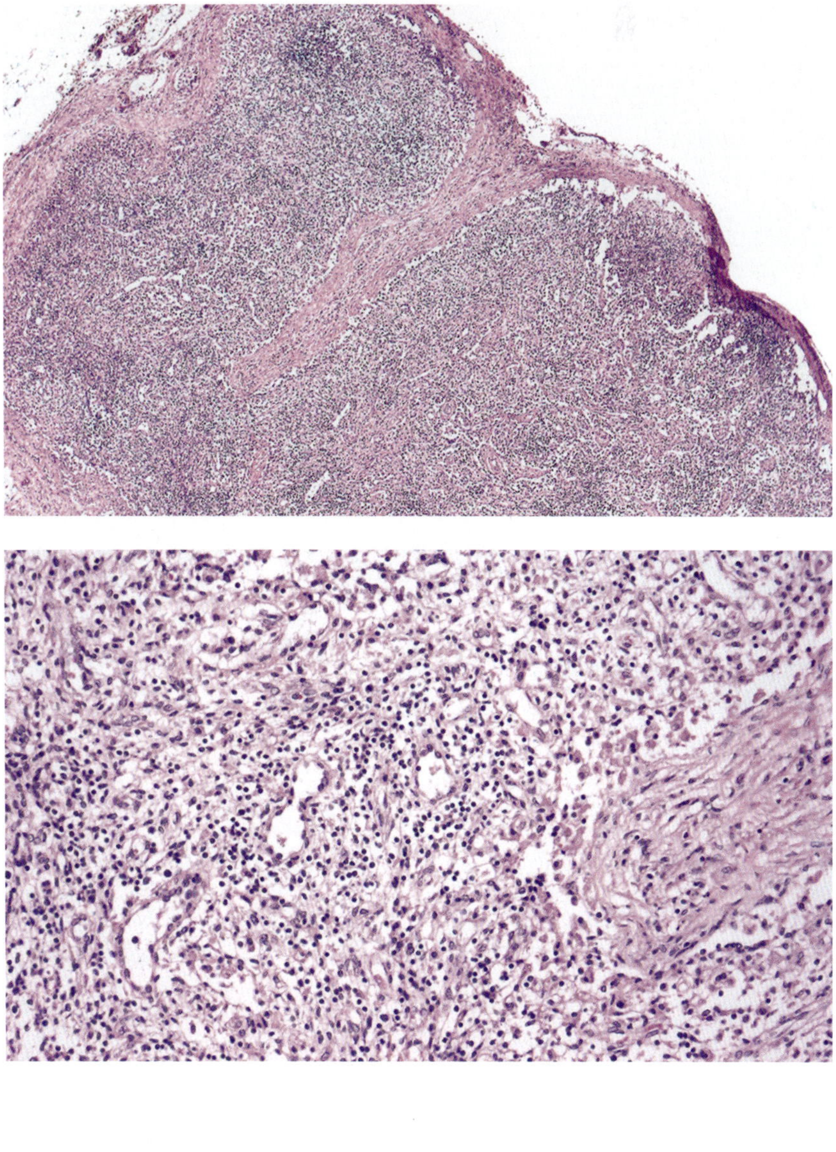

Figure 7-7

NEZELOF SYNDROME, LYMPH NODE

Top: A lymph node in this variant of severe combined immunodeficiency (SCID) shows marked depletion of lymphoid elements.

Bottom: Higher magnification shows the predominance of vascular and stromal elements.

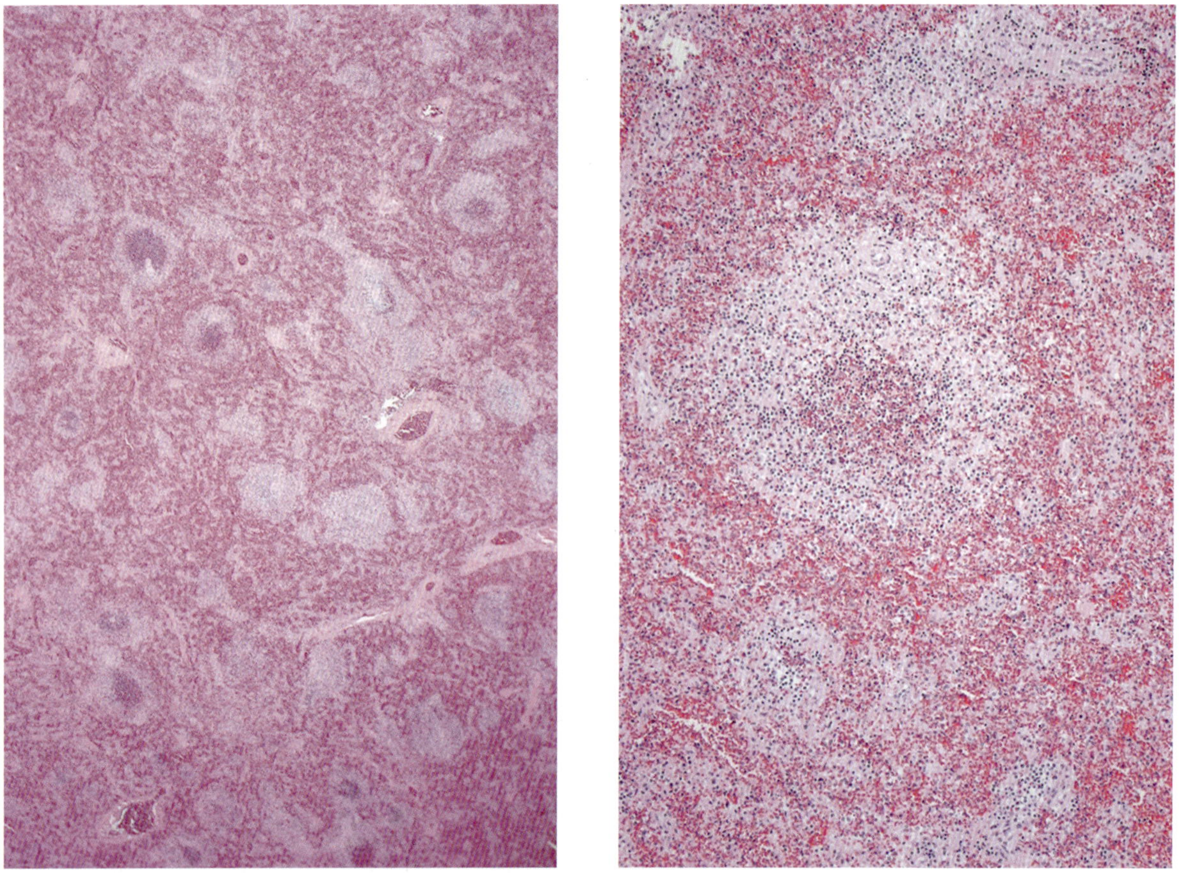

Figure 7-8

NEZELOF SYNDROME, SPLEEN

Although the red pulp appears normally formed (left), the white pulp is depleted of lymphocytes (right).

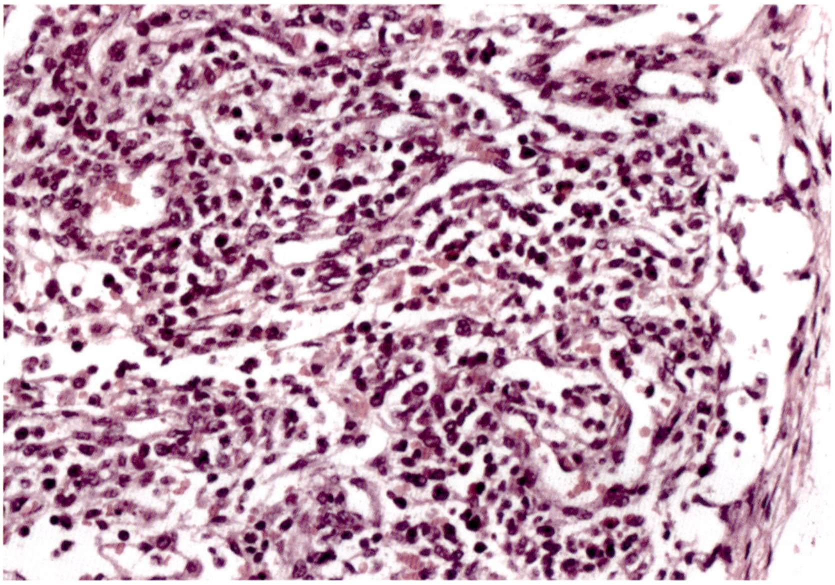

Figure 7-9

RETICULAR DYSGENESIS, LYMPH NODE

Lymph node biopsy of 3-month-old male after local antigenic stimulation. The lymph node consists only of minimal stromal elements. Only rare lymphoid elements are identified. (Courtesy of Ronald Jaffe, Pittsburgh, PA.)

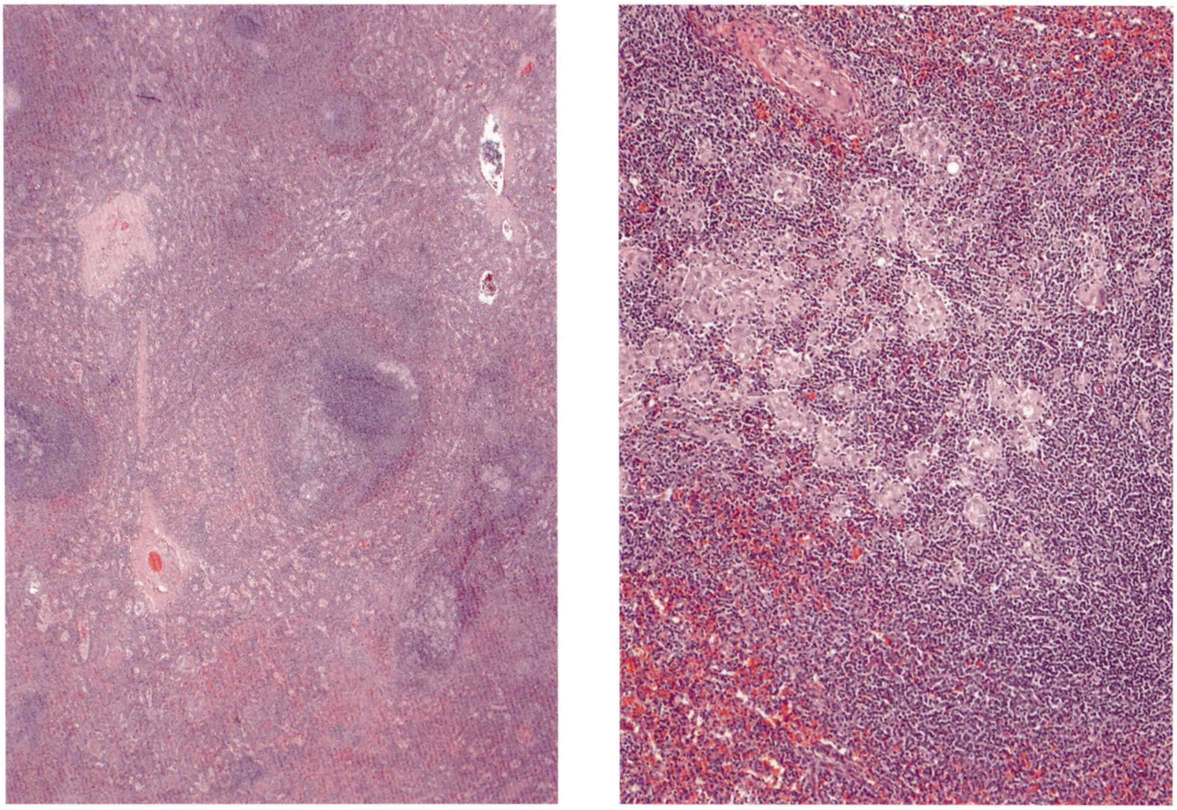

Figure 7-10

(VARIANT) DIGEORGE SYNDROME, SPLEEN

Left: In this partial variant of DiGeorge syndrome, the white pulp of the spleen is intact, although the periarteriolar lymphoid sheath (PALS) region appears small.

Right: On higher magnification, small granulomas are present adjacent to an arteriole.

only red pulp and vascular structures without associated white pulp.

In ADA-SCID, the splenic pathology parallels that of the lymph node. The white pulp is poorly developed, and typically, it is not possible to distinguish between the PALS and the germinal centers. If follicles are present, they are usually small primary follicles or atrophic follicles. In the red pulp, erythrophagocytosis is often prominent and hemosiderin deposition may be present. Periarteriolar fibrosis may also be seen, (18,116).

Omenn syndrome of the spleen has a lack of germinal centers and small atrophic PALS (fig. 7-11). Erythrophagocytosis and eosinophils are prominent in the red pulp (18).

Treatment and Prognosis. In many types of SCID, the patient's life span is limited (often less than 1 year) unless treatment is undertaken. At present, the therapy of choice in most disorders is bone marrow transplantation in an attempt to reconstitute the crippled immune system. Stem cell transplantation is successful in 75 to 90 percent of patients (109). Progress has been made with gene therapy, and it is likely that this therapy will become more prevalent (14).

The incidence of malignancies is increased in patients with SCID. Most commonly, lymphomas and gastrointestinal cancers are seen. Affected females have an incidence of lymphoma 300 times greater than affected males.

AUTOIMMUNE LYMPHOPROLIFERATIVE SYNDROME

Definition. Mutations or deficiencies in the fas/APO-1 receptor (CD95) are associated with different clinical spectrums of disease that include systemic lupus erythematosus, Canale-Smith syndrome, and, discussed here, the

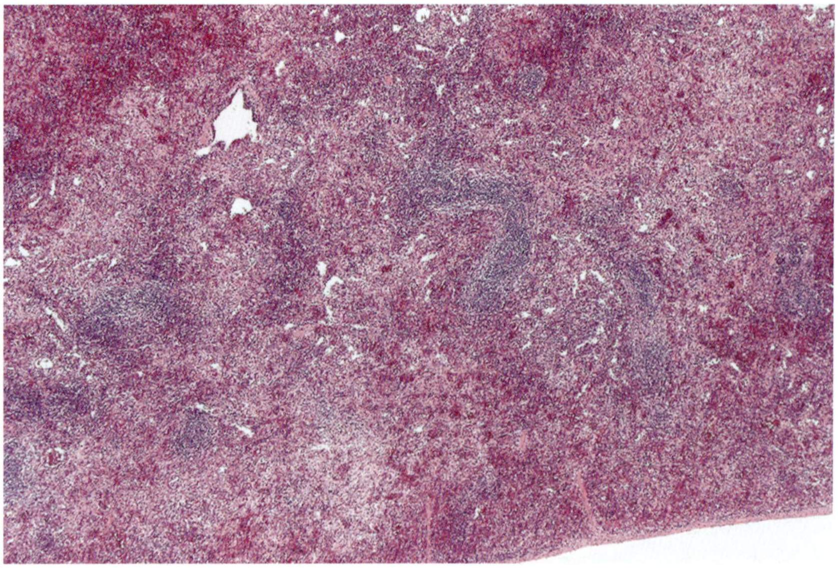

Figure 7-11

OMENN SYNDROME, SPLEEN

Expansion of the red pulp is seen with increased macrophages, depletion of the PALS, and no germinal centers.

autoimmune lymphoproliferative syndrome (ALPS) (32,41,81,144). ALPS I is a recently described disorder that is usually attributable to inherited mutations of CD95 (*fas* gene) and an inability to induce apoptotic cell death (22,86,133,134). ALPS type II and type III are clinically similar syndromes, without detectable mutations in CD95, and with mutations in *caspase 10* or presently undescribed mutations, respectively.

General Features. Loss of function of the *fas* gene has been reported in association with autoimmune phenomena, recurrent lymphadenopathies, and hepatosplenomegaly in mice (150). Deficiency of the fas apoptosis pathway without *fas* gene mutations has been reported to be a familial trait that predisposes to the development of autoimmune diseases, lymphadenopathy, and cancer (115).

Clinical Features. Patients are typically children, aged 6 months to 8 years, who present with symptoms of generalized persistent lymphadenopathy, with or without splenomegaly. Autoimmune phenomena, including hematologic disorders, are often present. These include hemolytic anemias, neutropenias, thrombocytopenias, and glomerulonephritis. These patients typically do not develop opportunistic infections, unlike those with other immune deficiency diseases. Penetrance and expression of clinical features are variable in individuals that share the same genetic defect.

Laboratory Findings. In almost all patients, autoantibodies directed against red blood cells and/or platelets are present (86). In addition, flow cytometry of the peripheral blood reveals increased numbers of T cells that are negative for both CD4 and CD8, the so-called double-negative T cells

Microscopic Features. The most frequent lymph node changes in ALPS I (86) are an intact, but distorted architecture and marked paracortical expansion (figs. 7-12–7-14). In these paracortical regions, immunoblasts are increased in number and are typically large in size, with prominent nucleoli and moderate amounts of deeply staining cytoplasm. Frequent mitoses are seen. Sheets of immunoblasts may simulate a large cell lymphoma. Mature lymphocytes and polyclonal plasma cells are also noted in the paracortex. An absence of tingible body macrophages and areas of necrosis have been reported (86). A polymorphic population of lymphocytes, plasma cells, and multinucleated giant cells (Warthin-Finkeldey or Reed-Sternberg-like cells) may be present.

The germinal centers show a spectrum of reactive changes, ranging from florid follicular hyperplasia with progressive transformation of germinal centers to atrophic, Castleman-like regressively transformed follicles. Prominent postcapillary venules are sometimes seen in the interfollicular region.

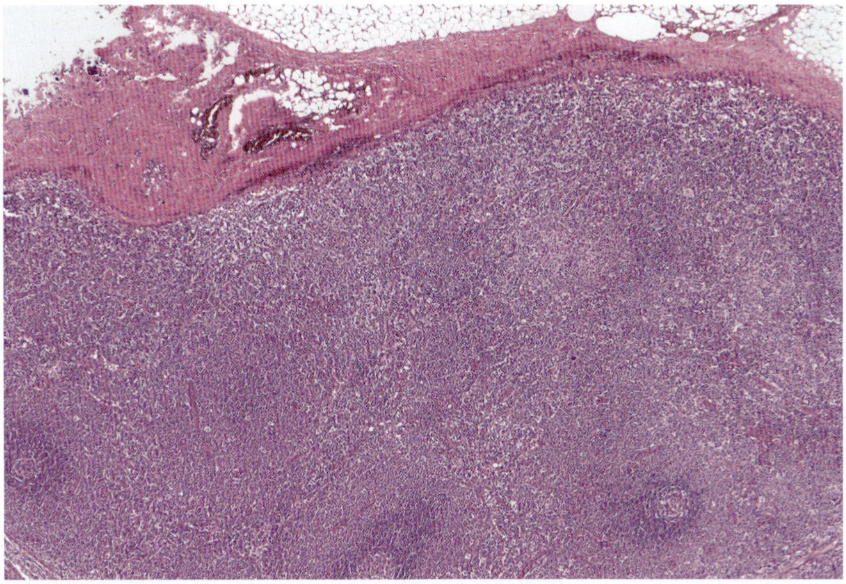

Figure 7-12

AUTOIMMUNE LYMPHOPROLIFERATIVE SYNDROME, LYMPH NODE

The interfollicular/paracortical areas are expanded, with small but normal-appearing follicles.

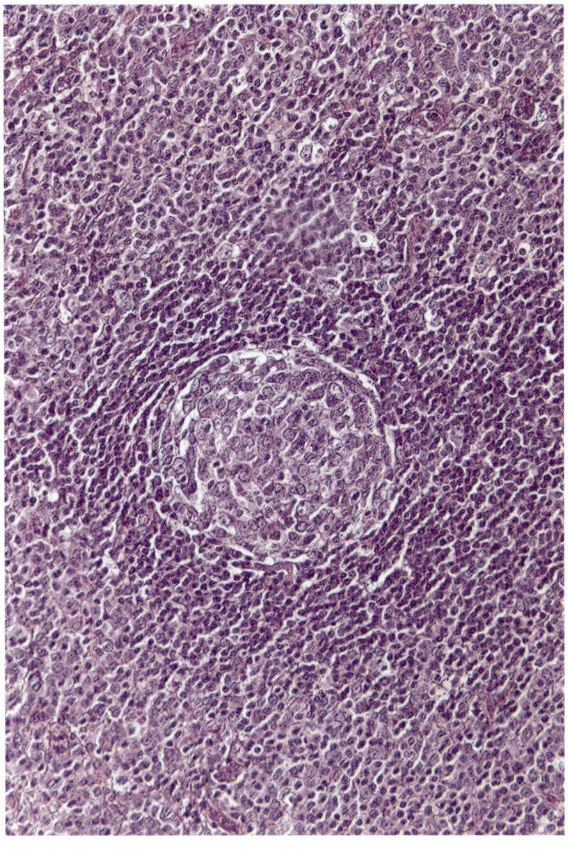

Figure 7-13

AUTOIMMUNE LYMPHOPROLIFERATIVE SYNDROME, LYMPH NODE

A relatively normal-appearing follicle, with massive expansion of the interfollicular areas by plasma cells.

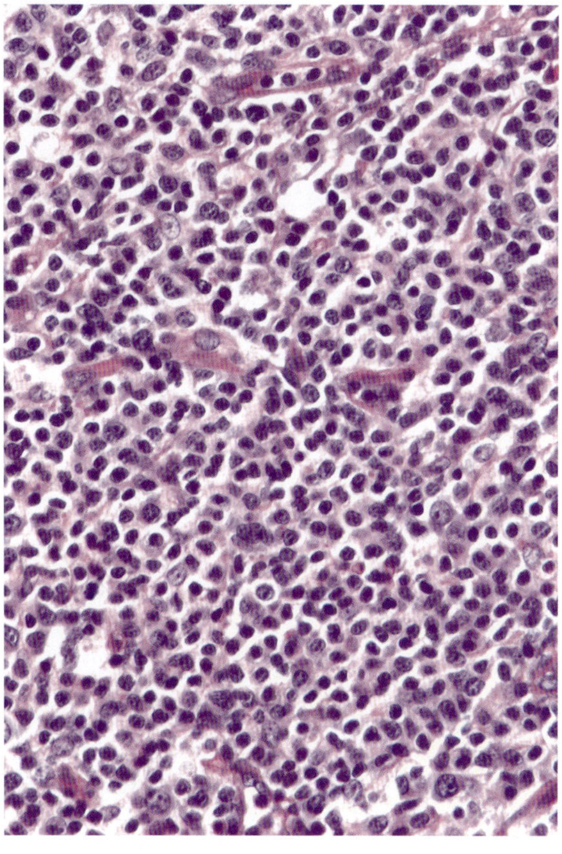

Figure 7-14

AUTOIMMUNE LYMPHOPROLIFERATIVE SYNDROME, LYMPH NODE

Plasmacytoid and monocytoid small lymphocytes are increased in number in the interfollicular region.

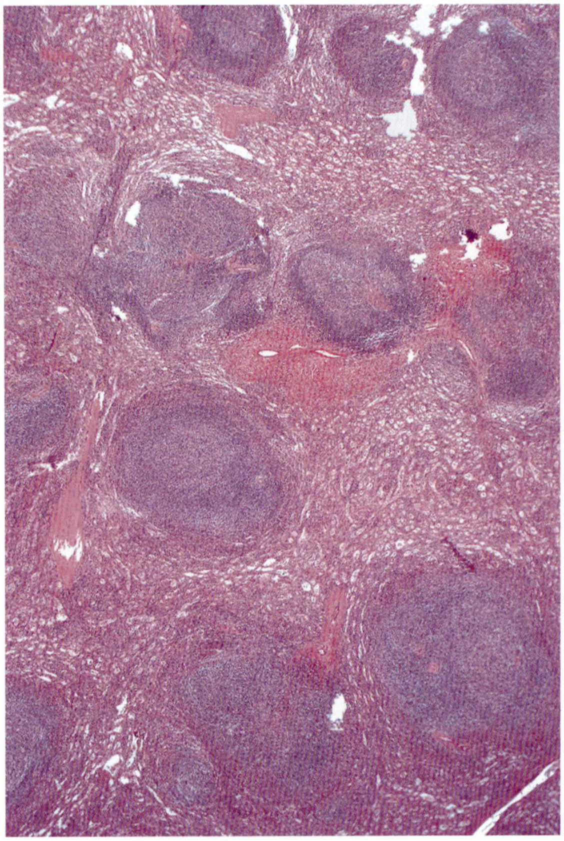

Figure 7-15

AUTOIMMUNE LYMPHOPROLIFERATIVE SYNDROME, SPLEEN

Marked follicular hyperplasia in the spleen.

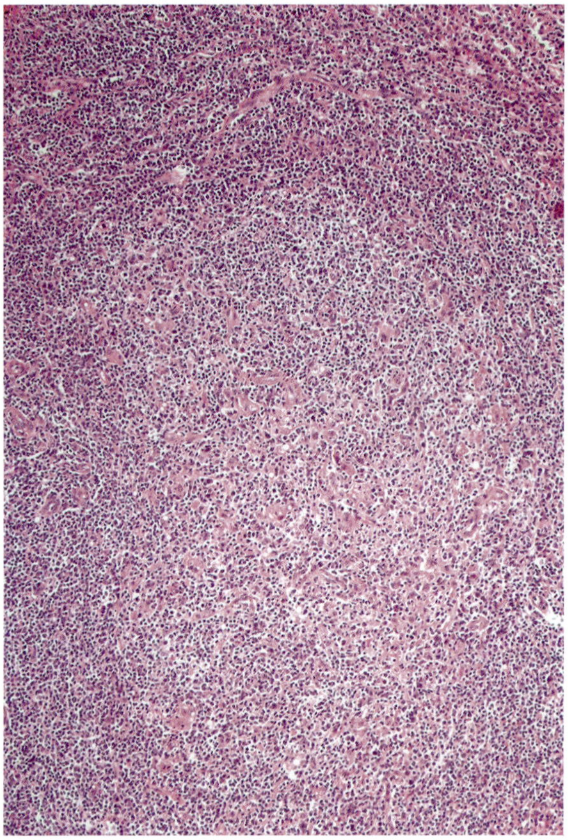

Figure 7-16

AUTOIMMUNE LYMPHOPROLIFERATIVE SYNDROME, SPLEEN

A poorly formed follicle with increased interfollicular fibrosis. The distinction between the germinal center and mantle region is difficult.

The histologic features of sinus histiocytosis with massive lymphadenopathy (Rosai-Dorfman disease) have been described in patients with ALPS (90). Of 44 patients with ALPS, 18 had proliferations of S-100–positive macrophages with emperipolesis.

The histologic changes in the spleen are similar to those in the lymph nodes (figs. 7-15, 7-16). Removed spleens are typically significantly enlarged beyond age-normal size, frequently up to 10 times normal. The PALS and red pulp are disproportionately expanded due to a marked increased in the number of T cells. These cells consist of a mixture of small lymphocytes and immunoblasts and are negative for both CD4 and CD8. In addition, the red pulp has an increased number of polyclonal plasma cells. The white pulp shows variable degrees of follicular hyperplasia, often with enlarged marginal zones. This finding is not seen in most patients because of previous treatment with steroids.

Ancillary Studies. Immunohistochemical evaluation of ALPS reveals several distinctive abnormalities. In both the lymph nodes and spleen, there are expanded populations of T cells that lack expression of both CD4 and CD8 (double-negative T cells). In addition, there is a striking lack of CD45RO in the lymphocytes, implying a naive or virgin phenotype of T cells. Rare CD30-positive cells are seen. There are increased numbers of lymphocytes positive for CD57, TIA-1, and perforin in both lymph nodes and spleen. There does not appear to be an increase in NK cells, however, as evidenced by no increase in the number of cells positive for CD56 and CD16.

In the peripheral blood, lymph nodes, and spleen, flow cytometry documents the presence of numerous double-negative T cells. These cells are of alpha/beta type and may show decreased CD7 expression. Flow cytometry also shows an increase in polyclonal B cells, with a disproportionate increase in B cells coexpressing CD5, a finding often seen in autoimmune disorders.

Diagnostic evaluation of lymph nodes and spleen is often suggestive of ALPS; however, to confirm the diagnosis, molecular studies are needed to evaluate for defects of the *fas* gene. In rare cases, gene rearrangement studies have shown clonal B-cell populations. In a case presented by Strobel (136), the adenopathy and clonal population disappeared without treatment, apparently representing transient clonal expansion.

Differential Diagnosis. In both the lymph nodes and spleen, there is a wide differential diagnosis. The presence of increased immunoblasts can suggest a large cell lymphoma of either B- or T-cell type, or possibly a viral-induced immunoblastic reaction as seen in infectious mononucleosis. Immunohistochemical analysis may suggest a T-cell lymphoma because of the aberrant phenotype of the T cells. The presence of significant plasmacytosis in either the lymph nodes or spleen can raise the possibility of the plasma cell variant of Castleman disease or another autoimmune disorder, or possibly a plasma cell dyscrasia. In all cases, correlation of the abnormal histology with the clinical history generally leads to a diagnosis of ALPS.

Treatment and Prognosis. Adenopathy and splenomegaly tend to resolve as patients reach adolescence or adulthood. Rare instances of both lymphoid and nonlymphoid malignancies have been associated with ALPS (68). Autoimmune phenomena tend to respond to steroid treatment, although this may have only a transient effect or no effect on the lymphadenopathy or splenomegaly. Prophylaxis for possible sepsis should be instituted in cases where splenectomy is performed.

COMMON VARIABLE IMMUNODEFICIENCY

Definition. *Common variable immunodeficiency* (CVID) is a heterogeneous group of disorders characterized by normal numbers of B cells, but abnormal levels of immunoglobulin subgroups (most often IgG and IgA) that do not form immunoglobulin to antigenic stimulus.

General Features. CVID is thought to represent a failure of B-cell differentiation, with impaired secretion of immunoglobulin. In some cases, there is abnormal synthesis or defective secretion of formed immunoglobulin proteins. There appear to be associated regulatory T-cell abnormalities with decreased cytokine production.

Clinical Features. CVID inheritance can be X-linked, autosomal recessive, or multifactorial. CVID is estimated to affect approximately 1/10,000 to 100,000 individuals. The patients display a marked reduction in serum levels of both IgG and IgA. In half of the patients, IgM is also reduced. The incidence of infections, thought to occur at the onset of the disease, shows two age peaks, one at 1 to 5 and the other at 16 to 20 years of age (28,56). The average age of patients at diagnosis, however, is the third decade of life.

The clinical spectrum of CVID is broad. The severity is variable, as is patient age at initial clinical presentation. Recurrent infection is the most common symptom. Upper and lower respiratory bacterial infections, including otitis, sinusitis, and pneumonia, are most frequent. Occasionally, opportunistic infections are seen.

Associated gastrointestinal disorders include diarrhea, malabsorption, and inflammatory bowel disease. There is an increased incidence of autoimmune disorders as well as hematologic problems such as immune thrombocytopenic purpura, hemolytic anemia, and pernicious anemia. Rheumatoid arthritis, hypothyroidism, and vitiligo are rare associated diseases. Patients often present with localized or generalized lymphadenopathy, prompting a lymph node biopsy.

Laboratory Findings. Low levels of immunoglobulins are found. IgG and IgA levels are typically reduced, with variable reductions in levels of other immunoglobulin isotypes. In spite of the decreased immunoglobulins, the number of B cells in the peripheral blood is often normal or only slightly decreased (79). In approximately 40 percent of cases, the response of T cells to mitogens is abnormally decreased.

Microscopic Findings. The morphologic findings can be quite variable in CVID. Four main patterns of lymph node pathology were

Table 7-7

HISTOLOGIC FINDINGS IN COMMON VARIABLE IMMUNODEFICIENCY[a]

Finding	Number of Cases	Percentage of Cases
Malignant lymphoma	2	7
Atypical lymphoid hyperplasia	8	27
Reactive lymphoid hyperplasia	14	47
Chronic granulomatous inflammation consistent with infection	6 (+4)[b]	33
Total Cases	30	

[a]Based on data from reference 125.
[b]Found in addition to reactive lymphoid hyperplasia.

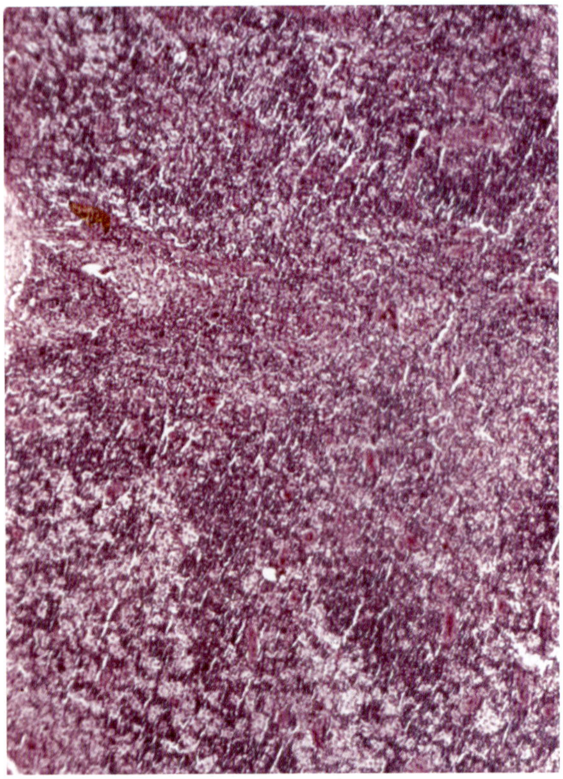

Figure 7-17

COMMON VARIABLE IMMUNODEFICIENCY, LYMPH NODE

Lymph node biopsy from 4-year-old male after local antigenic stimulation. Paracortical expansion is seen, with some follicle formation. (Courtesy of Ronald Jaffe, Pittsburgh, PA.)

identified by Sander et al. (79,125): malignant lymphoma, reactive lymphoid hyperplasia, atypical lymphoid hyperplasia, and chronic granulomatous inflammation (Table 7-7).

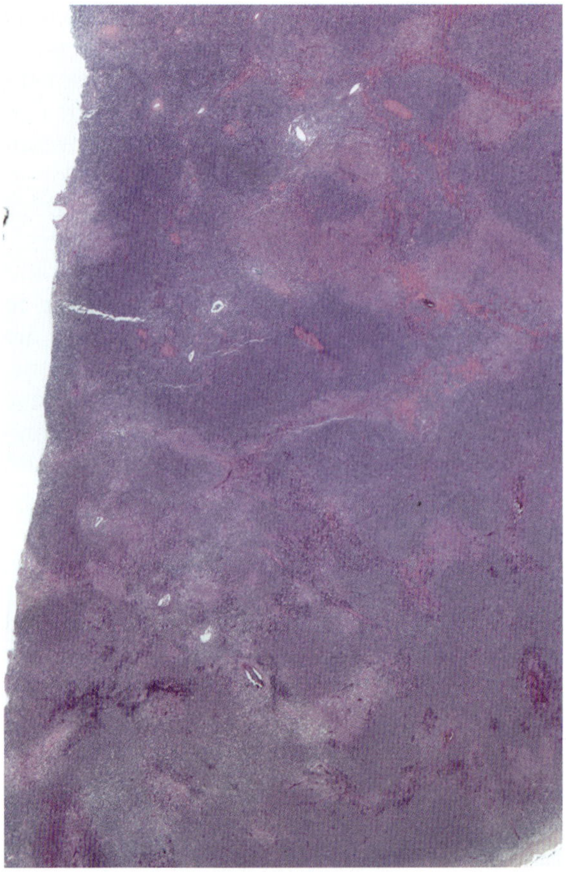

Figure 7-18

COMMON VARIABLE IMMUNODEFICIENCY, LYMPH NODE

No follicle formation is seen in this lymph node.

Reactive lymphoid hyperplasia has typical findings, with prominent follicular hyperplasia, paracortical hyperplasia, or a combination of both. The lymph node architecture is maintained.

Atypical lymphoid hyperplasia is characterized by a variable degree of effacement of the lymph node architecture, from focal to near complete effacement (figs. 7-17–7-20). Germinal centers are present, and may be hyperplastic, or most often, small. Germinal center cells are typically large, with centroblast morphology and prominent karyorrhexis and mitoses. Mantle zones are poorly formed or absent. Paracortical areas are expanded and have a polymorphous cellular appearance. Large transformed cells (immunoblasts) are seen in varying numbers. Marginal zone hyperplasia can be seen in some cases. Plasma cells are rare or absent.

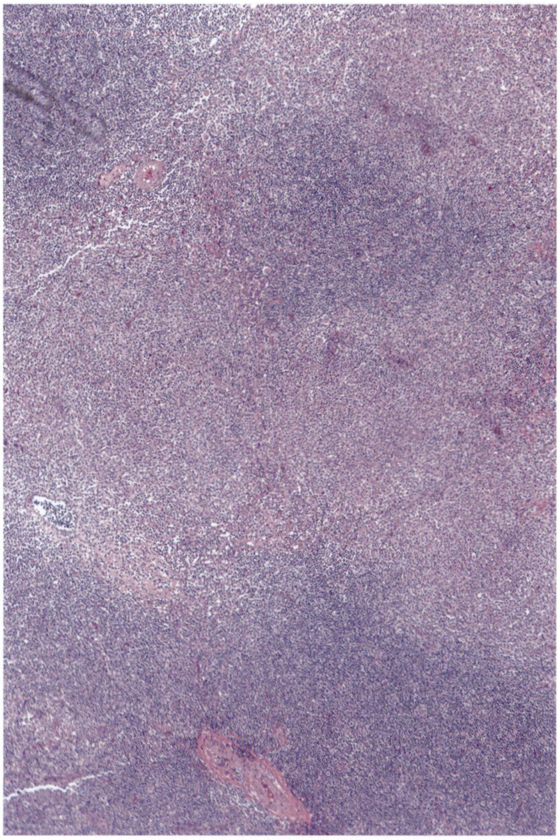

Figure 7-19

COMMON VARIABLE IMMUNODEFICIENCY, LYMPH NODE

Although no follicles are formed, small lymphocytes (blue) can be distinguished from other cell types (plasma cells, lymphoplasmacytoid cells).

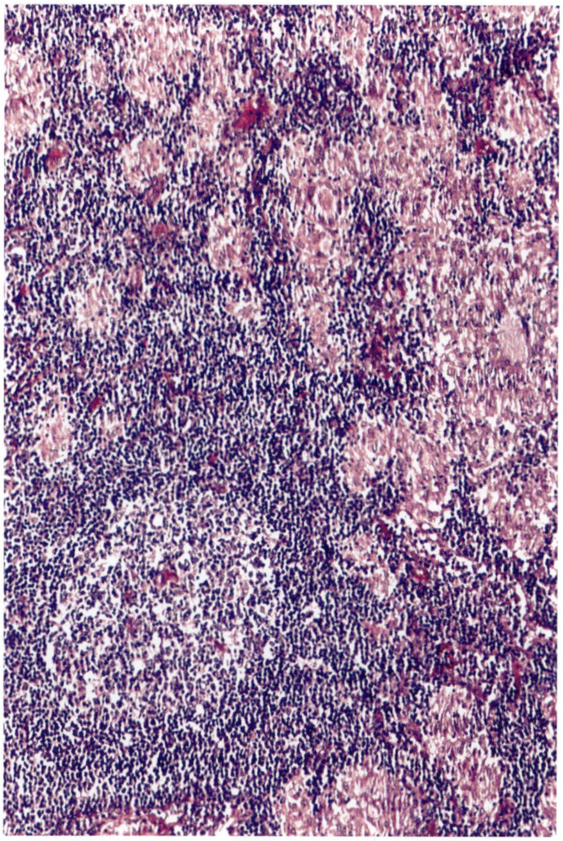

Figure 7-20

COMMON VARIABLE IMMUNODEFICIENCY, LYMPH NODE

Sarcoid-like epithelioid granulomas are present. They may be extensive enough to mimic sarcoidosis. (Courtesy of Ronald Jaffe, Pittsburgh, PA.)

Granuloma formation is common in CVID and is present in multiple body sites, including the lymph nodes. At this site, the granulomatous inflammation is diffuse. Giant cells are seen in the granulomas. Granuloma formulation is typically associated with central, coagulative necrosis and distortion of the normal lymph node architecture. The granulomas are often associated with infectious etiologies; special stains for organisms should be performed in all cases where granulomatous inflammation is seen.

As in the lymph nodes, a variety of patterns occurs in the spleen in CVID (figs. 7-21–7-23). Typically, the red pulp is unaffected. The white pulp may be hyperplastic, with associated splenomegaly. Although follicular hyperplasia with prominent germinal centers is the rule, atypical hyperplasia and chronic granulomatous inflammation occur as well. As in the lymph nodes, evaluation for infection, including EBV, may be appropriate.

Ancillary Studies. Because of the frequency of infections, special stains for organisms are recommended. Typical evaluations include an acid-fast bacillus (AFB) stain (for mycobacteria), a Gomori methenamine silver (GMS) and a periodic acid–Schiff (PAS) stain (for fungal forms), and in select cases, tissue Gram or silver stains for bacteria (e.g., Warthin-Starry). Tuberculosis, toxoplasmosis, and lymphogranuloma venereum are increased in association with CVID.

In situ stains for EBV should be considered in most cases of CVID. In a study by Sander (125), 50 percent of tested cases were positive for EBV

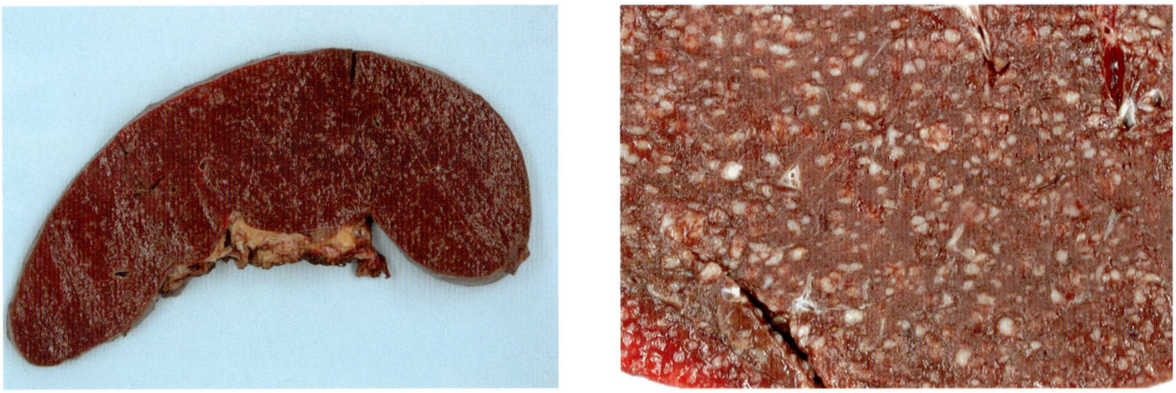

Figure 7-21

COMMON VARIABLE IMMUNODEFICIENCY, SPLEEN

An enlarged spleen (left) has prominent white pulp (right).

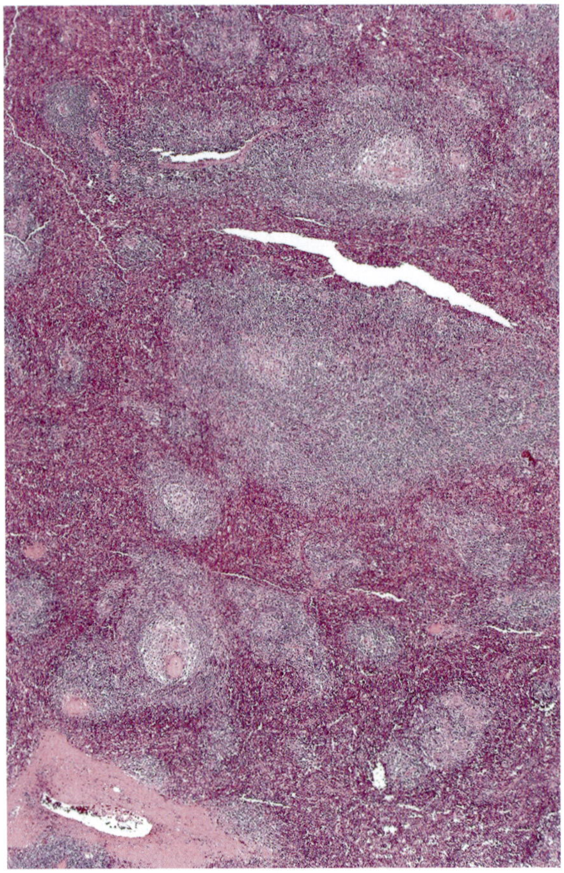

Figure 7-22

COMMON VARIABLE IMMUNODEFICIENCY, SPLEEN

The expanded white pulp includes prominent germinal centers and expanded PALS regions. Small collections of macrophages/granulomas are seen in occasional germinal centers.

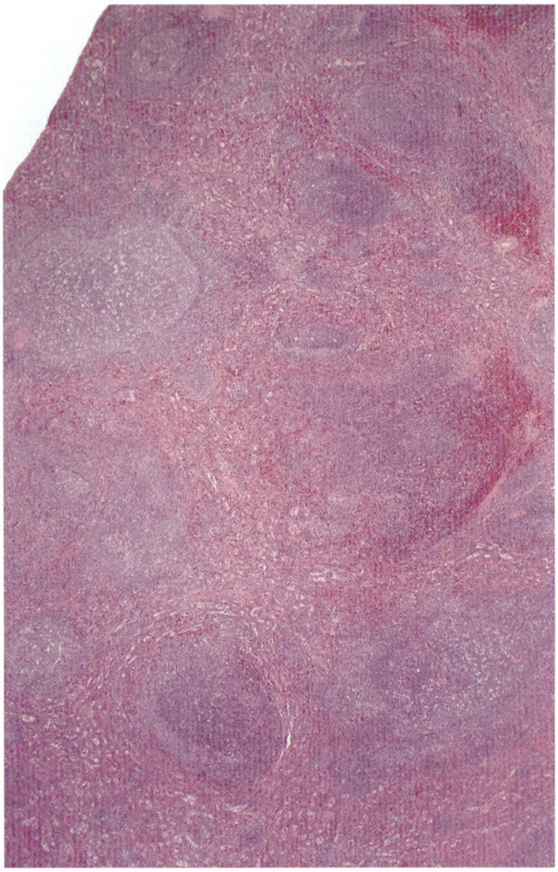

Figure 7-23

COMMON VARIABLE IMMUNODEFICIENCY, SPLEEN

Florid follicular hyperplasia, with normal red pulp.

by in situ methods. It is likely that EBV infection underlies many of the lymphoid proliferations associated with this disorder.

Differential Diagnosis. Atypical lymph node hyperplasia can be difficult to distinguish from lymphoma. In these cases, the use of immunohistochemical studies and gene rearrangement studies are helpful. In atypical lymphoid hyperplasia, the lymph node architecture usually is maintained, although distorted, while in lymphoma the architecture is effaced. Lymphomas typically have clonal IgH rearrangements. In cases with extensive granulomatous inflammation, CVID may clinically and pathologically mimic sarcoidosis.

Treatment and Prognosis. Although CVID is variable in severity, the mainstay of treatment is periodic infusions of intravenous immunoglobulin. This treatment decreases the incidence of recurrent infections. Most important is the significantly increased incidence of other neoplasms in CVID, estimated at 30 to 438 times normal. Non-Hodgkin lymphoma is the most common secondary malignancy identified; Hodgkin lymphoma is also frequent in CVID patients.

SELECTIVE IGA DEFICIENCY

Definition. *Selective IgA deficiency* is characterized by a lack of serum IgA associated with generally mild immunodeficiency.

General Features. The underlying pathology in selective IgA deficiency is a failure of terminal differentiation of B cells into IgA-producing cells. The underlying gene, *IGAD1*, has been mapped to 6p21, which is associated with *MHC* genes (148).

Clinical Features. Selective IgA deficiency is the most common of all primary immunodeficiencies, with a frequency of 1/700 Caucasians. Some patients are asymptomatic, while others have an increased incidence of bacterial infections. Patients with selective IgA deficiency have increased autoimmune phenomena including systemic lupus erythematosus, rheumatoid arthritis, immune thrombocytopenic purpura (ITP), autoimmune hemolytic anemia, Henoch-Schonlein purpura, vasculitis, dermatomyositis, and membranoproliferative glomerulonephritis (27). Celiac disease is commonly associated with selective IgA deficiency (3). Patients with IgA deficiency often have relatives with other immunoglobulin deficiencies, including CVID.

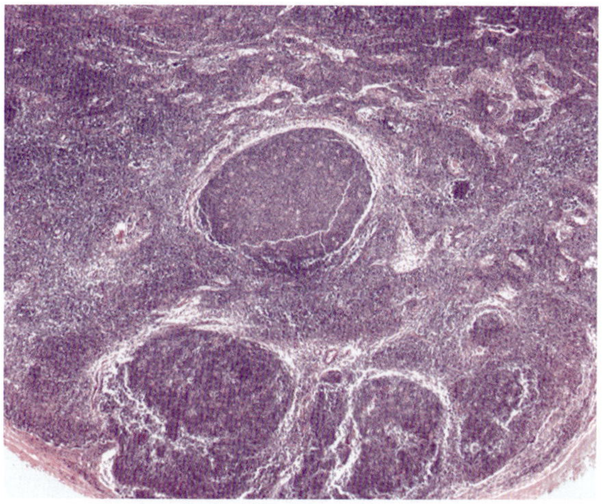

Figure 7-24

IGA DEFICIENCY, LYMPH NODE

Abnormal follicles are seen.

Dubowitz syndrome is an autosomal recessive complex of congenital abnormalities that include numerous dysmorphic features and retarded growth in addition to IgA deficiency. Patients with Dubowitz syndrome have an increased incidence of hematologic disorders, including aplastic anemia, acute lymphoblastic leukemia, and lymphomas.

Laboratory Findings. No serum IgA is detectable. The patients may produce antibodies directed against IgA, leading to severe anaphylactoid reactions when gammaglobulin or blood products are administered. Other autoantibodies are frequently identified, including rheumatoid factor, anticardiolipin antibodies, and antinuclear antibodies (3)

Microscopic Findings. A range of histologic findings may be seen in the lymph nodes or spleen of patients with selective IgA deficiency, although they are not specific (figs. 7-24–7-26). IgA-positive plasma cells are lacking. If infection is present, the features are compatible with those of the specific infectious agent.

HYPER-IGM SYNDROME

Definition. Immunodeficiency with elevated IgM levels, *hyper-Igm syndrome* is a combined primary immunodeficiency characterized by defective immunoglobulin isotype class switching, neutropenia, and frequent infections.

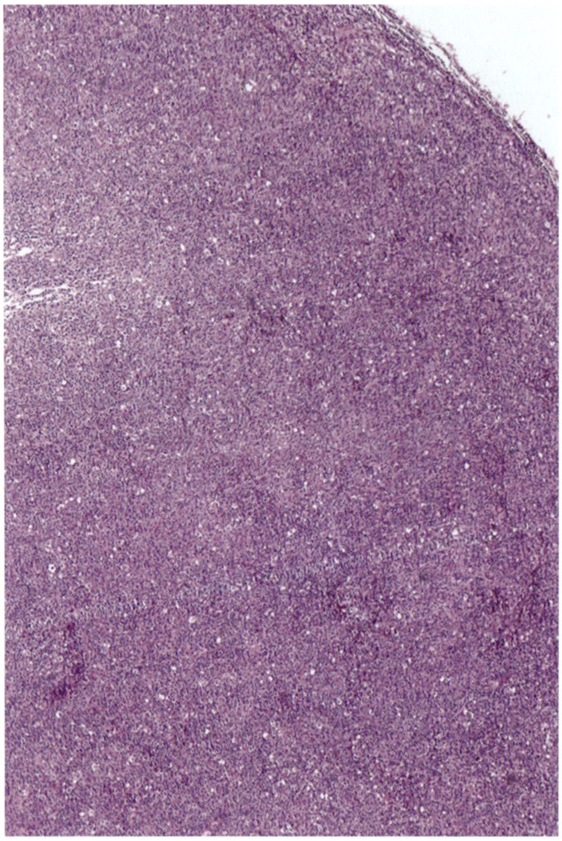

Figure 7-25

DUBOWITZ SYNDROME, LYMPH NODE

Lack of follicle formation and numerous immunoblasts are seen.

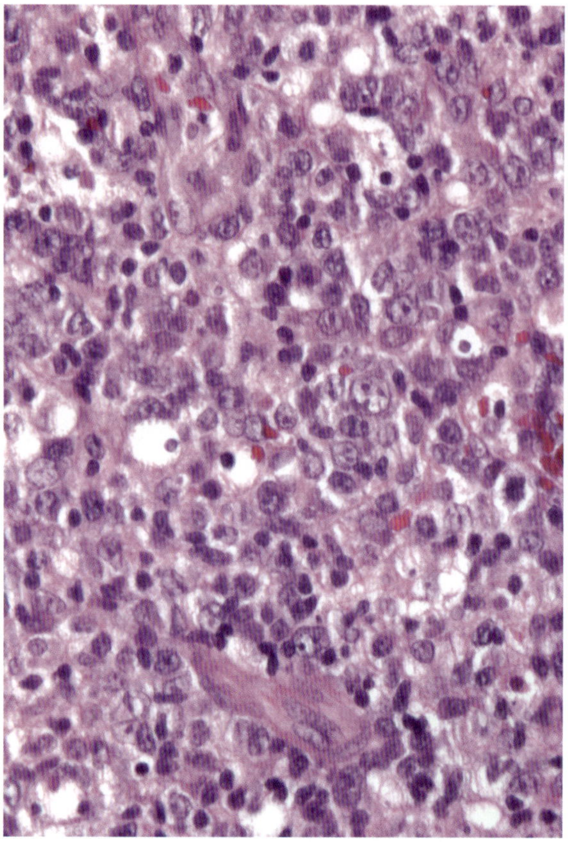

Figure 7-26

DUBOWITZ SYNDROME, LYMPH NODE

Large numbers of immunoblasts are present in this lymph node.

General Findings. The most common type of hyper-IgM syndrome is X-linked, but autosomal recessive and autosomal dominant forms are also described (108). Mutations involving at least five genes have been identified as causing this syndrome, including *CD40 ligand* (type 1) (2), *activation-induced cytidine deaminase* (type 2) (119), *CD40* (type 3)(39), *uracil DNA glycosylate* (type 5) (65), and *NF-kB essential modulator* (69) genes; the genetic defects associated with type 4 are not yet determined (30,65).

In type 1 hyper-IgM syndrome, inherited as an X-linked recessive trait, multiple mutations in the gene for *CD40 ligand*, located at Xq26.3-27, have been described (103). Mutations in the *CD40 ligand* gene (CD154, CD40L) prevent interaction of this T-lymphocyte surface molecule with CD40 present on the surface of B lymphocytes. This lack of interaction results in the inability to class switch from IgM to IgG, IgA, or IgE, resulting in normal or increased IgM levels (35,67,87). Humoral immunodeficiency is present, as shown by the pyogenic infections caused by encapsulated organisms in these patients. The presence of opportunistic infections caused by intracellular pathogens has suggested cellular immunity defects as well, with CD40 and CD40L playing roles in T-cell mediated immunity (84). Acquired hyper-IgM syndrome has been described in children following rubella infection (16), and in some adults without a clear etiology. One adult case was associated with T-cell lymphoma, another presented as recurrent pneumonia, and a third, as autoimmune hemolytic anemia (61,117,123).

Clinical Features. Recurrent pyogenic bacterial infections are the most common problems, starting during the first or second year of life.

Severe opportunistic infections, particularly *Cryptosporidium* enteritis and *Pneumocystis jiroveci* pneumonia, occur in patients with types 1 and 3 hyper-IgM syndrome (41). Patients with the autosomal recessive type 2 exhibit normal T-cell function and are not at risk for opportunistic infections (119). Many patients also have chronic neutropenia (15). Autoimmune diseases and hepatic carcinomas are increased in patients with type 1 hyper-IgM syndrome (84).

Laboratory Findings. Patients have markedly reduced levels of IgG, IgA, and IgE, with elevated or normal levels of IgM (84). Surprisingly, almost 50 percent of patients have normal levels of IgM (8,152). Isohemagglutinin levels are normal to increased (102). The numbers of circulating B cells are normal or increased, and T-cell numbers are normal. As expected, B cells are only IgM and IgD positive. Increased circulating gamma-delta T cells have been reported in a patient with hyper-IgM syndrome and central nervous system toxoplasmosis (82). In addition to neutropenia, autoantibodies and autoimmune hemolytic anemia have been described (15). Patients with CD40L deficiency have normal responses to mitogens, with defective in vitro T-lymphocyte proliferations (84). A recently described flow cytometry assay for CD40 ligand expression on CD4-positive T lymphocytes has been used to diagnose X-linked hyper-IgM syndrome (42).

Microscopic Findings. The lymph nodes may be normal to increased in size. Follicular hyperplasia is present in the cortex, but is composed of primary follicles with absent or abortive germinal centers and marked depletion of follicular dendritic cells (39,102). The paracortex may be expanded and include collections of plasmacytoid monocytes. Only rare to scant plasma cells are present in the medullary cords and interfollicular areas. The medullary sinuses are enlarged (38). An earlier case report of a 16-year-old boy with clinical features of hyper-IgM syndrome showed reactive follicular hyperplasia; however, well-developed follicles were apparent in all three lymph node biopsies and no plasma cells could be found (127).

Necrotizing granulomas have been described in a single patient with acquired hyper-IgM syndrome who did not have evidence of an underlying infection (48), and noncaseating granulomas have been reported in the lymph nodes and bone marrow in two other hyper-IgM patients (5,62). Infection of the lymph node may alter the histologic appearance described above, as seen in a patient with *Achromobacter xylosoxidans* lymph node infection which served as a source of bacteremia (151). This lymph node showed a polymorphous infiltrate consisting of plasma cells, small to large lymphocytes, and macrophages; flow cytometric findings showed a predominance of phenotypically normal T cells.

While specific splenic findings have not been described in patients with hyper-IgM syndrome, the findings should parallel those of the lymph nodes including the absence of germinal centers and follicular dendritic cells. Interestingly, one report of three infants described a primary immune deficiency with features of hyper-IgM syndrome, characterized by splenomegaly, anemia, and severe infections (36). The lymph node findings were typical of those seen in hyper-IgM syndrome. Gross splenomegaly was present. Microscopic examination showed depletion of the white pulp, which contained small primary follicles associated with malpighian corpuscles lacking germinal centers. No follicular dendritic cells were detected. The red pulp was congested, but otherwise normal in appearance.

Ancillary Studies. Primary follicles are composed of CD20- and bcl-2–positive B lymphocytes. If any abortive germinal centers are present, these will be bcl-2 negative with a high Ki-67 proliferative fraction. The lack of germinal centers correlates with a paucity of follicular dendritic cells. In addition to being reduced in number, the follicular dendritic cells express nerve growth factor receptor and lack Ki-M4p, with poor expression of CD21 and CD23. Paracortical T cells are without immunologic abnormalities and are admixed with S-100 protein–positive interdigitating reticulum cells. Intrafollicular T cells also appear unremarkable, with rare cells expressing CD3, CD43, CD45RO, and CD57. Scattered plasma cells express only µ-chain (38).

Differential Diagnosis. Other immunodeficiencies, such as X-linked agammaglobulinemia or SCID, are included in the differential diagnosis as these also lack follicular dendritic cell networks.

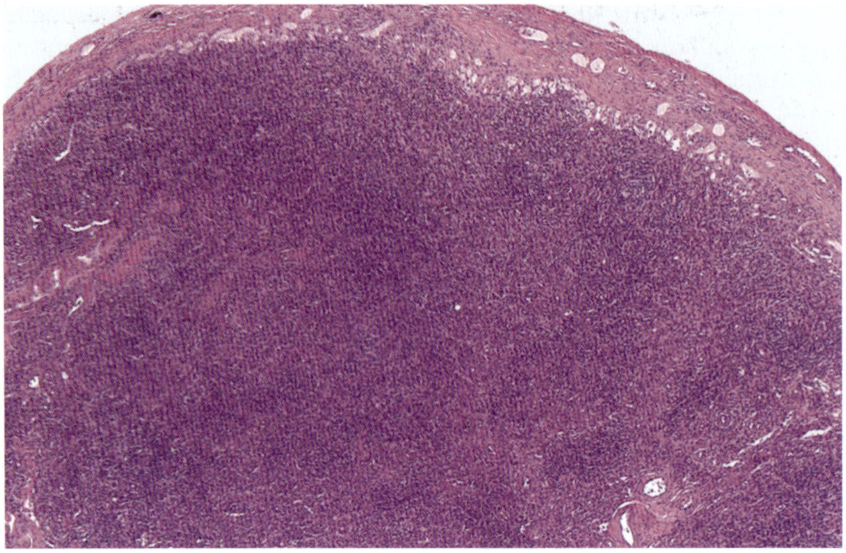

Figure 7-27

HYPER-IGE SYNDROME, LYMPH NODE

There is poor germinal center formation, with increased fibrosis and a thickened capsule.

Treatment and Prognosis. The treatment has focused on reducing infections using intravenous immunoglobulin and antibiotic prophylaxis. Many patients with severe neutropenia respond to granulocyte-colony stimulating factor (G-CSF). Only 20 percent of patients reach age 30 and a high percentage of these patients have hepatic complications; lymphoid malignancies are also increased (84). Chronic liver disease has been documented in a cohort of patients with hyper-IgM syndrome; 70 percent of the patients have chronic infection with *Cryptosporidium parvum* (58). This cohort also has an increased incidence of gastrointestinal cancers. While allogeneic bone marrow transplantation has been reported to cure X-linked hyper-IgM syndrome (141), it has typically been performed in patients without severe liver disease. Liver and bone marrow transplantation were reportedly successful in correcting the hyper-IgM syndrome in an 18-year-old male with end-stage chronic liver disease (54).

HYPER-IGE SYNDROME (JOB SYNDROME)

Definition. *Hyper-IgE syndrome* (HIES), also referred to as *Job syndrome*, is characterized by elevated serum levels of IgE, recurrent infections, and immunodeficiency.

General Features. The underlying molecular and gene defects are unknown, although the disorder has been mapped to 4q21. Defects in granulocyte chemotaxis are part of the causal mechanism (96).

Clinical Features. HIES is usually autosomal dominant, with variable expressivity, and less commonly, autosomal recessive (53). The diagnosis is often made in childhood; however, some cases go unrecognized until adulthood. In the Book of Job, it is stated that "Satan...smote Job with sore boils from the sole of his foot unto his crown" (Job 2:7). Such a clinical picture is related to the presence of frequent *Staphylococcus* skin abscesses and chronic dermatitis (131). Patients with HIES have recurrent bacterial infections, including recurrent pneumonia with pneumatocele, cryptococcal meningitis, and mucocutaneous candidiasis. In addition, they have recurrent fractures and hyperextensible joints. As they age, they develop coarse facial features.

Laboratory Findings. The cornerstone of the diagnosis of HIES is the demonstration of elevated serum IgE levels. Eosinophilic leukocytosis (over 0.7×10^9/L) is seen in many patients (37,96). The T-cell proliferation is decreased in response to mitogens.

Microscopic Findings. The microscopic features of HIES have not been well-described in the literature. Besides an increase in eosinophils, capsular thickening and fibrosis are common in lymph nodes (figs. 7-27–7-29). These changes are probably due to the effects of eosinophil proteins and cytokine signals. It is unclear whether there are significant changes in the follicles or interfollicular areas.

Treatment and Prognosis. The treatment of patients with HIES relies heavily on prophylactic

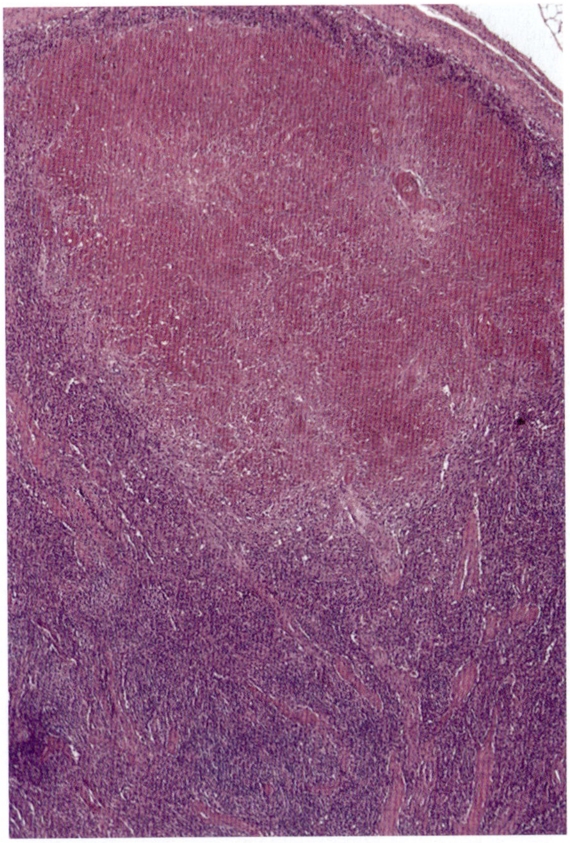

Figure 7-28

HYPER-IGE SYNDROME, LYMPH NODE

Focal necrosis, fibrosis, and lack of follicles are seen in this lymph node.

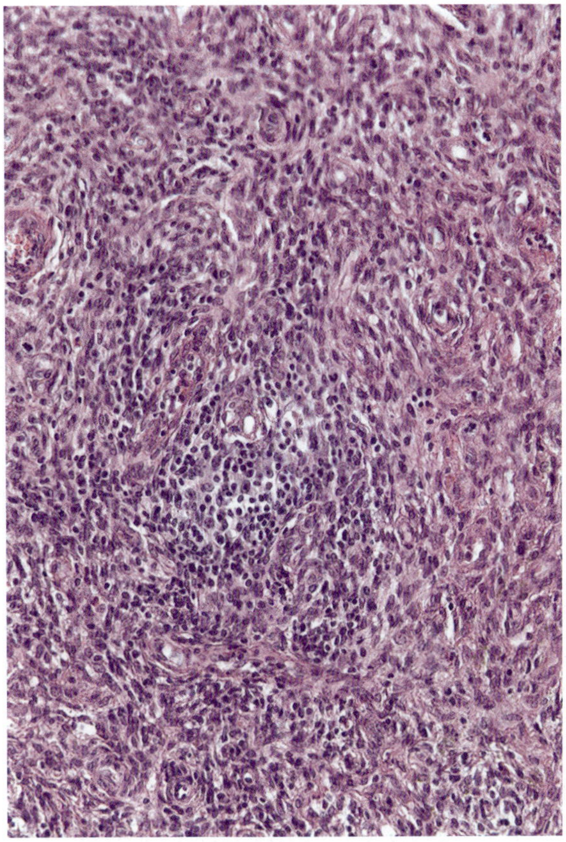

Figure 7-29

HYPER-IGE SYNDROME, LYMPH NODE

High magnification shows increased fibroblasts/stromal elements and decreased lymphocytes.

antibiotics to prevent infections. High-dose intravenous immunoglobulin, cyclosporine A, and interferon have been used with some benefit (96). Patients with HIES have an increased risk of the development of lymphomas.

X-LINKED AGAMMAGLOBULINEMIA (BRUTON AGAMMAGLOBULINEMIA) AND HYPOGAMMAGLOBULINEMIA

Definition. *X-linked agammaglobulinemia* (XLA), also known as *Bruton agammaglobulinemia,* is a severe defect of immunoglobulin production, resulting in immunodeficiency. In some cases, severe *hypogammaglobulinemia* is seen, in contrast to a complete lack of immunoglobulin.

General Features. XLA is due to a gene defect located at Xq21.3-q22, which encodes the B-cell tyrosine kinase (*Btk*) gene. The *Btk* gene is a key regulator of B-cell development, apparently controlling the maturation from pro-B cell to pre-B cell. It appears that *Btk* is involved in signaling through the pre-B-cell receptor (19).

Clinical Features. As implied in the name, XLA is an X-linked disorder. Affected males do not usually present clinically until 9 to 12 months, after loss of passive maternal antibody protection (124). There are varying degrees of severity associated with the disorder, and differing levels of immunoglobulin production recognized. Increased bacterial infections are a hallmark of the disease; recurrent or severe infections with encapsulated bacteria (*Staphylococcus aureus, Streptococcus pneumoniae* and *pyogenes, Haemophilus influenzae*) are the most common. Otitis, sinusitis, conjunctivitis, pneumonia, and pyoderma are all common types of infection (19). Chronic lung disease due to

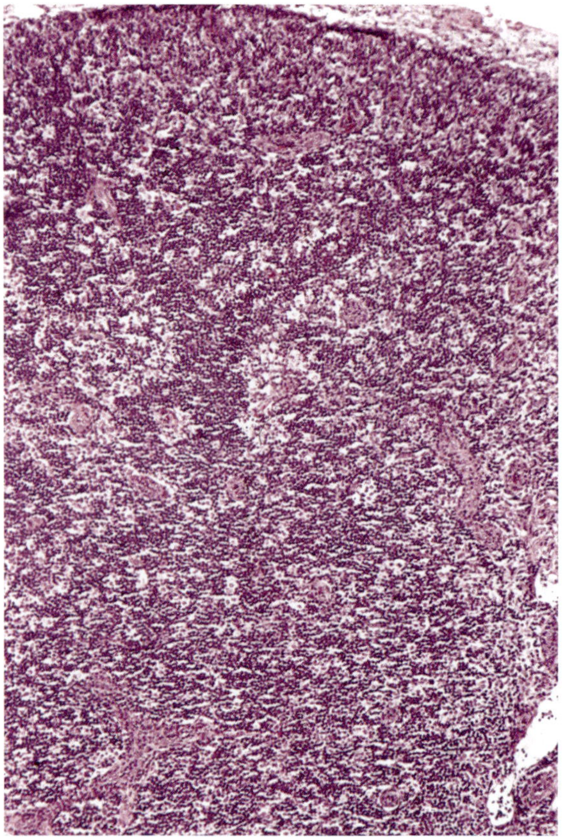

Figure 7-30

X-LINKED AGAMMAGLOBULINEMIA, LYMPH NODE

No follicles are present, although there is paracortical expansion. (Courtesy of Ronald Jaffe, Pittsburgh, PA.)

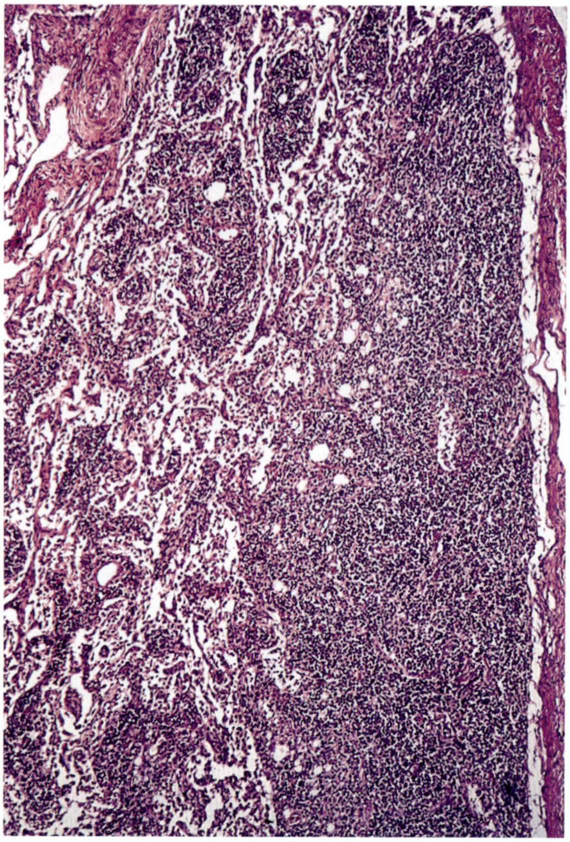

Figure 7-31

X-LINKED AGAMMAGLOBULINEMIA, LYMPH NODE

Follicles are not present, but lymph node cords and sinuses are. (Courtesy of Ronald Jaffe, Pittsburgh, PA.)

the destruction of lung tissue from recurrent infections is a major cause of morbidity. *Giardia* infections are common and may lead to chronic gastrointestinal symptoms and weight loss. Chronic enteroviral infections are also a frequent cause of gastrointestinal symptoms. A rheumatoid arthritis–like syndrome is frequently seen, and some arthritis symptoms are due to *Mycoplasma* infections. Female carriers are immunologically normal.

Laboratory Findings. In XLA, IgG levels are severely decreased (less than 100 mg/dL); other immunoglobulin levels are also markedly decreased. XLA patients do not make IgG in response to immunizations. In the peripheral blood, there is lymphocytopenia due to a profound decrease in circulating B cells; there are normal to increased numbers of T cells. Neutropenia is also seen, although this manifestation typically resolves rapidly upon treatment with intravenous immunoglobulin.

Gross Findings. Occasionally, patients with XLA are discovered through physical examination. Affected patients have small to almost absent lymph nodes, even in the face of infection. Lack of palpable lymph nodes, especially in the cervical region of a child with an active infection, may be a diagnostic clue for XLA. In addition, patients have severely hypoplastic or absent tonsils and adenoids.

Microscopic Findings. The lymph nodes in XLA have a distinctive appearance (figs. 7-30, 7-31) (26). They are small and lack normal architecture. Often, there are no germinal centers; when present, these are small and atretic. The paracortical areas are expanded, but in these areas and throughout the lymph node, there are no plasma cells.

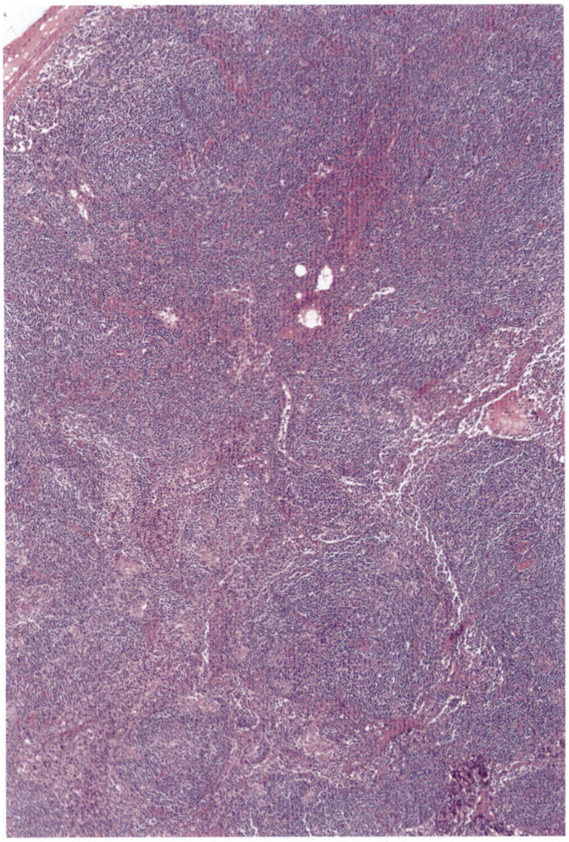

Figure 7-32

HYPOGAMMAGLOBULINEMIA, LYMPH NODE

Poor follicle formation, fibrosis, and vascular proliferation are seen.

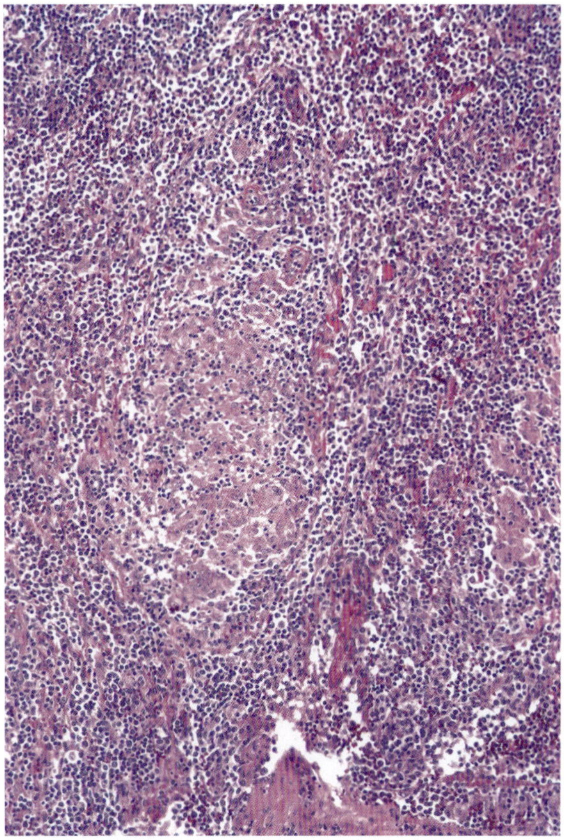

Figure 7-33

HYPOGAMMAGLOBULINEMIA, LYMPH NODE

There is a small granuloma.

XLA spleens show similar findings to lymph nodes, although they have not been thoroughly described (18). Germinal centers are not present and plasma cells are lacking. Expansion in the PALS may be seen. Splenomegaly due to red pulp hyperplasia is present in a subset of patients; this is sometimes referred to as *empty spleen syndrome* (18).

Ancillary Studies. A flow cytometric assay for Btk expression has been described (64). Individuals with XLA lack expression of Btk on their monocytes and platelets. Female carriers have populations of cells with and without expression of Btk.

Differential Diagnosis. Other disorders of gammaglobulin production may show similar clinical and pathologic findings (figs. 7-32, 7-33). The pathologic findings can be mimicked by other congenital immunodeficiencies.

Treatment and Prognosis. Large doses of intravenous immunoglobulin (IVIG) reduce the frequency and severity of infections.

X-LINKED LYMPHOPROLIFERATIVE DISEASE (DUNCAN SYNDROME)

Definition. *X-linked lymphoproliferative disease* (XLP), also known as *Duncan syndrome*, is a rare immunodeficiency characterized by a selective inability to respond appropriately to EBV infection and an increased susceptibility to lymphoma.

General Features. A spectrum of EBV-induced lymphoid proliferations caused by an underlying defect in response to EBV infection is found in patients with XLP (112). The associated lymphoproliferative disorders range from fatal infectious mononucleosis to non-Hodgkin lymphoma to dysgammoglobulinemia (55). Mutations in *SH2D1A* (SH2 domain–encoding gene, also known as *SAP, DSHP*) at Xq25 are responsible for XLP (17,98,99,126). Multiple functional mutations have been described in *SH2D1A*, including deletions, transcription/splicing mutations, nonsense mutations leading to premature protein termination, and missense mutations affecting function of SAP (signaling lymphocyte activation molecule protein) (138). The SAP protein interacts with a family of SLAM (signaling lymphocyte activation molecule) receptors expressed on the surface of T and B cells, thought to be important in bidirectional T- and B-cell stimulation (126). SAP-deficient cytotoxic T cells display a specific lytic defect against EBV-positive B cells, thus at least partially explaining the ineffective T-cell response in eliminating EBV-infected B cells (33).

Clinical Features. This rare immunodeficiency was initially described in one family in which three brothers died from infectious mononucleosis and investigation revealed four male cousins with lymphoma or unusual complications following EBV infection (112). Subsequently, several kindreds have been described (55).

The inheritance is always X-linked recessive with presentation occurring after EBV infection. Patients range in age from 5 months to 23 years. Phenotypes include acquired agammaglobulinemia, hypogammaglobulinemia, dysgammaglobulinemia, aplastic anemia or agranulocytosis, chronic or fatal infectious mononucleosis, and malignant B-cell lymphoma (111). A single patient may have multiple manifestations of disease (80). Lymphomas are predominantly extranodal and include primarily diffuse large B-cell lymphoma and Burkitt/Burkitt-like lymphomas; occasional diffuse mixed cell lymphomas (Working Formulation) have been reported (57). Rare cases of T-cell lymphoma and Hodgkin lymphoma have also occurred (129). Systemic lymphocytic vasculitis is an atypical presentation (72,83). More than half of the patients present with fulminant EBV hepatitis with hemophagocytosis. The majority of these individuals are dead within 1 month. Survivors usually have residual immune dysfunction and may develop fulminant hepatitis upon EBV reexposure.

Laboratory Findings. Lymphocytosis characterized by atypical plasmacytoid lymphocytes is present in the peripheral blood of patients with XLP. Other hematologic manifestations include pancytopenia and agranulocytosis. Some patients show partial IgA deficiency or mild hypogammaglobulinemia before EBV infection; however, following infection there is increased IgM, polyclonal hypergammaglobulinemia, or agammaglobulinemia (113). EBV serology may not be indicative of active infection in these individuals and other studies may be necessary (EBV-encoded DNA [EBER] in situ hybridization, immunohistochemistry, viral cultures, and/or polymerase chain reaction [PCR]) (110).

Microscopic Findings. In the lymph nodes, the morphologic features of fatal infectious mononucleosis are characterized by three phases and are similar in patients with XLP and sporadic disease: hyperplastic, necrotic, and lymphocyte-depleted phases (89,114). In the earliest phases, the morphologic appearance is similar to primary acute infectious mononucleosis/EBV infection. The lymph nodes are typically enlarged and the paracortex expanded. These paracortical areas have increased numbers of large immunoblasts, small and large lymphocytes, and polyclonal plasma cells. In the necrotic phase, single cell necrosis is frequent, giving an appearance of hypocellularity. This stage is followed by larger areas of more confluent necrosis, typically in B-cell areas. In the later stages, the necrosis resolves, and the lymph node is often depleted of lymphocytes and markedly hypocellular. Erythrophagocytosis is also usually seen.

In the spleen, necrosis is seen in the white pulp in the PALS and may be quite extensive (figs. 7-34–7-37). Plasma cells can be seen in association with the necrotic areas. Hemophagocytosis is also common and usually disseminated. As in acute EBV infections, vascular and capsular invasion by lymphocytes can be seen (111).

Ancillary Studies. The initial viral infection in XLP results in an expansion of cytotoxic CD8-positive T cells and infection of CD20-positive B lymphocytes. Plasmacytoid cells may show light chain restriction (89). In situ hybridization studies for EBER are positive and abundant EBV DNA may be demonstrated by PCR. B-cell clonality studies may be positive, but often are negative in patients with fatal infectious mononucleosis. A mechanism similar to that seen in post-transplant lymphoproliferative disorders is thought to occur, wherein immune suppression leads to proliferation of

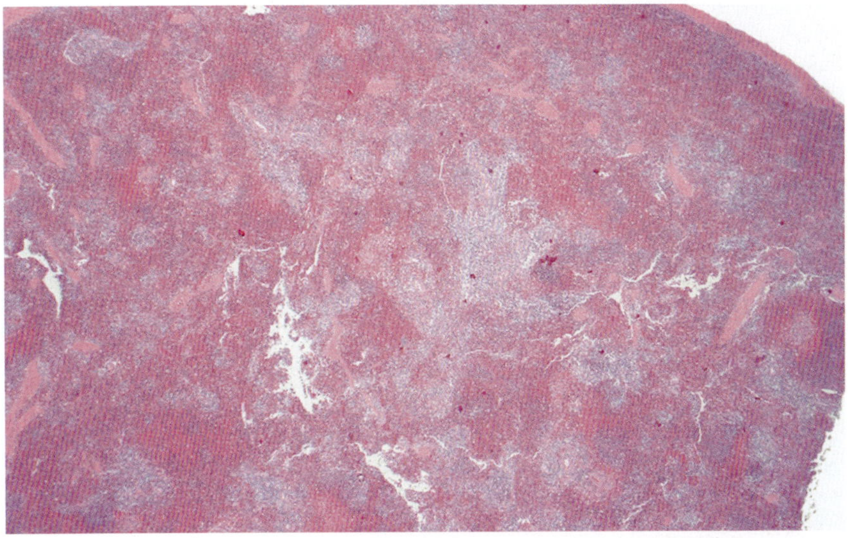

Figure 7-34

X-LINKED LYMPHOPROLIFERATIVE DISORDER, SPLEEN

Hemorrhagic, congested red pulp, with disordered, atrophic white pulp. (Courtesy of Chris Garwacki, Charlotte, NC.)

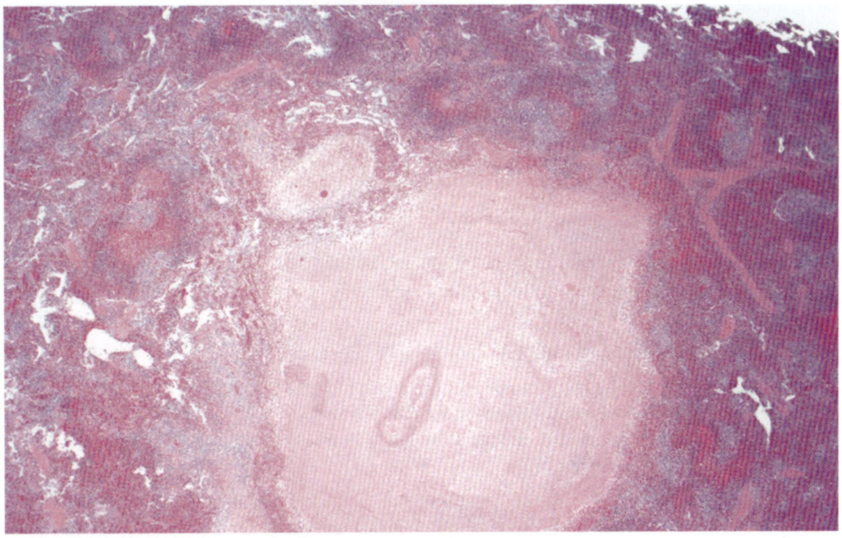

Figure 7-35

X-LINKED LYMPHOPROLIFERATIVE DISORDER, SPLEEN

A large, geographic area of necrosis is associated with a splenic vessel (center of necrosis). (Courtesy of Chris Garwacki, Charlotte, NC.)

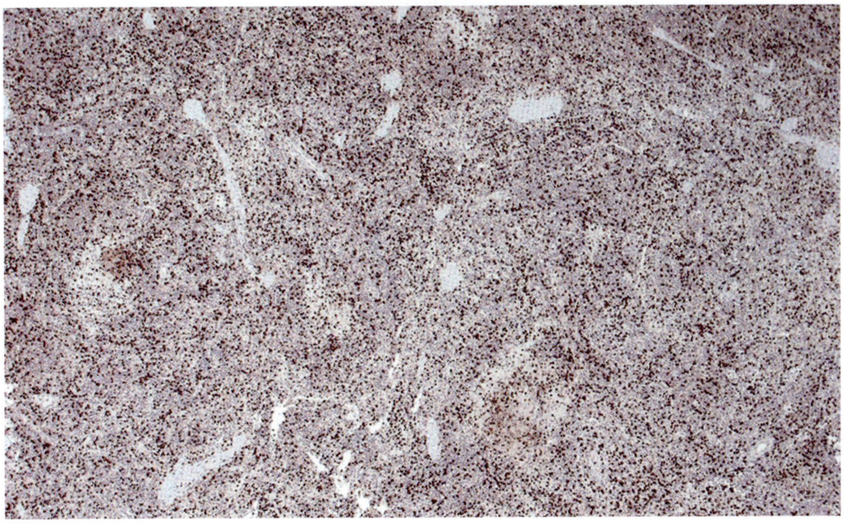

Figure 7-36

X-LINKED LYMPHOPROLIFERATIVE DISORDER, SPLEEN

The CD3 immunohistochemical stain shows scattered T cells in the spleen. The PALS regions have fewer T cells than expected. (Courtesy of Chris Garwacki, Charlotte, NC.)

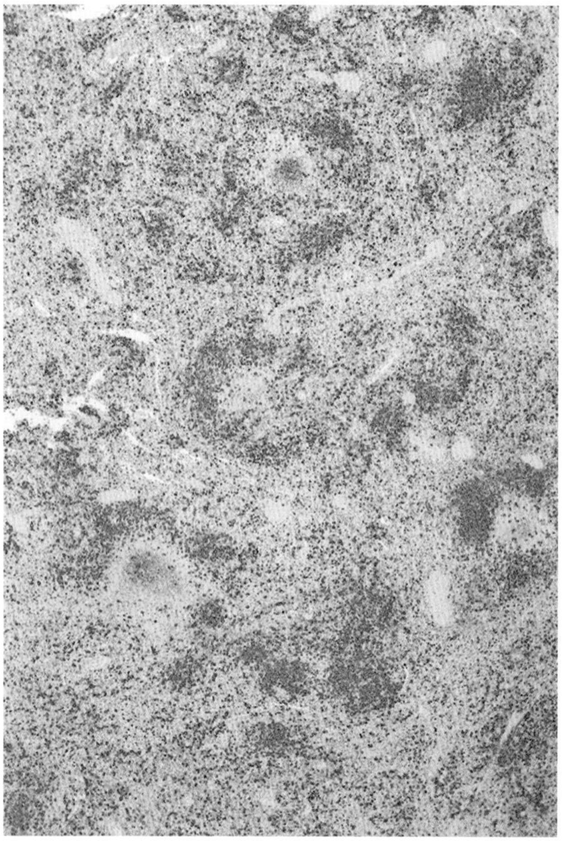

Figure 7-37

X-LINKED LYMPHOPROLIFERATIVE DISORDER, SPLEEN

The CD20 immunohistochemical stain highlights follicles that have decreased numbers of B cells, and other large foci of B cells that are not within follicles. (Courtesy of Chris Garwacki, Charlotte, NC.)

EBV-infected cells. These cells expand initially in a polyclonal manner from which a single clone or clones may emerge. The rapid course of fatal infectious mononucleosis precludes the development of a single clone in most cases.

Differential Diagnosis. The differential diagnosis of fatal infectious mononucleosis in XLP patients includes hemophagocytic syndrome. In hemophagocytic syndrome, erythrophagocytosis is present, but does not include the polymorphous proliferation of B cells seen in XLP with fatal infectious mononucleosis. Hemophagocytic syndromes may be primary, as in familial hemophagocytic lymphohistiocytosis, or secondary to systemic infections, typically viruses and often EBV. Secondary hemophagocytic syndromes are also described with both B- and T-cell lymphoproliferative disorders. Familial hemophagocytic lymphohistiocytosis is an autosomal recessive disorder of infancy. Patients present with fever, pancytopenia, organomegaly, hypertriglyceridemia, and hypofibrinogenemia. *Perforin* gene mutations occur in a subset of patients.

Treatment and Prognosis. Antiviral agents and immunoglobulin have shown only marginal benefits in EBV-infected individuals. Etoposide and cyclosporine have been used with some success (60). More recently, anti-CD20 immunotherapy has been successfully used in two patients with acute primary EBV infection (94). The only cure for XLP is stem cell transplantation (149).

GRISCELLI SYNDROME AND CHEDIAK-HIGASHI SYNDROME

Definition. *Griscelli syndrome* and *Chediak-Higashi syndrome* are clinically related disorders of cellular mechanisms leading to abnormal pigmentation (partial or complete albinism) and immunodeficiency due to abnormalities of cytotoxic T cells and NK cells.

General Features. Griscelli syndrome includes disorders of melanin transport and abnormalities in perforin expression (92,93). Chediak-Higashi syndrome is a disorder of the *CHS1* gene, which regulates and controls lysosomal trafficking.

Clinical Features. Both Griscelli and Chediak-Higashi syndromes are rare, autosomal recessive disorders. Their onset is usually in infancy or early childhood. Partial or complete albinism is seen in both and affected patients have characteristic silver-gray hair.

In Griscelli syndrome, there are profound neurologic deficits. Hepatosplenomegaly is seen and is mainly due to systemic hemophagocytic syndrome. This hemophagocytosis is characterized by the acute onset of uncontrolled activation of T lymphocytes and macrophages.

The features of Chediak-Higashi syndrome are decreased pigmentation of hair and eyes (partial albinism), photophobia, nystagmus, large eosinophilic peroxidase-positive inclusion bodies in the myeloblasts and promyelocytes of the bone marrow, neutropenia, abnormal susceptibility to infection, and malignant lymphoma (73). Death often occurs before the age of 7 years.

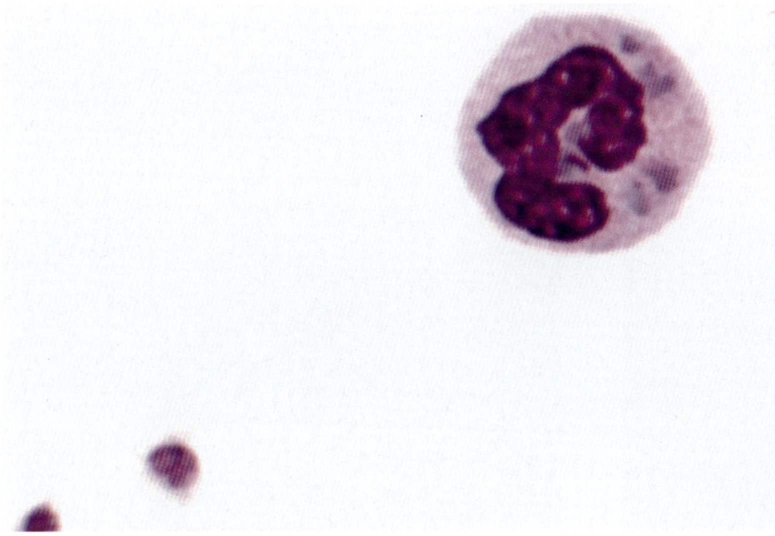

Figure 7-38

CHEDIAK-HIGASHI SYNDROME, PERIPHERAL BLOOD

Abnormal, large, fused cytoplasmic granules are seen. (Courtesy of Ronald Jaffe, Pittsburgh, PA.)

Laboratory Findings. In Griscelli syndrome, there are decreased T cells; those that are present are poorly responsive to T-cell mitogens. NK-cell activity is impaired. NK-cell function is abnormal in Chediak-Higashi syndrome. The most characteristic finding in Chediak-Higashi syndrome is the presence of large, abnormal granules in peripheral blood leukocytes (fig. 7-38). These granules are actually small granules that fuse because of underlying defects of microtubular function. They can be seen in granulocytes, monocytes, and lymphocytes.

Microscopic Findings. Lymph nodes in Griscelli syndrome are typically abnormal. Prominent hemophagocytosis is seen, and may be so extensive as to efface the entire lymph node (79). The lymph nodes in Chediak-Higashi syndrome tend to be at least partially depleted of lymphocytes, with increased dendritic cells and macrophages (fig. 7-39). Germinal centers are often absent (26). Lymphohistiocytic infiltration and hemophagocytosis can be seen in multiple organs.

In both syndromes, the spleen is normal or shows evidence of lymphohistiocytic infiltration. There may be focal or extensive hemophagocytosis.

Treatment and Prognosis. Bone marrow transplant is the only current treatment for Griscelli syndrome. Chediak-Higashi syndrome is associated with an increased incidence of lymphoma, often of NK-cell type, with aggressive clinical behavior.

WISKOTT-ALDRICH SYNDROME

Definition. *Wiskott-Aldrich syndrome* is an X-linked recessive immunodeficiency disease characterized by thrombocytopenia, eczema, and recurrent infections. Patients have an increased risk of lymphoproliferative disorders.

General Features. Wiskott-Aldrich syndrome is caused by mutations in the Wiskott-Aldrich syndrome protein gene (*WASP*) located at Xp11.22-23 (31). Hence, most patients are males. However, rare females with *WASP* mutations and suspected abnormal X-inactivation mechanisms and one family with an autosomal dominant inheritance pattern have been reported (88,121). The WAS protein is expressed only in hematopoietic cells and its function has been linked to the regulation of the actin cytoskeleton (11,154). Thus, loss of function mutations that occur in the *WASP* gene are thought to deregulate the actin cytoskeleton in response to external stimuli. WAS protein-deficient B cells, T cells, and dendritic cells show defects in cell migration or cell surface cytoarchitecture (142). While specific mutations do not predict an exact clinical phenotype, a mild form of the disease is associated with decreased WAS protein expression, while a severe form of the disease is associated with absent protein (66).

Clinical Features. This rare congenital disorder was first described in three boys with thrombocytopenia, eczema, and frequent infections (153). Now more than 300 kindreds have been reported (137).

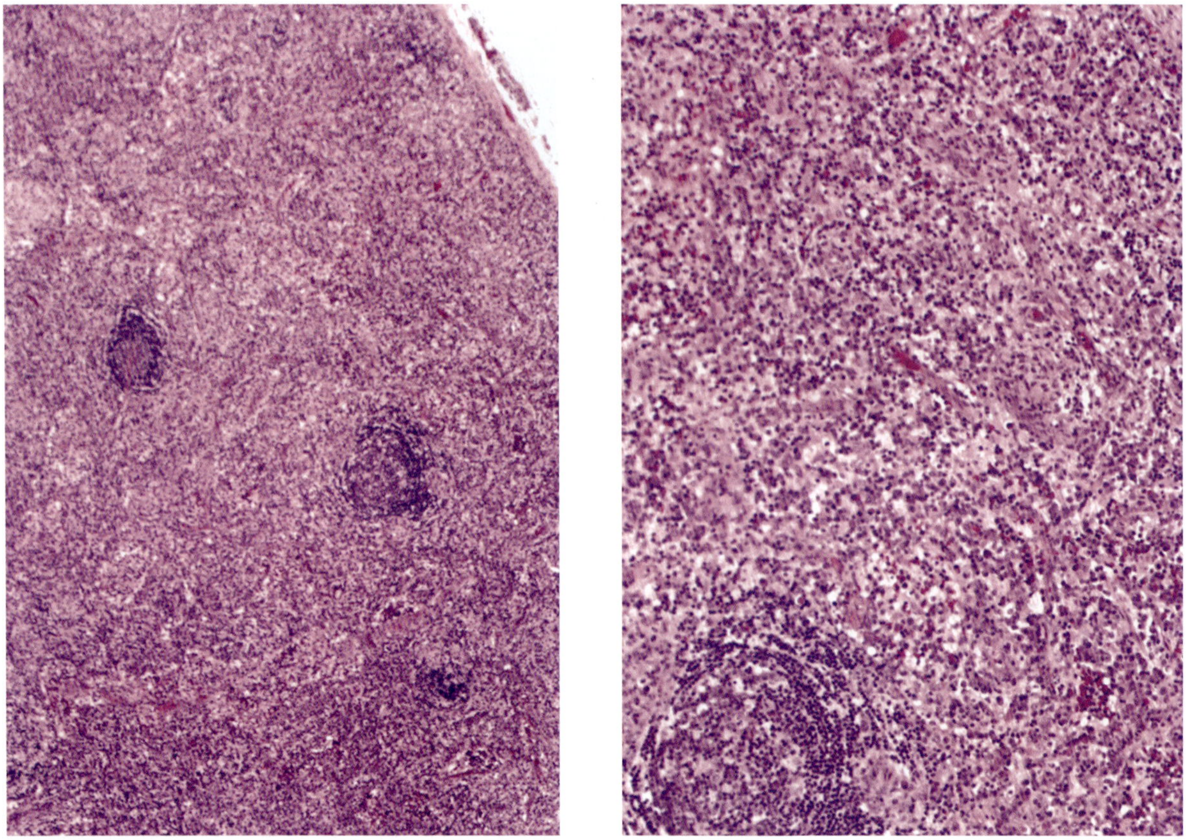

Figure 7-39

CHEDIAK-HIGASHI SYNDROME, LYMPH NODE

Left: Lymph node biopsy from 2-year-old male after local antigenic stimulation. Increased macrophages are in the interfollicular regions. Small follicles are present.

Right: Higher magnification shows numerous macrophages. (Courtesy of Ronald Jaffe, Pittsburgh, PA.)

Clinically, patients present with bleeding secondary to thrombocytopenia, recurrent infections, and eczema of varying severity. The main cause of morbidity in these patients is bleeding (137). Both bacterial and opportunistic infections are common. More than 40 percent of patients, typically those with a severe Wiskott-Aldrich phenotype (34,137), also have autoimmune disorders. There is a marked increase in the development of lymphoproliferative disorders, particularly at extranodal sites (25,130).

The diagnosis of Wiskott-Aldrich syndrome is established by the presence of congenital thrombocytopenia (less than 70 x 10^9/L), small platelets (with either a mutation in *WASP* or absent *WASP* mRNA or protein), or maternal cousins, uncles, or nephews with microthrombocytopenia (20).

Laboratory Findings. Prominent hematologic findings include significant thrombocytopenia, usually below 50 x 10^9/L, with platelets of unusually small size (mean platelet volume 3.8 to 5.0 fl) (104). Because of platelet abnormalities, the patients may have a prolonged bleeding time. Lymphopenia is common, and about half of the patients have decreased in vitro lymphocyte responses to nonspecific mitogens (104). A marked decrease in the number of microvillus projections and abnormal cytoskeletal responses upon in vitro activation are seen in the lymphocytes (46,75). Decreased CD8 alpha/beta heterodimer expression is seen in peripheral blood T cells, suggesting aberrant differentiation of CD8-positive T cells. (74). Delayed-type hypersensitivity skin testing is abnormal in the majority of patients (137). Neutrophils are normal in

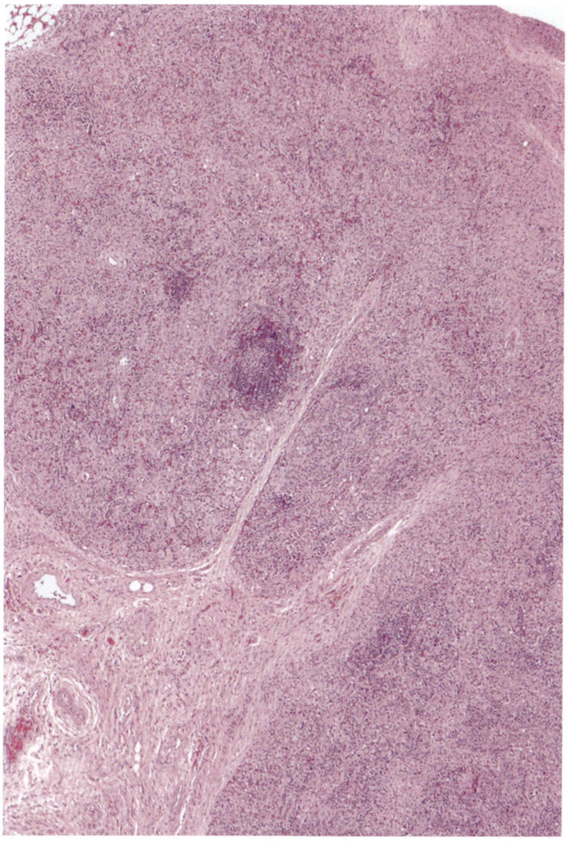

Figure 7-40

WISKOTT-ALDRICH SYNDROME, LYMPH NODE

Small, hypocellular lymph node with only rare lymphocytes and numerous macrophages.

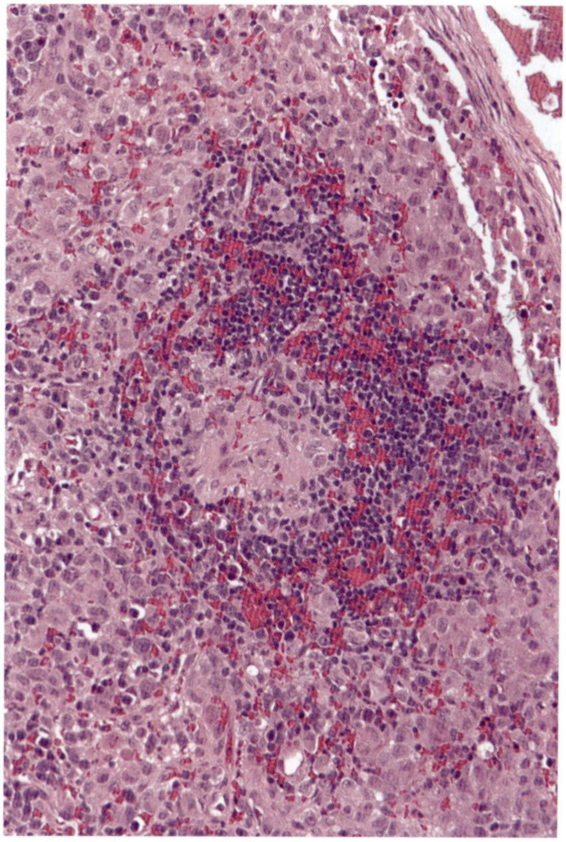

Figure 7-41

WISKOTT-ALDRICH SYNDROME, LYMPH NODE

High magnification of a small, atrophic follicle.

number with appropriate phagocytic activity, but with reduced chemotactic responses (104). Peripheral eosinophilia is a common finding. Patients have hemolytic or iron deficiency anemia. Although IgG levels are typically normal, IgA and IgE levels are increased while IgM is reduced (7). Serum monoclonal gammopathies are common (25). Patients also have elevated erythrocyte sedimentation rates and C-reactive protein levels.

Microscopic Findings. The lymph nodes in patients with Wiskott-Aldrich syndrome are hypocellular, making the stromal components appear more prominent. This hypocellularity is mostly due to the depletion of the T-cell zones (paracortical regions) within the lymph node (figs. 7-40, 7-41) (21,135). The germinal centers have variable features: most commonly, they are absent to atrophic, although occasionally, they are hyperplastic. Atrophic or burned-out germinal centers sometimes impart an appearance of granulomas or hyalinization to the lymph node. The interfollicular areas sometimes have prominent plasmacytosis. The plasma cells are polyclonal, and are often atypical, including large and multinucleated forms. Extramedullary hematopoiesis is frequently seen in the interfollicular areas and sinuses, and consists of varying numbers of myeloid, erythroid, and megakaryocytic elements. In some cases, eosinophilia is prominent. The sinuses of the lymph nodes appear normal or expanded, and contain increased numbers of foamy macrophages or macrophages with prominent hemophagocytosis.

The findings in the spleen parallel those in the lymph nodes. There is significant depletion of total white pulp (including T-cell areas, follicles, and marginal zones) (48,135,147). The spleen is of normal size or slightly enlarged. Like in the lymph nodes, the T-cell zones of the spleen are typically depleted. This is characterized by absent to severe depletion of PALS. The arterioles lack their characteristic cuff of lymphocytes. The collapsed and empty stromal framework can be seen with a reticulin stain which highlights collapsed fibers surrounding the arterioles. Germinal centers are most often absent or atrophic, but may occasionally be hyperplastic. The splenic marginal zone is typically diminished to absent, resulting in follicles surrounded by mantle lymphocytes but lacking the rim of marginal zone B cells. Polyclonal plasmacytosis is present in the red pulp, including atypical forms, although it is often less prominent than in the lymph nodes. Extramedullary hematopoiesis is also less prominent than in the lymph nodes. Hemophagocytosis, particularly erythrophagocytosis, may be prominent in the red pulp cords and sinuses. In some cases, prominent eosinophilia is seen in the red pulp.

Ancillary Studies. Clonal populations may be seen in Wiskott-Aldrich syndrome. The presence of clonal B-cell populations is of uncertain significance. Since there is an increased incidence of lymphoid malignancies in patients with the syndrome, the possibility of an overt or evolving lymphoma must be considered when a clonal population is present.

Immunohistochemistry may highlight the depletion of T and B cells by demonstrating regressed germinal centers containing predominantly CD21-positive follicular dendritic cells and only a few CD20-positive centroblasts. The reduction of the marginal zone in splenic B follicles may be seen as few $IgM^{hi}IgD^{lo}$ CD20-positive lymphocytes surrounding the mantle zone. Aberrant expression is not seen in either B or T lymphocytes (147).

Differential Diagnosis. While other primary immunodeficiencies may be considered, correlation with the history and peripheral blood smear (i.e., platelet size) remains critical in establishing a diagnosis of Wiskott-Aldrich syndrome.

Treatment and Prognosis. The thrombocytopenia may be improved by splenectomy (23); however, bone marrow transplantation is considered to be the only definitive treatment (95). Recently, anti-CD20 immunotherapy has been used to successfully treat an EBV-associated lymphoproliferative disease in a child with Wiskott-Aldrich syndrome (128).

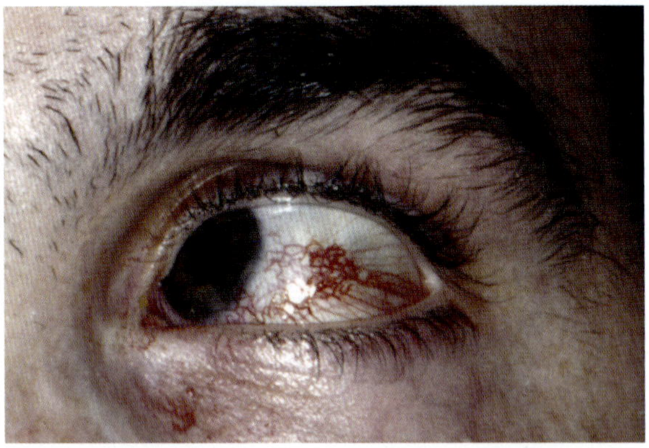

Figure 7-42

ATAXIA-TELANGIECTASIA, OCULAR FINDINGS

A clinical photograph of conjunctival telangiectasia. (Courtesy of Valerie Purvin, Indianapolis, IN.)

ATAXIA-TELANGIECTASIA (INCLUDING NIJMEGEN BREAKAGE SYNDROME AND BERLIN BREAKAGE SYNDROME)

Definition. *Ataxia-telangiectasia* (AT) is characterized by immunodeficiency and neurological deficits, including cerebellar degeneration and oculocutaneous telangiectasia. *Nijmegen breakage syndrome* (NBS) and *Berlin breakage syndrome* (BBS) are considered variants of AT (AT variant-1, AT variant-2, respectively). Clinically, NBS and BBS are identical.

General Features. The function of the defective gene in AT, *ATM* (11q22-q23), is unknown. Abnormalities in *ATM* lead to defective DNA repair and chromosomal instability. The genes in NBS and BBS (*NBS1, LIG4, nibrin/p95*; 8q21) are proposed to have similar functions. The chromosomal breaks that occur in AT are random, and the genetic defect underlying the disorder is not the result of chromosomal breakage.

Clinical Features. AT is a rare autosomal recessive disorder. The onset of disease is usually in infancy or early childhood. Cerebellar ataxia is usually the presenting symptom. It is typically severe and progressive. Telangiectasia typically begins on the conjunctiva, and progresses to involve the nose and ears, as well as hands, feet, and antecubital and popliteal areas (fig. 7-42) (79). The patients are susceptible to infections,

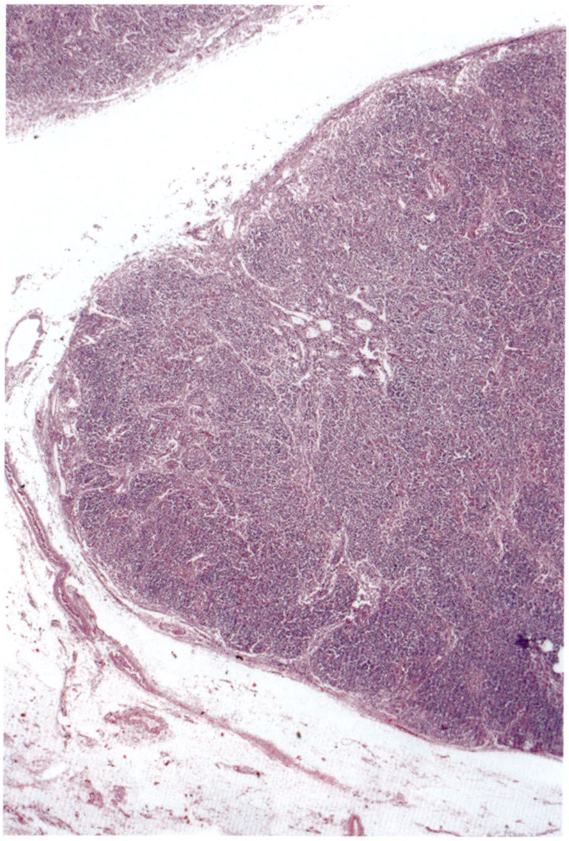

Figure 7-43

ATAXIA-TELANGIECTASIA, LYMPH NODE

Small lymph node with no germinal centers. (Courtesy of Peter Banks, Charlotte, NC.)

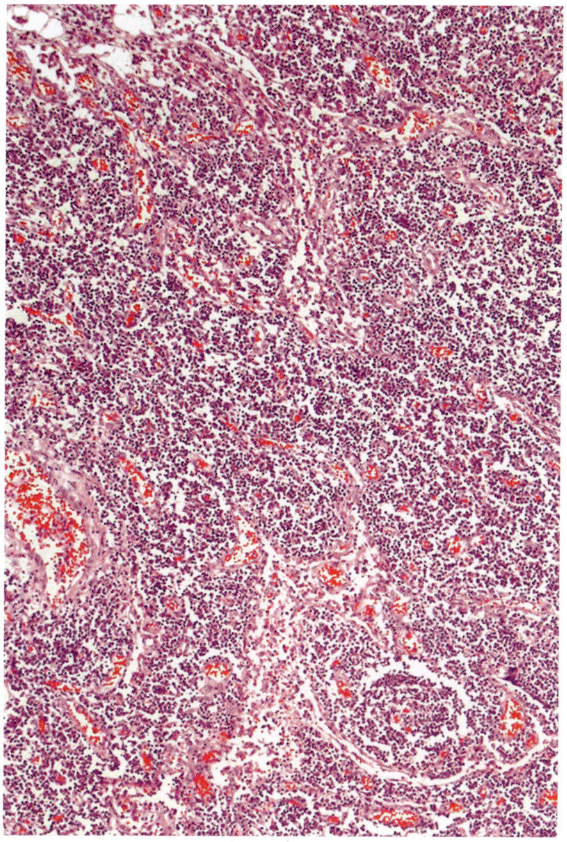

Figure 7-44

ATAXIA-TELANGIECTASIA, LYMPH NODE

Intact sinuses, with some vascular proliferation and no germinal centers. (Courtesy of Peter Banks, Charlotte, NC.)

both bacterial and viral, with recurrent sinopulmonary infections being most common.

The immunologic defects are of variable severity. AT patients have thymic hypoplasia as well as hypogonadism. NBS and BBS are clinically identical autosomal recessive disorders that are characterized by growth retardation, microcephaly, immunodeficiency, and chromosomal breakage.

Laboratory Findings. In AT, flow cytometry shows no characteristic findings in the peripheral blood lymphocytes; however, the number of gamma-delta T cells is often increased (13). Lymphocytopenia, predominantly due to decreases in CD4-positive lymphocytes, and eosinophilia are seen. The T cells respond abnormally to mitogens. Almost all AT patients have elevated alpha-fetoprotein levels, in the absence of liver disease or malignancy. IgA deficiency is seen in 70 percent.

Patients with NBS and BBS have an increased incidence of autoimmune hemolytic anemia and immune thrombocytopenic purpura. Like AT, there are decreased total lymphocytes and CD4-positive lymphocytes. In contrast to AT, the alpha-fetoprotein levels are normal.

Microscopic Features. The lymph nodes in AT are variable in size, but tend to be hypoplastic, with depletion of B lymphocytes in the follicles (figs. 7-43–7-45) (79). The junction between the follicles and paracortical areas is poorly defined. Progressive reduction in lymphocytes (especially CD4-positive T cells) is seen, with a relative increase in CD8-positive cells. Germinal centers vary from large and reactive to small and fibrotic. There is often a lack of follicular

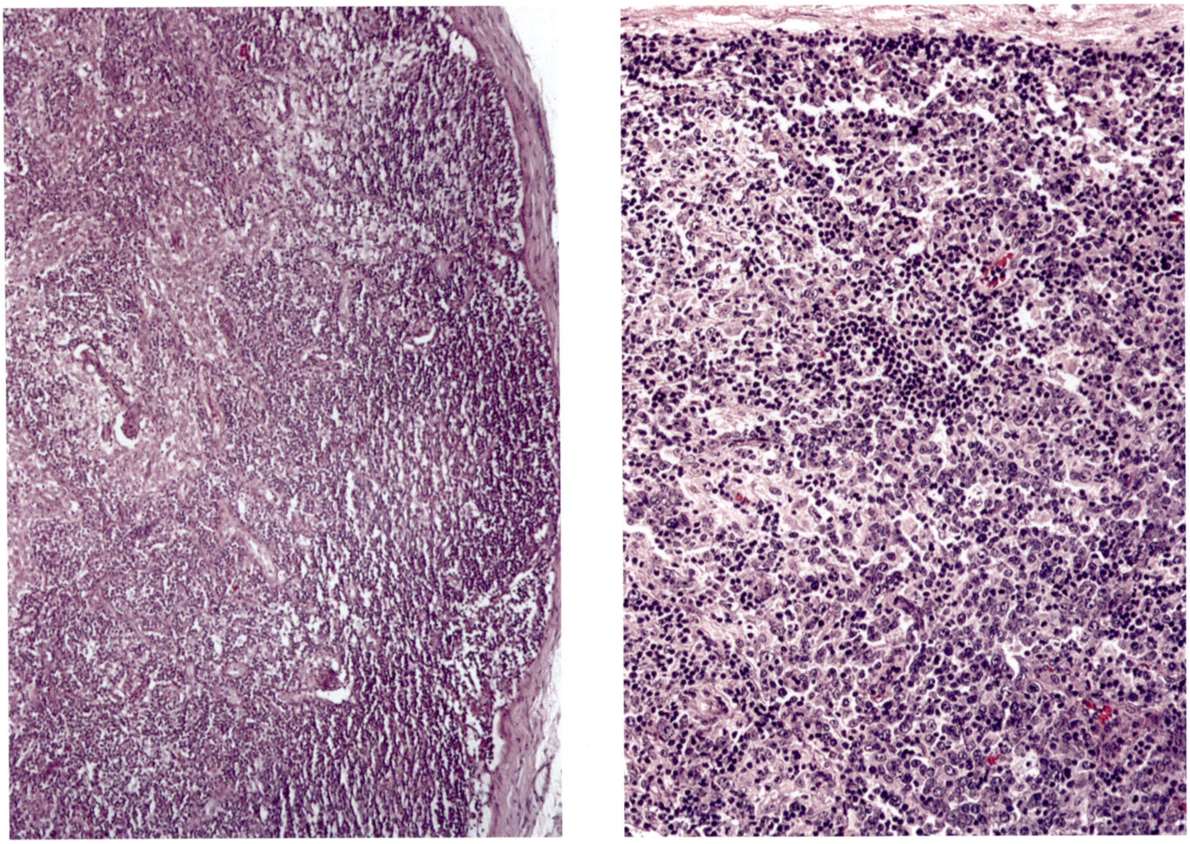

Figure 7-45

ATAXIA-TELANGIECTASIA, LYMPH NODE

Left: The lymph node has both germinal centers and paracortical areas.

Right: Higher magnification shows increased immunoblasts in the paracortical region. (Courtesy of Ronald Jaffe, Pittsburgh, PA.)

hyperplasia after antigenic stimulation. Plasma cells are frequently decreased in number.

As in the lymph nodes, AT in the spleen shows decreased or absent T cells. The germinal centers and plasma cells are normal or decreased (18).

Ancillary Studies. In approximately 10 percent of AT cases, the T cells show chromosomal translocations involving T-cell receptor antigen genes (14q11-12, 7q32-35, 7p15) and the immunoglobulin genes (14q32, 2p11, 22p11) (37). This finding may be used as a diagnostic criterion of the disease, in the appropriate context.

Differential Diagnosis. Since the findings are relatively nonspecific, the differential diagnosis includes benign reactive conditions and other primary immunodeficiency disorders. The cytogenetic findings of multiple T- and B-cell gene rearrangements may be of diagnostic benefit.

Treatment and Prognosis. In AT, it is more common to have a T-cell, rather than B-cell, lymphoma, unlike all other congenital immunodeficiencies. This may be due to the frequency of T-cell gene rearrangements seen in the circulating T-cell population. Lymphomas have been reported as early as 10 years of age in AT patients (37). T-cell prolymphocytic leukemia is particularly common. Other nonlymphoid malignancies, such as leukemia, are also increased. Exposure to ionizing radiation leads to chromosomal breakage. The use of conventional doses of radiation to treat AT may be lethal.

CHRONIC GRANULOMATOUS DISEASE

Definition. *Chronic granulomatous disease* (CGD) is a spectrum of disorders caused by an absent oxidative-burst generating function of

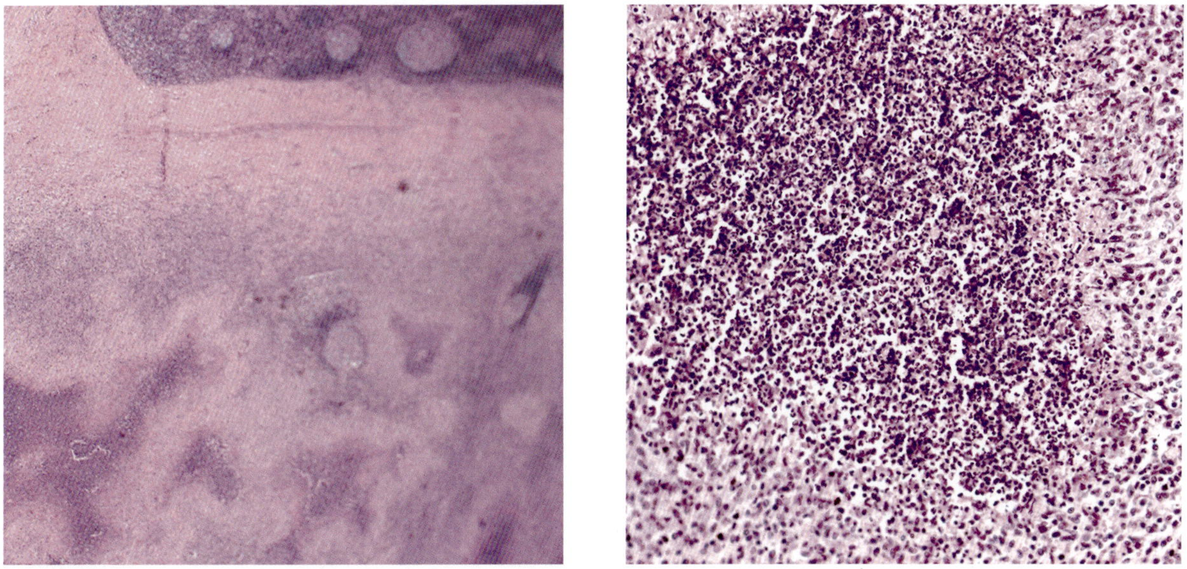

Figure 7-46

CHRONIC GRANULOMATOUS DISEASE, LYMPH NODE

Large geographic areas of necrosis are seen in this lymph node.

neutrophils, which causes a severe defect in bacterial and fungal killing.

General Features. Intracellular killing of bacterial and fungal organisms is impaired due to a failure to produce oxidative-burst products, such as superoxide radicals. The lack of this function is due to fundamental defects in the NADPH oxidase system, which generates the toxic byproducts used to kill microbes. There are a variety of molecular defects that have been identified, including abnormalities of the gp21phox, p67phox, and p22phox components of the NADPH oxidase system (70).

Clinical Features. CGD has both autosomal recessive and X-linked forms, which have essentially identical clinical manifestations. CGD occurs in approximately 1/200,000 births. It is characterized by recurrent bacterial and fungal infections, most notably pneumonia, infectious dermatitis, and recurrent or severe cutaneous abscesses. Organisms that produce catalase are particularly pathogenic in CGD patients. These include *Staphylococcus aureus*, gram-negative enteric bacteria, *Pseudomonas*, yeasts, fungi, and *Nocardia*. *Burkholderia cepacia* infections are a common cause of death in CGD patients and *Aspergillus* infections are frequent (70). The mean age of diagnosis is 3 years, with an average survival period of only 20 years. Patients and relatives appear to have an increased incidence of systemic lupus erythematosus. Lymphadenopathy, especially in the cervical area, is a common finding, and may prompt a biopsy.

Laboratory Findings. The diagnostic test for CGD is the nitroblue tetrazolium (NBT) reduction test. NBT tests the activity of the oxidase-producing capacity of neutrophils. In affected males, none of the cells are positive while female carriers have normal-stained cells and a subset of negative cells. The granulocytes of the peripheral blood are morphologically normal.

Microscopic Findings. The architecture is distorted, but not usually effaced. Often, there is a background of follicular hyperplasia. Numerous macrophages, which contain pigmented material, are in the interfollicular areas and lymph node sinuses. Granulomas form in portions of the lymph nodes (figs. 7-46, 7-47). These granulomas are composed of epithelioid macrophages with varying numbers of giant cells. Central necrosis, either caseous or coagulative, is common. There may be abscess formation with suppuration.

Necrosis, suppuration, and granuloma formation are seen in the spleen as well (18,139). These are often infection-related findings,

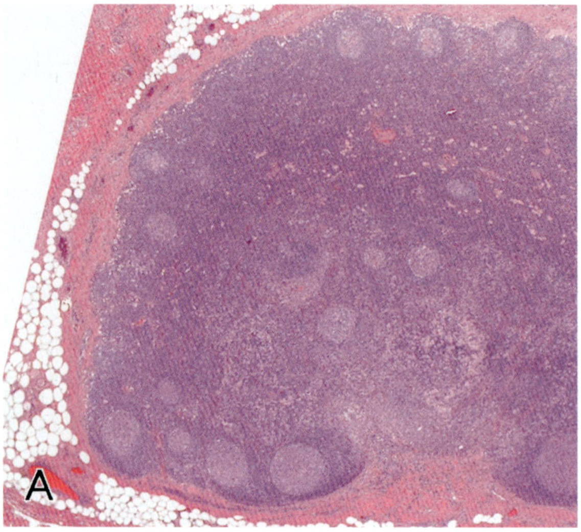

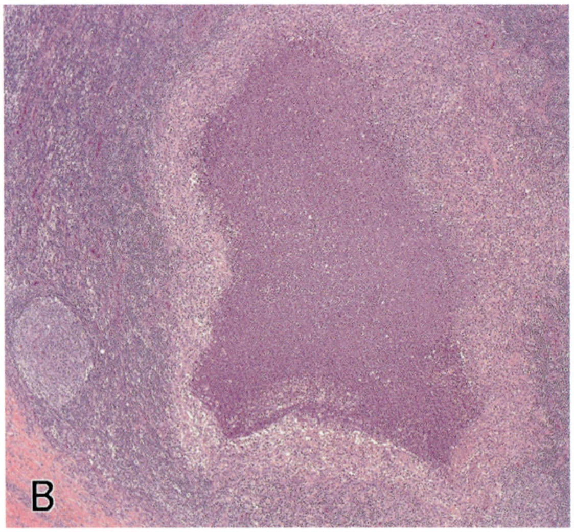

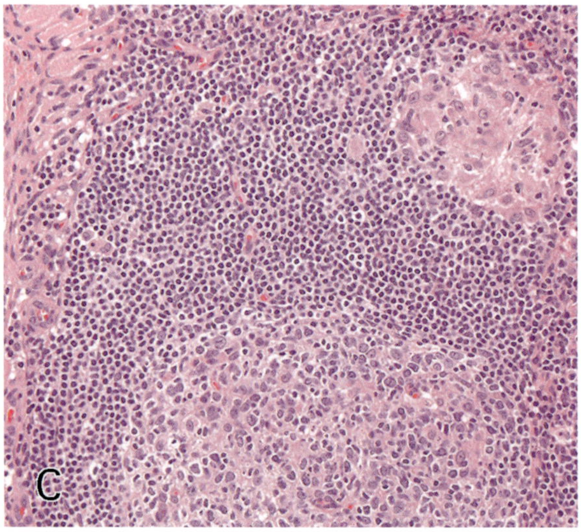

Figure 7-47

CHRONIC GRANULOMATOUS DISEASE, LYMPH NODE

Combinations of necrosis and granulomas are seen. (Courtesy of Steve Kroft, Milwaukee, WI.)

although organisms may be difficult to identify. The red pulp shows the presence of numerous histiocytes/macrophages with yellow-brown granules in the cytoplasm. When stained with Giemsa type stains, these macrophages have the classic sea blue appearance. These macrophages are also seen in the bone marrow of patients with CGD.

Ancillary Studies. Special histologic stains for organisms (AFB, PAS, GMS, Gram, and others), should be used in almost all cases, since infections are common in these patients. Because of the nature of the disease, only small numbers of organisms may be responsible for extensive infection, and organisms may not be identified. Flow cytometric techniques have been used in the diagnosis of CGD (64). Flow cytometric methods measure neutrophil fluorescence of a laser-sensitive dye that responds to the stimulus of an oxidative burst. In patients with GCD, the oxidative burst does not occur, and there is no increase in fluorescence. Carriers show two populations of neutrophils, one with increased fluorescence and one without.

Differential Diagnosis. The gastrointestinal findings in CGD closely mimic those of Crohn disease. The formation of granulomas, with or without central necrosis or abscess formation, may be confused with a variety of infectious causes. The morphologic findings are not unique to CGD and should be taken in the context of the clinical, microbiologic, and other laboratory findings.

Treatment and Prognosis. Management of patients with CGD involves appropriate treatment of infections. Prophylactic administration of antibiotics, especially trimethoprim-sulfamethoxazole, is important to control symptoms. Interferon treatment also appears to reduce serious infections. Bone marrow transplantation has been successful in many cases. Gene therapy is an area of current investigation.

TUBEROUS SCLEROSIS

Definition. *Tuberous sclerosis* is an inherited neurocutaneous disorder characterized by multiple benign neoplasms primarily involving the kidney, skin, and brain, but not limited to these organs.

General Features. Mutations in two genes, *TSC1* and *TSC2*, have been described in 60 to 80 percent of patients with tuberous sclerosis (38,71,100,145). *TSC1*, located at chromosome 9q34, encodes hamartin, a protein expressed widely in normal tissues (78,145). Hamartin and tuberin protein complexes are encoded by *TSC2* located at chromosome 16p13.3 (38). Tuberin is important in normal brain development and terminal differentiation of the cardiomyocyte (107,118). The hamartin-tuberin complex acts as a negative cell cycle regulator (140,145,146). *TSC1* and *TSC2* are thought to function as tumor suppressor genes; loss of heterozygosity at these sites is associated with the benign tumors (hamartomas, angiofibromas, and lymphangioleiomyomas) seen in patients with tuberous sclerosis (12,13,51,59).

A wide variety of mutation types are found in each gene, including deletions, rearrangements, insertions, and point mutations, with the majority resulting in loss of function of the proteins (71,76,100). Genotype-phenotype correlations suggest that a milder neurologic phenotype is seen in patients with *TSC1* mutations (71). A subset of patients have large deletions which inactivate the polycystic kidney disease 1 (*PKD1*) gene as well as *TSC2*, resulting in severe early onset of cystic renal disease (10,91).

Clinical Features. An autosomal dominant disorder, tuberous sclerosis has an incidence of 1/5,000 to 10,000 live births (85,106). One third of the cases are familial in origin, but the majority are nonfamilial and result from spontaneous mutations or mosaicism (77,122).

Table 7-8

DIAGNOSTIC CRITERIA FOR TUBEROUS SCLEROSIS[a]

Major Criteria[b]
Facial angiofibromas/forehead plaques
Connective tissue nevus
Hypomelanotic macules (three or more)
Ungula or periungual fibromas (nontraumatic)
Lymphangioleiomyomatosis
Renal angiomyolipoma
Cardiac rhabdomyoma
Retinal nodular hamartomas
Cortical tuber
Subependymal nodules
Subependymal giant cell astrocytoma
Minor Criteria
Multiple 1-2 mm hypomelanotic macules
Gingival fibromas
Multiple random pits in dental enamel
Hamartomatous rectal polyps
Multiple renal cysts
Nonrenal hamartomas
Bone cysts
Retinal achromic patch
Cerebral white matter radial migration lines

[a]Modified from table 2 from reference 120.
[b]Definite tuberous sclerosis: 2 major or 1 major + 2 minor criteria; probable tuberous sclerosis: 1 major + 1 minor criteria; possible tuberous sclerosis: 1 major or 2+ minor criteria.

While the penetrance of the disease is complete, the severity of tuberous sclerosis varies widely from individual to individual, even within the same family (101).

The diagnosis of tuberous sclerosis is clinically based on major and minor criteria: a definite diagnosis requires two major criteria or one major and two minor criteria. If only one major and one minor criteria are present, this is probable tuberous sclerosis, while only one major criteria or two or more minor criteria suggest possible tuberous sclerosis. These criteria were developed by a consensus conference, as shown in Table 7-8 (120). Vogt triad, seen in a minority of patients with tuberous sclerosis, is characterized by seizures, mental retardation, and facial angiofibromas (120).

The relative risk of malignancy in children with tuberous sclerosis is higher than in children without tuberous sclerosis. Malignant tumors occur in brain, kidneys, and soft tissues (97). Adults are also at increased risk for malignant tumors, particularly renal cell carcinoma (132). The increased morbidity in tuberous sclerosis has been attributed to neurologic disease (status epilepticus and subependymal giant cell

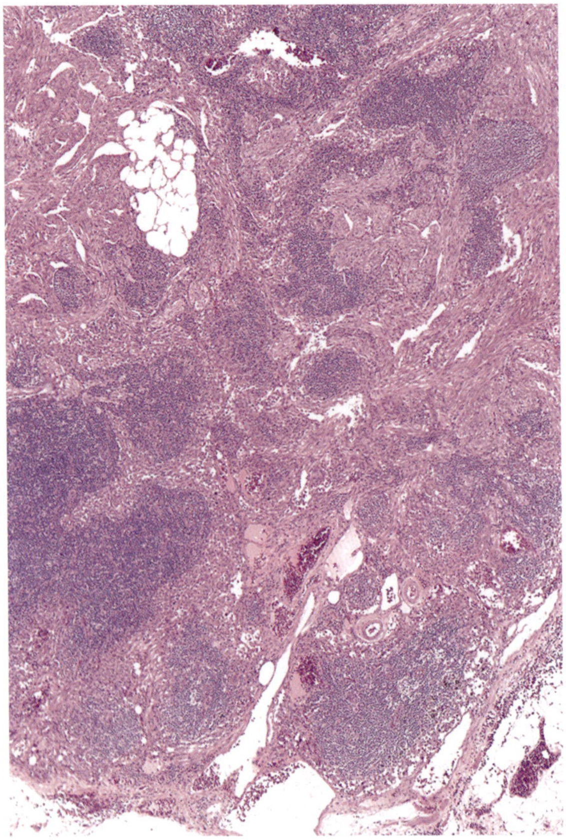

Figure 7-48

TUBEROUS SCLEROSIS, LYMPH NODE

A lymph node in a patient with tuberous sclerosis shows fat, smooth muscle, and vascular elements, suggesting a diagnosis of angiomyolipoma.

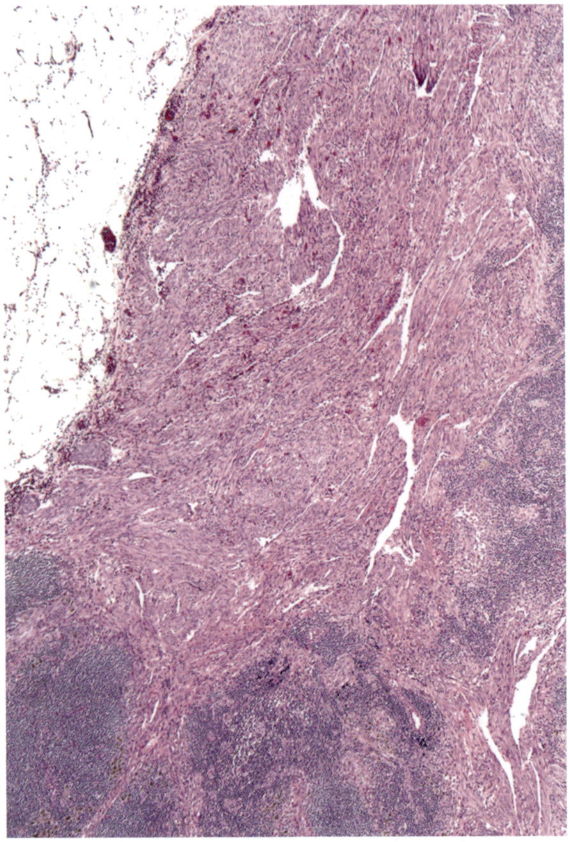

Figure 7-49

TUBEROUS SCLEROSIS, LYMPH NODE

Smooth muscle elements arise in the region of the lymph node and expand into it.

tumors), renal disease (carcinoma, renal failure, and hemorrhage into angiomyolipoma), and less commonly, pulmonary disease (pneumonia, lymphangioleiomyomatosis) and cardiac rhabdomyoma.

Laboratory Findings. Molecular testing, including prenatal testing, may be performed for mutations in the *TSC1* and *TSC2* genes, but detect only 60 to 80 percent of mutations; thus, a negative test does not exclude the diagnosis of tuberous sclerosis (71,100). Other laboratory findings are not specific for tuberous sclerosis.

Gross and Microscopic Findings. While lymph node involvement has not been specifically described in tuberous sclerosis, several authors have speculated whether lymphangiomyomatosis represents a forme fruste of tuberous sclerosis (figs. 7-48–7-50) (24). Grossly, the lymph nodes are spongy and pale tan or white. A sinusoidal pattern of involvement is typical, with smooth muscle cells forming a network around endothelial cells. Smooth muscle cells are plump with pale to clear cytoplasm, without atypia or mitoses, and with cigar-shaped oval nuclei.

Splenic involvement in tuberous sclerosis is rare, but includes hamartoma (29), angiomyolipoma (1,4,63), and collections of histiocytoid cells primarily described in the spleens of neonates (6,143). Of the reported splenic angiomyolipomas, only one presented clinically as a chronic expanding hematoma caused by repeated bleeding from a small angiomyolipoma (4). This patient also had large bilateral renal angiomyolipomas. Adjacent to the organized hematoma was a small area of fibroadipose tissue with a small number of smooth muscle

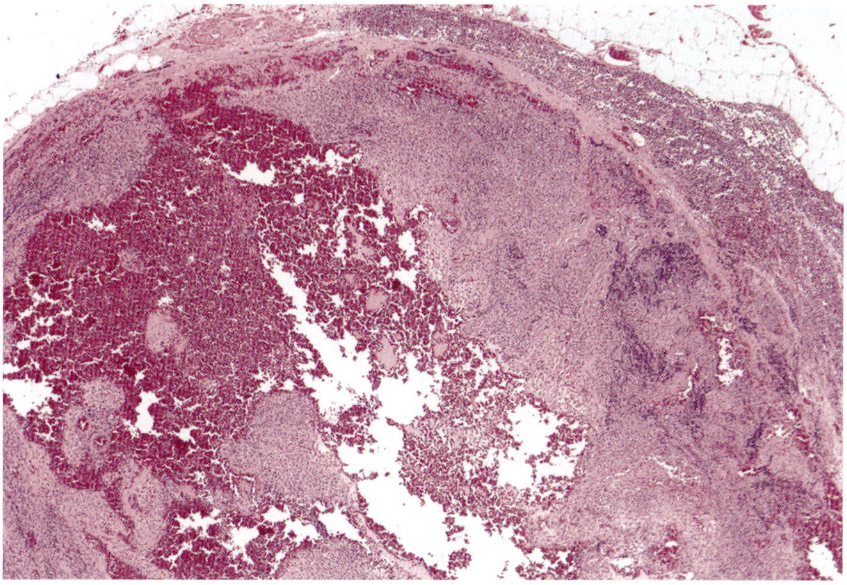

Figure 7-50

TUBEROUS SCLEROSIS, LYMPH NODE

Mature, vascular elements within a lymph node are associated with proliferating smooth muscle elements.

bundles and blood vessels of varying size, likely representing an angiomyolipoma. A second case showed the typical elements of mature adipose tissue, atypical blood vessels, and smooth muscle involving both spleen and regional lymph nodes (63). A third case was in a patient with multiple angiomyolipomas involving liver, spleen, and lungs (1). There were severe nuclear pleomorphism, significant mitotic activity, and necrosis. Collections of the histiocytoid cells of tuberous sclerosis in the spleen have been described in a small number of neonates and a fetus (6,143). These focal collections of large cells have abundant eosinophilic cytoplasm and resemble the cells seen in brain lesions of tuberous sclerosis.

Ancillary Studies. Splenic angiomyolipomas are positive for smooth muscle actin in the smooth muscle component and for HMB45 (1,4). The collections of histiocytoid cells found in the spleen of neonates are positive for CD68, negative for glial fibrillary acidic protein (GFAP), and contain membrane-bound cytoplasmic bodies of 90 to 270 nm in diameter, ultrastructurally resembling macrophages (6,143).

Differential Diagnosis. Metastatic well-differentiated leiomyosarcoma may mimic lymphangiomyomatosis that can be seen in tuberous sclerosis. Greater cellular atypia, mitoses, and HMB45 negativity are seen in metastatic sarcoma.

Metastatic well-differentiated leiomyosarcoma may also mimic angiomyolipoma, particularly if a smooth muscle component predominates, but the spleen is not a site of metastases for leiomyosarcoma. Similarly, vascular tumors of the spleen should be investigated for smooth muscle and adipose components to exclude angiomyolipoma. Splenic hamartomas show similar features to splenic hemangiomas and may be difficult to distinguish. Splenic hamartomas contain irregular sinuses admixed with cord-like elements and endothelial cells are CD8 positive; those of hemangioma are not (155). Splenic hemangiomas may also contain lymphoid tissue, not seen in splenic hamartomas.

Treatment and Prognosis. While there is no cure, the guidelines provided by the Tuberous Sclerosis Consensus Conference (1), suggest treatment for some complications. Careful surveillance is recommended to evaluate the potential malignancies discussed above.

REFERENCES

1. Abdulla M, Bui HX, del Rosario AD, et al. Renal angiomyolipoma, DNA content and immunohistochemical study of classic and multicentric variants. Arch Pathol Lab Med 1994;118:735-9.
2. Allen RC, Armitage RJ, Conley ME, et al. CD40 ligand gene defects responsible for X-linked hyper-IgM syndrome. Science 1993;259:990-3.
3. Arkwright PD, Abinun M, Cant AJ. Autoimmunity in primary immunodeficiency diseases. Blood 2002;99:2694-702.
4. Asayama Y, Fukuya T, Honda H, et al. Chronic expanding hematoma of the spleen caused by angiomyolipoma in a patient with tuberous sclerosis. Abdom Imaging 1998;23:527-30.
5. Beall GN, Ashman RF, Miller ME, et al. Hypogammaglobulinemia in mother and son. J Allergy Clin Immunol 1980;65:471-81.
6. Bender BL, Yunis EJ. Splenic involvement in tuberous sclerosis. Report of three cases. Virchows Arch A Pathol Anat Histol 1981;391:363-9.
7. Blaese RM, Strober W, Brown RS, Waldmann TA. The Wiskott-Aldrich syndrome. A disorder with a possible defect in antigen processing or recognition. Lancet 1968;1:1056-61.
8. Bonilla FA, Geha RS. CD154 deficiency and related syndromes. Immunol Allergy Clin North Am 2001;21:65-90.
9. Brasch RC, Royal S, Ammann AJ, Crowe J. Pseudolymphoma in two immunodeficient children. AJR Am J Roentgenol 1979;132:844-7.
10. Brook-Carter PT, Peral B, Ward CJ, et al. Deletion of the TSC2 and PKD1 genes associated with severe infantile polycystic kidney disease. A contiguous gene syndrome. Nat Genet 1994;8:328-32.
11. Burns S, Cory GO, Vainchenker W, Thrasher AJ. Mechanisms of WASP-mediated hematologic and immunologic disease. Blood 2004;104:3454-62.
12. Carbonara C, Longa L, Grosso E, et al. 9q34 loss of heterozygosity in a tuberous sclerosis astrocytomas suggests a growth suppressor-like activity also for the TSC1 gene. Hum Mol Genet 1994;3:1829-32.
13. Carbonari M, Cherchi M, Paganelli R, et al. Relative increase of T cells expressing the gamma/delta rather than alpha/beta receptor in ataxia-telangiectasia. N Engl J Med 1990;322:73-6.
14. Cavazzana-Calvo M, Lagresle C, Hacein-Bey-Abina S, Fischer A. Gene therapy for severe combined immunodeficiency. Annu Rev Med. 2005;56:585-602.
15. Cham B, Bonilla MA, Winkelstein J. Neutropenia associated with primary immunodeficiency syndromes. Semin Hematol 2002;39:107-12.
16. Claman HN, Suvatte V, Githens JH, Hathaway WE. Histiocytic reaction in dysgammaglobulinemia and congenital rubella. Pediatrics 1970;46:89-96.
17. Coffey AJ, Brooksbank RA, Brandau O, et al. Host response to EBV infection in X-linked lymphoproliferative disease results from mutations in an SH2-domain encoding gene. Nat Genet 1998;20:129-35.
18. Collins RD. Spleen. In: Collins RD, Swerdlow SH, eds. Pediatric hematopathology. Philadelphia: Churchill Livingstone; 2001:343-60.
19. Conley ME, Notarangelo LD, Etzioni A. Diagnostic criteria for primary immunodeficiencies. Representing PAGID (Pan-American Group for Immunodeficiency) and ESID (European Society for Immunodeficiencies). Clin Immunol 1999;93:190-7.
20. Cooper MD, Chae HP, Lowman JT, Krivit W, Good RA. Wiskott-Aldrich syndrome. An immunologic deficiency disease involving the afferent limb of immunity. Am J Med 1968;44:499-513.
21. Cooper MD, Lanier LL, Conley ME, Puck JM, Sneller MC. ALPS: an autoimmune human lymphoproliferative syndrome associated with abnormal lymphocyte apoptosis. Semin Immunol 1997;9:77-84.
22. Cooper MD, Lanier LL, Puck JM, Conley ME. Immunodeficiency disorders. Hematology (Am Soc Hematol Educ Program) 2003;314-30.
23. Corash L, Shafer B, Blaese RM. Platelet-associated immunoglobulin, platelet size, and the effect of splenectomy in the Wiskott-Aldrich syndrome. Blood 1985;65:1439-43.
24. Corrin B, Liebow AA, Friedman PJ. Pulmonary lymphangiomyomatosis. A review. Am J Pathol 1975;79:348-82.
25. Cotelingam JD, Witebsky FG, Hsu SM, Blaese RM, Jaffe ES. Malignant lymphoma in patients with the Wiskott-Aldrich syndrome. Cancer Invest 1985;3:515-22.
26. Cottier H, Kraft R, Meister F. Primary immunodeficiency syndromes and their manifestations in lymph nodes. Curr Top Pathol 1991;84(Pt 2):81-155.
27. Cunningham-Rundles C. Hematologic complications of primary immune deficiencies. Blood Rev 2002;16:61-4.
28. Cunningham-Rundles C, Bodian C. Common variable immunodeficiency: Clinical and immunological features of 248 patients. Clin Immunol 1999;92:34-48.

29. Darden JW, Teeslink R, Parrish A. Hamartoma of the spleen: a manifestation of tuberous sclerosis. Am Surg 1975;41:564-6.
30. Darlow JM, Farrell AM, Stott DI. Non-functional immunoglobulin G transcripts in a case of hyper-immunoglobulin M syndrome similar to type 4. Immunology 2004;111:212-22.
31. Derry JM, Ochs HD, Francke U. Isolation of a novel gene mutated in Wiskott-Aldrich syndrome. Cell 1994;78:635-44.
32. Drappa J, Vaishnaw AK, Sullivan KE, Chu JL, Elkon KB. Fas gene mutations in the Canale-Smith syndrome, an inherited lymphoproliferative disorder associated with autoimmunity. N Engl J Med 1996;335:1643-9.
33. Dupre L, Andolfi G, Tangye SG, et al. SAP controls the cytolytic activity of CD8+ T cells against EBV-infected cells. Blood 2005;105:4383-9.
34. Dupuis-Girod S, Medioni J, Haddad E, et al. Autoimmunity in Wiskott-Aldrich syndrome: risk factors, clinical features, and outcome in a single-center cohort of 55 patients. Pediatrics 2003;111:622-7.
35. Durandy A, Revy P, Imai K, Fischer A. Hyper-immunoglobulin M syndromes caused by intrinsic B-lymphocyte defects. Immunol Rev 2005;203:67-79.
36. Eisenstein EM, Aker M, Savoldi G, Jaffe R, Prus D. A primary immunodeficiency disorder associated with absence of lymphoid germinal centers. J Clin Immunol 2002;22:297-305.
37. Elenitoba-Johnson KS, Jaffe ES. Lymphoproliferative disorders associated with congenital immunodeficiencies. Semin Diagn Pathol 1997;14:35-47.
38. European Chromosome 16 Tuberous Sclerosis Consortium. Identification and characterization of the tuberous sclerosis gene on chromosome 16. Cell 1993;75:1305.
39. Facchetti F, Appiani C, Salvi L, Levy J, Notarangelo LD. Immunohistologic analysis of ineffective CD40-CD40 ligand interaction in lymphoid tissues from patients with X-linked immunodeficiency with hyper-IgM. Abortive germinal center cell reaction of severe depletion of follicular dendritic cells. J Immunol 1995;154:6624-33.
40. Ferrari S, Giliani S, Insalaco A, et al. Mutations of CD40 gene causes an autosomal recessive form of immunodeficiency with hyper IgM. Proc Natl Acad Sci U S A 2001;98:12614-9.
41. Fisher GH, Rosenberg FJ, Straus SE, et al. Dominant interfering Fas gene mutations impair apoptosis in a human autoimmune lymphoproliferative syndrome. Cell 1995;81:935-46.
42. Fontana S, Moratto D, Mangal S, et al. Functional defects of dendritic cells in patients with CD40 deficiency. Blood 2003;102:4099-106.
43. Freyer DR, Gowans LK, Warzynski M, Lee WI. Flow cytometric diagnosis of X-linked hyper-IgM syndrome: application of an accurate and convenient procedure. J Pediatr Hematol Oncol 2004;26:363-70.
44. Frizzera G. Atypical lymphoproliferative disorders. In: Knowles DM, ed. Neoplastic hematopathology, 2nd ed. Philadelphia: Lippincott Williams & Wilkins; 2001:569-622.
45. Frizzera G, Rosai J, Dehner LP, Spector BD, Kersey JH. Lymphoreticular disorders in primary immunodeficiencies: new findings based on an up-to-date histologic classification of 35 cases. Cancer 1980;46:692-9.
46. Gallego MD, Santamaria M, Pena J, Molin IJ. Defective actin reorganization and polymerization of Wiskott-Aldrich T cells in response to CD3-mediated stimulation. Blood 1997;90:3089-97.
47. Gatti RA, Good RA. Occurrence of malignancy in immunodeficiency states. A literature review. Cancer 1971;28:89-98.
48. Gerwin N, Friedrich C, Perez-Atayde A, Rosen FS, Gutierrez-Ramos JC. Multiple antigens are altered on T and B lymphocytes from peripheral blood and spleen of patients with Wiskott-Aldrich syndrome. Clin Exp Immunol 1996;106:208-17.
49. Goldstein MF, Kornstein MJ, Talbot S, Levinson AI. Acquired hyper-IgM syndrome with necrotizing granuloma. J Allergy Clin Immunol 1985;75:472-8.
50. Gosseye S, Diebold N, Griscelli C, Nezelof C. Severe combined immunodeficiency disease: a pathological analysis of 26 cases. Clin Immunol Immunopathol 1983;29:58-77.
51. Green AJ, Smith M, Yates JR. Loss of heterozygosity on chromosome 16p13.3 in hamartomas from tuberous sclerosis patients. Nat Genet 1994;6:193-6.
52. Grierson H, Purtilo DT. Epstein-Barr virus infections in males with the X-linked lymphoproliferative syndrome. Ann Intern Med 1987;106:538-45.
53. Grimbacher B, Holland SM, Puck JM. Hyper-IgE syndromes. Immunol Rev 2005;203:244-50.
54. Hadzic N, Pagliuca A, Rela M, et al. Correction of the hyper-IgM syndrome after liver and bone marrow transplantation. N Eng J Med 2000;342:320-4.
55. Hamilton JK, Paquin LA, Sullivan JL, et al. X-linked lymphoproliferative syndrome registry report. J Pediatr 1980;96:669-73.
56. Hammarstrom L, Smith CI. Genetic approach to common variable immunodeficiency and IgA deficiency. In: Ochs HD, Smith CIE, Puck JM, eds. Primary immunodeficiency diseases: a molecular and genetic approach. New York: Oxford University Press; 1999:250-62.

57. Harrington DS, Weisenburger DD, Purtilo DT. Malignant lymphoma in the X-linked lymphoproliferative syndrome. Cancer 1987;59:1419-29.
58. Hayward AR, Levy J, Facchetti F, et al. Cholangiopathy and tumors of the pancreas, liver, and biliary tree in boys with X-linked immunodeficiency with hyper-IgM. J Immunol 1997;158:977-83.
59. Henske EP, Neumann HP, Scheithauer BW, Herbst EW, Short MP, Kwiatkowski DJ. Loss of heterozygosity in the tuberous sclerosis (TSC2) region of chromosome band 16p13 occurs in sporadic as well as TSC-associated renal angiomyolipomas. Genes Chromosomes Cancer 1995;13:295-8.
60. Henter JI, Samuelsson-Horne A, Arico M, et al. Treatment of hemophagocytic lymphohistiocytosis with HLH-94 immunochemotherapy and bone marrow transplantation. Blood 2002;100:2367-73.
61. Hinz CF, Boyer JT. Dysgammaglobulinemia in the adult manifested as autoimmune hemolytic anemia. Serologic and immunochemical characterization of an antibody of unusual specificity. N Engl J Med 1963;269:1329-35.
62. Hobbs JR, Russell A, Worlledge SM. Dysgammaglobulinemia type IV. Clin Exp Immunol 1967;2:589-99.
63. Hulbert JC, Graf R. Involvement of the spleen by renal angioimyolipoma: metastasis or multicentricity? J Urol 1983;130:328-9.
64. Illoh OC. Current applications of flow cytometry in the diagnosis of primary immunodeficiency diseases. Arch Pathol Lab Med 2004;128:23-31.
65. Imai K, Catalan N, Plebani A, et al. Hyper-IgM syndrome type 4 with a B lymphocyte-intrinsic selective deficiency in Ig class-switch recombination. J Clin Investig 2003;112:136-42.
66. Imai K, Morio T, Zhu Y, et al. Clinical course of patients with WASP gene mutations. Blood 2004;103:456-64.
67. Imai K, Slupphaug G, Lee WI, et al. Human uracil-DNA glycosylase deficiency associated with profoundly impaired immunoglobulin class-switch recombination. Nat Immunol 2003;4:1023-8.
68. Jackson CE, Puck JM. Autoimmune lymphoproliferative syndrome, a disorder of apoptosis. Curr Opin Pediatr 1999;11:521-7.
69. Jain A, Ma CA, Liu S, Brown M, Cohen J, Strober W. Specific missense mutations in NEMO result in hyper-IgM syndrome with hypohydrotic ectodermal dysplasia. Nat Immunol 2001;2:223-8.
70. Johnston RB Jr. Clinical aspects of chronic granulomatous disease. Curr Opin Hematol 2001;8:17-22.
71. Jones AC, Shyamsundar MM, Thomas MW, et al. Comprehensive mutation analysis of TSC1 and RSC2- and phenotypic correlations in 150 families with tuberous sclerosis. Am J Hum Genet 1999;64:1305-15.
72. Kanegane H, Ito Y, Ohshima K, et al. X-linked lymphoproliferative syndrome presenting with systemic lymphocytic vasculitis. Am J Hematol 2005;73:130-3.
73. Karim MA, Suzuki K, Fukai K, et al. Apparent genotype-phenotype correlation in childhood, adolescent, and adult Chediak-Higashi syndrome. Am J Med Genet 2002;108:16-22.
74. Kawabata K, Nagasawa M, Morio T, Okawa H, Yata J. Decreased alpha/beta heterodimer among CD8 molecules of peripheral blood T cells in Wiskott-Aldrich syndrome. Clin Immunol Immunopathol 1996;81:129-35.
75. Kenney D, Cairns L, Remold-O'Donnell E, Peterson J, Rosen FS, Parkman R. Morphological abnormalities in the lymphocytes of patients with the Wiskott-Aldrich syndrome. Blood 1986;68:1329-32.
76. Kwiatkowska J, Jozwiak S, Hall F, et al. Comprehensive mutational analysis of the TSC1 gene: observations on frequency of mutation, associated features, and nonpenetrance. Ann Hum Genet 1998;62:277-85.
77. Kwiatkowska J, Wigowska-Sowinska J, Napierala D, Slomski R, Kwiatkowski DJ. Mosaicism in tuberous sclerosis as a potential cause of the failure of molecular diagnosis. N Engl J Med 1999;340:703-7.
78. Lamb RF, Roy C, Diefenbach TJ. The TSC1 tumour suppressor hamartin regulates cell adhesion through ERM proteins and the GTPase Rho. Nat Cell Biol 2000;2:281-7.
79. Larson RS. Immunodeficiency disorders. In: Pediatric hematopathology. Collins RD, Swerdlow SH, eds. New York: Churchill Livingstone; 2001:21-41.
80. Latour S, Veillette A. Molecular and immunological basis of X-linked lymphoproliferative disease. Immunol Rev 2003;192:212-24.
81. Le Deist F, Emile JF, Rieux-Laucat F, et al. Clinical, immunological, and pathological consequences of Fas-deficient conditions. Lancet 1996;348:719-23.
82. Leiva LE, Junprasert J, Hollenbaugh D, Sorensen RU. Central nervous system toxoplasmosis with an increased proportion of circulating gamma delta T cells in a patient with hyper-IgM syndrome. J Clin Immunol 1998;18:283-90.
83. Loeffel S, Chang CH, Heyn R, et al. Necrotizing lymphoid vasculitis in X-linked lymphoproliferative syndrome. Arch Pathol Lab Med 1985;109:546-50.
84. Levy J, Espanol-Boren T, Thomas C, et al. Clinical spectrum of X-linked hyper-IgM syndrome. J Pediatr 1997;131:47-54.

85. Levy M, Feingold J. Estimating prevalence in single-gene kidney diseases progressing to renal failure. Kidney Int 2000;58:925-43.
86. Lim MS, Straus SE, Dale JK, et al. Pathological findings in human autoimmune lymphoproliferative syndrome. Am J Pathol 1998;153:1541-50.
87. Lougaris V, Badolato R, Ferrari S, Plebani A. Hyper immunoglobulin M syndrome due to CD40 deficiency: clinical, molecular, and immunological features. Immunol Rev 2005;203:48-66.
88. Lutskiy MI, Sasahara Y, Kenney DM, Rosen FS, Remold-O'Donnell E. Wiskott-Aldrich syndrome in a female. Blood 2002;100:2763-8.
89. Maia DM, Garwacki CP. X-linked lymphoproliferative disease: pathology and diagnosis. Pediatr Dev Pathol 1999;2:72-7.
90. Maric I, Pittaluga S, Dale JK, et al. Histologic features of sinus histiocytosis with massive lymphadenopathy in patients with autoimmune lymphoproliferative syndrome. Am J Surg Pathol 2005;29:903-11.
91. Martignoni G, Bonetti F, Pea M, Tardanico R, Brunelli M, Eble JN. Renal disease in adults with RSC2/PKD1 contiguous gene syndrome. Am J Surg Pathol 2002;26:198-205.
92. Menasche G, Fischer A, de Saint Basile G. Griscelli syndrome types 1 and 2. Am J Hum Genet 2002;71:1237-8.
93. Menasche G, Pastural E, Feldmann J, et al. Mutations in RAB27A cause Griscelli syndrome associated with haemophagocytic syndrome. Nat Genet 2000;25:173-6.
94. Milone MC, Tsai DE, Hodinka RL, et al. Treatment of primary Epstein-Barr virus infection in patients with X-linked lymphoproliferative disease using B-cell-directed therapy. Blood 2005;105:994-6.
95. Mullen CA, Anderson KD, Blaese RM. Splenectomy and/or bone marrow transplantation in the management of the Wiskott-Aldrich syndrome: long-term follow-up of 62 cases. Blood 1993;82:2961-6.
96. Murray JC, Strong GB, Murphey DK. Clinical pathology case: hyperimmunoglobulin E syndrome (Job's syndrome). Pediatr Pathol Mol Med 2001;20:223-6.
97. Narod SA, Stiller C, Lenoir GM. An estimate of the heritable fraction of childhood cancer. Br J Cancer 1991;63:993-9.
98. Nichols KE, Harkin DP, Levitz S, et al. Inactivating mutations in an SH2 domain-encoding gene in X-linked lymphoproliferative syndrome. Proc Natl Acad Sci U S A 1998;95:13765-70.
99. Nichols KE, Ma CS, Cannons JL, Schwartzberg PL, Tangye SG. Molecular and cellular pathogenesis of X-linked lymphoproliferative disease. Immunol Rev 2005;203:180-99.
100. Niida Y, Lawrence-Smith N, Banwell A, et al. Analysis of both TSC1 and TSC2 for germline mutations in 126 unrelated patients with tuberous sclerosis. Hum Mutat 1999;14:412-22.
101. Northrup H, Wheless JW, Bertin TK, Lewis RA. Variability of expression in tuberous sclerosis. J Med Genet 1993;30:41-3.
102. Notarangelo LD, Duse M, Ugazio AG. Immunodeficiency with hyper-IgM (HIM). Immunodef Rev 1992;3:101-21.
103. Notarangelo LD, Peitsch MD. CD40lbase: a database of CD40L gene mutations causing X-linked hyper-IgM syndrome. Immunol Today 1996;17:511-6.
104. Ochs HD, Slichter SJ, Harker LA, Von Behrens WE, Clark RA, Wedgwood RJ. The Wiskott-Aldrich syndrome: studies of lymphocytes, granulocytes, and platelets. Blood 1980;55:243-52.
105. Okano M, Mizuno F, Osato T, Takahashi Y, Sakiyama Y, Matsumoto S. Wiskott-Aldrich syndrome and Epstein-Barr virus-induced lymphoproliferation. Lancet 1984;2:933-44.
106. Osborne JP, Fryer A, Webb D. Epidemiology of tuberous sclerosis. Ann NY Acad Sci 1991;615:125-7.
107. Pajak L, Jin F, Xiao GH, Soonpa MH, Field LJ, Yeung RS. Sustained cardiomyocyte DNA synthesis in whole embryo cultures lacking the TSC2 gene product. Am J Physiol 1997;273:H1619-27.
108. Primary immunodeficiency diseases: Report of a WHO scientific group. Clin Exp Immunol 1995;99(suppl 1):1-24.
109. Puck JM. Immunodeficiency disorders. II. Severe combined immunodeficiency update. Hematology (Am Soc Hematol Educ Program) 2003;314-30.
110. Purtilo DT. Epstein-Barr virus induced-oncogenesis in immune-deficient individuals. Lancet 1980;1:300-3.
111. Purtilo DT. X-linked lymphoproliferative syndrome. An immunodeficiency disorder with acquired agammaglobulinemia, fatal infectious mononucleosis, or malignant lymphoma. Arch Pathol Lab Med 1981;105:119-21.
112. Purtilo DT, Cassel CK, Yang JP, Harper R. X-linked recessive progressive combined variable immunodeficiency (Duncan's disease). Lancet 1975;1:935-40.
113. Purtilo DT, Paquin L, DeFlorio D, Virzi F, Sakhuja R. Immunodiagnosis and immunopathegenesis of the X-linked recessive lymphoproliferative syndrome. Semin Hematol 1979;16:309-43.
114. Purtilo DT, Strobach R, Okano M, Davis JR. Epstein-Barr virus-associated lymphoproliferative disorders. Lab Invest 1992;67:5-23.

115. Ramenghi U, Bonissoni S, Migliaretti G, et al. Deficiency of the Fas apoptosis pathway without Fas gene mutations is a familial trait predisposing to development of autoimmune diseases and cancer. Blood 2000;95:3176-82.
116. Ratech H, Hirschhorn R, Greco MA. Pathologic findings in adenosine deaminase deficient-severe combined immunodeficiency. II Thymus, spleen, lymph node and gastrointestinal tract lymphoid tissue alterations. Am J Pathol 1989;135:1145-56.
117. Raziuddin S, Assaf HM, Teklu B. T cell malignancy in Richter's syndrome presenting as hyper IgM. Induction and characterization of a novel CD3+, CD4-, CD8+ T cell subset from phytohemagglutinin-stimulated patient's CD3+, CD4+, CD8+ leukemic T cells. Eur J Immunol 1989;19:469-74.
118. Rennebeck G, Kleymenova EV, Anderson R, Yeung RS, Artzt K, Walker CL. Loss of function of the tuberous sclerosis 2 tumor suppressor gene results in embryonic lethality characterized by disrupted neuroepithelial growth and development. Proc Natl Acad Sci U S A 1998;95:15629-34.
119. Revy P, Muto T, Levy Y, et al. Activation-induced cytidine deaminase (AID) deficiency causes the autosomal recessive form of the hyper-IgM syndrome (HIGM2). Cell 2000;102:565-75.
120. Roach ES, Gomez MR, Northrup H. Tuberous sclerosis complex consensus conference: revised clinical diagnostic criteria. J Child Neurol 1998;13:624-8.
121. Rocca B, Bellacosa A, De Cristofaro R, et al. Wiskott-Aldrich syndrome: report of an autosomal dominant variant. Blood 1996;87:4538-43.
122. Rose VM, Au KS, Pollom G, Roach ES, Prashner HR, Northrup H. Germ-line mosaicism in tuberous sclerosis: how common? Am J Hum Genet 1999;64:986-92.
123. Rosen FS, Bougas JA. Acquired dysgammaglobulinemia. Elevation of the 19S gamma globulin and deficiency of the 7S gamma globulin in a woman with chronic progressive bronchiectasis. N Engl J Med 1963; 269:1336-40.
124. Rosen FS, Cooper MD, Wedgwood RJ. The primary immunodeficiencies. N Engl J Med 1984;311:235-42.
125. Sander CA, Medeiros LJ, Weiss LM, Yano T, Sneller MC, Jaffe ES. Lymphoproliferative lesions in patients with common variable immunodeficiency syndrome. Am J Surg Pathol 1992;16:1170-82.
126. Sayos J, Wu C, Morra M, et al. The X-linked lymphoproliferative-disease gene product SAP regulates signals induced through the co-receptor SLAM. Nature 1998;395:462-9.
127. Schulte-Wissermann H, Lemmel EM, Opferkuch W, et al. [Immunologic deficiency syndrome with dysgammaglobulinemia and lymphatic hyperplasia.] Helv Paediatr Acta 1973;28:569-81. [German]
128. Sebire NJ, Haselden S, Malone M, Davies EG, Ramsay AD. Isolated EBV lymphoproliferative disease in a child with Wiskott-Aldrich syndrome manifesting as cutaneous lymphomatoid granulomatosis and responsive to anti-CD20 immunotherapy. J Clin Pathol 2003;56:555-7.
129. Seemayer TA, Grierson H, Pirruccello SJ, et al. X-linked lymphoproliferative disease. Am J Dis Child 1993;147:1242-5.
130. Shcherbina A, Candotti F, Rosen FS, Remold-O'Donnel E. High incidence of lymphomas in a subgroup of Wiskott-Aldrich syndrome patients. Br J Haematol 2003;121:529-30.
131. Shemer A, Weiss G, Confino Y, Trau H. The hyper-IgE syndrome. Two cases and review of the literature. Int J Dermatol 2001;40:622-8.
132. Shepherd CW, Gomez MR, Lie JT, Crowson CS. Causes of death in patients with tuberous sclerosis. Mayo Clin Proc 1991;66:792.
133. Sneller MC, Wang J, Dale JK, et al. Clinical, immunologic, and genetic features of an autoimmune lymphoproliferative syndrome associated with abnormal lymphocyte apoptosis. Blood 1997;89:1341-8.
134. Sneller MC, Straus SE, Jaffe ES, et al. A novel lymphoproliferative/autoimmune syndrome resembling murine lpr/gld disease. J Clin Invest 1992;90:334-41.
135. Snover DC, Frizzera G, Spector BD, Perry GS 3rd, Kersey KH. Wiskott-Aldrich syndrome: histopathologic findings in the lymph nodes and spleens of 15 patients. Hum Pathol 1981;12:821-31.
136. Strobel P, Nanan R, Gattenlohner S, et al. Reversible monoclonal lymphadenopathy in autoimmune lymphoproliferative syndrome with functional FAS (CD95/APO-1) deficiency. Am J Surg Pathol 1999;23:829-37.
137. Sullivan KE, Mullen CA, Blaese RM, Winkelstein JA. A multiinstitutional survey of the Wiskott-Aldrich syndrome. J Pediatr 1994;125:876-85.
138. Sumegi J, Seemayer TA, Huang D, et al. A spectrum of mutations in SH2D1A that causes X-linked lymphoproliferative disease and other Epstein-Barr virus-associated illnesses. Leuk Lymphoma 2002;43:1189-201.
139. Tanaka T, Takahashi K, Morita H, et al. Chronic granulomatous disease of childhood and sea-blue histiocytosis. A pathologic study of an autopsy case. Acta Pathol Jpn 1984;34:1385-401.

140. Tee AR, Fingar DC, Manning BD, Kwiatkowski DJ, Cantley LC, Blenis J. Tuberous sclerosis complex-1 and –2 gene products function together to inhibit mammalian target of rapamycin (mTOR)-mediated downstream signaling. Proc Natl Acad Sci U S A 2002;99:13571-6.
141. Thomas C, de Saint Basile G, Le Deist F, et al. Brief report: correction of X-linked hyper-IgM syndrome by allogeneic bone marrow transplantation. N Engl J Med 1995;333:426-9.
142. Thrasher AJ, Jones GE, Kinnon C, Brickell PM, Katz DR. Is Wiskott-Aldrich syndrome a cell trafficking disorder? Immunol Today 1998;19:537-9.
143. Tunali N, Gumurdulu D, Zorludemir S. Splenic involvement in a stillborn fetus with tuberous sclerosis and multiple cardiac rhabdomyomas. Turk J Pediatr 2004;46:357-61.
144. Vaishnaw AK, Toubi E, Ohsako S, et al. The spectrum of apoptotic defects and clinical manifestations, including systemic lupus erythematosus, in humans with CD95 (Fas/APO-1) mutations. Arthritis Rheum 1999;42:1833-42.
145. Van Slegtenhorst M, de Hoogt R, Hermans C, et al. Identification of the tuberous sclerosis gene TSC1 on chromosome 9q34. Science 1997;277:805-8.
146. Van Slegtenhorst M, Nellist M, Nagelkerkern B, et al. Interactin between hamartin and tuberin, the TSC1 and TSC2 gene products. Hum Mol Genet 1998;7:1053-7.
147. Vermi W, Blanzuoli L, Kraus MD, et al. The spleen in the Wiskott-Aldrich syndrome: histopathologic abnormalities of the white pulp correlate with the clinical phenotype of the disease. Am J Surg Pathol 1999;23:182-91.
148. Vorechovsky I, Cullen M, Carrington M, Hammarstrom L, Webster AD. Fine mapping of IGAD1 in IgA deficiency and common variable immunodeficiency: identification and characterization of haplotypes shared by affected members of 101 multiple-case families. J Immunol 2000;164:4408-16.
149. Vowels MR, Tang RL, Berdoukas V, et al. Correction of X-linked lymphoproliferative disease by transplantation of cord-blood stem cells. N Engl J Med 1993;329:1623-5.
150. Watanabe-Fukunaga R, Brannan CI, Copeland NG, Jenkins NA, Nagata S. Lympholiferation disorder in mice explained by defects in Fas antigen that mediates apoptosis. Nature 1992;356:314-7.
151. Weitkamp JH, Tang YW, Haas DW, Midha NK, Crowe JE Jr. Recurrent Achromobacter xylosoxidans bacteremia associated with persistent lymph node infection in a patient with hyper-immunoglobulin M syndrome. Clin Infect Dis 2000;31:1183-7.
152. Winkelstein JA, Marino MC, Ochs H et al. The X-linked hyper-IgM syndrome: clinical and immunologic features of 79 patients. Medicine (Baltimore) 2003;82:373-84.
153. Wiskott A. Familiarer, angeobren Morbus Werlhofi? Monatsschrift fur Kinderheilkinde 1937;68:212-216.
154. Zhu Q, Watanabe C, Liu T, et al. Wiskott-Aldrich syndrome/X-linked thrombocytopenia: WASP gene mutation, protein expression, and phenotype. Blood 1997;90:2680-9.
155. Zukerberg LR, Kaynor BL, Silverman ML, Harris NL. Splenic hamartoma and capillary hemangioma are distinct entities: immunohistochemical analysis of CD8 expression by endothelial cells. Hum Pathol 1991;22:1258-61.

8 BACTERIAL INFECTIONS

Most infectious organisms primarily or secondarily involve the lymph nodes or spleen because of the important role these organs play in the body's immune system. Many of these infections result in nonspecific cellular and architectural changes, while others cause changes that are characteristic of a specific organism. In general, the tissue response to infection in a lymph node mimics the inflammatory response that is seen at other anatomic sites. Although some infections, such as cat-scratch disease, primarily affect the lymph nodes, most bacterial infections involve lymph nodes or spleen as a secondary site of dissemination.

Pyogenic bacteria such as *Staphylococcus*, *Streptococcus*, or *Neisseria* may cause acute inflammation in the lymph nodes that drain primary sites of infection or the spleen. The histopathologic changes caused by these organisms are similar and include focal or diffuse infiltration by polymorphonuclear leukocytes, often with the formation of suppurative microabscesses (fig. 8-1). Capsular edema and neutrophilic infiltration of the perinodal tissue, with suppuration, also occur in the early stages of infection (fig. 8-2). Sinus formation, in untreated cases, may be a late sequela of the infection. The spleen may be a site of abscess formation (fig. 8-3). Resolution of a bacterial abscess may ultimately lead to the formation of a cyst. As the acute inflammation subsides, chronic inflammatory cells, including lymphocytes, plasma cells, and phagocytic macrophages, replace the neutrophilic granulocytes (103).

The term *splenitis* has historically been used to refer to a group of changes in the spleen associated with infectious processes (46). Unfortunately, this term is of little use; it does not refer specifically to any histologic or clinical findings and has no proven association with splenic infection. As such, its use should be avoided.

GRAM-POSITIVE BACTERIAL INFECTIONS

The range of bacteria that can involve the human lymph nodes and spleen is only limited by the number of species that are seen in humans. Those that are common are covered in individual sections below.

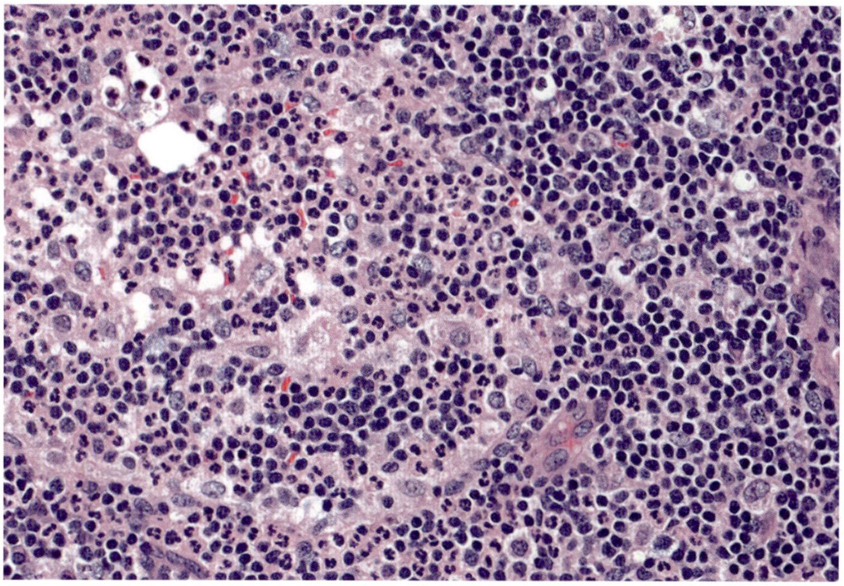

Figure 8-1

INFECTION, MICROABSCESSES, LYMPH NODE

Small foci of bacteria in this lymph node suggest the possibility of early bacterial infection. Typically, a specific etiology is not identified without microbiologic studies.

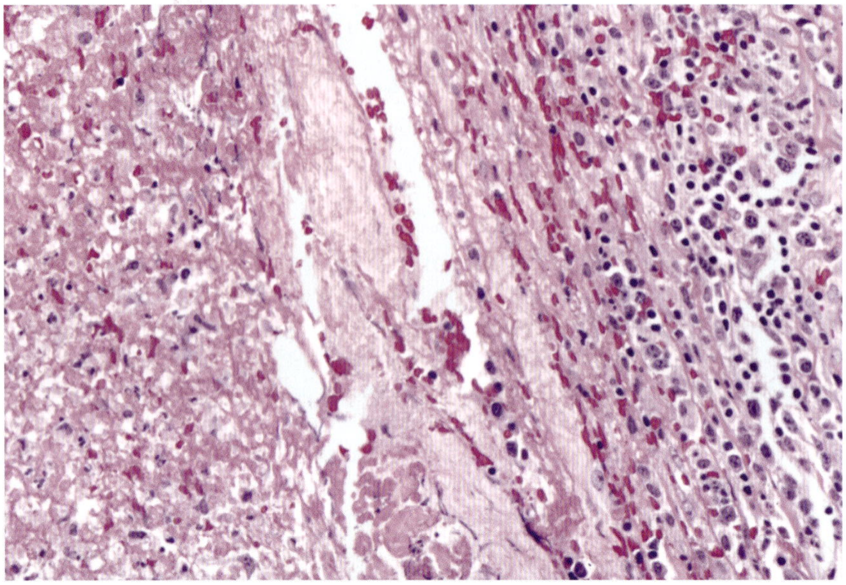

Figure 8-2

INFECTION, CAPSULAR EDEMA AND NEUTROPHILIC INFILTRATION

An early stage of acute streptococcal lymphadenitis shows a suppurative, edematous exudate in the perinodal tissue.

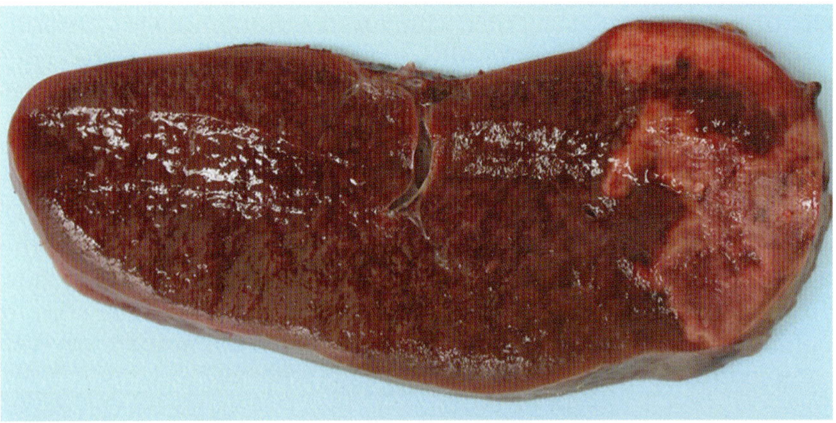

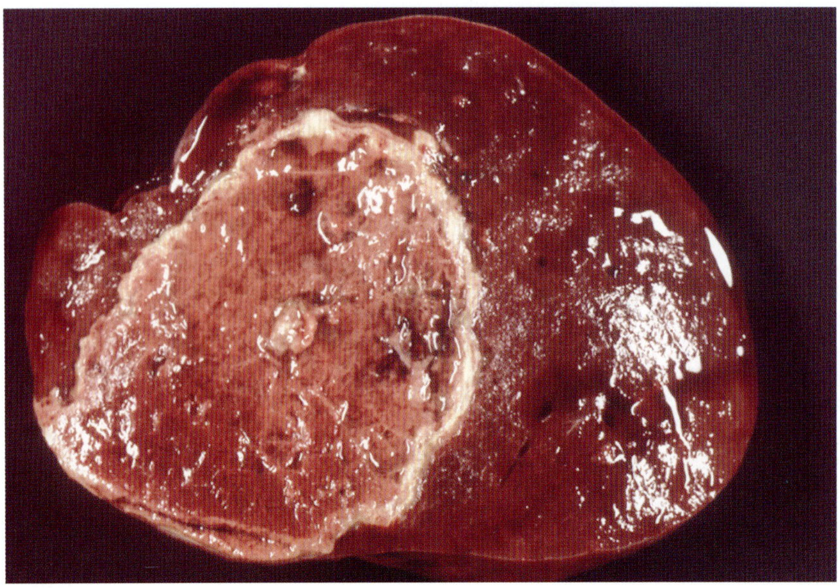

Figure 8-3

BACTERIAL ABSCESS, SPLEEN

The abscess has irregular borders. The red-yellow color contrasts with the adjacent, uninvolved spleen. (Bottom figure courtesy of Peter Banks, Charlotte, NC.)

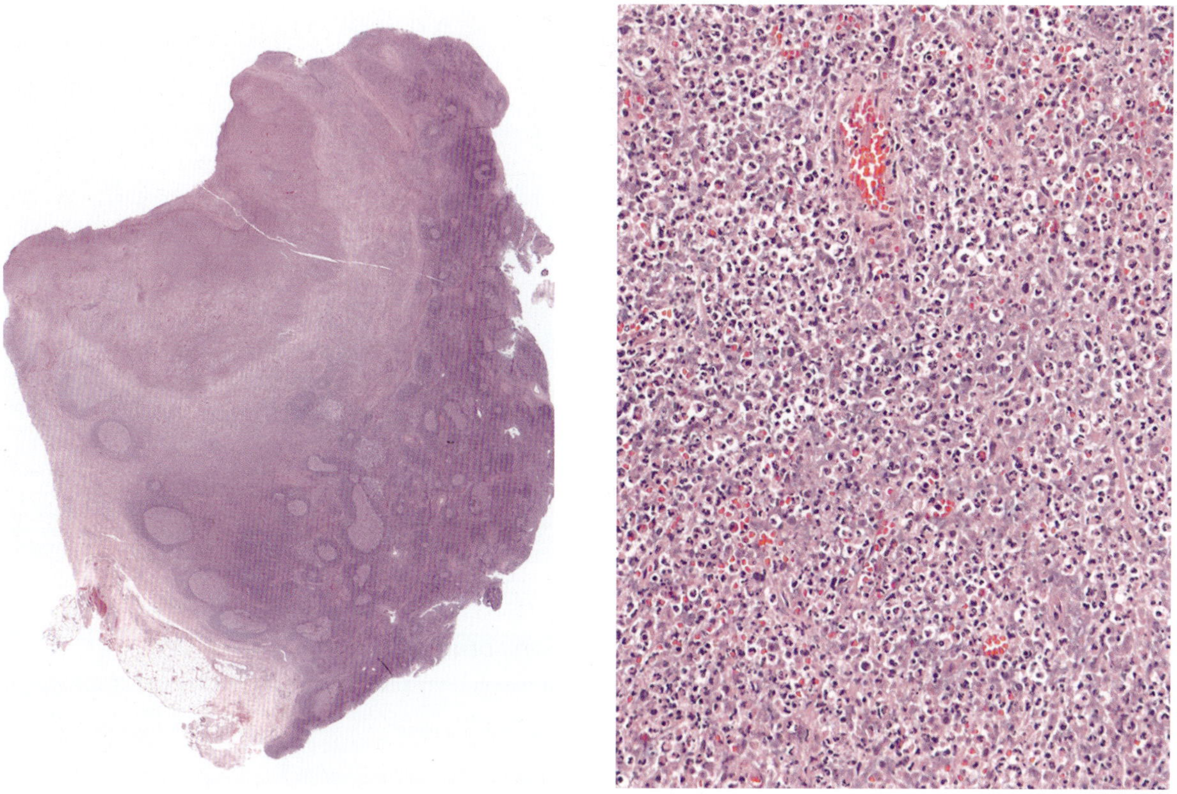

Figure 8-4

STAPHYLOCOCCAL LYMPHADENITIS

A case of culture-proven staphylococcal lymphadenitis shows areas of necrosis (left) and abscess formation (right).

Staphylococcus and *Streptococcus*

Definition. *Staphylococcus* and *Streptococcus* organisms are common causes of localized or regional suppurative lymphadenitis.

General Features. Pyogenic infections, especially those of the skin, scalp, and oropharynx, are often caused by gram-positive organisms. *Staphylococcus aureus* and group A beta-hemolytic streptococci are the most common etiologic agents (106). The draining lymph nodes may become involved and subsequently enlarge. Enlarged nodes are often fluctuant, swollen, and tender.

Streptococcal organisms primarily cause two clinical forms of disease: spreading suppurative infections (*Streptococcus pyogenes* or beta-hemolytic *Streptococcus*) or poststreptococcal hypersensitivity disease. *S. aureus* is the usual cause of skin abscesses in the form of furuncles or carbuncles, and the regional lymphadenitis it produces is seldom as severe as the primary infection (103).

Microscopic Findings. The histopathologic appearance of suppurative infection is inflammation of the lymph node capsule, and possible abscess formation, with central necrotic material and acute inflammatory cells (figs. 8-4–8-6). Abscesses are often surrounded by increased numbers of macrophages, and occasionally, a localized immunoblastic reaction. The organisms are identified in some cases using tissue Gram stains. Tissue culture typically positively identifies the causative organisms.

Corynebacterium

Definition. There are numerous *Corynebacterium* species, but only two are covered here: *C. diphtheriae* and *C. pseudotuberculosis* (also known as *C. ovis*). Both can cause significant lymphadenopathy.

General Features. *Diphtheria,* caused by *C. diphtheriae,* is uncommon in developed countries because of frequent vaccination. In

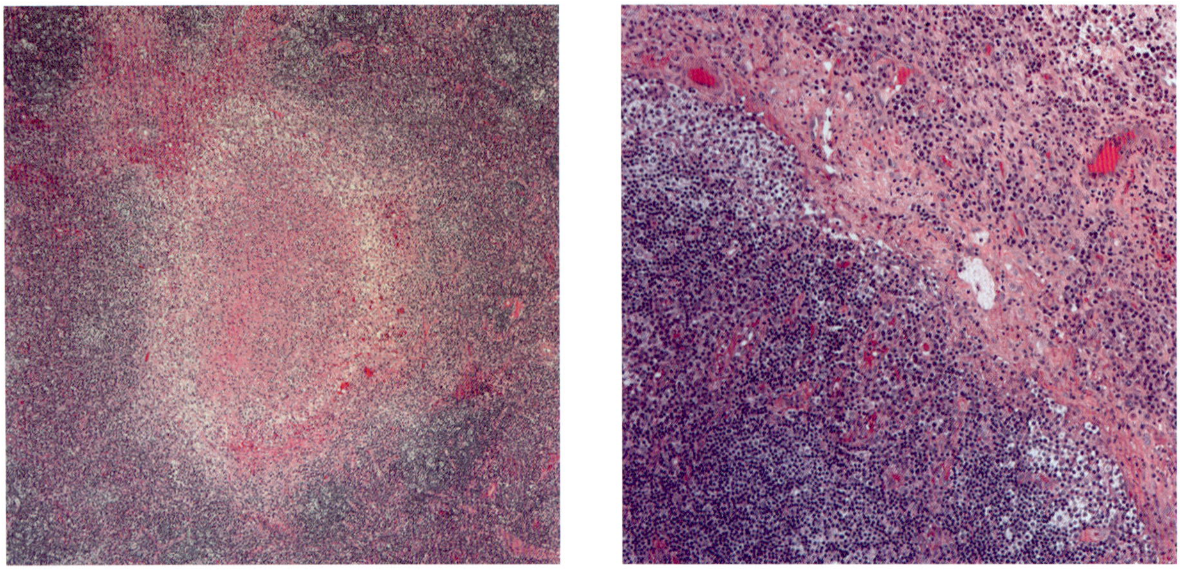

Figure 8-5

STREPTOCOCCAL LYMPHADENITIS

Culture-proven streptococcal lymphadenitis shows abscess formation (left) and neutrophilic infiltration of the lymph node capsule (right).

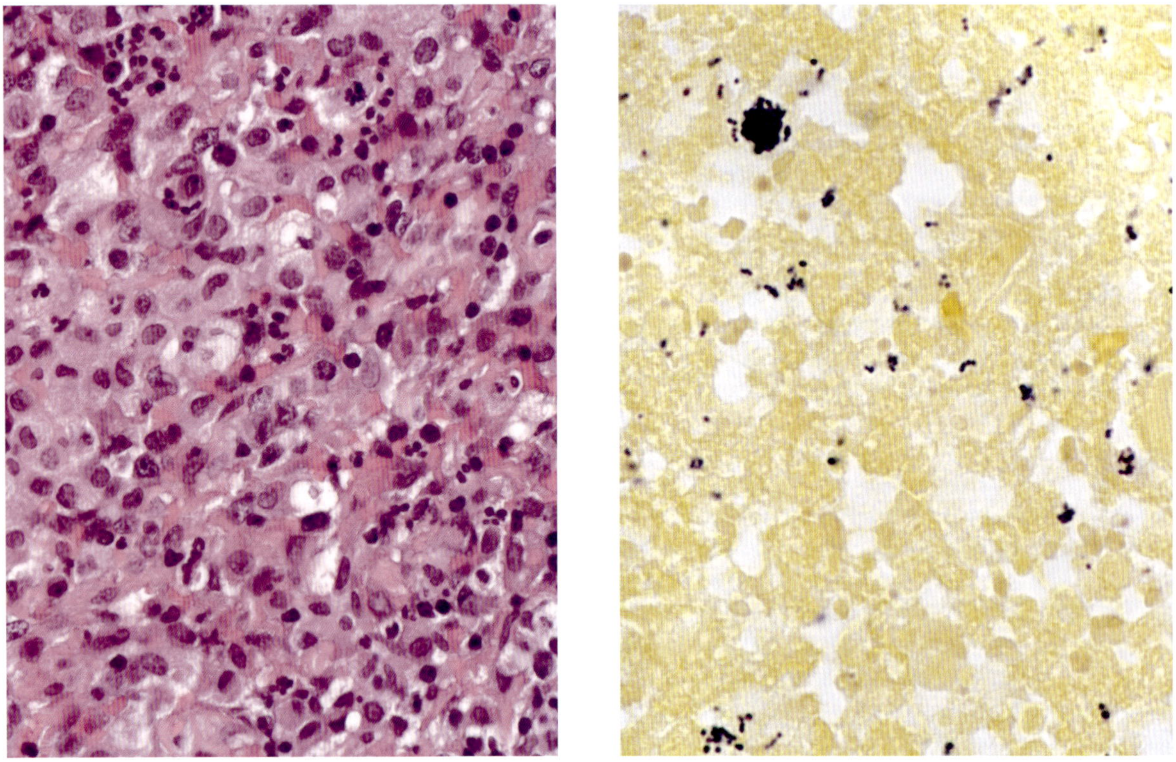

Figure 8-6

STREPTOCOCCAL LYMPHADENITIS

A neutrophilic infiltrate (left) and a tissue Gram stain showing numerous bacteria (right).

less-developed parts of the world, however, the disease remains a threat. Diphtheria presents in the upper respiratory tract. Production of a toxin by the organism leads to the production of a pseudomembranc which covers the upper respiratory tract. At this stage, cervical and submandibular lymphadenopathy is common. The term "bull neck" has been sometimes applied to the prominent adenopathy associated with diphtheria. The diphtheria toxin may cause additional dangerous symptoms in other organ systems, including heart, gastrointestinal tract, liver, kidney, and peripheral nervous system.

C. pseudotuberculosis is a relatively common pathogen of sheep, and the related infection is given the name "cheesy gland" by Australian sheep farmers. Human infections are seen in those who have close contact with sheep. Most cases have been in Australia, but exceptional cases have been seen in the United States and South America (14,55,87).

Microscopic Findings. The lymph node changes due to *C. diphtheriae* are most likely not due to direct infection, but to the distant effects of the infection caused by the diphtheria toxin (125). Hemorrhage, necrosis, and thrombosis are seen in lymph nodes. The necrosis occurs in the parenchyma of the node and within the germinal centers. Marked edema, with proteinaceous fluid and fibrin deposition, is also seen. Splenic abscess has been reported as part of disseminated disease (67).

The changes in *C. pseudotuberculosis* infection are different. As the species name implies, the findings are similar to those seen with tuberculosis. Granuloma formulation with epithelioid macrophages, giant cells, and prominent central caseation is the most striking feature (14,55,87). Smears of the purulent fluid show varying numbers of gram-positive bacteria.

Listeria Monocytogenes

Definition. *Listeria monocytogenes* is a rare cause of suppurative lymphadenitis.

General Features. *L. monocytogenes*, a gram-positive motile rod-shaped organism, is the causative agent of *listeriosis*, which results in acute gastroenteritis. It is transmitted by contaminated milk products and has serious implications for the infected fetus or immunocompromised host. In these patients, acute, exudative leptomeningitis is the primary manifestation of the disease, although widespread systemic involvement of any organ, including lymph nodes, may occur. Rare cases of focal, node-based listeriosis have been reported (99). The diagnosis depends on culture and microbiologic identification.

Microscopic Findings. *Listeria* involvement in lymph node or spleen shows an exudative pattern of inflammation, with neutrophilic infiltration and microabscess formation. Granuloma formation may also be seen. The intracellular aggregates of organisms are termed "Chinese character" formations (106).

Actinomyces, Nocardia, and *Rhodococcus Equi*

Definition. *Actinomyces* and *Nocardia* are filamentous bacteria that are seen in association with human infections, particularly acute exudative lymphadenitis. *Rhodococcus equi* infections appear "diphtheroid" (club-shaped, similar to *Corynebacterium diphtheriae*), and cause lymphadenitis in immunocompetent and immunocompromised patients.

General Features. *Actinomyces* organisms are gram-positive bacteria that show some similarity to fungi (formation of mycelia and branching patterns of growth). They are non-acid fast and strictly anaerobic. *Actinomyces* organisms are normally found within the oral cavity, gastrointestinal tract, or vagina, and become invasive following trauma to the tissue. Species that are commonly associated with human disease include: *A. israelii, A. meyeri, A. naeslundii, A. odonontolyticus, A. gerencseriae,* and *A. viscosus*. Splenic abscesses due to *Actinomyces* organisms have been reported (54,93). *Actinomyces* is a normal constituent of oropharyngeal bacterial flora, and in contrast to *Nocardia*, is pathogenic in nonimmunocompromised hosts (103). Actinomycotic splenic abscesses have been reported (93). Confirmatory diagnosis relies upon culturing the organism in the appropriate media. *Actinomycosis* is a chronic infection that primarily manifests as cervico-facial, abdominal, or thoracic infection (18).

Nocardia is an aerobic, filamentous gram-positive bacterium that forms branching chains and is weakly acid fast. Although the exact mode of transmission is unclear, *Nocardia* organisms are known to be widespread in nature and typically affect immunocompromised or chronically ill patients. The skin and lungs are the primary

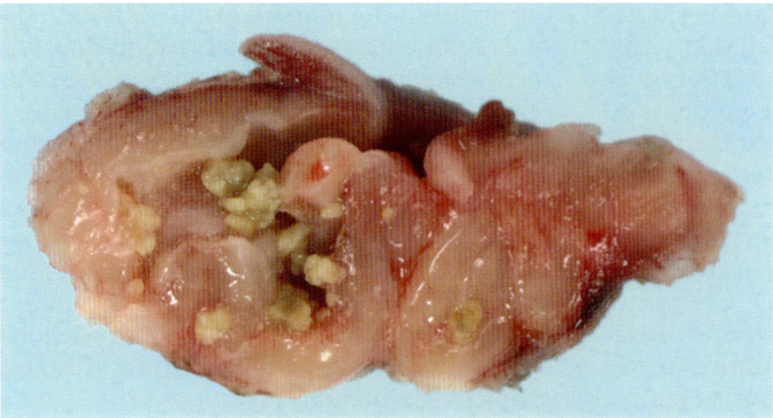

Figure 8-7

SULFUR GRANULES, TONSIL

Several small yellow nodules (sulfur granules) are present in the tonsil.

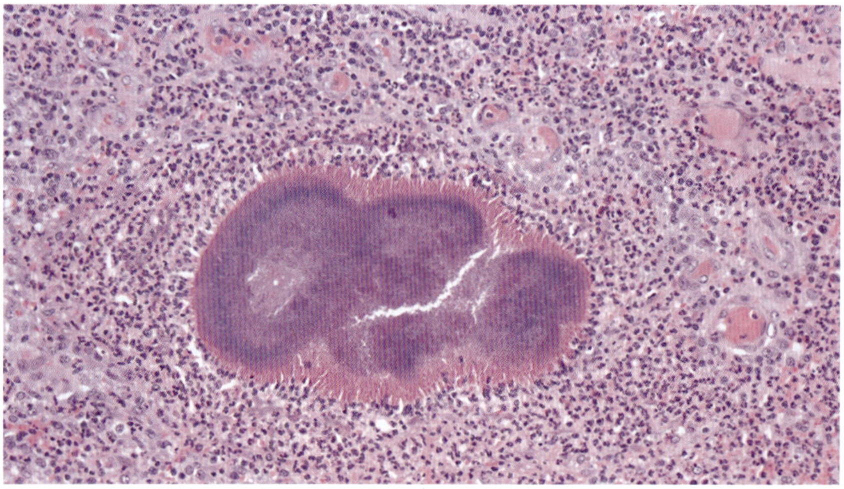

Figure 8-8

ACTINOMYCOSIS, LYMPH NODE

A nidus of *Actinomyces* organisms is surrounded by neutrophils. (Figs. 8-8 and 8-9 are from the same patient.)

infectious sites, and secondary lymphadenitis or splenic abscess may subsequently develop (66,110).

Rhodococcus equi is a widely distributed bacterium that is closely related phylogenetically to *Nocardia*. Infections are most often found in immunocompromised patients (30). The common presentation is a pulmonary cavitary lesion, but lymphadenitis also occurs (26,37,57,106).

Gross Findings. "Sulfur granules" are small (a few millimeters in size), yellow or yellow-brown nodules. They are bacterial colonies with adherent granulocytes seen in actinomycotic infections (fig. 8-7).

Microscopic Findings. In the lymph nodes, the histopathologic changes are similar to those described above for the pyogenic bacteria (figs. 8-8, 8-9). In tissue sections, the organisms do not stain with hematoxylin and eosin (H&E) and can be visualized, instead, with a modified acid-fast stain or tissue Gram stain.

When the infection involves the regional lymph nodes, the histopathologic findings are similar to those produced by the organisms in other organs and include central suppurative necrosis surrounded, at first, by neutrophils and, later, by granulation tissue and subsequent fibrosis. Plasma cells and foamy macrophages (histiocytes) may be prominent, especially within the germinal centers (5). The characteristic histologic feature of *Actinomyces*, which is often noted incidentally in routine tonsillectomy specimens, is the diagnostic mycelial masses or sulfur granules, which are large bacterial colonies. They appear as radiating filaments surrounded by eosinophilic hyaline material (fig. 8-10). The inflammatory cell infiltrate in these cases includes primarily plasma cells and reactive lymphocytes.

Actinomyces and *Nocardia* organisms are gram positive and about 1 μm in diameter. *Actinomyces* is not acid fast, in contrast to *Nocardia*, which stains

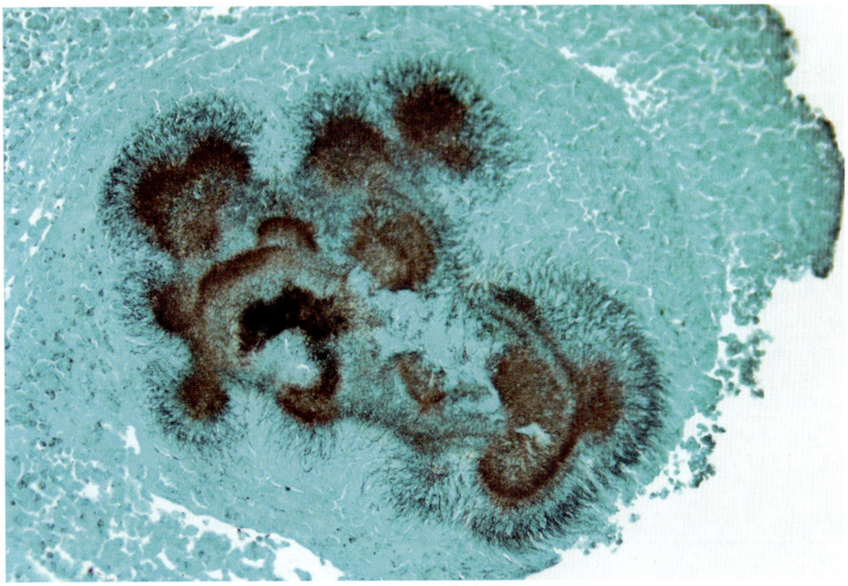

Figure 8-9

ACTINOMYCOSIS, LYMPH NODE

Gomori methenamine silver (GMS) stain.

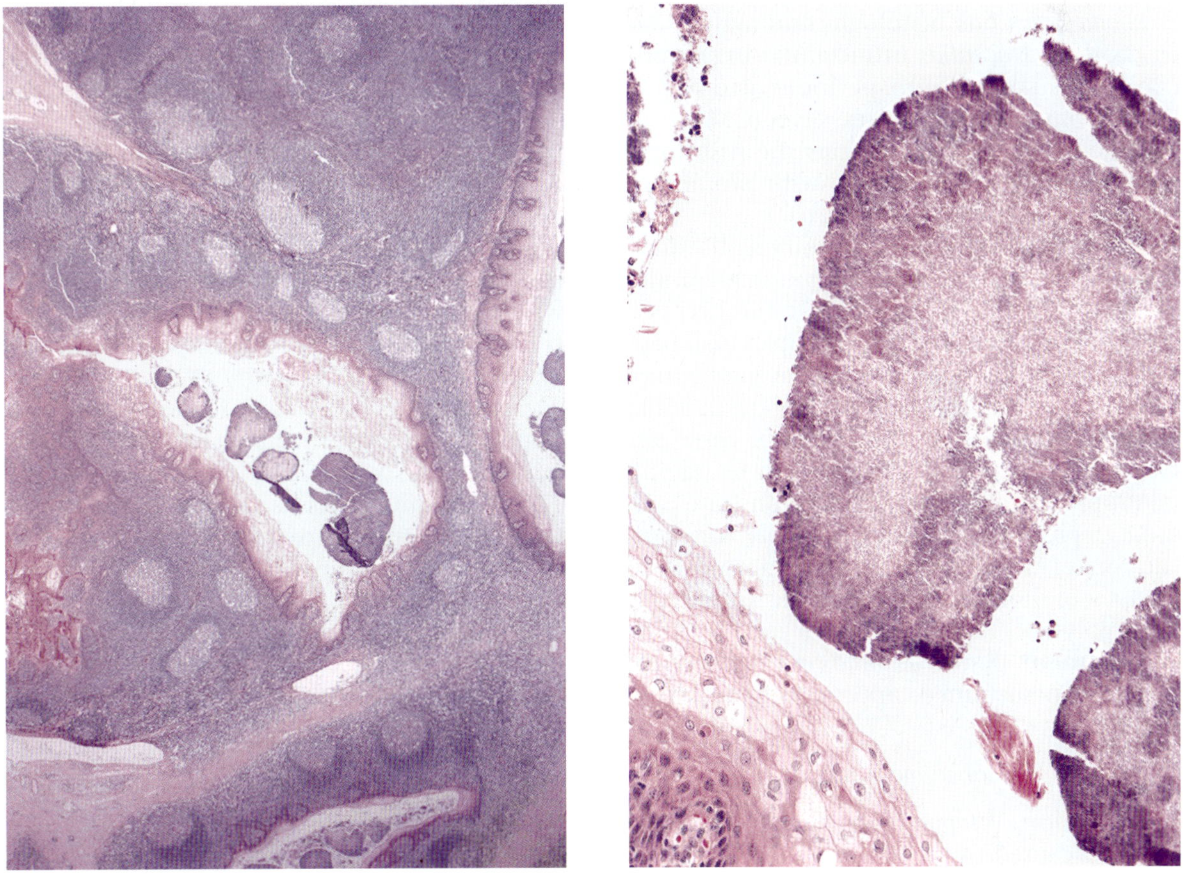

Figure 8-10

ACTINOMYCOSIS, TONSIL

Actinomyces are frequently found in tonsil, where they are not invasive and do not elicit a tissue response.

Figure 8-11

WHIPPLE DISEASE

Lymphadenopathy in Whipple disease is characterized by prominent sinusoidal dilatation (left) and epithelioid macrophages containing periodic acid–Schiff (PAS)-positive organisms (right).

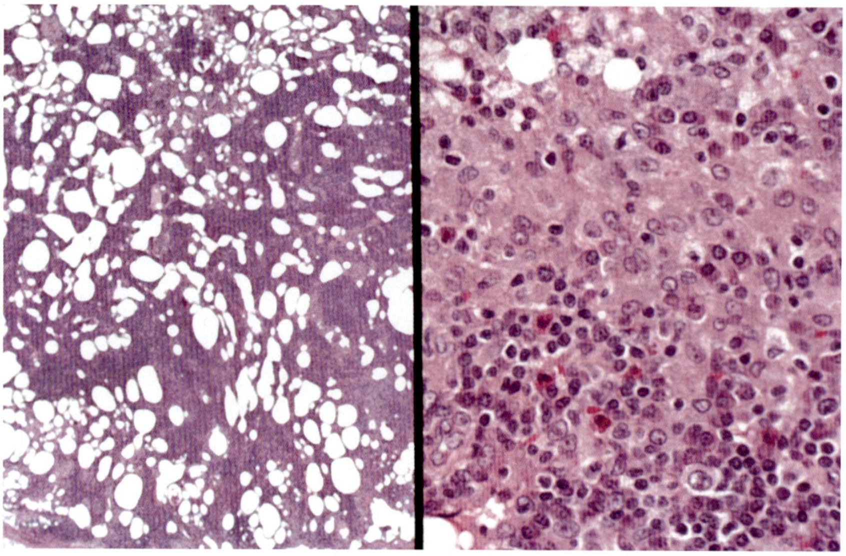

with an acid-fast bacillus (AFB) stain. Sinus tract formation may be seen in these infections.

Rhodococcus has histologic findings similar to those of *Nocardia*. Intracellular organisms can be visualized with periodic acid–Schiff (PAS), Gomori methenamine silver (GMS), and AFB stains. Rarely, *R. equi* has the histologic appearance of malakoplakia, with prominent Michaelis-Gutman bodies (30,107).

Differential Diagnosis. The differential diagnosis of the acute, exudative lymphadenitides includes viral infections, which cause necrosis, such as Epstein-Barr and herpes simplex (see chapter 9), and the so-called suppurative granulomas, such as cat-scratch disease and lymphogranuloma venereum (see later in this chapter). These last two entities, however, in addition to having neutrophilic infiltration, also demonstrate palisading epithelioid macrophages that surround the foci of necrosis. Kikuchi-Fujimoto disease (chapter 6) shows similar histologic features but lacks polymorphonuclear leukocytes.

Treatment. Both *Nocardia* and *Actinomyces* respond to sustained, appropriate antibiotic therapy.

Tropheryma Whipplei

Definition. *Whipple disease* is a multisystem disorder caused by infection with *Tropheryma whipplei.* Although the disease most commonly presents as gastrointestinal manifestations, lymph node and splenic involvement are seen as well.

General Features. Whipple disease primarily affects the small bowel mucosa, as well as other organs including lymph nodes. It usually presents as a malabsorption syndrome and is considered to be more common in males in the 4th to 5th decades of life. The abdominal, or even peripheral, lymph nodes may be involved in patients with gastrointestinal Whipple disease. Generalized lymphadenopathy occurs in about 50 percent of patients. The clinical findings are often nonspecific and include fatigue, weight loss, polyarthralgia, and diarrhea. Less commonly, the initial manifestation of the disease is lymphadenopathy (4). The causative bacterium has recently been identified and classified as *T. whipplei* (the name has been recently revised from "whippleii" to "whipplei") (97). The bacterium cannot be cultured using routine techniques, and the diagnosis is usually based on histologic examination, with other ancillary studies for confirmation.

Gross Findings. The cut surface of lymph nodes extensively involved by Whipple disease is described as yellow and "spongy" (89).

Microscopic Findings. The characteristic histopathologic features include dilatation of lymph node sinuses by large lipid vacuoles and multinucleated giant cells, and macrophages with abundant vacuolated cytoplasm, imparting a "Swiss cheese" appearance (fig. 8-11). An occasional non-necrotizing (sarcoid-like) granuloma is noted. Splenic involvement shows similar histologic features. The macrophages contain

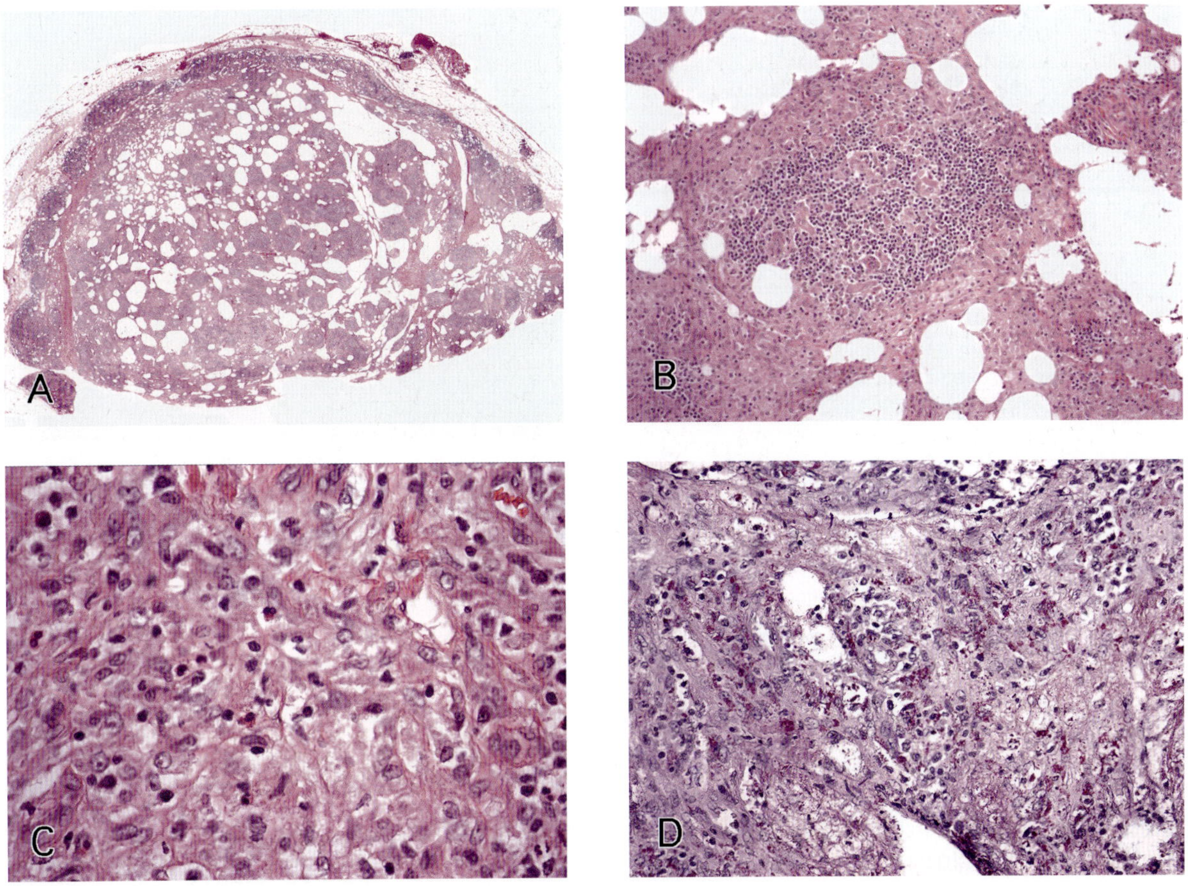

Figure 8-12

WHIPPLE DISEASE

The massive sinusoidal dilatation seen in Whipple disease is highlighted.

diastase-resistant PAS-positive, rod-shaped bacilli that can be seen by light microscopy (fig. 8-12) (35,80). These bacteria are negative for AFB stains. The organisms are identified by electron microscopy, but more recently, conformation is by immunohistochemical or polymerase chain reaction (PCR) study (9,42,56,77,136).

Differential Diagnosis. The differential diagnosis includes lymphangiogram effect (which lacks organisms in similar-appearing foamy macrophages), and other infectious agents, especially the atypical mycobacterium, *Mycobacterium avium-intracellulare,* and *Rhodococcus equi* (42).

Treatment and Prognosis. Whipple disease is an important condition to recognize since it is promptly cured by appropriate antibiotic therapy. A case report of concurrent B-cell lymphoma and Whipple disease in lymph nodes raised the possibility that *T. whipplei* may initiate lymphomagenesis in a similar manner to *Helicobacter pylori* in extranodal marginal zone lymphoma; however, the rarity of this combination suggests that this may be a chance occurrence (132).

Bacillus Anthracis

Definition. *Anthrax,* caused by the gram-positive bacterium, *Bacillus anthracis,* is a cause of adenopathy and, rarely, splenic involvement in disseminated disease.

General Features. *B. anthracis,* the etiologic agent of anthrax, is an encapsulated, gram-positive, spore-bearing organism found in many animal species, and transmitted to man primarily by contact with infected animal hides or carcasses. Anthrax has more recently gained

Table 8-1

BIOTERRORISM AGENTS WITH POSSIBLE LYMPH NODE FINDINGS

CDC[a] Category	Disease/Agent	Chapter Discussed
A	Anthrax (*Bacillus anthracis*)	This
	Plague (*Yersinia pestis*)	This
	Smallpox (variola major)	9
	Tularemia (*Francisella tularensis*)	This
	Hemorrhagic fever viruses (including Marburg, Ebola, and Lassa)	9
B	Brucellosis (*Brucella* species)	This
	Q fever (*Coxiella burnetii*)	This
	Typhus fever (*Rickettsia prowazekii*)	This
	Glanders (*Burkholderia mallei*)	This

[a]CDC = Centers for Disease Control.

notoriety for its use as a bioterrorism agent and through accidental infection from military or research stores (Table 8-1) (1,10,62).

The primary lesion is a cutaneous hemorrhagic pustule that eventually ruptures to form a black eschar (fig. 8-13). There is secondary, tender regional lymphadenopathy due to spread along the lymphatic channels. In inhalational anthrax, involvement includes lungs, mediastinal lymph nodes, pleural cavities, and frequently, the heart. Hemorrhagic thoracic lymphadenitis and hemorrhagic mediastinitis are cardinal signs of inhalation anthrax. Sites that are involved in disseminated anthrax infection are the gastrointestinal tract, skin, spleen, and liver.

In all circumstances of possible anthrax infection, public health authorities should be consulted. Confirmational tests including enzyme-linked immunosorbent assay (ELISA) serology, immunohistochemistry, or PCR should be performed, usually at specialized labs.

Microscopic Findings. The lymph nodes may show hemorrhagic necrosis and edema in the interstitial regions, and bacilli both within macrophages and free-floating in the lymphatic vessels (58,60,125). Neutrophils and prominent immunoblasts may infiltrate the nodes (fig. 8-14). Splenic white pulp shows necrosis, with fragmented cellular debris, changes more prominent in the periarterial lymphatic sheaths (PALS) than the germinal centers (58). The red pulp shows expanded cords with macrophages containing numerous ingested bacteria. Vasculitis is rarely seen.

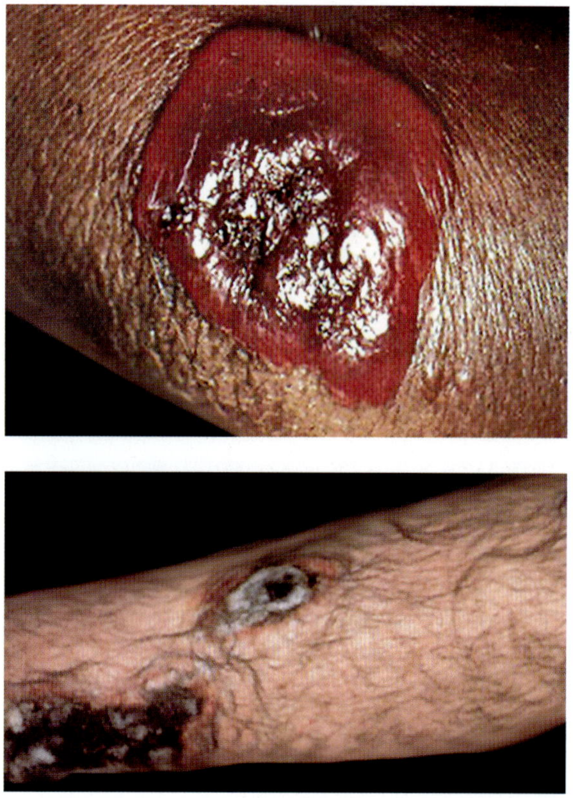

Figure 8-13

ANTHRAX, ESCHAR

The cutaneous lesions of anthrax are seen. (Courtesy of Mark Wick, Charlottesville, VA.)

A Gram, Giemsa, or silver stain (Steiner, Dieterle) helps to visualize the organisms (60,125). Immunohistochemical or DNA-based studies (PCR) confirm the presence of the organisms.

GRAM-NEGATIVE BACTERIAL INFECTIONS

As with gram-positive bacteria, the range of gram-negative bacteria that cause either lymph nodal or splenic infections is broad. Several are covered briefly below, while others are covered more extensively.

Gonococcal infection, caused by *Neisseria gonococcus,* is a venereal disease that begins with urethritis, proctitis, or pharyngitis depending upon the mode of sexual transmission. Regional lymphadenitis may result from local or systemic dissemination. Tissue Gram stains (Brown-Hopps, Brown-Brenn) help identify the causative gram-negative

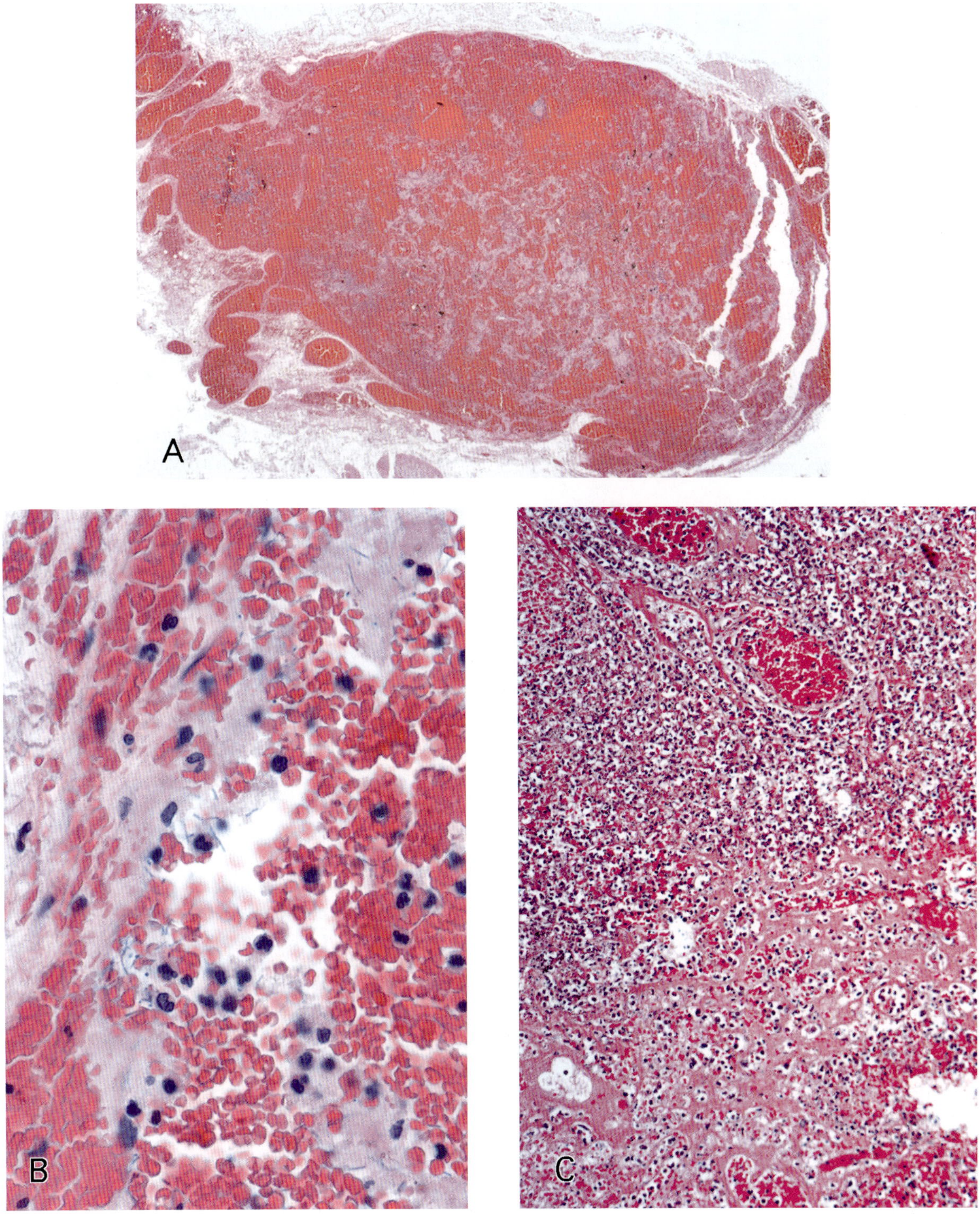

Figure 8-14

ANTHRAX, LYMPH NODE

A lymph node from an experimentally infected primate shows hemorrhage and necrosis (A,B). A lymph node from a fatal human case of anthrax shows similar findings. (A and B courtesy of Keith Steele, LTC, Frederick, MD; C courtesy of Mary G. Ripple, Baltimore, MD.)

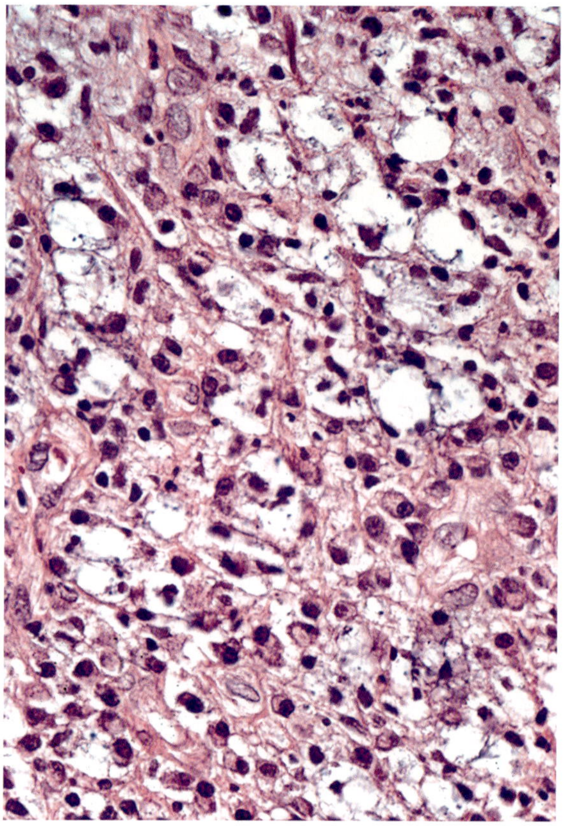

Figure 8-15

RHINOSCLEROMA, LYMPH NODE

Small organisms are seen in the cytoplasm of macrophages. (Courtesy of Luis Fajardo, Palo Alto, CA.)

Neisseria diplococci, but bacterial culture results and biochemical characteristics are the most important methods of diagnosis for bacterial lymphadenitis. *N. gonorrhea* is demonstrated within host phagocytes, most often on smears taken from the primary infective exudate. Histologic changes include necrotizing granulomatous lymphadenitis (31). Regional lymphadenitis associated with a primary bacterial infection usually responds well to appropriate antibiotic therapy for the primary lesion.

Haemophilus ducreyi, the etiologic agent of *chancroid*, causes secondary, tender regional lymphadenitis. Histologically, this is characterized by neutrophilic microabscesses and acute suppuration. Capsular edema and inflammation may result in perforation with sinus tract formation (103). Although clinically similar to lymphogranuloma venereum, the lymphadenitis secondary to *H. ducreyi* lacks the characteristic stellate microabscesses that are associated with lymphogranuloma venereum. Positive culture results and skin test confirm a diagnosis of chancroid.

Another sexually-transmitted bacterial disease is *granuloma inguinale*, caused by *Calymmatobacterium granulomatis*. Most commonly a tropical disease, granuloma inguinale, also called *donovanosis*, is most common in young adults. Most frequently, it presents as ulcerated, necrotizing skin lesions in the anogenital region. The lymph nodes are not initially enlarged, but ultimately increase in size and form "pseudobuboes." Both suppuration and granulomas are seen. The characteristic and diagnostic finding is the presence of *C. granulomatis* within the cytoplasm of enlarged macrophages. Single organisms or clusters (Donovan bodies) are in the cystic spaces in the cytoplasm. Donovan bodies stain poorly with H&E, but are apparent on Gram or Wright/Wright-Giemsa stains.

Stenotrophomonas maltophilia causes infection in immunocompromised, and rarely, immunocompetent, hosts (106). Granulomatous inflammation may be seen in lymph nodes. *Klebsiella rhinoscleromatis* may cause a foamy macrophage reaction in lymph nodes; this results in the characteristic pathologic findings of *rhinoscleroma* (fig. 8-15) (8,21). Exudative inflammation may also be seen in association with *Pseudomonas aeruginosa*, *Escherichia coli*, *Streptococcus faecalis*, and *Streptomyces madurae*. *Pasteurella multocida* may cause granulomatous lymphadenitis.

Legionella pneumophila and related species are most known for outbreaks of an acute respiratory disease, *Legionnaire disease* (137). Lymphadenopathy and splenic pathology are rarely seen (fig. 8-16). In involved lymph nodes, there is hyperplasia with sinus histiocytosis. The causative bacteria are rarely identified. Splenic changes are most often red pulp congestion and expansion, but little change in the white pulp. Rarely, *Legionella* organisms are associated with splenic rupture (36).

Bartonella Henselae and *B. Quintana:* Cat-Scratch Disease

Definition. A common and well-characterized cause of necrotizing granulomatous lymphadenitis, *cat-scratch disease*, is caused most commonly by *Bartonella henselae*. Splenic involvement, although rare, can be seen.

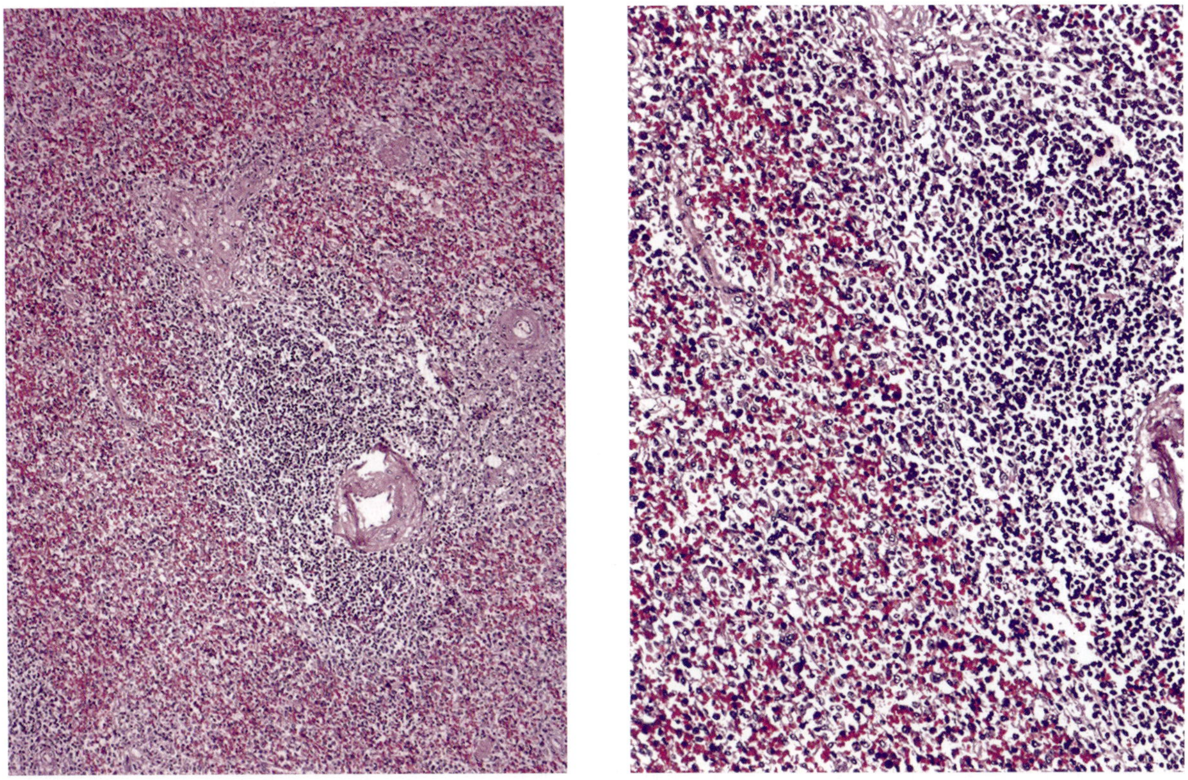

Figure 8-16

LEGIONELLA, SPLEEN

No specific histologic changes are seen, although this spleen was culture positive for *Legionella*. (Courtesy of California Tumor tissue Registry, Loma Linda, CA.)

General Features. Cat-scratch disease is a bacterial infection that classically results in localized lymphadenopathy proximal to the bite or scratch of a cat. It occurs in both children and adults, and is usually self-limited (41,90,133). In approximately half of the cases, regional lymphadenitis, most often in the cervical, axillary, epitrochlear, or supraclavicular region is the only sign of the disease (82). This is usually seen 10 days to 2 weeks after primary inoculation of organisms in the skin. If systemic symptoms do occur, they frequently include fever, malaise, and anorexia. Laboratory findings include elevation of the sedimentation rate and mild neutrophilia or eosinophilia. About 10 percent of patients develop complications including hepatic granulomas, splenic abscesses, or encephalitis (34,98,130). Over a period of weeks or months, the lymph nodes become suppurative or spontaneously regress. In most cases, full resolution occurs within 1 month even without treatment.

Wear et al. (133) at the Armed Forces Institute of Pathology were the first to isolate the causative bacterium of cat-scratch disease, a pleomorphic gram-negative rod. Subsequent studies have shown that *B. henselae* is visualized by the Warthin-Starry silver impregnation method (fig. 8-17) (41,86), immunohistochemistry, or electron microscopy. The organism was initially referred to as *Afipia felis* sp.nov., but has since been reclassified as *B. henselae* (16,17). *B. quintana* also causes cat-scratch disease, and more rarely, atypical lymph node hyperplasia (fig. 8-18).

Microscopic Findings. The histopathologic changes in the lymph nodes depend on the duration/stage of the disease. Initially, there is reactive follicular hyperplasia with focal areas of necrosis and cellular debris showing neutrophilic infiltration (fig. 8-19). Subcapsular infiltration by a sinusoidal monocytoid B-cell infiltrate is often present. In later stages, there are giant cells and palisading epithelioid macrophages, which

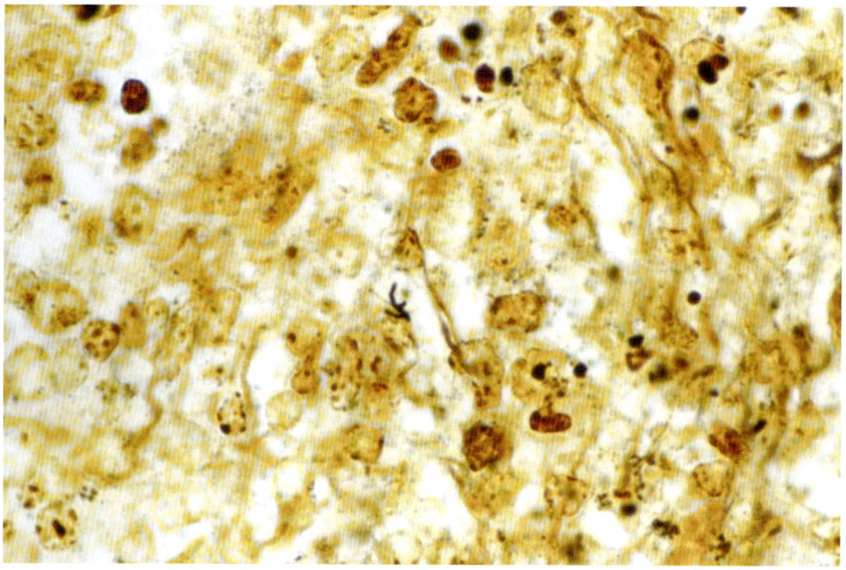

Figure 8-17

CAT-SCRATCH DISEASE

The causative agent of cat-scratch disease, *Bartonella henselae*, is highlighted by the Warthin-Starry stain.

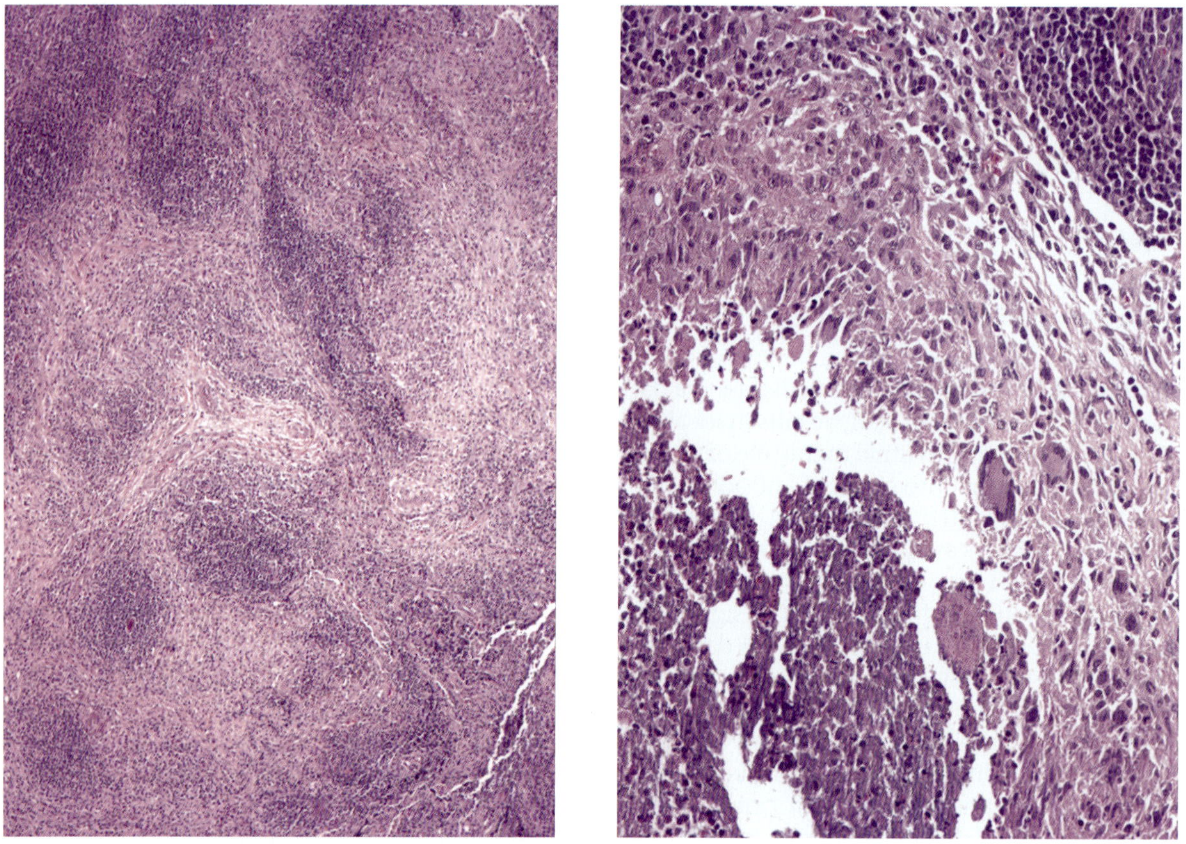

Figure 8-18

BARTONELLA QUINTANA, LYMPH NODE

A rare causative agent of necrotizing granulomatous lymphadenitis, *B. quintana* has a histologic appearance similar to *B. henselae*. Low magnification (left) shows necrosis and granulomatous inflammation, while higher magnification (right) highlights necrosis and macrophages. Culture or other microbiologic studies are required to distinguish the two organisms. (Courtesy of Peter Banks, Charlotte, NC.)

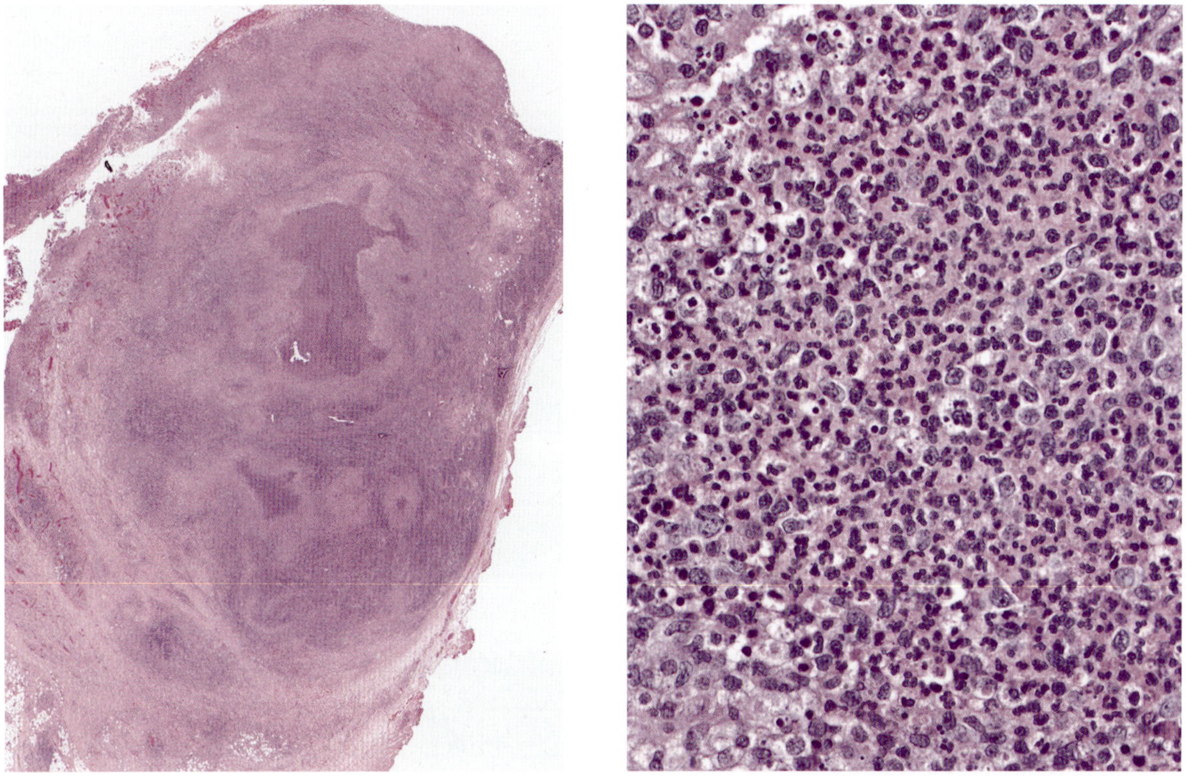

Figure 8-19

CAT-SCRATCH DISEASE

A stellate granuloma (left) and details of an abscess (right) in this case of cat-scratch disease.

surround larger areas of suppurative necrosis, forming the "stellate microabscesses" (figs. 8-20, 8-21) (19,86). The same lymph node may show other lesions varying from small, well-formed granulomas with small foci of necrosis, to large areas of suppuration. Plasmacytoid dendritic cells, which are identified by staining for CD123, are increased (71). Splenic involvement shows similar necrotizing, granulomatous reactions (fig. 8-22) (78). *B. henselae* infection has been associated with splenic rupture (32). Immunohistochemistry is used to confirm the diagnosis.

Differential Diagnosis. Other causes of necrotizing granulomatous lymphadenitis should be considered in the differential diagnosis. Lymphogranuloma venereum, discussed later in this chapter, may have an identical histologic appearance. Clinical information can usually distinguish the two entities.

Treatment and Prognosis. There is no definitive treatment for cat-scratch disease although oral and intravenous (in systemic cases) antibiotics have been used successfully (19). Azithromycin has been suggested as an effective therapeutic approach (43). Local drainage of the lymph node, if there is abscess formation, may also be therapeutic. In the majority of cases, however, the disease has a benign, self-limited course with an excellent prognosis, primarily requiring reassurance for the patient.

Bartonella Henselae and *B. Quintana*: Bacillary Angiomatosis

Definition. *Bacillary angiomatosis* is a vascular proliferation which is associated with localized infection by *Bartonella henselae*, or more rarely, *B. quintana*.

General Features. Bacillary angiomatosis is typically seen in patients with human immunodeficiency virus (HIV)/acquired immunodeficiency disease syndrome (AIDS) and other immunocompromised patients. Often, patients have had previous exposure to cats. Exposure can occur at any site, with skin being most

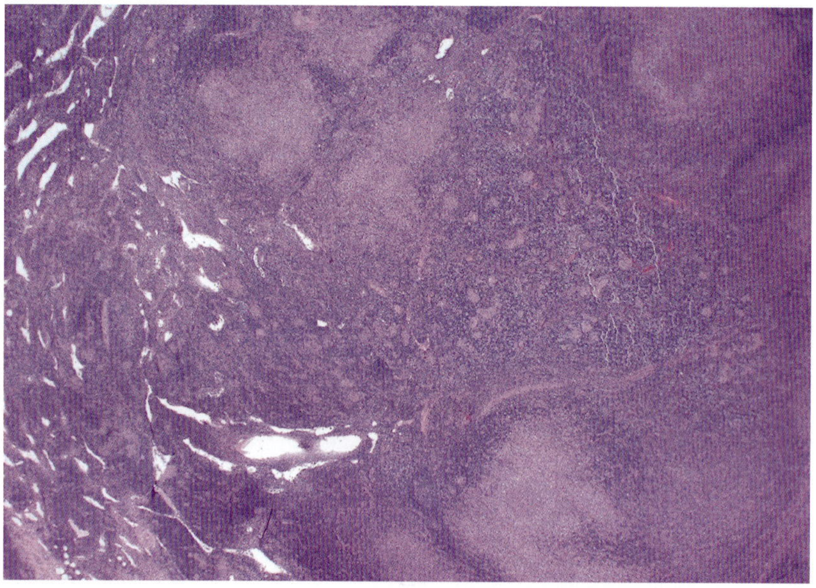

Figure 8-20

CAT-SCRATCH DISEASE

Cat-scratch lymphadenitis with multiple palisading granulomas.

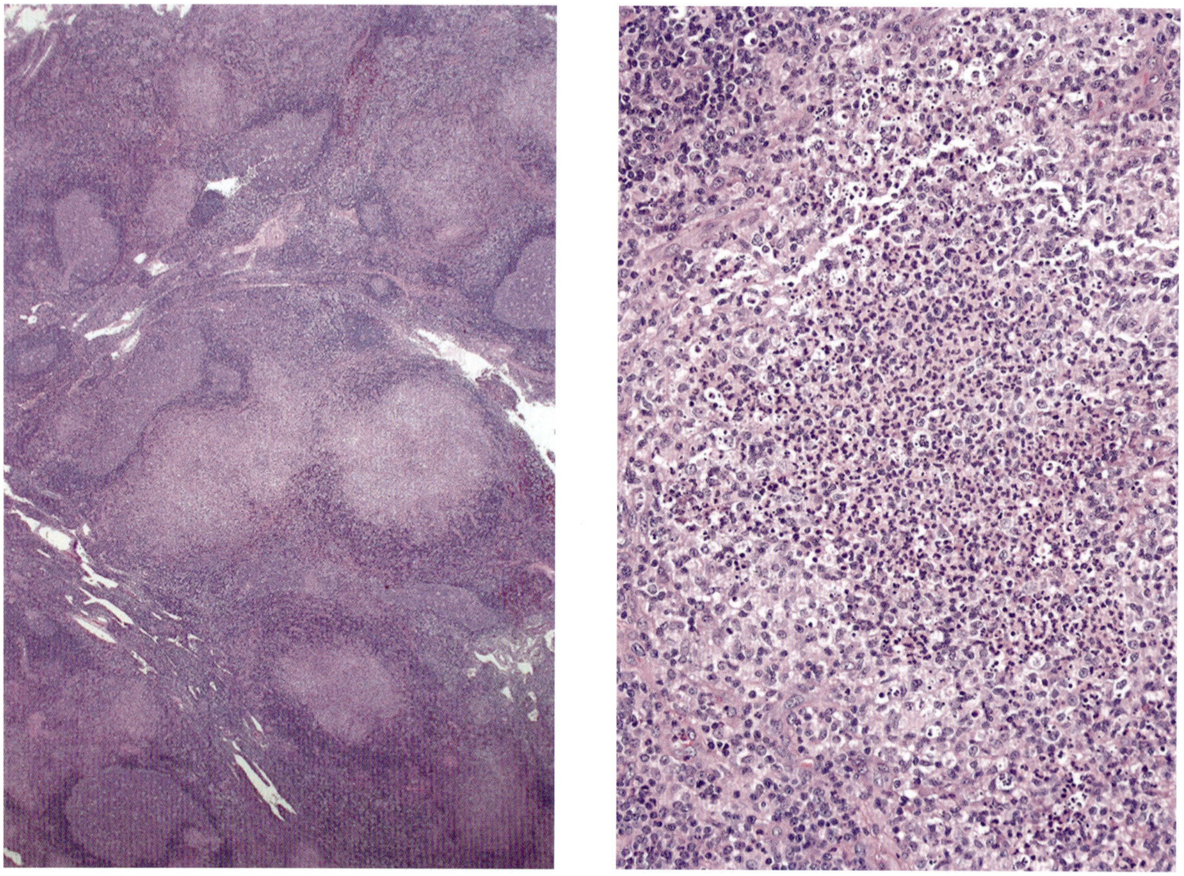

Figure 8-21

CAT-SCRATCH DISEASE

Classic suppurative granulomas with palisading epithelioid macrophages surround central areas of necrosis.

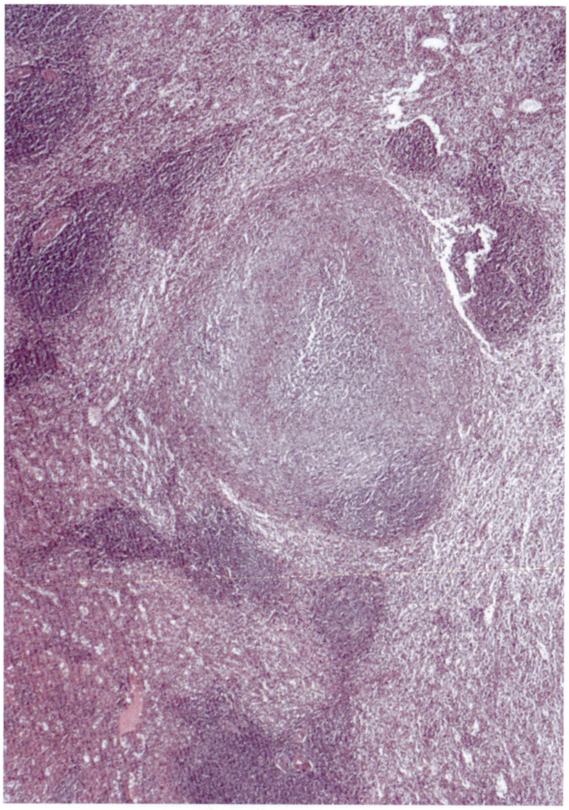

Figure 8-22

CAT-SCRATCH DISEASE, SPLEEN

Although rare, the findings of cat-scratch disease can also be seen in the spleen.

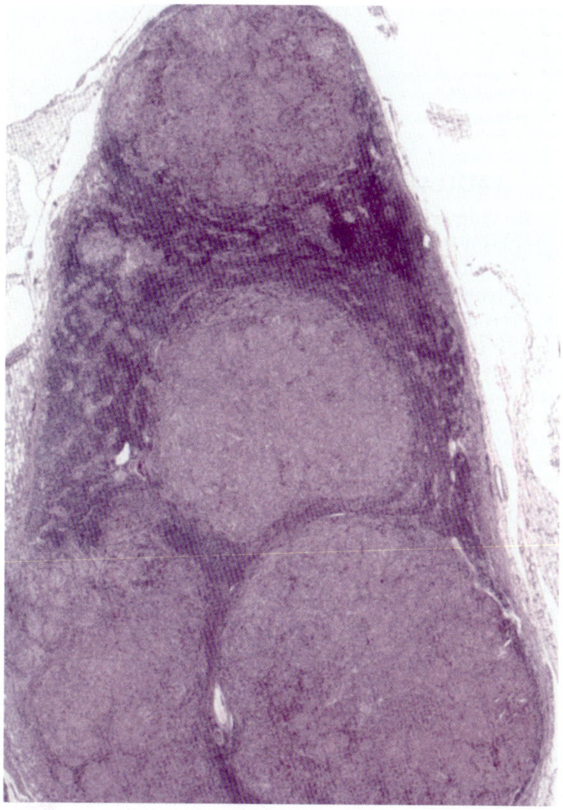

Figure 8-23

BACILLARY ANGIOMATOSIS, LYMPH NODE

The normal architecture is replaced by well-demarcated, pale-staining nodules.

common. The reservoir of *B. henselae* is fleas and ticks, as well as cats.

A recently described infectious process, bacillary angiomatosis is associated with HIV-related lymphadenopathy. Bacillary angiomatosis is an important entity to recognize because of its similarity to vascular neoplasms and its potential for complete cure by the appropriate antibiotic therapy (see chapter 17). This disease has been described as a "pseudoneoplastic" process and was initially reported in the clinical literature as a cutaneous lesion in HIV-positive patients (118) and referred to as epithelioid angiomatosis (28). An infectious agent was identified that shows similarities to the cat-scratch bacillus, including positive staining by the Warthin-Starry method and immunoreactivity with antisera raised against cultured cat-scratch bacilli. Both organisms also show a similar electron microscopic appearance. The question was whether the same organism was involved in both cat-scratch disease and bacillary angiomatosis, the latter of which could therefore be regarded as the "cat-scratch disease of AIDS" (6,75). Bacillary angiomatosis was soon reported to occur in other organs, including the lymph nodes of immunosuppressed patients (22).

It was originally thought that the cause of bacillary angiomatosis was a rickettsia-like organism closely related to *Rochalimaea quintana* (97). Upon further study, the organism has been reclassified as *B. henselae* (17,134). It is usually responsive to antibiotic treatment, especially erythromycin

Microscopic Findings. The histopathologic changes of the lymph nodes include pale nodules (fig. 8-23) composed of vessels lined by plump endothelial cells with finely vacuolated cytoplasm and interspersed spindle cells (fig. 8-24). There is prominent interstitial amphophilic

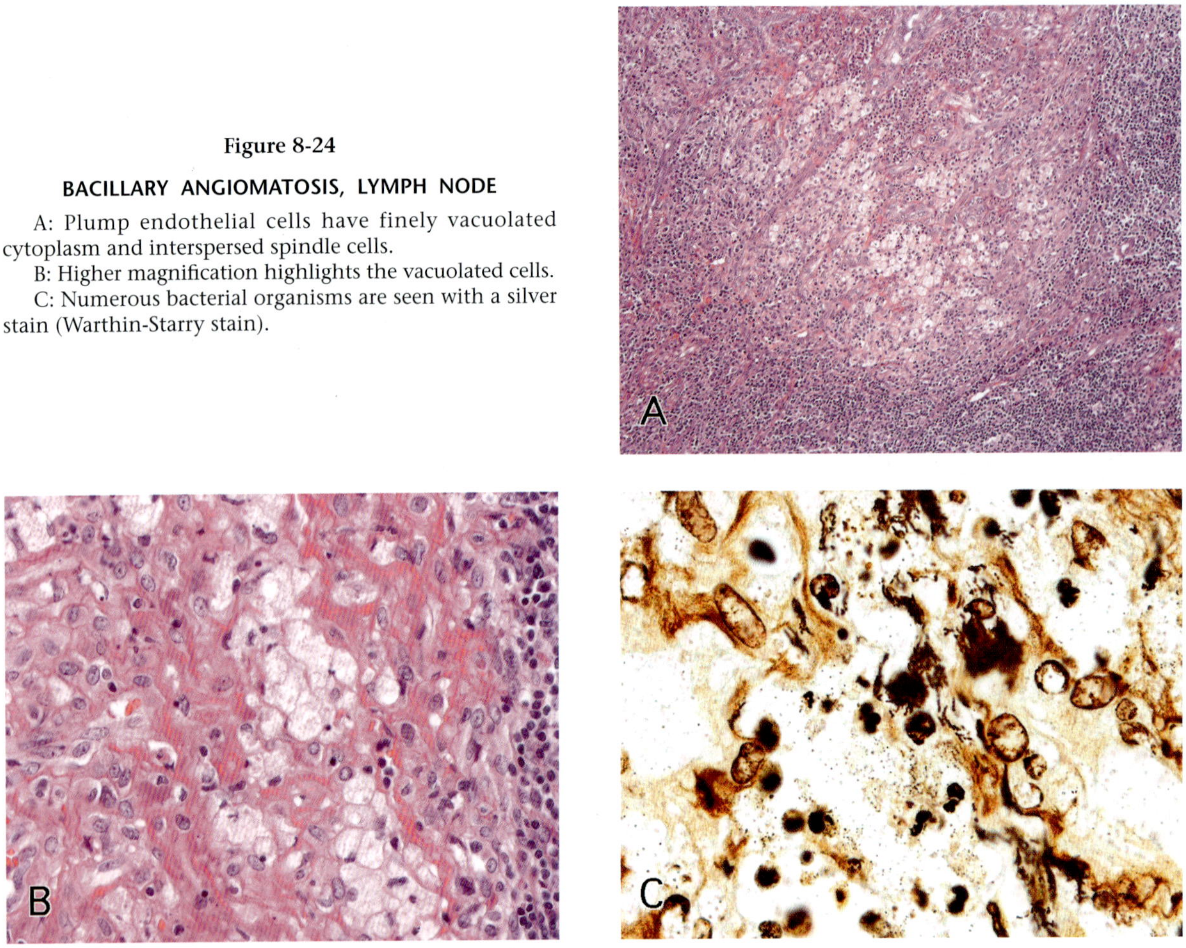

Figure 8-24

BACILLARY ANGIOMATOSIS, LYMPH NODE

A: Plump endothelial cells have finely vacuolated cytoplasm and interspersed spindle cells.

B: Higher magnification highlights the vacuolated cells.

C: Numerous bacterial organisms are seen with a silver stain (Warthin-Starry stain).

material between the endothelial channels (fig. 8-25), which represents large numbers or clumps of bacilli. Focally, there are clusters of bacterial organisms, associated with and often surrounded by neutrophils. Striking stromal edema may be present in other areas of the lymph node, as well as collections of foamy macrophages and extravasated red blood cells.

Only rare mitoses or atypical nuclei are present, helping to differentiate this lesion from a malignant vascular neoplasm such as Kaposi sarcoma or angiosarcoma. The Warthin-Starry stain best demonstrates these organisms (fig. 8-26). The bacteria are weakly gram negative.

Salmonella Typhi and *Salmonella Enteritidis*

Definition. *Salmonella typhi* and *Salmonella enteritidis* are the causative agents of *typhoid fever*. Lymphadenopathy and splenic involvement are rarely seen in typhoid fever.

General Features. Typhoid fever is a severe systemic infection caused by *Salmonella* species. Typhoid fever is endemic where there are poor sanitary conditions. Fever, headache, diarrhea, abdominal pain, respiratory symptoms, and prominent hepatosplenomegaly are common clinical findings. Typhoid fever is rare in North America. The gold standard of diagnosis is culture of the causative gram-negative bacilli, although the Widal test or newer, PCR-based assays are also used. The mesenteric lymph nodes are most often involved. A *mesenteric lymphadenitis syndrome*, mimicking appendicitis or infection by *Yersinia* species (see below), has been reported associated with nontyphoidal *Salmonella* species (53).

Microscopic Findings. Nonspecific findings, including marked follicular hyperplasia, plasmacytosis, and sinus histiocytosis, may be seen in Peyer patches, lymph nodes, and spleen (figs. 8-27, 8-28) (106). Macrophages, filled with bacteria, cellular

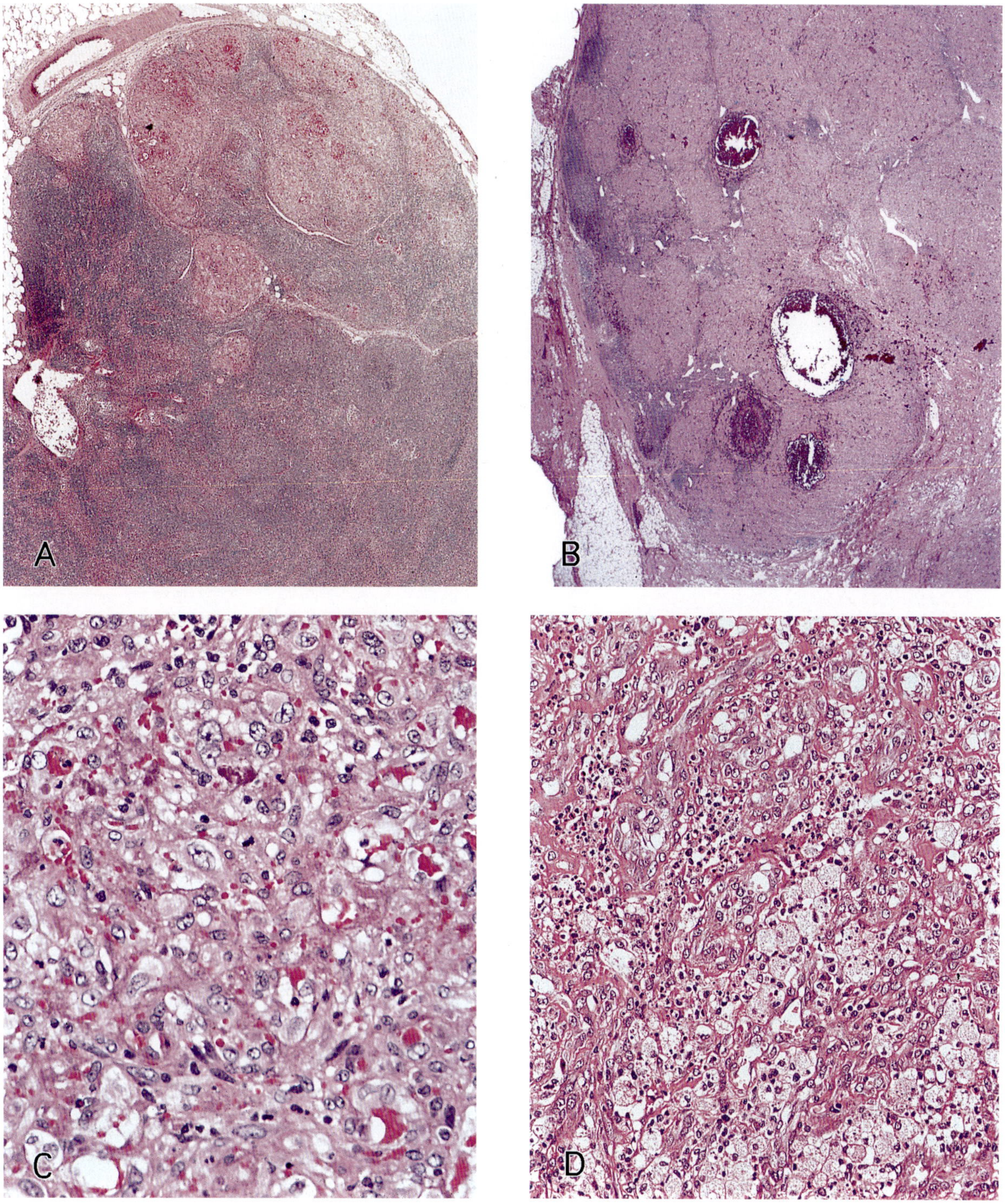

Figure 8-25

BACILLARY ANGIOMATOSIS, LYMPH NODE

A: Lymph node shows a multinodular pattern of involvement.

B: Extensive replacement of the nodal parenchyma by confluent nodules. There are also peliotic spaces.

C: Barely canalized blood vessels are lined by plump cells with atypical nuclei. Neutrophils are sparse, but amphophilic interstitial material is evident.

D: Foamy macrophages are found between blood vessels. (Figs. 21-54, 21-57, and 21-61 from Fascicle 14, Third Series.)

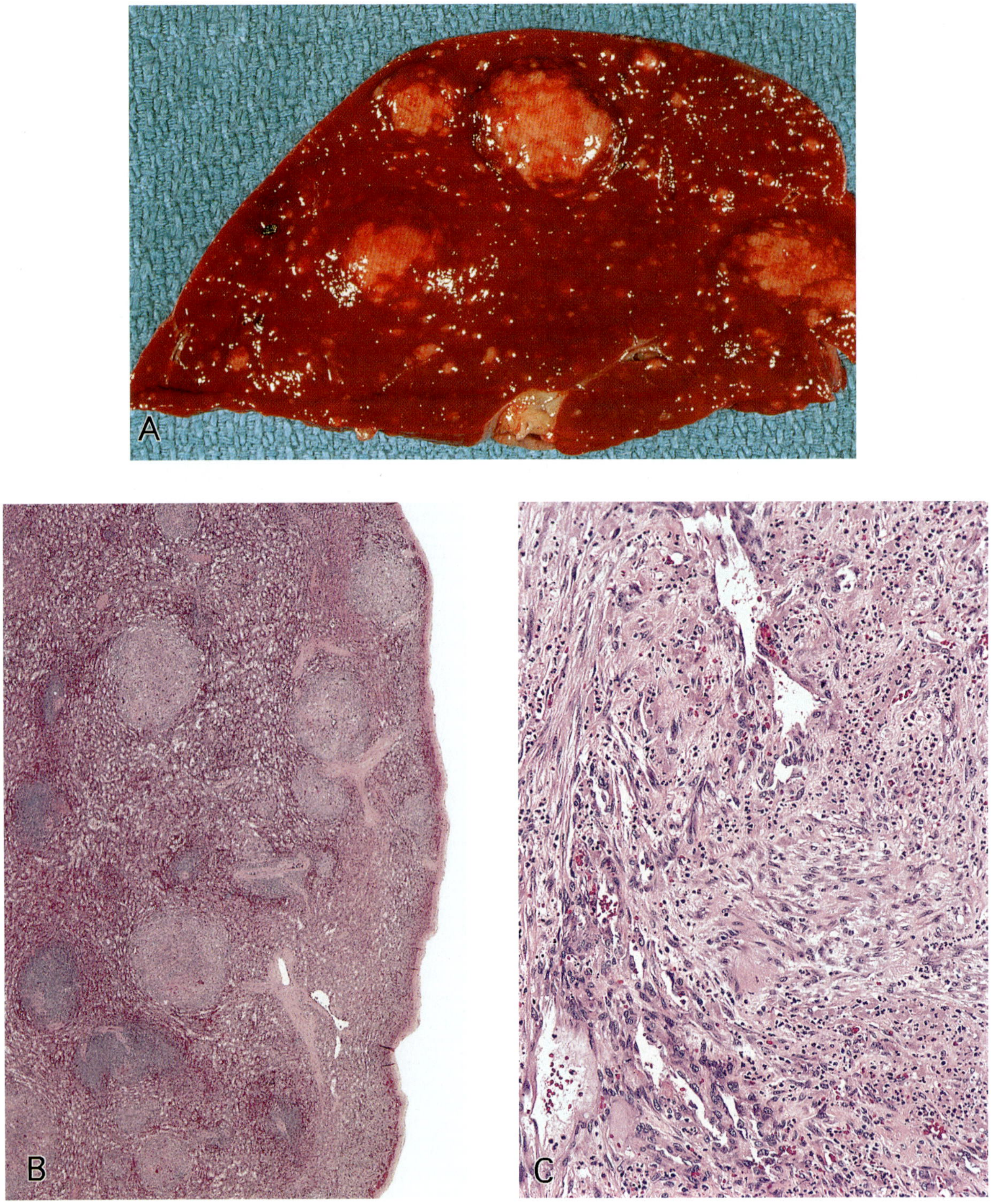

Figure 8-26

BACILLARY ANGIOMATOSIS, SPLEEN

A: The cut surface of the spleen is studded with small and large fleshy nodules of bacillary angiomatosis.

B: These nodules are haphazardly distributed in the splenic parenchyma.

C: Irregular, branching, narrow vascular channels are separated by a fibrous stroma containing amphophilic interstitial deposits and neutrophils. (Figs. 21-55 and 21-58 from Fascicle 14, Third Series.)

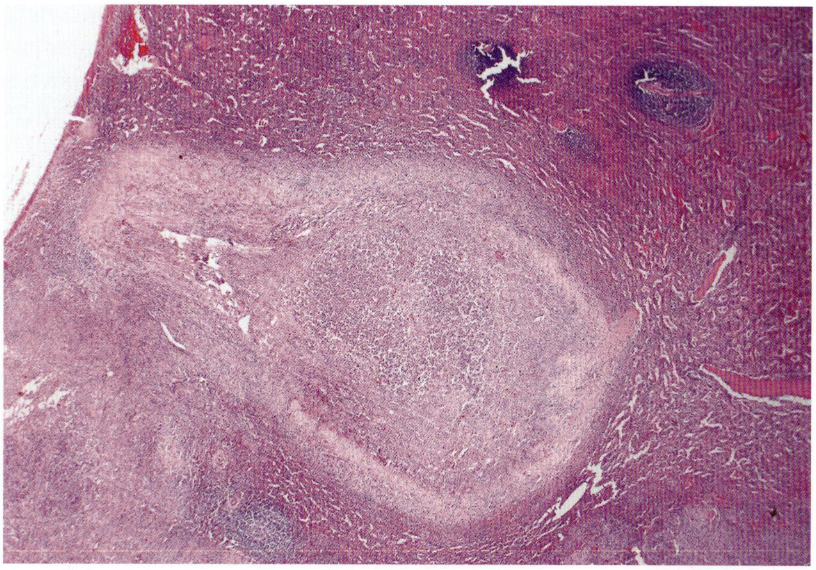

Figure 8-27

TYPHOID, SPLEEN

Large area of necrosis are associated with typhoid. (Courtesy of Thomas Davis, Indianapolis, IN.) (Figs. 8-27 and 8-28 are from the same patient.)

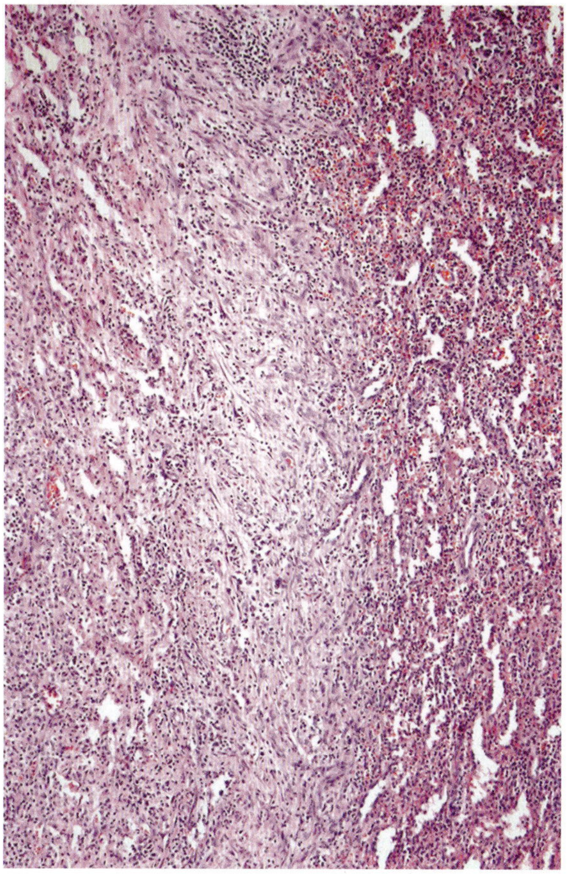

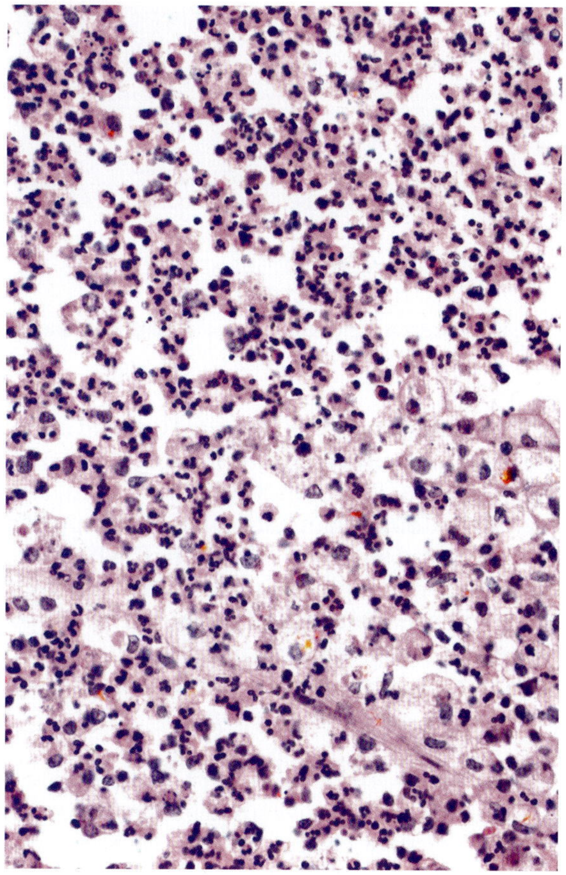

Figure 8-28

TYPHOID, SPLEEN

The wall of the granuloma is composed of organized macrophages and vascular elements (left), while the central portion is composed of neutrophils, macrophages, and cellular debris (right). (Courtesy of Thomas Davis, Indianapolis, IN.)

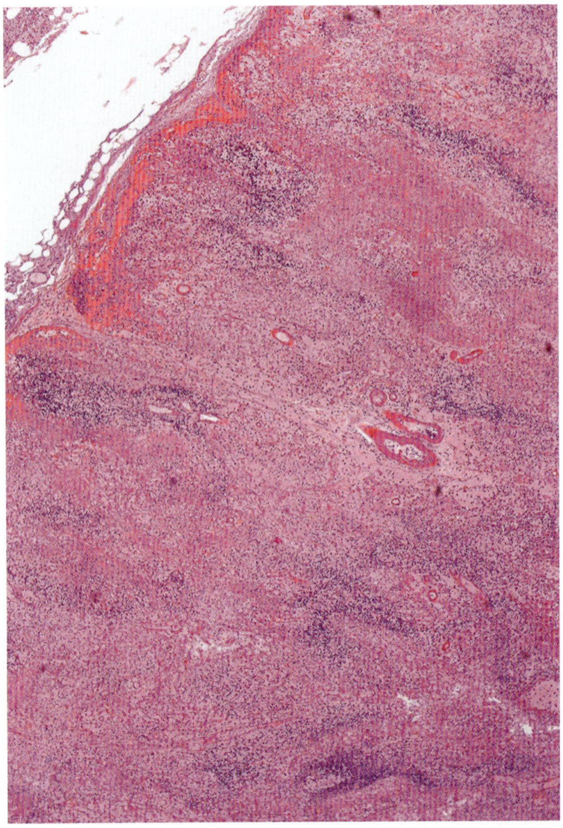

Figure 8-29

PLAGUE, LYMPH NODE

Confluent areas of necrosis and hemorrhage are apparent in this lymph node infected with *Y. pestis*.

debris, and erythrocytes (so-called typhoid cells), are often prominent. Erythrophagocytosis may be prominent. Foci of necrosis may be seen, and granulomatous inflammation has been reported on rare occasion. Typhoid nodules, which are clusters of macrophages with central necrosis, are seen in the spleen, and rarely, in the lymph nodes. Splenic changes include white pulp hyperplasia and red pulp congestion. Splenic rupture is a rare complication (3).

Yersinia Pestis: Plague

Definition. *Plague* is caused by *Yersinia pestis*, a gram-negative bacillus. It may cause significant suppurative lymphadenitis.

General Features. Plague is primarily a disease of wild rodents, which carry *Y. pestis*, a gram-negative bacillus that has a characteristic bipolar or "safety pin" appearance. The disease is found in many parts of the world (especially Asia), including the western United States where it is, fortunately, uncommon. Fleas transmit the disease to rodents and subsequently to man. When *Y. pestis* enters the body, it is rapidly conveyed to regional lymph nodes, resulting in the most common form of the disease, bubonic plague. *Y. pestis* is a potential bioterrorism agent (see Table 8-1).

Microscopic Findings. The histopathologic changes in the lymph nodes include an early mononuclear cell response followed by pronounced neutrophilic infiltration with suppurative microabscesses (figs. 8-29, 8-30) (62). Lymphocyte depletion, necrosis, edema, and foamy macrophages are also seen (61). Hemorrhagic edema and nodal infarction, with subsequent rupture to the skin, are responsible for the characteristic "bubo." The spleen may have multiple abscesses, with increased macrophages in the red pulp (61). Immunohistochemical stains, as well as PCR or direct fluorescent antibody (DFA) assays are available for confirmation of the diagnosis (62).

Treatment and Prognosis. Rapid antibiotic treatment has greatly reduced mortality from this disease. A vaccine is available that offers protection to those who may be exposed to the disease (103).

Other *Yersinia* Infections

Definition. Beside *Yersinia pestis*, the causative agent of plague (see above), other *Yersinia* species have been associated with mostly *mesenteric lymphadenitis*.

General Features. *Yersinia* species are common causes of acute mesenteric lymphadenitis. *Yersinia* enteritis, most often due to *Y. enterocolitica* or *Y. pseudotuberculosis,* is usually a self-limited disease in children or adults, although death may occur if the incorrect diagnosis or treatment is rendered (15). The disease is caused by zoonotic, gram-negative, pleomorphic coccobacilli that can be demonstrated by a tissue Gram stain in histologic sections. Definitive diagnosis relies upon culture of the organism or hemagglutinin test results. Although mesenteric lymph nodes are most often affected by *Yersinia* organisms, pharyngeal lymph nodes may also be involved (15).

Microscopic Findings. The mesenteric lymphadenitis caused by *Y. enterocolitica* (15) or *Y. pseudotuberculosis* (40) shows histopathologic

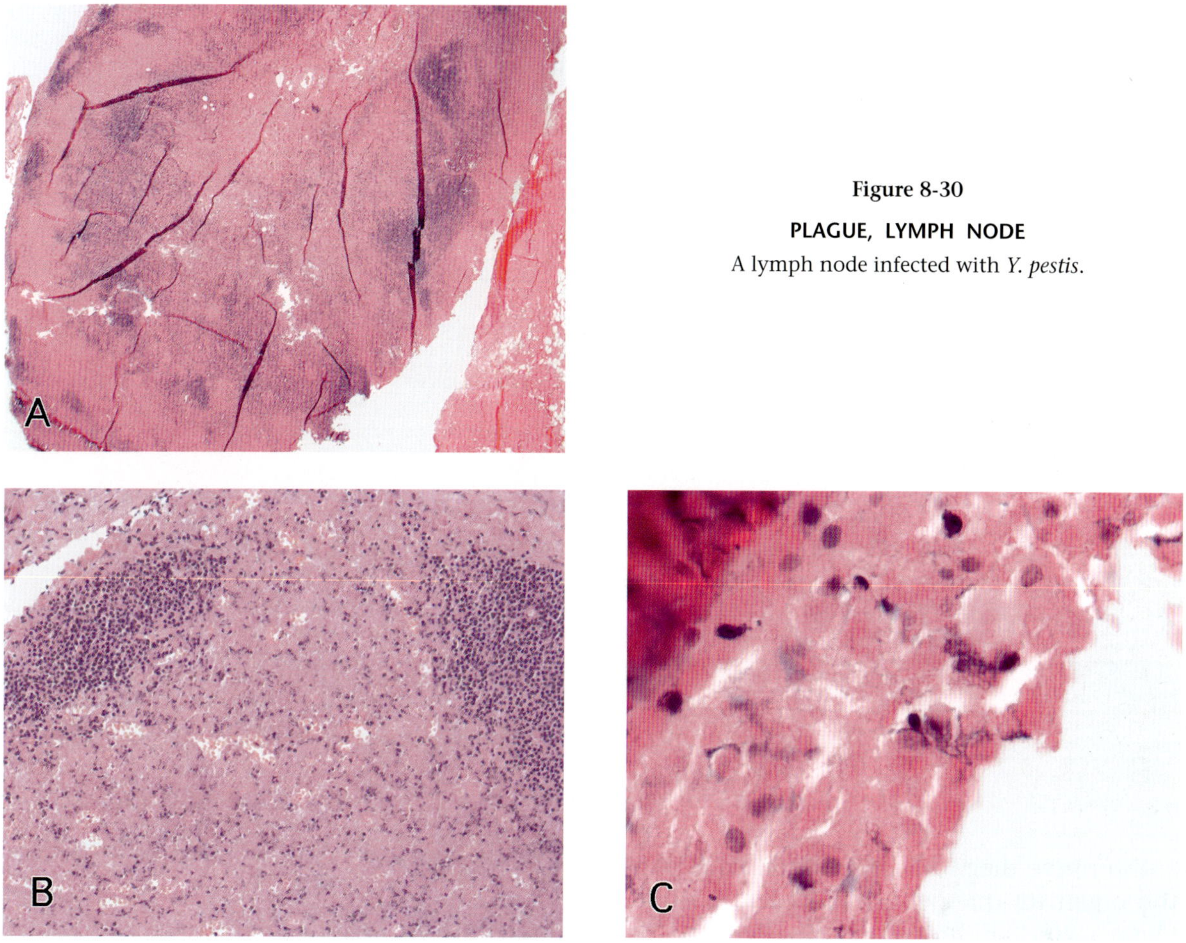

Figure 8-30

PLAGUE, LYMPH NODE

A lymph node infected with *Y. pestis*.

features similar to those described for cat-scratch disease and lymphogranuloma venereum. The histopathologic changes include epithelioid granulomas in various stages of development, with extensive central necrosis associated with neutrophils and eosinophils. Suppurative granulomas with identifiable organisms may be noted within the germinal centers (fig. 8-31). This localization is different than cat-scratch lymphadenitis in which the granulomas typically do not occur within the germinal centers. Reactive follicular hyperplasia with subcapsular infiltration by sinusoidal lymphocytes, paracortical immunoblastic proliferation, and capsular thickening are other nonspecific findings (105).

Francisella Tularensis

Definition. *Tularemia* is a zoonotic disease caused by *Francisella tularensis*; it is a rare cause of lymphadenitis.

General Features. *Francisella tularensis* is an intracellular, gram-negative bacillus that is transmitted by ticks, other insects, or handling of infected animals. Tularemia has a worldwide distribution and 5 percent morbidity. Man is often primarily inoculated by handling rabbits or their skins. Lymphadenopathy is a prominent feature in three of the four major clinical forms of the disease, namely, ulceroglandular, oculoglandular, and glandular types, of which the ulceroglandular is the most common (50,123). The lymph nodes that drain the primary inoculation site become enlarged and fluctuant.

The peripheral blood may show a leukemoid reaction (increase in granulocytes, probably with a left shift) and intracellular organisms (gram-negative bacilli) in the late stages. The bone marrow shows multiple necrotizing, epithelioid granulomas in disseminated disease. *F. tularensis* is a potential bioterrorism agent (see Table 8-1).

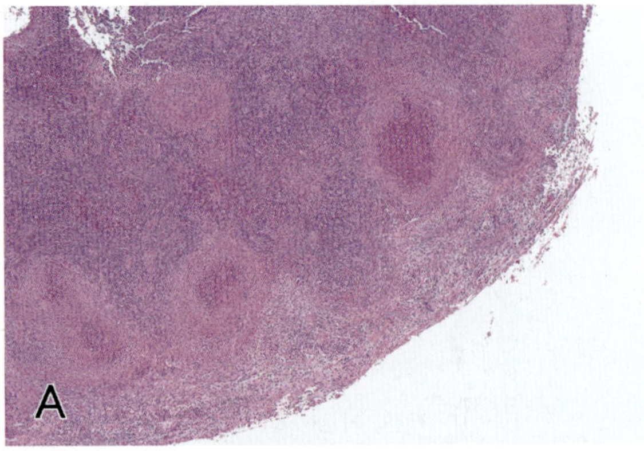

Figure 8-31

***YERSINIA*, MESENTERIC LYMPHADENITIS**

A mesenteric lymph node infected with *Yersinia* has germinal center-based abscesses.

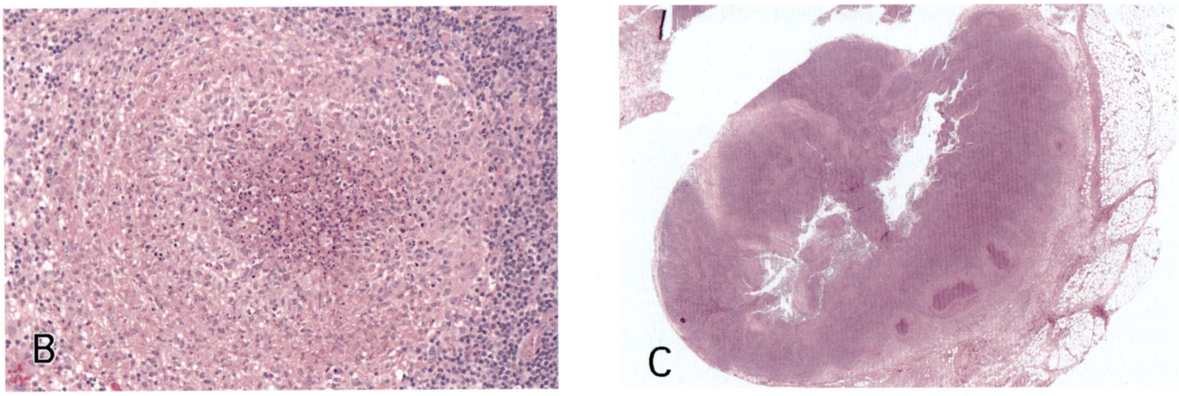

Definitive diagnosis relies upon culture of the organism on special media and positive heme agglutination test results. There are few ways to confirm this diagnosis, and most rely on identification of the agent in other tissue by means such as serology or PCR studies. *F. tularensis* is considered to be a significant biohazard, and culture should not be attempted under routine conditions. Although antibiotic treatment is beneficial, especially in the acute phase of tularemia, it must be sustained in order to prevent relapse.

Microscopic Findings. The histopathologic changes of the lymph nodes and spleen include follicular hyperplasia and epithelioid cell granulomas, with or without giant cells or necrosis (figs. 8-32, 8-33) (74). Increased neutrophils associated with microabscess formation and palisading suppurative granulomas eventually occur, similar to those lesions already discussed. Ulceration of the infected skin via sinus tracts may occur. The causative coccobacillus may be demonstrated by methylene blue or silver staining of lymph node aspirate smears. Immunohistochemical stains and DFA assays are available (62).

Brucella

Definition. *Brucellosis* is a bacterial infection, caused by *Brucella* organisms, that typically results from animal exposure. It is an infrequent cause of *granulomatous lymphadenitis*.

General Features. Although brucellosis may have varied clinical manifestations, most cases present as an acute febrile, systemic illness in those who work in veterinary medicine, meat processing plants, or animal husbandry, or in consumers of contaminated milk products. The disease is most prevalent in countries that lack meat inspections or pasteurized milk products. *Brucella* is also a potential bioterrorism agent (see Table 8-1).

Of the four species of *Brucella* that affect humans, *B. abortus* predominates in the United States. The organism is a gram-negative, aerobic, intracellular coccobacillus whose growth rate is inhibited by macrophage activation. The infection may be inapparent, acute, or chronic with fever of unknown origin (142). Chronic hepatosplenic abscesses can be seen (29). After a brief period of bacteremia, *Brucella* can cause

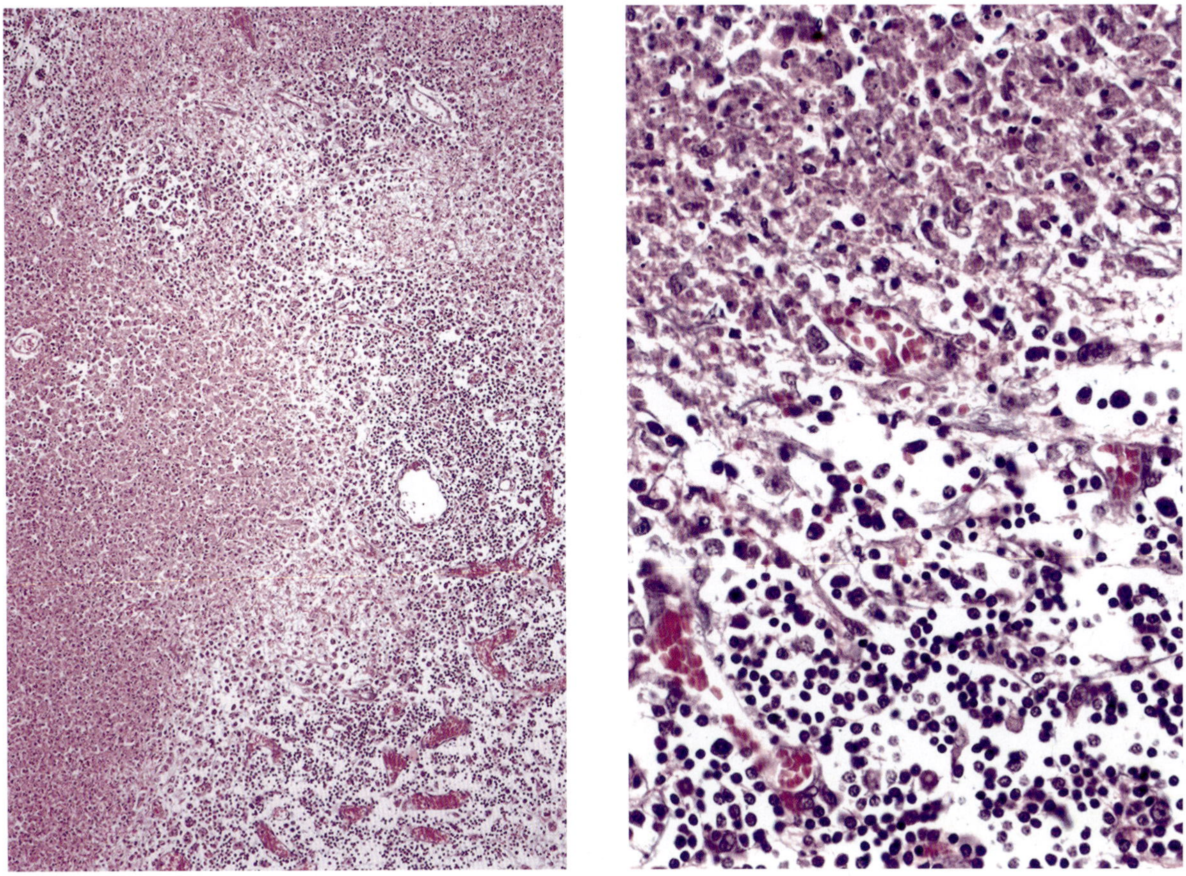

Figure 8-32

TULAREMIA, LYMPH NODE

Necrosis and granuloma formation in this lymph node with *Francisella* infection.

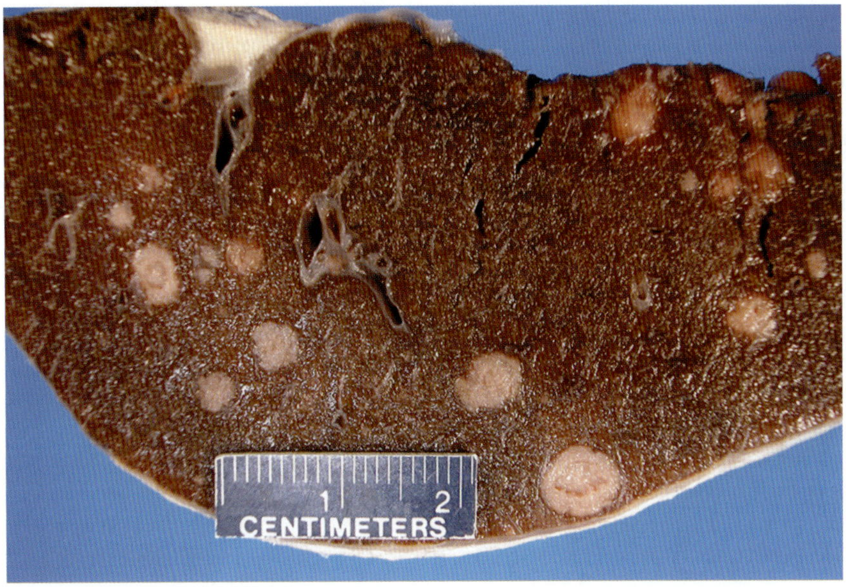

Figure 8-33

TULAREMIA, SPLEEN

Well-circumscribed firm nodules are seen. The areas of central depression probably represent foci of necrosis.

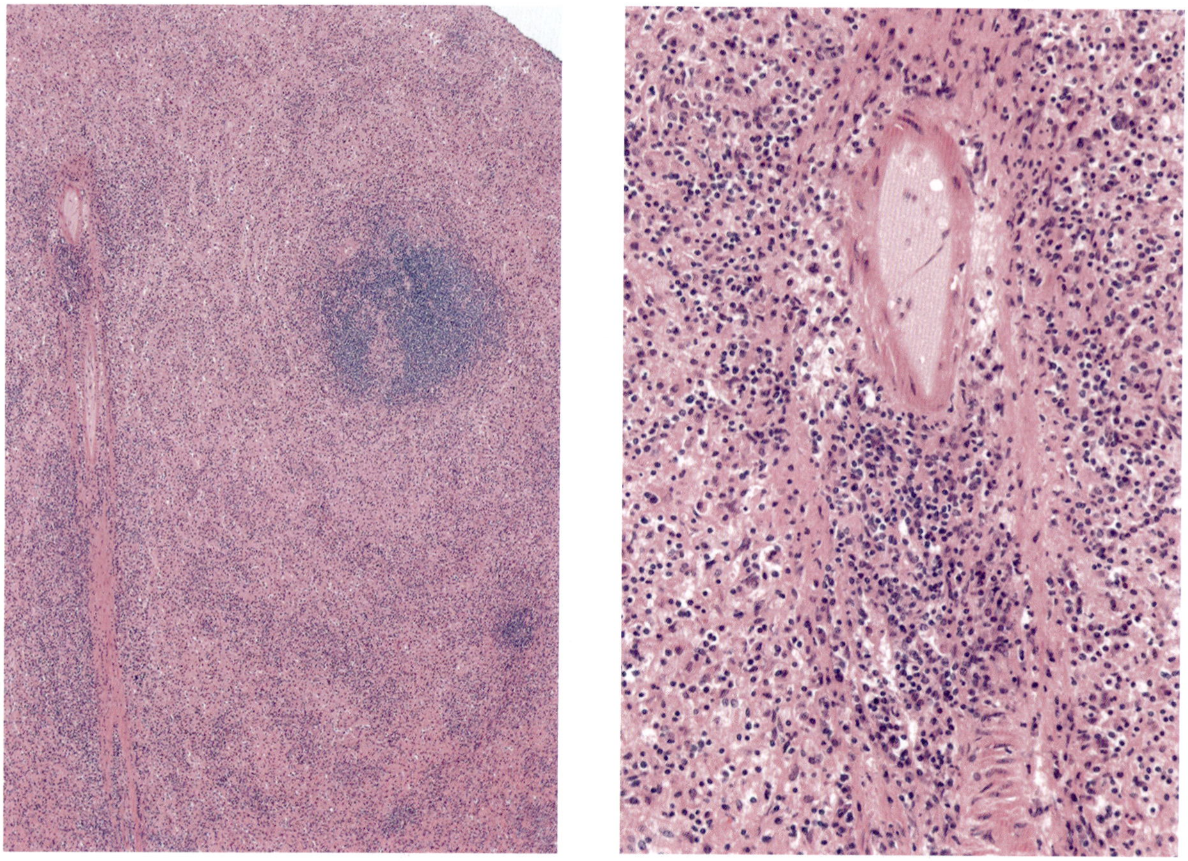

Figure 8-34

BRUCELLOSIS, SPLEEN

Congested red pulp (left) and vasculitis (right) are seen in a spleen infected with *Brucella*.

widespread granulomatous inflammation in many organs, which, grossly, results in a spotted yellow appearance.

Brucella is extremely difficult to identify in tissue sections and definitive diagnosis relies upon culturing the organism from blood, bone marrow, or specific organs. Serologic studies may show evidence of infection by a four-fold rise in immunoglobulin (Ig)M antibody titer or a single titer of 1/160. The infection is usually treated with prolonged antibacterial medications (103).

Microscopic Findings. Lymph node involvement, especially in the hilar region, is common, and the disease may be difficult to distinguish from tuberculosis by histomorphologic criteria. *Brucella* lymphadenitis shows a pattern of granulomatous inflammation that is either necrotic or sarcoid-like. Calcific deposits as well as fibrosis or scarring may eventually result, and are demonstrated radiologically. Splenic involvement includes abscesses with peripheral fibrosis, central necrosis, and granuloma formation (fig. 8-34) (29). Plasma cells and lymphocytes may rim the affected areas. Although gram negative, the organisms are very difficult to identify in routine histologic preparations.

Burkholderia Pseudomallei

Definition. *Melioidosis*, also known as *Whitmore disease*, is a tropical infection caused by the gram-negative bacteria *Burkholderia pseudomallei*, which occasionally involves lymph nodes and spleen.

General Features. Melioidosis has a wide range of clinical manifestations including asymptomatic infection, abscess formation, chronic (localized) infection, severe disseminated infection, and acute pneumonia (83,106). It is most common in Southeast Asia and other tropical

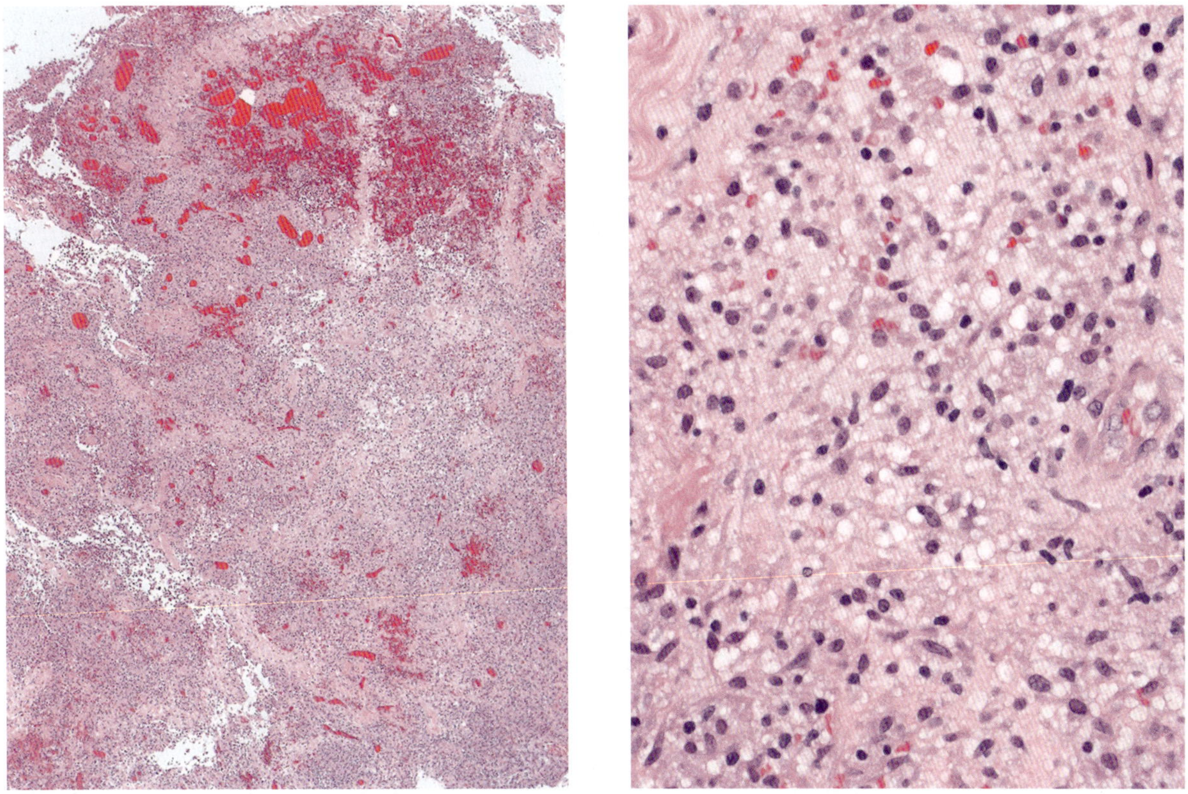

Figure 8-35

MELIOIDOSIS, LYMPH NODE

Lymphoid depletion (left) and proliferation of foamy macrophages (right) in this case of melioidosis. (Courtesy of Marie-Claire Marroum, Charlotte, NC.) (Figs. 8-35 and 8-36 are from the same patient.)

locations. A related species, *B. mallei*, causes infections in horses and humans referred to as glanders (pulmonary) and farcy (lymph node).

In melioidosis, the primary infection is usually introduced through a cutaneous wound, and localized lymph node involvement is common. Splenic abscess is common in disseminated disease (135). Severe infections are often associated with underlying immunodeficiency.

Microscopic Findings. Infection by *B. pseudomallei* is associated with suppurative inflammation, abscess with necrosis, acute inflammatory cells, and macrophages (figs. 8-35, 8-36) (92, 119). A Gram stain shows numerous gram-negative bacilli. These can also be highlighted with a Warthin-Starry stain. Another pattern, more commonly associated with chronic infection, is loose granulomas with necrosis. Giant cells with clusters of bacilli may also be seen. This latter pattern is more common in the spleen.

MYCOPLASMA, TREPONEMA PALLIDUM, BORRELIA, AND *RICKETTSIA* INFECTIONS

This section covers a wide variety of infectious organisms with diverse biochemical and clinical features. *Mycoplasma* are obligate intracellular parasites. The only representative of the spirochetes discussed is *Treponema pallidum. Borrelia burgdorferi*, the causative agent of *Lyme disease*, is an exceptionally rare causative agent of lymphadenitis (fig. 8-37).

Coxiella Burnetii

Definition. Lymphadenitis has rarely been associated with infection by *Coxiella burnetii*, the causative agent of *Q fever*.

General Features. Q Fever is a zoonosis, with only half of infected patients becoming symptomatic. Manifestations include febrile illness, pneumonia, hepatitis, and endocarditis. The morphologic finding of ring (or donut)

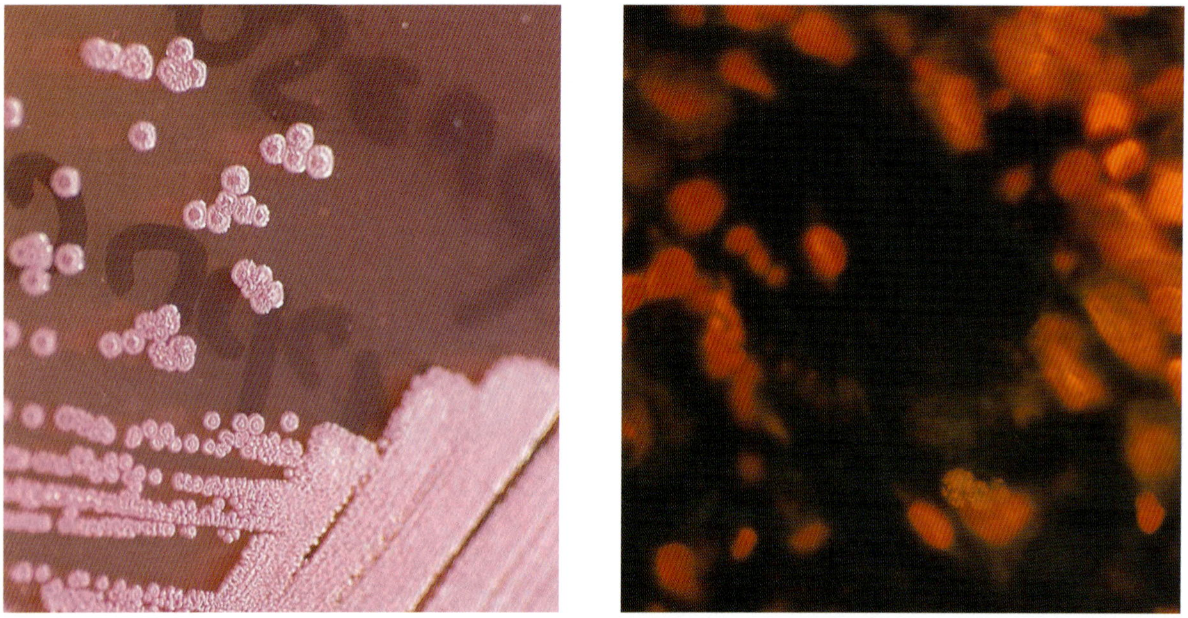

Figure 8-36

MELIOIDOSIS, LYMPH NODE

Results of culture (left) and fluorescent staining (right) are shown, confirming the presence of *B. pseudomallei*. (Courtesy of Marie-Claire Marroum, Charlotte, NC.)

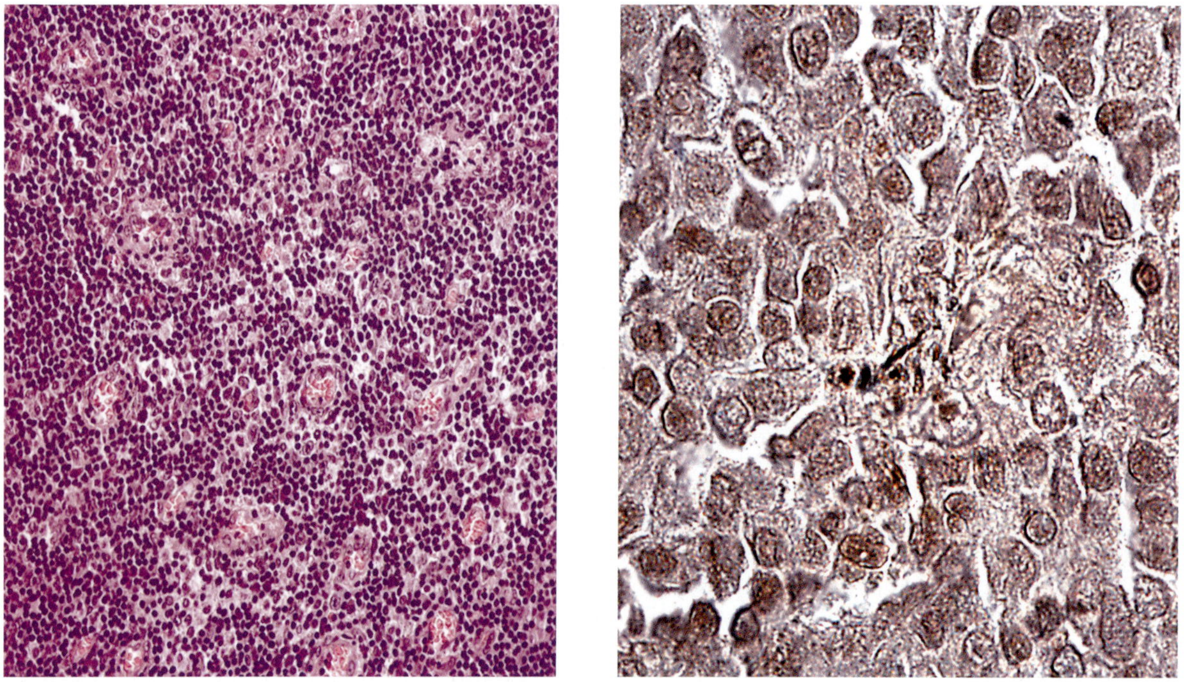

Figure 8-37

LYME DISEASE, LYMPH NODE

The histologic changes (left) and organisms (right, Warthin-Starry stain) are seen in those rare cases of Lyme disease in which lymph node biopsies are performed. (Courtesy of Peter Banks, Charlotte, NC.)

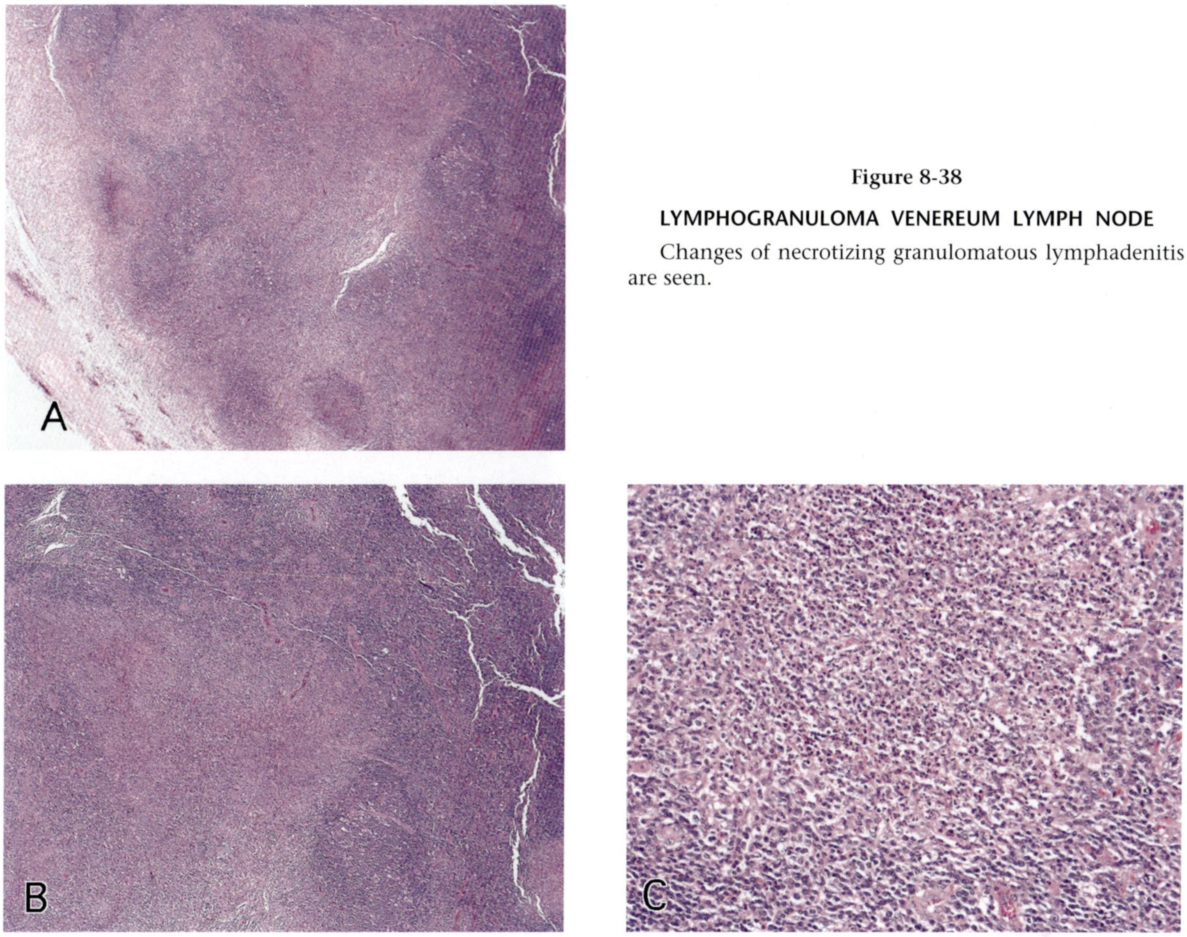

Figure 8-38

LYMPHOGRANULOMA VENEREUM LYMPH NODE

Changes of necrotizing granulomatous lymphadenitis are seen.

granulomas in the bone marrow is suggestive, but by no means specific, for Q fever. Lymphadenitis is rare, but has been reported (7,48). The diagnosis is confirmed by culture, but because of the danger of contamination (biosafety level 3), serologic techniques are recommended. There are currently no specific antibodies for immunohistochemistry. Specific PCR is available but only as a research tool. *C. burnetii* is a potential bioterrorism agent (see Table 8-1).

Microscopic Findings. The histologic findings associated with *C. burnetii* include granulomas with or without central necrosis, inflammation, and areas of geographic necrosis.

Chlamydia Trachomatis

Definition. *Lymphogranuloma venereum* is a sexually transmitted disease caused by *Chlamydia trachomatis,* which also causes *necrotizing granulomatous lymphadenitis*.

General Features. Lymphogranuloma venereum occurs most frequently (but not exclusively) in the inguinal region (113,131). Patients returning from endemic tropical countries have contracted most of the cases that are seen in the United States. A primary inoculation lesion is followed by regional, fluctuant, tender lymphadenopathy.

A definitive diagnosis is based upon clinicopathologic correlation, culture results, and demonstration of characteristic intracytoplasmic inclusion bodies, best demonstrated by Giemsa or immunofluorescent staining.

Microscopic Findings. The non-necrotizing granulomatous lymphadenitis of lymphogranuloma venereum with central suppuration, often confluent, eventually results in the formation of stellate microabscesses (figs. 8-38, 8-39). These histologic findings are exactly the same as those seen in cat-scratch disease (see above). Large vacuoles that demonstrate Warthin-Starry–positive

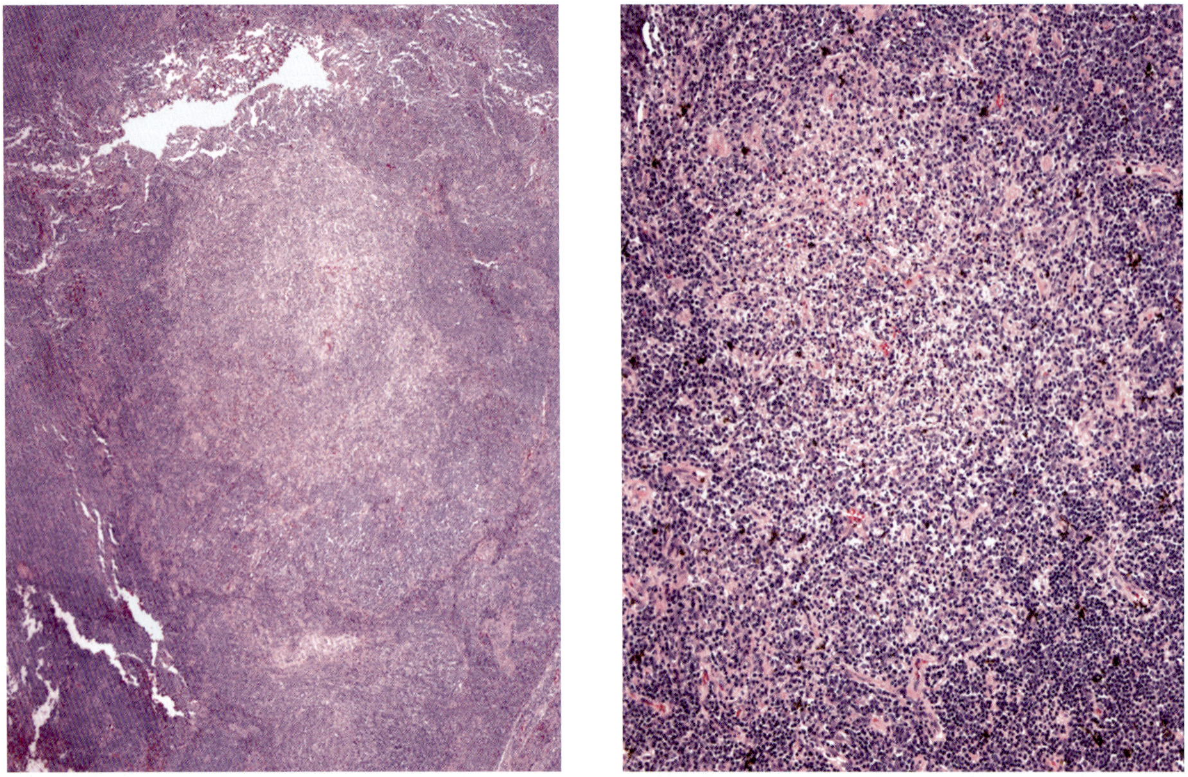

Figure 8-39

LYMPHOGRANULOMA VENEREUM, LYMPH NODE

Left: An early case, with vague granuloma formation and only minimal necrosis.
Right: Higher magnification highlights the clustering of macrophages.

organisms may also be noted and confirmed by electron microscopy.

Differential Diagnosis. Necrotizing granulomatous lymphadenitis has a relatively limited differential diagnosis. Cat-scratch disease is by far the more common cause, although in the appropriate clinical circumstances, lymphogranuloma venereum must be considered. Other infections with similar histopathologic findings include brucellosis and tularemia. The acute stage of autoimmune-associated lymphadenitis, especially lupus lymphadenitis, may have a similar appearance. In all circumstances, correlation with clinical findings, microbiologic studies, and appropriate stains for organisms (such as Warthin-Starry) help distinguish these entities.

Treponema Pallidum

Definition. *Syphilis,* caused by the spirochete *Treponema pallidum,* is a venereal disease that may present with either localized or generalized lymphadenopathy, depending upon the stage of the disease.

General Features. *T. pallidum* is a 10- to 13-μm cork-screw–shaped spirochete that is transmitted by sexual intercourse or other types of intimate contact. Transplacental fetal infection is a potentially devastating sequela in the pregnant woman. Downward modulation of the host's lymphocytic response by a serum factor is thought to weaken the immune reactivity and contribute to the latency and chronicity of infection, which is characteristic of this disease (52).

Syphilis presents with localized or generalized lymphadenopathy, depending upon the stage of disease (129). Formerly a rare infection, syphilis is now on the increase. Mostly, this parallels the rise in HIV/AIDS. Primary infection by syphilis takes place through sexual contact and produces the characteristic lesion, the chancre. This is a painless ulcer on the genitalia. The infection then spreads to the regional

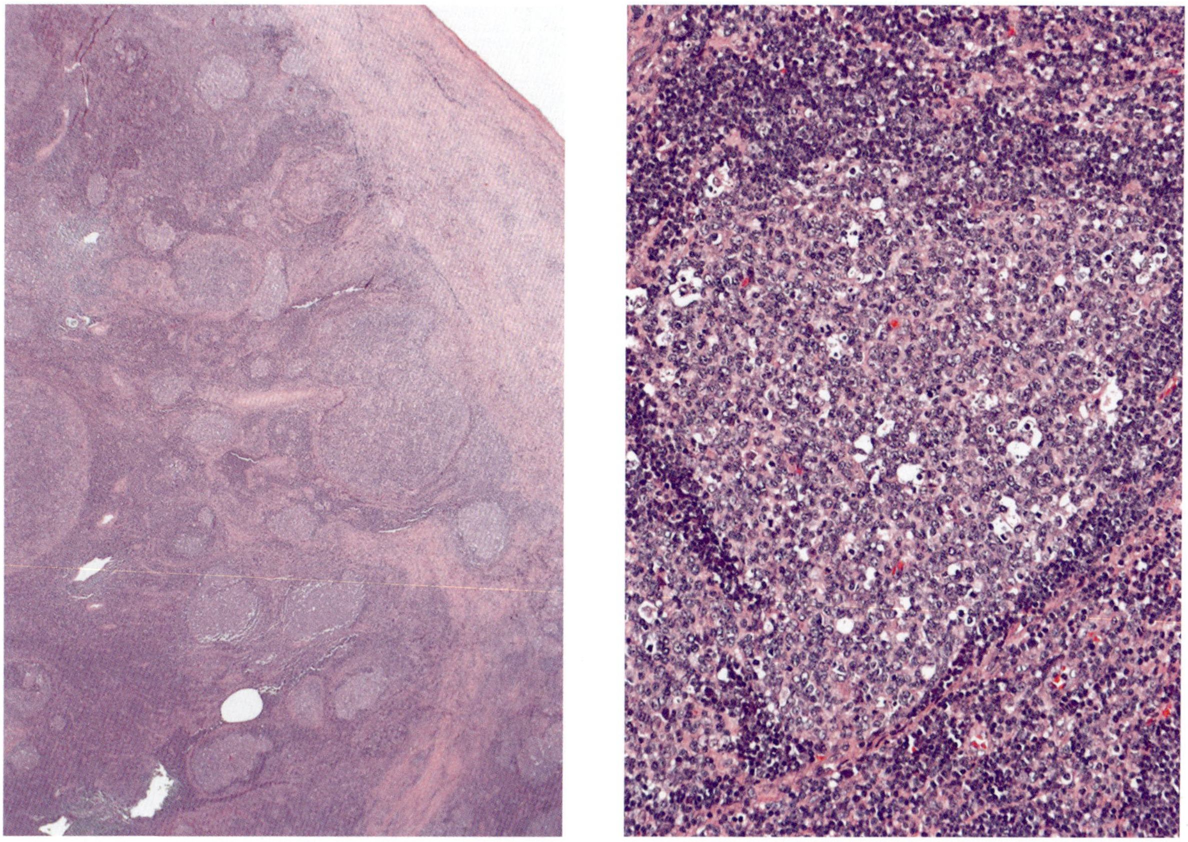

Figure 8-40

SYPHILIS, LYMPH NODE

A thickened capsule (left) and hyperplastic follicles (left, right) are seen in syphilitic lymphadenitis.

lymph nodes. The secondary phase of syphilis lasts up to a few months and consists of florid proliferation of the organisms. In this phase, rash, fever, generalized lymphadenopathy, and malaise are present. A variety of organs may be involved. The later stages of syphilis are notable for the rarity of organisms; however, the effects can be devastating. Central nervous system and cardiovascular disease are significant causes of morbidity and mortality. Tumorous masses due to infection, called gummas, may be seen in almost any site.

While culture is considered the gold standard for the diagnosis of syphilis, it is a difficult, expensive, and time-consuming process. Serologic testing is the cornerstone of diagnosis. Screening tests such as the Venereal Disease Research Laboratory (VDRL) or rapid plasma reagin (RPR) tests, which are based on identifying a lipid product produced as a result of syphilis infection, are commonly used. For confirmation, more specific treponemal tests, such as the fluorescent treponemal antibody-absorption (FTA-ABS) test, are used. Currently, more specific immunoassays and DNA-based tests are being developed.

Microscopic Findings. Follicular hyperplasia is probably the most consistent reactive pattern seen in either primary or secondary syphilis (fig. 8-40). The follicular hyperplasia, which may be prominent, is often associated with intense interfollicular polyclonal plasmacytosis. Capsular thickening with plasma cell infiltration (fig. 8-41) and nonspecific perivascular thickening with inflammatory cells are seen in secondary syphilitic lymphadenitis (65). Well-formed granulomas or epithelioid macrophages (single or in clusters) may be present (fig. 8-42).

This lesion presents with a variety of inflammatory changes such as reactive follicular and interfollicular hyperplasia, stromal/vascular

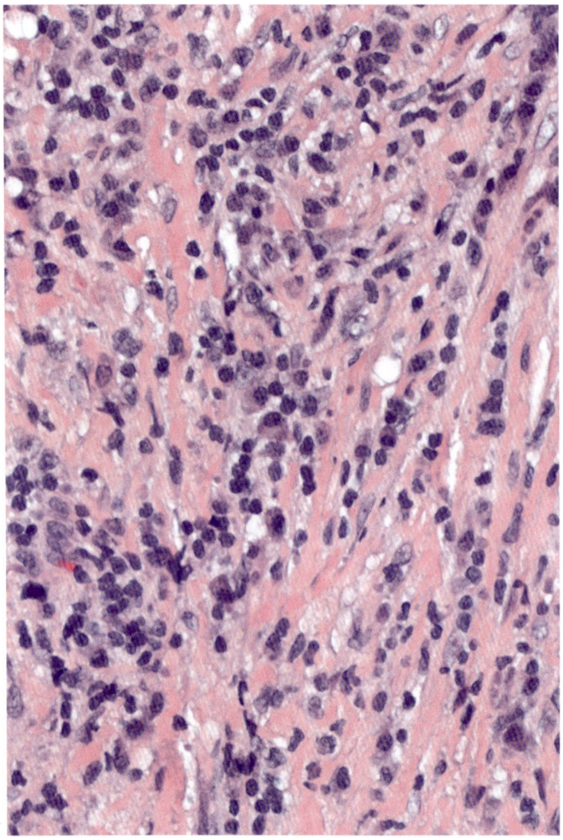

Figure 8-41

SYPHILIS, LYMPH NODE

Polyclonal plasmacytosis is seen within the thick capsule.

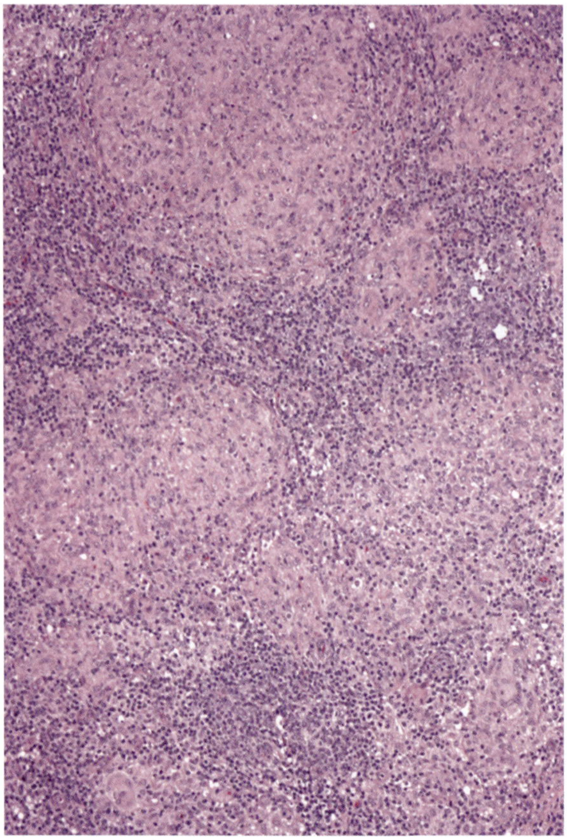

Figure 8-42

SYPHILIS, LYMPH NODE

Granuloma formation is a feature of syphilitic lymphadenitis.

hyperplasia, and granulomatous lymphadenitis. It characteristically affects the interstitial structures, including the framework (capsule, blood vessels) of the lymph node (fig. 8-43). Although there are no pathognomonic histopathologic features of secondary syphilis, reactive follicular hyperplasia, capsular thickening, obliterative vasculitis, and prominent plasma cell infiltration that may extend to the capsule, are characteristically seen in syphilitic lymphadenitis (Table 8-2) (45,65,129). A study comparing syphilitic lymphadenitis in HIV-positive and -negative patients showed essentially identical histologic features (45).

After the secondary stage, the patient may enter a period of latent, or tertiary, syphilis that can last for decades. Fortunately, this complication is less common today due to successful recognition and treatment of the disease by penicillin and other antibiotics. During this stage, localized destructive lesions form in different organs, including gummatous lymphadenitis, in which most (or all) of a lymph node is replaced by necrotic material. The necrotic material consists of cellular and stromal remnants, surrounded by a rim of epithelioid macrophages and multinucleated giant cells. Softening of the node and formation of a sinus tract to the skin causes gummatous ulceration. Treponemes are difficult to visualize in gummatous lesions. A miliary form of gummatous lymphadenitis demonstrates small, scattered gummas that may be surrounded by multinucleated giant or epithelioid cells (124).

Lymphadenitis in congenital syphilis shows features similar to those described in early syphilis except that there may be lymphoid atrophy rather than follicular hyperplasia. Minute foci of necrosis may be surrounded by epithelioid

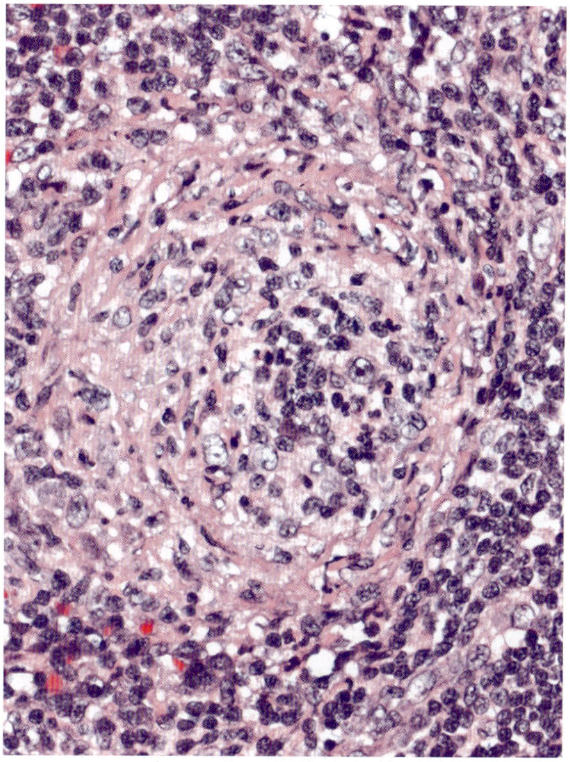

Figure 8-43

SYPHILIS, LYMPH NODE

Vasculitis is characteristic of syphilis.

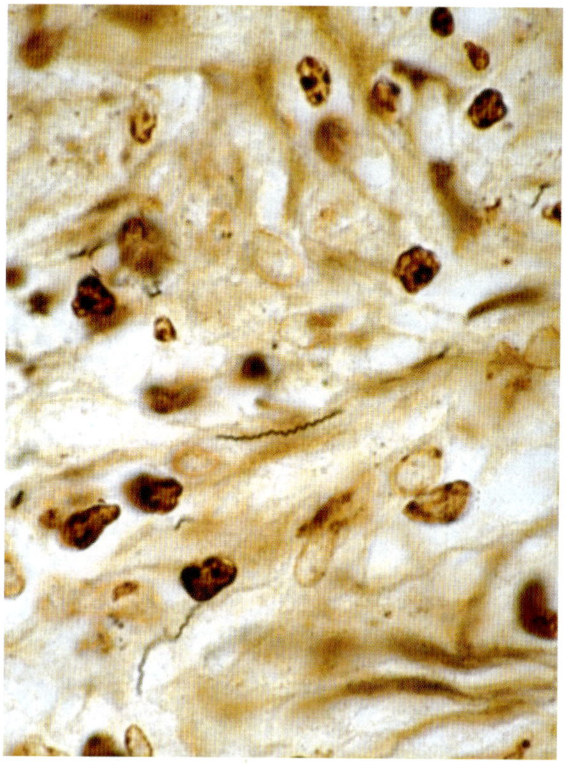

Figure 8-44

SYPHILIS, LYMPH NODE

Warthin-Starry silver stain highlights the classic morphology of the tightly coiled *Treponema pallidum* organisms, the causative spirochete of syphilis.

Table 8-2

MORPHOLOGIC FEATURES OF SYPHILIS (LUETIC) LYMPHADENITIS

Capsular thickening
Polyclonal plasmacytosis
Vascular proliferation
Vasculitis
Follicular hyperplasia
Identification of organisms by silver stain or immunohistochemistry

macrophages. The differential diagnosis of syphilitic granulomatous lymphadenitis includes tuberculosis, sarcoidosis, and other diseases associated with necrotizing or non-necrotizing lymphadenitis caused by infectious agents.

The causative spirochetes are usually located within the blood vessel walls, necrotic areas, or giant-cell granulomas and are demonstrated by Warthin-Starry staining (fig. 8-44). Using specific antisera to *T. pallidum* and immunofluorescent staining, spirochetes are demonstrated in histologic sections and imprints of lymph nodes (27). Immunohistochemical stains are available and show greater sensitivity and specificity than the traditional histologic stains (fig. 8-45).

Rickettsia

Definition. *Rickettsia* organisms cause a variety of human diseases. There may be lymphadenopathy and splenic involvement but typically the features are nonspecific.

General Features. *Rickettsia* organisms are obligate intracellular parasites, typically carried by an insect vector. Regional lymphadenopathy may be seen near inoculation sites of the rickettsial organisms, such as in scrub typhus (*R. tsutsugamushi*). In epidemic typhus (*R. prowazekii*), adenopathy and splenic involvement are only minor features of the disease. *R. rickettsii* is the causative agent of Rocky Mountain spotted fever (RMSF).

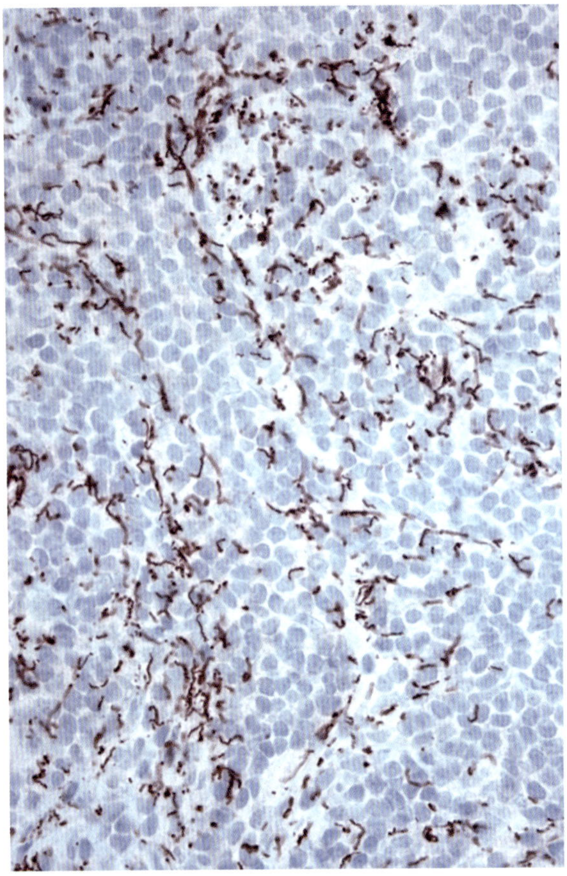

Figure 8-45

SYPHILIS, LYMPH NODE

Immunohistochemical staining for *Treponema pallidum* reveals the causative organisms. Immunohistochemical staining is more sensitive and specific than silver staining techniques.

Rickettsia is an obligate intracellular parasite, with a reservoir in ticks. *R. rickettsii* infects endothelial cells and adjacent vascular smooth muscle cells. Generalized adenopathy is a frequent clinical finding in RMSF. *R. sibirica* infections are associated with lymphadenopathy, but the specific histologic findings are not reported (49). Vasculitis is a frequent finding in rickettsial infections, as endothelial cells are a primary site of infection.

Microscopic Findings. Rickettsial infections all have similar histologic findings in the lymph nodes. There is an increase in acute inflammation, especially in the sinuses (125). There is activation of paracortical lymphocytes, leading to increases in immunoblasts. Plasma cells may be increased. More characteristic of rickettsial infection, in general, is involvement of vascular elements. In severe infection, inflammatory cells infiltrate and thicken blood vessels, causing edema.

Table 8-3

HISTOCHEMICAL FEATURES OF MYCOBACTERIA

	Ziehl-Neelsen or Kinyoun Stain (AFB)[a]	Fite-Faraco Stain (Modified AFB)	PAS Stain	Auramine or Auramine-Rhodamine (Fluor-) escent) Stain
M. tuberculosis	+	+	–	+
M. avium-intracellulare	+	+	+	+
M. leprae	–	+	–	+
Atypical mycobacteria	+/–	+	–/+	+/–

[a]AFB = acid-fast bacillus; PAS = periodic acid–Schiff.

MYCOBACTERIAL INFECTIONS

There are about 30 species of mycobacteria that affect man. Certain species, such as *M. tuberculosis,* are considerable worldwide health problems, while others are most known as opportunistic organisms, such as *M. avium-intracellulare*. In any case, mycobacterial infections in lymph nodes and spleen share a variety of histologic features, including a combination of granulomatous and acute inflammation (51).

The histochemical staining characteristics of representative mycobacterial species are summarized in Table 8-3. In most circumstances, it is difficult to identify a particular mycobacterial species in histologic sections. Newer PCR-based tests provide definitive identification, even in paraffin-embedded tissue. In most cases, however, correlation with microbiology studies and culture results is the most appropriate approach (51).

Mycobacterium Tuberculosis

Definition. *Tuberculosis* has been a scourge of humanity, both historically and presently. The causative agent, *Mycobacterium tuberculosis,* is supremely adapted to evade human immunologic defenses. Although rare in North America, it is a common cause of adenopathy and splenic lesions in other parts of the world.

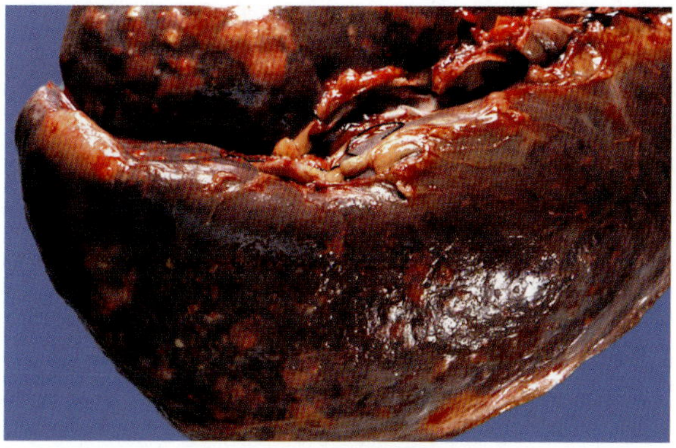

Figure 8-46

TUBERCULOSIS, SPLEEN

The surface of a spleen involved by tuberculosis. (Courtesy of Luis Fajardo, Palo Alto, CA.)

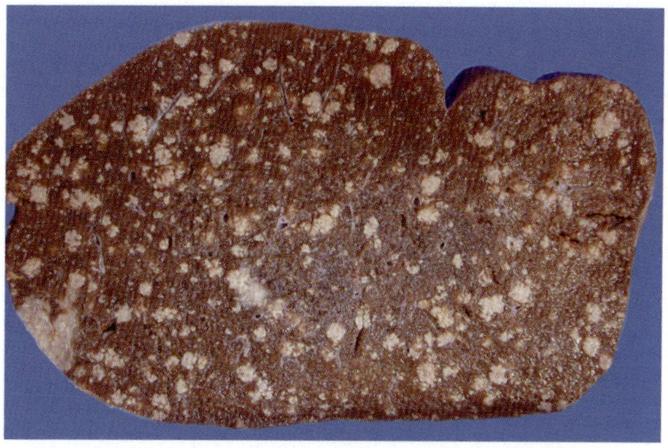

Figure 8-47

TUBERCULOSIS, SPLEEN

The cut surface of the spleen shows multiple variably sized, slightly irregular nodules in a miliary pattern (i.e., granulomas).

General Features. Tuberculosis is a chronic world-wide disease that is caused by the species of *M. tuberculosis*. In the United States and other developed countries, the disease is most often caused by *M. tuberculosis hominis* and transmitted via inhalation of aerosolized infective droplets. *M. tuberculosis bovis*, which is uncommon in developed countries, is ingested in milk from infected cows. In Africa and Asia, tuberculosis is still a significant cause of lymphadenopathy, and can account for as much as 25 percent of biopsied lymph nodes (108).

Most individuals affected by *M. tuberculosis* develop an asymptomatic primary infection that can be reactivated if the host becomes immunocompromised, or, less commonly, by repeated exposure to exogenous organisms. The disease has become increasingly more prevalent since the advent of the AIDS epidemic. Although the primary manifestation of tuberculosis occurs in the lungs, systemic dissemination characteristically results in hilar lymph node involvement. The major immune response to tuberculosis includes macrophage activation, T-cell–mediated reactivity, and the formation of granulomas (141), although nonimmunologic mechanisms result in the transformation of macrophages into epithelioid cells (126).

Involved lymph nodes are typically painless and matted. Patients have constitutional symptoms including night sweats, fever, malaise, and weight loss. These symptoms are not specific and can be seen in nontuberculous causes of lymphadenitis (23). *Tuberculous lymphadenitis* is the most common form of extrapulmonary reactivation of tuberculosis, and is a frequent cause of cervical lymphadenitis in endemic regions (23,63). The anterior and posterior triangle nodes of the neck are most commonly involved, with dissemination from pulmonary sites. Splenic involvement is typically seen as part of disseminated disease; however, rare cases of isolated splenic tuberculosis have been reported (84).

Gross Findings. The classic gross appearance of tuberculous involvement in lymph node is gray-white, soft foci that vary in size. These areas may have central cheesy-white soft material, which is known as caseation (from the Latin word for cheese). The central portions of the granulomas may also have liquid, suppurative degeneration. Another pattern of involvement, seen less commonly, is miliary tuberculosis. This is so named for the characteristic small (1 to 4 mm), yellow, white, or gray nodules that are scattered throughout the tissue and resemble millet seeds.

Splenic involvement in disseminated tuberculosis is characterized by miliary involvement (figs. 8-46, 8-47). Occasionally, there are large macronodules, which have a similar appearance, and may have caseous regions, similar to those described in the lymph nodes. These may be seen in the intact spleen as subcapsular, irregular yellow masses. In addition, cystic degeneration with suppuration and microabscess formation are also seen in splenic tuberculosis (24).

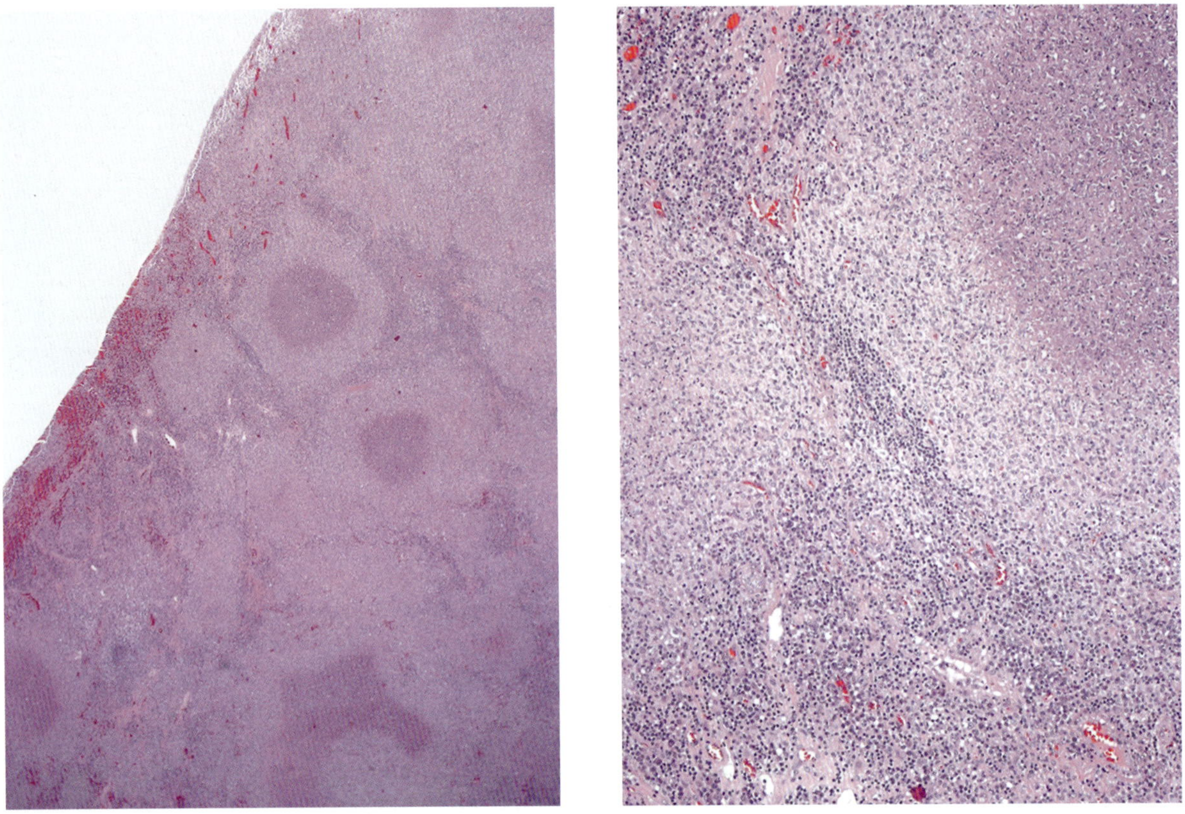

Figure 8-48

TUBERCULOSIS, LYMPH NODE

Centrally necrotic granulomas are seen in this case of tuberculous lymphadenitis.

Microscopic Findings. The histopathologic changes in lymph nodes involved by tuberculosis are considered the prototype for granulomatous lymphadenitis. The characteristic granuloma, or tubercle, is composed of plump epithelioid macrophages and occasional Langerhans multinucleated giant cells formed by the fusion of macrophages (fig. 8-48). A peripheral collar of fibroblasts, lymphocytes, and plasma cells surrounds the granuloma, which, in the absence of central necrosis, is referred to as a "hard tubercle" (fig. 8-49). Granulomas with central, coagulative necrosis (grossly described as caseous) are noted in tuberculous lymphadenitis, and are referred to as "soft tubercles." These granulomatous areas are often confluent (fig. 8-50).

In primary tuberculosis, the combination of a single lung lesion and involvement of the tracheobronchial lymph nodes is referred to as the "Ghon complex." Eventually, most lymph nodes involved by primary disease develop areas of fibrosis with calcific deposits and scarring in which bacilli may be demonstrated, even many years later (101). Secondary tuberculosis represents reactivation of the primary disease or, less commonly, exposure to exogenous organisms. The histologic appearance of the lymph nodes is dependent on the host response (Table 8-4) (95).

Splenic involvement in disseminated tuberculosis is common and is typically seen as a miliary pattern. Although rare, macronodular masses in the spleen, and spleen as a primary site of infection, have been reported (12,39,127).

The identification of beaded, rod-shaped acid-fast bacilli by Ziehl-Neelsen or Fite-Faraco special stains is essential for a definitive diagnosis. Organisms may be exceedingly difficult to demonstrate in cases of tuberculous lymphadenitis although they are usually abundant in HIV-associated mycobacterial infections.

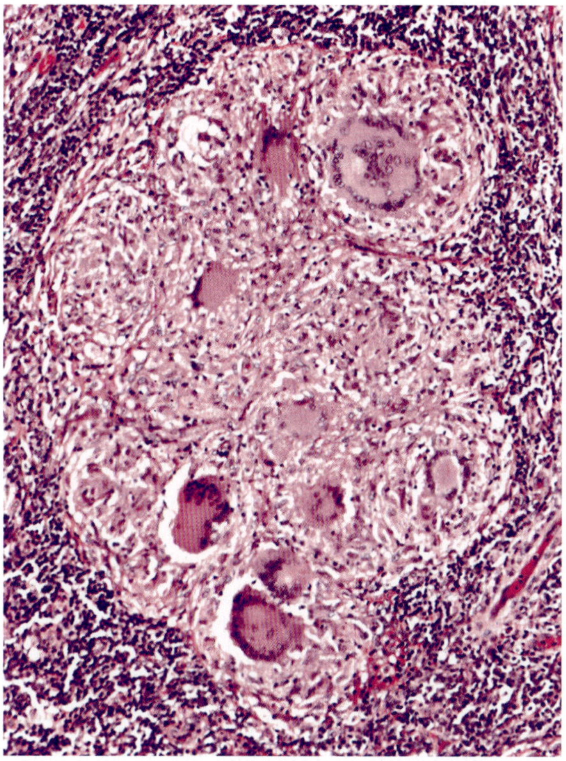

Figure 8-49

TUBERCULOSIS, LYMPH NODE

The granuloma has many multinucleated giant cells but no central caseation.

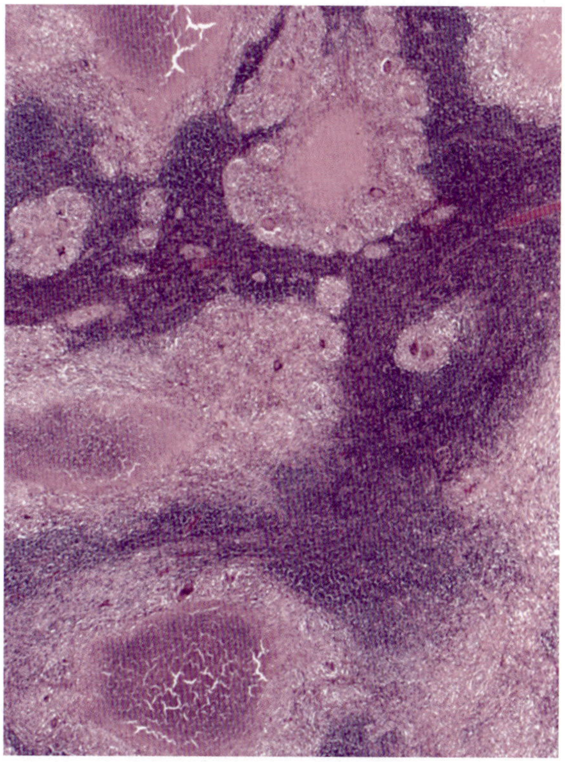

Figure 8-50

TUBERCULOSIS, LYMPH NODE

Caseation is highlighted in this case of tuberculous lymphadenitis.

Table 8-4

HISTOLOGIC RESPONSES IN TUBERCULOUS LYMPHADENITIS[a]

Response Type	Histology	Organisms/AFB[b]
Hyperplastic	Well-organized granuloma, few giant cells, inflammation mostly lymphocytic, none or minimal necrosis	Rare[c]
Reactive	Well-organized granuloma, giant cells common, lymphocytes and plasma cells, +/- neutrophils, central eosinophilic necrosis	Variable
Hyporeactive	Poorly defined granuloma, macrophages, rare giant cells, mixed lymphocytes and plasma cells, extensive basophilic necrosis (caseation)	Common
Nonreactive	No distinct granuloma, rare giant cells, macrophages with lymphocytes and plasma cells, necrosis, and karyorrhexis without caseation	Common

[a]Modified from table I from Ramanathan VD, Jawahar MS, Paramasivan CN, Rajaram K, et al. A histological spectrum of host responses in tuberculous lymphadenitis. Indian J Med Res 1999;109:214.

[b]AFB = acid-fast bacillus.

[c]Rare = 1/100 high-power fields; common = 1-10/10 high-power fields.

The characteristic acid-fast beaded organism is usually demonstrated at the periphery of necrotic areas or within the epithelioid macrophages (fig. 8-51). Ultraviolet microscopy following auramine-rhodamine staining is also useful. Culturing the organism and correlating the laboratory findings with the clinicopathologic features, especially the tuberculin skin test result, is confirmative (23). PCR identifies *M. tuberculosis* in paraffin-embedded tissues (81).

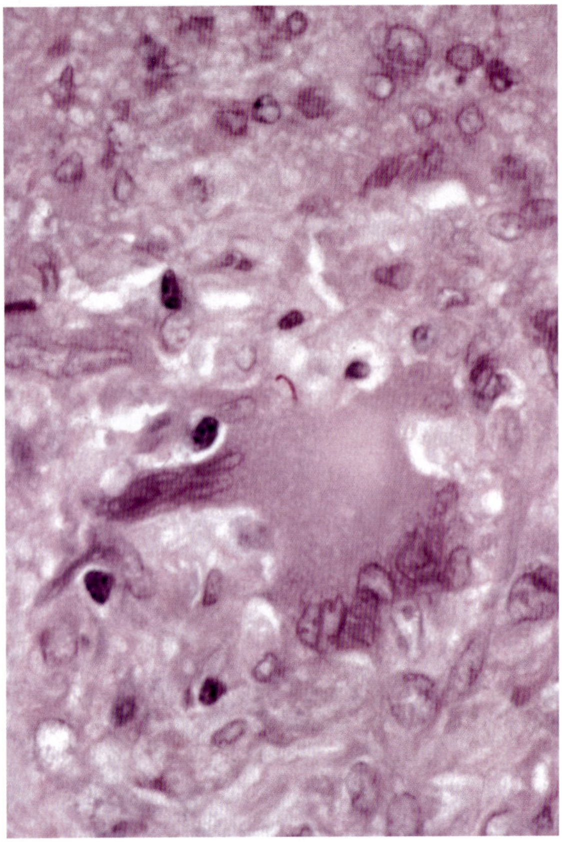

Figure 8-51

TUBERCULOSIS, LYMPH NODE

An acid-fast stain shows the morphology of a rare *Mycobacterium*.

Differential Diagnosis. The differential diagnosis of tuberculous lymphadenitis includes sarcoidosis, histoplasmosis (and other fungal infections), and cat-scratch disease. Sarcoidosis is a multisystem granulomatous disease, which often presents with bilateral hilar adenopathy on chest roentgenogram (138). Although the histologic features of sarcoidal lymphadenopathy are not pathognomonic, they are highly suggestive of this disorder. The granulomas are usually well formed and better organized than those of tuberculous lymphadenitis, and do not have central necrosis. Schaumann and asteroid bodies may be noted in the absence of acid-fast bacilli.

Treatment. Combination drug therapy is essential for the treatment of tuberculosis and the prevention of resistant strains. The drugs, which include isoniazid, rifampicin, paraaminosalicylates, and streptomycin, are usually effective if the patient is compliant.

Mycobacterium Avium-Intracellulare

Definition. Mycobacterial infection caused by *Mycobacterium avium-intracellulare* (MAI) has become relatively common since the onset of AIDS. Sites of involvement vary widely, but include lymph nodes and spleen. *Mycobacterial spindle cell tumor* is an unusual histologic presentation of MAI infection in which macrophages filled with bacteria have a distinct spindle cell appearance.

General Features. MAI has been associated with HIV infection since the beginning of the epidemic (96). In severely immunocompromised patients, MAI infection may involve the entire lymphoreticular system including lymph nodes, bone marrow, and spleen, as well as other solid organs. A definitive diagnosis of MAI depends upon the results of biochemical tests and culture characteristics on specialized media.

Microscopic Findings. In the lymph nodes, there is focal or diffuse sinusoidal infiltration by bland-appearing macrophages with vacuolated cytoplasm, usually in a lymphoid-depleted background (figs. 8-52, 8-53). In some cases, there may be diffuse sheets of these cells occupying all, or a large portion, of a lymphoid-depleted node (109). Well-formed granulomas are rarely noted. Neutrophils and macrophages are associated with the granuloma formation (72).

In a study of AIDS patients, spleens harboring MAI organisms had a variety of histologic features, including depletion of white pulp (probably due to HIV/AIDS), and proliferations of macrophages, plasma cells, and immunoblastics (70). Splenic involvement is similar in cytologic appearance to that of the lymph node. Clusters or sheets of macrophages are seen, and may be extensive enough to mimic a storage disease (fig. 8-54). The appearance of the macrophages has been described as Gaucher-like, or pseudo-Gaucher, cells. Although red pulp involvement is most common, involvement of the white pulp also occurs. A single case has been reported of a splenic abscess due to MAI in an immunocompromised child (116).

In some cases, the engorged macrophages have a spindle cell or pseudosarcomatous appearance, which is termed *mycobacterial spindle cell tumor* (fig. 8-55) (79,109,122,139,140). The

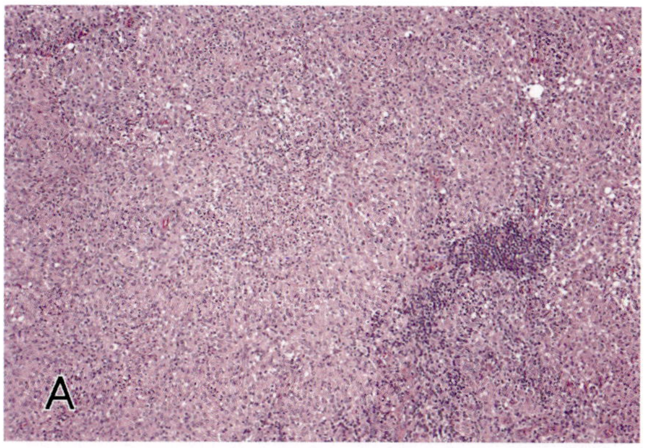

Figure 8-52

***MYCOBACTERIUM AVIUM-INTRACELLULARE* (MAI), LYMPH NODE**

Low magnification shows generalized effacement by plump macrophages (A), with abundant granular cytoplasm (B). An acid fast stain highlights many mycobacterial organisms (C).

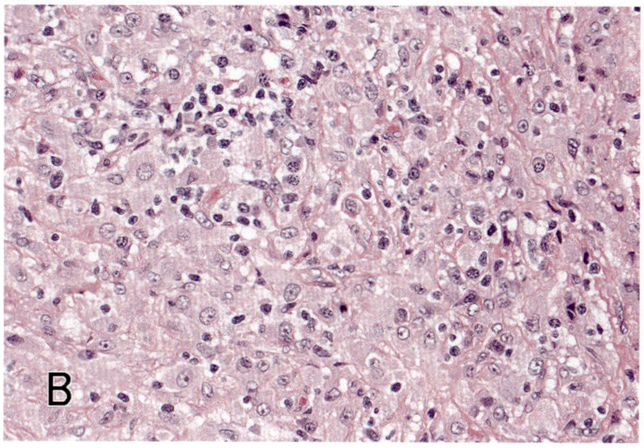

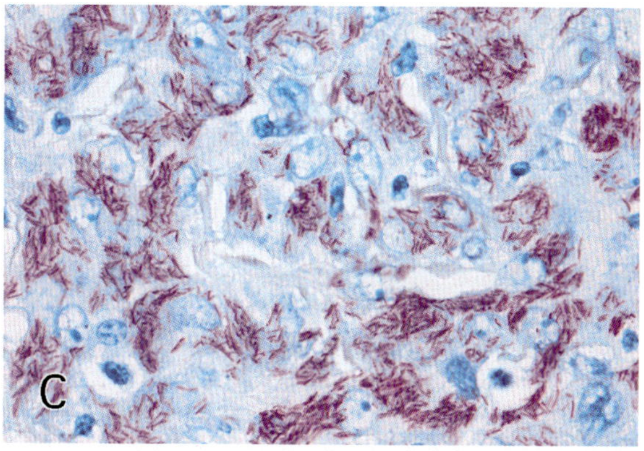

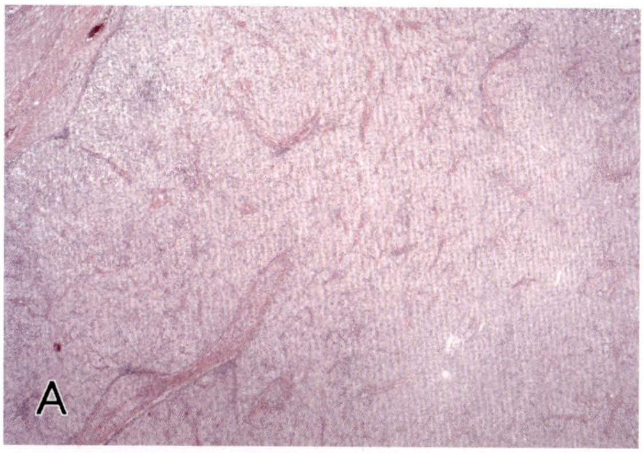

Figure 8-53

***MYCOBACTERIUM AVIUM-INTRACELLULARE,* LYMPH NODE**

This lymph node is diffusely replaced by foamy macrophages filled with organisms.

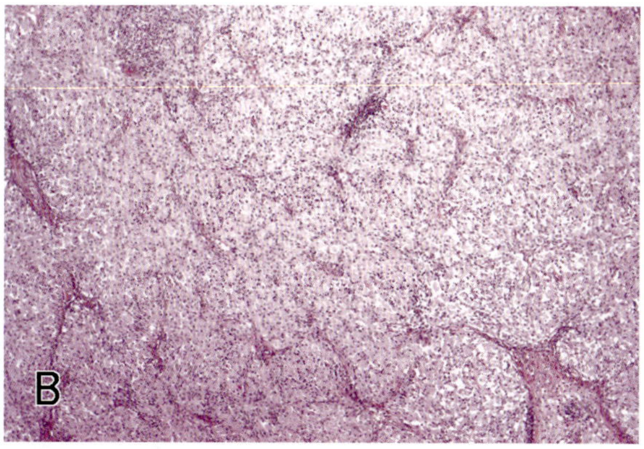

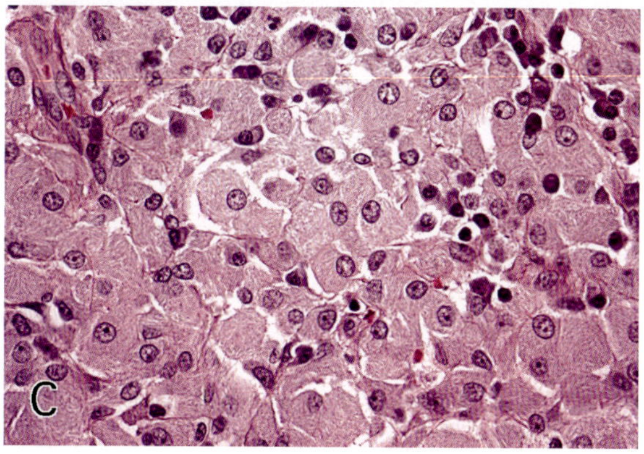

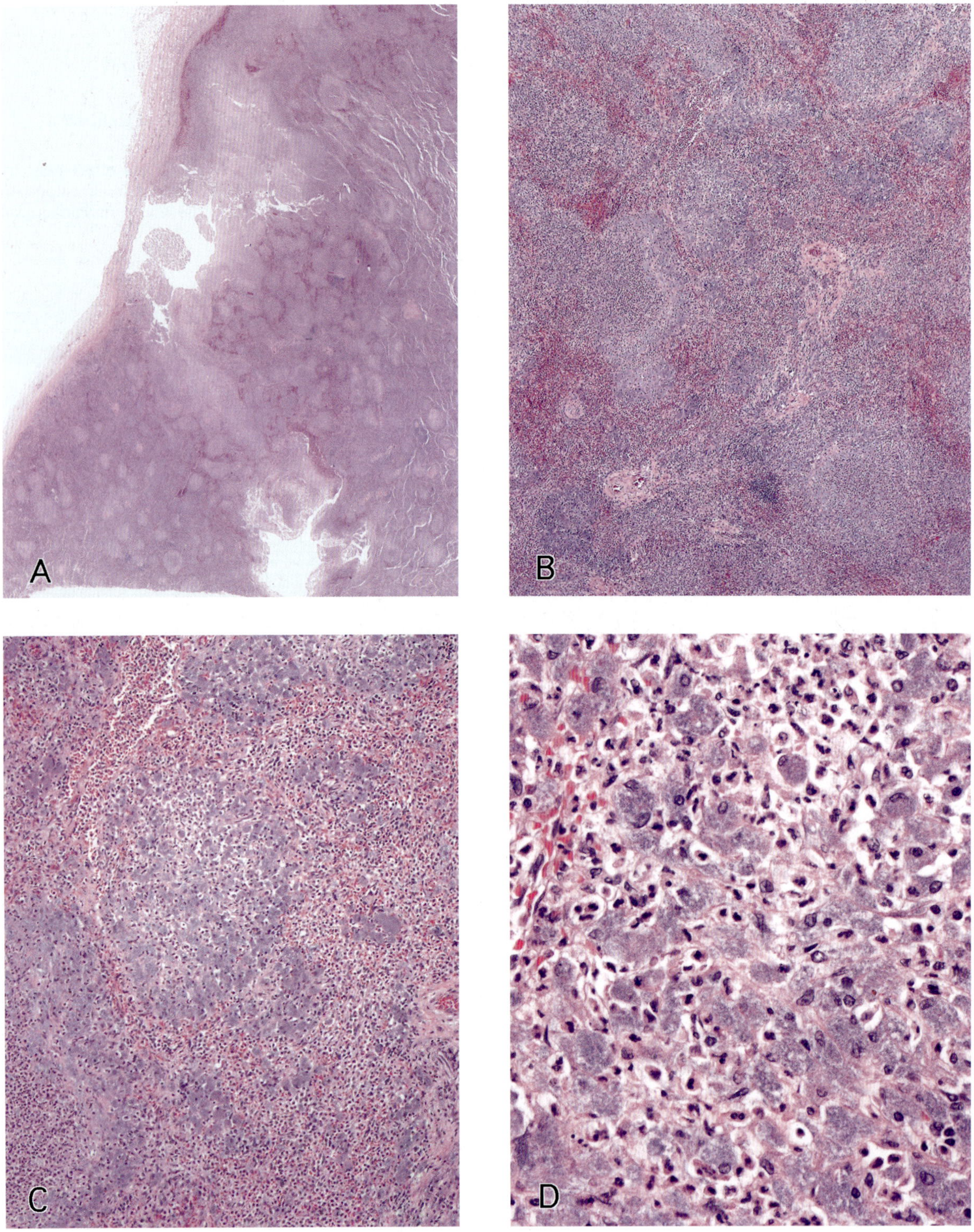

Figure 8-54

***MYCOBACTERIUM AVIUM-INTRACELLULARE,* SPLEEN**

Splenic involvement by disseminated MAI is common. In this case, the macrophages filled with mycobacteria take on a pale, bluish appearance.

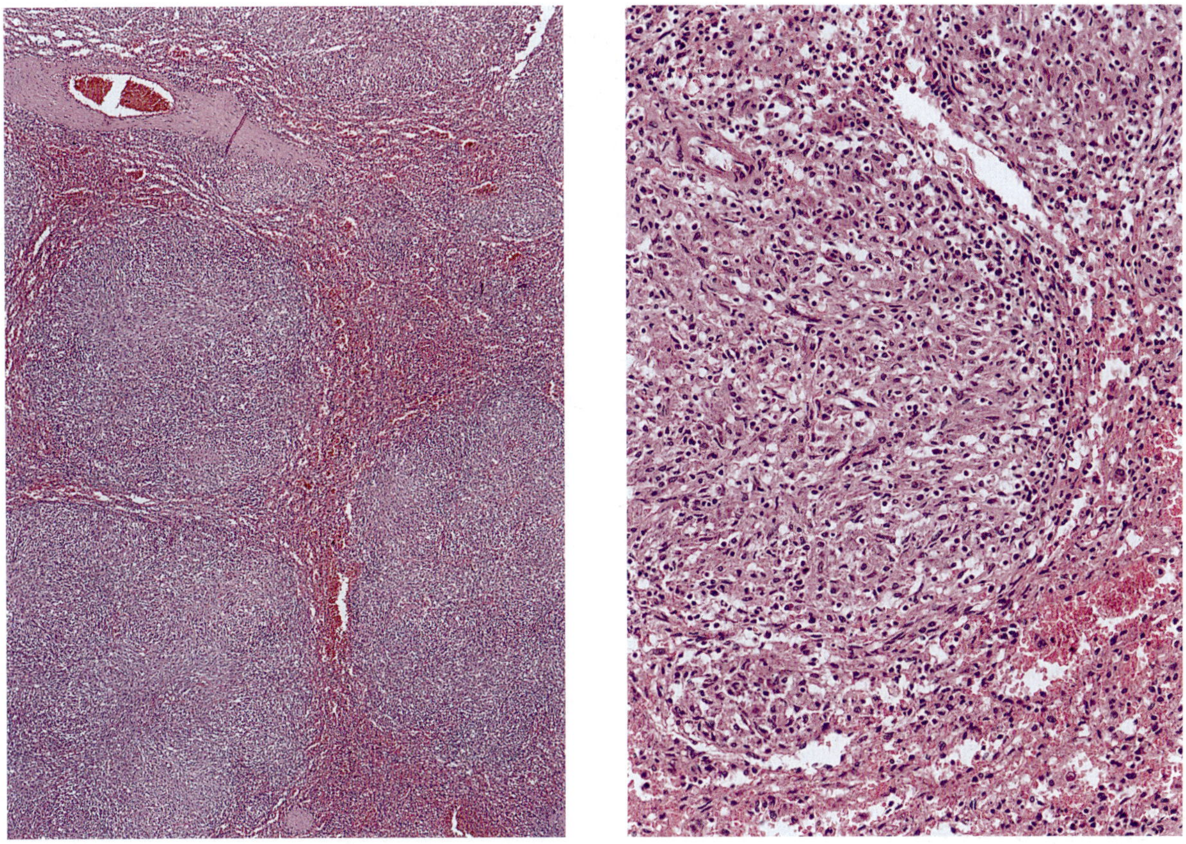

Figure 8-55

MYCOBACTERIAL SPINDLE CELL TUMOR, SPLEEN

Left: Multiple spindle cell nodules are found in the splenic parenchyma.

Right: The expansile nodules are composed of spindled cells and mononuclear cells. (Fig. 21-16 from Fascicle 14, Third Series.)

cells are cytologically bland, with rounded nuclei with blunt ends, and are arranged in short fascicles or a storiform pattern. This lesion may occur in lymph nodes, spleen, skin, or bone marrow. It is important to distinguish this lesion from Kaposi sarcoma in these sites, and also to recognize that the two may occur in one tissue simultaneously (79). Although MAI is most frequently identified, other mycobacterial species are associated with mycobacterial spindle cell tumors, although rarely.

The staining characteristics of MAI are well described. The mycobacterial organisms are visualized in the pale, foamy macrophages as beaded rod-like structures and easily seen with AFB or modified AFB stains. In contrast to most other mycobacteria species, they also stain for PAS (fig. 8-56) (13). In comparison to all but the most florid cases of tuberculosis, visualized MAI organisms are numerous compared to other mycobacterial infections.

Differential Diagnosis. In the lymph node or spleen, the masses of foamy macrophages raise a differential diagnosis of storage disease, infections associated with granulomas, or rarely, nonhematopoietic neoplasm. Correlation with the history, especially of HIV/AIDS, suggest MAI infection. In these cases, appropriate histochemical stains (PAS, AFB) clarify the diagnosis. Mycobacterial spindle cell tumor may be confused with inflammatory pseudotumor, smooth muscle tumors, or even Kaposi sarcoma. Appropriate ancillary studies, such as an AFB stain, confirm the diagnosis.

Treatment. Patients with MAI infection are treated with antituberculous and/or antibiotic

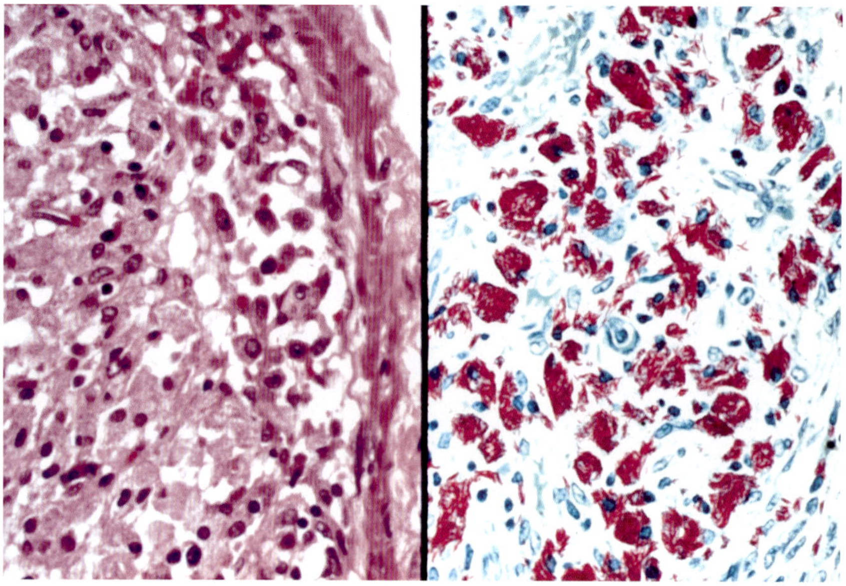

Figure 8-56

***MYCOBACTERIUM AVIUM-INTRACELLULARE* LYMPHADENITIS**

The foamy cytoplasmic appearance of sinusoidal macrophages (left) is due to red, rod-like organisms visualized with a modified acid-fast stain (Fite).

drugs. MAI lymphadenitis has been associated with activation of antiretroviral protease inhibitors (e.g., indinavir), which may serve to "unmask" a previously clinically silent infection (94).

Mycobacterium Leprae

Definition. In advanced stages, *leprosy*, also called *Hanson disease*, caused by *Mycobacterium leprae*, is associated with adenopathy. The changes may be characteristic, and nodal biopsies are often performed for diagnosis, for evaluation of treatment, and for evaluating immune response. The disease spectrum ranges from the tuberculoid to the lepromatous type.

General Features. *Lepromatous leprosy* is a slowly progressive chronic disease caused by *M. leprae*, a gram-positive intracellular acid-fast bacillus. Leprosy primarily involves the coolest parts of the body such as the skin and peripheral nerves. If untreated, it may spread to other organs, including the lymph nodes. Certain lymph nodes are affected more than others and are listed in descending order: inguinal, axillary, cervical, epitrochlear (68). Man and armadillos appear to be the only naturally susceptible hosts. There is direct transmission of the disease from active cases, usually through skin contact or inhalation of aerosolized droplets. Cellular immunity and not antibody formation is the method of host resistance, and the correlation between T-lymphocyte reactivity and subsequent clinical course provides insight into the so-called polar ends of the disease spectrum, namely tuberculoid and lepromatous types, with an intermediate (borderline) type (85).

Tuberculoid leprosy begins with macular skin lesions that histologically show perineural granulomatous inflammation. Eventually, many organs, including lymph nodes, demonstrate hard tuberculoid granulomas in which bacilli are difficult to identify. Rheumatic manifestations are rare but well-described complications of tuberculoid leprosy (104).

The histologic features of the lymph nodes in tuberculoid and lepromatous leprosy are reflective of the polar ends of a disease spectrum and depends upon the patient's immunologic condition. The Ridley-Jopling classification (bacterial morphology), bacterial index (BI), and granuloma fraction (GF) are all methods to classify the degree of the disease and the host immunologic response. Their application and applicability vary widely (111).

Gross Finding. The lymph nodes are grossly enlarged and firm in lepromatous leprosy. The size of the lymph nodes is proportional to the duration of the disease (68). On cut section, they are yellow-white in the cortical area and pink-gray in the background in more central portions of the node.

Microscopic Findings. The histopathologic features of leprosy depend on the stage of the disease, which is modified by host immune response and treatment (Table 8-5). Histopathologic changes include reactive follicular hyperplasia and aggregates of pale foamy macrophages, primarily in the paracortical area (figs. 8-57, 8-58). These macrophages usually contain large numbers of bacilli that can be visualized with a modified AFB stain such as the Fite-Faraco method (fig. 8-59) (85). It is important to note that *M. leprae* may be negative for the Ziehl-Neelsen variant of the AFB stain, due to the more aggressive decoloration step.

Table 8-5

HISTOLOGIC FEATURES OF LEPROSY INVOLVEMENT OF LYMPH NODES OR SPLEEN[a]

	Lepromatous	Tuberculous
Capsular thickening	+++	++
Follicular changes	++	+/–
Lepra cells in sinuses	++/+++	–
Granulomas; foamy macrophages	+++	–
Granulomas; epithelioid macrophages, giant cells	–	+++
Plasma cells	++	–
Fibrosis	+	+

[a]Data from reference 68.

The lymph nodes in tuberculoid leprosy commonly show discrete epithelioid cell granulomas with multinucleated giant cells, which may be confluent and without necrosis. Fibrosis and hyalinization also occur. Bacilli are rarely demonstrable at this stage since the host is able to mount a vigorous T-cell–mediated immune response. This is in contrast to lepromatous leprosy in which there is poor host resistance due to a lack of T-cell–mediated immunity. In lepromatous leprosy, affected lymph nodes show a focal or diffuse accumulation of foamy macrophages with vacuolated cytoplasm containing large numbers of bacilli, so-called lepra cells (76). This histologic picture contrasts with the discrete or confluent granulomas seen in the tuberculoid type. In lepromatous leprosy,

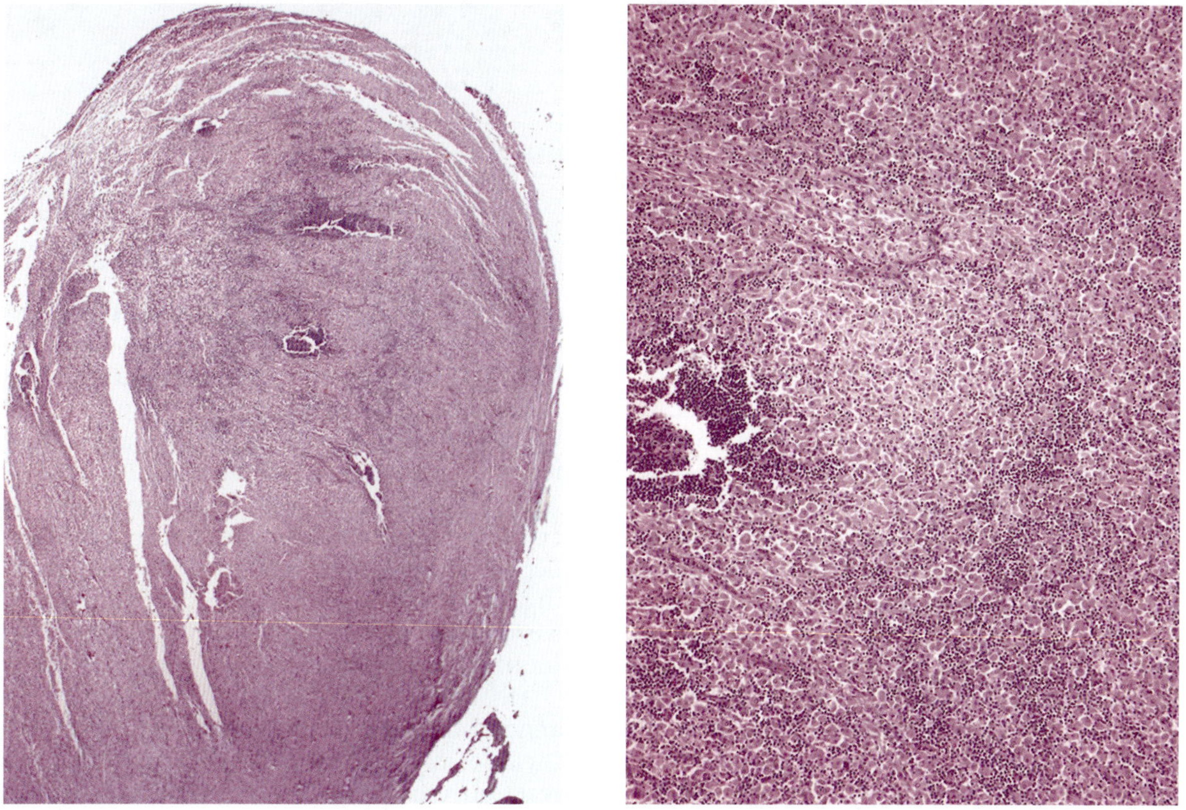

Figure 8-57

LEPROSY, LYMPH NODE

Like MAI, infection with leprosy often diffusely effaces the lymph node with a proliferation of foamy macrophages.

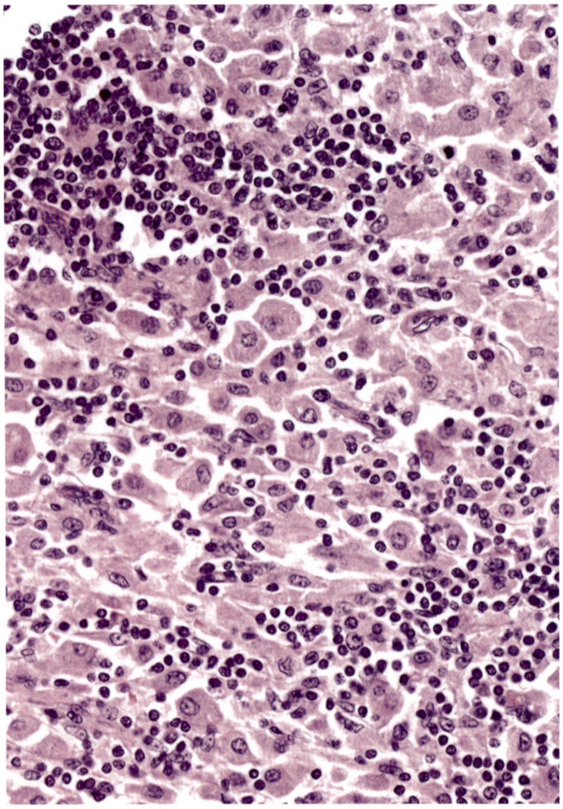

Figure 8-58

LEPROSY, LYMPH NODE

Details of the lepra cells in this lymph node with leprosy.

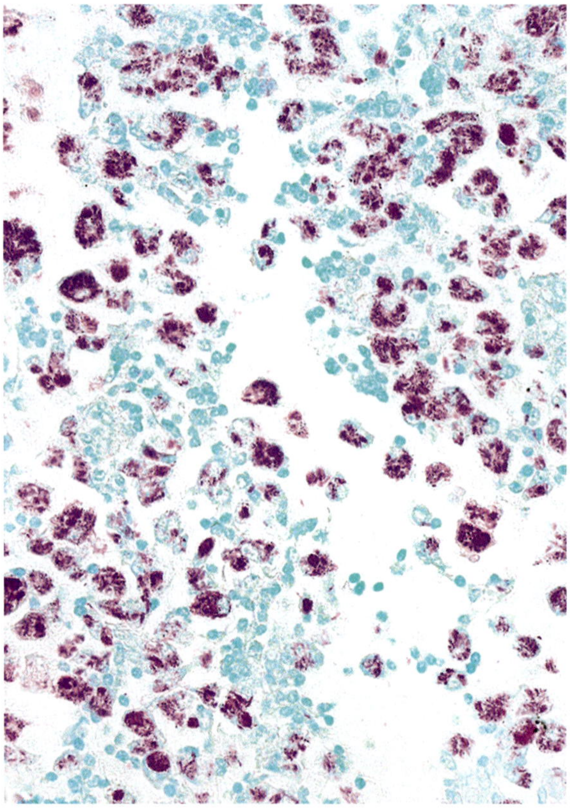

Figure 8-59

LEPROMATOUS LEPROSY LYMPHADENITIS

Macrophages contain numerous organisms, which are visualized with the Fite-Faraco stain.

rounded structures referred to as "globi" may also be noted, and represent coalesced masses of bacilli. Occasionally, multinucleated lepra cells are present and resemble Touton giant cells. Necrosis is seldom seen in the lymph nodes of lepromatous leprosy. In the lepromatous stage, follicles are depleted or replaced. In tuberculoid leprosy, follicles are hyperplastic and increased in number. A good clinical history in conjunction with the light microscopic findings, including the results of special stains, should help distinguish the two.

In cases of borderline leprosy, the clinical and histologic features are intermediate between the tuberculoid and lepromatous types. Involved lymph nodes show changes that are characteristic of both types, although tuberculoid granulomas usually predominate. Since this form of leprosy is unstable (unlike the polar forms of the disease which do not transform) and capable of deteriorating into the lepromatous type, it is essential to examine the lymph nodes of borderline leprosy to note the presence of interspersed lepra cells, an ominous finding.

The splenic findings in leprosy are similar to those seen in the lymph nodes (fig. 8-60). A rare finding in patients affected by leprosy is erythema nodosum leprosum, a reaction which occurs in the skin, or rarely, lymph nodes, during treatment. It is characterized by neutrophils surrounding foamy macrophages, and less commonly, necrotizing vasculitis (47).

Differential Diagnosis. The differential diagnosis of tuberculoid leprosy lymphadenitis includes other causes of foamy macrophage reaction, especially silicone lymphadenopathy. In borderline leprosy cases, the differential diagnosis includes other mycobacterial infections or other granulomatous processes such as sarcoidosis.

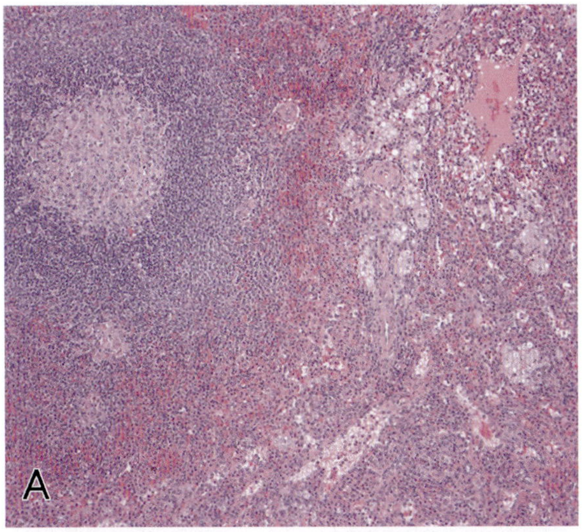

Figure 8-60

LEPROSY, SPLEEN

Clusters of foamy macrophages are seen in this spleen with leprosy (A,B). Numerous organisms are highlighted with a modified acid-fast stain (C). (Courtesy of California Tumor Tissue Registry, Loma Linda, CA.)

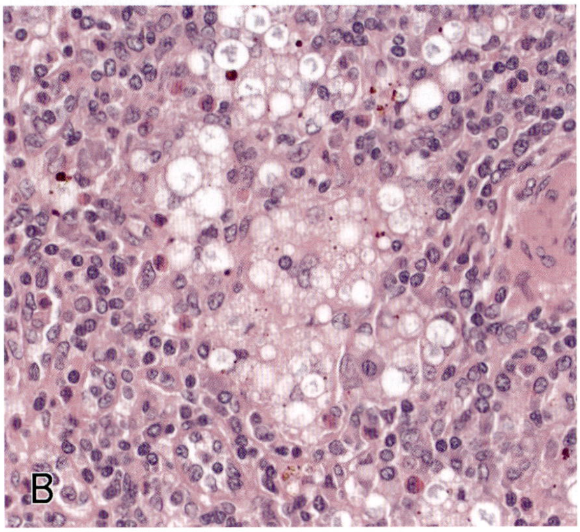

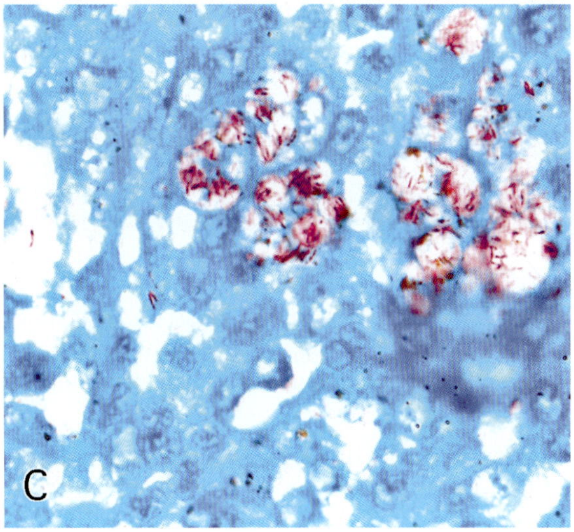

Treatment. Drug therapy, especially dapsone, has been the treatment of choice for patients with leprosy and must be sustained for many years to prevent relapse. One of the medications used in the treatment of leprosy, clofazimine, may cause an unusual proliferation of macrophages with cytoplasmic crystals (120). This is discussed in more detail in chapter 14.

Bacille Calmette-Guerin

Definition. *Bacille Calmette-Guerin* (BCG) is an attenuated strain of *Mycobacterium bovis*, which is used as an antituberculous vaccine in many parts of the world. In rare circumstances, particularly in immunosuppressed patients, BCG vaccinations lead to localized lymphadenitis, splenitis, or disseminated disease.

General Features. Vaccination with BCG is associated with complications in about 2 percent of cases and these include: regional lymphadenopathy, subcutaneous abscess at vaccination site, osteomyelitis, arthritis, and hepatic granulomas (2,69). Enlargement of the lymph nodes is a typical finding in BCG vaccination, and indicates an appropriate immunologic response to the avirulent mycobacterial strain. Severe infection occurs in rare patients, typically those with known or previously undescribed immunodeficiencies (112). A large study found that over 50 percent of cases of disseminated BCG infection were associated with either severe combined immunodeficiency, DiGeorge syndrome, chronic granulomatous disease, or HIV/AIDS (20). Microbiologic culture proves the presence of *M. bovis*, BCG strain.

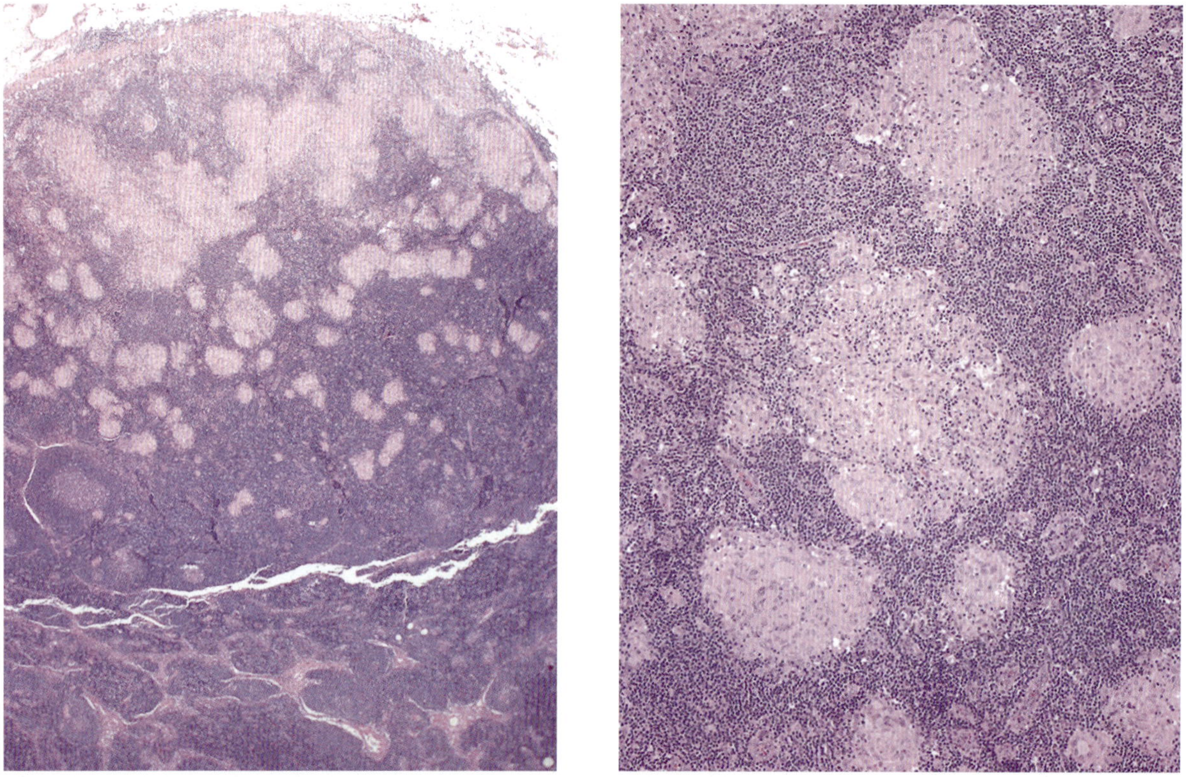

Figure 8-61

BACILLE CALMETTE-GUERIN (BCG), LYMPH NODE

Left: Numerous granulomas are seen in this lymph node adjacent to a bladder that was treated with BCG therapy. Right: Higher magnification of the granulomas. (Courtesy of John Eble, Indianapolis, IN.)

Microscopic Findings. Lymph nodes affected by BCG infection have multiple epithelioid granulomas with Langerhans giant cells (fig. 8-61) (2,11). Central caseation may be seen as well as focal suppuration and even sinus tract formation. Extensive necrosis is sometimes present. In occasional macrophages in touch preparations or cytologic specimens, negative images of mycobacteria can be seen (73). These macrophages may have the appearance of Gaucher cells, but are filled with mycobacteria. If there is a severe underlying immunodeficiency, the histologic picture may be altered depending on the type and severity of the underlying disorder. The microscopic findings of BCG infection are indistinguishable from those of tuberculosis. As with tuberculosis, BCG stains with AFB and modified AFB stains.

Treatment. Antimycobacterial/antituberculous therapy should be instituted in patients with severe BCG-related infection. Although the outcome is typically good, rare fatal cases have been recorded (2).

Atypical Mycobacterial Infections

Definition. Many other species of mycobacteria are associated with human infection. These infections may result in lymph node or splenic lesions.

General Features. Mycobacterial organisms have many features in common with ordinary bacteria, but also have distinctive cell walls composed of phosphoglycolipids, phospholipids, and waxes that are responsible for their acid-fastness. *Mycobacterium tuberculosis* and *M. leprae* comprise the so-called typical mycobacteria. In addition, there are at least 30 other types of so-called atypical mycobacteria which are classified according to their reactions to light, growth rate, and pigment production on culture media. Many of these have been known to cause lymphadenopathy (25,33,44,59,88,91,

114,115,117,121,128). A partial list of mycobacteria associated with human disease is seen in Table 8-6. Immunocompromised patients have a propensity for infection with atypical mycobacteria and therefore these organisms have shown an increase in incidence with the advent of the AIDS epidemic.

Although the most common presentation is that of an isolated enlarged cervical lymph node in a child, chronic adenopathy due to atypical mycobacteria is also seen in adults (25). Primary mycobacterial lymphadenitis ("scrofulaceum," or "scrofula") is a chronic granulomatous process that is seen most often in the cervical lymph nodes of children. It is due to atypical mycobacteria, especially *M. scrofulaceum*, *M. kansasii*, or MAI, most often as a result of dermal trauma to the oropharyngeal mucosa (38,102,121,124,140). Eighty percent of cases occur between the ages of 1 and 5 years. Infection is limited to single or groups of nodes. The submandibular and parotid lymph nodes are most often affected and their nontender enlargement may interfere with swallowing or breathing.

Microscopic Findings. The histopathologic change in lymphadenitis secondary to *M. scrofulaceum*, namely, granulomatous inflammation, is virtually indistinguishable from tuberculous lymphadenitis. In atypical mycobacterial infections, either in the spleen or lymph node, the histologic picture usually consists of various combinations of granulomatous and suppurative inflammation (fig. 8-62). Necrosis is variable; giant cells and associated fibrosis depend not only on the type of bacteria, but also on the host immunologic responses.

Table 8-6

ATYPICAL MYCOBACTERIAL SPECIES REPORTED IN ASSOCIATION WITH LYMPHADENOPATHY

M. abscessus	*M. gordonae*
M. bohemicum	*M. kansasii*
M. celatum	*M. interjectum*
M. chelonae	*M. malmoense*
M. fortuitum	*M. scrofulaceum*
M. genavense	*M. tusciae*

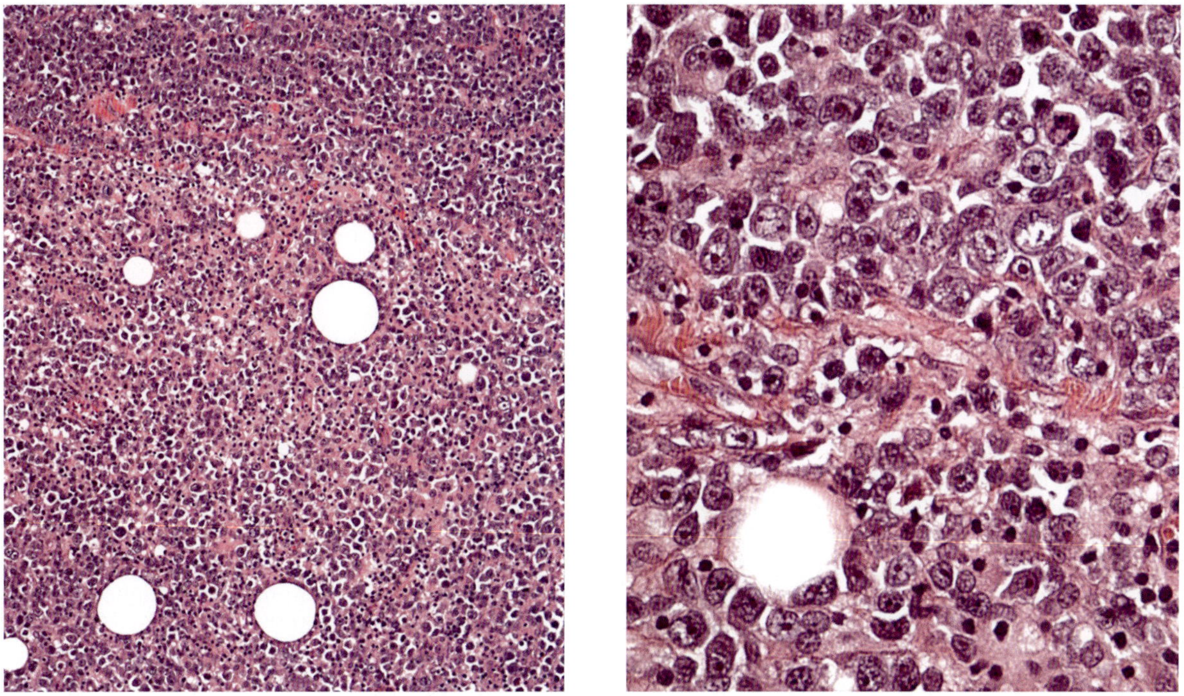

Figure 8-62

MYCOBACTERIUM FORTUITUM, LYMPH NODE

One of the family of "atypical" mycobacteria, the lymphadenitis in this case includes proliferation of immunoblasts, but no granuloma formation. (Courtesy of Peter Banks, Charlotte, NC.)

The histology may be like that of MAI infection, leprosy, or tuberculosis, or combinations of these. Organisms may be rare, as in tuberculosis, or common, as in MAI infections. In all circumstances, microbiologic studies, either culture or DNA-based assays, are required to identify the involved mycobacterial species.

Treatment. Cervical lymphadenitis due to atypical mycobacteria is treated by complete surgical excision of the involved lymph nodes and skin, and postoperative drug therapy with antituberculous drugs (102).

POSTSPLENECTOMY INFECTIONS

The critical role of the spleen in preventing infection is well known and has been discussed previously (see chapter 1). It is also well known that splenectomy or hyposplenism from any cause increases susceptibility to certain infections. Overwhelming sepsis is the most dreaded complication of the postsplenectomy state. Although it is more often encountered in young patients, any age may be affected. Clinically, patients present with the typical manifestations of fever, chills, nausea, vomiting, multiorgan failure, disseminated intravascular coagulation, seizures, and rapid death.

Postsplenectomy infections are usually due to encapsulated bacteria, including *Streptococcus pneumoniae, Haemophilus influenzae* type b, and *Neisseria meningitidis*. Other unusual pathogens may be associated with severe infections, including bacteria, viruses, and protozoa (100). The risk of overwhelming infection after splenectomy is the highest within 2 years after removal of the spleen (100).

The cornerstone of management of postsplenectomy patients is immunization against encapsulated bacteria. Immunizations for *S. pneumoniae, H. influenzae*, and *N. meningitidis* are readily available. In cases where splenectomy is planned, presurgical immunization is recommended for optimal response. Antibiotic prophylaxis is recommended by some; however, there are no long-term controlled trials evaluating its effectiveness. In spite of this, most recommendations are that prophylactic penicillin be given to children for at least the first 2 years after splenectomy.

When traumatic damage to the spleen necessitates splenectomy, attempts should be made at splenic preservation. Autotransplantation of splenic tissue, accessory spleens, or partial splenectomy allow retention of the immunologic function of the spleen. In any circumstance, postsplenectomy or hyposplenic patients should be treated early and aggressively when there is suspicion of infection. Finally, it is recommended that any asplenic individuals should wear medical alert bracelets to warn medical professionals and allow for appropriate treatment.

REFERENCES

1. Abramova FA, Grinberg LM, Yampolskaya OV, Walker DH. Pathology of inhalational anthrax in 42 cases from the Sverdlovsk outbreak of 1979. Proc Natl Acad Sci U S A 1993;90:2291-4.
2. al-Bhlal LA. Pathologic findings for bacille Calmette-Guerin infections in immunocompetent and immunocompromised patients. Am J Clin Pathol 2000;113:703-8.
3. Ali G, Kamili MA, Rashid S, Mansoor A, Lone BA, Allaqaband GQ. Spontaneous splenic rupture in typhoid fever. Postgrad Med J 1994;70:513-4.
4. Alkan S, Beals TF, Schnitzer B. Primary diagnosis of Whipple disease manifesting as lymphadenopathy: use of polymerase chain reaction for detection of Tropheryma whippelii. Am J Clin Pathol 2001;116:898-904.
5. Amrikachi M, Krishnan B, Finch CJ, Shahab I. Actinomyces and actinobacillus actinomycetemcomitans—Actinomyces-associated lymphadenopathy mimicking lymphoma. Arch Pathol Lab Med 2000;124:1502-5.
6. Angritt P, Tuur SM, Macher AM, et al. Epithelioid angiomatosis in HIV infection: neoplasm or cat-scratch disease? Lancet 1988;1:996.
7. Ariga T, Nagaoka H, Miyanoshita A, et al. Coxiella burnetii lymphadenitis: a possible fever focus in acute Q fever. Pediatr Int 2000;42:711-4.

8. Badrawy R, el-Shennawy M. Affection of cervical lymph nodes in rhinoscleroma. J Laryngol Otol 1974;88:261-9.
9. Baisden BL, Lepidi H, Raoult D, Argani P, Yardley JH, Dumler JS. Diagnosis of Whipple disease by immunohistochemical analysis: a sensitive and specific method for the detection of Tropheryma whipplei (the Whipple bacillus) in paraffin-embedded tissue. Am J Clin Pathol 2002;118:742-8.
10. Barakat LA, Quentzel HL, Jernigan JA, et al. Anthrax Bioterrorism Investigation Team. Fatal inhalational anthrax in a 94-year-old Connecticut woman. JAMA 2002;287:863-8.
11. Barouni AS, Augusto C, Queiroz MV, Lopes MT, Zanini MS, Salas CE. BCG lymphadenopathy detected in a BCG-vaccinated infant. Braz J Med Biol Res 2004;37:697-700.
12. Bastounis E, Pikoulis E, Varelas P, Cirochristos D, Aessopos A. Tuberculoma of the spleen: a rare but important clinical entity. Am Surg 1999;65:131-2.
13. Biberfeld P, Ost A, Porwit A, et al. Histopathology and immunohistology of HTLV-III/LAV related lymphadenopathy and AIDS. Acta Pathol Microbiol Immunol Scand [A] 1987;95:47-65.
14. Blackwell JB, Smith FH, Joyce PR. Granulomatous lymphadenitis caused by Corynebacterium ovis. Pathology 1974;6:243-9.
15. Bradford WD, Noce PS, Gutman LT. Pathologic features of enteric infection with Yersinia enterocolitica. Arch Pathol 1974;98:17-22.
16. Brenner DJ, Hollis DG, Moss CW, et al. Proposal of Afipia gen. nov., with Afipia felis sp. nov. (formerly the cat scratch disease bacillus), Afipia clevelandensis sp. nov. (formerly the Cleveland Clinic foundation strain), Afipia broomeae sp. nov., and three unnamed genospecies. J Clin Microbiol 1991;29:2450-60.
17. Brenner DJ, O'Connor SP, Winkler HH, Steigerwalt AG. Proposals to unify the genera Bartonella and Rochalimaea, with descriptions of Bartonella quintana comb. nov., Bartonella vinsonii comb. nov., Bartonella henselae comb. nov., and Bartonella elizabethae comb. nov., and to remove the family Bartonellaceae from the order of Rickettsiales. Int J Syst Bacteriol 1993;43:777-86.
18. Brown JR. Human actinomycosis. A study of 181 subjects. Hum Pathol 1973;4:319-30.
19. Campbell JA. Cat-scratch disease. Pathol Annu 1977;12:277-92.
20. Casanova JL, Blanche S, Emile JF, et al. Idiopathic disseminated bacillus Calmette-Guerin infection: a French national retrospective study. Pediatrics 1996;98:774-8.
21. Chakravarti A, Goyal A, Vishwakarma SK, Arora VK. Affection of cervical lymph nodes in rhinoscleroma. Trop Doct 2000;30:110-1.
22. Chan JK, Lewin KJ, Lombard CM, Teitelbaum S, Dorfman RF. Histopathology of bacillary angiomatosis of lymph node. Am J Surg Pathol 1991;15:430-7.
23. Chao SS, Loh KS, Tan KK, Chong SM. Tuberculous and nontuberculous cervical lymphadenitis: a clinical review. Otolaryngol Head Neck Surg 2002;126:176-9.
24. Chen CH, Fang YH, Chiang PM, Lin DT, Huang LM. Disseminated tuberculosis presenting as multiple hepatosplenic microabscesses and pancytopenia in a teenage boy. J Formos Med Assoc 2004;103:939-42.
25. Chetchotisakd P, Mootsikapun P, Anunnatsiri S, et al. Disseminated infection due to rapidly growing mycobacteria in immunocompetent hosts presenting with chronic lymphadenopathy: a previously unrecognized clinical entity. Clin Infect Dis 2000;30:29-34.
26. Chiewchanvit S, Mahanupab P, Baosoung V, Khamwan C. Uncommon manifestations of opportunistic infections in an HIV infected patient. J Med Assoc Thai 1998;81:923-6.
27. Choi YJ, Reiner L. Syphilitic lymphadenitis: immunofluorescent identification of spirochetes from imprints. Am J Surg Pathol 1979;3:553-5.
28. Cockerell CJ, Webster GF, Whitlow MA, Friedman-Kien AE. Epithelioid angiomatosis: a distinct vascular disorder in patients with the acquired immunodeficiency syndrome or AIDS-related complex. Lancet 1987;2:654-6.
29. Colmenero Jde D, Queipo-Ortuno MI, Maria Reguera J, Angel Suarez-Munoz M, Martin-Carballino S, Morata P. Chronic hepatosplenic abscesses in Brucellosis. Clinico-therapeutic features and molecular diagnostic approach. Diagn Microbiol Infect Dis 2002;42:159-67.
30. Cornish N, Washington JA. Rhodococcus equi infections: clinical features and laboratory diagnosis. Curr Clin Top Infect Dis 1999;19:198-215.
31. Dahl R, Dans PE. Gonococcal lymphadenitis. Arch Intern Med 1974;134:116-7.
32. Daybell D, Paddock CD, Zaki SR, et al. Disseminated infection with Bartonella henselae as a cause of spontaneous splenic rupture. Clin Infect Dis 2004;39:e21-4.
33. den Broeder AA, Vervoort G, van Assen S, Verduyn Lunel F, de Lange WC, de Sevaux RG. Disseminated Mycobacterium gordonae infection in a renal transplant recipient. Transpl Infect Dis 2003;5:151-5.
34. Destuynder O, Vanlemmans P, Mboyo A, et al. Systemic cat scratch disease: hepatic and splenic involvement about 3 pediatric cases. Eur J Pediatr Surg 1995;5:365-8.

35. Dobbins WO 3rd, Ruffin JM. A light-and electron-microscopic study of bacterial invasion in Whipple's disease. Am J Pathol 1967;51:225-42.
36. Domingo P, Rodriguez P, Lopez-Contreras J, Rebasa P, Mota S, Matias-Guiu X. Spontaneous rupture of the spleen associated with pneumonia. Eur J Clin Microbiol Infect Dis 1996;15:733-6.
37. Donisi A, Suardi MG, Casari S, Longo M, Cadeo GP, Carosi G. Rhodococcus equi infection in HIV-infected patients. AIDS 1996;10:359-62.
38. Dooley JR. Other mycobacterial diseases. In: Binford CH, Connor DH, eds. Pathology of tropical and extraordinary diseases, Vol. 1. Washington DC: Armed Forces Institute of Pathology; 1976:235-43.
39. Drevelengas A. The spleen in infectious disorders. JBR-BTR 2000;83:208-10.
40. El-Maraghi NR, Mair NS. The histopathology of enteric infection with Yersinia pseudotuberculosis. Am J Clin Pathol 1979;71:631-9.
41. English CK, Wear DJ, Margileth AM, Lissner CR, Walsh GP. Cat-scratch disease. Isolation and culture of the bacterial agent. JAMA 1988; 259:1347-52.
42. Enzinger FM, Helwig EB. Whipple's disease: a review of the literature and report of fifteen patients. Virchows Arch Pathol Anat Physiol Klin Med 1963;336:238-69.
43. Estrada B. Azithromycin and cat-scratch disease. Infect Med 1998;15:517.
44. Evans MJ, Smith NM, Thornton CM, Youngson GG, Gray ES. Atypical mycobacterial lymphadenitis in childhood—a clinicopathological study of 17 cases. J Clin Pathol 1998;51:925-7.
45. Farhi DC, Wells SJ, Siegel RJ. Syphilitic lymphadenopathy. Histology and human immunodeficiency virus status. Am J Clin Pathol 1999;112:330-4.
46. Feig JA, Cina SJ. Evaluation of characteristics associated with acute splenitis (septic spleen) as markers of systemic infection. Arch Pathol Lab Med 2001;125:888-91.
47. Fiallo P, Pesce C, Lenti E, Nunzi E. Short report: erythema nodosum leprosum lymphadenitis. Am J Trop Med Hyg 1995;52:297-8.
48. Foucault C, Lepidi H, Poujet-Abadie JF, et al. Q fever and lymphadenopathy: report of four new cases and review. Eur J Clin Microbiol Infect Dis 2004;23:759-64.
49. Fournier PE, Gouriet F, Brouqui P, Lucht F, Raoult D. Lymphangitis-associated rickettsiosis, a new rickettsiosis caused by Rickettsia sibirica mongolotimonae: seven new cases and review of the literature. Clin Infect Dis 2005;40:1435-44.
50. Francis E, Callender GR. Tularemia: the microscopic changes of the lesions in man. Archives of Pathology and Laboratory Medicine 1927;3:577-607.
51. Freidig EE, McClure SP, Wilson WR, Banks PM, Washingon JA 2nd. Clinical-histologic-microbiologic analysis of 419 lymph node biopsy specimens. Rev Infect Dis 1986;8:322-8.
52. Friedman PS, Turk JL. A spectrum of human lymphocyte responsiveness in human syphilis. Clin Exp Immunol 1975;21:59-64.
53. Garcia-Corbeira P, Ramos JM, Aguado JM, Soriano F. Six cases in which mesenteric lymphadenitis due to non-typhi Salmonella caused an appendicitis-like syndrome. Clin Infect Dis 1995;21:231-2.
54. Garduno E, Rebollo M, Asencio MA, Carro J, Pascasio JM, Blanco J. Splenic abscesses caused by Actinomyces meyeri in a patient with autoimmune hepatitis. Diagn Microbiol Infect Dis 2000;37:213-4.
55. Goldberger AC, Lipsky BA, Plorde JJ. Suppurative granulomatous lymphadenitis caused by Corynebacterium ovis (pseudotuberculosis). Am J Clin Pathol 1981;76:486-90.
56. Gras E, Matias-Guiu X, Garcia A, et al. PCR analysis in the pathological diagnosis of Whipple's disease: emphasis on extraintestinal involvement or atypical morphological features. J Pathol 1999;188:318-21.
57. Gray KJ, French N, Lugada E, Watera C, Gilks CF. Rhodococcus equi and HIV-1 infection in Uganda. J Infect 2000;41:227-31.
58. Grinberg LM, Abramova FA, Yampolskaya OV, Walker DH, Smith JH. Quantitative pathology of inhalational anthrax I: quantitative microscopic findings. Mod Pathol 2001;14:482-95.
59. Guarner J, Bartlett J, Whitney EA, et al. Histopathologic features of Mycobacterium ulcerans infection. Emerg Infect Dis 2003;9:651-6.
60. Guarner J, Jernigan JA, Shieh WJ, et al. Inhalational Anthrax Pathology Working Group. Pathology and pathogenesis of bioterrorism-related inhalational anthrax. Am J Pathol 2003;163:701-9.
61. Guarner J, Shieh WJ, Greer PW, et al. Immunohistochemical detection of Yersinia pestis in formalin-fixed, paraffin-embedded tissue. Am J Clin Pathol 2002;117:205-9.
62. Guarner J, Zaki SR. Histopathology and immunohistochemistry in the diagnosis of bioterrorism agents. J Histochem Cytochem 2006;54:3-11.
63. Gupta SN, Flaherty JP, Shaw JC. Erythema nodosum associated with reactivation tuberculous lymphadenitis (scrofula). Int J Dermatol 2002;41:173-5.
64. Haase G, Skopnik H, Batge S, Bottger EC. Cervical lymphadenitis caused by Mycobacterium celatum. Lancet 1994;344:1020-1.
65. Hartsock RJ, Halling LW, King FM. Luetic lymphadenitis: a clinical and histologic study of 20 cases. Am J Clin Pathol 1970;53:304-14.

66. Idriss ZH, Cunningham RJ, Wilfert CM. Nocardiosis in children: report of three cases and review of the literature. Pediatrics 1975;55:479-84.
67. Isaac-Renton JL, Boyko WJ, Chan R, Crichton E. Corynebacterium diphtheriae septicemia. Am J Clin Pathol 1981;75:631-4.
68. Kar HK, Mohanty HC, Mohanty GN, Nayak UP. Clinico-pathological study of lymph node involvement in leprosy. Lepr India 1983;55:725-38.
69. Karadeniz C, Oguz A, Ezer U, Ozturk G, Dursun A. The etiology of peripheral lymphadenopathy in children. Pediatr Hematol Oncol 1999;16:525-31.
70. Klatt EC, Jensen DF, Meyer PR. Pathology of Mycobacterium avium-intracellulare infection in acquired immunodeficiency syndrome. Hum Pathol 1987;18:709-14.
71. Kojima M, Morita Y, Shimizu K, Itoh H, Masawa N, Nakamura S. Plasmacytoid monocytes in cat scratch disease with special reference to the histological diversity of suppurative lesions. Pathol Res Pract 2006;202:17-22.
72. Kraus M, Benharroch D, Kaplan D, et al. Mycobacterial cervical lymphadenitis: the histological features of non-tuberculous mycobacterial infection. Histopathology 1999;35:534-8.
73. Kumar PV, Monabati A, Kadivar R, Soleimanpour H. Peripheral blood and marrow findings in disseminated bacille Calmette-Guerin infection. J Pediatr Hematol Oncol 2005;27:97-9.
74. Lamps LW, Havens JM, Sjostedt A, Page DL, Scott MA. Histologic and molecular diagnosis of tularemia: a potential bioterrorism agent endemic to North America. Mod Pathol 2004;17:489-95.
75. LeBoit PE, Berger TG, Egbert BM, et al. Epithelioid haemangioma-like vascular proliferation in AIDS: manifestation of cat scratch disease bacillus infection? Lancet 1988;1:960-3.
76. Lele VR, Raichur BS, Grover S. Study of lymph node biopsies in lepromatous leprosy patients under treatment. Lepr India 1983;55:739-42.
77. Lepidi H, Costedoat N, Piette JC, Harle JR, Raoult D. Immunohistological detection of Tropheryma whipplei (Whipple bacillus) in lymph nodes. Am J Med 2002;113:334-6.
78. Liston TE, Koehler JE. Granulomatous hepatitis and necrotizing splenitis due to Bartonella henselae in a patient with cancer: case report and review of hepatosplenic manifestations of bartonella infection. Clin Infect Dis 1996;22:951-7.
79. Logani S, Lucas DR, Cheng JD, Ioachim HL, Adsay NV. Spindle cell tumors associated with mycobacteria in lymph nodes of HIV-positive patients: 'Kaposi sarcoma with mycobacteria' and 'mycobacterial pseudotumor.' Am J Surg Pathol 1999;23:656-61.
80. Mansbach CM 2nd, Shelburne JD, Stevens RD, Dobbins WO 3rd. Lymph-node bacilliform bodies resembling those of Whipple's disease in a patient without intestinal involvement. Ann Intern Med 1978;89:64-6.
81. Marchetti G, Gori A, Catozzi L, et al. Evaluation of PCR in detection of Mycobacterium tuberculosis from formalin-fixed, paraffin-embedded tissues: comparison of four amplification assays. J Clin Microbiol 1998;36:1512-7.
82. Margileth AM, Wear DJ, English CK. Systemic cat scratch disease: report of 23 patients with prolonged or recurrent severe bacterial infection. J Inf Dis 1987;155:390-402.
83. Meier FA. Melioidosis. In: Connor DH, Chandler FW, Schwartz DA, Manz HJ, Lack EE, eds. Pathology of infectious diseases. Stamford, CT: Appleton & Lange; 1997:647-56.
84. Menakuru SR, Singh R, Sharma N, Verma S. Isolated splenic TB report of three cases. Trop Doct 2005;35:246-7.
85. Meyers WM. Leprosy. Dermatol Clin 1992;10:73-96.
86. Miller-Catchpole R, Variakojis D, Vardiman JW, Loew JM, Carter J. Cat scratch disease. Identification of bacteria in seven cases of lymphadenitis. Am J Surg Pathol 1986;10:276-81.
87. Mills AE, Mitchell RD, Lim EK. Corynebacterium pseudotuberculosis is a cause of human necrotising granulomatous lymphadenitis. Pathology 1997;29:231-3.
88. Monill JM, Franquet T, Sambeat MA, Martinez-Noguera A, Villalba J. Mycobacterium genavense infection in AIDS: imaging findings in eight patients. Eur Radiol 2001;11:193-6.
89. Muir-Padilla J, Myers JB. Whipple disease: a case report and review of the literature. Arch Pathol Lab Med 2005;129:933-6.
90. Naji AF, Carbonell F, Barker HJ. Cat scratch disease. A report of three new cases, review of the literature, and classification of the pathologic changes in the lymph nodes during various stages of the disease. Am J Clin Pathol 1962;38:513-21.
91. Palca A, Aebi C, Weimann R, Bodmer T. Mycobacterium bohemicum cervical lymphadenitis. Pediatr Infect Dis J 2002;21:982-4.
92. Piggott JA, Hochholzer L. Human melioidosis. A histopathologic study of acute and chronic melioidosis. Arch Pathol 1970;90:101-11.
93. Quintero-Del-Rio AI, Trujillo M, Fink CW. Actinomycotic splenic abscesses presenting with arthritis. Clin Exp Rheumatol 1997;15:445-8.

94. Race EM, Adelson-Mitty J, Kriegel GR, et al. Focal mycobacterial lymphadenitis following initiation of protease-inhibitor therapy in patients with advanced HIV-1 disease. Lancet 1998;351:252-5.
95. Ramanathan VD, Jawahar MS, Paramasivan CN, et al. A histological spectrum of host responses in tuberculous lymphadenitis. Indian J Med Res 1999;109:212-20.
96. Reichert CM, O'Leary TJ, Levens DL, Simrell CR, Macher AM. Autopsy pathology in the acquired immune deficiency syndrome. Am J Pathol 1983;112:357-82.
97. Relman DA, Schmidt TM, MacDermott RP, Falkow S. Identification of the uncultured bacillus of Whipple's disease. N Engl J Med 1992;327:293-301.
98. Rolain JM, Chanet V, Laurichesse H, Lepidi H, Beytout J, Raoult D. Cat scratch disease with lymphadenitis, vertebral osteomyelitis, and spleen abscesses. Ann N Y Acad Sci 2003;990:397-403.
99. Rosenthal R, Vogelbach P, Gasser M, Zimmerli W. Cervical lymphadenitis—a rare case of focal listeriosis. Infection 2001;29:170-2.
100. Rushton TC, Gorse GJ, Bowdler AJ. The relationship of the spleen to infection. In: Bowdler AJ, ed. The complete spleen: structure, function and clinical disorders, 2nd ed. Totowa, NJ: Humana Press; 2002:175-92.
101. Said J. AIDS-related lymphadenopathies. Semin Diagn Pathol 1988;5:365-75.
102. Salyer KE, Votteler TP, Dorman GW. Surgical management of cervical adenitis due to atypical mycobacteria in children. JAMA 1968;204:1039-40.
103. Samuelson J, von Lichtenberg F. Infectious diseases. In: Cotran RS, Robbins SL, Kumar V, Schoen FJ. Pathologic basis of disease, 5th ed. Philadelphia, PA: W.B. Saunders; 1994:305-77.
104. Satti MB, al-Mohaya S, Omer AS. Hansen's disease: a cause of lymphadenopathy in endemic areas. Trop Geogr Med 1989;41:80-4.
105. Schapers RF, Reif R, Lennert K, Knapp W. Mesenteric lymphadenitis due to Yersinia enterocolitica. Virchows Arch A Pathol Anat Histol 1981;390:127-38.
106. Scott MA. Infections involving lymph nodes. In: Pediatric hematopathology. Collins RD, Swerdlow SH, eds. New York: Churchill Livingstone; 2001;289-312.
107. Scott MA, Graham BS, Verrall R, Dixon R, Schaffner W, Tham KT. Rhodococcus equi—an increasingly recognized opportunistic pathogen. Report of 12 cases and review of 65 cases in the literature. Am J Clin Pathol 1995;103:649-55.
108. Sibanda EN, Stanczuk G. Lymph node pathology in Zimbabwe: a review of 2194 specimens. Q J Med 1993;86:811-7.
109. Siegel RJ. Human immunodeficiency virus- associated lymphoid disease. In: Connor DH, Chandler FW, Schwartz DA, Manz HJ, Lack EE, eds. Pathology of infectious diseases, Vol. I. Stamford, CT: Appleton & Lange; 1997:161-8.
110. Simpson GL, Stinson EB, Egger MJ, Remington JS. Nocardial infections in the immunocompromised host: a detailed study in a defined population. Rev Infect Dis 1981;3:492-507.
111. Singh N, Manucha V, Bhattacharya SN, Arora VK, Bhatia A. Pitfalls in the cytological classification of borderline leprosy in the Ridley-Jopling scale. Diagn Cytopathol 2004;30:386-8.
112. Skinner R, Appleton AL, Sprott MS, et al. Disseminated BCG infection in severe combined immunodeficiency presenting with severe anaemia and associated with gross hypersplenism after bone marrow transplantation. Bone Marrow Transplant 1996;17:877-80.
113. Smith EB, Custer RP. Histopathology of lymphogranuloma venereum. J Urol 1950; 63:546-63.
114. Smith MB, Molina CP, Schnadig VJ, Boyars MC, Aronson JF. Pathologic features of Mycobacterium kansasii infection in patients with acquired immunodeficiency syndrome. Arch Pathol Lab Med 2003;127:554-60.
115. Smith MB, Schnadig VJ, Boyars MC, Woods GL. Clinical and pathologic features of Mycobacterium fortuitum infections. An emerging pathogen in patients with AIDS. Am J Clin Pathol 2001;116:225-32.
116. Smith MD Jr, Nio M, Camel JE, Sato JK, Atkinson JB. Management of splenic abscess in immunocompromised children. J Pediatr Surg 1993;28:823-6.
117. Springer B, Kirschner P, Rost-Meyer G, Schroder KH, Kroppenstedt RM, Bottger EC. Mycobacterium interjectum, a new species isolated from a patient with chronic lymphadenitis. J Clin Microbiol 1993;31:3083-9.
118. Stoler MH, Bonfiglio TA, Steigbigel RT, Pereira M. An atypical subcutaneous infection associated with acquired immune deficiency syndrome. Am J Clin Pathol 1983;80:714-8.
119. Sukpanichnant S. Leishmaniasis, melioidosis, penicilliosis and typhoid fever. In: Collins RD, Swerdlow SH, eds. Pediatric hematopathology. New York: Churchill Livingstone; 2001:312-7.
120. Sukpanichnant S, Hargrove NS, Kachintorn U, et al. Clofazimine-induced crystal-storing histiocytosis producing chronic abdominal pain in a leprosy patient. Am J Surg Pathol 2000;24:129-35.

121. Suskind DL, Handler SD, Tom LW, Potsic WP, Wetmore RF. Nontuberculous mycobacterial cervical adenitis. Clin Pediatr (Phila) 1997;36:403-9.
122. Suster S, Moran CA, Blanco M. Mycobacterial spindle-cell pseudotumor of the spleen. Am J Clin Pathol 1994;101:539-42.
123. Sutinen S, Syrjala H. Histopathology of human lymph node tularemia caused by Francisella tularensis var palaearctica. Arch Pathol Lab Med 1986;110:42-6.
124. Symmers WStC. Lymphadenitis caused by infection and infestation. In: Henry K, Symmers WStC, ed. Systemic pathology, 3rd ed. New York: Churchill Livingstone; 1992:326-492.
125. Symmers WStC. The lymphoreticular system. In: Lewis ML, Lucas RB, McMenem WH, et al, eds. Systemic pathology by 38 authors, 2nd. Edniburgh: Churchill Livingstone; 1978:504-891.
126. Tanaka A, Emori K, Nagao S, et al. Epithelioid granuloma formation requiring no T-cell function. Am J Pathol 1982;106:165-70.
127. Thomson SR, Ghimenton F. Splenic tuberculosis. Postgrad Med J 1999;75:578.
128. Tortoli E, Kroppenstedt RM, Bartoloni A, et al. Mycobacterium tusciae sp. nov. Int J Syst Bacteriol 1999;49:1839-44.
129. Turner DR, Wright DJ. Lymphadenopathy in early syphilis. J Pathol 1973;110:305-9.
130. Ventura A, Massei F, Not T, Massimetti M, Bussani R, Maggiore G. Systemic Bartonella henselae infection with hepatosplenic involvement. J Pediatr Gastroenterol Nutr 1999:29:52-6.
131. Walzer PD, Armstrong D. Lymphogranuloma venereum presenting as superclavicular and inguinal lymphadenopathy. Sex Transm Dis 1977;4:12-4.
132. Wang S, Ernst LM, Smith BR, et al. Systemic Tropheryma whippleii infection associated with monoclonal B-cell proliferation: a Helicobacter pylori-type pathogenesis? Arch Pathol Lab Med 2003;127:1619-22.
133. Wear DJ, Margileth AM, Hadfield TL, Fischer GW, Schlagel CJ, King FM. Cat scratch disease: a bacterial infection. Science 1983;221:1403-5.
134. Welch DF, Pickett DA, Slater LN, Steigerwalt AG, Brenner DJ. Rochalimaea henselae sp. nov., a cause of septicemia, bacillary angiomatosis, and parenchymal bacillary peliosis. J Clin Microbiol 1992;30:275-80.
135. White NJ. Melioidosis. Lancet 2003;361:1715-22.
136. Wilcox GM, Tronic BS, Schecter DJ, Arron MJ, Righi DF, Weiner NJ. Periodic acid-Schiff-negative granulomatous lymphadenopathy in patients with Whipple's disease. Localization of the Whipple bacillus to noncaseating granulomas by electron microscopy. Am J Med 1987;83:165-70.
137. Winn WC Jr, Myerowitz RL. The pathology of the Legionella pneumonias. A review of 74 cases and the literature. Hum Pathol 1981;12:401-22.
138. Winterbauer RH, Belic N, Moores KD. Clinical interpretation of bilateral hilar adenopathy. Ann Intern Med 1973:78:65-71.
139. Wolf DA, Wu CD, Medeiros LJ. Mycobacterial pseudotumors of lymph node. A report of two cases diagnosed at the time of intraoperative consultation using touch imprint preparations. Arch Pathol Lab Med 1995;119:811-4.
140. Wolinsky E. Mycobacterial lymphadenitis in children: a prospective study of 105 nontuberculous cases with long-term follow-up. Clin Infect Dis 1995;20:954-63.
141. Youmans GP. Mechanisms of immunity in tuberculosis. Pathobiol Annu 1979;9:137-62.
142. Young EJ. Human brucellosis. Rev Infect Dis 1983;5:821-42.

9 VIRAL LYMPHADENOPATHIES

GENERAL VIRAL-ASSOCIATED LYMPHADENOPATHY

Many cases of viral-associated lymphadenitis show the typical pattern of diffuse paracortical immunoblastic hyperplasia that was described in chapter 5. The features of some commonly encountered viral adenopathies are discussed in Table 9-1. Occasionally, however, certain viral infections cause a diffuse atypical or pseudoobliterative pattern of hyperplasia that may be difficult to recognize as a benign process (figs. 9-1, 9-2) (71). To avoid misinterpretation, a lymph node biopsy in known viral infections, such as infectious mononucleosis, is not recommended (29,81,108,125).

The patterns of nodal distortion can often be distinguished from typical paracortical hyperplasia by the greater disruption of the nodal architecture, with foci of necrosis and numerous, large immunoblasts. These atypical cells may mask the benign nature of the lesion and simulate a large cell lymphoma (33). When atypical cells are noted in a sinusoidal location, they may simulate an anaplastic large cell lymphoma (fig. 9-3). Reactivity for CD30 has been reported in the immunoblasts of infectious mononucleosis lymphadenitis, and this also may erroneously support a diagnosis of anaplastic large cell lymphoma (2). An increased number of high endothelial venules are also present in such cases (120).

INFECTIOUS MONONUCLEOSIS/ ACUTE EPSTEIN-BARR VIRUS

Definition. Acute, primary infection by *Epstein-Barr virus* (EBV) causes the classic clinical syndrome of *infectious mononucleosis*. This may lead to lymphadenopathy and splenomegaly, with characteristic histopathologic findings.

General Features. EBV, a member of the herpes group of viruses, is perhaps the most ubiquitous virus associated with hematologic disorders. It is present in a wide range of

Table 9-1

SUMMARY OF FINDINGS IN FREQUENTLY ENCOUNTERED VIRAL LYMPHADENOPATHIES

Type of Lymphadenopathy	Nodal Compartment Involved	Key Histologic Findings	Differential Diagnosis	Key Factors in Establishing Diagnosis
Epstein-Barr, acute (infectious mononucleosis	Diffuse, paracortical	Atypical immunoblastic proliferation with "mottled" appearance; polymorphous background; proliferation of endothelium; variable necrosis, often focal	Large cell non-Hodgkin lymphoma; Hodgkin lymphoma	Distorted but intact nodal architecture; open sinuses; polymorphic background; staining for EBV-LMP[a]
Herpes simplex	Diffuse, paracortical	Findings similar to IM; rare intranuclear inclusions; discrete foci of necrosis, frequently extensive	Kikuchi disease; necrotic viral, bacterial, and fungal lymphadenitis	Immunostaining; in situ hybridization
Cytomegalovirus	Diffuse, paracortical	Follicular hyperplasia; marginal zone hyperplasia; characteristic viral inclusions	Other viral adenopathies; Hodgkin lymphoma	CD15 staining; in situ hybridization; immunostaining
Postvaccinial	Diffuse, paracortical	Follicular (after 15 days) or diffuse (before 15 days) immunoblastic proliferation; polymorphic background	Hodgkin lymphoma; non-Hodgkin lymphoma	History of recent immunization critical
HIV[b]	Follicular	Follicular hyperplasia with or without fragmentation; follicular regression with eventual lymphoid depletion	Other viral adenopathies; Castleman disease	History; viral serology

[a]EBV = Epstein-Barr virus; LMP = latent membrane protein; IM = infectious mononucleosis.
[b]HIV = human immunodeficiency virus.

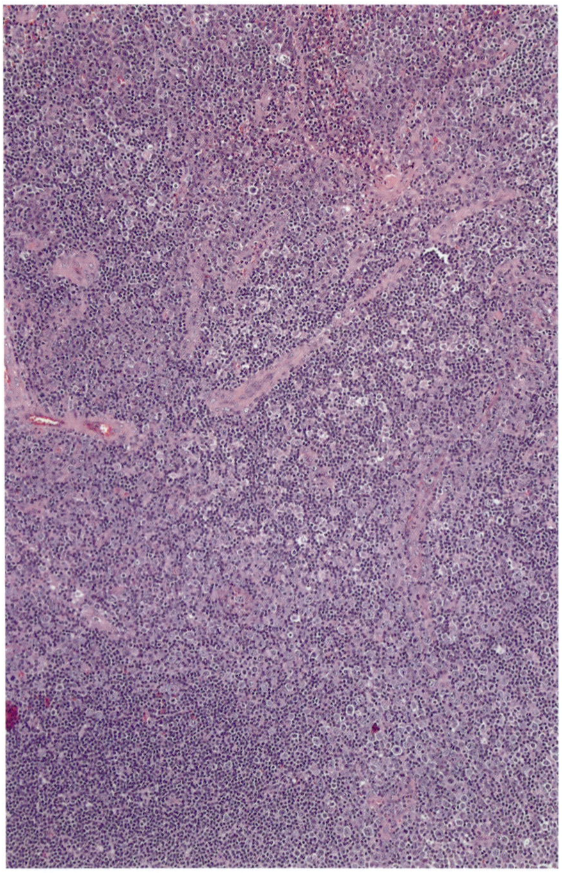

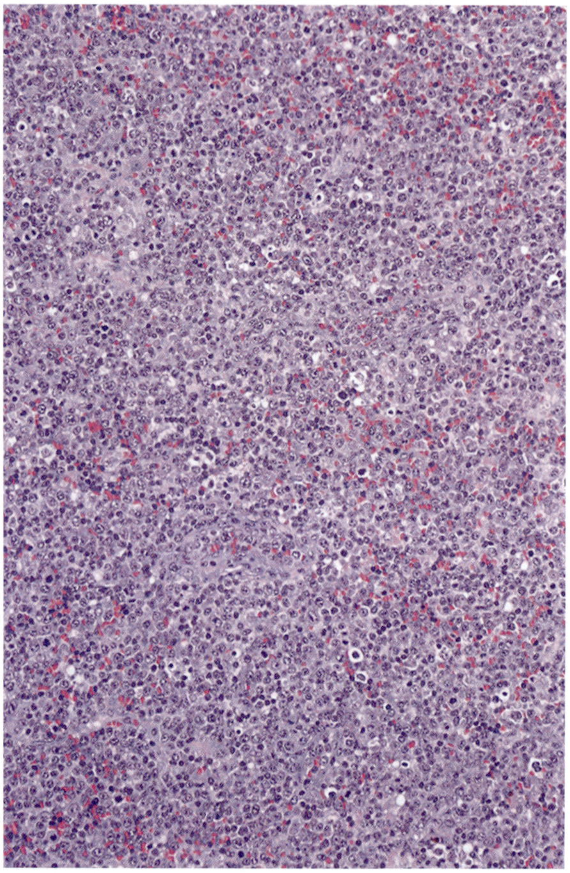

Figure 9-1

VIRAL LYMPHADENOPATHY

An immunoblastic proliferation is the earliest sign of viral lymphadenitis.

Figure 9-2

VIRAL LYMPHADENOPATHY

Diffuse atypical paracortical hyperplasia with no recognizable germinal centers.

Figure 9-3

ANAPLASTIC LARGE CELL LYMPHOMA

Sinusoidal localization of large atypical immunoblasts in infectious mononucleosis simulates an anaplastic large cell lymphoma.

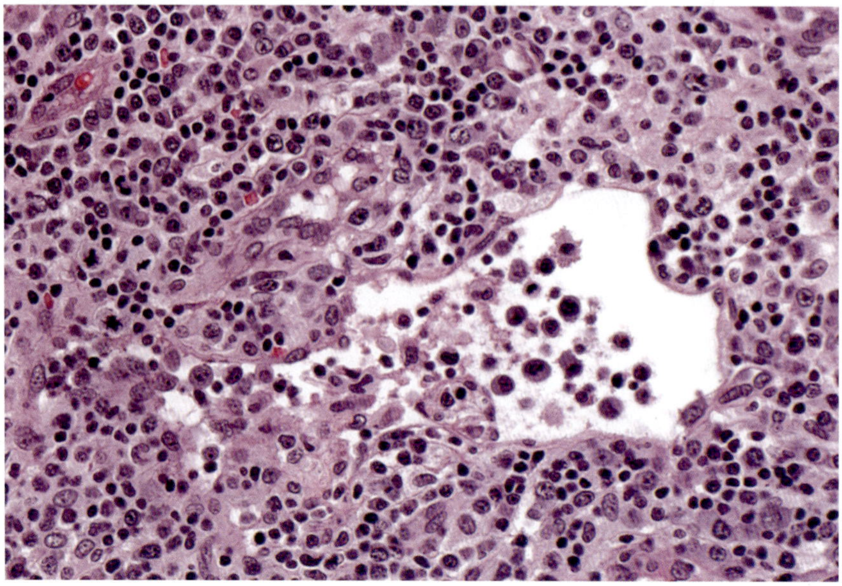

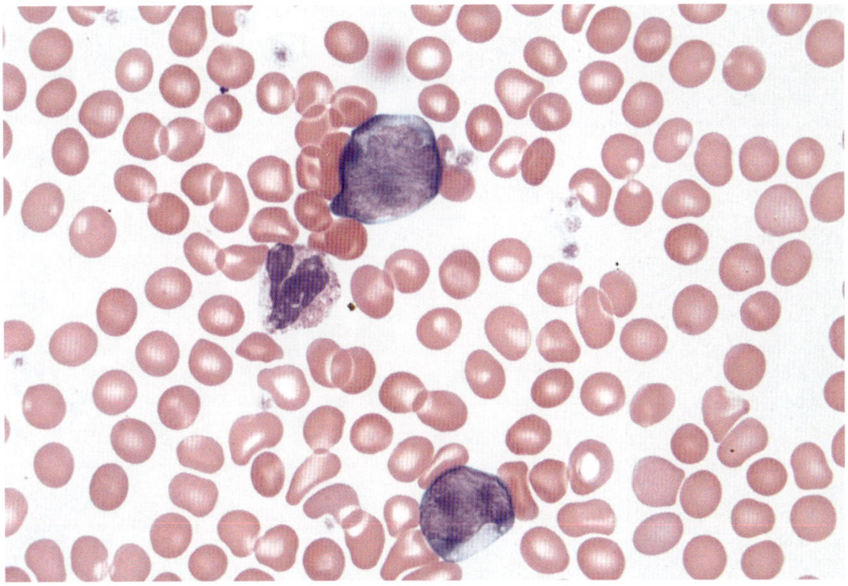

Figure 9-4

INFECTIOUS MONONUCLEOSIS, PERIPHERAL BLOOD

Circulating activated/atypical lymphocytes are seen in the peripheral blood.

hematologic disorders, including benign adenopathies, congenital and immunodeficiency-related disorders, post-transplant lymphoid proliferations, and lymphomas. It is also associated with nonhematopoietic malignancies, such as nasopharyngeal carcinoma.

EBV is transmitted primarily through contact with virally contaminated saliva. After replication within the salivary gland cells, the virions enter the B lymphocytes that have receptors (CD21) for the virus and subsequently disseminate. The infected B cells develop virus-directed membrane antigen, which evokes a killer T-cell response manifested both as atypical circulating lymphocytes and as stimulation of the T cells responsible for the lymphadenopathy and hepatosplenomegaly (36,104).

Clinical Features. Infectious mononucleosis is a viral syndrome that is most often caused by EBV. The clinicopathologic syndrome usually has an acute onset and a benign, self-limited course characterized by pharyngitis, fever, cervical or generalized lymphadenopathy, and atypical lymphocytosis (52). The disease most often affects children and young adolescents.

Lymph node biopsies are not recommended in this disorder because the worrisome histopathologic features may be misinterpreted as non-Hodgkin or Hodgkin lymphoma. Occasional cases may require lymph node biopsy, however, to rule out other causes of lymphadenopathy, including malignancy.

Infectious mononucleosis is a relatively common cause of splenic rupture (see also chapter 17) (7). Splenomegaly is common in infectious mononucleosis, and due to the histologic changes outlined below, the spleen is more susceptible to rupture. Although not "spontaneous," infectious mononucleosis–associated splenic rupture may be associated with insignificant trauma.

Laboratory Findings. The diagnosis of infectious mononucleosis primarily depends upon the correlation of signs and symptoms with serologic and laboratory findings; the latter include atypical lymphocytosis and a positive mono-spot test (fig. 9-4). Additional serodiagnostic studies include the presence of heterophile antibodies (Paul and Bunnell test) and antibodies to viral capsid antigen and virus-directed B-cell membrane antigens.

Microscopic Findings. Infectious mononucleosis lymphadenitis is the prototype of the group of reactive lymphadenopathies with diffuse paracortical involvement. The histologic features of the viral-associated lymphadenopathy have been well described in the literature, especially in association with EBV in cases of infectious mononucleosis (24). The histopathologic changes in EBV-related lymphadenopathy include paracortical expansion with diffuse hyperplasia (fig. 9-5), prominent vascularity, and a "mottled" appearance due to the presence of large immunoblasts (fig. 9-6).

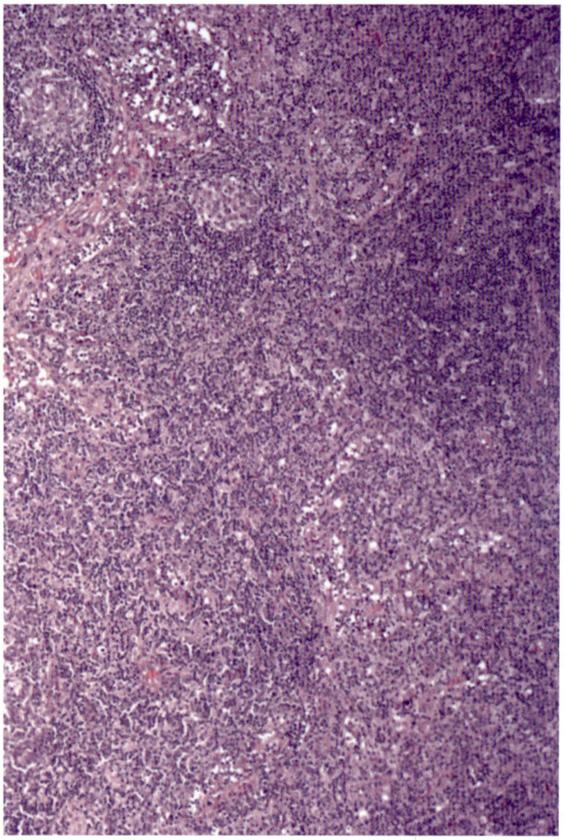

Figure 9-5

INFECTIOUS MONONUCLEOSIS, LYMPH NODE

Diffuse paracortical expansion with an inconspicuous residual germinal center in Epstein-Barr virus (EBV)-associated lymphadenitis.

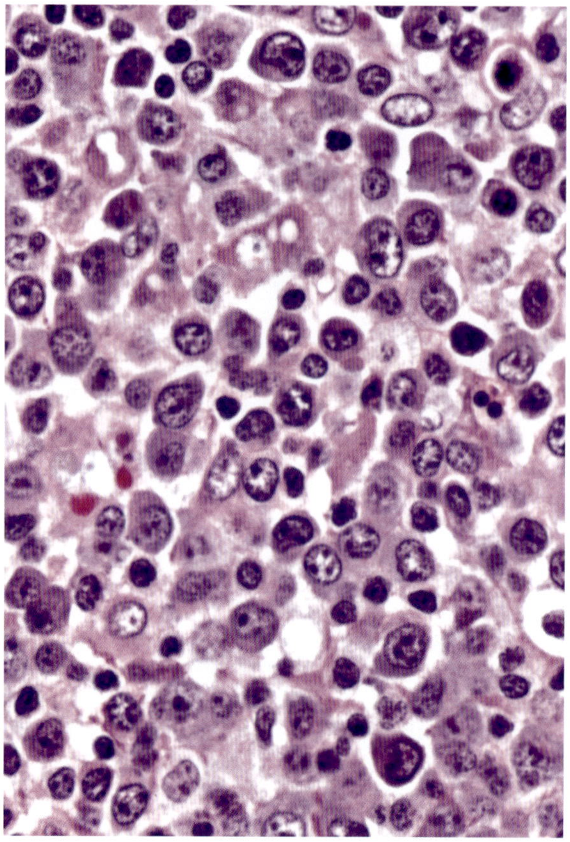

Figure 9-6

INFECTIOUS MONONUCLEOSIS, LYMPH NODE

EBV-associated lymphadenitis with immunoblasts.

Although follicular hyperplasia is occasionally noted (108), the germinal centers are usually inconspicuous (45). Numerous high endothelial venules may also be present (fig. 9-7). These changes are similar to those seen in dilantin-associated lymphadenopathy (1), which is in the differential diagnosis. Necrosis, either single cell type (apoptosis) or larger foci, may be present, as well as sinusoidal immunoblastic proliferation and marginal zone/monocytoid B-cell hyperplasia (Table 9-2, fig. 9-8) (24,33,39,45,70).

Occasional large, atypical cells with polylobated nuclei and prominent nucleoli, "Reed-Sternberg-like" cells, are present, which may add to the difficulty in distinguishing this lesion from Hodgkin lymphoma (fig. 9-9) (125). The presence of large, atypical immunoblasts in the lymph node sinuses may simulate an anaplastic large cell lymphoma (116), especially since these cells are CD30 positive in infectious mononucleosis (2). In infectious mononucleosis, the nodal sinuses are typically patent and filled with reactive immunoblasts, while in lymphomas the sinuses are inapparent. The normal nodal architecture is intact but distorted in infectious mononucleosis, rather than effaced as in lymphoma, which serves as an important diagnostic clue.

The normal lymph node architecture is preserved in atypical paracortical hyperplasia associated with a viral infection. There is a merging of the expanded paracortex with abnormal or "dissolved" germinal centers. The sinuses may be filled with activated immunoblasts, some with atypical features.

The splenic findings are also fairly characteristic. They include the histologic features mentioned above in relation to the lymph node histopathology. Reactive follicular hyperplasia,

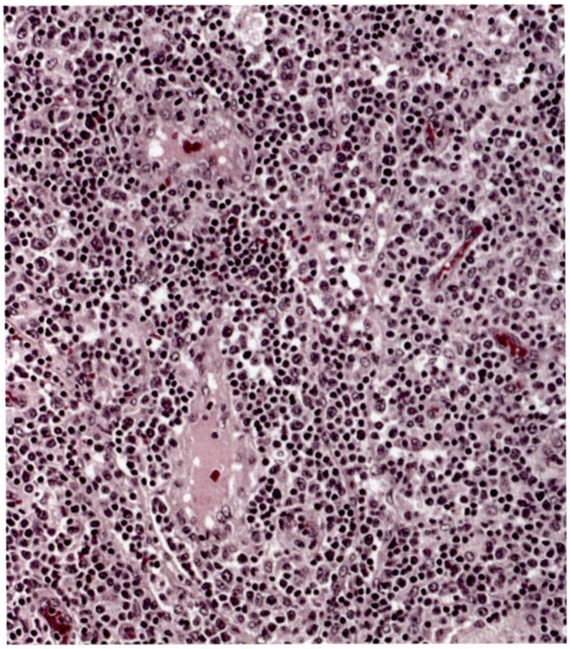

Figure 9-7

INFECTIOUS MONONUCLEOSIS, LYMPH NODE

Infectious mononucleosis lymphadenitis expands the paracortex and accentuates the vascularity.

without germinal center formation, which is characteristic of infectious mononucleosis as well as herpes simplex and other viral infections, is seen (89,96). This may resemble the immunologically unstimulated spleen (figs. 9-10, 9-11). High-power examination, however, reveals reactive changes such as the presence of lymphocytes in varying stages of transformation, including small and large lymphocytes and immunoblasts in the germinal centers (7).

Table 9-2

BENIGN ADENOPATHIES ASSOCIATED WITH MARGINAL ZONE (MONOCYTOID B-CELL) HYPERPLASIA

Frequent
Toxoplasmosis
Cytomegalovirus
HIV[a]-related lymphadenopathy
Occasional
Acute EBV/IM
Cat-scratch disease
Lymphogranuloma venereum
Herpes simplex virus

[a]HIV = human immunodeficiency virus; EBV = Epstein-Barr virus; IM = infectious mononucleosis.

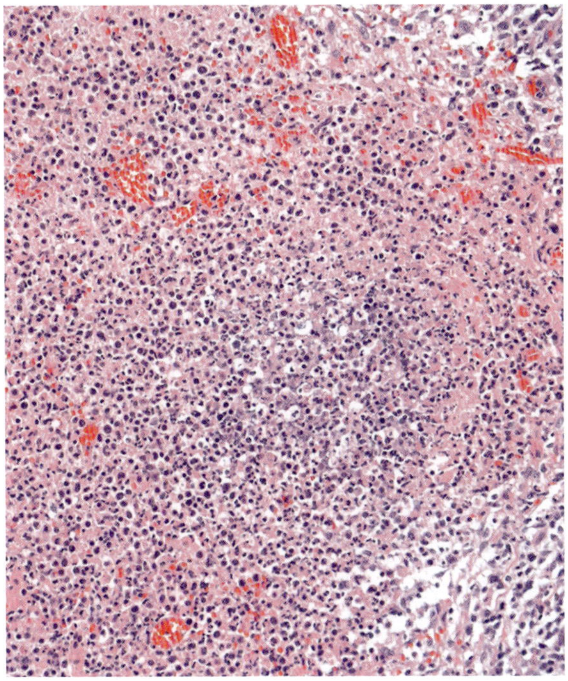

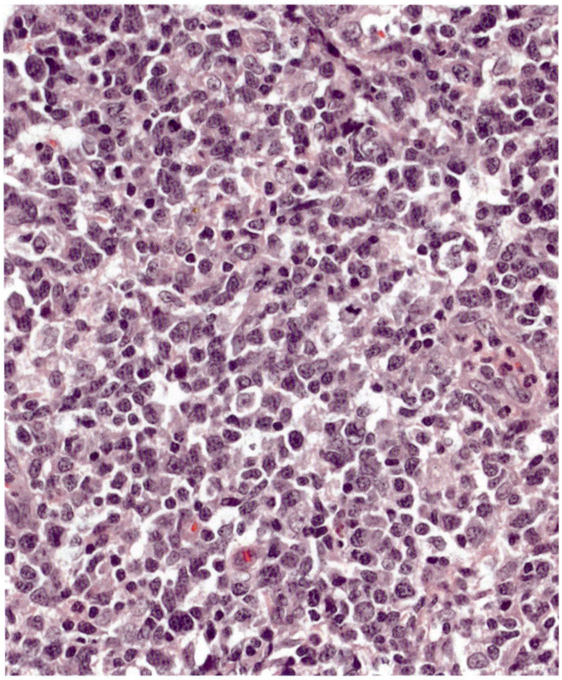

Figure 9-8

INFECTIOUS MONONUCLEOSIS, LYMPH NODE

Necrosis (left) and immunoblastic proliferation (right) in infectious mononucleosis.

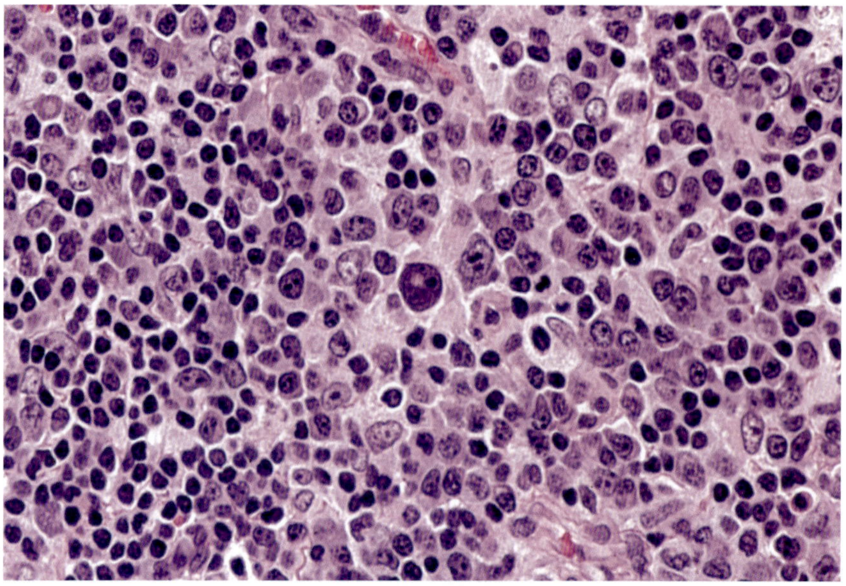

Figure 9-9

INFECTIOUS MONONUCLEOSIS, LYMPH NODE

A Reed-Sternberg–like cell in infectious mononucleosis.

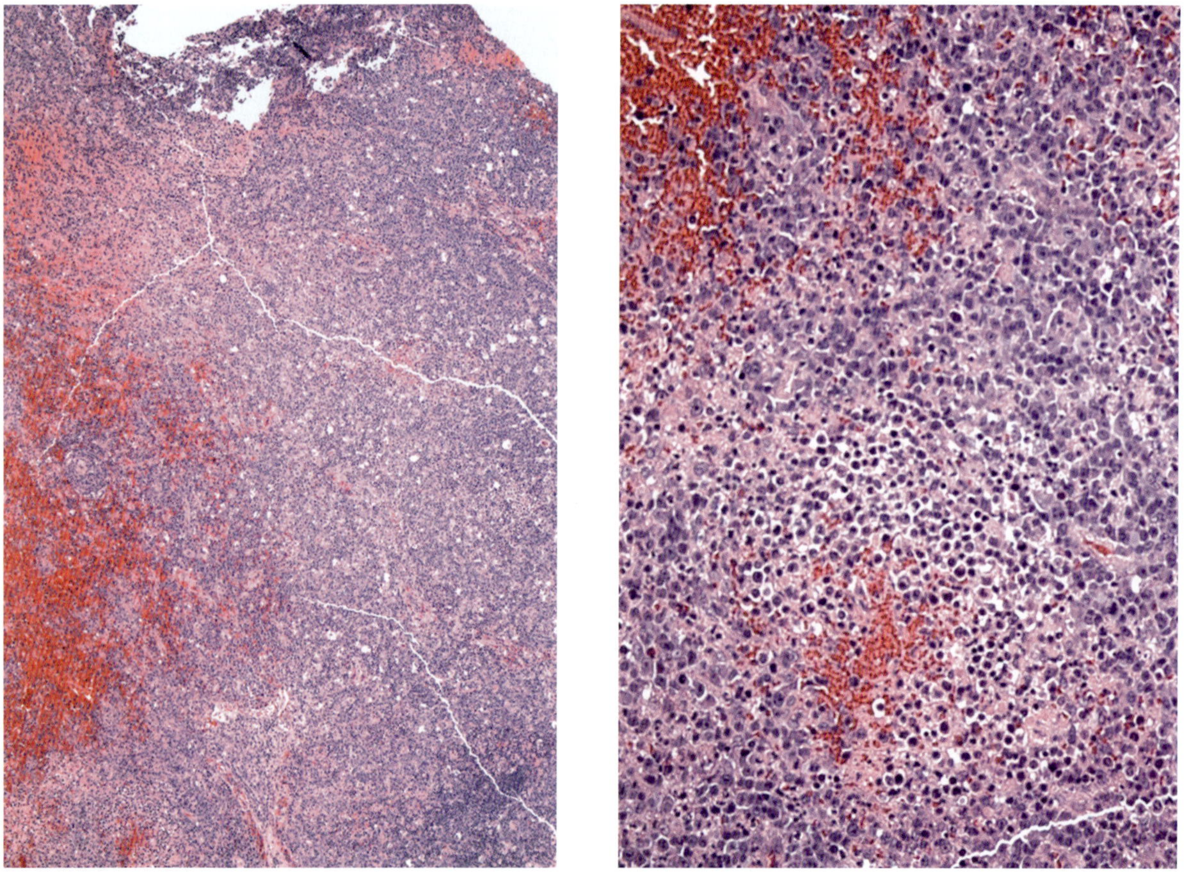

Figure 9-10

INFECTIOUS MONONUCLEOSIS, SPLEEN

Immunoblastic proliferation and hemorrhage (left) and necrosis (right) are seen.

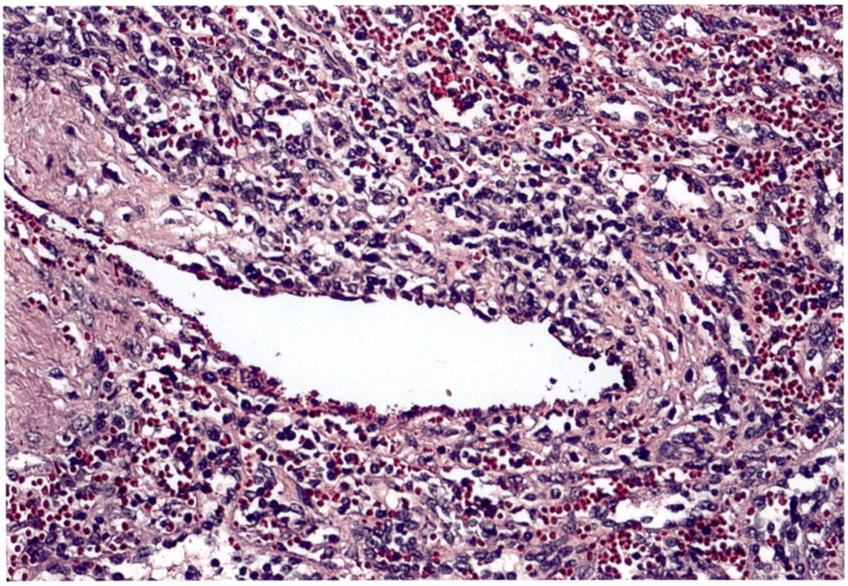

Figure 9-11

INFECTIOUS MONONUCLEOSIS, SPLEEN

Vasculitis is a hallmark of the histologic findings of splenic infectious mononucleosis.

Transformed lymphocytes/immunoblasts also proliferate around the splenic arterioles and may infiltrate the trabecular veins, the connective tissue framework, and the splenic capsule, resulting in splenic rupture in extreme cases. These morphologic findings are rarely seen in malignant lymphoma.

Ancillary Studies. The cellular composition of infectious mononucleosis lymphadenitis is heterogeneous and includes EBV-infected B cells, which are reactive with CD20 and may express latent membrane protein or EBV-encoded RNA (fig. 9-12). These cells may also show reactivity with CD30, raising the possibility of anaplastic large cell lymphoma (2). Surrounding reactive lymphocytes are predominantly T cells that react with T-cell markers such as CD3, CD45RO, and CD43. Immunohistochemical analysis for CD21/CD35 highlights the residual follicular network. The immunoblasts that are reactive for latent membrane protein of EBV are primarily B cells (90). The presence of intact sinuses supports a reactive rather than a neoplastic process (109). Lack of reactivity for CD15 helps in the distinction from Hodgkin lymphoma. In situ hybridization studies have demonstrated an interfollicular pattern of EBV infection in activated B immunoblasts in lymphoid tissues (91,111), especially in human immunodeficiency virus (HIV)-positive patients (6). Immunoreactivity of the immunoblasts in infectious mononucleosis lymphadenitis with

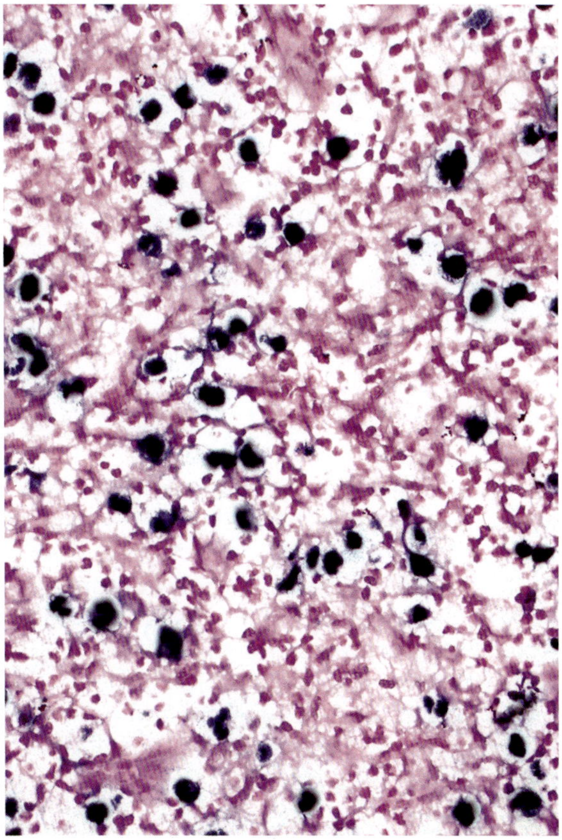

Figure 9-12

IN SITU HYBRIDIZATION REACTIVITY FOR EBV IN INFECTIOUS MONONUCLEOSIS

Numerous large transformed cells are strongly positive for EBV-encoded RNA (EBER).

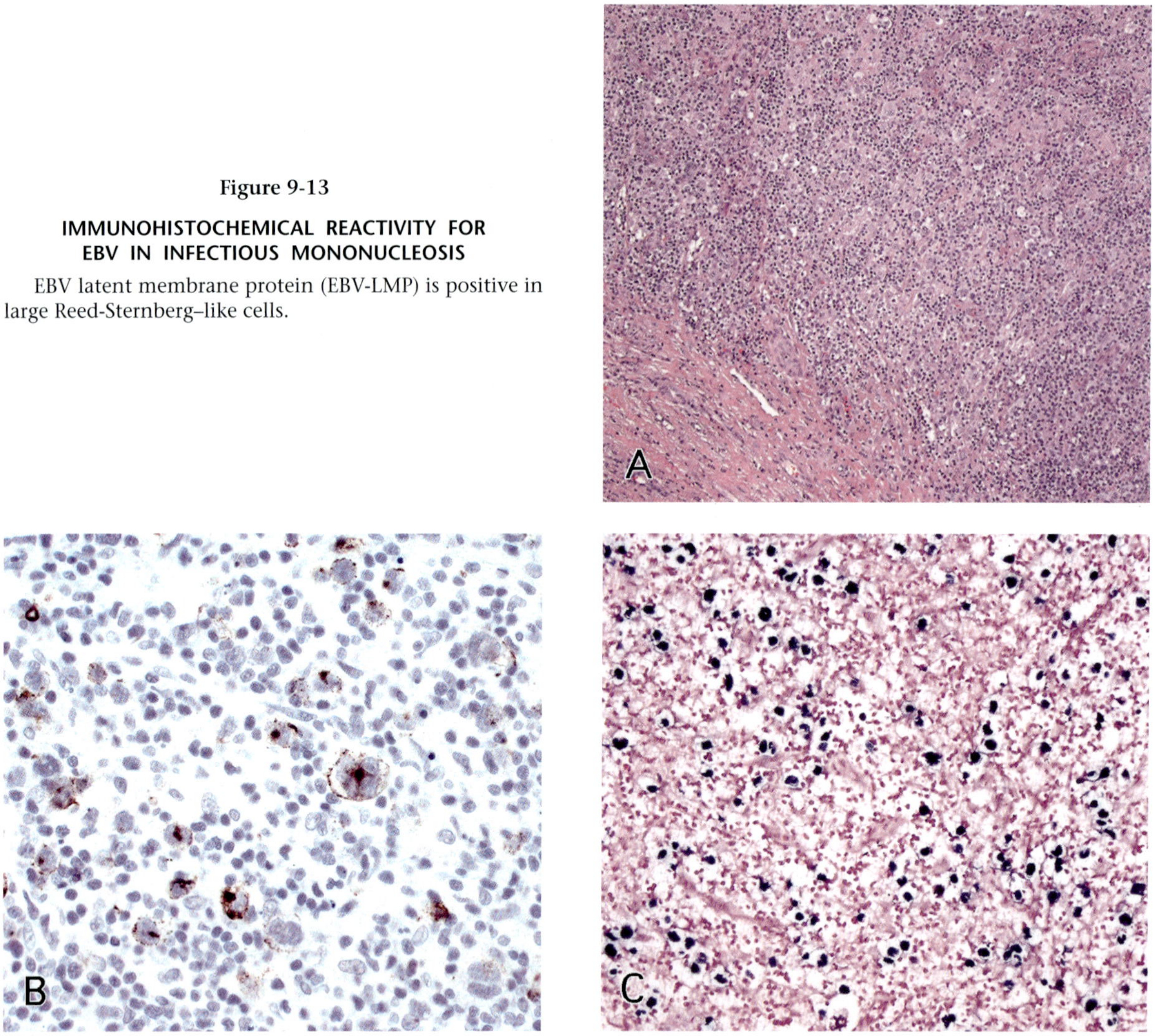

Figure 9-13

IMMUNOHISTOCHEMICAL REACTIVITY FOR EBV IN INFECTIOUS MONONUCLEOSIS

EBV latent membrane protein (EBV-LMP) is positive in large Reed-Sternberg–like cells.

an immunohistochemical antibody to EBV-latent membrane protein (LMP) helps confirm the diagnosis (fig. 9-13).

Flow cytometric findings show immunophenotypic abnormalities of T cells, in particular, significant downregulation of CD7 expression, and less commonly, CD5 (132). Without an appropriate clinical context, these findings could suggest a diagnosis of T-cell lymphoma, due to the "aberrant" immunophenotype.

Differential Diagnosis. The differential diagnosis of EBV-infected lymph nodes, based on the histologic features, includes other viral lymphadenitides, postvaccinial lymphadenitis, and malignant lymphoma (99,123,124). Other viral infections such as cytomegalovirus (60,109) or herpes simplex lymphadenitis (40,61,123,124) result in a similar pattern of diffuse paracortical expansion (see chapter 7, figs. 7-5, 7-6). A detailed clinical history with pertinent laboratory findings and a complete physical examination often help to support a diagnosis of diffuse atypical paracortical hyperplasia rather than malignant lymphoma.

The most important feature distinguishing EBV lymphadenitis from lymphoma is the overall preservation of the nodal architecture (33), even though the cellular infiltrate may extend into the capsule (108). Reed-Sternberg-like cells are commonly seen in EBV-related lymphadenitis and may result in a misdiagnosis of Hodgkin lymphoma (fig. 9-14). Features that help to identify Reed-Sternberg-like cells as simulators of their malignant counterpart are

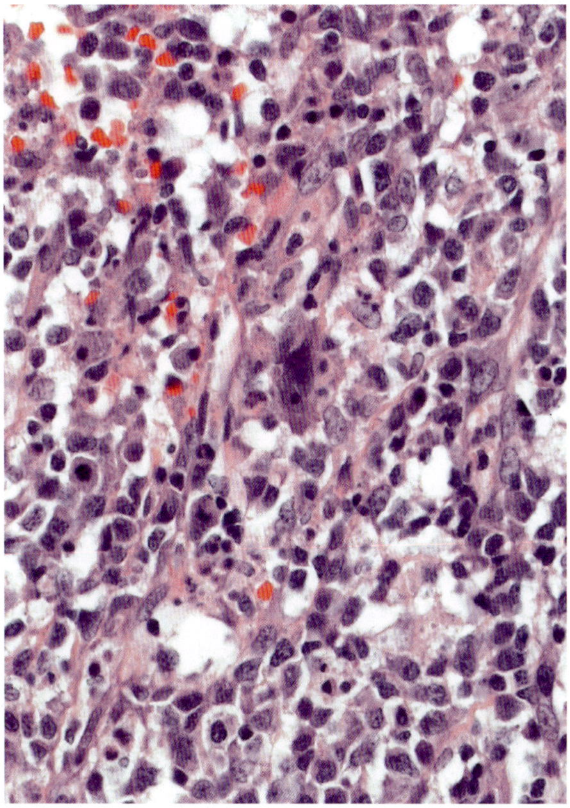

Figure 9-14

INFECTIOUS MONONUCLEOSIS, LYMPH NODE

Reed-Sternberg–like cells are common in cases of infectious mononucleosis.

basophilic rather than acidophilic nucleoli and a prominent paranuclear hof (33). Prominent eosinophilia, which is an important finding in most cases of Hodgkin lymphoma, is not a common feature of EBV lymphadenitis. Careful morphologic and immunohistochemical analyses, in conjunction with the clinical presentation and laboratory findings, are important for arriving at the correct diagnosis.

EBV-infected lymph nodes occasionally show reactive follicular hyperplasia and scattered microgranulomas, raising the possibility of toxoplasmic lymphadenitis. In toxoplasmic lymphadenitis, however, the microgranulomas are within or near the germinal centers, and sinusoidal monocytoid B-cell hyperplasia is consistently present (32).

Treatment and Prognosis. Infectious mononucleosis is typically a self-limited disease that does not require specific treatment.

Table 9-3

POST-TRANSPLANT LYMPHOPROLIFERATIVE DISORDERS[a]

Early Lesions
Reactive plasmacytic hyperplasia
Infectious mononucleosis-like
Polymorphic Post-Transplant Lymphoproliferative Disorder (PTLD)
Monomorphic PTLD
B-cell neoplasms
Diffuse large B-cell lymphoma (immunoblastic, centroblastic, anaplastic)
Burkitt/Burkitt-like lymphoma
Plasma cell myeloma
Plasmacytoma-like lesions
T-cell neoplasms
Peripheral T-cell lymphoma, not otherwise specified
Other types
Hodgkin Lymphoma and Hodgkin-Like PTLD

[a]Data from Table 9.02 from reference 49.

OTHER EPSTEIN-BARR VIRUS–ASSOCIATED LYMPHOID PROLIFERATIONS

Definition. Besides infectious mononucleosis (see previous section), EBV is associated with a variety of other lymphoid proliferations of both T and B cells, including *post-transplant lymphoproliferative disorder* (PTLD), *immunosuppression-related proliferation*, and other atypical EBV-related proliferations. *Postinfectious mononucleosis T-cell proliferation* (PIMTP), *severe chronic active EBV infection* (SCAEBV), and *fatal infectious mononucleosis* (FIM) are also described.

Clinical Features. PTLD represents a spectrum of lymphoid proliferations associated with immunosuppression in patients with transplanted organs or bone marrow (Table 9-3). The scope of this spectrum ranges from benign polyclonal disorders to malignant monoclonal disorders (e.g., lymphoma). The frequency of PTLD varies with the type of transplant, the degree of immunosuppression, and patient factors. In almost all circumstances, PTLD is associated with EBV infection. EBV-negative cases tend to occur late after transplantation (over 5 years), and their underlying etiology is not fully understood at this time.

Other types of immunosuppression are associated with EBV-driven lymphoid proliferations. These include immunosuppressive therapies, such as methotrexate (see chapter 14), primary immunodeficiency disorders (see chapter 7), HIV infection (see later, this chapter), and others (38,46).

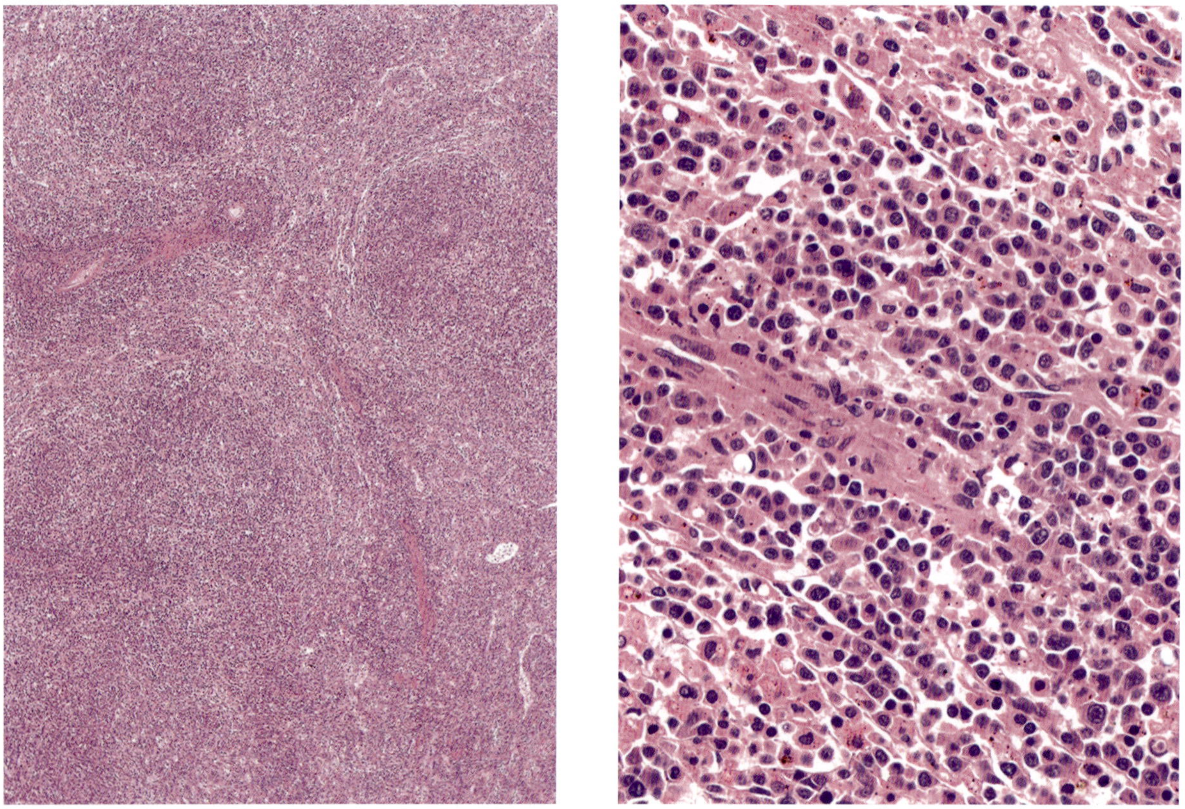

Figure 9-15

POST-TRANSPLANT LYMPHOPROLIFERATIVE DISORDER (PTLD), PLASMA CELL TYPE, SPLEEN

Plasma cell PTLD is a massive proliferation of plasma cells, as seen in this spleen (left, low magnification; right, high magnification).

PIMTP most often occurs after acute EBV infection, although rare cases occur during the course of chronic infection. Cytotoxic T cells that are infected by EBV proliferate; these are clonal and may be overt T-cell lymphomas or more atypical T-cell proliferations. This rare complication of EBV infection has a fulminant course and typically occurs in Asian patients, but has been reported in non-Asians (88,101).

The features of FIM and PIMTP may overlap and it can be difficult to distinguish them on clinical grounds. FIM is characterized by a severe sensitivity to EBV infection, with a fatal course (27,100). In most patients, FIM is due to X-linked lymphoproliferative syndrome (Duncan disease) (see chapter 7), although rare cases are seen in other forms of immunosuppression (134).

SCAEBV is thought to result from a defective immunologic response to EBV infection. The diagnostic criteria for SCAEBV include clinical signs (prolonged or recurrent fever or exanthem, hepatosplenomegaly and/or lymphadenopathy, chronic hepatitis and/or interstitial pneumonitis, pancytopenia and/or infection-associated hemophagocytic syndrome, hypersensitivity to mosquito bite, and large granular lymphocytic disease and/or an increase in human leukocyte antigen [HLA]-DR positive T cells) and abnormally high levels of anti-EBV antibodies with high copy numbers of EBV genomes (88).

Laboratory Findings. As with infectious mononucleosis, serologic studies of EBV help evaluate these viral infections.

Microscopic Findings. The plasmacytic hyperplasia type PTLD consists of focal increases of polyclonal, morphologically normal plasma cells (fig. 9-15). These more often involve lymph nodes than extranodal sites, in contrast to other types of PTLD.

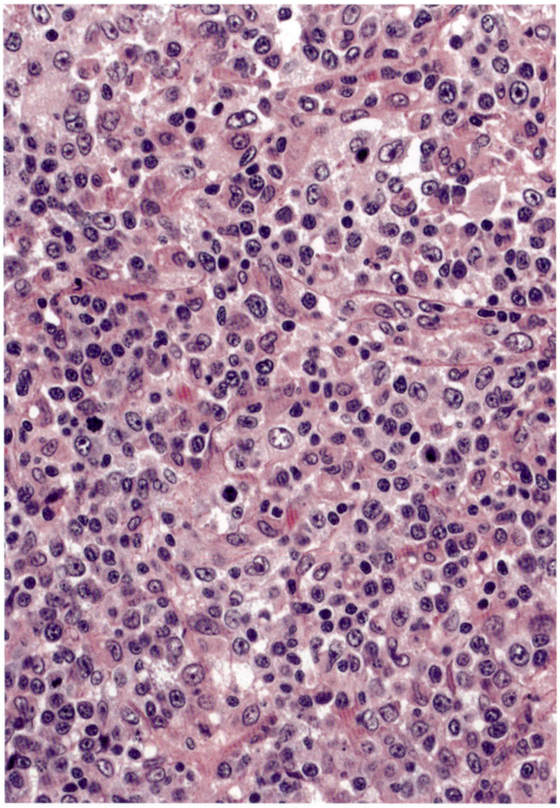

Figure 9-16

PTLD, POLYMORPHOUS TYPE, SPLEEN

The cellular infiltrate in the spleen is polymorphous. Additional studies are necessary to determine whether this proliferation was polyclonal or monoclonal.

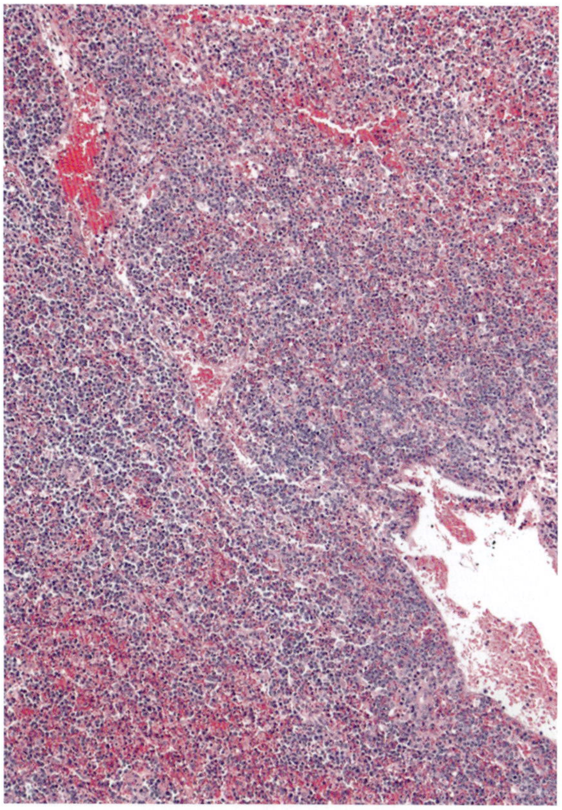

Figure 9-17

PTLD, T-CELL TYPE, SPLEEN

T-cell PTLD is seen in rare situations.

Infectious mononucleosis-like PTLD has features similar to those described in the previous section for infectious mononucleosis. This PTLD lesion is more likely to occur in tonsils and adenoids than other types, but may occur in other sites as well. In both lesions, the normal lymphoid architecture is spared.

Polymorphous PTLD is a more aggressive variant than those previously mentioned. As expected, the lesion consists of a mixture of immunoblasts, plasma cells, and intermediate-sized cells (fig. 9-16). These often form masses or destructive local lesions in extranodal sites. Other PTLD lesions are similar to lymphomas, and the reader is referred to other specialized texts for further descriptions (23,49).

PIMTP shows significant splenic pathology, and in some cases, significant changes in the lymph nodes (51,101). In the spleen, the white pulp is depleted and increased lymphocytes are in the red pulp sinuses (fig. 9-17). Necrosis may be seen. Hemophagocytosis can be prominent. The lymphocytes in the red pulp are predominantly T cells; B cells are decreased in number. Evaluation for clonal T-cell gene rearrangements shows polyclonal, monoclonal, or a combination of both populations. Lymph nodes are not well described but include changes such as granulomas, hemophagocytosis, and sinus histiocytosis.

SCAEBV may show follicular hyperplasia and plasmacytosis, and/or paracortical T-cell proliferations in the lymph nodes. In the spleen, the periarterial lymphatic sheath (PALS) area is expanded with small to intermediate-sized T lymphocytes, but relatively intact follicles (88,94). The red pulp is typically unremarkable.

The histologic appearance in FIM is characterized by polymorphous lymphoid infiltrates consisting of immunoblasts and polyclonal plasma cells, necrosis, lymphoid depletion, and

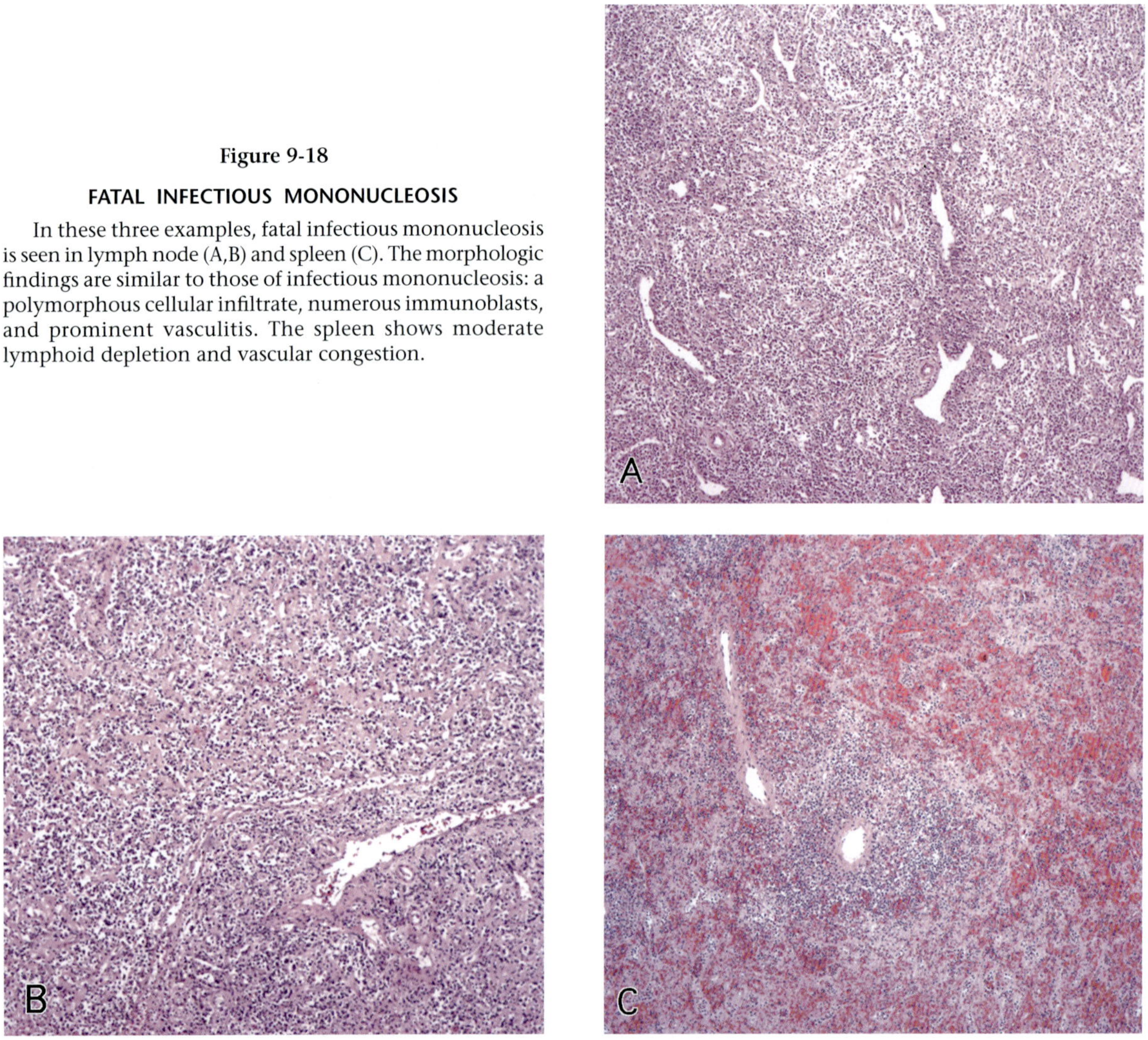

Figure 9-18

FATAL INFECTIOUS MONONUCLEOSIS

In these three examples, fatal infectious mononucleosis is seen in lymph node (A,B) and spleen (C). The morphologic findings are similar to those of infectious mononucleosis: a polymorphous cellular infiltrate, numerous immunoblasts, and prominent vasculitis. The spleen shows moderate lymphoid depletion and vascular congestion.

histiocytosis with or without hemophagocytosis (fig. 9-18). This infiltration is often present in a variety of organs, including lymph nodes and spleen.

Ancillary Studies. As mentioned previously, EBV can be detected by immunohistochemical and in situ techniques. In addition, it is possible to determine whether EBV viral DNA has been integrated into the genome of infected cells (93).

Differential Diagnosis. Lymphoid proliferations due to EBV can mimic a variety of infectious and neoplastic disorders, as discussed previously.

Treatment and Prognosis. The treatment of patients with EBV-related lymphoid proliferations is dependent on the establishment of appropriate memory cytotoxic T cells and control of the B-cell proliferation (46). A variety of therapies have been tested with EBV infections including interferon-alpha, cytotoxic therapy, intravenous immunoglobulin, and others.

The recognition of PTLD is important because reduction of immunosuppression may induce regression of the lymphoid lesions. It is unlikely that cases of frank lymphoma that develop in a post-transplant setting would regress with reduction in immunosuppression, whether EBV positive or not. The use of rituximab in the treatment of PTLD is effective in many cases, and it has been suggested that rituximab should be used before chemotherapy in all cases of PTLD (25,41).

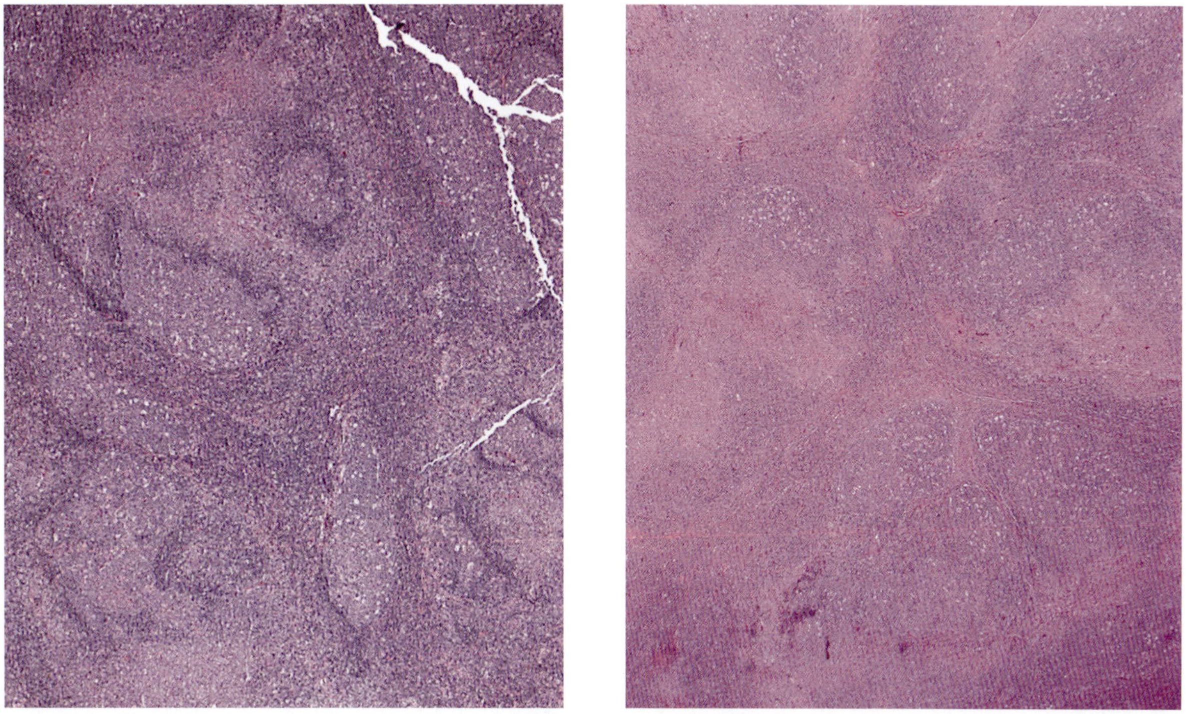

Figure 9-19

CYTOMEGALOVIRUS, LYMPH NODE

Follicular hyperplasia and marginal zone hyperplasia are seen in cases of cytomegalovirus lymphadenitis.

CYTOMEGALOVIRUS

Definition. *Cytomegalovirus* (CMV) is a ubiquitous viral infection. Although several clinical presentations are possible, lymphadenopathy due to CMV is most often seen in immunocompromised hosts.

General Features. CMV is a DNA virus, and is a member of the herpesvirus family. It is one of the largest animal viruses (42). It has a characteristic cytopathic effect consisting of massively swollen cells with familiar intranuclear inclusions.

Clinical Features. The clinical syndromes associated with CMV are variable and include: 1) severe congenital infections, 2) infectious mononucleosis-like illness, 3) limited, influenza-like illness, 4) immunosuppression/post-transplant infections (often disseminated), and most commonly, 5) asymptomatic infection (13,42,103). Infectious mononucleosis–like infection, with a negative mono-spot test, is often due to CMV infection.

Post-transplant and immunosuppression-related CMV infection is due to primary infection, reactivation, reinfection, or a combination of the latter two. Hepatitis, pneumonitis, encephalitis, retinitis, and colitis may all be caused by CMV. Lymphadenopathy is rare.

Laboratory Findings. In infectious mononucleosis–like infections, atypical lymphocytosis, similar to that of EBV-related infectious mononucleosis, may be seen (48). Serologic testing is useful in diagnosing whether the CMV infection is primary or a reactivation.

Microscopic Findings. CMV lymphadenitis displays histopathologic changes that are similar to those already described for other viral agents and include paracortical expansion and "mottling" due to immunoblastic and histiocytic proliferations. Classically, there is localized lymphadenopathy with follicular hyperplasia and sinusoidal or marginal zone proliferations of monocytoid/marginal zone cells (fig. 9-19; see Table 9-2).

The splenic changes associated with CMV are similar to those in lymph nodes (e.g., follicular hyperplasia, marginal zone hyperplasia). In addition, the spleen may have features such

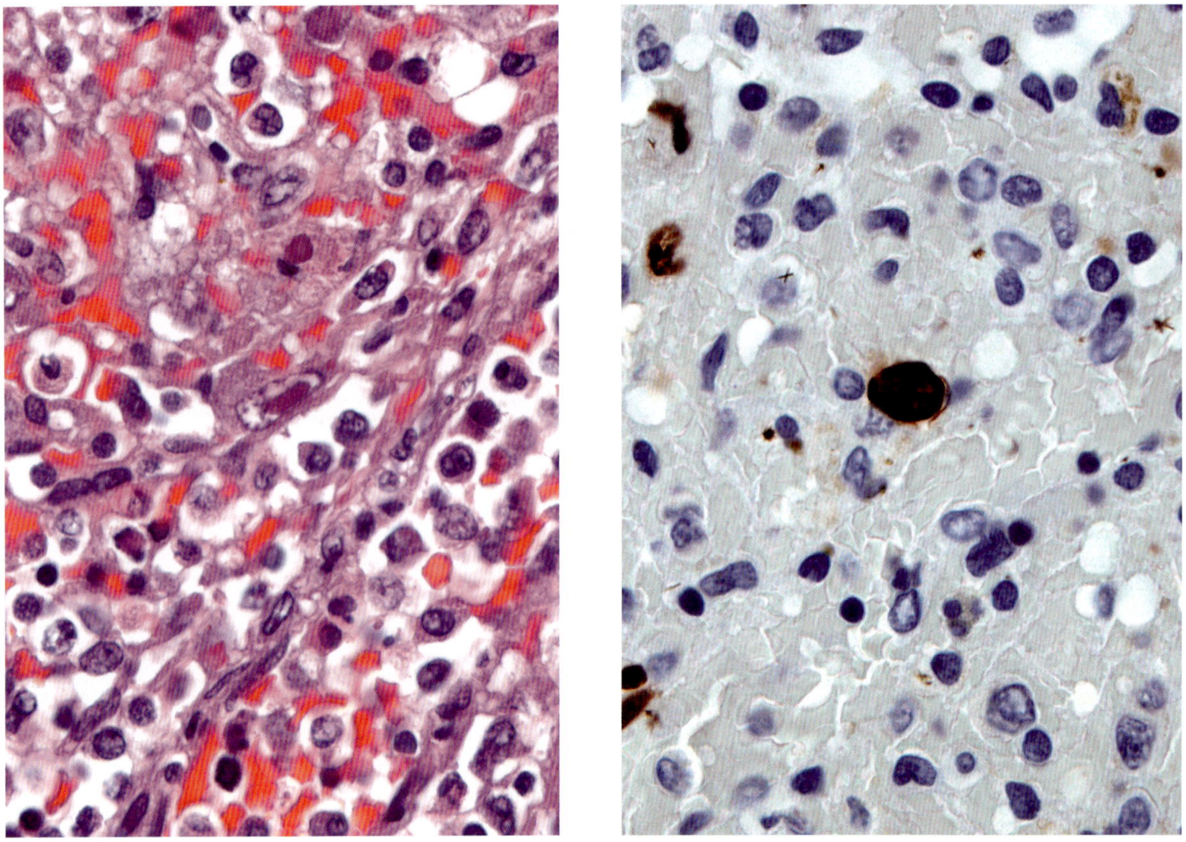

Figure 9-20

CYTOMEGALOVIRUS, SPLEEN

Although less commonly diagnosed, cytomegaloviral infections also affect the spleen. In this case, a hematoxylin and eosin (H&E) stain (left) and immunohistochemical stain (right) show evidence of viral infection in the red pulp.

as vasculitis, necrosis, and lymphoid depletion, indistinguishable from those seen in acute EBV infection/infectious mononucleosis. In some cases, the white pulp is depleted, and lymphocytic vasculitis/capsulitis is seen (fig. 9-20).

The striking cell enlargement (cytomegaly) with pleomorphic nuclei that contain characteristic intranuclear inclusions, surrounded by clear vacuolar spaces, is occasionally noted (fig. 9-21). There may be smaller, multiple basophilic cytoplasmic inclusions containing DNA and polysaccharides; these stain with the Feulgen and periodic acid–Schiff (PAS) stains.

Ancillary Studies. Some infected large lymphocytes stain for CD15 and may cause confusion with the Reed-Sternberg cells of classic Hodgkin lymphoma. The former do not stain for CD30, in contrast to Hodgkin/Reed-Sternberg cells. An immunoperoxidase antibody is available to identify viral antigens in infected CMV cells (fig. 9-22) (35). Immunohistochemical studies have shown that the characteristic cytomegalic cells that contain intranuclear and intracytoplasmic inclusions are T cells, stromal cells, or endothelial cells (138). In situ hybridization with biotinylated probes in formalin-fixed paraffin-embedded tissue sections is a highly specific technique that has been employed in the identification of CMV (86).

Differential Diagnosis. The differential diagnosis of CMV lymphadenitis includes other viral lymphadenitides, drug-induced lymphadenopathy, and malignant lymphoma, emphasizing the need for a good clinical history and clinicopathologic correlation.

Treatment and Prognosis. Ganciclovir is most effective in treating patients who are immunosuppressed or have life-threatening

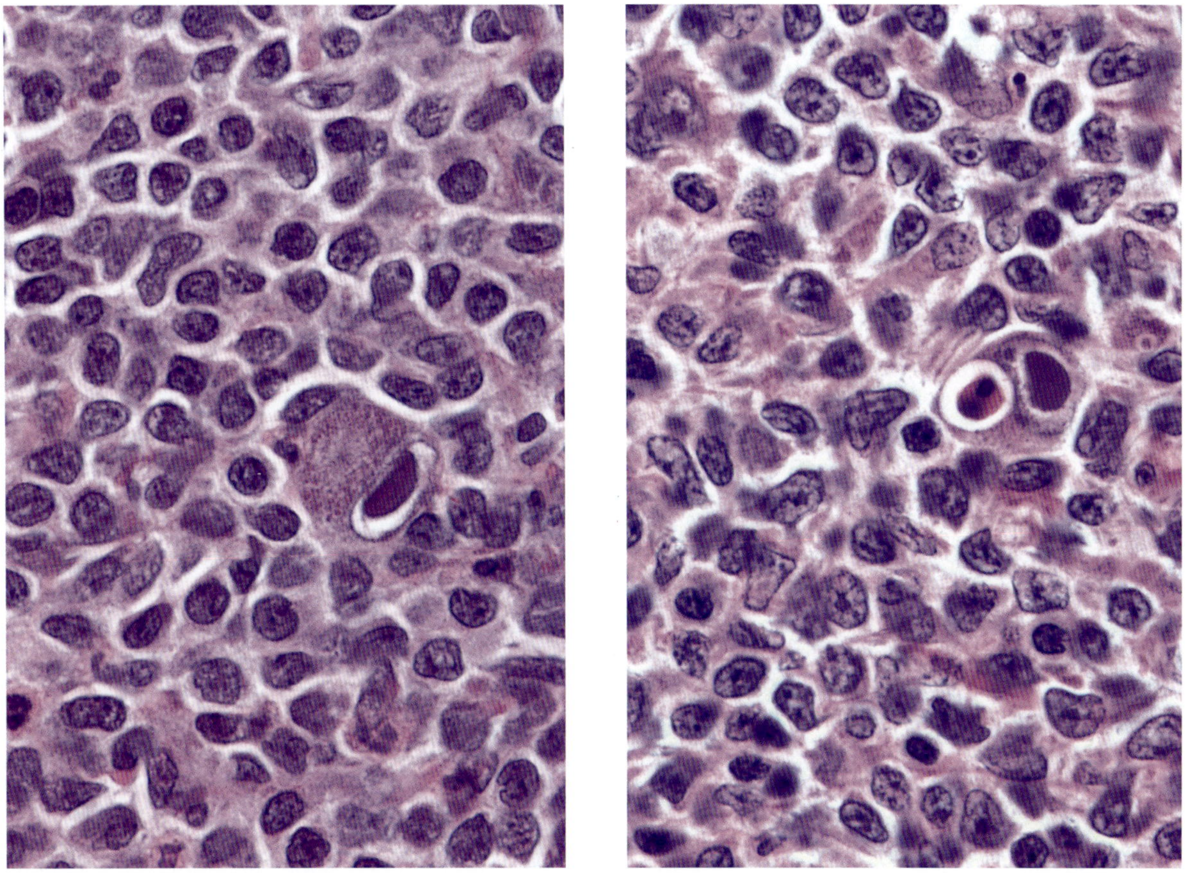

Figure 9-21

CYTOMEGALOVIRUS, VIRAL INCLUSION

High magnification of cytomegalovirus inclusions in lymph nodes.

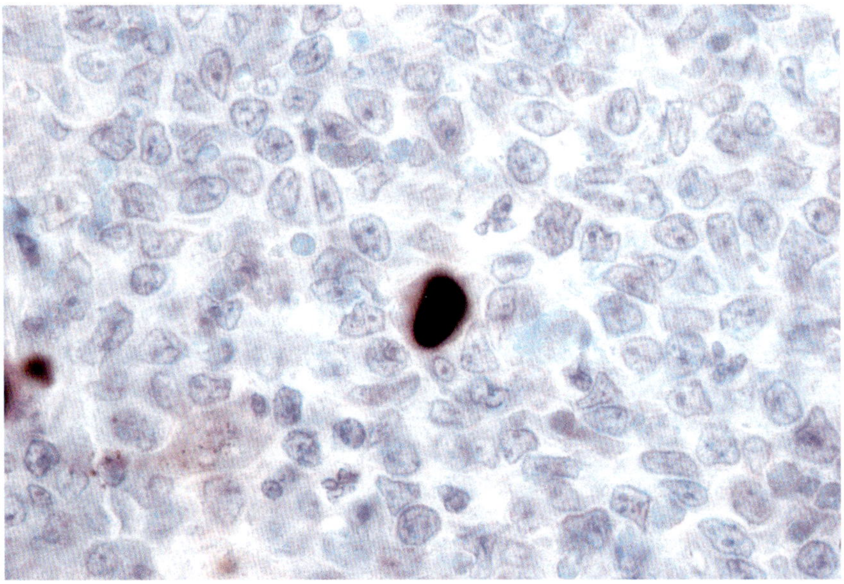

Figure 9-22

IMMUNOHISTOCHEMICAL REACTIVITY FOR CYTOMEGALOVIRUS

An immunohistochemical stain for cytomegalovirus is often effective in finding the rare infected cells.

illness. In cases of known immunosuppression, CMV infection can be a serious disorder. In the immunocompetent patient, illness typically resolves spontaneously. However, if the presentation is atypical or especially severe, it should prompt evaluation for underlying immunodeficiency.

HERPES SIMPLEX VIRUS

Definition. *Herpes simplex virus* (HSV) infection may rarely be associated with lymphadenitis, which is characterized by areas of necrosis and the viral inclusions typical of herpesvirus. Splenic involvement is rare, but the findings are similar to those in the lymph node.

General Features. HSV is a member of the alpha herpesviruses, with two distinct serotypes, HSV-1 and HSV-2 (115). HSV-1 is most often associated with oropharyngeal lesions (mouth, lips, skin), while HSV-2 is most often associated with genital infection. HSV has the capacity to invade and replicate in the nervous system, and establish latent infection. Subsequent reactivation causes symptomatic disease.

Clinical Features. The most typical and common infections associated with HSV are cutaneous lesions (cold sores, genital ulcers). The oropharyngeal and genital sites are typical for primary and reactivated infection. Disseminated disease can include skin, eye, oral, respiratory, and neurologic lesions (associated with a high rate of fatality) (115).

Lymphadenitis is rare and most frequently occurs in association with immune suppression. HSV lymphadenitis is seen with disseminated infection, generalized lymphadenopathy with rash, and generalized or local lymphadenopathy without rash (135). This includes cases of lymphoid neoplasms, such as chronic lymphocytic leukemia (CLL) (53,65) and primary and acquired immunodeficiencies (135). Exceptional cases have been reported in immunocompetent patients.

The skin lesions of HSV infection are so characteristic that lymph node biopsy is rare. HSV lymphadenitis presents clinically as rapidly enlarging, tender lymph nodes. Patients with preexisting lymphoid neoplasms may have persistent, slowly enlarging lymph nodes, compatible with their neoplasm. Interestingly, HSV lymphadenopathy tends to only involve regional lymph nodes; the presence of isolated HSV lymphadenitis is often associated with hematopoietic malignancies. Tonsillitis with a histologic pattern similar to herpetic lymphadenitis can be seen and is usually sexually transmitted (HSV-2 associated) (131).

Laboratory Findings. HSV antibody is detected by a number of methods, including serologic studies, viral culture, and polymerase chain reaction (PCR). The Tzanck smear, which has been supplanted by DNA-based methodologies, has historically been used to identify herpesvirus infections. In this technique, the base of an ulcer is scraped. The resulting slide is stained and examined for the presence of multinucleated giant cells, with the characteristic "ground-glass" chromatin.

Microscopic Features. HSV lymphadenitis shows histopathologic changes that are similar to the viral lymphadenitides already discussed. Discrete, focal areas of necrosis are characteristic of this infection, and often occur in paracortical regions (fig. 9-23) (40,56,123,124). These necrotic areas may enlarge and form geographic areas of necrosis. Cowdry type A intranuclear inclusions, which are large, acidophilic inclusions separated from the nuclear rim by a vacuole, may be demonstrated in paracortical immunoblasts (fig. 9-24). The inclusion-bearing cells are often within the areas of necrosis. Multinucleated giant cells may rarely be seen. The histologic changes of HSV lymphadenitis are primarily cytopathic rather than cytomegalic. Sinus histiocytosis may be prominent in HSV lymphadenitis. Rare cases lack necrosis, and occasionally have increased monocytoid/marginal zone B cells (85). Splenic involvement is rare, but the findings are similar (fig. 9-25).

HSV may be more difficult to recognize when associated with an underlying lymphoproliferative disorder. There is partial or complete effacement of the lymph node with the characteristic features of the underlying lymphoproliferative disorder (e.g., CLL); foci of necrosis are seen (fig. 9-26). Near and within these areas of necrosis are virally infected cells typical of HSV infections (53).

Ancillary Studies. Immunohistochemistry and in situ hybridization techniques for the detection of HSV (HSV-1 and -2) are routinely available. Because of the relatively nonspecific histologic features of viral infection and viral

Figure 9-23

HERPES SIMPLEX VIRUS, LYMPH NODE

Areas of necrosis (A) and immunoblastic proliferation (B) are clues to a diagnosis of herpes lymphadenitis. Occasionally, careful searching is required to find characteristic viral inclusions. Immunohistochemical staining highlights infected cells (C). (Courtesy of Dale Selby, San Antonio, TX.)

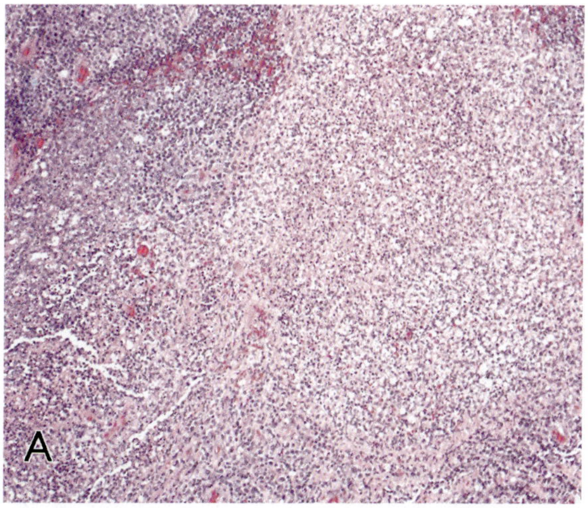

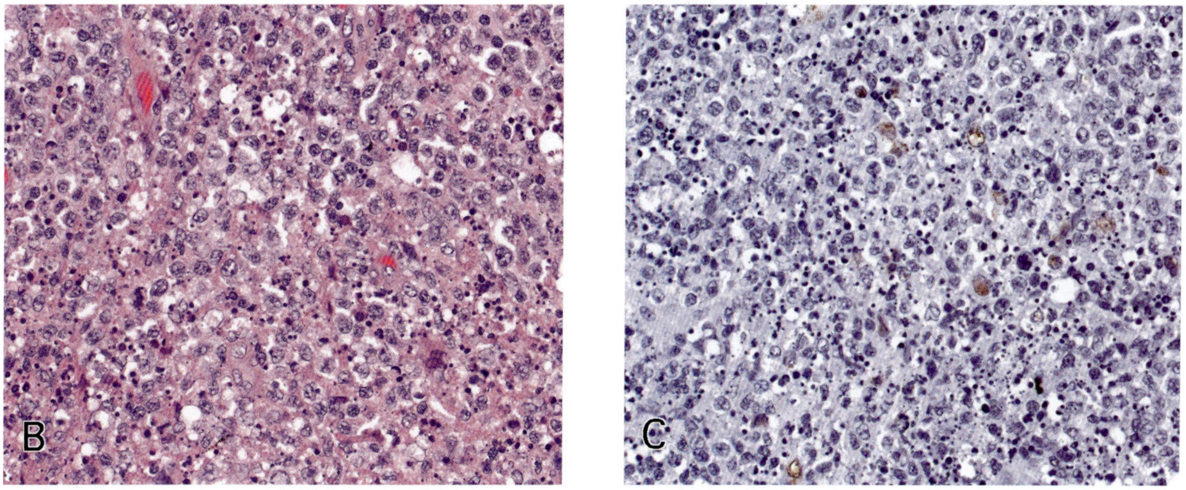

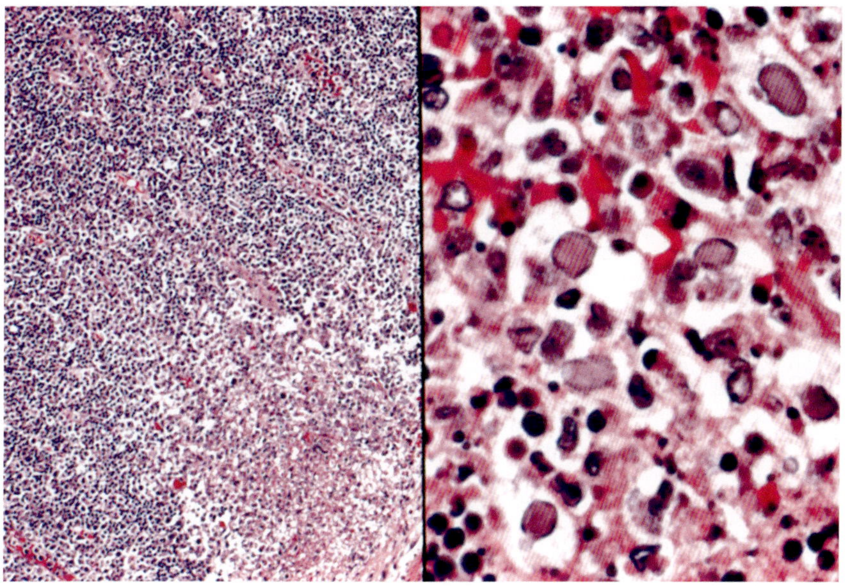

Figure 9-24

HERPES SIMPLEX VIRUS, LYMPH NODE

Herpes lymphadenitis (left) in which nuclear clearing due to viral inclusions (right) is seen.

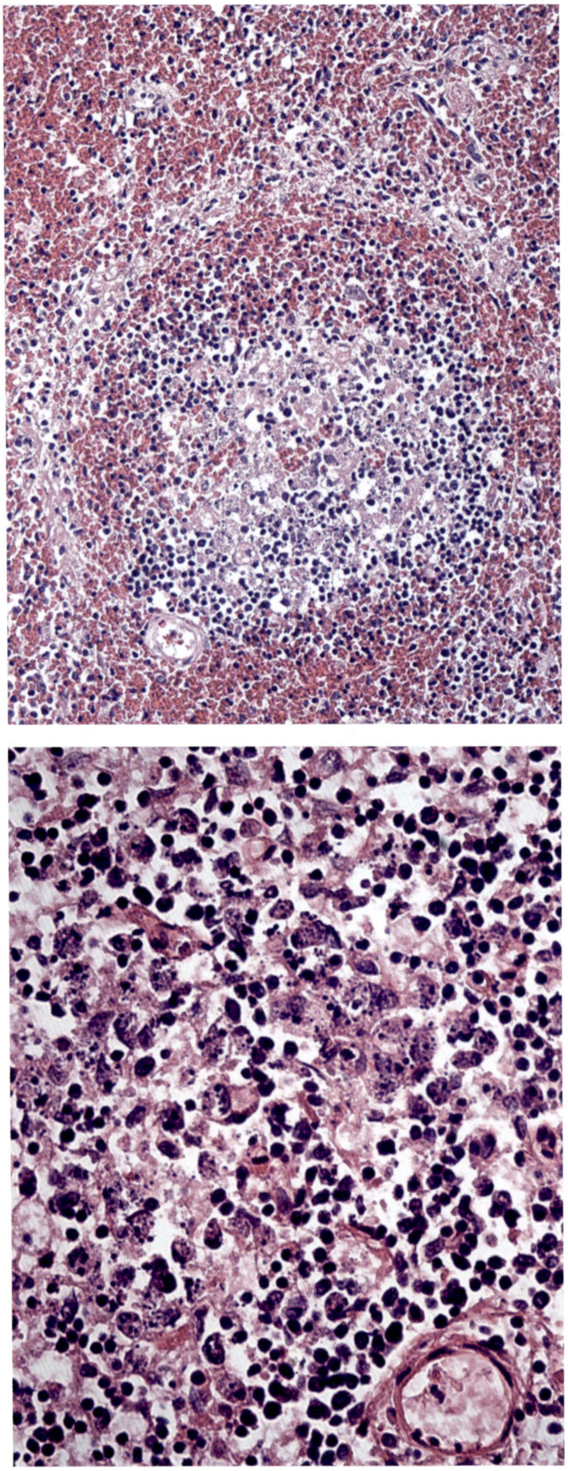

Figure 9-25

HERPES SIMPLEX VIRUS, SPLEEN

In this case of fatal, perinatal herpes simplex virus, changes in the spleen include lymphoid depletion (top) and necrosis with hemophagocytosis (bottom).

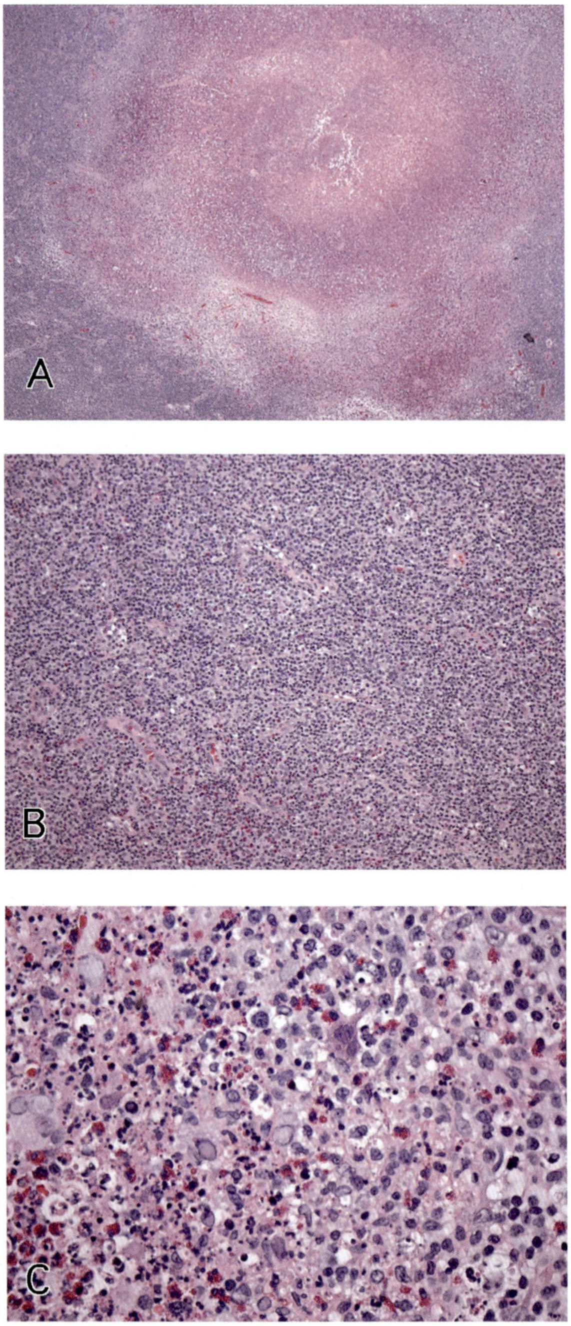

Figure 9-26

CHRONIC LYMPHOCYTIC LEUKEMIA/SMALL LYMPHOCYTIC LYMPHOMA WITH HERPES SIMPLEX VIRUS, LYMPH NODE

In cases of lymphoma with necrosis, careful attention should be paid to the areas of necrosis. The presence of herpes simplex virus infection has been reported in several types of lymphoma, especially small lymphocytic lymphoma, as in this case. (Courtesy of Peter Banks, Charlotte, NC.)

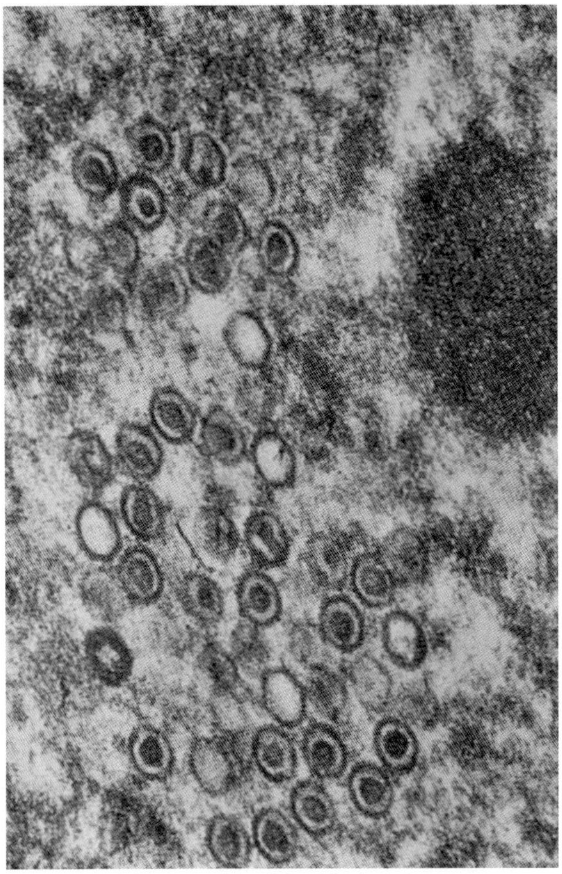

Figure 9-27

HERPES SIMPLEX VIRUS, TRANSMISSION ELECTRON MICROSCOPY

Occasionally, transmission electron microscopy is a useful adjunct to the diagnosis of viral infections, as in this case. (Courtesy of Gary Mierau, Denver CO.)

inclusions, these or other immunologic methods should be used to confirm a possible diagnosis of herpetic lymphadenitis (123).

Transmission electron microscopy confirms the presence of HSV (fig. 9-27). Viral particles are demonstrated in the nucleus or cytoplasm, consistent with herpes viral particles. However, the specific features of HSV are complex and should be referred to experts in viral morphology.

Differential Diagnosis. The primary entities in the differential diagnosis of HSV lymphadenitis are other causes of necrotizing lymphadenitis, such as Kikuchi disease; other infectious lymphadenopathies; and high-grade lymphomas (because of the associated necrosis). If associated skin lesions are present, they may suggest HSV lymphadenitis. The use of immunohistochemistry to detect HSV, or PCR for gene rearrangements to rule out lymphoma, may be necessary.

Treatment and Prognosis. Antiviral medications may be used, particularly in severe cases. Vidarabine or acyclovir has been shown to be effective. In patients with lymphoproliferative disorders, as suggested by Higgins and Warnke (53), HSV may lead a self-limited course and not require specific treatment.

VARICELLA-ZOSTER VIRUS

Definition. *Varicella-zoster virus* (VZV), a member of the herpesvirus family, is the causative agent of both *varicella (chickenpox)* and *herpes zoster*. It is occasionally associated with significant adenopathy, most commonly in immunocompromised hosts.

General Features. VZV is an alpha herpesvirus, and is in the same family as HSV. Primary infection typically results in latency in the sensory ganglia of the spinal cord. The virus may remain latent for years or even decades before recurrence (133).

Clinical Features. Varicella is an acute, contagious systemic infection that results in a vesicular, generalized maculopapular rash which is self-limited in children with normal immune systems. It is usually transmitted via the respiratory route and has a 2- to 3-week incubation period. In the immunocompromised patient, it can cause severe systemic disease. Herpes zoster refers to the recurrent form of viral infection which results from reactivation of the latent virus in previously infected adults. The cutaneous lesions resemble those of varicella except that they are usually limited to one sensory dermatome.

Lymphadenopathy may occur in either primary VZV or recurrent infection. The nodes most commonly affected are cervical, supraclavicular, and axillary (133). The enlarged lymph nodes are typically tender. In such cases, a good clinical history and appropriate laboratory studies are essential for the correct diagnosis.

Laboratory Findings. Direct immunofluorescence of skin vesicle fluid or a fresh lymph node touch preparation with fluorescein-conjugated VZV antiserum shows strong nuclear fluorescence, confirming the diagnosis (99). The finding of multinucleated virally infected cells from vesicle fluid (Tzanck smear) has largely been

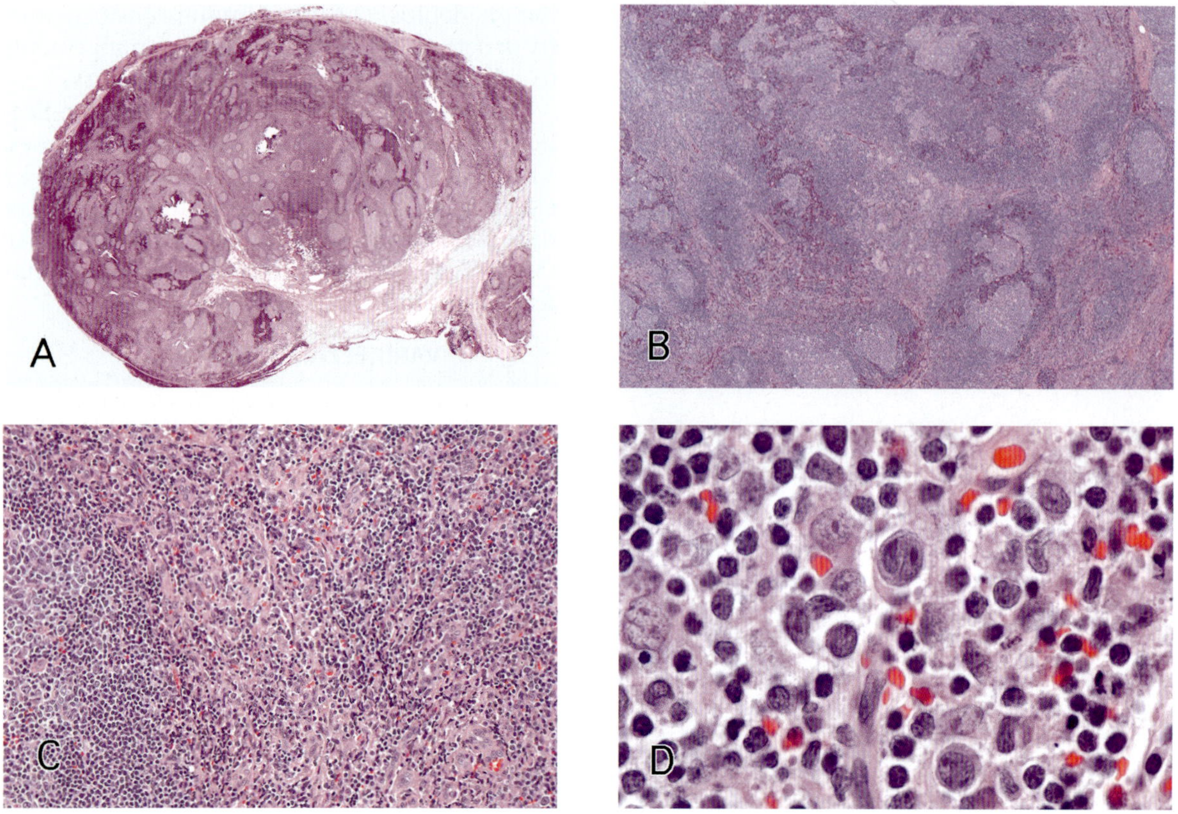

Figure 9-28

VARICELLA-ZOSTER VIRUS, LYMPH NODE

The immunosuppressed patient's lymphadenopathy showed follicular hyperplasia (A), paracortical expansion (B), and vascular proliferation (C). High magnification shows large cells with prominent intranuclear inclusions that likely represent viral inclusions (D).

supplanted by fluorescent antibody techniques. Serologic studies are also helpful in confirming a diagnosis of VZV infection.

Microscopic Findings. VZV infection causes diffuse paracortical hyperplasia with the characteristic nuclear inclusions in the acute phase (fig. 9-28). In later stages, however, the paracortical hyperplasia may be replaced by follicular hyperplasia with mild plasmacytosis (62,68,99). Large, atypical mononuclear cells with a characteristic inclusion-like nucleolus within an intranuclear vacuole may be noted. The capsule may be involved. The histopathologic changes are very similar to those described in EBV lymphadenitis.

Ancillary Studies. Ultrastructural examination has shown that the inclusions are multiple, spherical virus particles, 90 to 105 nm in diameter. These are typical of herpesviruses (61,99).

Differential Diagnosis. Other viral lymphadenitides, especially EBV, are commonly mistaken for VZV infection. Correlation with clinical and serologic studies is necessary to confirm a diagnosis. Rarely, VZV infection is mistaken for large cell lymphoma. As in other circumstances, correlation of clinical findings is important; the use of gene rearrangements or other studies to evaluate clonality may be necessary in some cases.

Treatment and Prognosis. The relatively recent approval of a varicella vaccine will undoubtedly reduce the incidence of VZV adenopathy. The administration of the VZV vaccine, however, also leads to occasional cases of postvaccinial lymphadenitis (see later this chapter). Acyclovir is an effective treatment, but must be administered early in the course of infection.

HUMAN HERPESVIRUS-8

Definition. *Human herpesvirus-8* (HHV-8), sometimes known as *Kaposi sarcoma–associated herpesvirus* (KSVH), is associated with several types of lymphoid proliferation, including plasma cell Castleman disease, primary effusion lymphoma, plasma cell malignancies, and other reactive adenopathies. It has also been suggested that HHV-8 may play a role in sarcoidosis.

General Features. HHV-8 is a gamma herpesvirus and is most closely related to EBV (75,78, 84). HHV-8 is well documented as causing all forms of Kaposi sarcoma. HHV-8 is known to infect endothelial cells (as in Kaposi sarcoma), bone marrow stromal cells, and neoplastic cells of lymphoma. Plasma cell disorders appear to be associated with the production large amounts of interleukin (IL)-6 by virally infected cells. IL-6 is associated with growth and proliferation of plasma cells. HHV-8 is associated with the tissues involved in sarcoidosis, although its relationship with this disease is unclear at this time (84).

Clinical Features. HHV-8 infection is most frequently associated with HIV infection, as well as several specific types of lymphoid proliferation. Plasma cell Castleman disease, a clinical entity characterized by systemic symptoms and angiofollicular hyperplasia with plasmacytosis, is discussed in chapter 6.

Primary effusion lymphoma, which is associated with HHV-8 infection, is typically found in patients with HIV, although it is seen in patients with other types of immunosuppression or, rarely, in immunocompetent individuals (fig. 9-29). It is composed of immunoblastic/plasmablastic-appearing abnormal lymphocytes in body cavities (9). The abnormal lymphocytes are positive for plasma cell–related antigens, such as CD38 and CD138, but they may lack other B-cell–associated markers such as CD19, CD20, and surface immunoglobulin light chains. Coinfection with EBV is present in most cases.

A range of plasma cell disorders, including monoclonal gammopathy of undetermined significance (MGUS), Waldenstrom macroglobulinemia, plasma cell myeloma, and plasmablastic lymphoma are associated with HHV-8 infection. The plasma cell proliferations range from atypical to frankly malignant. A rare variant of T-cell lymphoma has been described in association with HHV-8 infection (28).

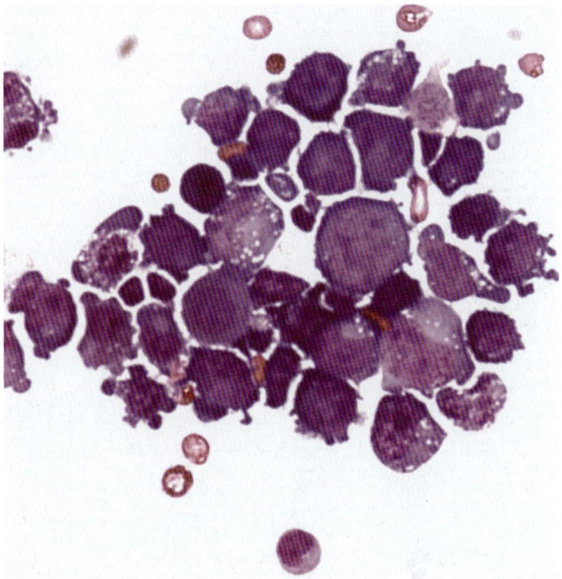

Figure 9-29

PRIMARY EFFUSION LYMPHOMA

A cytologic preparation of the large abnormal lymphocytes seen in primary effusion lymphomas.

Microscopic Findings. As mentioned, there are a variety of benign lymphoid proliferations associated with HHV-8 infection (75). Splenomegaly may be seen, but the pathologic findings have not been well described (78). It is possible that the complete spectrum of disorders associated with this virus has not been fully characterized. HHV-8 infection should be considered when there are: 1) unusual lymphoid proliferations in patients with acquired immunodeficiency syndrome (AIDS); 2) proliferations of plasma cells or plasmablasts in AIDS or immunosuppressed patients; and 3) coincident lymphoid proliferations in patients with known Kaposi sarcoma. Other HHV-8–associated proliferations may be indicated by clinical history or morphologic findings.

Florid follicular hyperplasia with vascular proliferation is associated with HHV-8 infection in the lymph nodes (fig. 9-30) (75,126). Nuclear localization of HHV-8–positive cells is seen in the interfollicular areas, within germinal centers, and in mantle zones. In the study of Lazzi et al. (75), the infected cells were B lymphocytes.

The HHV-8 (KSHV)-associated germinotropic lymphoproliferative disorder described by Du et al. (34), showed atypical plasmablasts that were

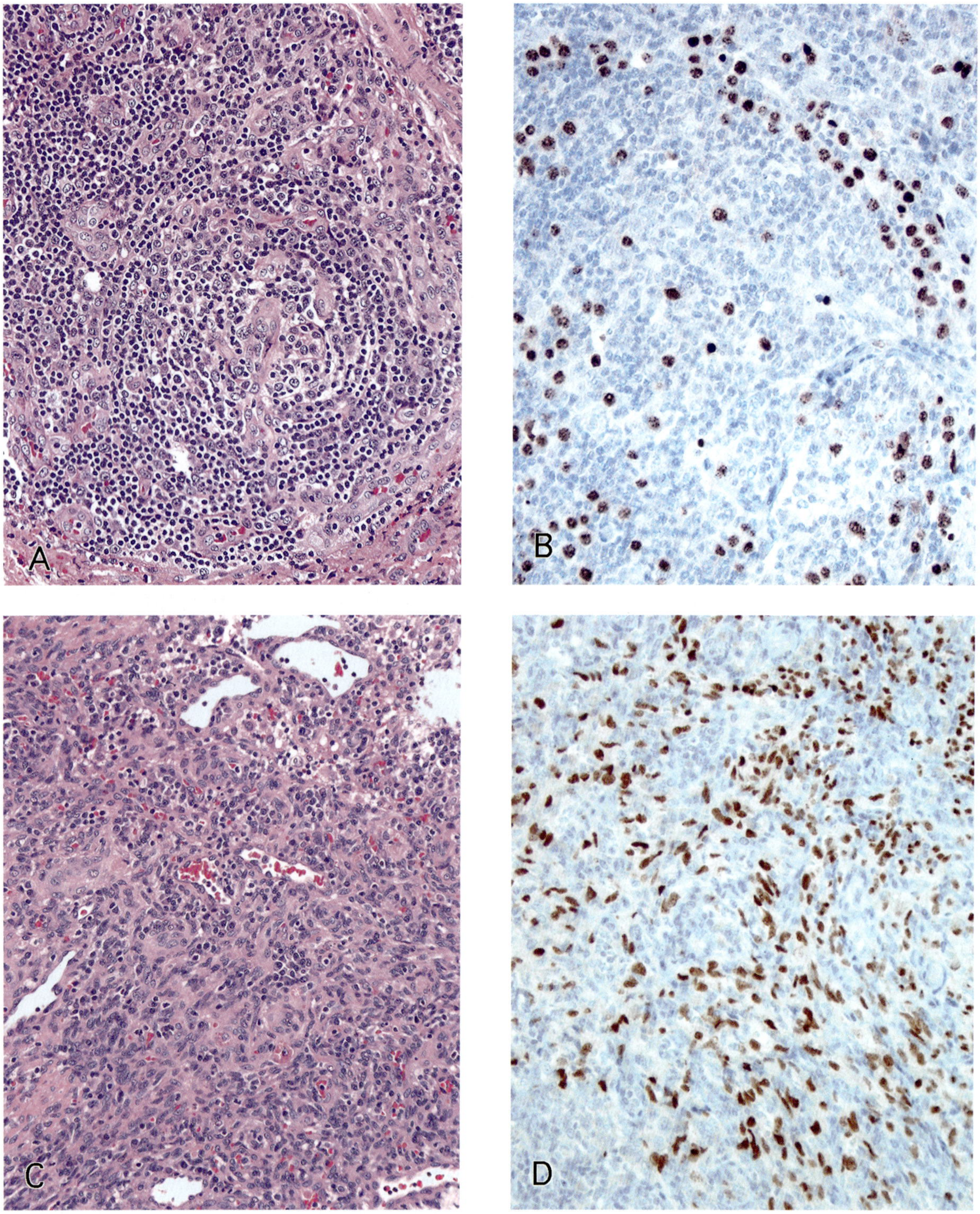

Figure 9-30

HUMAN HERPESVIRUS-8, LYMPH NODE

A lymph node in an immunocompromised patient shows plasma cell Castleman disease (A,B) and Kaposi sarcoma (C,D) simultaneously. Both were reactive for human herpesvirus-8 (HHV-8) immunohistochemical stains (B,D). (Courtesy of Anselm Hii, Irvine, CA.)

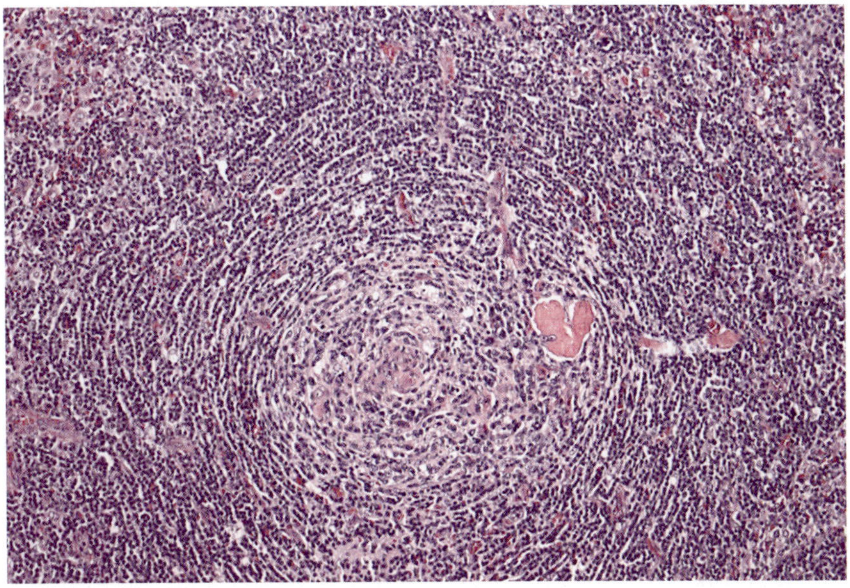

Figure 9-31

HUMAN HERPESVIRUS-8, SPLEEN

In cases of suspected HHV-8 infection in the spleen, the features are most commonly those of Castleman disease, as in this case.

preferentially located in germinal centers. The patients were immunocompetent, had localized adenopathy, and had a good response to therapy. The plasmablasts had restricted light chain expression, suggesting a neoplastic proliferation. A polymorphous lymphoid proliferation resembling plasmacytic hyperplasia PTLD has also been reported, with HHV-8 positivity seen in a subset of patients (87).

The combination of Kaposi sarcoma and HHV-8–associated lymphoid proliferations is common in the same lymph node. Plasma cell Castleman disease and Kaposi sarcoma is probably the most frequent combination, although a wide range of plasma cell proliferations are present in nodes with Kaposi sarcoma (fig. 9-31). Awareness of the possibility of multiple HHV-8–related proliferations/neoplasms in the same sample leads to more frequent recognition of this pathology.

Ancillary Studies. Immunohistochemical staining is available for HHV-8 and is useful for identifying virally infected cells. In situ hybridization studies for the virus are also available, and have increased sensitivity. EBV may coinfect the same cells that harbor HHV-8; in situ staining for EBV-encoded RNA (EBER) may highlight this finding. Coinfection by HHV-8 and EBV is seen in primary effusion lymphoma and has also been reported in benign lymphoid proliferations (75).

Differential Diagnosis. Plasma cell neoplasms, without associated HHV-8 infection, including plasmablastic lymphomas and plasma cell dyscrasia, may mimic the abnormalities associated with HHV-8–associated proliferations. Careful attention to the clinical history, including a history of HIV/AIDS, is helpful. Immunohistochemical or in situ hybridization staining for HHV-8 can characterize difficult cases.

Treatment and Prognosis. Antiviral treatments for HHV-8 have been tested with mixed results. Cidofovir, ganciclovir, and foscarnet have some effect in clinical trials. The prognosis depends on the type of lymphoid proliferation. Both immune-competent and -suppressed patients with plasmablastic neoplasms have a poor prognosis.

HUMAN HERPESVIRUS-6

Definition. *Human herpesvirus*-6 (HHV-6) is a ubiquitous member of the herpesvirus family. It is responsible for several distinctive types of lymphadenopathy in immune-competent and -compromised individuals and may also be associated with the development of lymphomas.

General Features. HHV-6 is the causative agent of *exanthem subitum* (also known as *roseola infantum* or *sixth disease*), a viral infection associated with generalized rash and fever, seen in children 4 to 24 months old (26,121). This infection typically resolves rapidly without sequelae.

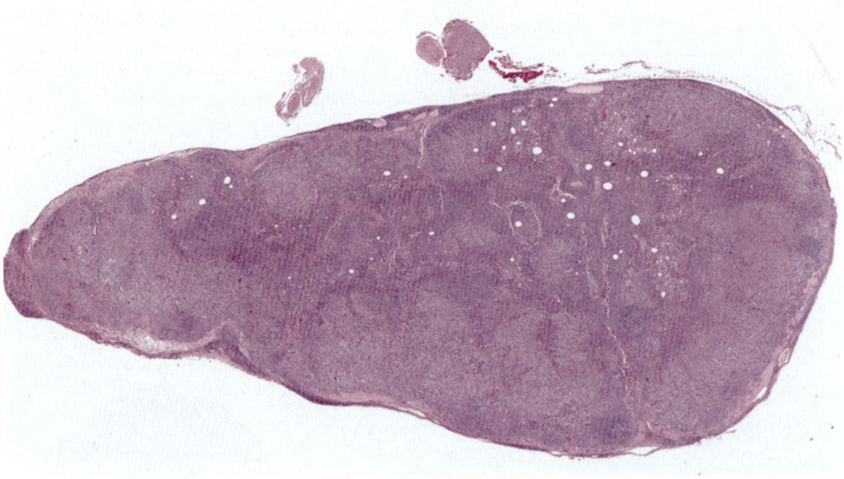

Figure 9-32

HUMAN HERPESVIRUS-6, LYMPH NODE

The normal lymph node architecture is distorted.

HHV-6 is a beta herpesvirus, and is most similar to CMV. Two variants of HHV-6, A and B, have been identified based on genetic differences (26). The B variant appears to be responsible for most symptomatic infections (130). The HHV-6 virus induces cytopathic effects and is tropic for CD4-positive T cells, although a variety of cell types can be infected in vivo, and latently infected cells include plasma cells and macrophages (26). CD46 is the cellular receptor for HHV-6.

Clinical Features. In primary infection or reactivation/reinfection by HHV-6, there is a variety of clinical presentations: classic exanthem subitum, infectious mononucleosis–like syndrome, fever with generalized adenopathy, immunocompromised opportunistic infection, and lymphoma-associated infection (3,15,26). The clinical findings are variable and include: encephalitis and encephalopathy, chronic fatigue, adenopathy, seizures, rashes, and splenomegaly (79,118). HHV-6 infections are becoming more recognized in the post-transplant setting. Transplant recipients with HHV-6 infection have encephalitis, pneumonitis, thrombotic thrombocytopenic purpura, graft failure, and bone marrow suppression (26). The virus may have a role as a cofactor or as an opportunistic infection in patients with HIV (26).

Lymphadenopathy and a variety of lymphoproliferative disorders are associated with HHV-6 infection. B-cell lymphomas (including Burkitt lymphoma), Hodgkin lymphoma, T-cell lymphomas (including angioimmunoblastic T-cell lymphoma and S-100 protein–positive T-cell lymphoproliferative disorder), and Rosai-Dorfman disease have all been associated with HHV-6 infection (15,16,26,76).

Laboratory Findings. Lymphocytosis with atypical lymphocytes, similar to that seen in infectious mononucleosis, is seen in the peripheral blood of patients with HHV-6 infections. Seroconversion occurs early in life after primary infection, with 72 to 100 percent positivity in the healthy population (130). Increasing viral titers, especially IgM levels, indicates active infection.

Microscopic Findings. Patients with HHV-6 infection have been described as having "reactive processes indicative of viral infection" (15). These "generic" viral changes include: paracortical hyperplasia and proliferation of large transformed lymphocytes (immunoblasts, centroblasts) in clusters or cohesive sheets (figs. 9-32–9-34). Increased numbers of high endothelial venules/vascular proliferations and increased follicular dendritic cell meshworks are seen (15,79). Eosinophils and plasma cells are increased in the paracortical regions. Mitotic figures are frequent in these regions. Small foci of monocytoid (marginal zone) cells are also present (121). Rare reports have suggested that there is follicular hyperplasia with prominent centroblasts (121), although small residual follicles are described in most reports. Similar to herpesvirus infections in other sites and lymphadenopathy due to HSV, focal (coagulative) necrosis is present.

Features similar to those of angioimmmunoblastic lymphadenopathy with dysproteinemia (AILD) can be seen in HHV-6 infection, and abnormal proliferations of T cells (such as S-100 protein–positive T-cell lymphoproliferative

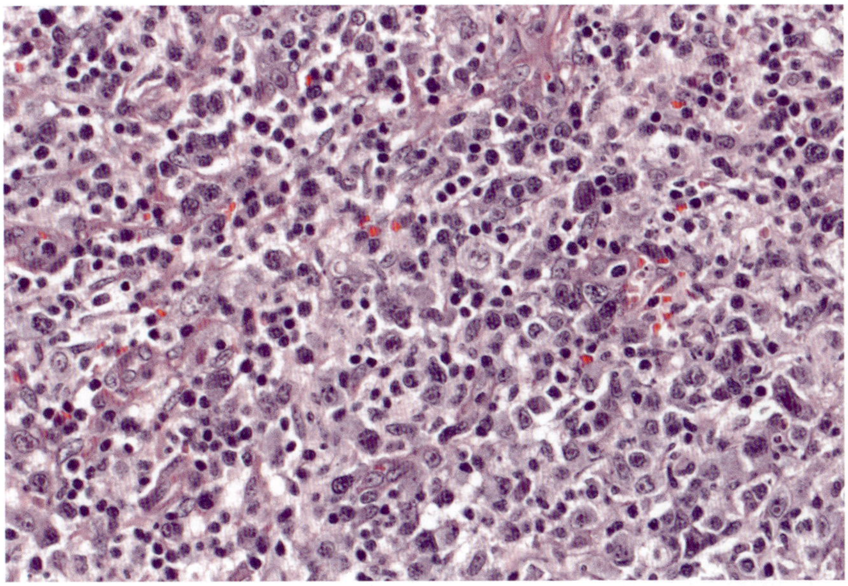

Figure 9-33

HUMAN HERPESVIRUS-6, LYMPH NODE

Large, atypical lymphocytes, many with a prominent nucleolus/viral inclusion, are seen.

Figure 9-34

HUMAN HERPESVIRUS-6, LYMPH NODE

Clusters of lymphocytes have prominent viral inclusions (A,B). Immunohistochemical staining for the gp60/110 kD HHV-6 viral protein is seen (C). (C courtesy of Stefania Pittlauga, Bethesda, MD.)

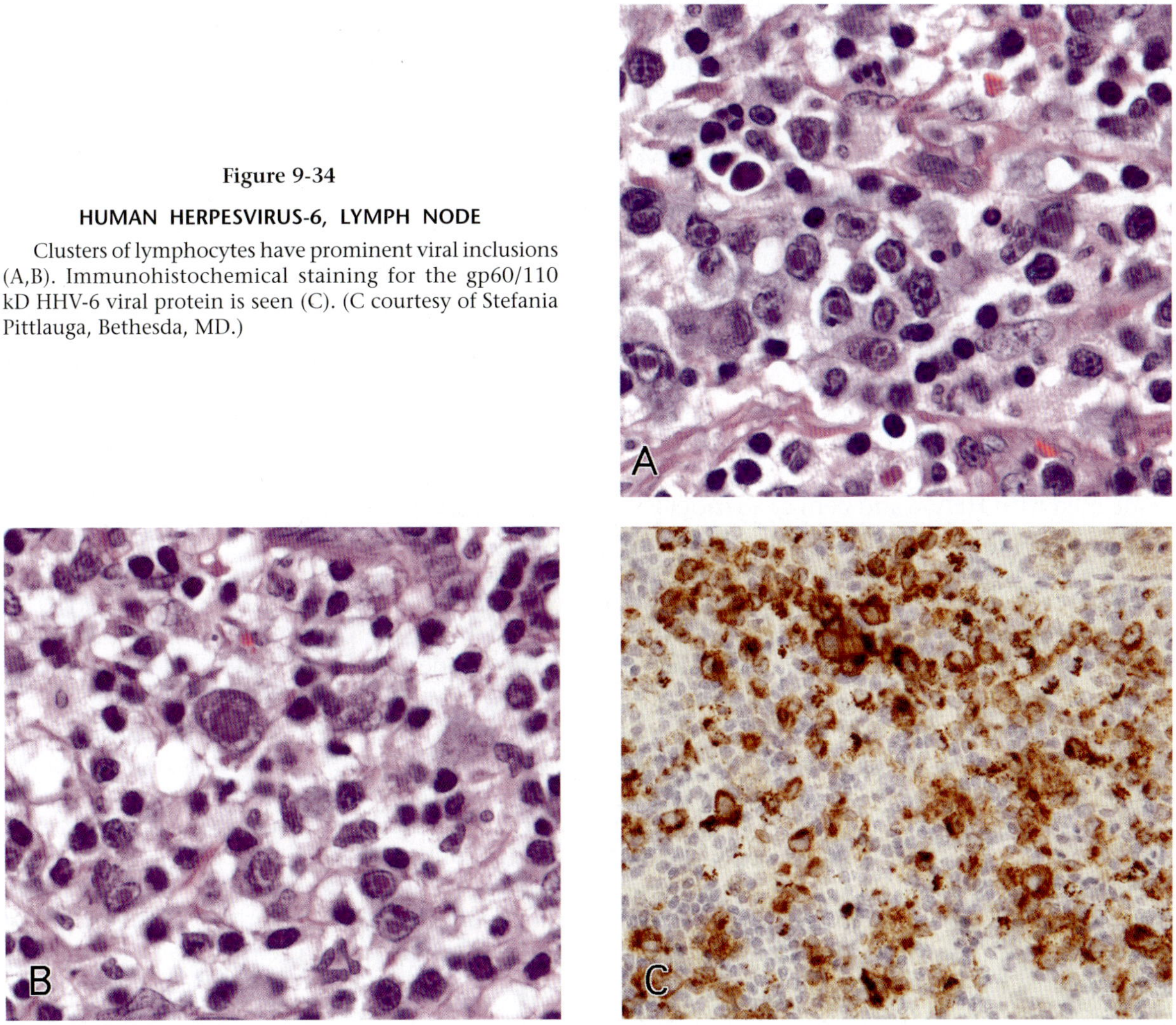

disorder) have been noted (16). Many of the histologic features described in HHV-6–associated lymphoid proliferations (large transformed T cells, vascular proliferation, increased in follicular dendritic cell networks) are seen in AILD and in angioimmunoblastic T-cell lymphoma.

Ancillary Studies. In cases with viral inclusions, the immunohistochemically reactive cells are CD4-positive T cells (79). An immunohistochemical stain for HHV-6 is available but only as a research tool. It is possible that as this infection is more frequently detected, the antibody will be more available.

Transmission electron microscopy of virally infected cells reveals typical herpesvirus particles (79). Although HHV-6 has subtle differences from other herpesviruses, these differences can only be appreciated by expert reviewers.

Differential Diagnosis. Acute EBV/infectious mononucleosis is very similar to HHV-6 in both clinical presentation and morphologic appearance. The presence of histologically identifiable viral inclusions suggests a non-EBV virus. Serologic, immunohistochemical, and PCR studies help distinguish HHV-6 from EBV. Both CMV and other herpesvirus infections are similar to HHV-6. HHV-6 does not have the cytomegaly seen in CMV, which also typically infects endothelial cells. As in other cases, serologic and other immunologic detection methods may be necessary to distinguish HHV-6 infection.

HHV-6–associated lymphomas have been reported (15); however, it is unclear whether HHV-6 plays an etiologic role in the malignant transformation. Differentiation of a lymphoma associated with HHV-6 and benign adenopathy should be based on multifactorial analysis of clinical, histologic, and ancillary studies including gene rearrangements in selected cases.

Treatment and Prognosis. There have been no controlled studies of antiviral agents on HHV-6. However, antiviral agents that are active against CMV appear to have similar potency against HHV-6 (26). Acyclovir has little or no effect on HHV-6.

MEASLES VIRUS

Definition. *Measles (rubeola)* is a now an uncommon childhood disease associated with a classic rash and viral syndrome, and occasionally with adenopathy. Measles may also be seen in association with immunosuppression. Now, more commonly, adenopathy is associated with administration of live, attenuated viral vaccines.

General Features. Measles is caused by an RNA paramyxovirus that is highly contagious by either droplet aspiration or placental transmission (14). The measles virus infects and is latent in a variety of white blood cell types.

Clinical Features. The measles virus is highly infectious, with a worldwide distribution. Since humans are the only reservoirs for the measles virus, it has been almost eliminated because of vaccination (14). The incubation period lasts 10 to 12 days, with a prodrome of 3 days. This is followed by fever and a generalized morbilliform rash, and clearance after several days. Other findings include coryza, pharyngitis, photophobia, conjunctivitis, and lymphadenopathy. Regional lymphadenopathy may also develop following the administration of live, attenuated virus for immunization purposes (postvaccinial lymphadenopathy, see later this chapter) (4,31,117). Severe postmeasles disorders include postinfectious encephalitis and subacute sclerosing panencephalitis (14). Immunocompromised individuals, including those with AIDS, transplantation, and iatrogenic immunosuppression, have an increased incidence of measles infection.

Laboratory Findings. Serologic responses are very specific for the diagnosis of the measles. Viral culture is difficult; however, PCR tests are rapid and effective.

Microscopic Findings. The histopathologic changes include a "mottled" paracortex and diffuse, immunoblastic hyperplasia. Occasionally, a reactive follicle is seen. The characteristic feature of measles infection is the presence of Warthin-Finkeldey type giant cells, or polykaryocytes, in the lymphoreticular organs (especially lymph nodes, thymus, tonsils, appendix), which usually occurs in the prodromal phase (31,33). These are large cells with numerous, darkly stained nuclei in grape-like clusters ("mulberry cells"), and abundant acidophilic cytoplasm (fig. 9-35). Occasionally, cellular inclusions are noted in the cytoplasm of giant cells or endothelial cells (119). Electron microscopy may reveal the relatively characteristic findings of coiled microtubules and dense fibrillar or granular bodies, usually in the endothelial cells (117).

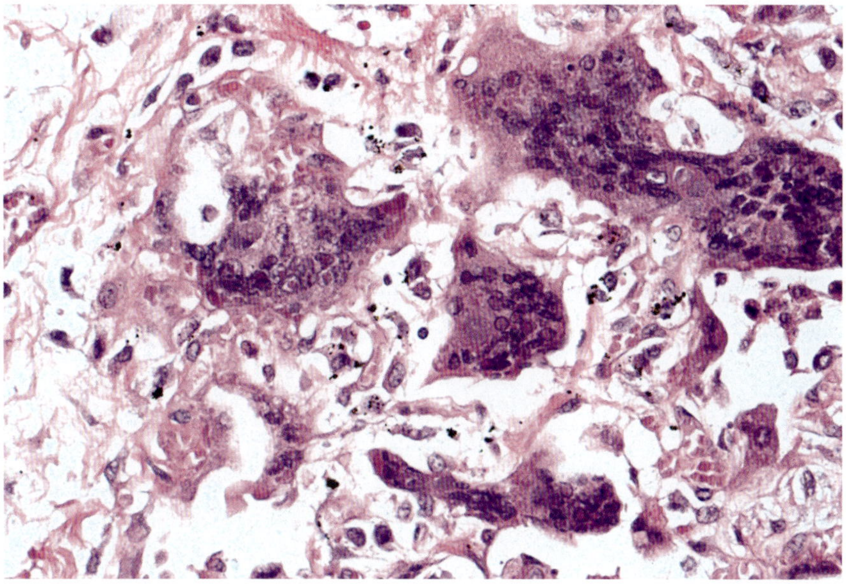

Figure 9-35

MEASLES VIRUS

Although this histologic sample is from the lung, similar multinucleated cells are seen in lymph nodes and spleen affected by measles virus.

Differential Diagnosis. The differential diagnosis includes other viral lymphadenitides, including HIV infection. In HIV-infected lymphoid tissues, polykaryocytes may be seen. In contrast to measles, in HIV these cells are likely derived from follicular dendritic cells, rather than lymphocytes.

Treatment and Prognosis. Measles infection is usually self-limited. Postmeasles vaccinial lymphadenitis also tends to resolve spontaneously.

RUBELLA VIRUS

Definition. *Rubella* is a virus that may be associated with lymphadenopathy and splenomegaly. The lymph nodes are rarely biopsied, and there are no specific morphologic findings.

Clinical Features. Rubella is an enveloped RNA virus, and is classified as a togavirus. Rubella infection is a generally mild viral illness associated with fever, lymphadenopathy, and generalized rash. Up to 50 percent of infections are subclinical (55). The clinical significance of rubella lies in the risks associated with congenital infection. *Congenital rubella syndrome* includes cataracts, other ocular abnormalities, cardiac defects, deafness, microcephaly, and mental retardation. Rubella may be associated with acute mesenteric lymphadenitis (122). Joint involvement is common, especially in adults.

The institution of regular vaccination for rubella has dramatically reduced the incidence of this disease. The majority of young adults in the United States have serologic evidence of immunity (55). It is typical that very specific lymph nodes are involved in rubella infection. The posterior auricular, suboccipital, and posterior cervical nodes are involved and may precede other symptoms by up to 1 week. Generalized adenopathy may also be seen (67).

Microscopic Findings. No specific microscopic features have been reported in rubella lymphadenopathy. It is likely that the histologic changes resemble those of other viral adenopathies (fig. 9-36). In congenital rubella infection, lymphoid depletion of both the spleen and lymph nodes has been reported (72). Transient splenomegaly may be seen in rubella infection (54), and cases of splenic rupture have also been reported (92,137).

HUMAN IMMUNODEFICIENCY VIRUS/ ACQUIRED IMMUNODEFICIENCY SYNDROME

Definition. *Human immunodeficiency virus* (HIV)/*acquired immunodeficiency syndrome* (AIDS) *lymphadenitis* is a distinctive and complex category of lymphadenopathy. Throughout the course of HIV infection and AIDS, there is a progression of lymph node changes that is fairly characteristic. Distinctive splenic changes are also present.

General Features. The virus responsible for AIDS is HIV, an RNA retrovirus. There are several subtypes of the HIV virus, with subtype B being the most commonly encountered in the United States. There are three general groups of genes

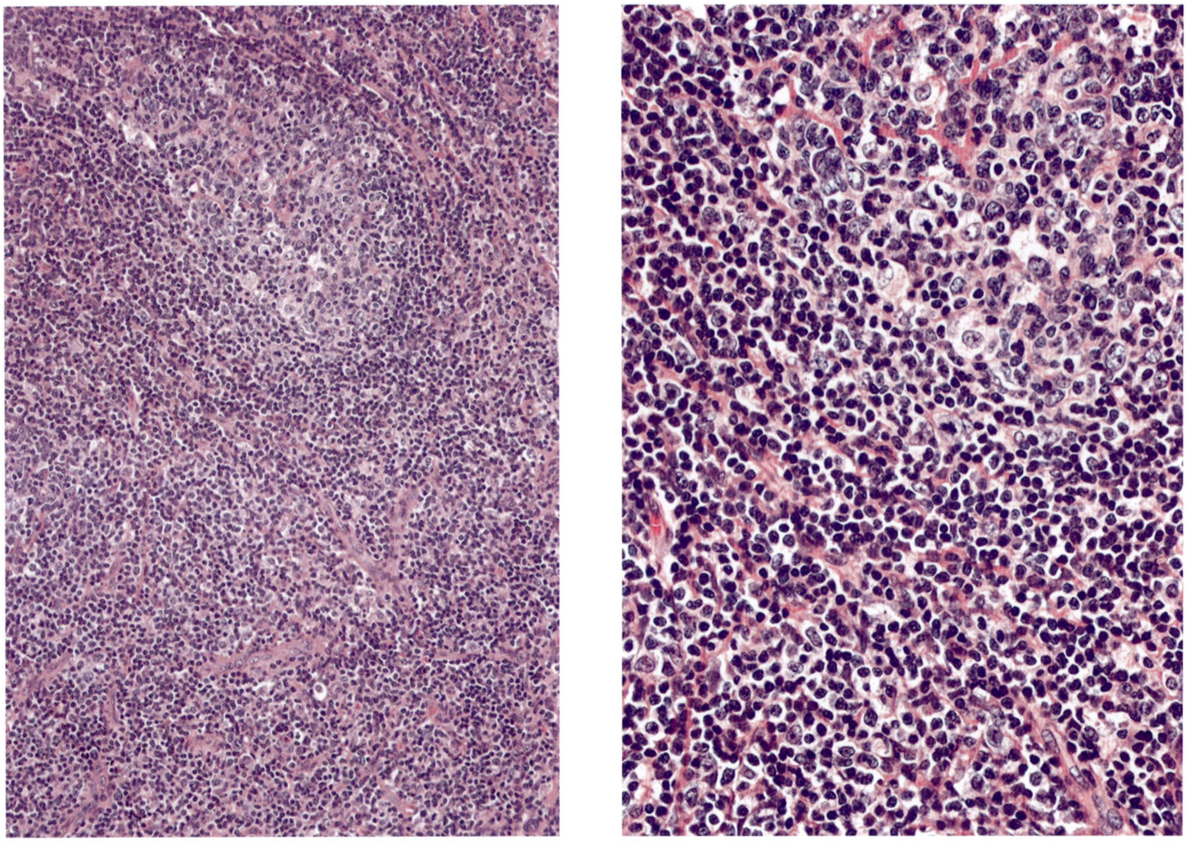

Figure 9-36

RUBELLA VIRUS, LYMPH NODE

An increase in immunoblasts (left) and vascular proliferation (right) are seen.

in HIV: group specific antigen/core (*GAG*), polymerase (*POL*), and envelope (*ENV*). The ability of HIV to vary its antigenic makeup is central to the difficulty in eradicating the virus. The virus is particularly tropic to CD4-positive T cells, although several other cells types act as viral reservoirs and are directly infected by the virus.

Clinical Features. Generally, histopathologic findings are nonspecific, and it is not wise to try and diagnose HIV/AIDS based on lymph node pathology alone. However, the constellation of lymphoid findings can be distinctive, and it is important to recognize these findings since they can mimic other benign adenopathies and lymphomas. It is important to remember, however, that HIV/AIDS is also associated with opportunistic infectious agents and intercurrent neoplasms (lymphomas, Kaposi sarcoma, etc.), which must be considered in any lymph node evaluation.

AIDS-related lymphadenopathy is one of the earliest signs of infection by HIV. The lymphadenopathy is often a generalized process that has been referred to as persistent (or progressive) generalized lymphadenopathy (127). The lymph nodes that are associated with HIV infection are often tender and may present in multiple anatomic sites. A recent comprehensive review of primary HIV infection reported the most frequent nodal sites as cervical, axillary, and inguinal (129).

The syndrome caused by HIV, which we refer to as AIDS, was first recognized in the male homosexual community (19,21,44), but has since been described among intravenous drug abusers, recipients of infected blood products, heterosexual partners of high-risk individuals, and infants of HIV-positive mothers. From the earliest pathologic reports of autopsied patients,

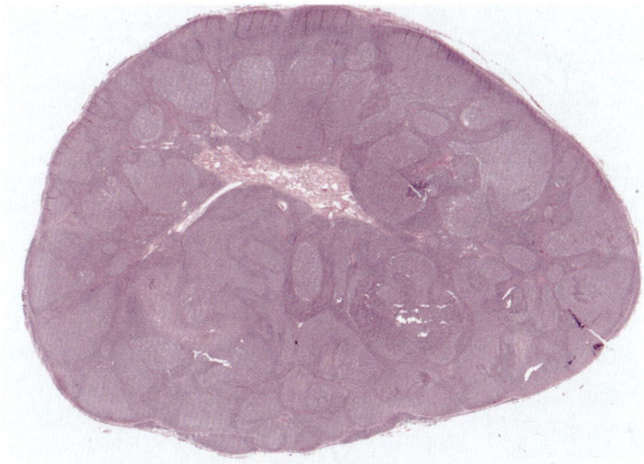

Figure 9-37

HUMAN IMMUNODEFICIENCY VIRUS (HIV)/ACQUIRED IMMUNODEFICIENCY SYNDROME (AIDS), LYMPH NODE

An enlarged lymph node with florid follicular hyperplasia. The follicles are massive in size, with irregular shapes and poorly formed or absent mantle zones.

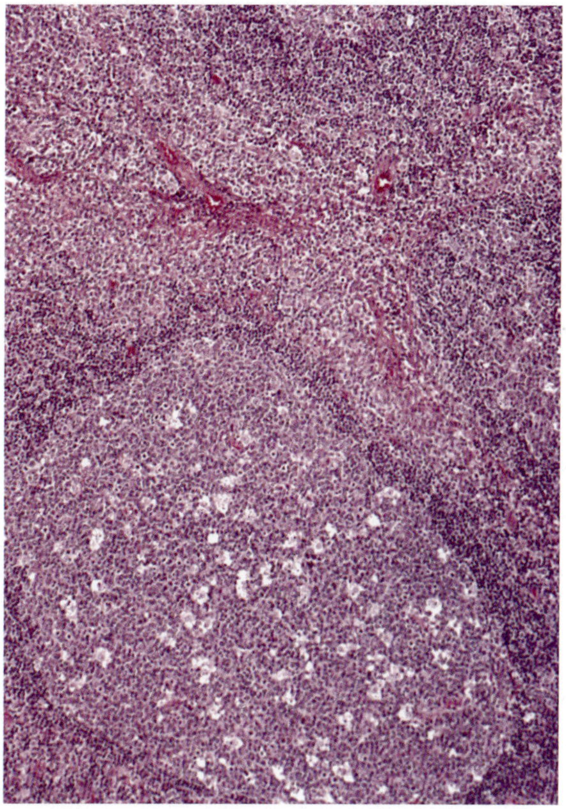

Figure 9-38

HIV/AIDS, LYMPH NODE

The reactive follicles of follicular hyperplasia show a very high proliferation rate and increased apoptosis as evidenced by numerous tingible body macrophages and mitotic figures.

it has been recognized that this disease has a devastating impact on the body's hematopoietic system, culminating in profound lymphoid depletion in the lymph nodes and spleen (103). One of the first names given to the retrovirus associated with AIDS was lymphadenopathy-associated virus, or LAV (11). Persistent generalized lymphadenopathy has long been recognized as an important early clinical finding in AIDS patients, and there have been extensive descriptions of the histopathologic changes in the lymph nodes of AIDS patients and successful attempts to correlate the histologic changes with the clinical course of the disease (18,22,43,58,95,127). Persistent generalized lymphadenopathy is defined as lymph node enlargement at two or more sites (excluding inguinal) that persists for at least 3 months without any other identifiable etiology.

Microscopic Findings. The histologic changes represent a temporal progression from florid, reactive follicular hyperplasia, to a mixed pattern with small, hyalinized follicles and larger ones, to an eventual lymphoid-depleted stage. At this point, opportunistic infections and/or malignancies are commonly seen (10,22,37,59,87,127).

The most striking change in the early stages is spectacular ("explosive") follicular hyperplasia, generally with very large follicles. Associated with this is a general loss of well-defined mantle zones, described as "naked" germinal centers, making the distinction from follicular lymphoma more difficult. The germinal centers have a prominent starry-sky appearance with numerous tingible body macrophages (figs. 9-37, 9-38). Follicle lysis, or invagination of small reactive mantle zone lymphocytes within the germinal centers, is an important finding in the hyperplastic phase of HIV-related lymphadenopathy (fig. 9-39) (106,136). These findings may not be affected by highly active antiretroviral therapy (HAART) (97).

Nonspecific hemorrhage, unrelated to the biopsy procedure, may be present (95). Prominent polyclonal plasmacytosis, scattered immunoblasts, and increased vascularity are characteristically noted in the interfollicular region. Focal Warthin-Finkeldey–like multinucleated giant cells, epithelioid macrophages, and neutrophils,

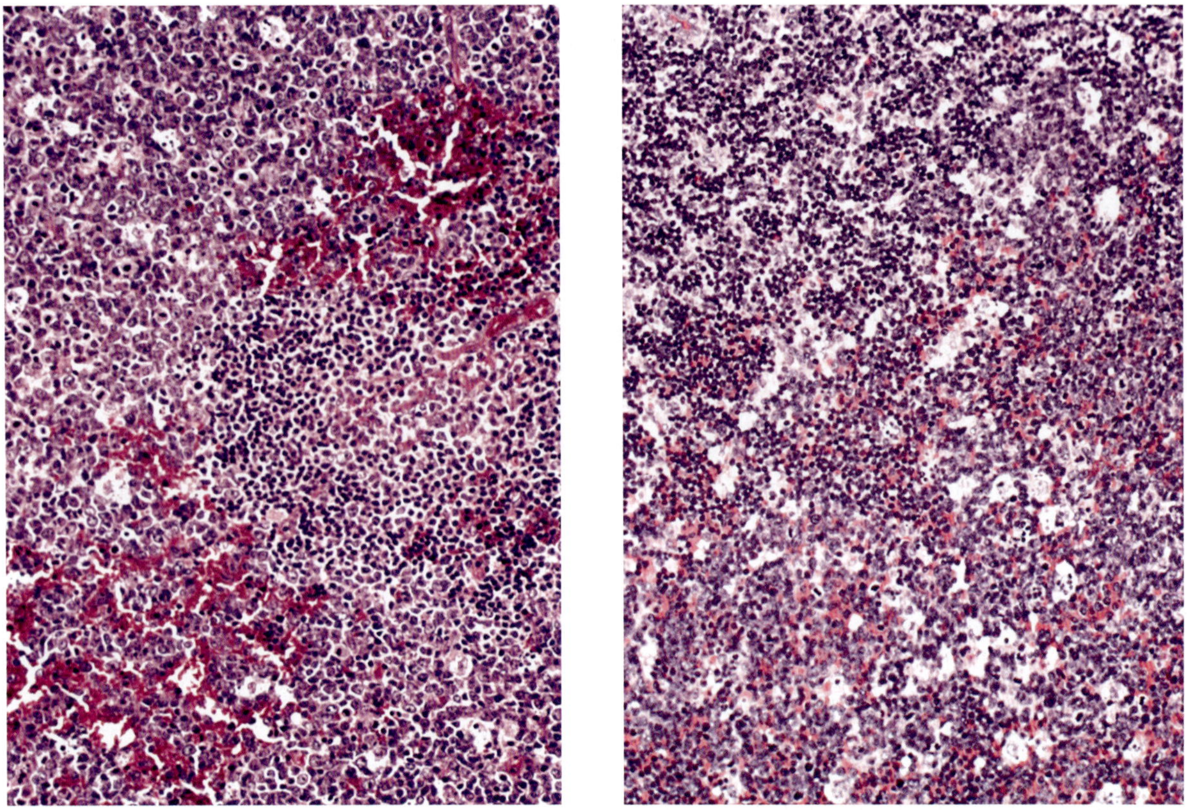

Figure 9-39

HIV/AIDS, LYMPH NODE

The structure of the follicles becomes disrupted, leading to follicular lysis. This destruction of the follicles may be due to viral effects on the follicular dendritic cells and other elements of the structural framework of the follicle.

usually within foci of sinusoidal monocytoid B-cell hyperplasia, are often seen (106,114). This finding is due in part to direct infection of follicular dendritic cells by the HIV virus. Follicular dendritic cells serve as a reservoir of virus and are the cell types that form the multinucleated giant cells (5,66). In this stage, there is also proliferation of small blood vessels in the germinal centers and paracortical high endothelial venules, similar to the changes seen in Castleman disease. There are also interfollicular aggregates of monocytoid B lymphocytes, which are seen in other viral infections.

Follicular fragmentation may be seen, which is marked by hemorrhage in germinal centers, foci of necrosis, and small lymphocyte infiltration of the necrotic foci (136). During the follicular fragmentation stage, there is a reduction in the number of CD4-positive T cells and an increase in the number of CD8-positive T cells, accompanied by follicular lysis and dissolution of the follicular dendritic cell network. Follicular fragmentation may represent an early regressive change of the lymph node and is associated with thinning of the mantle zones.

As the disease progresses, the lymph nodes show a mixed follicular hyperplasia/involution pattern consisting of reactive and regressively transformed germinal centers (fig. 9-40) and interfollicular plasmacytosis which is reminiscent of Castleman disease. There may be paracortical hyperplasia with prominent vascularity. The follicular involution stage shows small, atrophic germinal centers that may be hyalinized or show deposition of proteinaceous material (fig. 9-41).

The final stage is profound lymphoid depletion in which the nodes become completely devoid of recognizable paracortex or follicles (fig. 9-42). There is increased vascularity. Lymphoid-depleted nodes are most often seen at autopsy

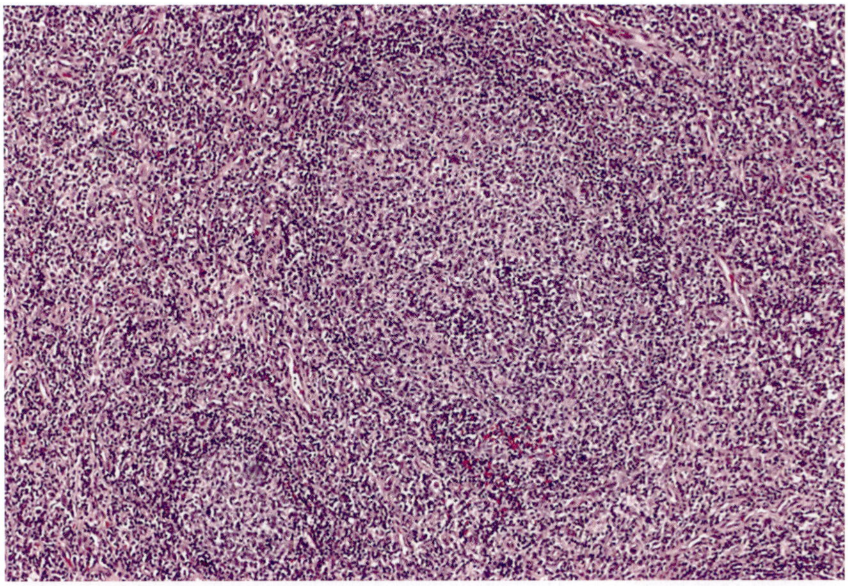

Figure 9-40

HIV/AIDS, LYMPH NODE

In later stages of untreated HIV/AIDS, there is a mixture of large, hyperplastic follicles and small, regressed follicles. As the disease progresses untreated, more follicles become small and regressed.

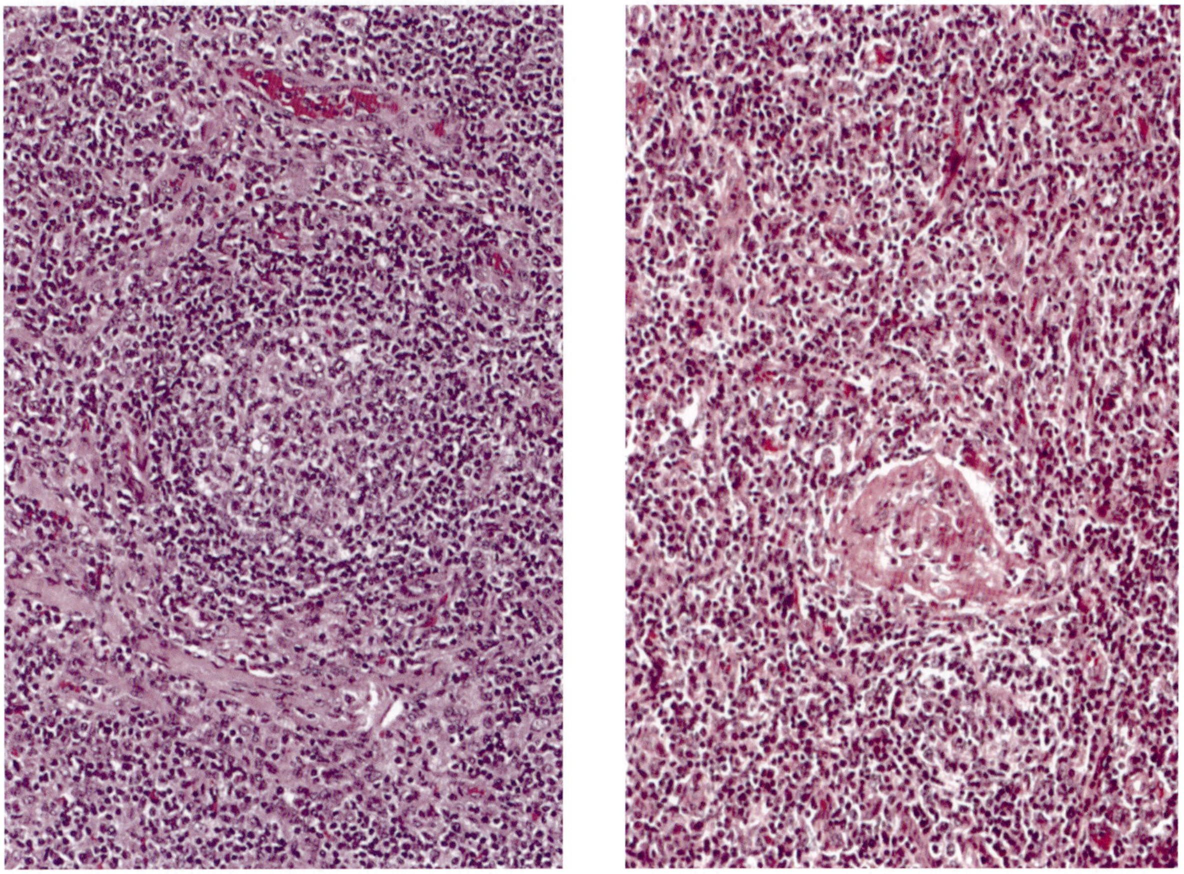

Figure 9-41

HIV/AIDS, LYMPH NODE

Vascular proliferation (left) and hyaline protein deposition (right) are seen in lymph nodes in the more advanced stages of HIV/AIDS.

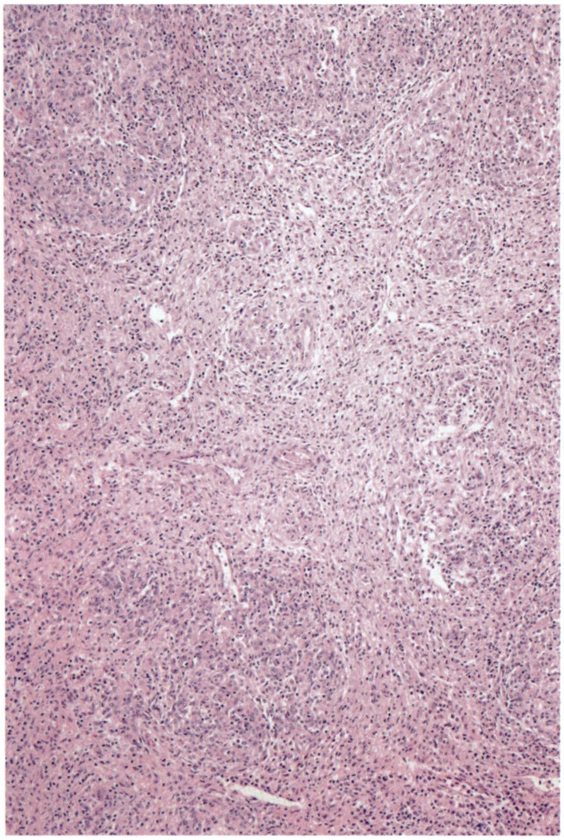

Figure 9-42

HIV/AIDS, LYMPH NODE

In the advanced stages of HIV/AIDS, there is severe lymphoid depletion. Stromal and vascular proliferations are the predominant findings in these lymphoid-depleted nodes.

(103). The medullary cords and sinuses comprise the major components, with scattered residual plasma cells and macrophages predominating. Erythrophagocytosis may be prominent at this stage (103). Studies have shown that these histologic changes represent a dynamic evolution of the disease with its progressive deleterious effect upon the body's immune system (22,58,127). These advanced changes in lymph node architecture may be reversible with the institution of HAART or other multiagent therapies (97).

Opportunistic infections, especially atypical mycobacteria, *Pneumocystis carinii*, CMV, and fungi, may totally replace the lymph nodes at this later stage of disease. The typical appearance of *Mycobacterium avium-intracellulare* (MAI) in lymph nodes is interpreted as a superimposition of sheets of foamy macrophages on the lymphoid-depleted pattern (see chapter 10).

Nador et al. (87) have reported the rare finding of polymorphic lymphoid proliferations in AIDS, resembling the findings seen in PTLD. These lymphoid proliferations are variable mixtures of lymphocytes, plasma cells, epithelioid macrophages, immunoblasts, and plasmablasts. Although most of their reported cases were clonal, some had no evidence of clonality, analogous to the "plasmacytic hyperplasia" stages of PTLD.

The two most common malignancies in AIDS, namely Kaposi sarcoma and non-Hodgkin lymphoma, usually occur at the lymphoid-depletion stage of the disease. Kaposi sarcoma is also seen in association with Castleman-like changes in the follicular involution stage. Although none of the histologic changes in HIV-related lymphadenopathy are pathognomonic for the disease, they are characteristic enough to suggest HIV as a possible etiology.

In summary, HIV-related lymphadenopathy shows a spectrum of histopathologic patterns ranging from follicular hyperplasia, to follicular involution, to eventual lymphoid depletion. At different stages, especially the lymphoid-depleted stage, the lymphadenopathy may be associated with opportunistic infections. Reports have documented the presence of HHV-6 encoded antigens by in situ immunohistochemistry in lymph node biopsies from AIDS patients (69). This virus is associated with both benign and malignant lymphadenopathies (see earlier this chapter).

Splenomegaly is common in AIDS patients (40 to 72 percent), although clinically significant splenomegaly is rare (30,80). The findings in the spleen include: white pulp depletion, amyloid-like protein deposition, perivascular hyalinization, infarcts, necrosis, hemosiderin deposition, plasma cell infiltrates, neutrophilic microabscesses, spindle cell infiltrates, extramedullary hematopoiesis, and granulomas (fig. 9-43) (30). These findings are similar in patients who are treated with HAART therapy and those who are not. The lymphoid depletion is primarily due to a reduction in the number of T cells in both the PALS and white pulp. Reductions in B cells are also seen, including small, regressed or even absent germinal centers. For patients not receiving newer, combined therapies, there

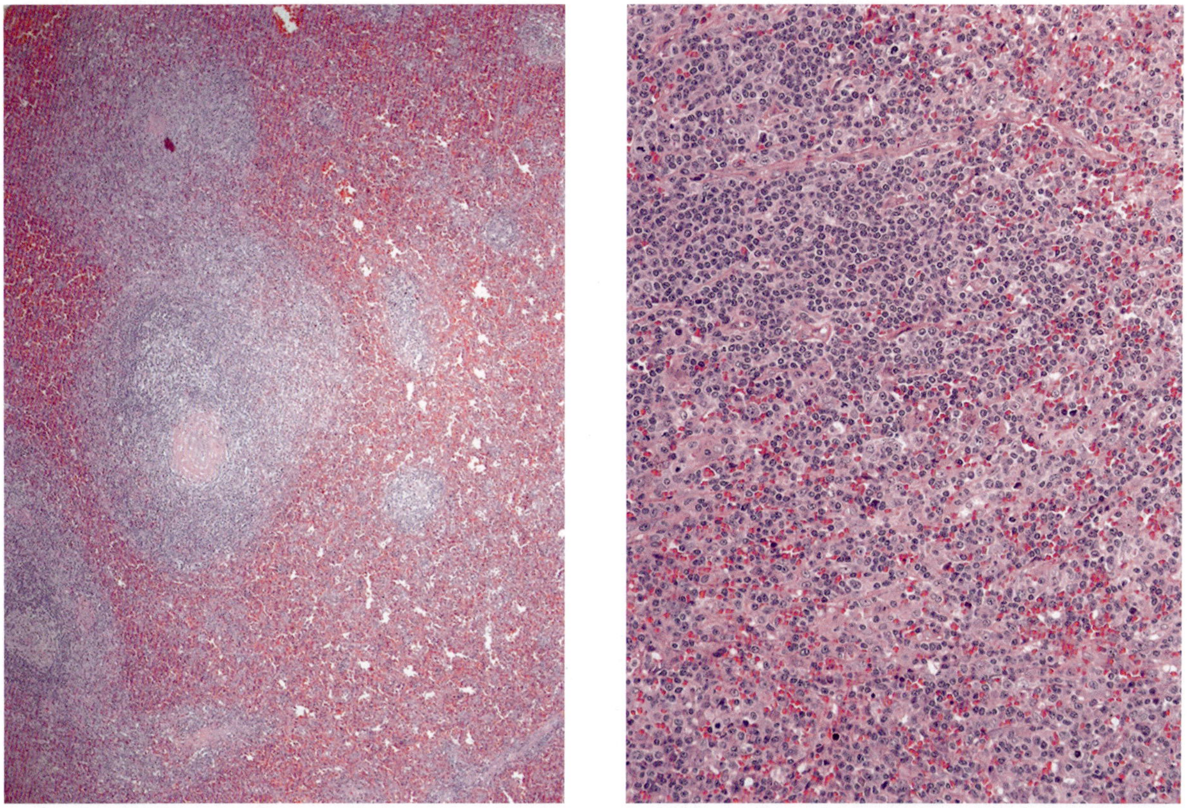

Figure 9-43

HIV/AIDS, SPLEEN

In this spleen of an AIDS patient, the white pulp is expanded by large lymphocytes, with a decrease in the size of the PALS.

is an increased frequency of splenic infection: CMV, MAI, various bacterial abscesses, and *Pneumocystis* (30,80). Neoplasms including lymphomas and Kaposi sarcoma are seen rarely in the AIDS spleen.

Another benign lymphoid lesion that is associated with AIDS is the cystic lymphoepithelial lesion of the salivary gland, particularly the parotid gland (fig. 9-44) (77). The lymph nodes of the salivary gland in HIV-positive patients may be unilaterally or bilaterally enlarged and represent a major site of infection. The histologic features, which resemble the changes that are seen in HIV-related lymph nodes in other anatomic sites, vary from florid follicular hyperplasia with follicle lysis and monocytoid B-cell hyperplasia to follicular involution or depletion. Foci of inflammation may be noted around the salivary gland ducts. Ductal squamous metaplasia and the formation of characteristic epimyoepithelial islands are commonly seen. Obliteration of the duct lumens and accumulation of keratin as a result of the newly formed squamous epithelium produces keratin-filled cystic structures. A foreign body giant cell reaction to extravasated keratin occurs in a background of acute and chronic inflammatory cells.

The differential diagnosis of HIV-related lymphoepithelial parotid gland cysts includes autoimmune processes that are associated with the formation of lymphoepithelial lesions such as Sjögren and Mikulicz syndromes. Because of the clinical and histologic similarities between the HIV-related and Sjögren syndrome salivary gland lesions, care must be taken in their evaluation (128).

Ancillary Studies. Immunohistochemical reactivity for a viral protein such as the p24 gag protein may be demonstrated in the follicles and interfollicular region (fig. 9-45). The follicular dendritic cells in HIV are highlighted by immunohistochemical staining with fascin, or the more specific markers, CD21 and CD35 (107).

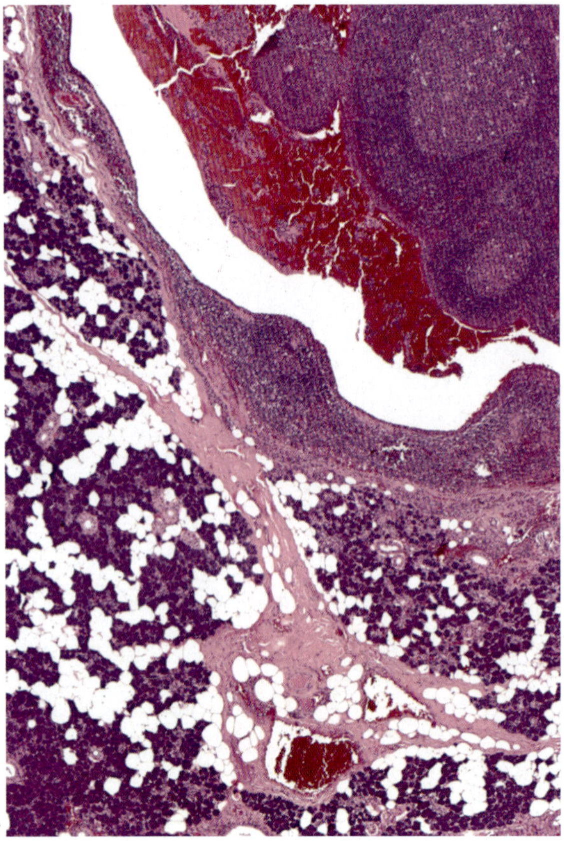

Figure 9-44

HIV/AIDS, SALIVARY GLAND

Squamous epithelial cysts with prominent lymphoid proliferations are often found in the salivary glands of HIV/AIDS patients.

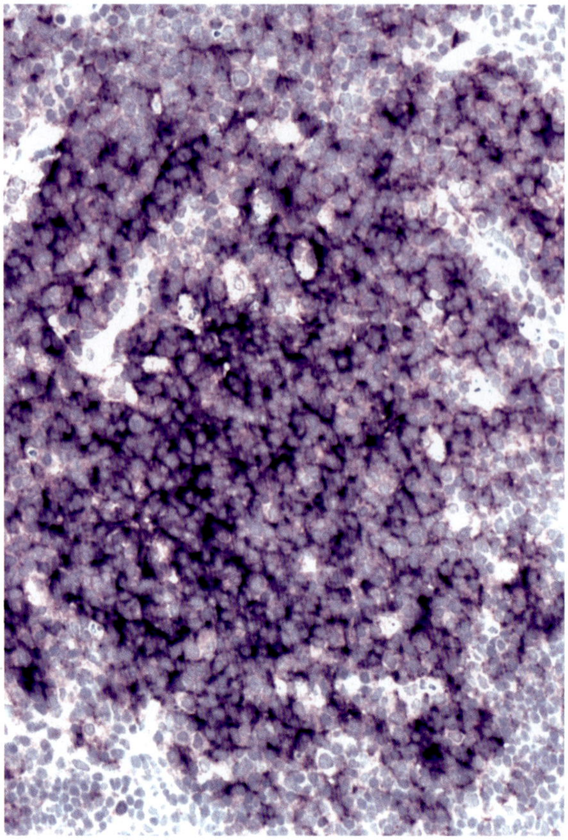

Figure 9-45

HIV/AIDS, LYMPH NODE

Immunohistochemical reactivity for p24 antigen in the AIDS virus.

Treatment and Prognosis. One of the most important new treatments for HIV infection is HAART. This therapy, which usually involves at least three antiviral drugs, including a protease inhibitor, is administered alone or with IL-2. Recently, patients receiving HAART have been reported to develop lymphadenitis due to MAI (102), referred to as HAART-associated lymphadenopathy (8). There is complete effacement of the normal nodal architecture by foamy macrophages in which MAI organisms are demonstrated. It is important to recognize this type of lymphadenopathy to ensure appropriate treatment.

ZOONOTIC VIRUSES

Definition. A wide variety of viruses are animal diseases that can be transmitted to humans, usually through insect vectors. Some of these are associated with lymphadenopathy.

General Features. The *zoonoses*, which include the arboviruses, arenaviruses, and filoviruses, typically require propagation by some arthropod vector (Table 9-4). These are mostly RNA viruses, although rare DNA arboviruses exist. The infections depend on the properties of the arthropod vector, the type of exposure humans have to the vector, and the presence of intermediate hosts (such as horses) (Table 9-5) (63,112,113). Incidence is highly variable depending on the virus involved, the geographic distribution of the virus, and other factors mentioned previously. The clinical syndromes vary widely and descriptions are best left to specialized texts (63,112,113). Laboratory diagnosis usually depends on serologic identification of the viral organism.

Table 9-4

PARTIAL LIST OF ZOONOTIC VIRUSES[a]

Filoviruses (African hemorrhagic fevers)
Marburg
Ebola
Arenaviruses
Lymphocytic choriomeningitis
Argentinean hemorrhagic fever
Bolivian hemorrhagic fever
Venezuelan hemorrhagic fever
Lassa fever
Arboviruses
Yellow fever
West Nile
Eastern equine encephalitis
Western equine encephalomyelitis
St. Louis encephalitis
California encephalitis
Colorado tick fever
Dengue
Rift valley fever
Japanese encephalitis
Murray Valley encephalitis
Chikungunya/O'Nyong nyong
Tick-borne encephalitis
Kyasanur Forest disease/Powassan
Crimean-Congo hemorrhagic fever
Venezuelan equine encephalitis

[a]Data from references 64, 112, and 113.

Table 9-5

PATTERN OF HOST RESPONSE IN ARBOVIRAL INFECTIONS IN MAN[a]

Asymptomatic infection	WEE[b], SLE, CE
Mild febrile illness	WEE, SLE, CE, yellow fever
Influenza-like illness with aching and joint pains	Dengue, chikungunya
Encephalitis, mild	CE, WEE, SLE
Encephalitis, severe	SLE, EEE, WEE, CE, tick-borne encephalitis
Jaundice, proteinuria	Yellow fever
Rash (+/- hemorrhagic manifestations)	Dengue
Shock syndrome	Dengue

[a]Data from reference 112.
[b]WEE = Western equine encephalomyelitis; SLE = St. Louis encephalitis; CE = California encephalitis; EEE = Eastern equine encephalomyelitis.

Microscopic Findings. The hemorrhagic fevers, particularly the African types, are associated with necrosis of lymphoid elements and hypertrophy of macrophages and vascular elements in lymph nodes and spleen (47,112).

PARVOVIRUS B19

Definition. *Parvovirus B19* is occasionally associated with lymphadenopathy or splenomegaly. It is more commonly associated with red cell aplasia.

General Features. Parvovirus B19 is a small DNA virus that is typically associated with a self-limited viral infection, *erythema infectiosum*, also known as *fifth disease* or *slapped cheek disease*. The virus infects a variety of cells types, but especially affects red blood cell precursors (17).

Clinical Features. The common viral illness associated with parvovirus is characterized by fever, coryza, headache, and mild gastrointestinal symptoms. The classic "slapped cheek" rash follows after a period of a few days. Congenital infection may lead to hydrops fetalis. Other systems affected by parvoviral infection include neurologic, arthritic, vasculitic, and cardiac (17, 98,105).

In hematopathology, parvovirus is known classically as the causative agent of pure red cell aplasia in susceptible individuals. The virus is particularly tropic for red blood cell precursors. In individuals with a shortened red blood cell life span, viral infection can cause a precipitous drop in hemoglobin. Chronic hematologic infections by parvovirus B19 also occur in immunosuppressed patients, leading to significant cytopenias.

There have been suggestions that parvoviral infection is associated with Kawasaki disease (see chapter 6), but these findings have not been validated by other studies. Other studies have suggested that parvovirus infection is associated with Kikuchi disease (64,83)

Laboratory Findings. Atypical lymphocytosis, similar to that seen in infectious mononucleosis and other viral infections, is seen in the acute phase of parvoviral infection. Serologic studies are a mainstay of diagnosis.

Microscopic Findings. Two distinct patterns of adenopathy are associated with parvoviral infection. The first is characterized by follicular hyperplasia with reactive germinal centers, paracortical expansion, increased vasculature, and expanded sinuses with neutrophils (105). No necrosis is seen.

The second pattern is that of necrotizing lymphadenitis, comparable to that seen in Kikuchi disease (see chapter 6). These cases have been reported

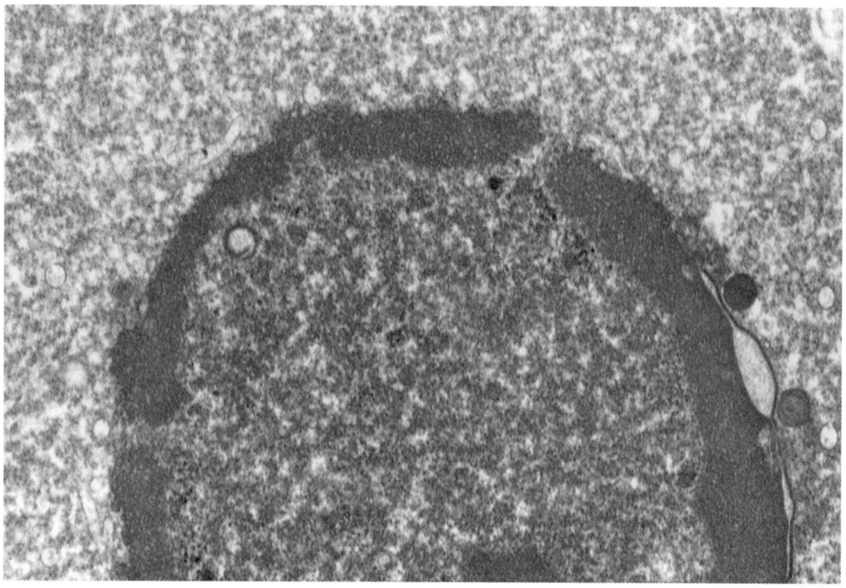

Figure 9-46

PARVOVIRUS B19, TRANSMISSION ELECTRON MICROSCOPY

Parvoviral inclusions are seen in the nucleus and cytoplasm of this cell. (Courtesy of Gary Mierau, Denver, CO.)

in patients with known systemic lupus erythematosus as well as healthy individuals (64,83,105). As mentioned previously, some feel that this represents Kikuchi disease, and that the parvovirus infection may be responsible. Further research is necessary to clarify this proposal.

Ancillary Studies. Immunohistochemical staining for parvovirus is available; however, no reports exist of positivity in lymph nodes or spleen, possibly due to the paucity of reported cases. The presence of virus is confirmed by PCR analysis and electron microscopy of affected tissues (fig. 9-46) (98,105).

SMALLPOX (VARIOLA VIRUS), COWPOX, MONKEYPOX

Definition. *Smallpox* is a highly contagious virus, typically associated with respiratory or cutaneous infection. Lymph nodes draining sites of infection may be enlarged.

General Features. Smallpox is caused by the *variola virus* (*Poxvirus variolae*); infection with variola major results in a high mortality rate, while variola minor, or alastrim, causes a milder form of disease (12,47). A closely related virus is the causative agent of *cowpox* (*Poxvirus bovis*). The *vaccinia virus* (*Poxvirus officinale*) is similar enough to the causative agent of smallpox to be used as a vaccination. Infection with vaccinia virus is covered in the section on postvaccinial lymphadenitis. *Monkeypox* is closely related to smallpox and has similar clinical findings with the exception of pronounced lymphadenopathy (12).

Clinical Features. Smallpox infection from a respiratory source is usually associated with fever, headache, vomiting, and low back pain, followed by skin lesions (47). Cutaneous lesions are typically the most easily acquired sample and show ballooning degeneration of epidermal cells and viral inclusions (Guarnieri bodies). Monkeypox is associated with lymphadenopathy in many cases, and may be the result of contact with prairie dogs or Gambian giant rats (which are kept as pets) (20).

Microscopic Findings. Regional lymph node involvement in smallpox is usually in sites draining skin lesions or other sites of infection. The lymph nodes show areas of necrosis, with or without suppuration. Rarely, intracellular viral inclusions similar to the Guarnieri bodies of skin lesions are seen within macrophages or within necrotic foci (122). Immunohistochemical stains and direct fluorescent antibodies are available for diagnosis (47,110).

SEVERE ACUTE RESPIRATORY SYNDROME

Definition. *Severe acute respiratory syndrome* (SARS) is a recently described syndrome associated with severe viral pneumonia. Lymphadenopathy and splenic changes are rarely seen.

Clinical Features. SARS was originally described after outbreaks in 2003 affected several thousand people in China, Taiwan, Hong Kong,

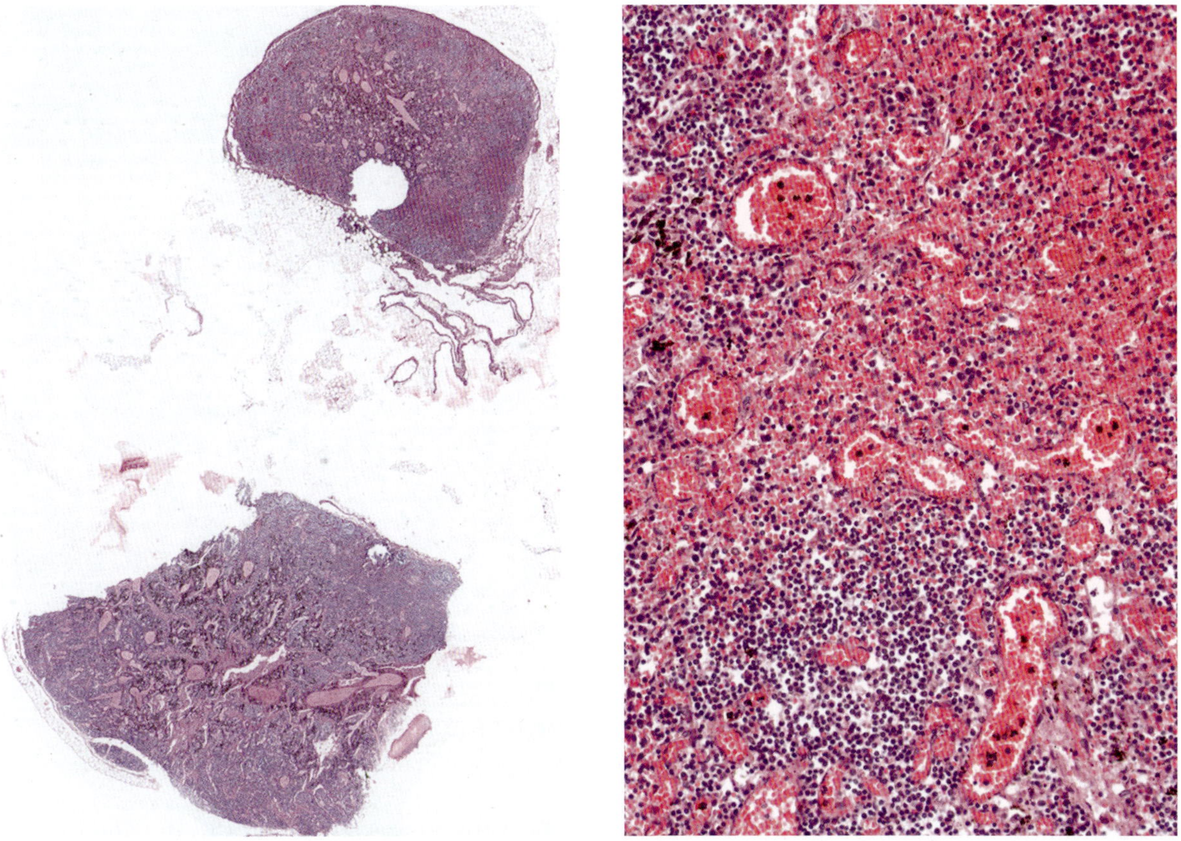

Figure 9-47

SEVERE ADULT RESPIRATORY DISTRESS SYNDROME (SARS)

Left: Lymph nodes from patient affected with SARS.
Right: Higher magnification reveals nonspecific hemorrhage and anthracotic pigment. (Courtesy of Ting Li, Beijing, China.)

Singapore, and Canada (73,74). The organism has been isolated and identified as a newly recognized coronavirus. SARS has an approximately 10 percent fatality rate. The majority of pathologic findings are in the lungs, including exudative and hemorrhagic pneumonia.

Distinctive laboratory findings include leucopenia (neutropenia and lymphopenia) and thrombocytopenia (73,74).

Microscopic Findings. Lymph node abnormalities are most likely seen in the hilar region. Lymphocyte depletion is the most common finding (fig. 9-47) (57,73,74). There are decreases in the cortical regions, and germinal centers are not seen. Expansion of sinuses with sinus histiocytosis is seen, particularly in the subcapsular area. Macrophages may contain small lipid vacuoles. Vascular proliferation may be seen. Splenic changes include depletion of lymphocytes in germinal centers, PALS, and the red pulp. There may be focal hemorrhage in both lymph nodes and spleen.

POLIOVIRUS

Definition. *Poliovirus* is a rare infection that is associated with lymphadenopathy. The histologic findings are nonspecific.

General Features. Poliovirus is a member of the group of enteroviruses. It is a type of RNA virus. As a group, enteroviruses cause a wide variety of diseases in man. Poliovirus exposure is usually oral. The virus first multiplies in the tonsils, then lymph nodes of the neck, and then spreads to other sites. Invasion of nerves follows, with subsequent symptoms.

There are four types of infection: inapparent infection without symptoms, mild viral type illness, aseptic meningitis, and paralytic poliomyelitis

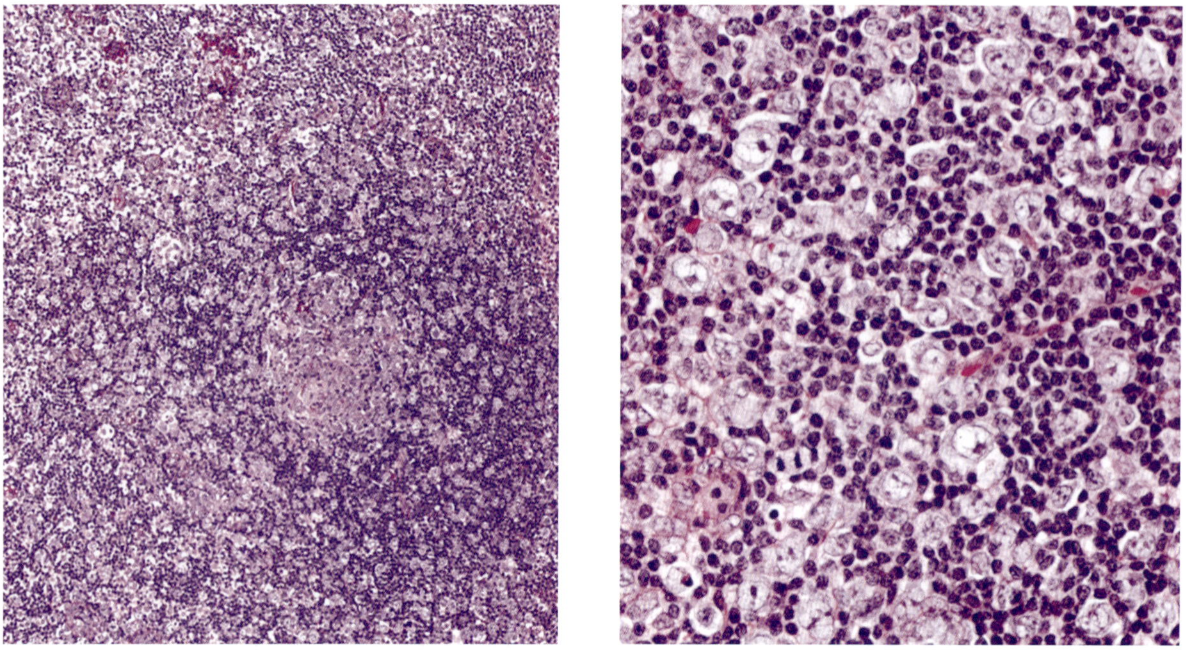

Figure 9-48

POSTVACCINIAL LYMPHADENITIS

Paracortical mottling and proliferation of immunoblasts are present in this postvaccination lymph node.

(82). The most well-known presentation of poliomyelitis affects the central nervous system. It results in the destruction of motor neurons of the spinal cord leading to paralysis. Poliovirus is rare since the advent of vaccination.

Microscopic Findings. Lymph nodes show nonspecific microscopic features consisting of vascular congestion, follicular hyperplasia, and increased neutrophils in sinuses (122). Multinucleated cells, presumably virally infected, are possibly derived from dendritic cells.

POSTVACCINIAL LYMPHADENITIS

Definition. Reactive changes in local lymph nodes, typically in the paracortical regions, are seen after the administration of a variety of vaccines, especially smallpox vaccine.

General Features. The changes seen in postvaccinial adenopathy are a natural consequence of the immune process associated with the vaccine administration. The administered viral antigen is transported to the lymph node by antigen presenting/processing cells. At this point the viral antigens activate the complex T- and B-cell response, resulting in the characteristic early histologic appearance. Development of the antibody response leads to the appearance of the later histologic stages

Clinical Features. The reactive changes of postvaccinial lymphadenitis occur 1 to 3 weeks after the smallpox vaccination (or in response to other vaccines). The involved lymph nodes typically drain the vaccination site (axillary, supraclavicular, or cervical). They are usually tender. Postvaccinial lymphadenitis was previously considered to be a relatively rare cause of nodal enlargement, associated with the administration of a variety of vaccines, including MMR (measles, mumps, rubella) and other attenuated virus vaccines. Now, with the reinstitution of vaccination for smallpox, it is likely that this will become a more prevalent cause of lymphadenitis. Postvaccinial lymphadenopathy is a common side effect. Historical information is critical in this diagnosis.

Microscopic Findings. The most characteristic, early histopathologic change is diffuse paracortical hyperplasia with mottling of the paracortex, imparting a "moth-eaten" appearance (figs. 9-48, 9-49). The germinal centers are usually small or inconspicuous at this stage, and may appear as inactive primary follicles. A follicular or a mixed

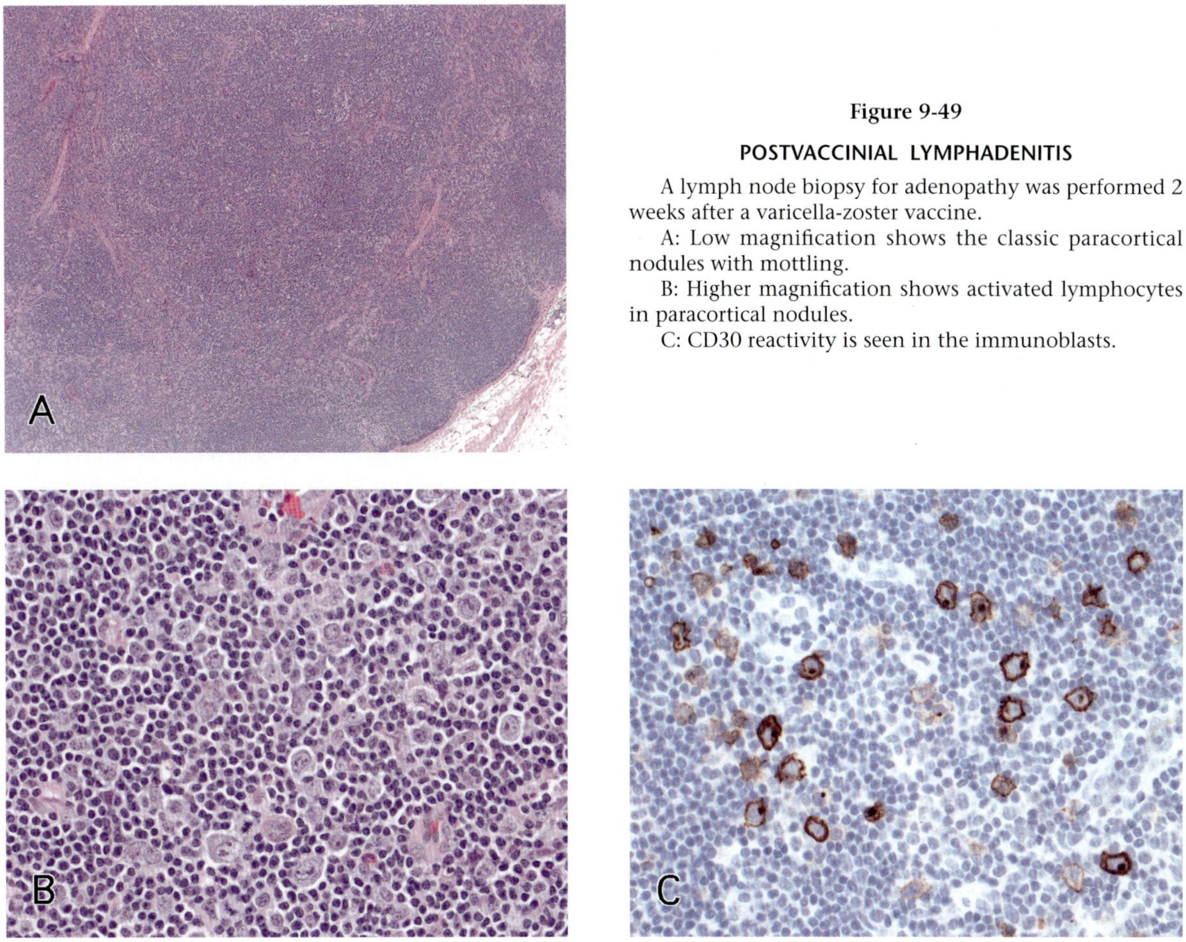

Figure 9-49

POSTVACCINIAL LYMPHADENITIS

A lymph node biopsy for adenopathy was performed 2 weeks after a varicella-zoster vaccine.

A: Low magnification shows the classic paracortical nodules with mottling.

B: Higher magnification shows activated lymphocytes in paracortical nodules.

C: CD30 reactivity is seen in the immunoblasts.

pattern of hyperplasia, with varying numbers of plasma cells, eosinophils, and mast cells, may be seen in a later biopsy (50). In the weeks after the immunization, there is an increase in plasma cells, signaling the development of an immune response to the vaccine. Lymph nodes biopsied after measles vaccination appear very similar but have increased numbers of plasma cells and Warthin-Finkeldey type giant cells

Ancillary Studies. No ancillary studies are required. In some cases, it is possible to identify viral reactivity by immunohistochemical stains or in situ hybridization for the administered virus.

Differential Diagnosis. Because of its morphologic features, postvaccinial lymphadenitis may be confused with lymphoma, particularly large cell lymphomas of B- or T-cell type. Other entities in the differential diagnosis are: interfollicular Hodgkin lymphoma, early involvement of lymph node by lymphoma, and acute EBV infection/infectious mononucleosis. Rare pathogens that are associated with this pattern of hyperplasia include cowpox, poliovirus, *Rickettsia*, and *Ehrlichia*.

Although postvaccinial lymphadenitis may suggest malignant lymphoma, lymph node biopsies are generally not performed if there is a suspicion of a viral etiology since the histopathologic changes may closely simulate a malignant process and could lead to an erroneous diagnosis if all of the clinical information is not known.

Treatment and Prognosis. No specific treatment is required. The adenopathy typically slowly resolves over several weeks or months. If revaccination is necessary, adenopathy may recur.

REFERENCES

1. Abbondanzo SL, Irey NS, Frizzera G. Dilantin-associated lymphadenopathy. Spectrum of histopathologic patterns. Am J Surg Pathol 1995;19:675-86.
2. Abbondanzo SL, Sato N, Straus SE, Jaffe ES. Acute infectious mononucleosis: CD30 (Ki-1) antigen expression and histologic correlations. Am J Clin Pathol 1990;93:698-702.
3. Akashi K, Eizuru Y, Sumiyoshi Y, et al. Brief report: severe infectious mononucleosis-like syndrome and primary human herpesvirus 6 infection in an adult. N Engl J Med 1993;329:168-71.
4. Allen MS Jr, Talbot WH, McDonald RM. Atypical lymph-node hyperplasia after administration of attenuated, live measles vaccine. N Engl J Med 1966;274:677-8.
5. Alos L, Navarrete P, Morente V, et al. Immunoarchitecture of lymphoid tissue in HIV-infection during antiretroviral therapy correlates with viral persistence. Mod Pathol 2005;18:127-36.
6. Arber DA, Shibata D, Chen YY, Weiss LM. Characterization of the topography of Epstein-Barr virus infection in human immunodeficiency virus-associated lymphoid tissues. Mod Pathol 1992;5:559-66.
7. Asgari MM, Begos DG. Spontaneous splenic rupture in infectious mononucleosis: a review. Yale J Biol Med 1997;70:175-82.
8. Ball SC, Chadburn A. HAART-associated lymphadenopathy. AIDS Read 1999;9:11-27.
9. Banks PM, Warnke RA. Primary effusion lymphoma. In: Jaffe ES, ed. World Health Organization Classification of Tumours. Pathology and genetics. Tumours of haematopoietic and lymphoid tissues. Lyon: IARC Press; 2001:179-80.
10. Baroni CD, Uccini S. Lymph nodes in HIV-positive drug abusers with persistent generalized lymphadenopathy: histology, immunohistochemistry, and pathogenetic correlations. Prog AIDS Pathol 1990;2:33-50.
11. Barre-Sinoussi F, Chermann JC, Rey F, et al. Isolation of a T-lymphotropic retrovirus from a patient at risk for acquired immune deficiency syndrome (AIDS). Science 1983;220:868-71.
12. Beneson AS. Smallpox: "The end of the story"? In: Evans AS, Kaslow RA, eds. Viral infections of humans: epidemiology and control, 4th ed. New York: Plenum Medical Book Co.; 1997:861-3.
13. Betts RF. Syndromes of cytomegalovirus infection. Adv Intern Med 1980;26:447-66.
14. Black FL. Measles. In: Evans AS, Kaslow RA, eds. Viral infections of humans: epidemiology and control, 4th ed. New York: Plenum Medical Book Co.; 1997:507-29.
15. Borisch B, Ellinger K, Neipel F, et al. Lymphadenitis and lymphoproliferative lesions associated with the human herpes virus-6 (HHV-6). Virchows Arch B Cell Pathol Incl Mol Pathol 1991;61:179-87.
16. Braun DK, Pellett PE, Hanson CA. Presence and expression of human herpesvirus 6 in peripheral blood mononuclear cells of S100-positive, T cell chronic lymphoproliferative disease. J Infect Dis 1995;171:1351-5.
17. Brown KE, Young NS. Parvovirus B19 infection. In: Evans AS, Kaslow RA, eds. Viral infections of humans: epidemiology and control, 4th ed. New York: Plenum Medical Book Co.; 1997;865-92.
18. Burns BF, Wood GS, Dorfman RF. The varied histopathology of lymphadenopathy in the homosexual male. Am J Surg Pathol 1985;9:287-97.
19. Centers for Disease Control (CDC). Kaposi's sarcoma and Pneumocystis pneumonia among homosexual men—New York City and California. MMWR Morb Mortal Wkly Rep 1981;30:305-8.
20. Centers for Disease Control (CDC). Multistate outbreak of monkeypox—Illinois, Indiana and Wisconsin. 2003. MMWR Morb Mortal Wkly Rep 2003;52:537-40.
21. Centers for Disease Control (CDC). Pneumocystis pneumonia—Los Angeles. MMWR Morb Mortal Wkly Rep 1981;30:250-2.
22. Chadburn A, Metroka C, Mouradian J. Progressive lymph node histology and its prognostic value in patients with acquired immunodeficiency syndrome and AIDS-related complex. Hum Pathol 1989;20:579-87.
23. Chan JK, Lewin KJ, Lombard CM, Teitelbaum S, Dorfman RF. Histopathology of bacillary angiomatosis of lymph node. Am J Surg Pathol 1991;15:430-7.
24. Childs CC, Parham DM, Berard CW. Infectious mononucleosis. The spectrum of morphologic changes simulating lymphoma in lymph nodes and tonsils. Am J Surg Pathol 1987;11:122-32.
25. Choquet S, Leblond V, Herbrecht R, et al. Efficacy and safety of rituximab in B-cell post-transplant lymphoproliferative disorders: results of a prospective multicentre phase 2 study. Blood 2006;107:3053-7.
26. Clark DA, Griffiths PD. Human herpesvirus 6: relevance of infection in the immunocompromised host. Br J Haematol 2003;120:384-95.
27. Coffey AJ, Brooksbank RA, Brandau O, et al. Host response to EBV infection in X-linked lymphoproliferative disease results from mutations in an SH2-domain encoding gene. Nat Genet 1998;20:129-35.

28. Coupland SE, Charlotte F, Mansour G, Maloum K, Hummel M, Stein H. HHV-8-associated T-cell lymphoma in a lymph node with concurrent peritoneal effusion in an HIV-positive man. Am J Surg Pathol 2005;29:647-52.
29. Custer RP, Smith EB. The pathology of infectious mononucleosis. Blood 1948;3:830-57.
30. Diaz LK, Murphy RL, Phair JP, Variakojis D. The AIDS autopsy spleen: a comparison of the pre-anti-retroviral and highly active anti-retroviral therapy eras. Mod Pathol 2002;15:406-12.
31. Dorfman RF, Herweg JC. Live attenuated measles virus vaccine. Inguinal lymphadenopathy complicating administration. JAMA 1966;198:320-1.
32. Dorfman RF, Remington JS. Value of lymph node biopsy in the diagnosis of acute acquired toxoplasmosis. N Engl J Med 1973;289:878-81.
33. Dorfman RF, Warnke R. Lymphadenopathy simulating the malignant lymphomas. Hum Pathol 1974;5:519-50.
34. Du MQ, Diss TC, Liu H, et al. KSHV- and EBV-associated germinotropic lymphoproliferative disorder. Blood 2002;100:3415-8.
35. Eizuru Y, Minematsu T, Minamishima Y, et al. Rapid diagnosis of cytomegalovirus infections by direct immunoperoxidase staining with human monoclonal antibody against an immediate-early antigen. Microbiol Immunol 1991;35:1015-22.
36. Epstein MA, Achong BG. Pathogenesis of infectious mononucleosis. Lancet 1977;2:1270-3.
37. Ewing EP Jr, Chandler FW, Spira TJ, Brynes RK, Chan WC. Primary lymph node pathology in AIDS and AIDS-related lymphadenopathy. Arch Pathol Lab Med 1985; 109:977-81.
38. Frizzera G. Atypical lymphoproliferative disorders. In: Neoplastic hematopathology, 2nd ed. Knowles DM, ed. Philadelphia: Lippincott Williams & Wilkins; 2001:569-622.
39. Frizzera G. The clinico-pathological expressions of Epstein-Barr virus infection in lymphoid tissues. Virchows Arch B Cell Pathol Incl Mol Pathol 1987;53:1-12.
40. Gaffey MJ, Ben-Ezra JM, Weiss LM. Herpes simplex lymphadenitis. Am J Clin Pathol 1991;95:709-14.
41. Ganne V, Siddiqi N, Kamaplath B, et al. Humanized anti-CD20 monoclonal antibody (Rituximab) treatment for post-transplant lymphoproliferative disorder. Clin Transplant 2003;17:417-22.
42. Gershon AA, Gold E, Nankervis GA. Cytomegalovirus. In: Evans AS, Kaslow RA, eds. Viral infections of humans: epidemiology and control, 4th ed. New York: Plenum Medical Book Co.; 1997:229-51.
43. Gerstoft J, Pallesen G, Mathiesen L, et al. Stages in LAV/HTLV-III lymphadenitis II: correlation with clinical and immunological findings. Scand J Immunol 1987;25:93-9.
44. Gottlieb MS, Schroff R, Schanker HM, et al. Pneumocystis carinii pneumonia and mucosal candidiasis in previously healthy homosexual men: evidence of a new acquired cellular immunodeficiency. N Engl J Med 1981;305:1425-31.
45. Gowing NF. Infectious mononucleosis: histopathologic aspects. Pathol Annu 1975;10:1-20.
46. Greiner T, Armitage JO, Gross TG. Atypical lymphoproliferative diseases. Hematology (Am Soc Hematol Educ Program) 2000:133-46.
47. Guarner J, Zaki SR. Histopathology and immunohistochemistry in the diagnosis of bioterrorism agents. J Histochem Cytochem 2006;54:3-11.
48. Han XY, Lin P, Amin HM, Ferrajoli A. Post-splenectomy cytomegaloviral mononucleosis: marked lymphocytosis, TCRgamma gene rearrangements, and impaired IgM response. Am J Clin Pathol 2005;123:612-7.
49. Harris NL, Swerdlow SH, Frizzera G, Knowles DM. Post-transplant lymphoproliferative disorders. In: World Health Organization Classification of Tumours. Pathology and genetics. Tumours of haematopoietic and lymphoid tissues. Lyon: IARC Press; 2001:264-71.
50. Hartsock RJ. Postvaccinial lymphadenitis: hyperplasia of lymphoid tissue that simulates malignant lymphomas. Cancer 1968;21:632-49.
51. Hauptmann S, Meru N, Schewe C, et al. Fatal atypical T-cell proliferation assciociated with Epstein-Barr virus infection. Br J Haematol 2001; 112:377-80.
52. Henle W, Henle GE, Horwitz CA. Epstein-Barr virus specific diagnostic tests in infectious mononucleosis. Hum Pathol 1974;5:551-65.
53. Higgins JP, Warnke RA. Herpes lymphadenitis in association with chronic lymphocytic leukemia. Cancer 1999;86:1210-5.
54. Higgins PM. Splenomegaly in acute infections due to group A streptococci and viruses. Epidemiol Infect 1992;109:199-209.
55. Holmes SJ, Orenstein WA. Rubella. In: Viral infections of humans: epidemiology and control, 4th ed. Evans AS, Kaslow RA, eds. New York: Plenum Medical Book Co; 1997:839-60.
56. Howat AJ, Campbell AR, Stewart DJ. Genralized lymphadenopathy due to herpes simplex virus type I. Histopathology 1991;19:563-4.
57. Hsiao CH, Wu MZ, Hsieh SW, Chien LC, Hwang KC, Su IJ. Clinicopathology of severe acute respiratory syndrome: an autopsy case report. J Formos Med Assoc 2004;103:787-92.

58. Ioachim HL, Cronin W, Roy M, Maya M. Persistent lymphadenopathies in people at high risk for HIV infection: clinicopathologic correlations and long-term follow-up in 79 cases. Am J Clin Pathol 1990;93:208-18.
59. Ioachim HL, Lerner CW, Tapper ML. The lymphoid lesions associated with the acquired immunodeficiency syndrome. Am J Surg Pathol 1983;7:543-53.
60. Ioachim HL, Ratech H. Cytomegalovirus lymphadenitis. In: Ioachim HL, Ratech H, eds. Ioachim's lymph node pathology, 3rd ed. J.B. Philadelphia: Lippincott Williams & Wilkins; 2002:79-82.
61. Ioachim HL, Ratech H. Herpes simplex virus lymphadenitis. In: Ioachim HL, Ratech H, eds. Ioachim's lymph node pathology, 3rd ed. J.B. Philadelphia: Lippincott Williams & Wilkins; 2002;83-6.
62. Ioachim HL, Ratech H. Varicella-herpes zoster lymphadenitis. In: Ioachim HL, Ratech H, eds. Ioachim's lymph node pathology, 3rd ed. Philadelphia: Lippincott Williams & Wilkins; 2002:87-9.
63. Jahrling PB. Arenaviruses. In: Evans AS, Kaslow RA, eds. Viral infections of humans: epidemiology and control, 4th ed. New York: Plenum Medical Book Co; 1997:185-209.
64. Johnson LB, Pasumarthy A, Saravolatz LD. Parvovirus B19 infection presenting with necrotizing lymphadenitis. Am J Med 2003;114:340-1.
65. Joseph L, Scott MA, Schichman SA, Zent CS. Localized herpes simplex lymphadenitis mimicking large-cell (Richter's) transformation of chronic lymphocytic leukemia/small lymphocytic lymphoma. Am J Hematol 2001;68:287-91.
66. Kapadia SB, Wiley CA, Soontornniyomkij V, Wang G, Swerdlow SH. HIV-associated Waldeyer's ring lymphoid hyperplasias: characterization of multinucleated giant cells and the role of Epstein-Barr virus. Hum Pathol 1999;30:1383-8.
67. Karadeniz C, Oguz A, Ezer U, Ozturk G, Dursun A. The etiology of peripheral lymphadenopathy in children. Pediatr Hematol Oncol 1999;16:525-31.
68. Kasahara M, Mizoguchi Y, Kuroda M, et al. Adult-type systemic varicella in a female patient in course of treatment of her so-called reactive lymphocytic (T-cell) hyperplasia. Acta Pathol Jpn 1984;34:169-89.
69. Knox KK, Carrigan DR. Active HHV-6 infection in the lymph nodes of HIV-infected patients: in vitro evidence that HHV-6 can break HIV latency. J Acquir Immune Defic Syndr Hum Retrovirol 1996;11:370-8.
70. Kojima M, Nakamura S, Sugihara S, Sakata N, Masawa N. Lymph node infarction associated with infectious mononucleosis: report of a case resembling lymph node infarction associated with malignant lymphoma. Int J Surg Pathol 2002;10:223-6.
71. Krishnan J, Danon AD, Frizzera G. Reactive lymphadenopathies and atypical lymphoproliferative disorders. Am J Clin Pathol 1993;99:385-96.
72. Landing BH, Yutuc IL, Swanson VL. Infantile lymphoreticular tissue: effects of perinatal infections and infantile malnutrition. Perspect Pediatr Pathol 1979;5:63-92.
73. Lang Z, Zhang L, Zhang S, et al. Pathological study on severe acute respiratory syndrome. Chin Med J (Engl) 2003;116:976-80.
74. Lang ZW, Zhang LJ, Zhang SJ, et al. A clinicopathological study of three cases of severe acute respiratory syndrome (SARS). Pathology 2003;35:526-31.
75. Lazzi S, Bellan C, Amato T, et al. Kaposi's sarcoma-associated herpesvirus/human herpesvirus 8 infection in reactive lymphoid tissues: a model for KSHV/HHV-8-related lymphomas? Hum Pathol 2006;37:23-31.
76. Luppi M, Barozzi P, Garber R, et al. Expression of human herpesvirus-6 antigens in benign and malignant lymphoproliferative diseases. Am J Pathol 1998;153:815-23.
77. Maiorano E, Favia G, Viale G. Lymphoepithelial cysts of salivary glands: an immunohistochemical study of HIV-related and HIV-unrelated lesions. Hum Pathol 1998;29:260-5.
78. Malnati MS, Dagna L, Ponzoni M, Lusso P. Human herpesvirus 8 (HHV-8/KSHV) and hematologic malignancies. Rev Clin Exp Hematol 2003;7:375-405.
79. Maric I, Bryant R, Abu-Asab M, et al. Human herpesvirus-6-associated acute lymphadenitis in immunocompetent adults. Mod Pathol 2004;17:1427-33.
80. Mathew A, Raviglione MC, Niranjan U, Sabatini MT, Distenfeld A. Splenectomy in patients with AIDS. Am J Hematol 1989;32:184-9.
81. McMahon NJ, Gordon HW, Rosen RB. Reed-Sternberg cells in infectious mononucleosis. Am J Dis Child 1970;120:148-50.
82. Melnick JL. Poliovirus and other enteroviruses. In: Viral infections of humans: epidemiology and control, 4th ed. Evans AS, Kaslow RA, eds. New York: Plenum Medical Book; 1997:583-663.
83. Meyer O, Kahn MF, Grossin M, et al. Parvovirus B19 infection can induce histiocyte necrotizing lymphadenitis (Kikuchi's disease) associated with systemic lupus erythematosus. Lupus 1991;1:37-41.
84. Mikala G, Xie J, Berencsi G, et al. Human herpesvirus 8 in hematologic diseases. Pathol Oncol Res 1999;5:73-9.

85. Miliauskas JR, Leong AS. Localized herpes simplex lymphadenitis: report of three cases and review of the literature. Histopathology 1991;19:355-60.
86. Myerson D, Hackman RC, Nelson JA, Ward DC, McDougall JK. Widespread presence of histologically occult cytomegalovirus. Hum Pathol 1984;15:430-9.
87. Nador RG, Chadburn A, Gundappa G, Cesarman E, Said JW, Knowles DM. Human immunodeficiency virus (HIV)-associated polymorphic lymphoproliferative disorders. Am J Surg Pathol 2003;27:293-302.
88. Nakagawa A, Ito M, Saga S. Fatal cytotoxic T-cell proliferation in chronic active Epstein-Barr virus infection in childhood. Am J Clin Pathol 2002;117:283-90.
89. Neiman R, Orazi A. Reactive lymphoid hyperplasia. In: Neiman R, Orazi, eds. Disorders of the spleen, 2nd ed. Major problems in pathology. Philadelphia: W.B. Saunders; 1999:67-84.
90. Niedobitek G, Agathanggelou A, Herbst H, Whitehead L, Wright DH, Young LS. Epstein-Barr virus (EBV) infection in infectious mononucleosis: virus latency, replication and phenotype of EBV-infected cells. J Pathol 1997;182:151-9.
91. Niedobitek G, Hamilton-Dutoit S, Herbst H, et al. Identification of Epstein-Barr virus-infected cells in tonsils of acute infectious mononucleosis by in situ hybridization. Hum Pathol 1989;20:796-9.
92. Nishida T, Ku Y, Saitoh Y. Spontaneous splenic rupture during the course of a rubella infection: report of a case. Surg Today 1995;25:83-5.
93. Ohshima K, Suzumiya J, Kanda M, Kato A, Kikuchi M. Integrated and episomal forms of Epstein-Barr virus (EBV) in EBV associated disease. Cancer Lett 1998;122:43-50.
94. Okano M, Matsumoto S, Osato T, Sakiyama Y, Thiele GM, Purtilo DT. Severe chronic active Epstein-Barr virus infection syndrome. Clin Microbiol Rev 1991;4:129-35.
95. O'Murchadha MT, Wolf BC, Neiman RS. The histologic features of hyperplastic lymphadenopathy in AIDS-related complex are nonspecific. Am J Surg Pathol 1987;11:94-9.
96. Orazi A, O'Malley DP. Pathology of the spleen. In: Jaffe ES, Vardiman J, Harris NL, eds. Disorders of lymph nodes and spleen. 2008 (in press).
97. Orenstein JM, Feinberg M, Yoder C, et al. Lymph node architecture preceding and following 6 months of potent antiviral therapy: follicular hyperplasia persists in parallel with p24 antigen restoration after involution and CD4 cell depletion in an AIDS patient. AIDS 1999;13:2219-29.
98. Papadogiannakis N, Tolfvenstam T, Fischler B, Norbeck O, Broliden K. Active, fulminant, lethal myocarditis associated with parvovirus B19 infection in an infant. Clin Infect Dis 2002;35:1027-31.
99. Patterson SD, Larson EB, Corey L. Atypical generalized zoster with lymphadenitis mimicking lymphoma. N Engl J Med 1980;302:848-51.
100. Purtilo DT, Yang JP, Allegra S, et al. Hematopathology and pathogenesis of the X-linked recessive lymphoproliferative syndrome. Am J Med 1977;62:225-33.
101. Quintanilla-Martinez L, Kumar S, Fend F, et al. Fulminant EBV(+) T-cell lymphoproliferative disorder following acute/chronic EBV infection: a distinct clinicopathologic syndrome. Blood 2000;96:443-51.
102. Race EM, Adelson-Mitty J, Kriegel GR, et al. Focal myobacterial lymphadenitis following initiation of protease-inhibitor therapy in patients with advanced HIV-1 disease. Lancet 1998;351:252-5.
103. Reichert CM, O'Leary TJ, Levens DL, Simrell CR, Macher AM. Autopsy pathology in the acquired immune deficiency syndrome. Am J Pathol 1983;112:357-82.
104. Rickinson AB. Cellular immunological responses to the virus infection. In: Epstein MA, Achong BG, eds. The Epstein-Barr virus: recent advances. New York: Heinemann Medical Books; 1986:75-125.
105. Sadahira Y, Yoshimoto S, Manabe T. Parvovirus B19-associated transient pure red cell aplasia with lymphadenopathy: a case report. Pathol Int 1998;48:829-33.
106. Said J. AIDS-related lymphadenopathies. Semin Diagn Pathol 1988;5:365-75.
107. Said JW, Pinkus JL, Yamashita J, et al. The role of follicular and interdigitating dendritic cells in HIV-related lymphoid hyperplasia: localization of fascin. Mod Pathol 1997;10:421-7.
108. Salvador AH, Harrison EG Jr, Kyle RA. Lymphadenopathy due to infectious mononucleosis: its confusion with malignant lymphoma. Cancer 1971;27:1029-40.
109. Schnitzer B. Reactive lymphadenopathies. In: Knowles DM, ed. Neoplastic hematopathology, 2nd ed. Philadelphia: Lippincott Williams & Wilkins; 2001:537-68.
110. Schoepp RJ, Morin MD, Martinez MJ, et al. Detection and identification of variola virus in fixed human tissue after prolonged archival storage. Lab Invest 2004;84:41-8.
111. Shin SS, Berry GJ, Weiss LM. Infectious mononucleosis: diagnosis by in situ hybridization in two cases with atypical features. Am J Surg Pathol 1991;15:625-31.
112. Shope RE, Meegan JM. African hemorrhagic fevers caused by Marburg and Ebola viruses. In: Evans AS, Kaslow RA, eds. Viral infections of humans: epidemiology and control, 4th ed. New York: Plenum Medical Book; 1997:139-50.

113. Shope RE, Meegan JM. Arboviruses. In: Evans AS, Kaslow RA, eds. Viral infections of humans: epidemiology and control, 4th ed. New York Plenum Medical Book; 1997:151-83.
114. Sohn CC, Sheibani K, Winberg CD, Rappaport H. Monocytoid B lymphocytes: their relation to the patterns of the acquired immunodeficiency syndrome (AIDS) and AIDS-related lymphadenopathy. Hum Pathol 1985;16:979-85.
115. Stanberry LR, Jorgensen DM, Nahmias AJ. Herpes simplex viruses 1 and 2. In: Evans AS, Kaslow RA, eds. Viral infections of humans: epidemiology and control, 4th ed. New York: Plenum Medical Book; 1997:419-46.
116. Stein H, Mason DY, Gerdes J, et al. The expression of the Hodgkin's disease-associated antigen Ki-1 in reactive and neoplastic lymphoid tissue: evidence that Reed-Sternberg cells and histiocytic malignancies are derived from activated lymphoid cells. Blood 1985;66:848-58.
117. Stejskal J. Measles lymphadenopathy. Ultrastruct Pathol 1980;1:243-7.
118. Stettner-Gloning R, Jager G, Gloning H, Pontz BF, Emmrich P. Lymphadenopathy in connection with human herpes virus type 6 (HHV-6) infection. Clin Investig 1992;70:59-62.
119. Strano AJ. Measles (Rubeola). In: Binford CH, Connor DH, eds. Pathology of tropical and extraordinary diseases, Vol 1; Washington, D.C.: Armed Forces Institute of Pathology; 1976:73-5.
120. Strickler JG, Fedeli F, Horwitz CA, Copenhaver CM, Frizzera G. Infectious mononucleosis in lymphoid tissue. Histopathology, in situ hybridization, and differential diagnosis. Arch Pathol Lab Med 1993;117:269-78.
121. Sumiyoshi Y, Kikuchi M, Ohshima K, Takeshita M, Eizuru Y, Minamishima Y. A case of human herpesvirus-6 lymphadenitis with infectious mononucleosis-like syndrome. Pathol Int 1995;45:947-51.
122. Symmers WStC. The lymphoreticular system. In: Symmers WStC, ed. Systemic pathology, 2nd ed. New York: Churchill Livingstone; 1978:507-891.
123. Tamaru J, Mikata A, Horie H, et al. Herpes simplex lymphadenitis: report of two cases with review of the literature. Am J Surg Pathol 1990;14:571-7.
124. Taxy JB, Tillawi I, Goldman PM. Herpes simplex lymphadenitis. An unusual presentation with necrosis and viral particles. Arch Pathol Lab Med 1985;109:1043-4.
125. Tindle BH, Parker JW, Lukes RJ. "Reed-Sternberg cells" in infectious mononucleosis? Am J Clin Pathol 1972;58:607-17.
126. Trovato R, Luppi M, Barozzi P, et al. Cellular localization of human herpesvirus 8 in nonneoplastic lymphadenopathies and chronic interstitial pneumonitis by in situ polymerase chain reaction studies. J Hum Virol 1999;2:38-44.
127. Turner RR, Levine AM, Gill PS, Parker JW, Meyer PR. Progressive histopathologic abnormalities in the persistent generalized lymphadenopathy syndrome. Am J Surg Pathol 1987;11:625-32.
128. Ulirsch RC, Jaffe ES. Sjogren's syndrome-like illness associated with the acquired immunodeficiency syndrome-related complex. Hum Pathol 1987;18:1063-8.
129. Vanhems P, Toma E. Recognizing primary HIV-1 infection. Infect Med 1999;16:104-8.
130. Wang FZ, Dahl H, Ljungman P, Linde A. Lymphoproliferative responses to human herpesvirus-6 variant A and variant B in healthy adults. J Med Virol 1999;57:134-9.
131. Wat PJ, Strickler JG, Myers JL, Nordstrom MR. Herpes simplex infection causing acute necrotizing tonsillitis. Mayo Clin Proc 1994;69:269-71.
132. Weisberger J, Cornfield D, Gorczyca W, Liu Z. Down-regulation of pan-T-cell antigens, particularly CD7, in acute infectious mononucleosis. Am J Clin Pathol 2003;120:49-55.
133. Weller TH. Varicella-herpes zoster virus. In: Viral infections of humans: epidemiology and control. Evans AS, Kaslow RA, eds. New York: Plenum Medical Book Co; 1997:865-92.
134. Wick MJ, Woronzoff-Dashkoff KP, McGlennen RC. The molecular characterization of fatal infectious mononucleosis. Am J Clin Pathol 2002;117:582-8.
135. Witt MD, Torno MS, Sun N, Stein T. Herpes simplex virus lymphadenitis: case report and review of the literature. Clin Infect Dis 2002;34:1-6.
136. Wood GS, Garcia CF, Dorfman RF, Warnke RA. The immunohistology of follicle lysis in lymph node biopsies from homosexual men. Blood 1985;66:1092-7.
137. Wright PJ, Davies A. Traumatic rupture of the spleen in rubella. J R Army Med Corps 1955;101:235-6.
138. Younes M, Podesta A, Helie M, Buckley P. Infection of T but not B lymphocytes by cytomegalovirus in lymph node: an immunophenotypic study. Am J Surg Pathol 1991;15:75-80.

10 FUNGAL INFECTIONS

Fungal infections, although rare, have significant manifestations in the lymph nodes and spleen. The frequency of fungal infections varies depending on the geographic distribution of the organisms and the susceptibility of the host. Several types of fungal infection are more commonly seen in the United States: histoplasmosis, blastomycosis, and coccidioidomycosis. Other fungi are worldwide in their distribution: *Cryptococcus* and *Candida* species, among others. Usually, these fungal infections are disseminated, and are most commonly seen in patients who are immunosuppressed. Occasionally, however, primary infections spread to local or regional lymph nodes and present with unusual clinical manifestations. The differential diagnosis of fungal infections of the lymph nodes or spleen includes other types of infection (bacterial, viral, and parasitic) and, depending on the clinical circumstances, either primary hematolymphoid malignancies or metastatic malignancies.

Rarely, nonbiologic materials mimic fungi in tissue sections (2,12,21,22). Termed pseudofungi, these structures simulate hyphae or yeast forms (fig. 10-1). They may be associated with typical histologic responses to fungal infections, such as granulomas or acute inflammation. Filamentous fungal forms are mimicked by Gamna-Gandy

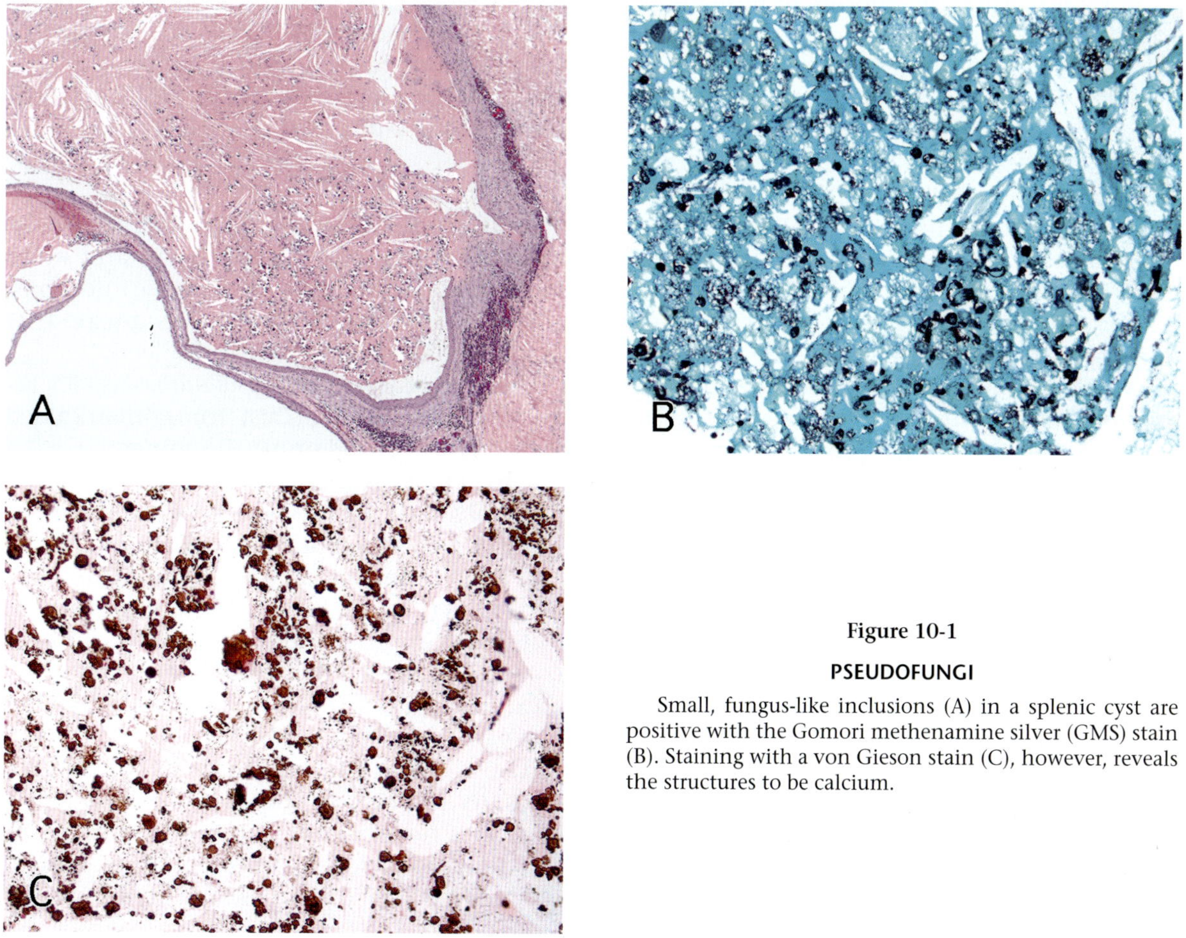

Figure 10-1

PSEUDOFUNGI

Small, fungus-like inclusions (A) in a splenic cyst are positive with the Gomori methenamine silver (GMS) stain (B). Staining with a von Gieson stain (C), however, reveals the structures to be calcium.

bodies, calcification, or iron encrustation of matrix structures or other nonbiologic materials. Yeast forms are mimicked by Hamazaki-Wesenberg bodies, myospherulosis, or small nodules of calcification. Careful correlation of morphology with the findings of ancillary techniques, such as special stains (von Kossa, periodic acid–Schiff [PAS], Gomori methenamine silver [GMS], Prussian blue) resolves most cases. Exotic techniques, such as dispersive X-ray elemental analysis, can be used in difficult cases (2).

CRYPTOCOCCUS NEOFORMANS

Definition. *Cryptococcus neoformans* is a yeast with a worldwide distribution. It can produce local and systemic infections, especially in immunocompromised hosts. Lymph nodal and splenic involvement are common in disseminated disease.

General Features. *C. neoformans* is endemic in soil and associated with bird feces (15). Exposure to dirt and dust that contain bird droppings is a common method of exposure in humans. *C. neoformans* is typically easy to see in histologic specimens because of the thick, gelatinous capsule. These capsules may be lost in culture or after partial treatment.

Clinical Features. Preceding the human immunodeficiency virus (HIV)/acquired immunodeficiency syndrome (AIDS) epidemic, cryptococcal infections were rare. In patients with HIV/AIDS, the infection is common, but is also seen in patients with other forms of immunosuppression. *Cryptococcus* infection may be an initial presentation of AIDS. As therapy for AIDS improves, a relative increase in cryptococcal infections in post-transplant patients has occurred.

Central nervous system and pulmonary involvement are the most common clinical presentations of cryptococcal infection. Disseminated or systemic infections are less common, but clinically serious (6). Any organ system or visceral location may be involved (10,23). The clinical symptoms include fever, malaise, weight loss, dyspnea, chest pain, and nausea and vomiting. Neurologic manifestations include mild headaches, symptoms of meningitis, mental status changes, delirium, and coma. Worsening neurologic symptoms suggest progressive disease.

Laboratory Findings. The latex agglutination test for cryptococcal antigen is useful for evaluating cerebrospinal fluid specimens. India ink is a traditional staining method, but lacks appropriate sensitivity and specificity. Microbiologic culture, including the use of selective media, definitively identifies *Cryptococcus*.

Gross Findings. Because of the thick capsules associated with *Cryptococcus*, tissues with extensive involvement may have glistening, slimy cut surfaces. The polysaccharide capsules impart a slippery feeling to the tissue.

Microscopic Findings. The yeast forms of *Cryptococcus* are 4 to 10 µm in diameter. The prominent capsule can be accentuated using certain staining techniques (such as India ink). Occasionally, associated granulomatous inflammation and hemophagocytosis make individual organisms harder to see (figs. 10-2–10-4). Cytochemical stains, most notably GMS and mucicarmine, are useful for identification.

Treatment and Prognosis. Treatment includes the antifungal agents fluconazole, itraconazole, and amphotericin B. HIV-associated cryptococcal infections have a high rate of recurrence (30 to 50 percent), and patients are often given prophylactic antifungal treatment (15).

HISTOPLASMA CAPSULATUM

Definition. *Histoplasma capsulatum* is a dimorphic fungus (both yeast form and mold form) that is associated with systemic infections. *Histoplasmosis* is a granulomatous disease that may involve lymph nodes and spleen.

General Features. *H. capsulatum* is usually acquired by inhalation of dust from contaminated soil containing bird or bat droppings.

Clinical Features. Histoplasmosis occurs primarily in the Ohio-Mississippi River basin in the United States, but is also found in Central and South America as well as Southeast Asia and Africa (17). It is the most common systemic fungal infection in the United States, and occurs in 2 to 5 percent of individuals in endemic areas. Histoplasmosis has become an increasing problem in AIDS patients (15).

The clinicopathologic findings are similar, in many respects, to those of coccidioidomycosis and tuberculosis. The host's response to the fungus depends upon the immunocompetency status. There may be latent asymptomatic

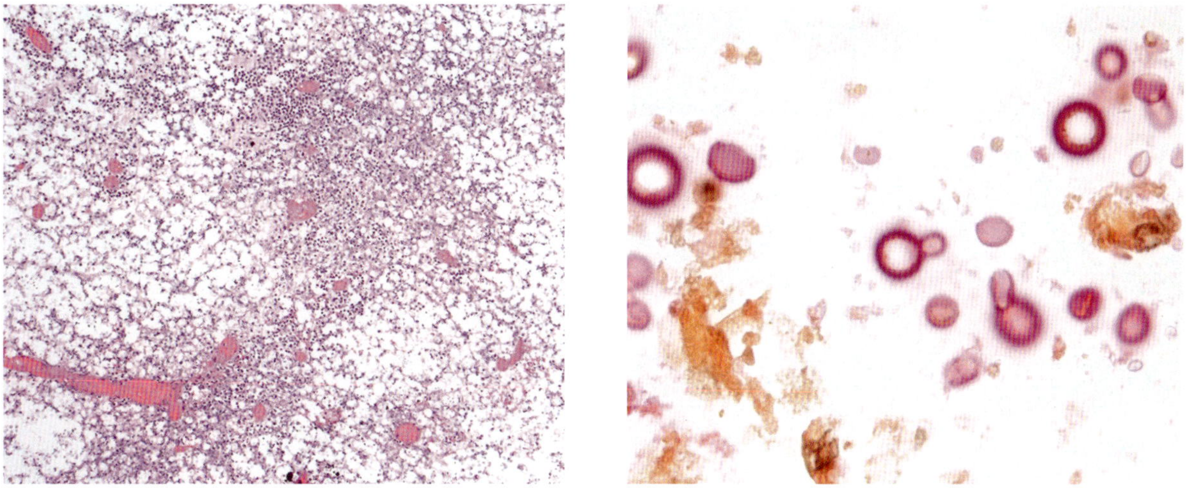

Figure 10-2

***CRYPTOCOCCUS,* LYMPH NODE**

The lymph node is partially replaced by clear-appearing structures, which displace the normal architecture (left) and are *Cryptococcus*, as shown by a mucin stain (right).

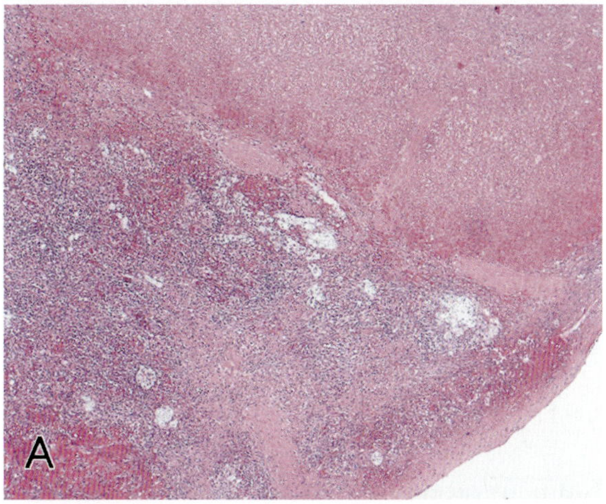

Figure 10-3

***CRYPTOCOCCUS,* SPLEEN**

A: A spleen with hemorrhage and necrosis.

B: Foci of macrophages with small intracellular and extracellular organisms which have a clear capsular structure.

C: High magnification highlights the organisms within their clear capsules.

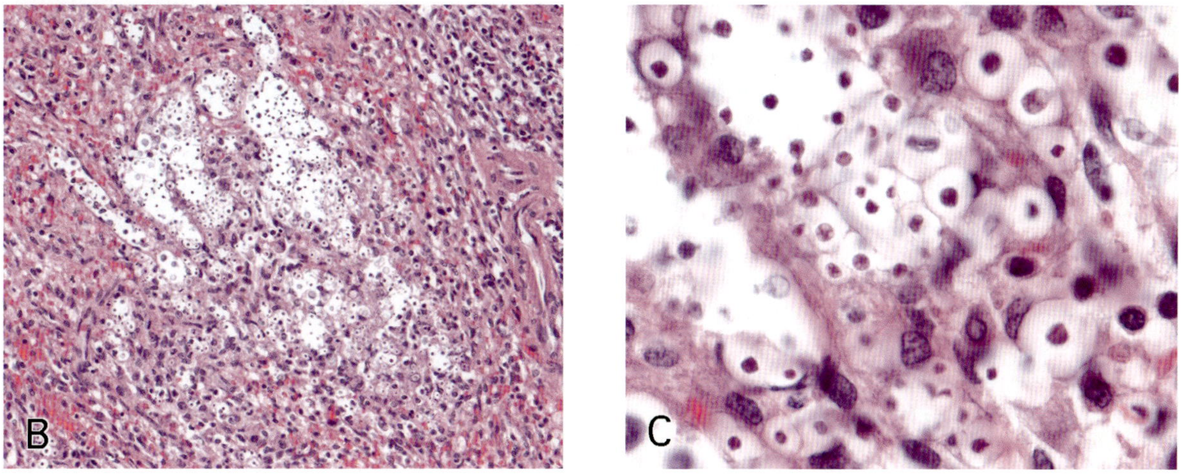

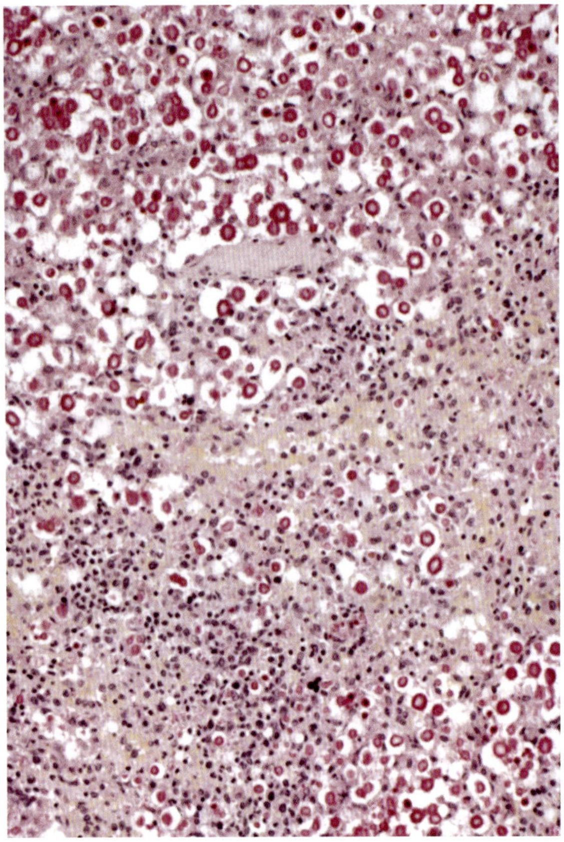

Figure 10-4

CRYPTOCOCCUS

Mucicarmine stains *Cryptococcus* organisms.

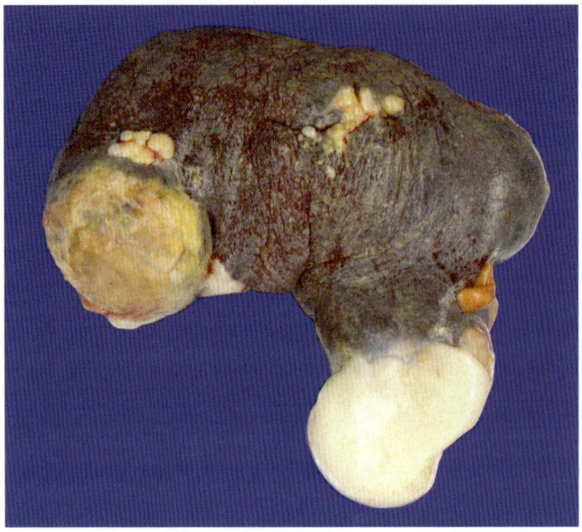

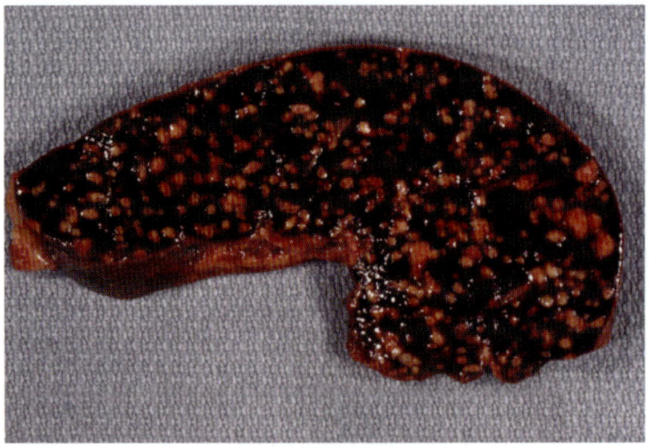

Figure 10-5

***HISTOPLASMA*, SPLEEN**

Splenic involvement by histoplasmosis. (Courtesy of John Eble, Indianapolis, IN.)

infection, self-limited or chronic progressive pulmonary disease, disseminated systemic disease, or solitary localized lesions. When seen in AIDS patients, the infection is disseminated in 95 percent of cases (15).

The clinical symptoms in disseminated cases may simulate those of other opportunistic infections such as *Pneumocystis jiroveci* and *Mycobacterium avium- intracellulare* (MAI) infections. Hilar lymph nodes are commonly involved in all of the clinical presentations.

Laboratory Findings. *Histoplasma* is positively identified by culture.

Microscopic Findings. The main histopathologic change in the lymph nodes and spleen is the presence of well-formed epithelioid cell granulomas that may undergo coagulative necrosis. Histologic differentiation from tuberculosis or coccidioidomycosis requires the identification of the causative organism. *H. capsulatum* is a 2- to 5-µm, intracellular yeast form, which has a thin cell wall but no true capsule, in spite of its name. The lesions of *H. capsulatum* infection eventually become fibrotic and calcified (figs. 10-5, 10-6). Fulminant, disseminated histoplasmosis in immunocompromised patients may not be associated with well-formed granulomas, but rather with collections of activated phagocytic macrophages that are filled with yeast forms, similar in appearance to kala-azar.

The definitive diagnosis of histoplasmosis is made by the demonstration of the characteristic yeast forms in smears or tissue sections highlighted by GMS (figs. 10-7, 10-8) and confirmed by culture results. They are also well visualized by Giemsa stains.

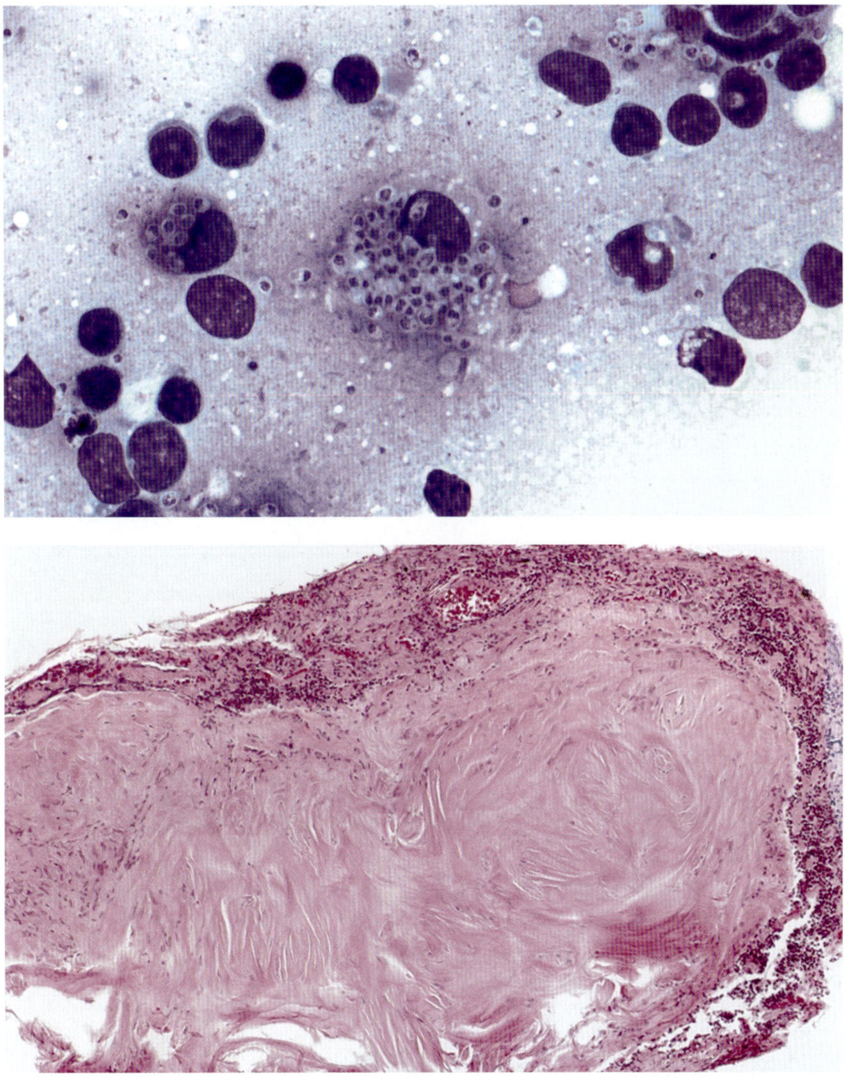

Figure 10-6

***HISTOPLASMA,* LYMPH NODE**

Top: Cytologic imprint of lymph node with histoplasmosis. The organisms are seen in the cytoplasm of the macrophages.

Bottom: Longstanding case of *H. capsulatum* lymphadenitis in a fibrotic, calcified hilar lymph node.

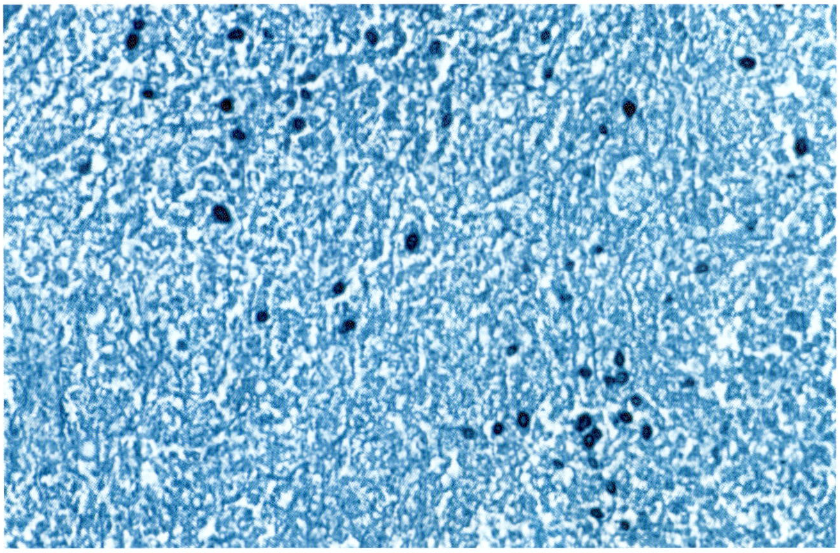

Figure 10-7

***HISTOPLASMA,* LYMPH NODE**

H. capsulatum yeast organisms are highlighted by the GMS stain.

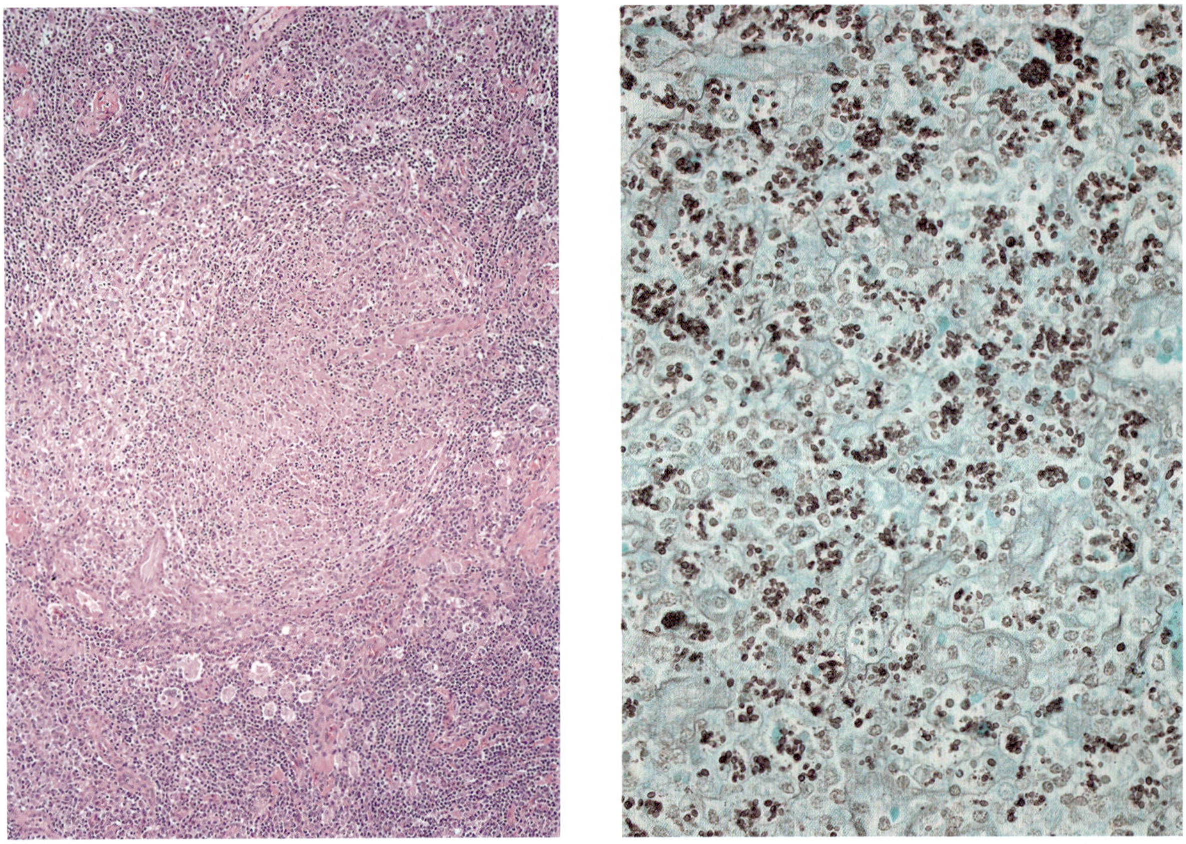

Figure 10-8

***HISTOPLASMA,* SPLEEN**

Left: Granuloma formation in the spleen.
Right: The organisms stain with GMS.

Differential Diagnosis. The differential diagnosis includes the yeast forms of *Candida albicans*, *Cryptococcus neoformans*, and *Pneumocystis jiroveci* (25). While *H. capsulatum* is most often intracellular, *C. neoformans* and *P. jiroveci* are not. *P. jiroveci* is a pulmonary pathogen that is frequently seen in AIDS patients. The organisms are identified by their characteristic "cup shape." They usually reside in an amorphous, foamy exudate and are best visualized by GMS. When the infection involves the lymph nodes, as it commonly does in AIDS patients, the exudate and organisms may be seen in the sinuses or within the lymph node parenchyma itself.

Treatment and Prognosis. Various antifungal treatments, including itraconazole, amphotericin B, and ketoconazole, have been used for the various forms of histoplasmosis.

BLASTOMYCES DERMATITIDIS

Definition. *Blastomyces dermatitidis* is a dimorphic fungus that typically infects either the skin or respiratory tract. Disseminated *blastomycosis* may result in organisms in the lymph nodes or spleen.

General Features. *B. dermatitidis* is found in moist soil that is often associated with rivers and other waterways.

Clinical Features. Blastomycosis is endemic in the Great Lakes region of the United States; rare cases are seen outside the United States. Blastomycosis has five distinct clinical forms: primary pulmonary infection, cutaneous disease, single organ system involvement, limited inoculation-associated disease, and a severe multisystem disseminated form. When the skin is involved, it may be an indication of disseminated

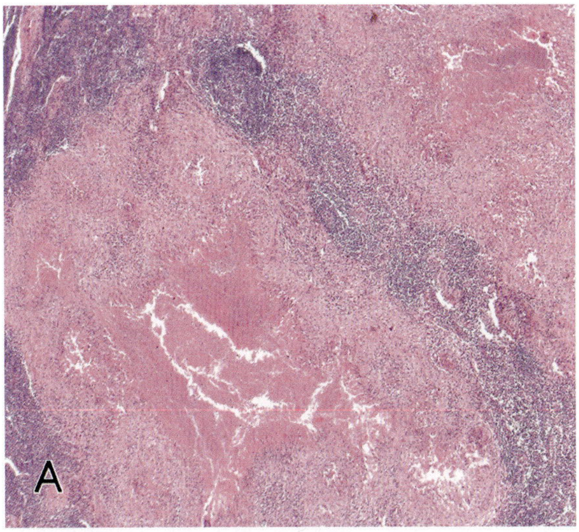

Figure 10-9

***BLASTOMYCES,* SPLEEN**

Caseating granulomas (A), multinucleated giant cells (B), and rare fungi with thick capsules (C) are seen in this spleen. (Courtesy of California Tumor Tissue Registry, Loma Linda, CA.)

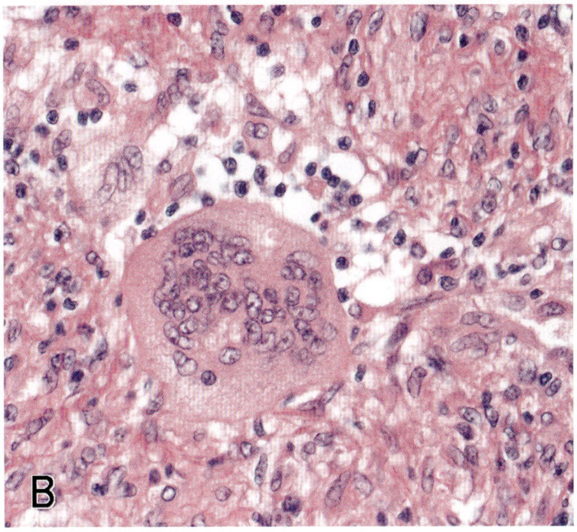

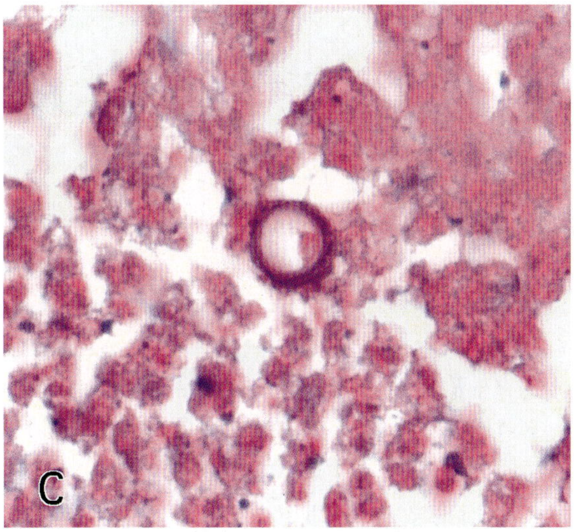

disease. Symptoms include cough, fever, chest pain, weight loss, night sweats, and malaise.

Laboratory Findings. Recovery of *B. dermatitidis* in blood cultures is rare.

Microscopic Findings. The yeast forms of *B. dermatitidis* are generally spherical with thick walls. They are 8 to 20 µm in diameter and have the characteristic "broad-based" budding of daughter forms. The histologic response is granulomatous and includes macrophages and giant cells (figs. 10-9, 10-10). Microabscesses associated with numerous neutrophils may be seen. Although they are often easily seen with hematoxylin and eosin (H&E) stains, the fungi can be highlighted with GMS and PAS stains.

Differential Diagnosis. The differential diagnosis includes other types of fungi that are seen in tissue sections. The size and characteristic findings, however, such as the broad-based budding, make most other fungi unlikely. Because occasional *Blastomyces* organisms overlap with *Coccidioides* in size, this is an important differential diagnostic consideration.

Treatment and Prognosis. Ketoconazole, fluconazole, amphotericin B, and other antifungal agents are used in treatment. Late relapses occur after treatment, so infected patients should have long-term follow-up.

COCCIDIOIDES IMMITIS

Definition. *Coccidioides immitis* is typically a pulmonary, dimorphic fungus, but rare disseminated cases of *coccidioidomycosis* involve the lymph nodes and spleen.

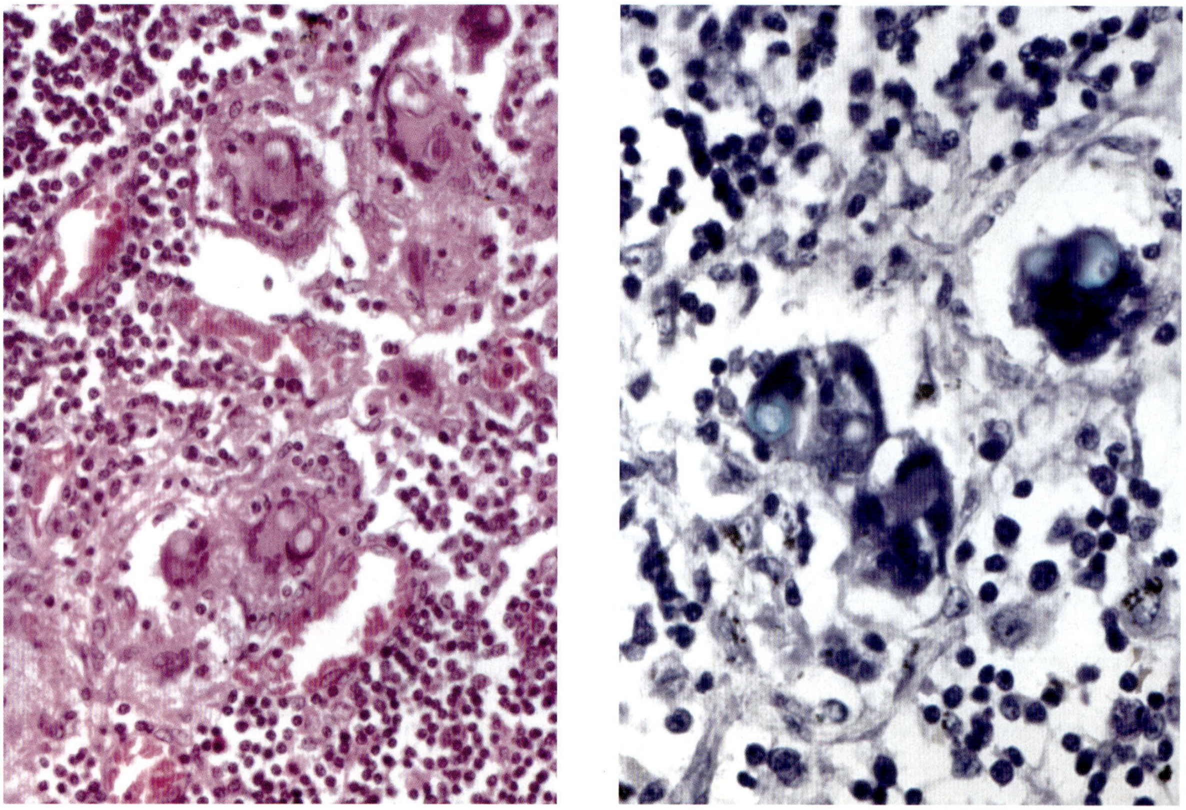

Figure 10-10

BLASTOMYCES, LYMPH NODE

The fungi are within the macrophages (Giemsa stain).

Clinical Features. The distribution of *C. immitis* is western United States, especially California, as well as Mexico and portions of Central and South America. Certain racial groups (Filipino, Asian, black) have increased sensitivity to infection (13). Pulmonary infection is the most common clinical presentation, although disseminated disease occurs. In disseminated cases, the inguinal lymph nodes are frequently involved (4). Immunosuppressed patients, especially those with HIV/AIDS, have increased susceptibility to infection.

Laboratory Findings. *Coccidioides* can be readily cultured; however, it can present great risk to laboratory personnel as the hyphae are especially infectious and easily become airborne. Serologic testing is readily available and confirms the histologic diagnosis.

Microscopic Findings. The classic histologic appearance of *C. immitis* is large spherules packed with smaller endospores. The spherules range from 10 to 60 µm, with the endospores measuring 2 to 4 µm. The spherules have relatively thin capsules (in contrast to the thick capsule of *Blastomyces*). There are often associated lymphoid aggregates and granulomas, with or without caseation (figs. 10-11–10-14). Giant cells, acute inflammation, and microabscesses are also associated with *C. immitis*. The organism stains well with fungal stains (GMS, PAS).

Differential Diagnosis. The endospores are similar in size to the yeast forms of *Histoplasma* and *Cryptococcus*. The spherules most resemble *Blastomyces*, which should be carefully considered in the differential diagnosis.

Treatment and Prognosis. Itraconazole, fluconazole, amphotericin B, and other antifungal agents are used in treatment. Late relapses occur after treatment, especially in HIV/AIDS patients, so infected patients should have long-term follow-up.

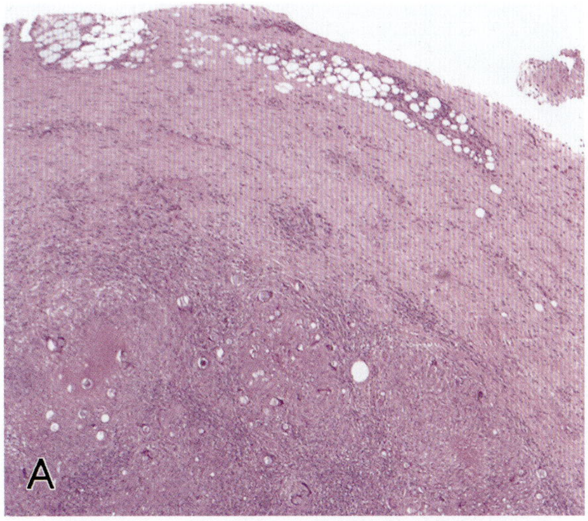

Figure 10-11

***COCCIDIOIDES,* LYMPH NODE**

Numerous spherules and a granulomatous reaction are seen in this lymph node. (Courtesy of Luis Fajardo, Palo Alto, CA.)

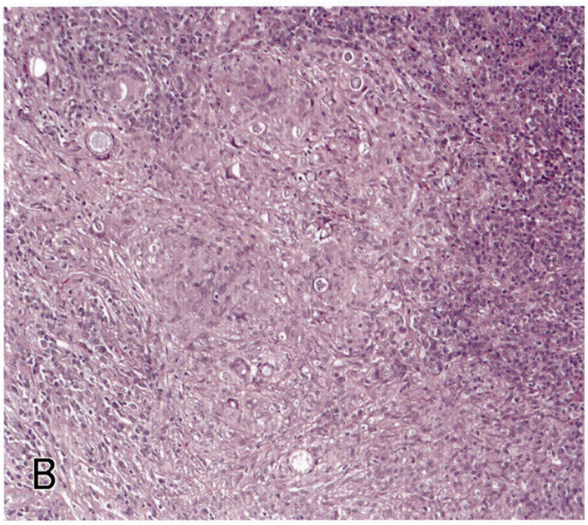

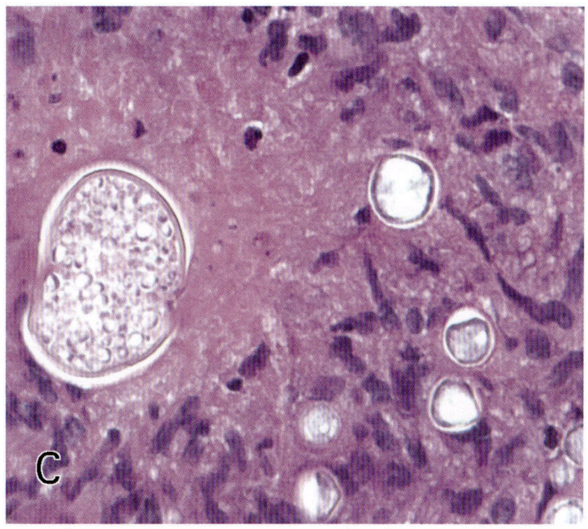

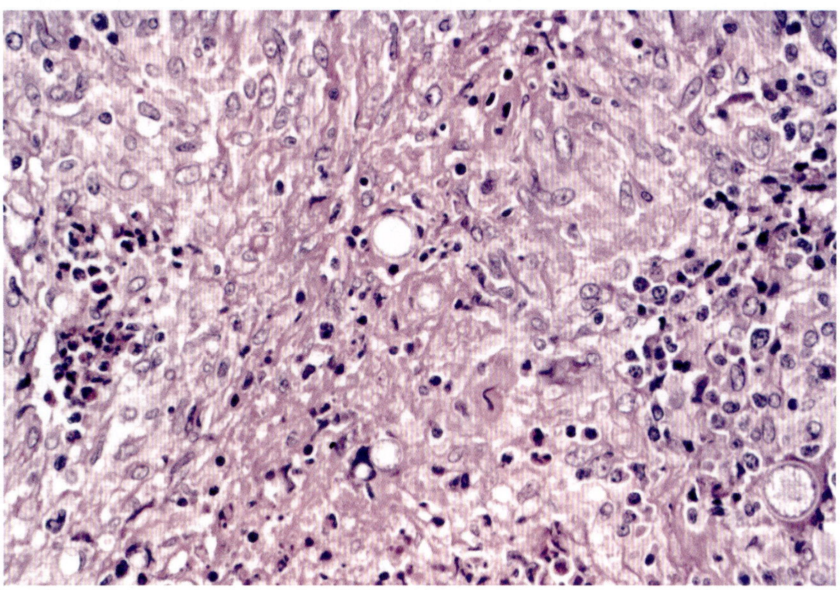

Figure 10-12

***COCCIDIOIDES,* LYMPH NODE**

Dense fibrosis, with entrapped spherules.

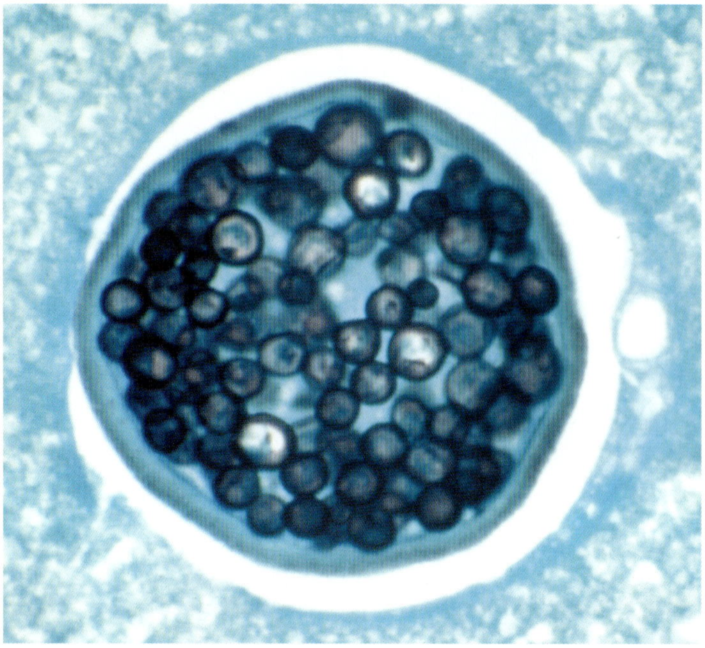

Figure 10-13

***COCCIDIOIDES,* LYMPH NODE**

The *C. immitis* capsule surrounds endospores that are highlighted by the GMS stain. (Courtesy of Ronald Neafie, Washington, DC.)

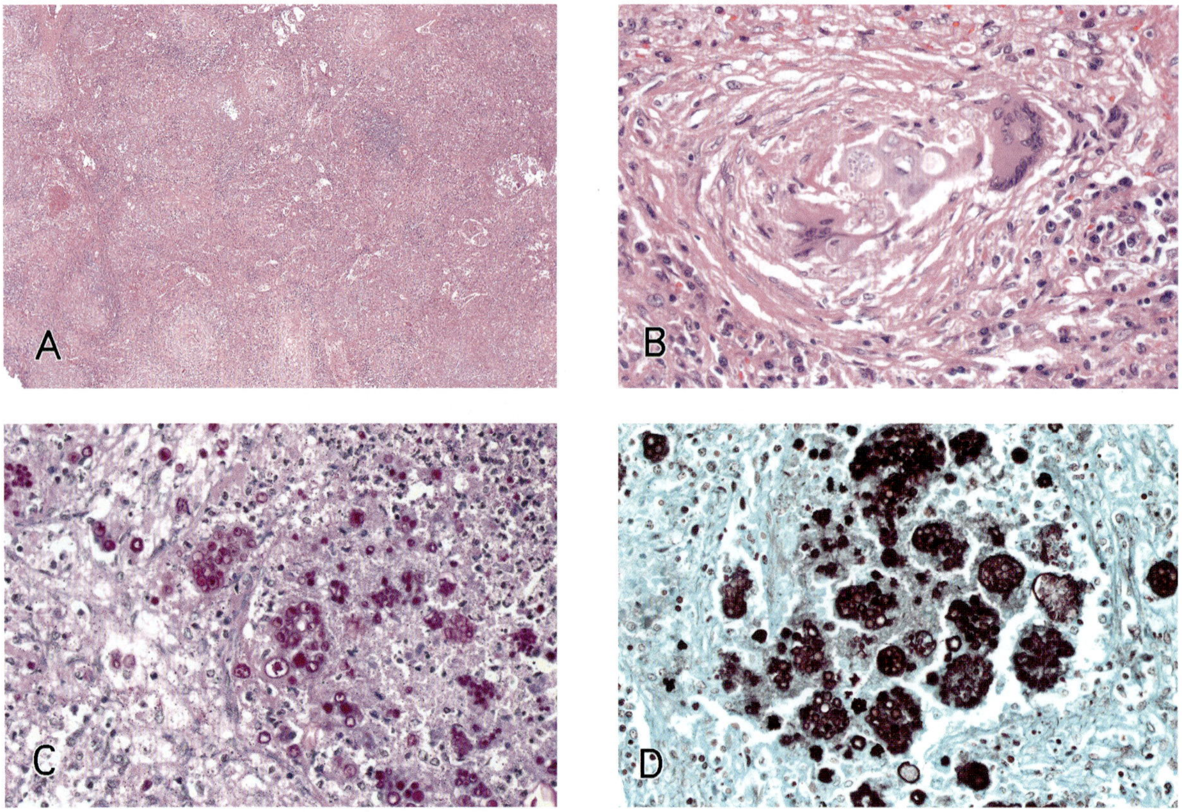

Figure 10-14

***COCCIDIOIDES,* SPLEEN**

Numerous spherules (A,B) stain with PAS (C) and GMS (D) stains.

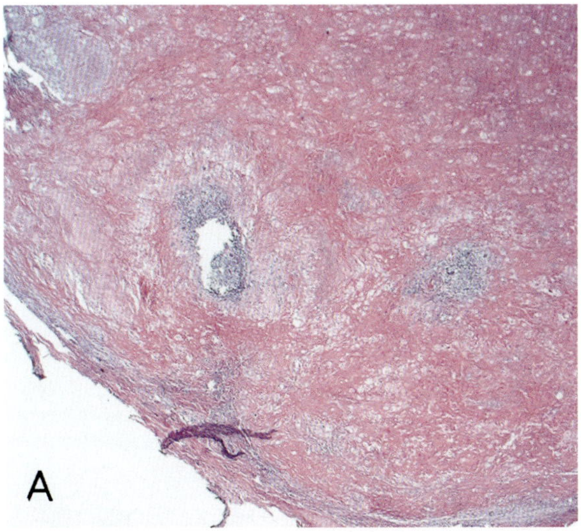

Figure 10-15

***PARACOCCIDIOIDES*, LYMPH NODE**

Hematoxylin and eosin (H&E) highlights the inflammatory reaction (A,B) and GMS highlights the classic "mariner's wheel" appearance.

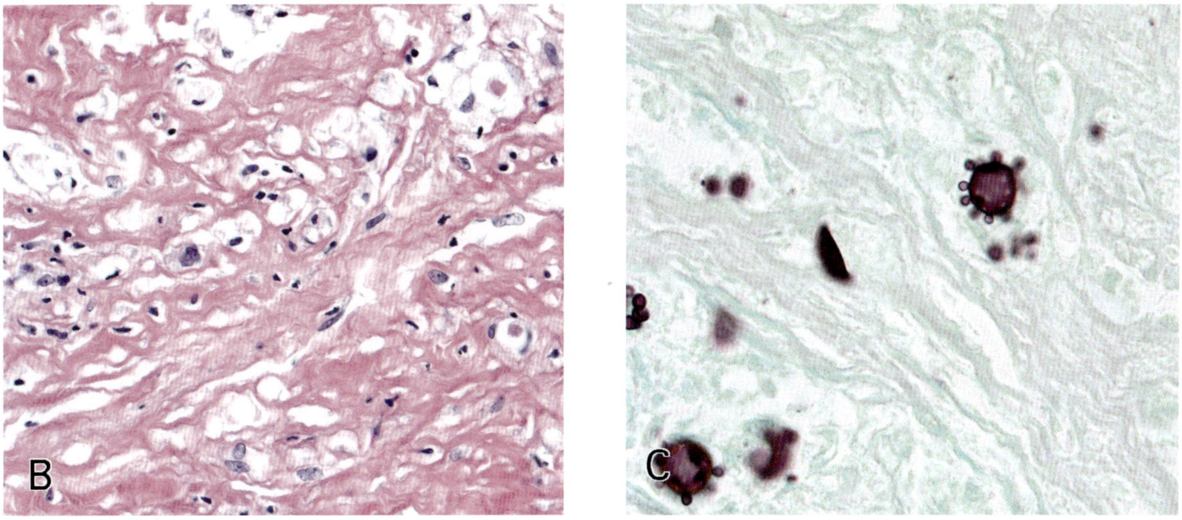

PARACOCCIDIOIDES BRASILIENSIS

Definition. *Paracoccidioides brasiliensis* is a dimorphic fungus, endemic in South and Central America. It most frequently produces pulmonary disease, but disseminated *paracoccioidomycosis* often involves the lymph nodes and spleen.

General Features. *P. brasiliensis* resides in soil, and human exposure is typically through inhalation of conidia.

Clinical Features. Chronic paracoccioidomycosis is slowly progressive and primarily consists of pulmonary manifestations. Symptoms include cough, sputum production, shortness of breath, fever, weight loss, and anorexia. Progressive pulmonary failure with fibrosis and right heart failure may lead to death. Progressive and disseminated disease occurs in about 5 percent of patients, most frequently children, young adults, and immunosuppressed persons.

Laboratory Findings. The histologic findings are often the cornerstone of the diagnosis. The organisms can be cultured or confirmed by polymerase chain reaction (PCR) testing.

Microscopic Findings. The yeast forms have walls of 10 to 30 μm in thickness. Each yeast may have several budding daughter yeasts, which have narrow bases and are arranged around the edges of the larger parent, in a pattern sometimes referred to as a "mariner's wheel" (figs. 10-15, 10-16) (11). The typical histologic appearance is of granulomas, with or without caseation. Acute inflammation and microabscesses may

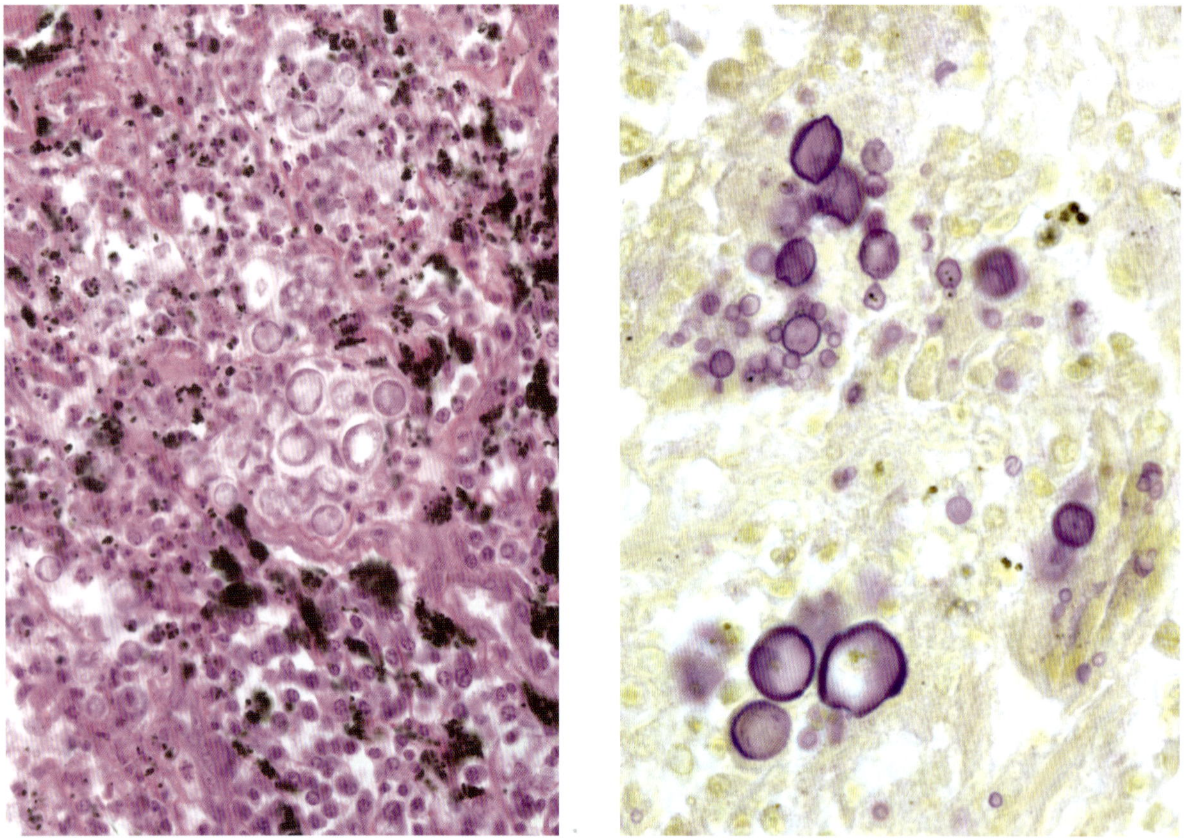

Figure 10-16

PARACOCCIDIOIDES, LYMPH NODE

H&E (left) and Gridley (right) stains. (Courtesy of Luis Fajardo, Palo Alto, CA.)

be present. Calcified fibrous nodules are found in older sites of involvement.

Yeast forms may be difficult to identify. As with other large yeasts, H&E stains are effective, but the organism can also be highlighted with PAS and GMS stains.

Treatment and Prognosis. Trimethoprim-sulfamethoxazole is an effective treatment for *P. brasiliensis*. Since this medication is often used for *Pneumocystis* prophylaxis, the incidence of paracoccidioidomycosis is not necessarily increased in AIDS patients. Ketoconazole and amphotericin B are also effective treatments. In spite of these treatments, the prognosis for patients with disseminated disease is poor.

PNEUMOCYSTIS JIROVECI

Definition. *Pneumocystis jiroveci,* formerly *P. carinii,* typically causes pneumonia, but also rarely involves the spleen and lymph nodes in disseminated disease.

General Features. The classification of *Pneumocystis* has historically been uncertain, but currently is placed as a fungus.

Clinical Features. *P. jiroveci* is worldwide in its distribution, with sporadic infections occurring in immunosuppressed individuals, especially those with HIV/AIDS. It is likely that subclinical infections occur in immunocompetent individuals, based on seroprevalence. Dyspnea, fever, cough, cyanosis, and hepatosplenomegaly are frequent clinical findings in patients with significant disease.

Laboratory Findings. Serologic evaluation may be performed, but many individuals have been exposed, so changes in titers may be necessary to confirm an active infection. PCR testing confirms the diagnosis.

Microscopic Findings. The organisms are associated with granulomas and macrophage aggregates (fig. 10-17). The cysts are small and often within macrophages. Occasionally, there is frothy extracellular material, similar to that seen in the lung. Other histologic features include granulomatous inflammation and vascular invasion (figs. 10-18, 10-19). The trophozoites are 2 to 4 µm, while the cysts measure 5 to 8 µm. The cyst forms have been likened to "crushed ping pong balls," "helmets," or a "ball in a cup," depending on the creativity of the writer. The cysts are difficult to visualize with the H&E or PAS stain. They can be visualized with Giemsa, Papanicolaou, and GMS stains as well as immunostains (see Differential Diagnosis).

Ancillary Studies. Monoclonal antibodies for *P. jiroveci* are available for both fluorescent stains and immunohistochemical techniques.

Differential Diagnosis. The differential diagnosis includes other fungal infections with small yeast forms including *Histoplasma*, or *Candida*. Erythrocytes stained with GMS look similar to

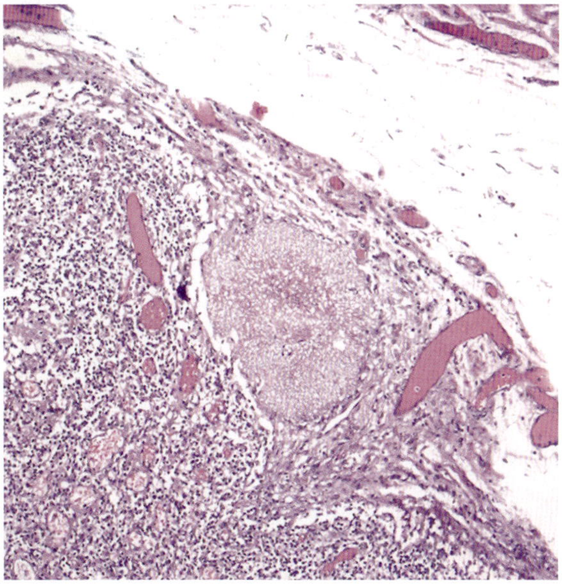

Figure 10-17

***PNEUMOCYSTIS,* LYMPH NODE**

A small nodule of foamy material near the capsule of a lymph node is *Pneumocystis*.

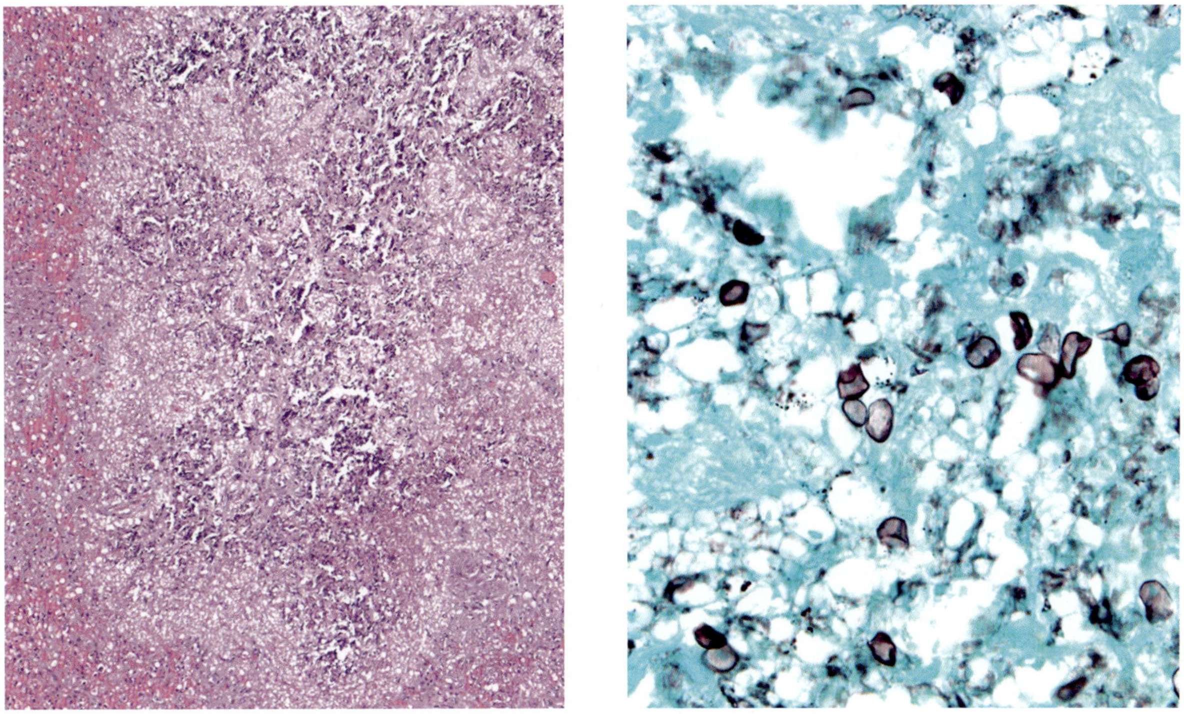

Figure 10-18

***PNEUMOCYSTIS,* SPLEEN**

Splenic *Pneumocystis* infection is seen as an area of necrosis and calcification (left), with GMS staining highlighting fungal organisms (right).

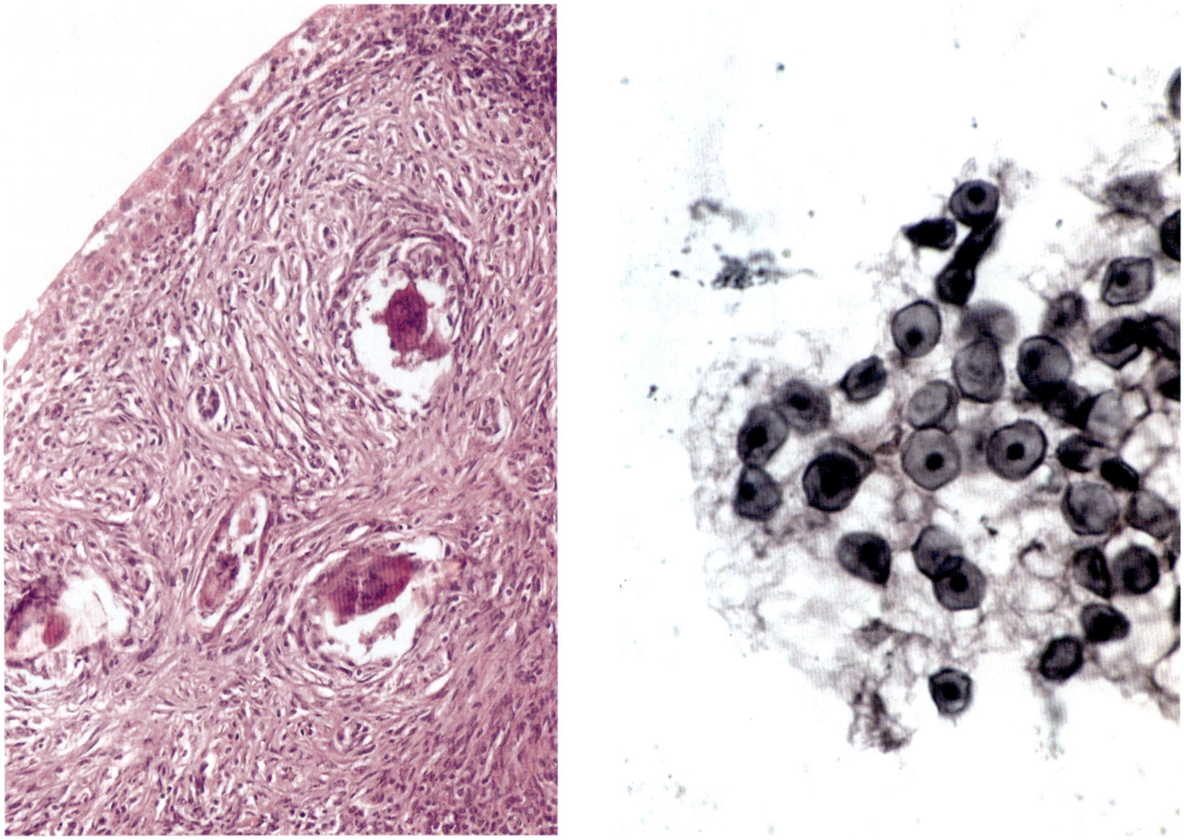

Figure 10-19

PNEUMOCYSTIS, LYMPH NODE

Left: High magnification of the foamy material of *Pneumocystis* infection.
Right: The "ball-in-cup" appearance is highlighted by the GMS stain. (Courtesy of Stefano Pileri, Bologna, Italy.)

Pneumocystis, and pathologists should be wary of this potential pitfall. The red blood cells lack the morphology of the cyst forms.

Treatment and Prognosis. Most cases are curable using trimethoprim-sulfamethoxazole or pentamidine. In immunosuppressed individuals, especially AIDS patients, trimethoprim-sulfamethoxazole prophylaxis markedly reduces the incidence of infection.

PENICILLIUM MARNEFFEI

Definition. Only relatively recently described, *Penicillium marneffei* is an opportunistic fungus that is endemic in Southeast Asia. Disseminated disease may occur, especially in immunocompromised individuals.

General Features. Bamboo rats are the reservoir for *P. marneffei,* which accounts for another name, "rat bite fever."

Clinical Features. Infections with *P. marneffei* are rare, and although frequent in immunocompromised individuals, more cases are seen sporadically in patients without predisposing features (about 75 percent) (26). Fever and generalized lymphadenopathy are frequent clinical findings. Skin lesions, splenomegaly, and peripheral blood cytopenias are also seen (19). The lymphadenopathy may be chronic and clinically mimic infection by tuberculosis (26).

Laboratory Findings. Both culture and serology diagnose *P. marneffei.* A definitive diagnosis relies on culture, although confirmation may also be made by PCR studies.

Microscopic Findings. Granulomatous inflammation and necrosis are the most prominent features associated with this disease. Individual yeast cells, 2 to 5 µm in size, are found within macrophages (fig. 10-20). Budding is not

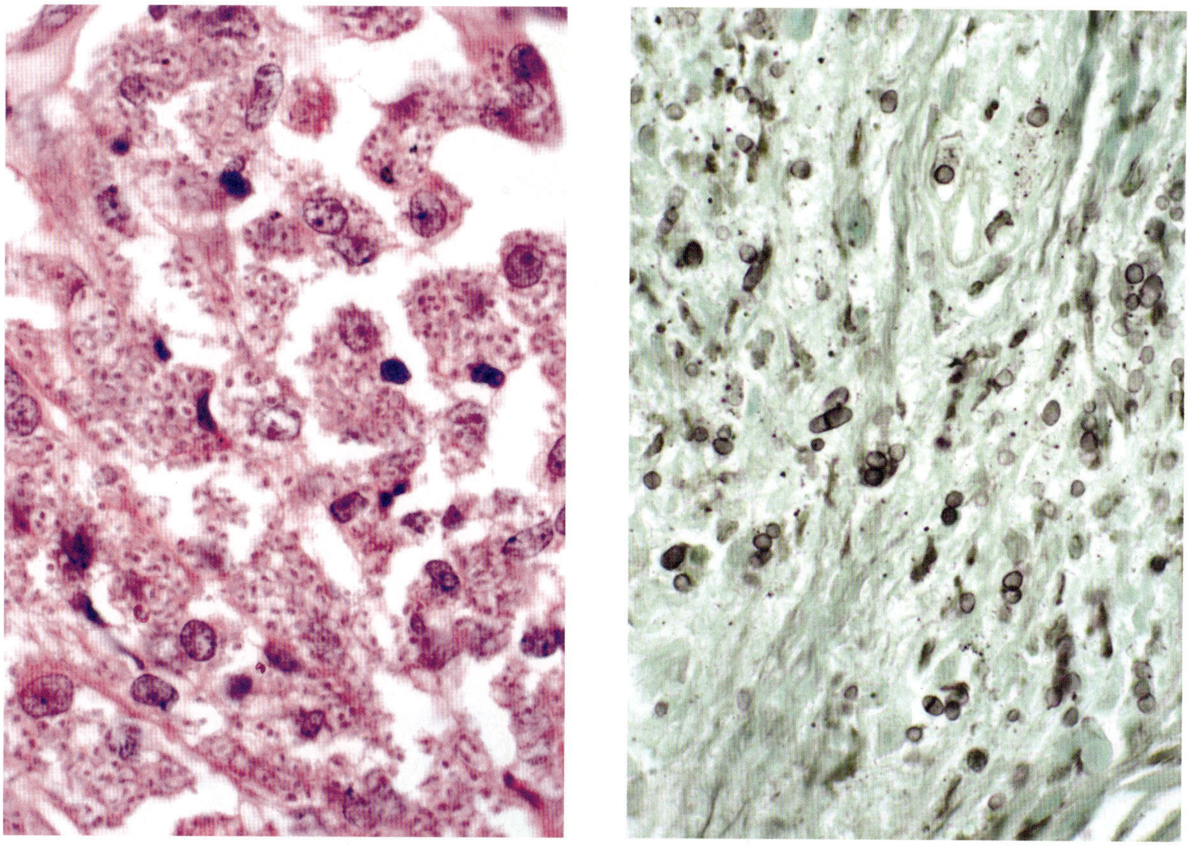

Figure 10-20

***PENICILLIUM MARNEFFEI*, LYMPH NODE**

Left: High magnification shows numerous fungal forms within macrophages.

Right: The organisms are highlighted with GMS stain. (Courtesy of Benjaporn Chaiwun, Chiang Mai University, Thailand.)

seen with *P. marneffei,* and if present, excludes the diagnosis. Rarely, septation is seen within the yeast and helps confirm the diagnosis.

Differential Diagnosis. *Histoplasma* is the closest mimic due to the similar size of the organisms. Close attention to morphologic features and clinical history (e.g., travel or residence in Asia) should help to differentiate the two.

Treatment and Prognosis. Both amphotericin B and ketoconazole are effective for treatment.

CANDIDA, TORULOPSIS GLABRATA, AND DERMATOPHYTES

Definition. Human infections with *Candida* species are common, although involvement of lymph nodes and spleen is rare. Included in this discussion is the closely related species, *Torulopsis glabrata.* Rarely, dermatophyte infections become disseminated and involve the lymph nodes and spleen.

General Features. Candidal infections are most commonly caused by *C. albicans, C. tropicalis, C. parapsilosis, C. krusei,* and *C. dubliniensis. T. glabrata,* formerly *C. glabrata,* has similar histologic and microbiologic features. Dermatophytes include the genuses *Epidermophyton, Microsporum,* and *Trichophyton.*

Clinical Features. In the United States, *Candida* infections are the most common fungal infections in hospitalized and immunosuppressed patients. Lymphadenitis typically only occurs with systemic infection, but rare reports exist of isolated nodal or splenic involvement (16,21,24). Cutaneous, vaginal, and mucocutaneous infections are the most common, and often precede disseminated infection. Oral

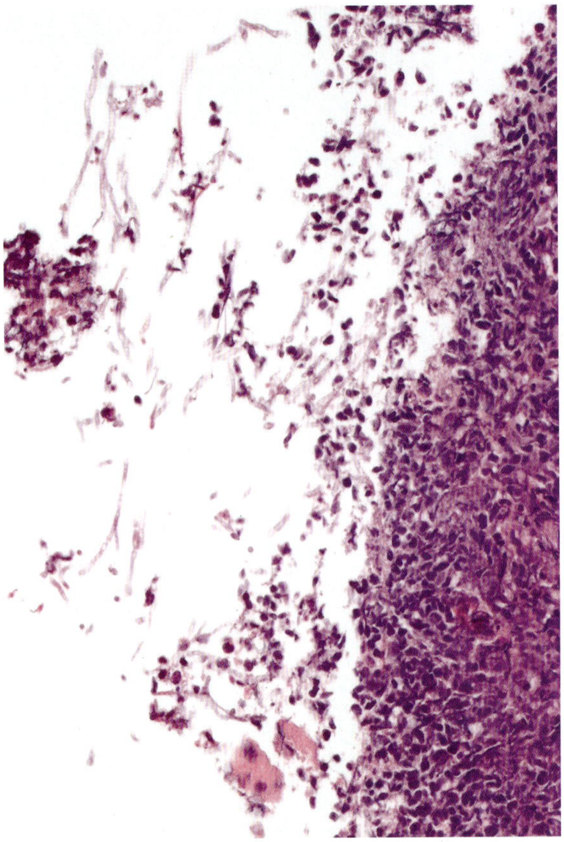

Figure 10-21

CANDIDA

Tissue infection with *Candida* shows numerous pseudohyphal forms.

candidiasis is a frequent finding in patients who are immunosuppressed. The clinical manifestations of *Candida* infection include fever, lymphadenopathy, skin lesions, endocarditis, and fungal abscesses. Systemic involvement in dermatophytic infections is rare.

Laboratory Findings. Candidal species are relatively easy to culture. Further, speciation of *Candida* can only be performed through culture. Identification of dermatophytes is also best performed through culture techniques.

Gross Findings. Lymph nodes affected with *Candida* infections show small miliary nodules that are 1 to 3 mm, tan, and friable (18). Rarely, splenic abscesses are associated with *Candida* species (20).

Microscopic Findings. The morphology is typical for *Candida* at other sites and includes both yeast forms and pseudohyphae. The yeast forms are ovoid and 3 to 6 µm. Numerous neutrophils are present in association with *Candida* infection (fig. 10-21). Multiple microabscesses are seen. Histochemical stains for fungi work well, but confirmation by culture is most appropriate for identification. Fungi are highlighted by GMS, PAS, and tissue Gram stains. Dermatophytes are identified by specific morphologic structures that develop and individually identify each species, but culture confirmation is advisable.

Treatment and Prognosis. Fluconazole is the primary choice for treatment of *Candida* infection. If systemic disease is present and resistant to fluconazole, itraconazole, caspofungin, or voriconazole may be effective.

ASPERGILLUS

Definition. *Aspergillus* is a relatively common fungal pathogen in humans. Although other forms exist, disseminated *aspergillosis* frequently involves the lymph nodes and spleen.

General Features. The commonly encountered species are *A. fumigatus*, *A. flavus*, and *A. niger*.

Clinical Features. *Aspergillus* organisms are worldwide in distribution. The main forms of aspergillosis are: allergic aspergillosis, invasive pulmonary aspergillosis, obstructing bronchial aspergillosis, and disseminated disease. When disseminated infection occurs, the mortality rate is high (1,5). Disseminated disease is common in immunosuppressed patients, especially those who are profoundly neutropenic.

Laboratory Findings. Culture, with morphologic identification of "fruiting bodies," identifies and speciates *Aspergillus*.

Microscopic Findings. The hyphae of *Aspergillus* are 3 to 6 µm wide, septate, and branch dichotomously (45 degrees). Angioinvasion is frequent and is often associated with hemorrhage and infarction (figs. 10-22, 10-23). In involved tissues, fungal forms are localized around affected vessels. Intense acute inflammation, predominantly neutrophilic, is common. Granulomatous inflammation may be present (9). The fungal hyphae stain well with the PAS and GMS stains.

Differential Diagnosis. Differentiation from zygomycetes is based on the presence of more frequent septations and dichotomous branching. The lack of pseudohyphae differentiates

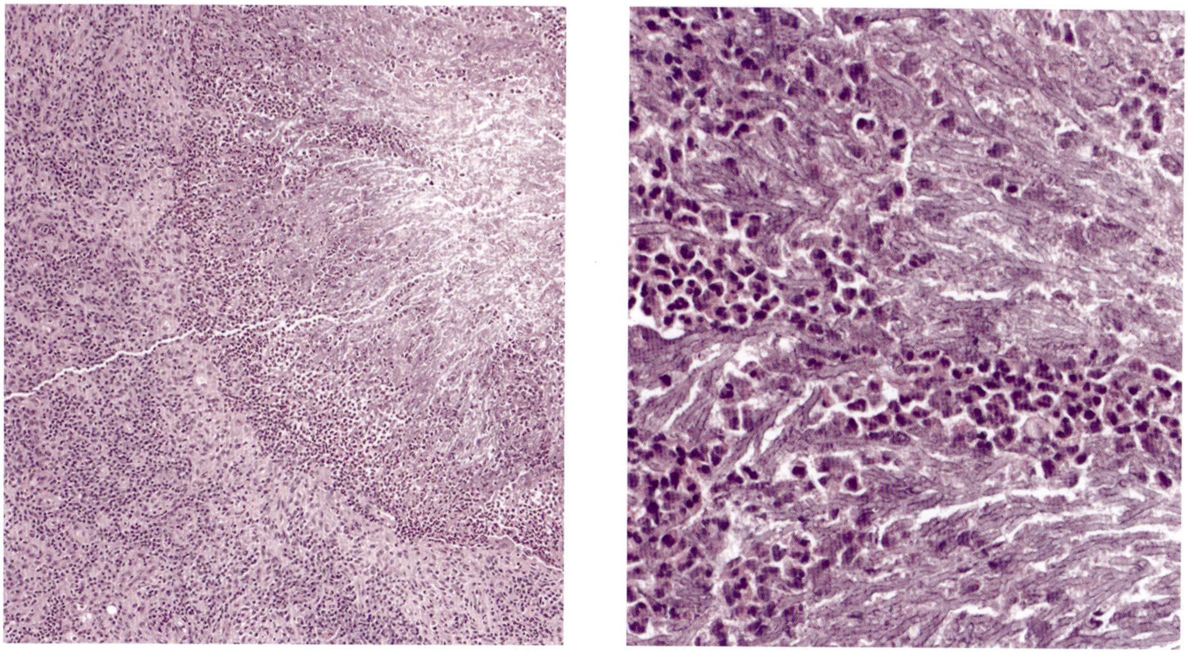

Figure 10-22

***ASPERGILLUS*, LYMPH NODE**

Left: A nodular aggregate of *Aspergillus* organisms in a lymph node with marked associated acute inflammation. Right: Higher magnification highlights the hyphal forms.

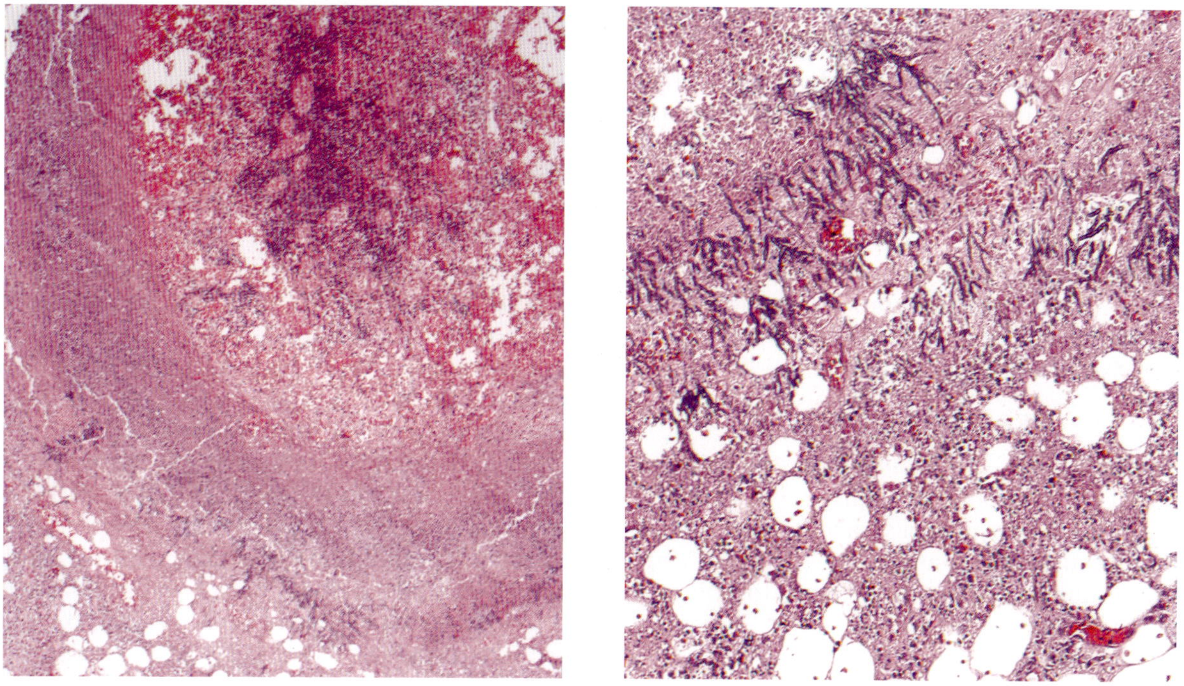

Figure 10-23

ASPERGILLUS

Numerous fungal hyphae (left) are positive for GMS (right). (Courtesy of Luis Fajardo, Palo Alto, CA.)

Aspergillus from *Candida* species. A single case of systemic infection due to *Chrysosporium zonatum* has been reported which closely mimicked *Aspergillus* infection (14).

Treatment and Prognosis. Amphotericin B and itraconazole are reasonable treatments, however, disseminated disease is typically fatal. Other, newer antifungal agents, such as voriconazole, may be more potent.

ZYGOMYCETES (INCLUDING *MUCOR* AND *RHIZOPUS*)

Definition. *Zygomycetes* are fungi with broad septate hyphae, and are associated with rhinocerebral or pulmonary infections. Lymph node or splenic involvement is seen in rare cases of disseminated infection.

General Features. Although *Rhizopus* and *Mucor* species are the most common, other causative forms of zygomycetes include *Rhizomucor, Absidia*, and *Cunninghamella*.

Clinical Features. These fungi are worldwide in distribution. Infection occurs through ingestion or inhalation of spores. Zygomycetes are opportunistic pathogens, and predisposing conditions for infection include diabetic ketoacidosis and hematologic malignancies. *Zygomycosis* is also seen in bone marrow transplant patients (8).

Microscopic Findings. The hyphae are broad (5 to 20 µm in width), with rare septation and rare right-angle branches (fig. 10-24). The walls are nonparallel, in contrast to *Aspergillus*. Vascular invasion, with subsequent hemorrhage and infarction, is common in zygomycosis. Hemorrhage, necrosis, acute inflammation, and abscess formation are common histologic findings. Zygomycetes stain with PAS and GMS, but are easily identified in H&E stains.

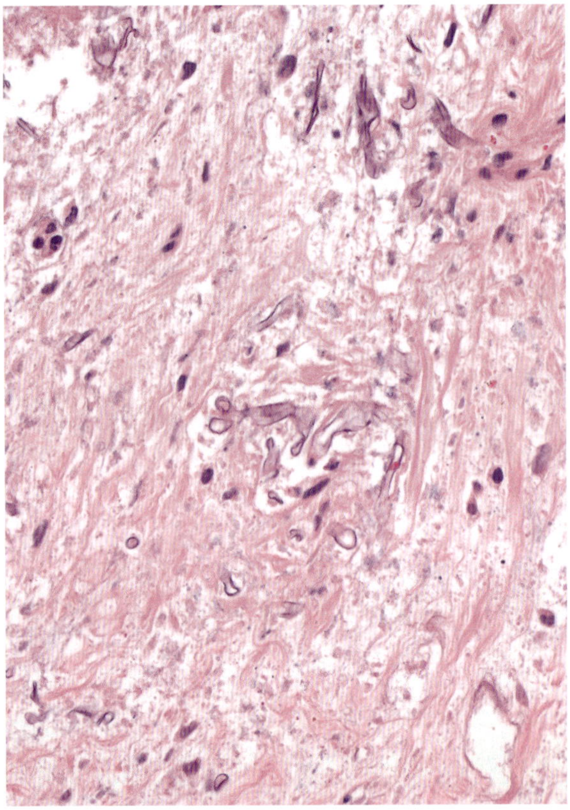

Figure 10-24

MUCOR

Necrotic tissue with irregular ribbon-like fungal forms of *Mucor* and adjacent necrotic tissue in an appendix.

CHROMOBLASTOMYCOSIS

Definition. *Chromoblastomycosis*, also referred to as *phaeohyphomycosis* or *chromomycosis*, is a chronic infection of skin and subcutaneous tissue caused by a variety of pigmented fungi. These dematiaceous fungi rarely involve regional lymph nodes.

General Features. The causative fungi of chromoblastomycosis are pigmented (dematiaceous) and reside in soil. Human infection is due to direct inoculation, typically in the lower extremities. Commonly encountered genuses are *Phialophora, Cladosporium, Fonsecaea, Exophiala, Alternaria, Bipolaris*, and *Wangiella*.

Clinical Features. Most commonly encountered in tropical climates, these fungi are also found in the southern United States. Infections are cutaneous, subcutaneous, or systemic. In cutaneous lesions, verrucous lesions overlie infected sites.

Microscopic Findings. Chromoblastomycosis is typically identified by the presence of dark brown, thick-walled fungi that are 5 to 12 µm in diameter (fig. 10-25). The deep brown pigment is caused by the presence of melanin, which may be identified by a Fontana-Masson stain. Short chains or clusters of dark brown yeasts are termed "Medlar bodies" or "copper pennies." Septation is seen within individual yeast forms. Granulomatous inflammation and microabscesses are also present, and extensive necrosis may be seen as well.

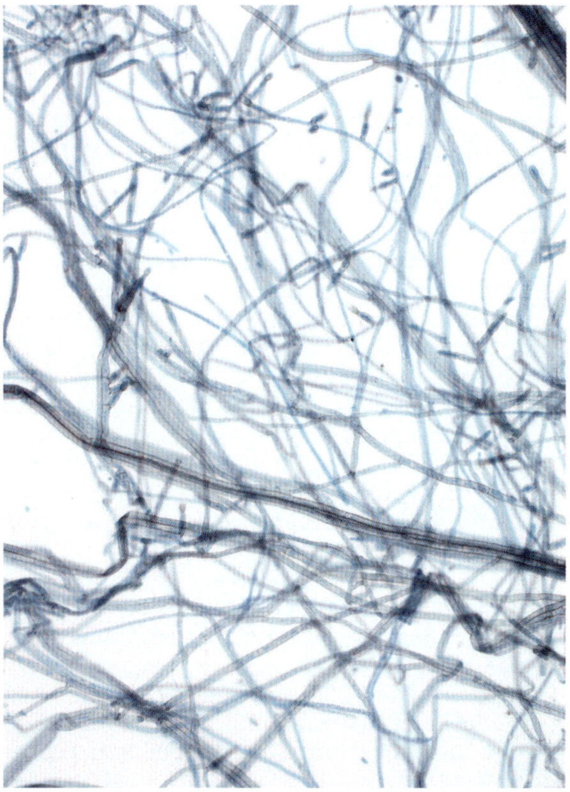

Figure 10-25

CHROMOBLASTOMYCOSIS

Slide culture of *Phialophora*, one of the causative fungi of chromoblastomycosis (lactophenol cotton blue stain). (Courtesy of Linda Marler, Indianapolis, IN.)

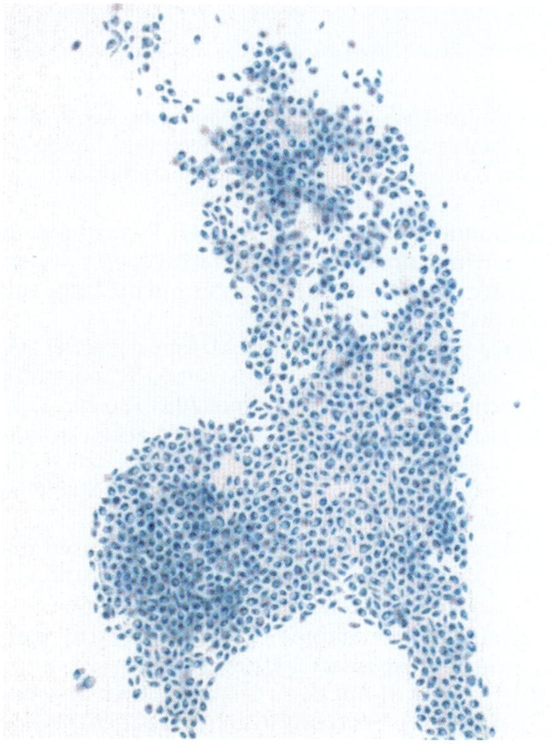

Figure 10-26

SPOROTHRIX

Slide culture of *Sporothrix* shows numerous fungal forms (lactophenol cotton blue stain). (Courtesy of Linda Marler, Indianapolis, IN.)

PSEUDOALLERICHIA AND *PETRIELLIDIUM*

Definition. *Pseudoallerichia* and *Petriellidium* are uncommon fungi, seen exclusively in immunocompromised patients. Disseminated disease is rare, but may have associated spleen and lymph node involvement (7). The fungi are found in soil.

Microscopic Findings. The features are identical to those seen in *Aspergillus* infections. Neutrophils, angioinvasion, hemorrhage, and necrosis are common. Distinction of *Pseudoallerichia* and *Petriellidium* from *Aspergillus* is accomplished by culture or antibody-based testing (18).

SPOROTHRIX SCHENCKII

Definition. *Sporothrix schenckii* is a fungus that can infect hosts without predisposing factors.

General Features. *Schenckii* occasionally causes enlargement of regional lymph nodes secondary to cutaneous infection, especially if the lesion is located close to a lymph node (3). The definitive diagnosis of *sporotrichosis* relies upon isolation of the organism in culture. Polyarticular arthritis is associated with disseminated infection. It is worldwide in distribution.

Microscopic Features. The histopathologic changes include suppurative granulomas with epithelioid macrophages and multinucleated giant cells that may become confluent (fig. 10-26). "Asteroids" are occasionally noted around the organism and can sometimes be visualized with special stains such as PAS or GMS. These asteroids are due to the Splendore-Hoeppli phenomenon, which is the deposition of proteinaceous material around fungal organisms. The yeast form of *S. schenckii* is cigar-shaped, 2 to 6 µm, yellow-brown, and only rarely seen in histologic sections.

REFERENCES

1. Callister ME, Griffiths MJ, Nicholson AG, et al. A fatal case of disseminated aspergillosis caused by a non-sporulating strain of Aspergillus fumigatus. J Clin Pathol 2004;57:991-2.
2. Connelly J, Ro JY, Cartwright J Jr. Pseudofungi in a lymph node. A case report with energy dispersive X-ray elemental analysis. Arch Pathol Lab Med 1991;115:1166-8.
3. Curi AL, Felix S, Azevedo KM, Estrela R, Villar EG, Saraca G. Retinal granuloma caused by Sporothrix schenckii. Am J Ophthalmol 2003;136:205-7.
4. Fish DG, Ampel NM, Galgiani JN, et al. Coccidioidomycosis during human immunodeficiency virus infection. A review of 77 patients. Medicine (Baltimore) 1990;69:384-91.
5. Hori A, Kami M, Kishi Y, Machida U, Matsumura T, Kashima T. Clinical significance of extra-pulmonary involvement of invasive aspergillosis: a retrospective autopsy-based study of 107 patients. J Hosp Infect 2002;50:175-82.
6. Khan ZU, Al-Anezi AA, Chandy R, Xu J. Disseminated cryptococcosis in an AIDS patient caused by a canavanine-resistant strain of Cryptococcus neoformans var. grubii. J Med Microbiol 2003;52:271-5.
7. Khurshid A, Barnett VT, Sekosan M, Ginzburg AS, Onal E. Disseminated Pseudallescheria boydii infection in a nonimmunocompromised host. Chest 1999;116:572-4.
8. Lee DG, Choi JH, Choi SM, et al. Two cases of disseminated mucormycosis in patients following allogeneic bone marrow transplantation. J Korean Med Sci 2002;17:403-6.
9. Mazzoni A, Ferrarese M, Manfredi R, Facchini A, Sturani C, Nanetti A. Primary lymph node invasive aspergillosis. Infection 1996;24:37-42.
10. Mohanty SK, Vaiphei K, Dutta U, Singh K. Granulomatous cryptococcal lymphadenitis in immunocompetent individuals: report of two cases. Histopathology 2003;42:96-7.
11. Restrepo A. Morphological aspects of Paracoccidioides brasiliensis in lymph nodes: implications for the prolonged latency of paracoccidioidomycosis? Med Mycol 2000;38:317-22.
12. Ro JY, Luna MA, Mackay B, Ramos O. Yellow-brown (Hamazaki-Wesenberg) bodies mimicking fungal yeasts. Arch Pathol Lab Med 1987;111:555-9.
13. Robinson MJ, Fogel R. Granulomatous lymphadenitis caused by Coccidioides immitis. J Am Osteopath Assoc 1994;94:578-2.
14. Roilides E, Sigler L, Bibashi E, Katsifa H, Flaris N, Panteliadis C. Disseminated infection due to Chrysosporium zonatum in a patient with chronic granulomatous disease and review of non-Aspergillus fungal infections in patients with this disease. J Clin Microbiol 1999;37:18-25.
15. Ruhnke M. Mucosal and systemic fungal infections in patients with AIDS: prophylaxis and treatment. Drugs 2004;64:1163-80.
16. Sang H, Wu B, Zhang X. Cervical lymphadenitis caused by Candida albicans. Mycoses 2003;46:422-4.
17. Severo LC, Oliveira FM, Irion K, Porto NS, Londero AT. Histoplasmosis in Rio Grande do Sul, Brazil: a 21-year experience. Rev Inst Med Trop Sao Paulo 2001;43:183-7.
18. Scott MA. Infections involving lymph nodes. In: Collins RD, Swerdlow SH, eds. Pediatric hematopathology. New York: Churchill Livingstone; 2001:289-311.
19. Sirisanthana V, Sirisanthana T. Disseminated Penicillium marneffei infection in human immunodeficiency virus-infected children. Pediatr Infect Dis J 1995;14:935-40.
20. Smith MD Jr, Nio M, Camel JE, Sato JK, Atkinson JB. Management of splenic abscess in immunocompromised children. J Pediatr Surg 1993;28:823-6.
21. Song DE, Kahn AG, Khang SK, Ro JY. Pseudofungi in pericolic lymph nodes. Arch Pathol Lab Med 2005;129:e97-100.
22. Teague MD, Tham KT. Hyphalike pseudofungus in a lymph node. Arch Pathol Lab Med 1994;118:95-6.
23. Trevenzoli M, Cattelan AM, Rea F, et al. Mediastinitis due to cryptococcal infection: a new clinical entity in the HAART era. J Infect 2002;45:173-9.
24. Vecchio R, Cacciola E, di Martino M, Cacciola RR, MacFadyen BV. A cause for conversion of laparoscopic splenectomy: splenic candidiasis. J Laparoendosc Adv Surg Tech A 2002;12:441-4.
25. Watts JC, Chandler FW. Pneumocystosis. In: Connor DH, Chandler FW, Schwartz DA, Manz HJ, Lack EE eds. Pathology of infectious diseases, Vol. II, Stamford, CT: Appleton & Lange; 1997:1241-51.
26. Yuen WC, Chan YF, Loke SL, Seto WH, Poon GP, Wong KK. Chronic lymphadenopathy caused by Penicillium marneffei: a condition mimicking tuberculous lymphadenopathy. Br J Surg 1986;73:1007-8.

11 PARASITIC AND MISCELLANEOUS INFECTIONS

Although the changes in infectious lymphadenitis may be nonspecific and similar to those elicited in other organ systems, there are important histologic features that often suggest an infectious organism. It is particularly difficult to categorize the changes seen in lymphadenitis due to parasites or other rare infectious organisms.

Most of the entities discussed in this chapter show a spectrum of histologic changes that depend on the stage of the disease or the status of the immune system. Aside from "typical" parasitic diseases, other unusual infections and agents (such as algae) are discussed, including those whose infectious potential and effects have only been partly described (such as prions).

TOXOPLASMA GONDII

Definition. *Toxoplasma* lymphadenitis is a manifestation of infection caused by the parasite *Toxoplasma gondii*. The characteristic histologic findings of *toxoplasmosis* in the lymph nodes include reactive follicular hyperplasia, clusters of epithelioid macrophages that occur within or near reactive germinal centers, and sinusoidal monocytoid B-cell hyperplasia.

General Features. The causative organism, *T. gondii*, is shed in the feces of cats in the form of oocysts, which are infective to humans. Other tissue forms, including tachyzoites and cysts containing bradyzoites, are transmitted primarily by the ingestion of uncooked meat. *Toxoplasma* has a high prevalence in warm and humid climates. Up to 40 percent of the adult population of the world has been infected by *Toxoplasma* (34,41).

Clinical Features. Toxoplasmosis is one of the most common human infections in the world. *Toxoplasma* has been estimated to cause 3 to 7 percent of clinically significant lymphadenopathy (41). Several clinical forms of toxoplasmosis are recognized: acute lymphadenopathy (with or without fever), severe acute systemic febrile illness, maternal infection during pregnancy with placental and fetal involvement, and in the immunocompromised, acute progressive encephalitis, myocarditis, pneumonitis, or retinochoroiditis. *Toxoplasma* lymphadenitis is the most common manifestation of infection in otherwise healthy adults. The average age of presentation is in the 3rd decade, although the age range is wide (41). The posterior cervical lymph nodes are usually involved.

Laboratory Findings. *Toxoplasma* infection is confirmed by serologic or microbiologic studies. *Toxoplasma* lymphadenitis is strongly suggested if the excised lymph node shows the appropriate histologic features.

Microscopic Findings. The characteristic triad of histopathologic features includes reactive follicular hyperplasia, scattered single or clusters of epithelioid macrophages within or in close proximity to germinal centers, and sinusoidal monocytoid B-cell hyperplasia (20,56). This triad of findings is reported as having a sensitivity of 44 to 63 percent and a specificity of 91 to 97 percent for the diagnosis of *Toxoplasma*, using the polymerase chain reaction (PCR) as the gold standard (21,37). Rarely, the cyst form is seen in a lymph node (3). In immunocompromised adults, toxoplasmosis may be associated with extensive necrotizing lymphadenitis and the presence of tachyzoites in cysts (figs. 11-1–11-3). The tachyzoites are 2 to 6 µm, and difficult to visualize on hematoxylin and eosin (H&E)-stained slides.

Ancillary Studies. Although immunohistochemical stains are commercially available to demonstrate the causative organism, definitive diagnosis currently relies upon the important correlation of serologic studies, clinical history, and classic histopathologic changes in the lymph nodes.

Differential Diagnosis. The main entity in the differential diagnosis of *Toxoplasma* lymphadenitis is human immunodeficiency virus (HIV)-associated lymphadenopathy, which can also cause reactive follicular hyperplasia, monocytoid B-cell hyperplasia, and scattered epithelioid macrophages. In HIV-infected hosts, however,

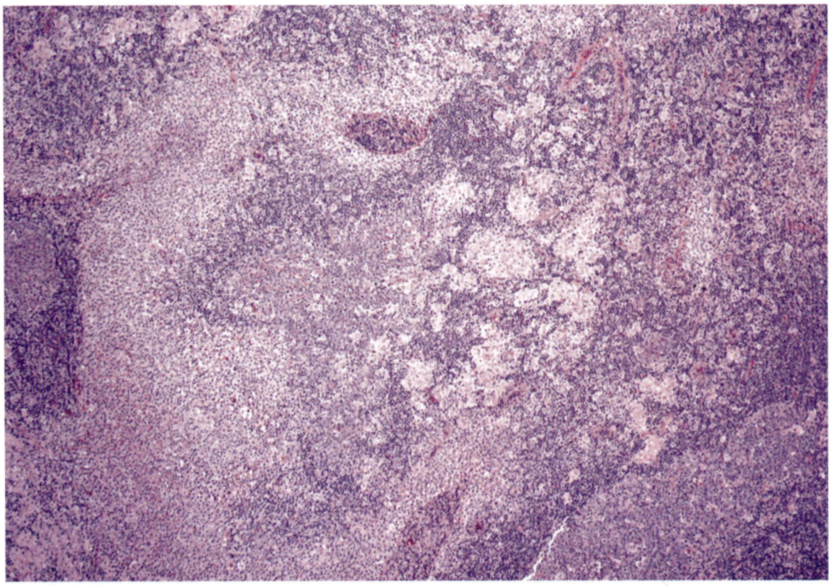

Figure 11-1

TOXOPLASMOSIS, LYMPH NODE

The cardinal features of *Toxoplasma* lymphadenitis include hyperplastic follicles, marginal zone hyperplasia, and granulomas.

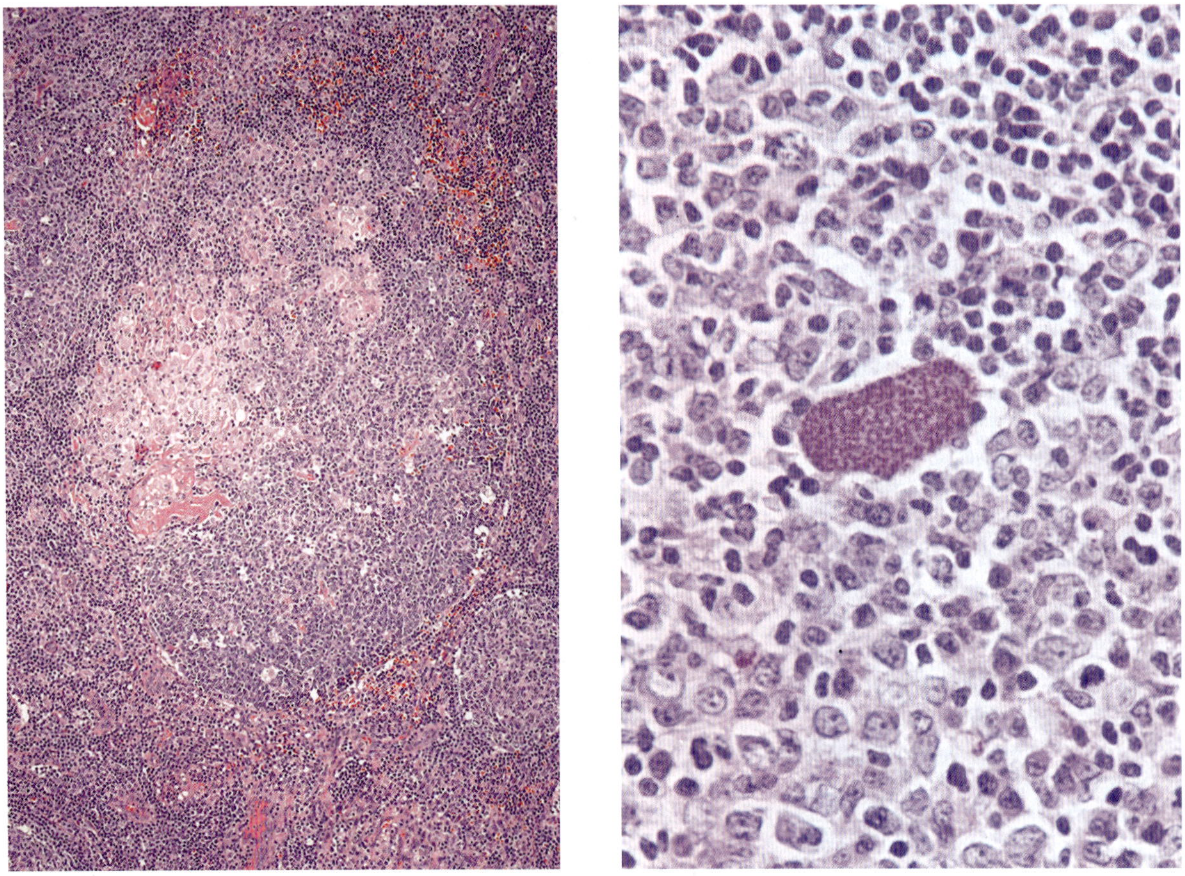

Figure 11-2

TOXOPLASMOSIS, LYMPH NODE

Granulomas, especially those that encroach upon germinal centers (left), are seen. Rarely, *Toxoplasma* cysts are seen in the infected lymphoid tissues (right). (Right figure courtesy of Dr. Karl Lennert, Kiel, Germany.)

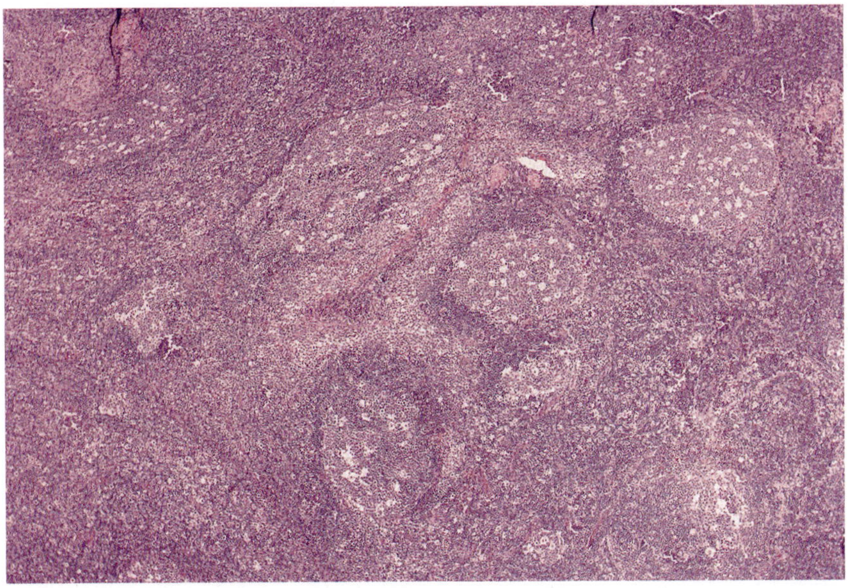

Figure 11-3

TOXOPLASMOSIS, LYMPH NODE

Marginal zone hyperplasia is seen in *Toxoplasma* lymphadenitis, although it is not specific for this diagnosis.

the epithelioid macrophages are not characteristically located within the germinal centers and the reactive germinal center hyperplasia tends to be more florid or explosive (55).

Occasionally, lymph nodes with prominent sinus histiocytosis show the formation of small groups of epithelioid cells without the reactive follicular hyperplasia and monocytoid B-cell hyperplasia associated with toxoplasmosis (46). The focal sinusoidal location of the monocytoid B cells and the absence of cellular atypia is consistent with a reactive rather than a neoplastic process (47).

Scattered microgranulomas are also seen in early syphilis in association with capsular fibrosis, perivascular plasmacytic infiltrates, interfollicular plasmacytosis, and microgranulomas. Visceral leishmaniasis may also demonstrate microgranulomatous lymphadenitis (60).

Treatment and Prognosis. Adult toxoplasmosis is responsive to combination drug therapy. If it is acquired during pregnancy and transmitted in utero, however, the damage to the fetus is irreversible.

ENTAMOEBA HISTOLYTICA

Definition. *Entamoeba histolytica* is well recognized as a pathogenic ameba, and associated with intestinal and extraintestinal infections. *Amebiasis* is present in lymph nodes draining sites of infection, and rarely, in the spleen.

General Features. Infection by *E. histolytica* occurs by ingestion of mature cysts in fecally contaminated food, water, or hands. The cysts develop and hatch in the small intestine, from which trophozoites are released and migrate to the large intestine. These ultimately produce cysts, which are passed in the feces. The cysts survive days to weeks in the external environment because of their durable outer coating. In some patients, the trophozoites travel through the bloodstream to extraintestinal sites such as the liver, brain, and lungs, with resultant histologic changes.

Clinical Features. The distribution of amebiasis is worldwide, with a higher incidence in developing countries. In the United States, groups with increased risk include male homosexuals, travelers, recent immigrants, and institutionalized populations. Many infections are asymptomatic; invasive intestinal amebiasis (diarrhea, colitis, appendicitis, amebomas) and extraintestinal amebiasis (liver abscess, peritonitis, pulmonary abscess, cutaneous and genital amebic lesions) are less common but are recognized more frequently.

Laboratory Findings. Microscopic identification of cysts and trophozoites in the stool is the common method for diagnosing *E. histolytica*. In addition, *E. histolytica* trophozoites are identified in aspirates or biopsy samples obtained during colonoscopy or surgery. *E. histolytica* must

Figure 11-4

AMEBIASIS

A: *Entameba histolytica* organisms are seen in large numbers in the fibrinopurulent exudate lining the ulcerated surface of the bowel.

B: The organisms are slightly larger than macrophages. Note the somewhat eccentric nuclei and the ingested red blood cells.

C: As the organisms invade the bowel wall they cause tissue necrosis. (Fig. 9-107D–F from Cooke RA. Infectious diseases: atlas, cases, text. Australia: McGraw Hill, Ltd; 2008:338.)

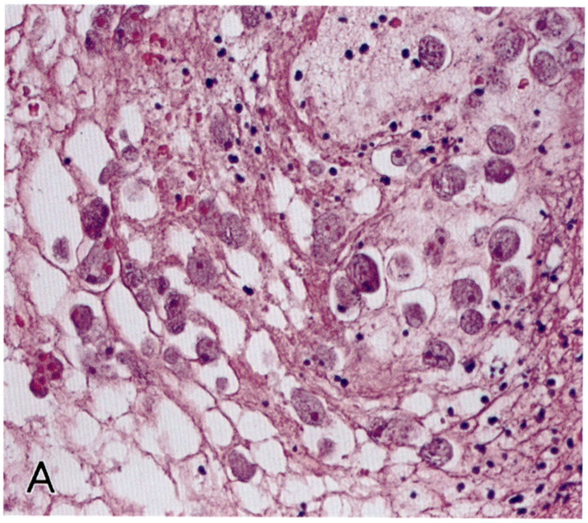

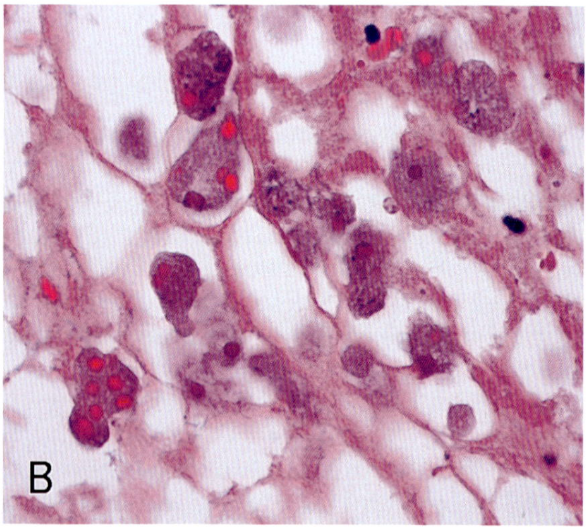

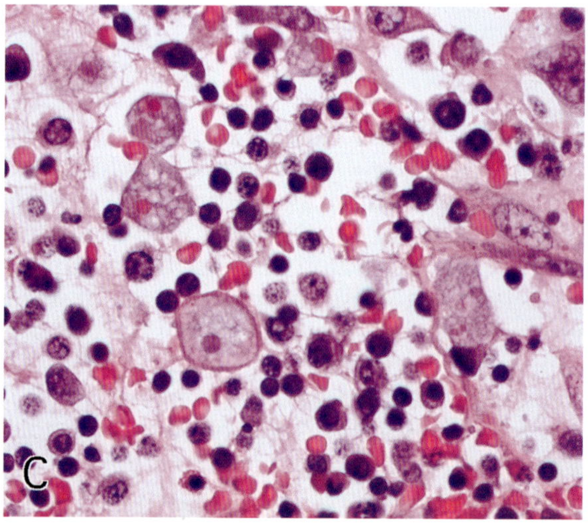

be differentiated from other intestinal protozoa and nonpathogenic amebae. Differentiation is based on the morphologic characteristics of the cysts and trophozoites. *E. dispar* is morphologically identical to *E. histolytica,* and differentiation is based on isoenzymatic or immunologic analysis. Molecular methods are also useful in distinguishing between *E. histolytica* and *E. dispar* and also identify *E. polecki.*

Microscopic Findings. When involving lymph nodes, the infectious amebae may be inapparent. They are most often found in sinuses and subcapsular spaces. They are usually associated with foci of necrosis. The size of the amebae (10 to 20 µm) is such that they may be easily confused with macrophages (fig. 11-4). The nucleus of the amoebae has a distinctive appearance with marginated chromatin. Also, amebae often have intracytoplasmic red blood cells or fragments. In experimental infections with *E. histolytica,* adjacent lymph nodes have shown progressive follicular hyperplasia, with an immunoblastic reaction and plasmacytosis (16). Later, there is lymphocyte depletion of the cords and histiocytosis. Follicular hyperplasia occurs in the spleen as well.

Differential Diagnosis. The primary difficulty is in initial identification of the pathologic ameba. Although several species exist which are not pathogenic (see above), it is unlikely that these would present in lymph node or spleen.

Treatment and Prognosis. For symptomatic infections by *E. histolytica* (e.g., hepatic abscess), the drug of choice is metronidazole or tinidazole, followed by treatment with iodoquinol, paromomycin, or diloxanide furoate.

OTHER PROTOZOA (*MICROSPORIDIUM, CRYPTOSPORIDIUM,* AND *ISOSPORA BELLI*)

Definition. *Coccidia* are a group of obligate intracellular protozoal parasites of humans. The entities in this group associated with human disease are *Cryptosporidium* species and *Isospora belli.* Another closely related group is the *Microsporidium* which includes *Encephalitozoon, Nosema, Pleistophora,* and *Enterocytozoon* genera. All are obligate intracellular parasites, and rarely involve the lymph nodes in disseminated disease.

General Features. Numerous species of microsporidia have been identified as human pathogens, although *Encephalitozoon intestinalis* is probably the most common. The infective form of microsporidia is the resistant spore, which can survive for some time in the environment. The spore infects the host cell, and once inside the cell, undergoes extensive multiplication. The spores have thick walls which allow them to survive for long periods in the environment. *Isospora belli* infects both humans and animals and has a similar life cycle.

Many species of *Cryptosporidium* infect humans: *C. parvum* and *C. hominis* are the most prevalent species causing disease in humans. Transmission of this group of protozoa occurs mainly through contact with contaminated water or food. Outbreaks of *Cryptosporidium* in the United States have occurred in water parks, community swimming pools, and daycare centers.

Clinical Features. Microsporidia, *I. belli,* and *Cryptosporidium* are increasingly recognized as opportunistic infectious agents worldwide, occurring mainly in patients with acquired immunodeficiency syndrome (AIDS). Additionally, cases have been seen in immunocompromised patients not infected with the human immunodeficiency virus (HIV) as well as in immunocompetent patients. A waterborne outbreak of *Cryptosporidium* occurred in Milwaukee, Wisconsin in 1993 and affected more than 400,000 people (40). Infections with these organisms have been reported in developed as well as in developing countries.

The clinical manifestations of microsporidia, *I. belli,* and cryptosporidia are diverse, with diarrhea the most common. Disseminated infection is rare, and most commonly seen in severely immunocompromised patients.

Laboratory Findings. Microscopic demonstration of the oocysts or spores in the stool is the basis for diagnosis. If stool examinations are negative, duodenal specimens should be examined by biopsy or string test. The oocysts can be visualized on wet mounts, with ultraviolet fluorescence, and are stained by a modified acid-fast stain. Immunofluorescence and PCR assays are available for some of these parasitic infections although usually only on a research basis. Peripheral blood eosinophilia may be present in *Isospora* infections

Microscopic Features. The spores of microsporidia, *I. belli,* and *Cryptosporidium* associated with human infection measure from 1 to 4 µm. In disseminated *Isospora* infection, numerous microgametocytes and macrogametocytes are seen within mesenteric lymph nodes (25,26,45,52). They are typically surrounded by a thick eosinophilic sheath. The organisms are associated with increased eosinophils and plasmacytosis. In splenic involvement, the organisms are present in the white pulp and red pulp (14). Studies have reported the presence of microsporidia within the macrophages of lymph nodes and spleen in disseminated cases (42,48,64). Other sites of involvement have extensive necrotic areas, surrounded by fibrosis and mixed inflammatory cells. The organisms are seen within the necrotic areas and in surrounding cells. Similar changes are seen with *Microsporidium* and *Cryptosporidium.* Many histochemical stains highlight the organisms, including Warthin-Starry, periodic acid–Schiff (PAS), and Giemsa, but they are less apparent with H&E stains.

Ancillary Studies. Transmission electron microscopy confirms the diagnosis of microsporidia, *I. belli,* and *Cryptosporidium* (42).

Treatment and Prognosis. Nitazoxanide improves the diarrhea caused by *Cryptosporidium* but is less effective in immunosuppressed patients. Improvement of the immune status reduces oocyst excretion and decreases the diarrhea. For infections caused by *Isospora,* trimethoprim-sulfamethoxazole is recommended. Albendazole is the drug of choice for the gastroenteritis caused by *E. intestinalis* and for disseminated microsporidiosis.

FILARIA

Definition. *Filarial infection* that involves the lymph nodes and spleen is due to filarial worms, parasitic nematodes that cause significant morbidity in tropical and subtropical countries.

General Features. The adult filariae are long, thin nematode worms which primarily inhabit the lymphatic vessels, testis, and epididymis. Fertilized females release microfilariae into the bloodstream, which are then taken up by biting mosquitoes; here the microfilariae metamorphose into infective third-stage larvae. The larvae then infect a new host via the mosquito's proboscis. Infective larvae subsequently enter the human host and migrate to a suitable location where they begin the slow process of maturing into adult worms (43).

Human filarial infections, which are endemic in tropical lowlands and coastal plains, are divided into *lymphatic filariasis* and *onchocerciasis* ("river blindness"). Lymphatic filariasis is a disease that results from infection by *Wucheria bancrofti* (most commonly in tropical and subtropical climates) or *Brugia malayi*; onchocerciasis is caused by *Onchocerca volvulus*. *W. bancrofti* is prevalent in Central and South America, Asia, and Africa while *B. malayi* is prevalent in Southeast Asia. *Loa loa* causes an asymptomatic infection and is commonly seen in Africa. A remarkable case of zoonotic lymphatic filariasis was reported in the United States in Michigan in 1993, most likely as a result of infection from the local animal population (22).

Onchocerca volvulus, which only causes disease in man, has a life cycle that involves the blackfly of the genus *Simulium* as its vector. Unlike brugian and malayan filariasis, the microfilariae inhabit the skin, not the blood, where they develop into infective larvae and are then deposited on the new host's skin. They course through the skin to the subcutaneous tissues where they mature to an adult worm in a nodular fibrous reaction known as an "onchocercoma." Worms can reside in these nodules for more than a decade and the females produce microfilariae, which migrate within the skin.

There are two major forms of onchocerciasis, each of which occurs in specific regions. In the Yemen Arab Republic, the organism causes a characteristic syndrome that is referred to as sowda, derived from the Arab word meaning black or dark. The clinical changes are often confined to one limb and include hyperpigmentation, edema, papular rash, and regional lymphadenopathy (28). The lymph nodes are characteristically large and soft, and histologically show follicular hyperplasia with an edematous, mucin-containing capsule. Microfilariae may be seen on H&E-stained slides.

Clinical Features. The clinical manifestations of lymphatic filariasis depend upon the susceptibility of the individual, the duration of infection, and the endemic location. Two distinct processes have been recognized. One results in lymphadenitis, lymphangitis, lymphedema, and elephantiasis from parasitic infestation of the lymphatic channels. The other process causes benign lymph node or spleen enlargement (*Meyers-Kouwenaar syndrome*) due to immunologic hyper-responsiveness of patients who live in certain areas of the Pacific or East Indies (figs. 11-5, 11-6) (30). The acute signs and symptoms of bancroftian and brugian filariasis include fever, malaise, nontender matted lymphadenopathy, and lymphangitis. *Loa loa* infection is known for its migration across the conjunctiva or eyelid, and is called the "eye worm."

Laboratory Findings. The definitive diagnosis of lymphatic filariasis is usually made by correlation of the clinical findings and identification of the microfilariae in the peripheral blood or in paraffin-embedded tissue sections. Peripheral blood eosinophilia is frequent.

Microscopic Findings. The histopathologic changes in filarial infection vary depending upon the stage of infection (35). Initially, the presence of the worm results in dilatation of the sinuses or lymphatic channels. This occurs in a background of lymphoid hyperplasia and a mixed inflammatory cell infiltrate. Occasionally, monocytoid B cells proliferate (23). Later, a granulomatous reaction, consisting of giant cells and epithelioid macrophages, develops, with eventual sclerosis, fibrosis, and calcific deposits (figs. 11-6–11-10). If the parasites are located in lymphatic channels that are exterior to the lymph node, they elicit a chronic inflammatory cell reaction with the formation of lymphoid follicles and aggregates.

Degenerating worms cause an acute inflammatory cell reaction consisting of neutrophils and eosinophils (43). Degenerating organisms may be noted in the center of discrete microabscesses or granulomatous necrotic foci. Lymph nodes containing dead organisms are necrotic

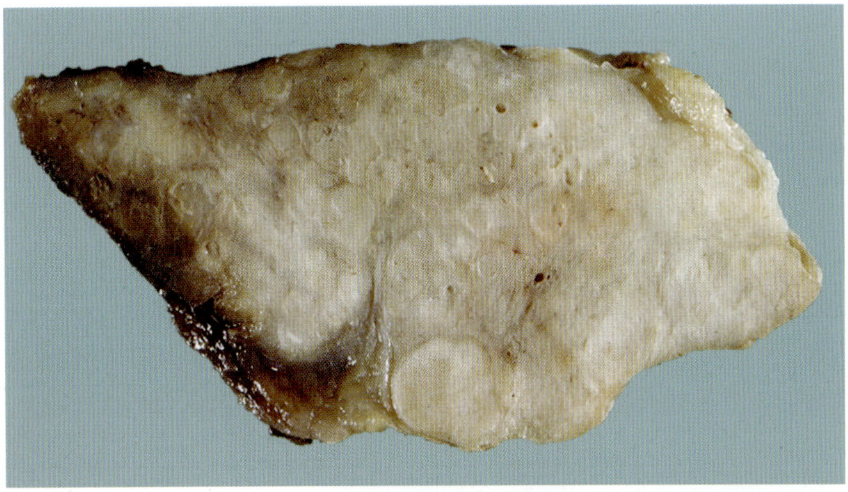

Figure 11-5

FILARIASIS, LYMPH NODE

An enlarged inguinal lymph node resulting from the presence of adult filarial worms. The architecture is markedly distorted by fibrosis. (Fig. 10-11 from Cooke RA. Infectious diseases: atlas, cases, text. Australia: McGraw-Hill, Ltd; 2008:360.)

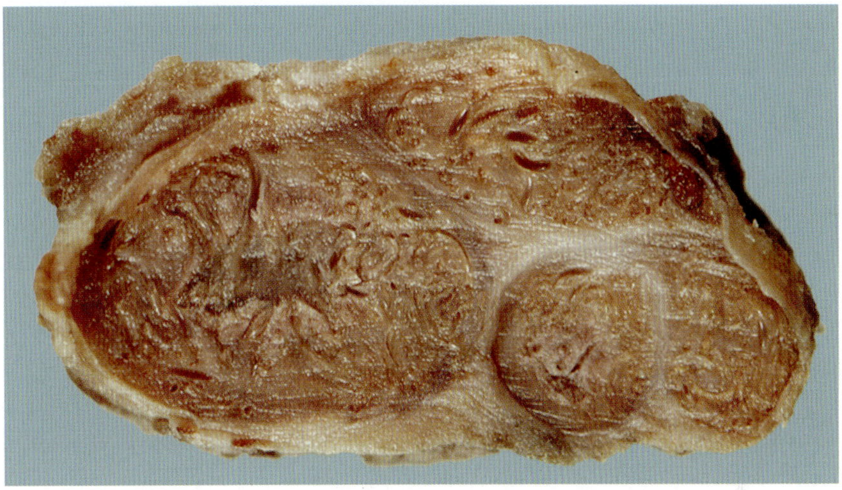

Figure 11-6

ONCHOCERCIASIS

Cut surface of a subcutaneous lump removed from the right hip region of an Australian male aged 30 years who had been working in Nigeria. (Fig. 10-27 from Cooke RA. Infectious diseases: atlas, cases, text. Australia: McGraw-Hill, Ltd; 2008:367.)

and have variable numbers of neutrophils, macrophages, giant cells, and granulomas that may contain parts of parasites. Eosinophils with Charcot-Leyden crystals and mineral deposits may also be noted.

Occasionally, a biopsy or autopsy specimen shows microfilariae within the blood or lymphatic channels. Focal vasculitis with thrombosis and occlusion may occur from blood vessel invasion. Lymphadenitis due to *Loa loa* has been described as having the following features: sinus histiocytosis with eosinophils, atrophic follicles, thickened capsule, increased numbers of mast cells and plasma cells with or without Russell bodies, and occasionally, microfilaria within capsular lymphatics (49).

The chronic stage of bancroftian and brugian filariasis develops 10 to 15 years after the initial infection in patients who are continuously infected. Elephantiasis develops in a small number of patients due to repeated episodes of lymphangitis and lymphedema resulting from the presence of dead or dying worms. The histopathologic changes are similar for both types of lymphatic filariasis. The size of the parasite, on cross section at midbody, and the thickness of the cuticle are features that help to distinguish *Wucheria* from *Brugia* (30). The female *Wucheria* has a maximum diameter of approximately 300 µm and a cuticle less than 1 µm thick. The female of *B. malayi* has a maximum diameter of approximately 170 µm, with a thick cuticle in relation to the diameter of the worm.

The African type of onchocercal lymphadenitis is characterized by large, firm, rubbery lymph nodes that histologically show capsular scarring and fibrosis of the pericapsular tissues and parenchyma of the nodes. There is a

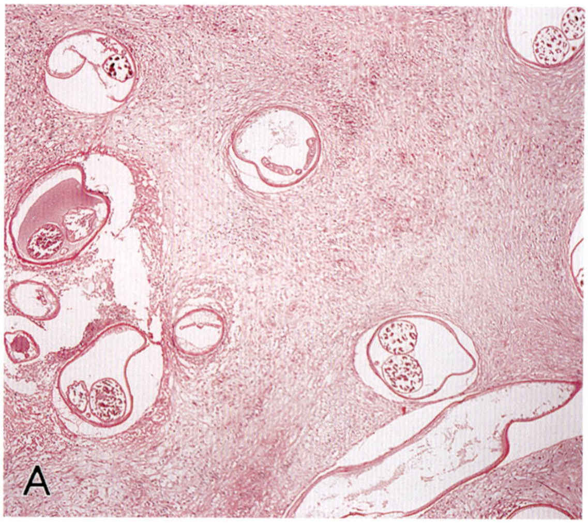

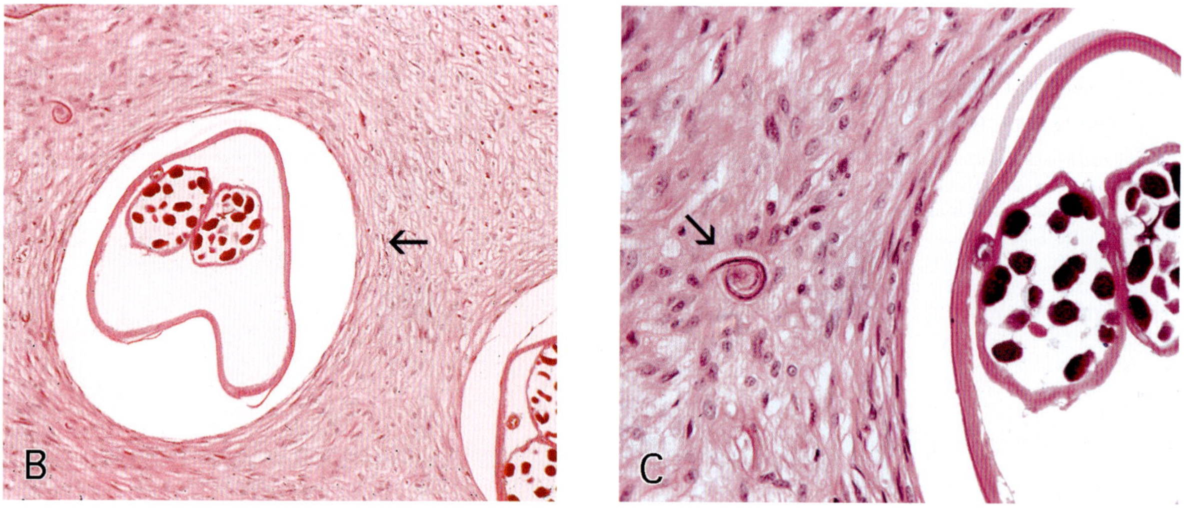

Figure 11-7

ONCHOCERCIASIS, LYMPH NODE

The microscopic section shows a fibrotic nodule throughout which are many adult *onchocerca* worms cut in transverse section. The morphology of these worms is similar to that of *W. bancrofti* but the adult worms are found in subcutaneous nodules and not in lymph nodes, and the microfilariae (arrow) are nonsheathed and are present in the dermis. (Fig. 10-28A–C from Cooke RA. Infectious diseases: atlas, cases, text. Australia: McGraw-Hill, Ltd; 2008:367.)

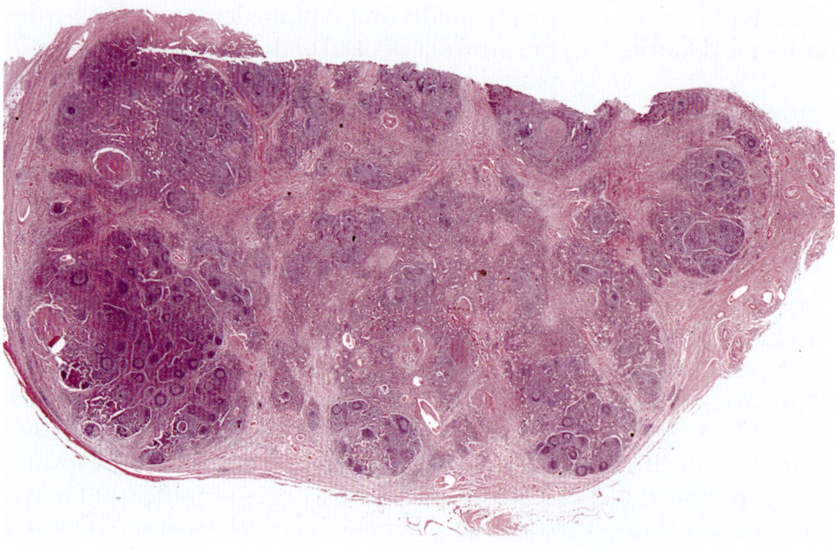

Figure 11-8

MICROFILARIAE, LYMPH NODE

The normal lymph node architecture is markedly distorted, with the blue-staining lymphoid tissue separated by broad bands of pink-staining fibrous tissue. The lymphatic sinusoids are considerably dilated. (Fig. 10-12 from Cooke RA. Infectious diseases: atlas, cases, text. Australia: McGraw-Hill, Ltd; 2008:360.)

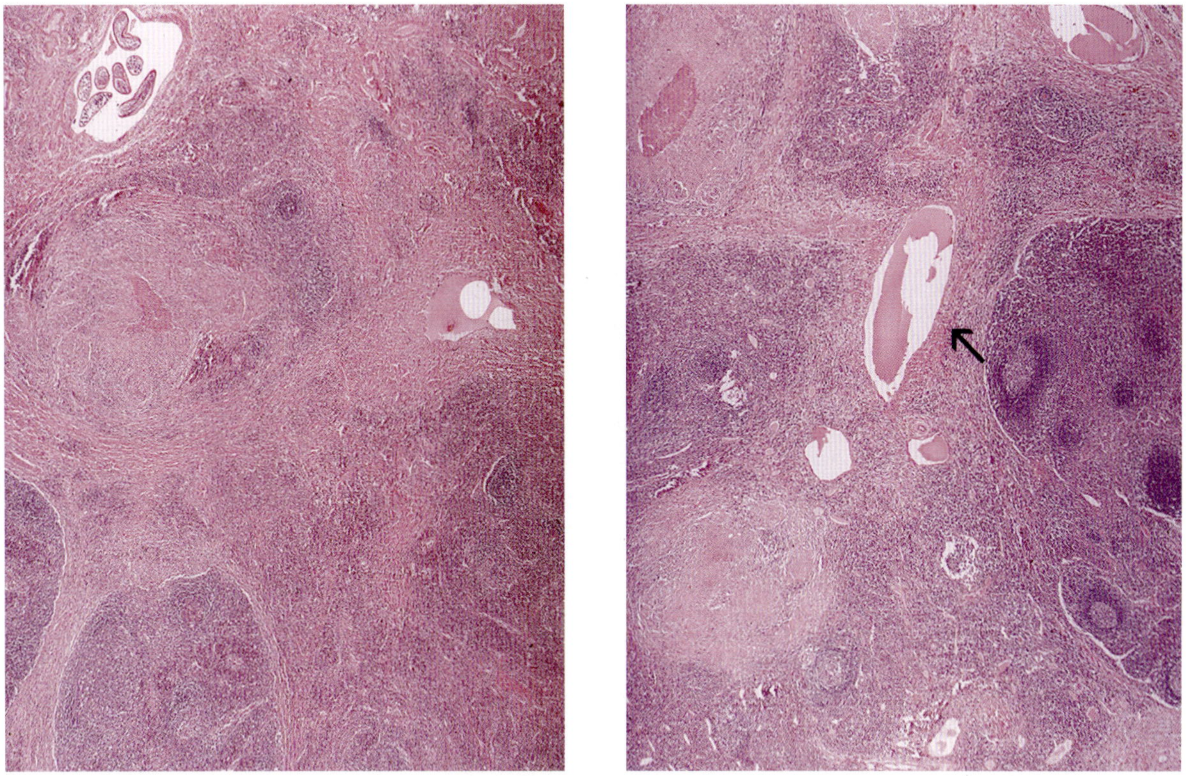

Figure 11-9

MICROFILARIAE, LYMPH NODE

Left: The dilated lymphatics are easily seen.

Right: Adult filarial worms are present in a dilated lymphatic vessel (arrow). (Fig. 10-13A,B from Cooke RA. Infectious diseases: atlas, cases, text. Australia: McGraw-Hill, Ltd; 2008:361.)

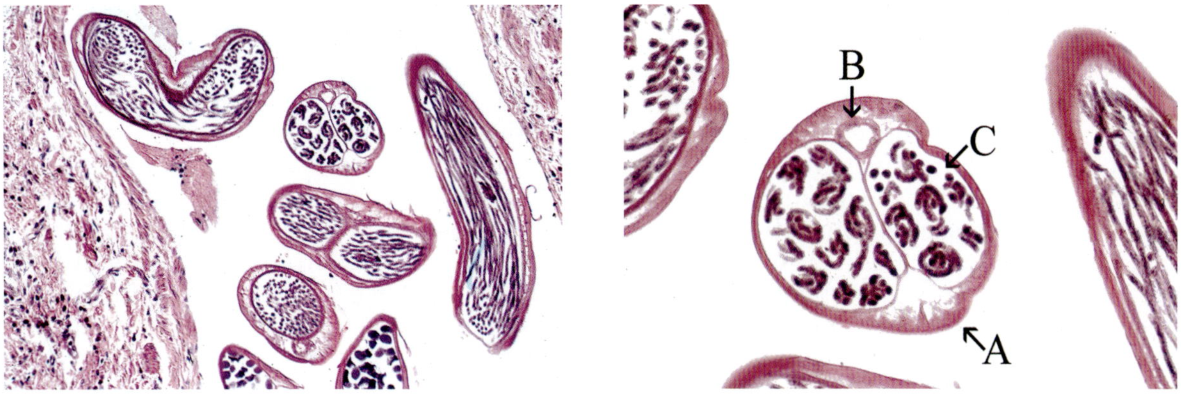

Figure 11-10

MICROFILARIAE, LYMPH NODE

Left: Adult female worms are cut in cross section.

Right: A high magnification view of a transverse section of an adult female worm is shown. The cuticle stains pink (A). There is an alimentary canal (B) and a bilobed uterus that contains microfilariae (C). (Fig. 10-14A,B from Cooke RA. Infectious diseases: atlas, cases, text. Australia: McGraw-Hill, Ltd; 2008:361.)

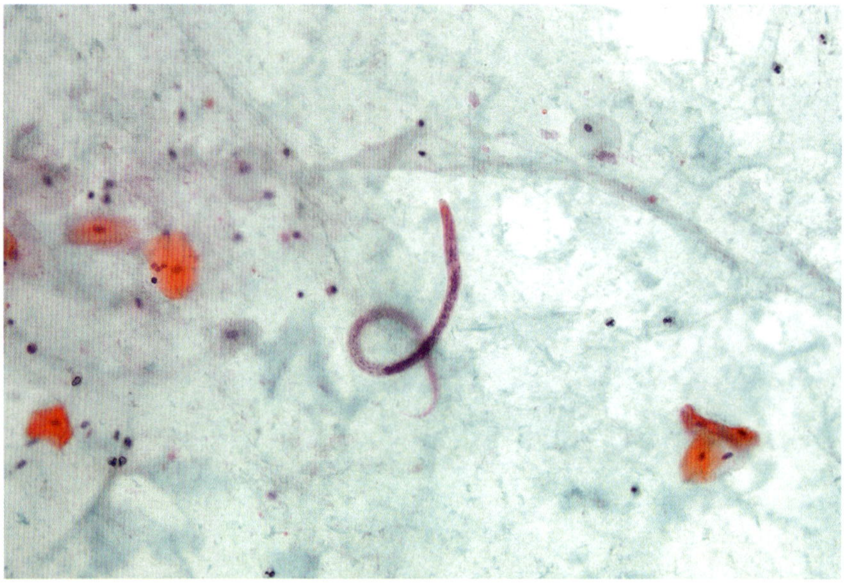

Figure 11-11

STRONGYLOIDES

The rhabditiform larvae of *Strongyloides stercoralis* are seen.

distinctive pattern of perivascular fibrosis with fibrinoid material. Other nonspecific findings include plasmacytosis with prominent eosinophilia, neutrophilia, and sinus histiocytosis, often in a background of lymphoid depletion. Deposition of melanin pigment may be noted in subcapsular macrophages. Russell bodies and giant cells may be seen in the medulla. Microfilariae are demonstrated in the fibrous capsule, interstitial connective tissue, perivascular fibrosis, and within lymphatic vessels. Eventually, elephantiasis develops as a chronic complication of the disease.

Differential Diagnosis. The differential diagnosis of lymphatic filariasis primarily includes onchocerciasis caused by *Onchocerca volvulus*. The diagnosis of onchocerciasis is made by correlating the clinical presentation with the identification of either the microfilariae or the adult worm in tissue sections. The definitive diagnosis relies upon the recognition of the organism's characteristic morphologic features and size (i.e., a maximum diameter of the adult male of 125 µm and 350 µm for the female). The cuticle measures 6 µm and appears two-layered in longitudinal sections. It contains discrete, regularly spaced ridges. *O. volvulus* is the largest human filarial organism and may measure up to 50 cm.

Treatment and Prognosis. Lymphatic filariasis is treated with diethylcarbamazine, a specific microfilarial drug (although adult worms are occasionally killed as well) (43). The fibrosis and lymphedema, however, are not reversible (58). The treatment for Onchocerca is diethylcarbamazine, which may cause painful lymphadenitis due to the degeneration of large numbers of microfilariae. Suramin has also been used to treat adult worms as well as the microfilariae.

NEMATODE INFECTIONS (INCLUDING *STRONGYLOIDES*) AND OTHER PARASITIC WORMS

Definition. *Nematodes* occasionally infect lymph nodes and spleen. Although *Strongyloides stercoralis* is the most frequent pathogen, there are several other species that may cause lymph node disease.

General Features. *Strongyloides* has a complex life cycle. The rhabditiform larvae pass in stool to become free living adult males and females that produce eggs from which rhabditiform larvae hatch. The larvae penetrate the human host skin through contaminated soil to initiate the parasitic cycle. They are transported to the lungs; carried through the bronchial tree to the pharynx; swallowed and then reach the small intestine. They then develop into adult females and produce eggs which yield rhabditiform larvae (fig. 11-11). The rhabditiform larvae may cause autoinfection.

Strongyloides stercoralis causes a worldwide parasitic infection of relatively high prevalence,

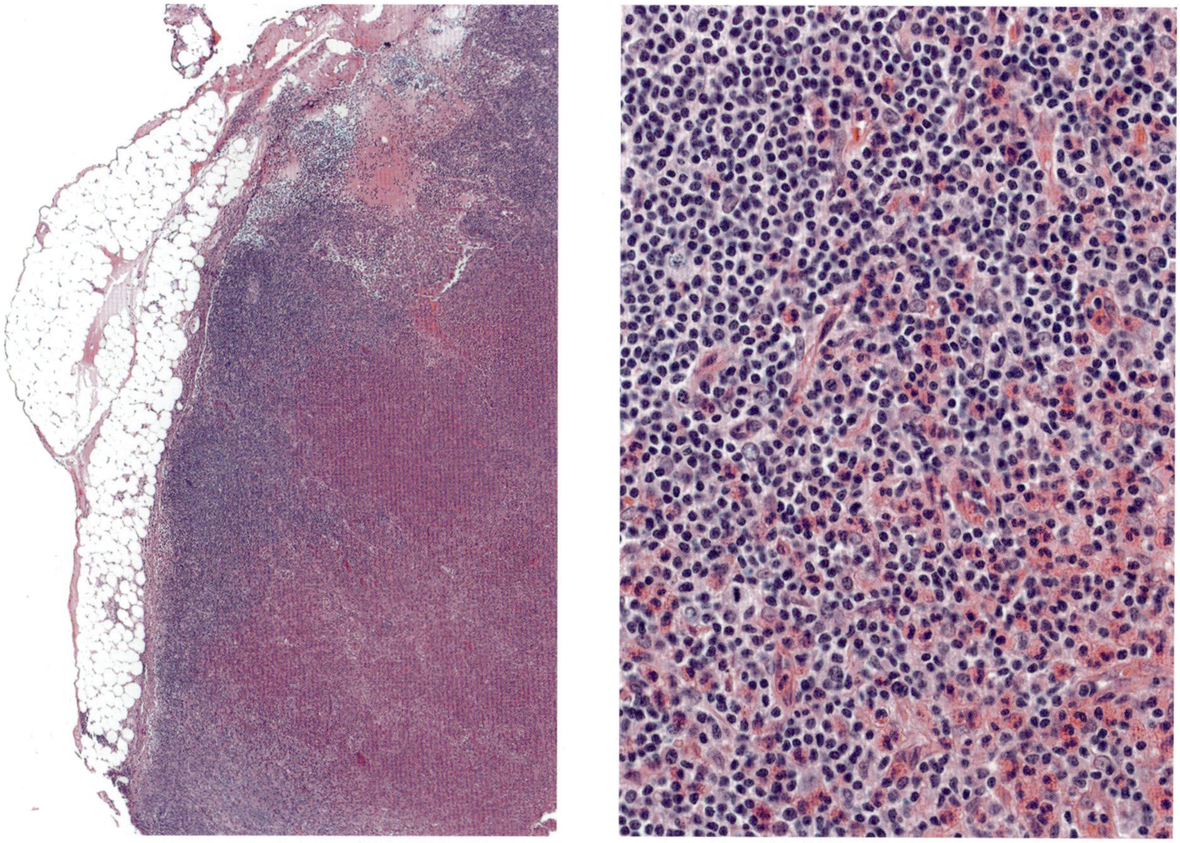

Figure 11-12

VISCERAL LARVA MIGRANS, LYMPH NODE

In this lymph node with *Toxocara*, there is massive eosinophilia, although no organisms are identified.

which is found in tropical and subtropical areas but also in temperate areas. In the United States, the parasite is most prevalent in Kentucky, Tennessee, Louisiana, and Texas and is more frequent in rural areas, institutional settings, and lower socioeconomic groups.

Clinical Features. *Strongyloides* infection is frequently asymptomatic. Gastrointestinal symptoms include abdominal pain and diarrhea. Pulmonary symptoms (including Loeffler syndrome) occur during pulmonary migration of the filariform larvae. Disseminated strongyloidiasis occurs in immunosuppressed patients, who present with abdominal pain, shock, and septicemia; disease in this population is frequently fatal (31).

Other parasitic nematodes seen in the lymph nodes are: *Ascaris, Trichuris* (whipworms), *Enterobius* (pinworms), *Trichinella*, and *Ancylostoma* (hookworms) (59). Roundworms of the species *Toxocara canis* or *T. catti* (visceral larva migrans) are also seen in lymph nodes (fig. 11-12).

Laboratory Findings. The diagnosis of *Strongyloides* rests on the microscopic identification of larvae in the stool or duodenal fluid using techniques such as the string test or duodenal aspiration. Larvae may be detected in sputum from patients with disseminated strongyloidiasis. Blood eosinophilia is generally present during the acute and chronic stages, but may be absent in disseminated disease.

Microscopic Findings. In the case of *Strongyloides*, the presence of larvae (most frequently seen), eggs, adult forms in lymph nodes distant from lung, gastrointestinal tract, or spleen, is evidence of disseminated disease. Larvae may be seen in the lymphoid sinuses, with little associated inflammatory reaction. If noncaseating granulomas are present, fragments of larvae may be seen within the granulomas. Eosinophils

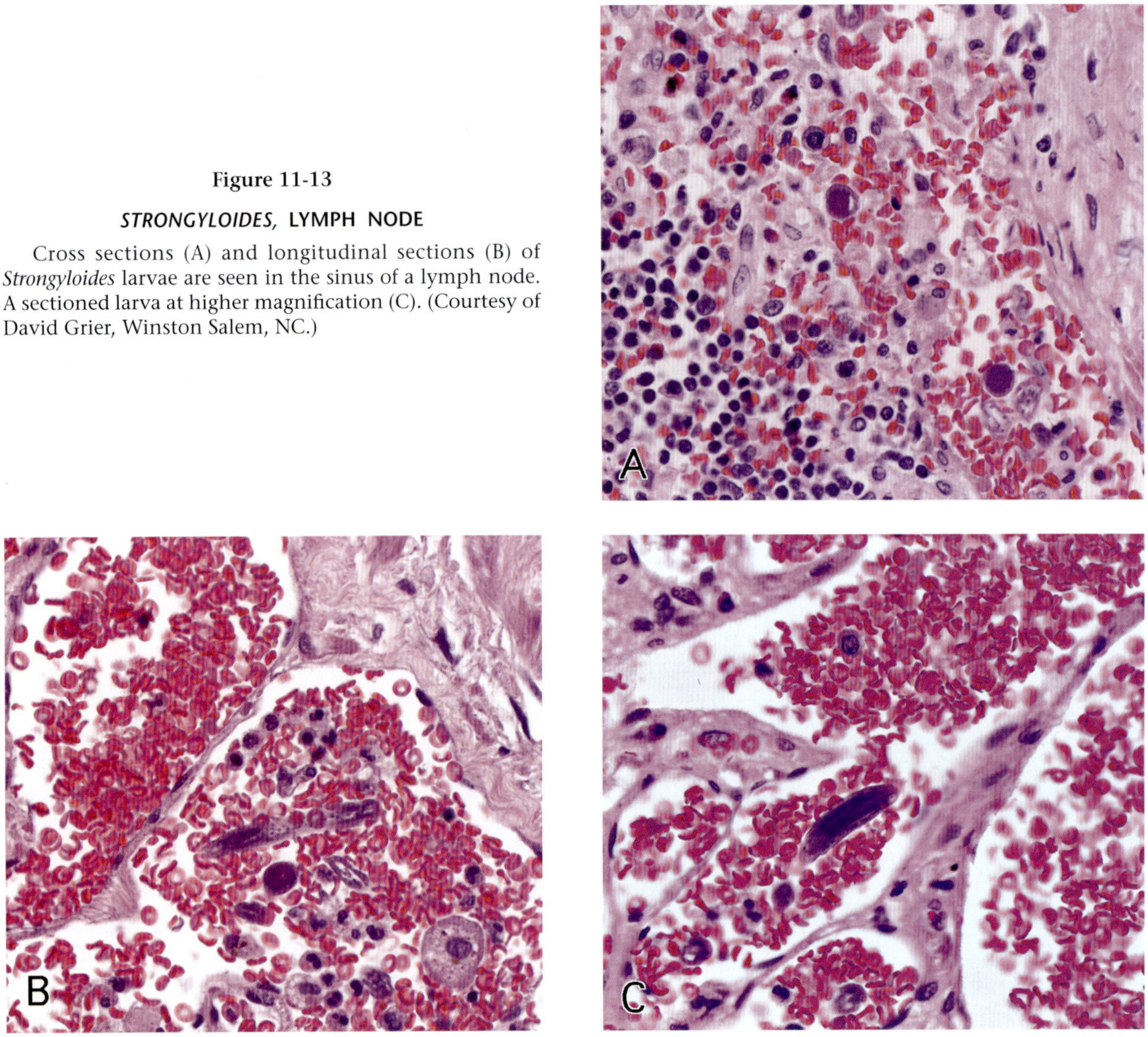

Figure 11-13

STRONGYLOIDES, LYMPH NODE

Cross sections (A) and longitudinal sections (B) of *Strongyloides* larvae are seen in the sinus of a lymph node. A sectioned larva at higher magnification (C). (Courtesy of David Grier, Winston Salem, NC.)

may be prominent, with varying numbers of lymphocytes, plasma cells, and macrophages.

Infestation of lymph nodes or spleen with other nematodes shows similar histologic features. Inflammation, with or without granulomas, is common. There are mixtures of acute and chronic inflammation, with prominent eosinophilia. Fragments of worms are often seen (fig. 11-13). Specific species are identified by the morphologic findings of size, surface structures (e.g., cuticle), and internal structures.

Differential Diagnosis. Infections by nematodes, roundworms, and hookworms are rare, and may be difficult or impossible to identify by morphology alone. Evaluation of the morphologic appearance of the fragmented worms may allow speciation. In these cases, reference to specialized texts or experts is recommended (9,44).

Treatment and Prognosis. The drug of choice for the treatment of uncomplicated strongyloidiasis is ivermectin, with albendazole as the alternative. All patients who are at risk of disseminated strongyloidiasis should be treated aggressively, given the high morbidity associated with this complication (31).

ECHINOCOCCUS

Definition. *Hydatid disease,* also known as *hydatidosis,* is caused by *Echinococcus* tapeworms. Most frequently seen as splenic cysts, rare lymph node changes are also encountered (see chapter 19).

General Features. *Echinococcus granulosus* is the most frequent cause of infections. Other

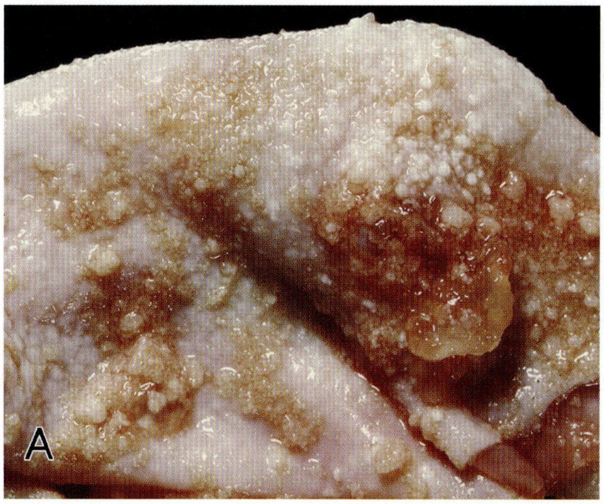

Figure 11-14

ECHINOCOCCUS

A: A view of the inner lining of the hydatid cyst. Multiple small nodules are on the surface.

B: View of the laminated membrane (A), the germinal epithelium (B), and the developing daughter cysts (C).

C: View of the edge of the hydatid cyst. A piece of laminated membrane adheres to the adjacent lung. Often, the laminated membrane is the only microscopic indication of the presence of a hydatid cyst, and is diagnostic. Nowadays patients are treated before surgical removal of the cysts and by the time the cyst is seen in the laboratory, the germinal epithelium has been destroyed. (Figs. 10-143, 10-144, 10-152) from Cooke RA. Infectious diseases: atlas, cases, text. Australia: McGraw-Hill, Ltd; 2008:417, 422.)

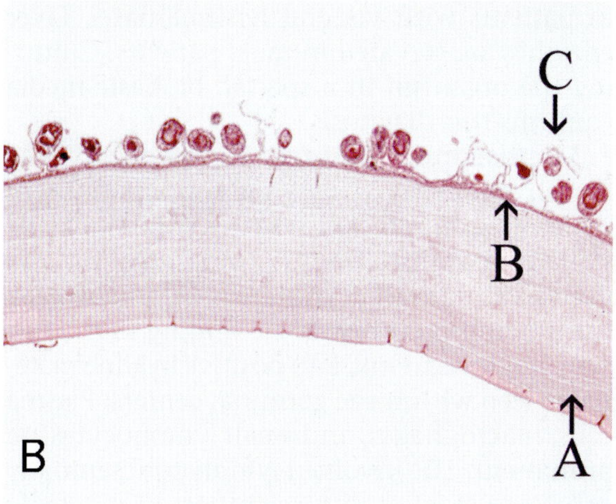

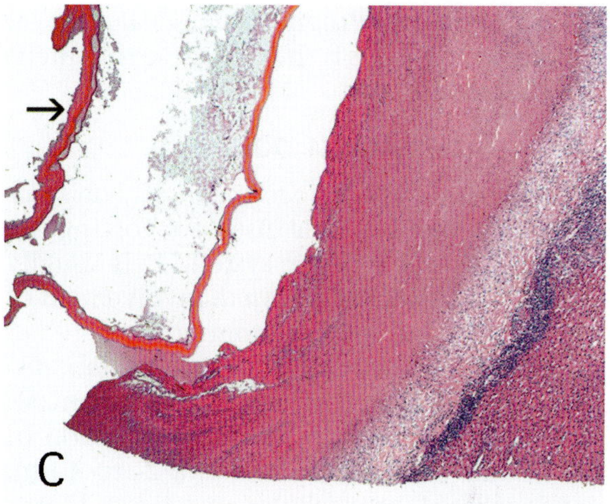

species (*E. multilocularis*, *E. vogeli*, *E. oligarthrus*) also cause human disease. The adult *Echinococcus* resides in the small bowel of the definitive hosts, usually dogs. These adults release eggs that are passed in the feces. Humans become infected by ingesting eggs, which hatch in the small bowel, enter the circulatory system, and migrate to the liver and lungs. In these organs, a cyst develops, producing protoscolices and daughter cysts that fill the cyst interior. *E. granulosus* occurs practically worldwide, and more frequently in rural, grazing areas where dogs ingest organs from infected animals.

Clinical Features. Echinococcal cysts of the spleen are rare, usually solitary, and have imaging characteristics similar to those of hepatic hydatid cysts. Radiologic studies are usually diagnostic. Serologic testing is more specific, but less sensitive, than most imaging modalities. Most patients are asymptomatic. Large cysts, however, may cause pressure symptoms owing to compression of other viscera. Severe complications occur because of secondary infection, rupture of the cyst into adjacent structures, or intraperitoneal anaphylaxis.

Gross Findings. Splenic cysts vary in size. Scolices develop on the inner aspect of the capsule, forming a sand-like material ("hydatid sand"). This becomes suspended in the cyst fluid.

Microscopic Findings. The microscopic features of echinococcal cysts are described in detail in chapter 19. Scolices are recognized in imprints of the cyst wall and, occasionally, in histologic sections. Each scolex is about 100 µm, and has suckers and a double row of hooklets (fig. 11-14). Lymph nodes adjacent to echinococcal cysts may be enlarged and show follicular hyperplasia, a paucicellular paracortical region, and marked plasmacytosis (66).

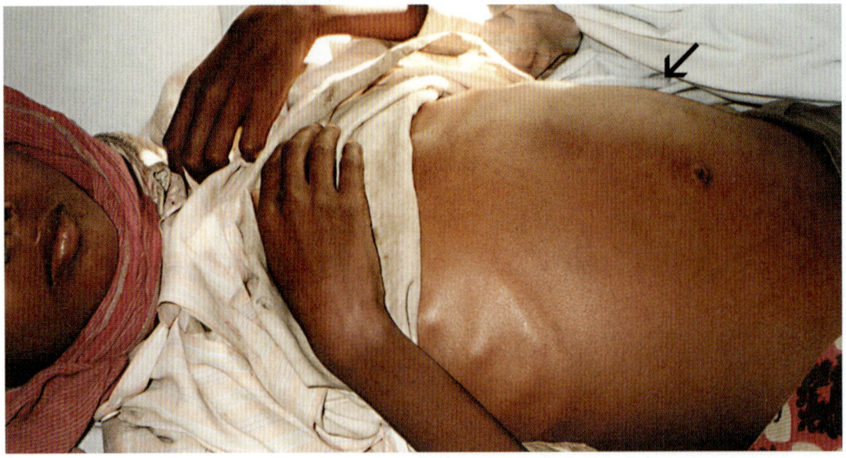

Figure 11-15

LEISHMANIASIS, SPLEEN

A sick child from Bihar state in northern India presented with fever, wasting, and splenomegaly. The clinical diagnosis was kala-azar. This diagnosis was confirmed by examining a Giemsa-stained smear made from a fine needle aspirate from the spleen. (Fig. 9-14 from Cooke RA. Infectious diseases: atlas, cases, text. Australia: McGraw-Hill, Ltd; 2008:296.)

Treatment and Prognosis. Surgical removal of *Echinococcus* cysts is the definitive treatment (see chapter 19).

LEISHMANIA DONOVANI

Definition. *Visceral leishmaniasis*, or *kala-azar*, is a severe systemic disease involving the mononuclear-phagocytic system. It is usually caused by *Leishmania donovani*. Involvement of lymph node and spleen is common.

General Features. Also known as *Black disease* and *Dum Dum fever*, visceral leishmaniasis is a relatively common protozoal infection in the Middle East. *L. donovani* is a 2- to 4-µm, nonflagellated, intracellular amastigote that is transmitted via the bite of a sandfly (33). Cutaneous leishmaniasis, also endemic in the Middle East, is due to infection by other species, such as *L. major, L. (vianna) braziliensis, L. tropica,* and *L. amazonensis* (4,18,27,57). These species less commonly cause visceral disease.

Clinical Features. The clinical presentation of visceral leishmaniasis includes weight loss, hepatomegaly, splenomegaly (over 95 percent of cases), fever, pancytopenia, and lymphadenopathy (over 50 percent of cases) (fig. 11-15). The inguinal, axillary, cervical, and epitrochlear lymph nodes are often enlarged (70). Nausea, vomiting, and diarrhea may also occur in affected patients. The latency period after the initial bite by an infected sandfly to the onset of clinical manifestations can be months or years. Ninety percent of cases of visceral leishmaniasis occur in Brazil, India, Sudan, Nepal, and Bangladesh (70).

Laboratory Findings. Anemia, leukopenia, and thrombocytopenia are common findings in patients with visceral leishmaniasis. Liver enzymes are elevated in most patients. Culturing the organism in a special, biphasic media confirms this diagnosis.

Microscopic Findings. Histologically, the lymph nodes show varying combinations of hyperplasia and foci of necrosis, which may be stellate in appearance (27,67). Caseating and noncaseating granulomas are seen, and become the predominant histologic finding as the disease progresses. Pink, PAS-positive hyaline material is seen within the germinal centers. Plasma cells, macrophages, and small lymphocytes are prominent. The involved lymph nodes initially consist of focal or diffuse clusters of markedly swollen phagocytic macrophages stuffed with *Leishmania* organisms (amastigotes). These organisms are visualized in H&E-stained tissue sections (fig. 11-16) or smears as two basophilic dots comprising the nucleus and kinetoplast; these are better visualized by Giemsa staining.

The initial presentation may be as a draining, suppurative lymph node (bubo). Necrosis and purulent acute inflammation are the dominant findings at this stage. The splenic changes include deposition of extracellular PAS-positive hyaline material, white pulp necrosis, and lymphocyte depletion of the white pulp (figs. 11-17, 11-18) (67).

Lymph node involvement may be seen with cutaneous leishmaniasis, with similar histopathologic features (18,27). The chronic changes in lymph nodes associated with cutaneous disease include fibrosis and capsular thickening.

Ancillary Studies. *Leishmania* amastigotes are PAS, Gomori methenamine silver (GMS),

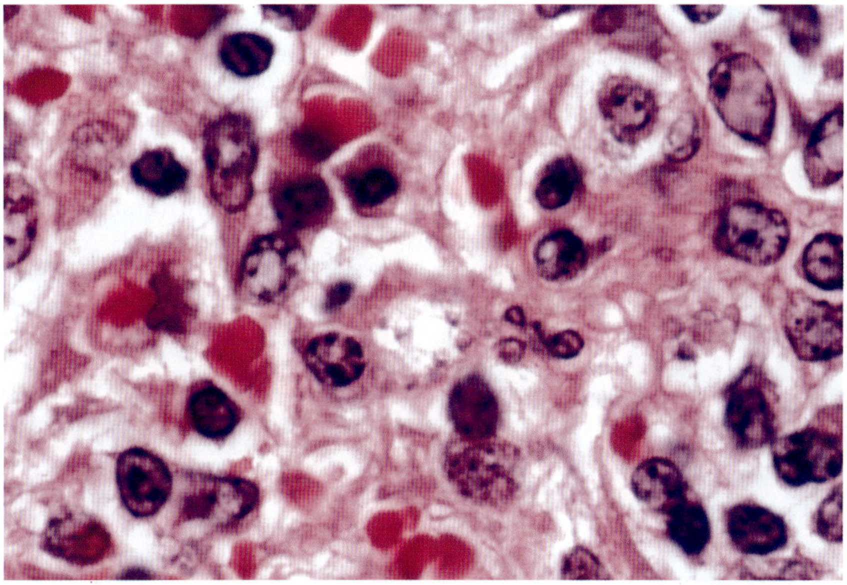

Figure 11-16

LEISHMANIASIS, LYMPH NODE

Leishmania donovani organisms in a macrophage in visceral leishmaniasis (kala-azar).

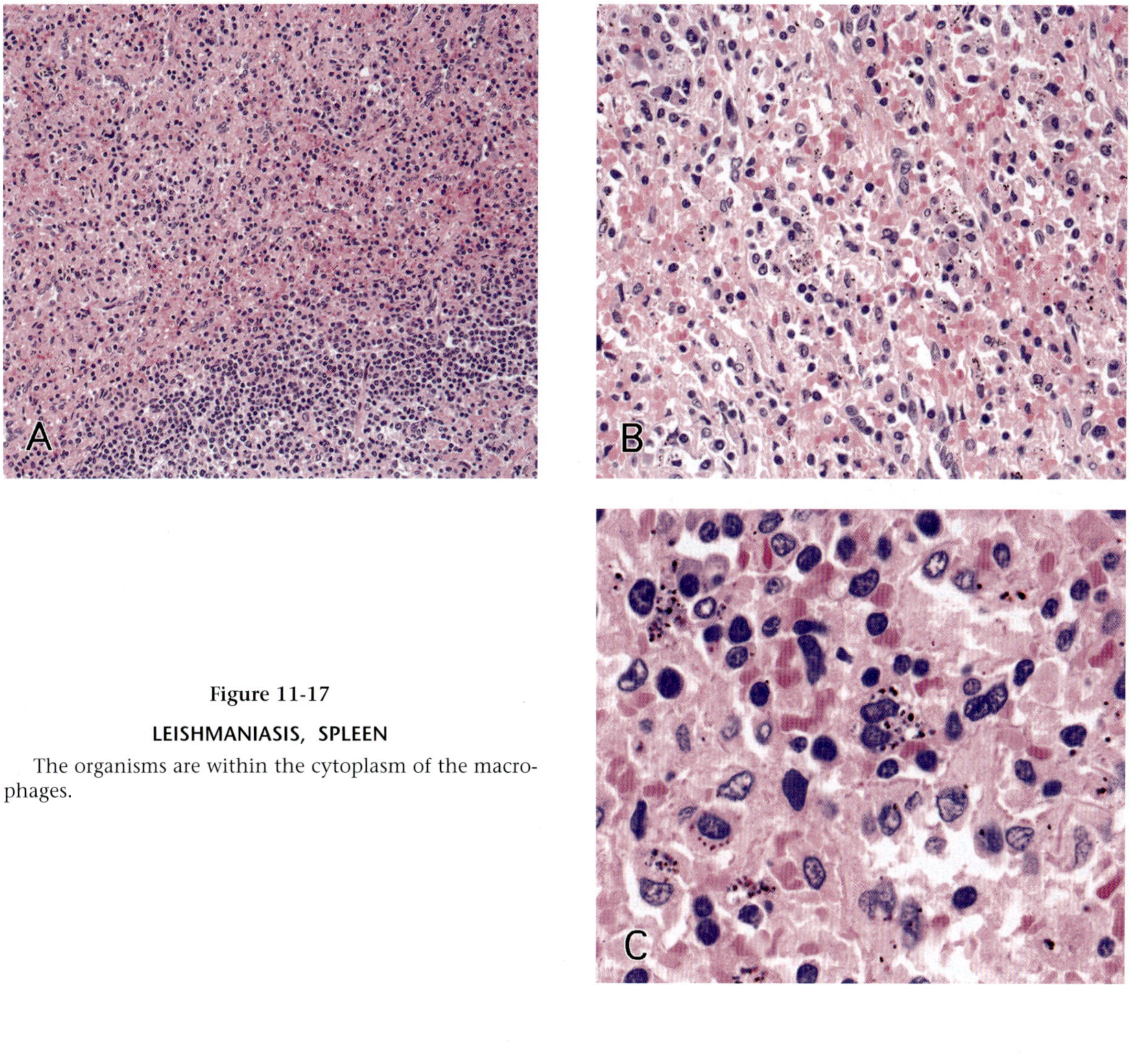

Figure 11-17

LEISHMANIASIS, SPLEEN

The organisms are within the cytoplasm of the macrophages.

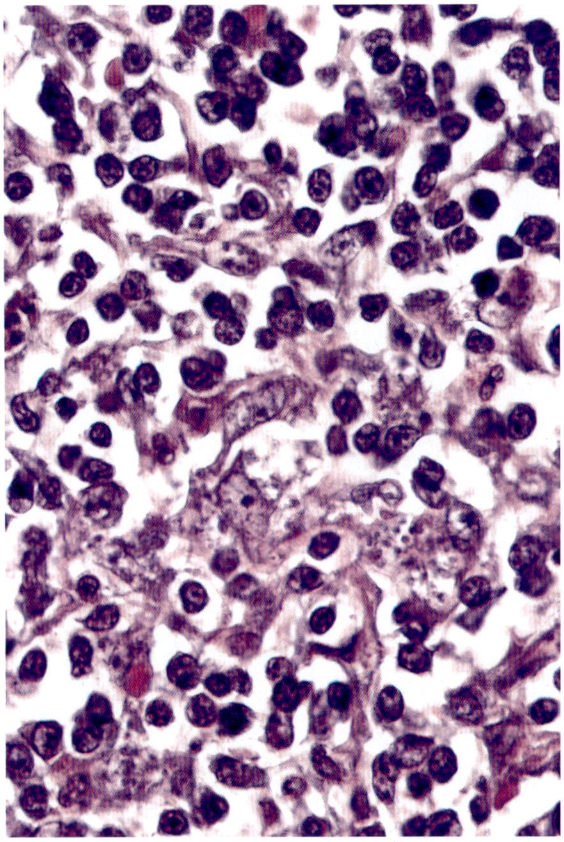

Figure 11-18

LEISHMANIASIS, SPLEEN

At high magnification, organisms are seen within a macrophage.

and mucicarmine negative. They are best visualized with a Giemsa stain which highlights the nucleus and kinetoplast.

Differential Diagnosis. The differential diagnosis of leishmaniasis includes fulminant disseminated histoplasmosis, cryptococcal infection, and American trypanosomiasis (Chagas disease). The yeast form of *Histoplasma capsulatum* is slightly larger than *L. donovani* and it lacks a kinetoplast. *Histoplasma* organisms are not as readily demonstrable by H&E staining and usually require methenamine silver staining for visualization. American trypanosomiasis is caused by *Trypanosoma cruzi* which uses the reduviid bug as its vector. *T. cruzi* enters the skin either through the insect's bite or abrasions caused by scratching, and usually causes acute, unilateral conjunctivitis and ipsilateral lymphadenitis. The histopathologic changes in the lymph node include multinucleated giant cells and macrophages stuffed with *T. cruzi* organisms, similar in appearance to *L. donovani*. They can easily be confused with *Histoplasma* or less commonly, *Cryptococcus*.

Treatment and Prognosis. Antimicrobicidal agents are used to treat leishmaniasis. Visceral leishmaniasis is treated with sodium stibogluconate (Pentostam) and meglumine antimoniate (Glucantime). Recent treatments include liposomal amphotericin-B.

TRYPANOSOMA CRUZI AND *T. BRUCEI*

Definition. Two distinct types of disease are caused by parasitic infection by trypanosome species: *Chagas disease* (*American trypanosomiasis*) and *African trypanosomiasis* (*sleeping sickness*). Both can involve lymph nodes and spleen.

General Features. Trypanosomiasis is caused by the protozoal species *Trypanosoma brucei*, which consists of two subspecies that are morphologically indistinguishable. These two subspecies cause distinctly different clinical diseases: *T. gambiense* causes West African sleeping sickness and *T. rhodesiense* causes East African sleeping sickness. Both *T. rhodesiense* and *T. gambiense* are transmitted via the tsetse fly vector.

The infected tsetse fly injects trypomastigotes into the skin, which enter the lymphatic system and pass into the bloodstream. They are carried to other sites throughout the body, reach other body fluids (e.g., lymph, spinal fluid), and replicate. The entire life cycle is extracellular. Humans are the main reservoir for *T. gambiense*, while animals are the main reservoir of *T. rhodesiense*.

The protozoal parasite, *T. cruzi*, causes Chagas disease, a zoonotic disease that is transmitted to humans by blood-sucking reduviid bugs. The reduviid bug takes a blood meal and releases trypomastigotes in its feces near the site of the bite wound. Trypomastigotes enter the host through the wound or through intact mucosal membranes, such as the conjunctiva. Inside the host, the trypomastigotes invade cells, where they differentiate and multiply, and are then released into the bloodstream. They then infect a variety of tissues.

Clinical Features. The disease caused by *T. rhodesiense* or *T. gambiense*, African trypanosomiasis, may clinically present as chronic, intermittent fever with splenomegaly and lymphadenopathy with pruritus. *T. rhodesiense* is more prevalent in the East African plains whereas *T. gambiense* is found predominantly in West Africa where it typically causes posterior cervical lymphadenopathy referred to as Winterbottom sign (17). A trypanosomal chancre develops at the site of the tsetse fly's bite. In the meningoencephalitic stage, invasion of the central nervous system causes headaches, somnolence, and abnormal behavior, leading to loss of consciousness and coma ("sleeping sickness"). The course of infection is much more acute with *T. rhodesiense* than with *T. gambiense*.

T. cruzi enters the skin either through insect bites or abrasions caused by scratching, and usually causes acute, unilateral conjunctivitis and ipsilateral lymphadenitis. *T. cruzi* infection is seen in the southern United States to southern Argentina, but occurs mostly in poor, rural areas of Central and South America. Chronic Chagas disease is a major health problem in many Latin American countries. *T. cruzi* can also be transmitted through blood transfusions, organ transplantation, and laboratory accidents as well as transplacentally.

Laboratory Findings. Typically, the diagnosis of infection by trypanosomes is accomplished by microscopic examination of chancre fluid, lymph node aspirates, blood, and bone marrow or cerebrospinal fluid. A wet preparation should be examined for motile trypanosomes, and a smear should be fixed, stained, and examined. Serologic detection of infection has sensitivity and specificity issues that prevent unequivocal diagnosis.

Microscopic Findings. Lymph nodes involved by African trypanosomiasis consist of reactive follicular hyperplasia with intense interfollicular polyclonal plasmacytosis. Macrophage lymphophagocytosis and reactive morular cells of Mott are characteristically noted. Although the organism is rarely visualized on histologic sections, trypanosomes can be demonstrated in fluid from aspirated lymph nodes, especially in the early stages of the disease. In later stages, considerable fibrosis develops in the lymph nodes.

Lymph nodes with Chagas disease show multinucleated giant cells and macrophages stuffed with *T. cruzii* organisms, similar in appearance to *L. donovani*. The splenic changes include lymphoid depletion and a decrease in the size of the follicles (50). Red pulp changes are dependent on the presence or absence of congestive heart failure, secondary to the Chagas disease. When heart failure is present, there is significant congestive splenomegaly associated with hyperplasia of the red pulp stromal components.

Treatment and Prognosis. In African trypanosomiasis, treatment should be started as soon as possible and is based on symptoms and laboratory results. The drug regimen depends on the infecting species and the stage of infection. Pentamidine and suramin are the drugs of choice to treat the hemolymphatic stage of *T. gambiense* and *T. rhodesiense*, respectively.

SCHISTOSOMA

Definition. *Schistosomiasis* is a trematodal infection caused by *Schistosoma* species. Splenomegaly due to portal hypertension is common and eggs or organisms are seen occasionally in lymph nodes and spleen.

General Features. Specific marine snails are the intermediate hosts of *Schistosoma*. These snails release infective cercariae into the water which then penetrate the skin of the human host. Human contact with water is thus necessary for infection by schistosomes. This parasitic stage migrates through several tissues and takes up residence in the veins and matures. *Schistosoma japonicum* parasites are more frequently found in the superior mesenteric veins, *S. mansoni* in the superior mesenteric veins draining the large intestine, and S. *haematobium* in the venous plexus of the bladder or the rectal venules. The eggs produced by the adult female are moved progressively toward the lumen of the intestine (*S. mansoni* and *S. japonicum*) and the bladder and ureters (*S. haematobium*), and are released with feces or urine. Various animals serve as reservoirs for different schistosome species.

Clinical Features. The three main species of *Schistosoma* infecting humans are *Schistosoma haematobium, S. japonicum,* and *S. mansoni;* rarer causes of human infections are *S. mekongi* and *S. intercalatum. S. mansoni* is found in parts of South America and the Caribbean, Africa, and the Middle East; *S. haematobium* in Africa and the Middle East; and *S. japonicum* in the Far East. *S. mekongi* and *S. intercalatum* are found in Southeast Asia and central West Africa, respectively.

Most infections are asymptomatic. Acute schistosomiasis may manifest as fever, cough, abdominal pain, diarrhea, hepatosplenomegaly, and eosinophilia. Occasionally, granulomatous central nervous system lesions occur.

Continuing infection may cause granulomatous reactions and fibrosis in the affected organs, which result in manifestations that include colonic polyposis with bloody diarrhea, portal hypertension, splenomegaly, cystitis, hematuria, pulmonary hypertension, and glomerulonephritis. *S. haematobium* has been associated with the development of squamous cell carcinoma of the bladder (60).

Laboratory Findings. Microscopic identification of eggs in stool or urine is the most practical method for diagnosis. Stool should be examined when infection with *S. mansoni* or *S. japonicum* is suspected, and urine examined if *S. haematobium* is suspected.

Microscopic Findings. Schistosomes may be found in the lymph nodes draining cutaneous sites of infection and other central lymph nodes (59). Schistosome eggs may be found in both lymph nodes and spleen. The number is variable, and the surface spines, which may indicate the species, may be intact. The eggs are variably calcified. In the early stages, eggs are surrounded by mixed inflammatory cells. Later, the inflammation becomes more granulomatous. Ultimately, the eggs are surrounded by dense, concentric fibrosis (fig. 11-19).

Adult schistosomes may migrate to the spleen from the liver (29,59). They may be present in larger tributaries of the splenic veins. Schistosome eggs may be found in the trabecular and hilar region of the spleen. The enlargement of the spleen is typically due to portal congestion as a result of liver involvement.

Treatment and Prognosis. The drug of choice is praziquantel for infections caused by all *Schistosoma* species.

PLASMODIUM

Definition. There are a variety of pathologic findings in the spleen associated with *malaria*, an infection caused by *Plasmodium* species. These findings include hyperreactive malarial splenomegaly (formerly known as tropical splenomegaly), splenic rupture, hypersplenism, splenic torsion, and the formation of splenic cysts.

General Features. There are over 170 species of *Plasmodium* that infect birds, reptiles, and mammals. Humans are the specific vertebrate host for certain *Plasmodium* species (*P. falciparum, P. ovale, P. malariae, P. vivax*), with the *Anopheles* mosquito as the only vector. The spleen plays a central role in the pathologic and physiologic response to malaria (24). Splenic removal of parasites and destruction of parasite-infected cells allow for the antigen presentation and development of an adaptive immune response (65).

Hyperreactive malarial splenomegaly (HMS) is a relatively common finding in endemic malarial areas. It is an abnormal immune response to malarial antigens, with the excessive production of immunoglobulin (Ig)M (1,12). This results in the formation of immune complexes which are removed by the reticuloendothelial system, massively expanding spleen and liver.

Clinical Features. Splenomegaly is present in 50 to 80 percent of the population in malaria-endemic areas (71). Massive splenomegaly is common in African countries and is present in 1 to 2 percent of the population (13), with approximately 40 percent being due to malaria. The spleen enlarges over the course of 2 to 5 days, and becomes tender with each febrile paroxysm. After the febrile episode, the splenomegaly may partially resolve, but eventually the enlargement is sustained.

Splenic rupture due to malaria occurs as either an acute or chronic effect of infection, although it is more common in acute infection, usually during the first paroxysm. It is associated with all four major species of *Plasmodium* (69,71), although it appears to be most common with *P. vivax*. The rate of occurrence of splenic rupture in malaria patients has been estimated at 0.4 percent (71).

HMS, more common in females, is characterized by major and minor criteria (1). The major criteria include: splenic enlargement of at least 10 cm below the costal margin, immunity to malaria, IgM elevated to at least two standard deviations above normal, and clinical and immunologic response to antimalarial therapy. The minor criteria include: hepatic sinusoidal lymphocytosis, normal phytohemagglutinin response, hypersplenism, peripheral blood lymphocytosis, and familial/genetic occurrence. Hemolytic

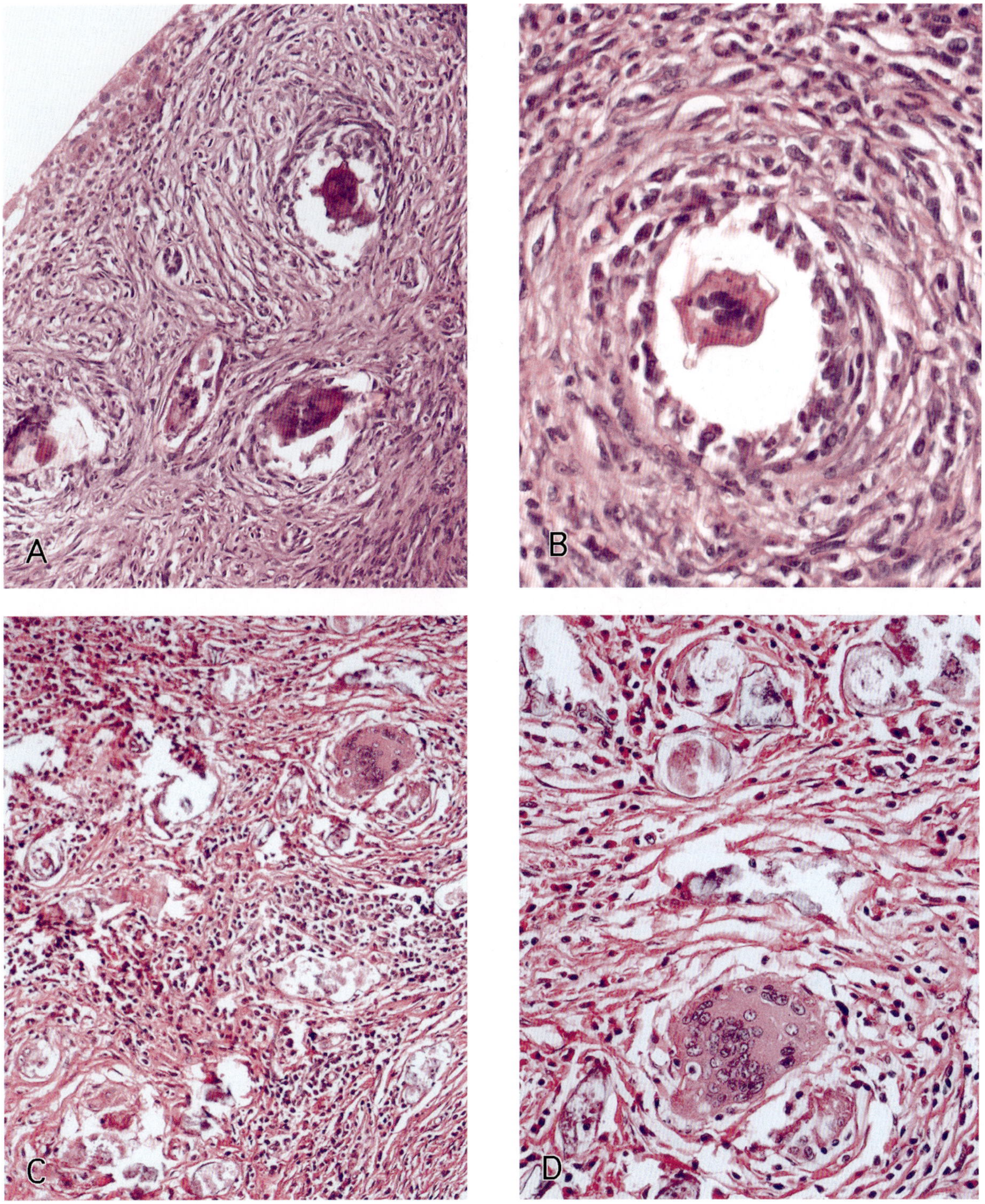

Figure 11-19

SCHISTOSOMIASIS

A,B: Tissue granulomas due to *Schistosoma mansoni* show the offending schistosomes in the center of the granuloma. (Courtesy of Linda Marler, Indianapolis, IN.)

C,D: Views of the inflammatory response in which degenerating schistosome ova are seen. ((Fig. 10-114A,B from Cooke RA. Infectious diseases: atlas, cases, text. Australia: McGraw-Hill, Ltd; 2008:403.)

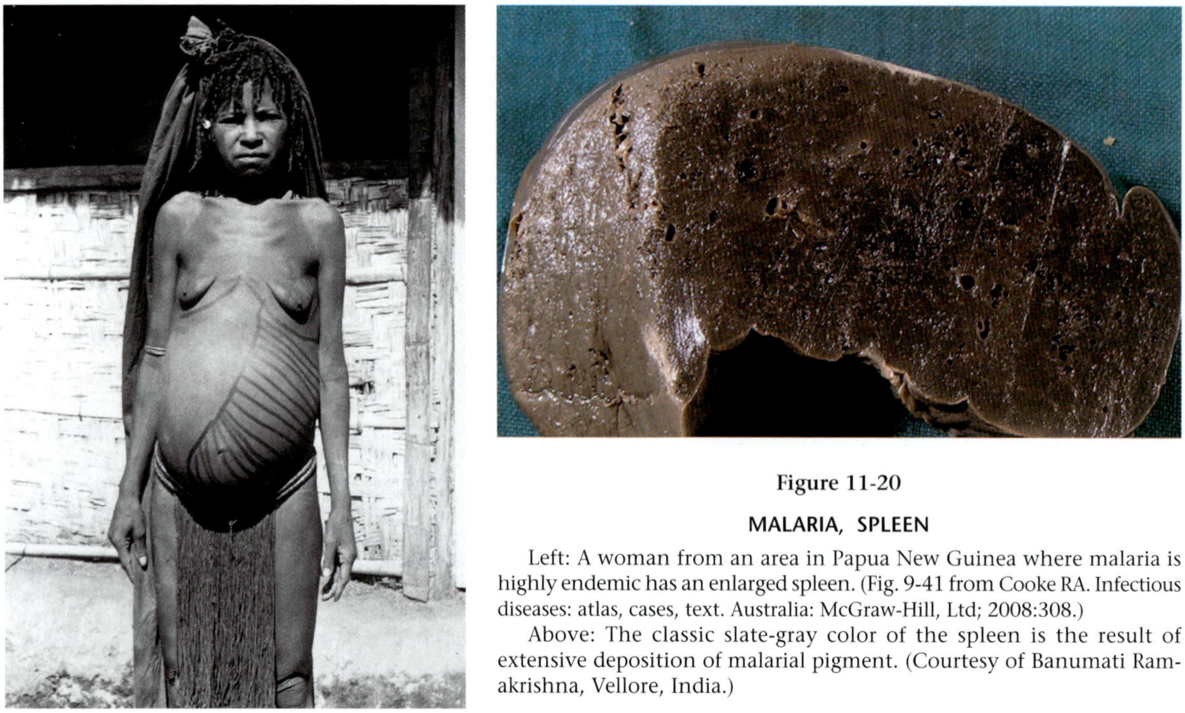

Figure 11-20

MALARIA, SPLEEN

Left: A woman from an area in Papua New Guinea where malaria is highly endemic has an enlarged spleen. (Fig. 9-41 from Cooke RA. Infectious diseases: atlas, cases, text. Australia: McGraw-Hill, Ltd; 2008:308.)

Above: The classic slate-gray color of the spleen is the result of extensive deposition of malarial pigment. (Courtesy of Banumati Ramakrishna, Vellore, India.)

anemia is present in virtually all patients, and is especially severe in pregnant patients.

In HMS, the lymphocytosis may be impressive enough that a lymphoproliferative disorder is simulated, so-called African chronic lymphocytic leukemia (CLL) (12). This lymphocytosis usually resolves upon treatment of the malaria. Some patients in malaria-endemic areas, however, develop splenic marginal zone lymphoma (SMZL) with villous lymphocytes (11), and it is possible that there is an etiologic link between malarial infection and SMZL in these patients.

Malarial infection can be more severe in splenectomized patients than in those with an intact spleen. This is especially true with *P. falciparum*, where levels of parasitemia can be higher. In *P. falciparum* infection, the presence of usual ring forms and trophozoites may be accompanied by other "intermediate" forms, which are not usually seen in the peripheral blood.

Laboratory Findings. Examination of the peripheral blood is a cornerstone in the diagnosis of malaria. Depending on the specific species, parasitemia and morphology vary. Because of clinical concerns, the important differentiation is between *P. falciparum*, which has a more aggressive clinical course, and the other species.

In HMS, lymphocytosis is common. The lymphocytes may be villous in appearance (up to 75 percent of peripheral blood lymphocytes) and show the same morphology as seen in SMZL with villous lymphocytes (12). IgM levels are elevated. Findings associated with hemolytic anemia, including elevated bilirubin, lactate dehydrogenase (LDH), and decreased haptoglobin, are seen. In spite of the clinical findings, malarial parasites are not usually detected in HMS.

Gross Findings. Spleens with chronic malarial infection have a characteristic slate gray-blue color due to extensive deposition of hemosiderin and malarial pigment (fig. 11-20). Chronic splenomegaly leads to an enlarged, firm organ. Acute splenic infection tends to show a red, hyperemic gross appearance, due to massive congestion. A ruptured spleen typically has a thin, friable capsule.

Microscopic Findings. Expansion of the red pulp with increased macrophages in the cords and expansion of the sinuses are commonly seen in malaria-affected spleens. There is often significant congestion, with increased red blood cells in the sinuses and cords (figs. 11-21, 11-22). Focal necrosis may be seen. Fibrosis and proliferation of fibroblasts are significant. Macrophages

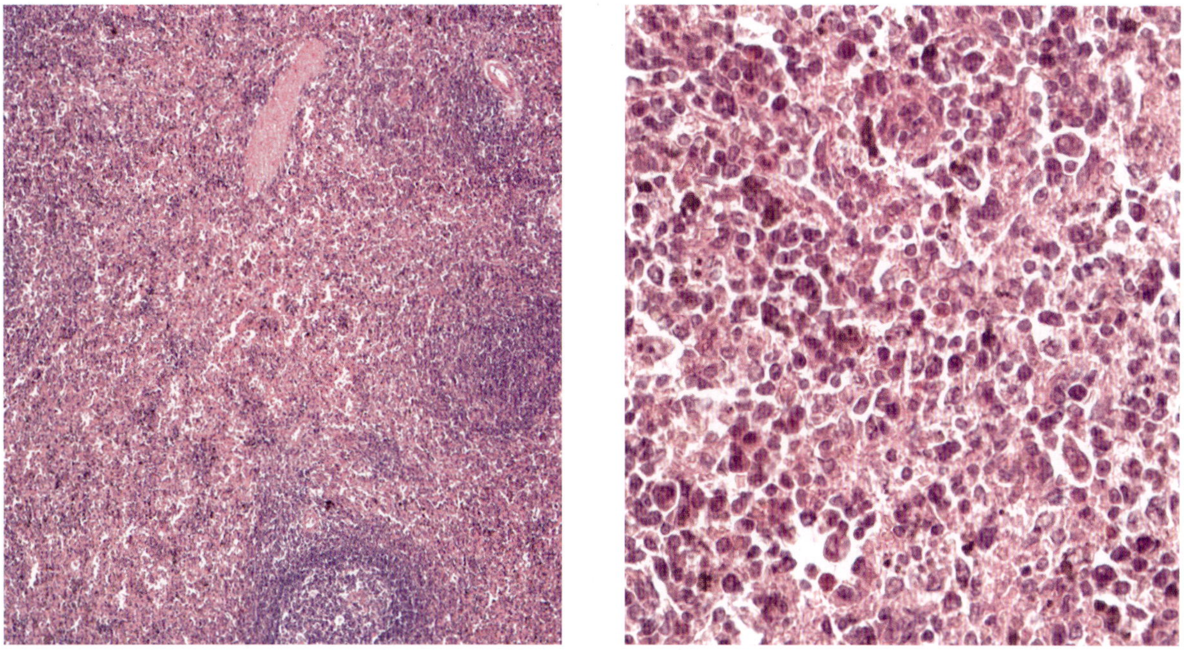

Figure 11-21

MALARIA, SPLEEN

Red pulp congestion and malarial pigment are seen in this spleen affected by plasmodia. In near-perfect histologic sections, organisms are seen within circulating red blood cells.

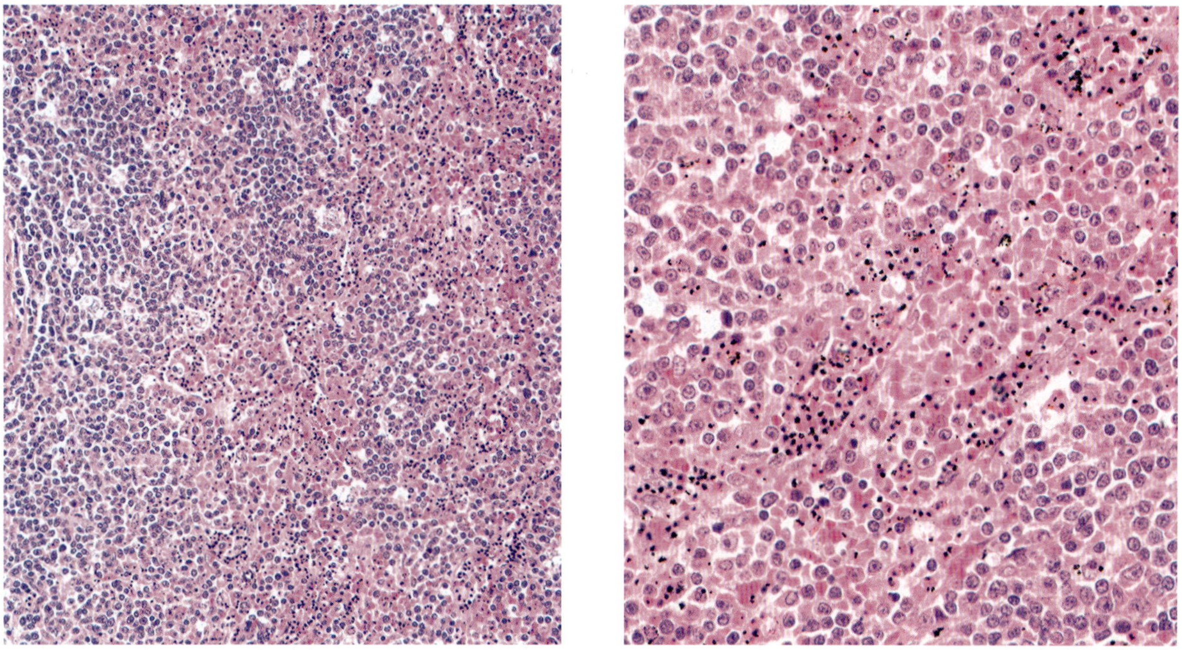

Figure 11-22

MALARIA, SPLEEN

This unfortunate patient had both a malarial infection in the spleen as well as prolymphocytic leukemia. Malarial pigment is prominent and rare parasitized red blood cells are seen.

are often greatly increased in number in the red pulp and may be large in size with pigment or granular material in their cytoplasm. In cases with significant parasitemia, the organisms may be seen within red blood cells, distributed throughout the spleen. The white pulp often lacks reactive germinal centers, and has a depleted marginal zone (65). Pigment deposition includes hemosiderin and hemazoin (malarial pigment; polymerized hemoglobin resulting from digestion by the parasite).

Ancillary Studies. Flow cytometry may be performed in cases with significant lymphocytosis. There should be no evidence of clonal populations (19). Cytogenetic studies do not reveal any abnormalities.

Differential Diagnosis. Although HMS is the most common cause of tropical splenomegaly, B-cell lymphomas still account for 12 percent of cases (13). Because of the similarities between SMZL with villous lymphocytes and HMS, thorough evaluation should be performed to rule out the former. The presence of clonality by flow or cytogenetic abnormalities suggests the diagnosis of lymphoma rather than HMS.

Treatment and Prognosis. In HMS, splenectomy should only be used for patients who fail medical therapy. Splenic rupture in association with malaria can be treated with splenectomy, however, in malaria-endemic areas, conservative, nonsurgical management is suggested (71). This may prevent severe complications such as increased risk of complicated or fatal malaria, lifelong malarial prophylaxis, latent malaria postoperatively, poor postoperative wound healing, and an increased risk of cerebral malaria (10,15,71).

BABESIA

Definition. *Babesiosis* is an infection caused by intraerythrocytic parasites of the genus *Babesia* (32,51). Although many infections are asymptomatic, occasionally there is a life-threatening hemolytic reaction. *Babesia* organisms can be found in the lymph nodes and spleen.

General Features. Only a few species have been identified as causing human infections including *Babesia microti* and *B. divergens*. The *Babesia* life cycle involves a definitive host (the deer tick, *Ixodes dammini*). Deer are the hosts upon which the adult ticks feed and when deer populations increase, the tick population also increases, increasing the possibility of transmission. Within the tick, gametes unite and form sporozoites. Humans are bitten by infected ticks. During a blood meal, the *Babesia*-infected tick introduces sporozoites into the human host. The sporozoites enter erythrocytes and undergo asexual replication (budding), which is responsible for the clinical manifestations of the disease. Humans are dead-end hosts and subsequent transmission is unlikely. Rare human to human transmission occurs through blood transfusions.

Clinical Features. In the United States, *B. microti* is the species most frequently identified (Northeast and Midwest), although the distribution of *Babesia* is worldwide (32,51). Most *Babesia* infections are asymptomatic. When there is symptomatic disease, the manifestations include fever, chills, sweating, myalgias, fatigue, hepatosplenomegaly, and hemolytic anemia. Symptoms typically occur after an incubation period of 1 to 4 weeks, and can last several weeks. The disease is more severe in patients who are immunosuppressed, splenectomized, or elderly (54).

Laboratory Findings. The diagnosis is made by microscopic examination of thick and thin blood smears stained with Giemsa. Isolation of the organisms by inoculation of patient blood into hamsters or gerbils also assists in diagnosis. Animals inoculated with infective blood typically develop parasitemia within 1 to 4 weeks.

Microscopic Findings. Babesial organisms are intraerythrocytic, and as such, do not cause a specific tissue reaction. The organisms have been described in spleen and lymph nodes (63). *Babesia* merozoites are 1.5 to 3.0 µm. These forms are shaped like rings, and may be single or paired pear-shaped trophozoites or assume a tetrad form, or "Maltese cross."

Ancillary Studies. Immunoassays (in both fresh and formalin-fixed tissue), PCR testing, and serologic testing are all available for *Babesia* species (32,51,63), although primarily as research tools.

Differential Diagnosis. Because of the morphologic similarity, *Babesia* may be confused with *Plasmodium* species. Although a clinical history should differentiate the two, specific serologic or immunohistochemical tests may be necessary.

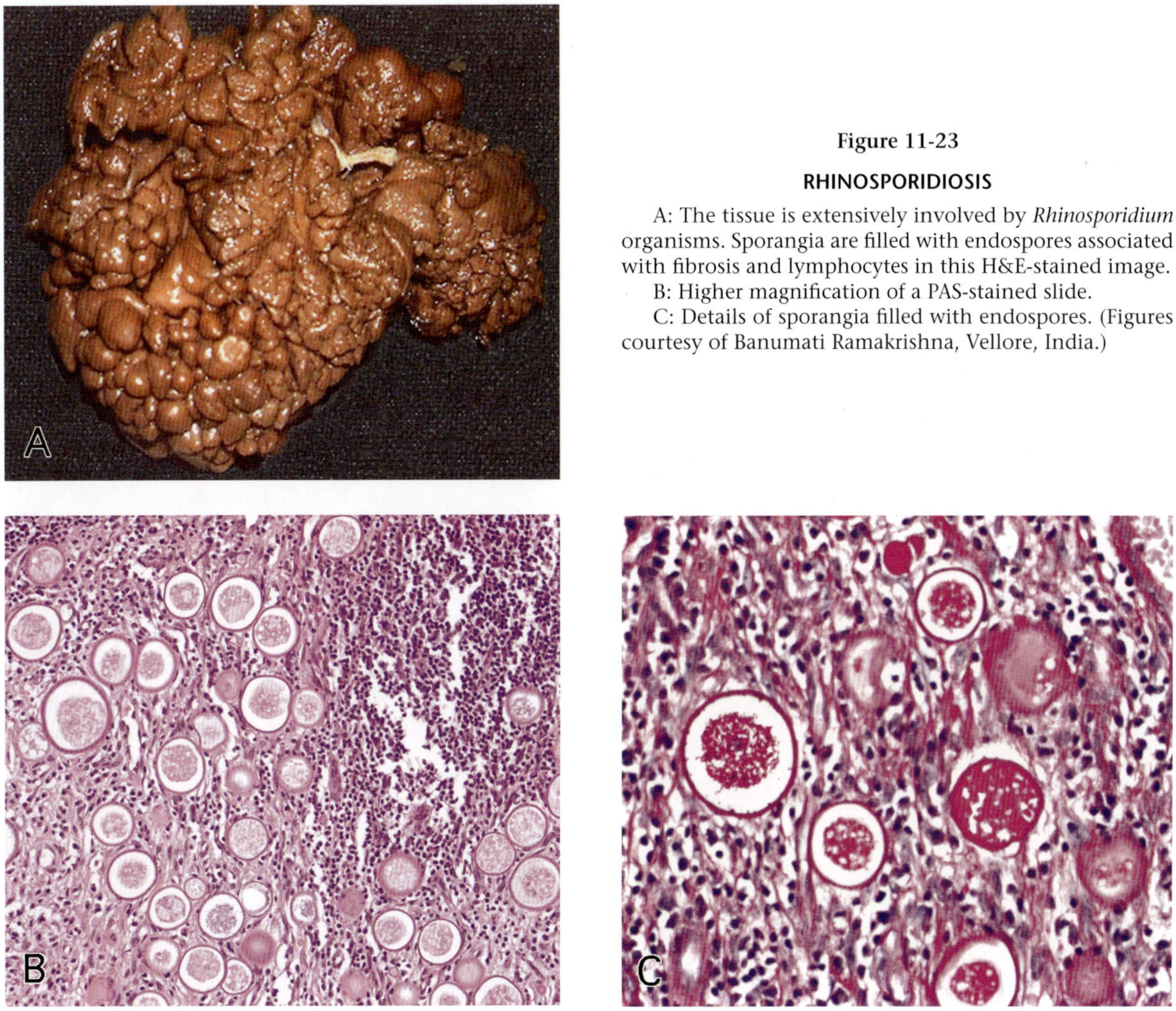

Figure 11-23

RHINOSPORIDIOSIS

A: The tissue is extensively involved by *Rhinosporidium* organisms. Sporangia are filled with endospores associated with fibrosis and lymphocytes in this H&E-stained image.

B: Higher magnification of a PAS-stained slide.

C: Details of sporangia filled with endospores. (Figures courtesy of Banumati Ramakrishna, Vellore, India.)

Treatment and Prognosis. Clindamycin is the most commonly used treatment. In rare cases, exchange transfusion is used in severely ill patients with high parasitemia.

RHINOSPORIDIUM SEEBERI

Definition. *Rhinosporidium seeberi* is the causative pathogen of human *rhinosporidiosis,* which is an endemic disease in South Asia.

General Features. Little is known about the life cycle of this organism and its taxonomic relationships, whether fungal or protozoan, are unclear (6–8). The diagnosis is histopathologic. Rhinosporidiosis is a chronic granulomatous disorder that typically involves skin, subcutaneous tissues, and mucous membranes (conjunctival, nasal); lymph nodes are rarely involved (fig. 11-23) (8,59).

Microscopic Findings. Infected tissue has minute cyst-like spaces. The sporangia (cyst-like capsules) range from 50 to 350 µm and are filled with endospores (5,8). The walls of the cyst measure approximately 5 µm. The organisms typically induce a fibrous or granulomatous tissue response with plasma cells and lymphocytes. The sporangia and endospores stain for PAS, mucicarmine, and GMS. An important differential diagnostic consideration is *Coccidioides immitis* (see chapter 10).

PROTOTHECA

Human infection by algae is due to only a single genus, *Prototheca.* Extraordinary cases have been described in the lymph nodes (36,53,61,62).

In the case described by Symmers (59), the pattern of lymph node involvement was

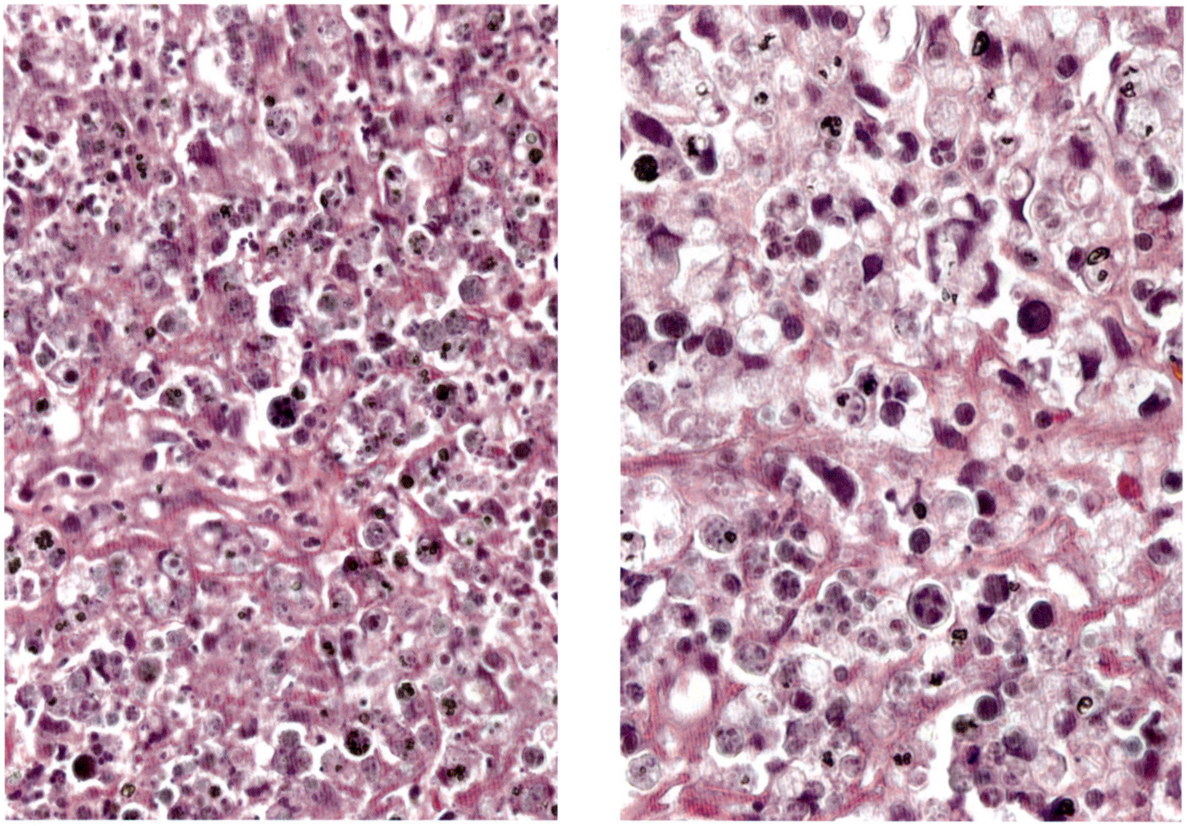

Figure 11-24

PROTOTHECA

Left: This sample from skin shows the *Prototheca* organisms.
Right: Higher magnification view. (Both figures courtesy of Luis Fajardo, Palo Alto, CA.)

granulomatous, with caseation. Within the granulomas were algae, which were 8 to 30 μm in diameter (fig. 11-24). Unlike similar-sized fungi, they may contain multiple daughter cells, and have flattened surfaces when adjacent to one another. *Prototheca* grows in standard culture media and stains well with PAS and GMS stains (36).

PRIONS

Prion diseases in humans, referred to under the grouping of *transmissible spongiform encephalopathies* (TSE), include *kuru, Creutzfeldt-Jakob disease* (CJD), *variant CJD* (vCJD), *Gerstmann-Straussler-Scheinker disease*, and *fatal familial insomnia*. These diseases are associated with conformational changes in a normal protein that is widely expressed in humans and animals, prion protein (PrP) (38). The development of prion disease is associated with changes in the secondary and tertiary molecular conformations of the PrP protein, which is referred to as PrP^{Sc}. This abnormal protein is thought to induce conformational changes in normal PrP.

The reticuloendothelial system plays a central role in the infection and propagation of PrP^{Sc} (2,38,39,68). The abnormal proteins appear to be transported from the site of exposure to local lymph nodes. The PrP^{Sc} then replicates within the follicular dendritic cells of the germinal centers. Infection spreads from the follicular dendritic cells to sympathetic nerves within lymphoid tissues and eventually to the brain. Although specific lymphadenopathy and splenic histopathologic changes are not noted, the lymphoid cells, associated follicular dendritic cells, and other supporting tissues play a pivotal role in the development and progression of prion diseases.

REFERENCES

1. Ackerman L. Hyperreactive malarial syndrome. J Am Board Fam Pract 1996;9:356-9.
2. Aguzzi A. Prions and the immune system: a journey through gut, spleen, and nerves. Adv Immunol 2003;81:123-71.
3. Aisner SC, Aisner J, Moravec C, Arnett EN. Acquired toxoplasmic lymphadenitis with demonstration of the cyst form. Am J Clin Pathol 1983;79:125-7.
4. Aleixo JA, Nascimento ET, Monteiro GR, et al. Atypical American visceral leishmaniasis caused by disseminated Leishmania amazonensis infection presenting with hepatitis and adenopathy. Trans R Soc Trop Med Hyg 2006;100:79-82.
5. Ali A, Flieder D, Guiter G, Hoda SA. Rhinosporidiosis: an unusual affliction. Arch Pathol Lab Med 2001;125:1392-3.
6. Angunawela P, De Tissera A, Dissanaike AS. Rhinosporidiosis presenting with two soft tissue tumors followed by dissemination. Pathology 1999;31:57-8.
7. Arseculeratne SN. Rhinosporidiosis: what is the cause? Curr Opin Infect Dis 2005;18:113-8.
8. Arseculeratne SN, Panabokke RG, Atapattu DN. Lymphadenitis, trans-epidermal elimination and unusual histopathology in human rhinosporidiosis. Mycopathologia 2002;153:57-69.
9. Ash LR, Orihel TC. Atlas of human parasitology, 4th ed. Chicago: ASCP Press; 1997.
10. Bach O, Baier M, Pullwitt A, et al. Falciparum malaria after splenectomy: a prospective controlled study of 33 previously splenectomized Malawian adults. Trans R Soc Trop Med Hyg 2005;99:861-7.
11. Bates I, Bedu-Addo G, Rutherford T, Bevan DH. Splenic lymphoma with villous lymphocytes in tropical West Africa. Lancet 1992;340:575-7.
12. Bates I, Bedu-Addo G, Rutherford TR, Bevan DH. Circulating villous lymphocytes—a link between hyperreactive malarial splenomegaly and splenic lymphoma. Trans R Soc Trop Med Hyg 1997;91:171-4.
13. Bedu-Addo G, Bates I. Causes of massive tropical splenomegaly in Ghana. Lancet 2002;360:449-544.
14. Bernard E, Delgiudice P, Carles M, et al. Disseminated isosporiasis in an AIDS patient. Eur J Clin Microbiol Infect Dis 1997;16:699-701.
15. Bidegain F, Berry A, Alvarez M, et al. Acute Plasmodium falciparum malaria following splenectomy for suspected lymphoma in 2 patients. Clin Infect Dis 2005;40:e97-100.
16. Chadee K, Meerovitch E. Entamoeba histolytica: lymphoreticular changes in gerbils (Meriones unguiculatus) with experimentally induced cecal amebiasis. J Parasitol 1985;71:566-75.
17. Connor DH, Neafie RC, Dooley JR. African trypanosomiasis. In: Binford CH, Connor DH, eds. Pathology of tropical and extraordinary diseases, Vol.1. Washington, D.C.: Armed Forces Institute of Pathology; 1976:252-7.
18. Dabiri S, Meymandi SS, Nadji M, Kharazmi A. A description of parasite-harbouring cells in localized lymphadenitis in dry type cutaneous leishmaniasis. Acta Trop 2001;79:129-33.
19. Dascalescu CM, Rosenzwajg M, Bonte H, et al. Bcl-2 and immunoglobulin gene rearrangements in patients with malaria related chronic splenomegaly. Leuk Lymphoma 2004;45:2093-7.
20. Dorfman RF, Remington JS. Value of lymph-node biopsy in the diagnosis of acute acquired toxoplasmosis. N Engl J Med 1973;289:878-81.
21. Eapen M, Mathew CF, Aravindan KP. Evidence based criteria for the histopathological diagnosis of toxoplasmic lymphadenopathy. J Clin Pathol 2005;58:1143-6.
22. Eberhard ML, DeMeester LJ, Martin BW, Lammie PJ. Zoonotic Brugia infection in western Michigan. Am J Surg Pathol 1993;17:1058-61.
23. Elenitoba-Johnson KS, Eberhard ML, Dauphinais RM, Lammie PJ, Khorsand J. Zoonotic Brugian lymphadenitis. An unusual case with florid monocytoid B-cell proliferation. Am J Clin Pathol 1996;105:384-7.
24. Engwerda CR, Beattie L, Amante FH. The importance of the spleen in malaria. Trends Parasitol 2005;21:75-80.
25. Frenkel JK, Silva MB, Saldanha J, et al. Isospora belli infection: observation of unicellular cysts in mesenteric lymphoid tissues of a Brazilian patient with AIDS and animal inoculation. J Eukaryot Microbiol 2003;50:682-4.
26. Frenkel JK, Silva MB, Saldanha JC, et al. [Extraintestinal finding of Isospora belli unizoic cysts in a patient with AIDS: case report.] Rev Soc Bras Med Trop 2003;36:409-12. [Portuguese]
27. Gaafar A, Ismail A, el Kadaro AY, Hashim E, Khalil EA, el Hassan AM. Necrotizing and suppurative lymphadenitis in Leishmania major infections. Trop Med Int Health 1996;1:243-50.
28. Gibson DW, Heggie C, Connor DH. Clinical and pathologic aspects of onchocerciasis. Pathol Annu 1980;15:195-240.

29. Guangjin S, Mingdao J, Qiyang L, Hui X, Jiangming H, Xiaomei Y. Study on histopathology, ultrasonography and some special serum enzymes and collagens for 38 advanced patients of schistosomiasis japonica. Acta Trop 2002;82:235-46.
30. Guttierrez Y. Filariae of lymphatics. In: Guttierrez Y, ed. Diagnostic pathology of parasitic infections with clinical correlations. Philadelphia: Lea & Febiger 1990:284-300.
31. Haque AK, Schnadig V, Rubin SA, Smith JH. Pathogenesis of human strongyloidiasis: autopsy and quantitative parasitological analysis. Mod Pathol 1994;7:276-88.
32. Homer MJ, Aguilar-Delfin I, Telford SR 3rd, Krause PJ, Persing DH. Babesiosis. Clin Microbiol Rev 2000;13:451-69.
33. Hutt MS, K`berle F, Salfelder K. Leishmaniasis and trypanosomiasis. In: Spencer H, ed. Tropical Pathology. New York: Springer-Verlag 1973:351-98.
34. Jayaram N, Ramaprasad AV, Chethan M, Sujay AR. Toxoplasma lymphadenitis. Analysis of cytologic and histopathologic criteria and correlation with serologic tests. Acta Cytol 1997;41:653-8.
35. Jungmann P, Figueredo-Silva J, Dreyer G. Bancroftian lymphadenopathy: a histopathologic study of fifty-eight cases from northeastern Brazil. Am J Trop Med Hyg 1991;45:325-31.
36. Leimann BC, Monteiro PC, Lazera M, Candanoza ER, Wanke B. Protothecosis. Med Mycol 2004;42:95-106.
37. Lin MH, Kuo TT. Specificity of the histopathological triad for the diagnosis of toxoplasmic lymphadenitis: polymerase chain reaction study. Pathol Int 2001;51:619-23.
38. Mabbott N, Turner M. Prions and the blood and immune systems. Haematologica 2005;90:542-8.
39. Mabbott NA, Bruce ME. Prion disease: bridging the spleen-nerve gap. Nat Med 2003;9:1463-4.
40. MacKenzie WR, Hoxie NJ, Proctor ME, et al. A massive outbreak in Milwaukee of cryptosporidium infection transmitted through the public water supply. N Engl J Med 1994;331:161-7.
41. McCabe RE, Brooks RG, Dorfman RF, Remington JS. Clinical spectrum in 107 cases of toxoplasmic lymphadenopathy. Rev Infect Dis 1987;9:754-74.
42. Mertens RB, Didier ES, Fishbein MC, Bertucci DC, Rogers LB, Orenstein JM. Encephalitozoon cuniculi microsporidiosis: infection of the brain, heart, kidneys, trachea, adrenal glands, and urinary bladder in a patient with AIDS. Mod Pathol 1997;10:68-77.
43. Meyers WM, Neafie RC, Connor DH. Bancroftian and Malayan filariasis. In: Binford CH, Connor DH, eds. Pathology of tropical and extraordinary diseases, Vol. 2. Washington DC: Armed Forces Institute of Pathology; 1976:340-55.
44. Meyers WM, Neafie RC, Marty AM, Wear DJ. Pathology of infectious diseases; Vol. I. Helminthiases. Washington DC: American Registry of Pathology; 2000.
45. Michiels JF, Hofman P, Bernard E, et al. Intestinal and extraintestinal Isospora belli infection in an AIDS patient. A second case report. Pathol Res Pract 1994;190:1089-94.
46. Miettinen M. Histological differential diagnosis between lymph node toxoplasmosis and other benign lymph node hyperplasias. Histopathology 1981;5:205-16.
47. Mohrmann R, Nathwani B, Brynes R, Taylor C, Hansmann M, Sheibani K. Morphologic criteria to distinguish malignant from reactive monocytoid B cell (MBC) proliferations. Mod Pathol 1991;4:79A.
48. Orenstein JM, Gaetz HP, Yachnis AT, Frankel SS, Mertens RB, Didier ES. Disseminated microsporidiosis in AIDS: are any organs spared? AIDS 1997;11:385-6.
49. Paleologo FP, Neafie RC, Connor DH. Lymphadenitis caused by Loa loa. Am J Trop Med Hyg 1984;33:395-402.
50. Pereira SA, Rodrigues DB, Castro EC, dos Reis MA, Teixeira Vde P. Morphometric study of the spleen in chronic Chagas' disease. Am J Trop Med Hyg 2002;66:401-3.
51. Pruthi RK, Marshall WF, Wiltsie JC, Persing DH. Human babesiosis. Mayo Clin Proc 1995;70:853-62.
52. Restrepo C, Macher AM, Radany EH. Disseminated extraintestinal isosporiasis in a patient with acquired immune deficiency syndrome. Am J Clin Pathol 1987;87:536-42.
53. Revisse P, de Bievre C, Campos Magalhaes M, Ramos I, Huerre M. Protothécose cutanée traitée avec succés par l'itraconazole: noveau cas et revue generale des protothécoses humaines [French]. J Mycologie Med 1993;3:84-94.
54. Rosner F, Zarrabi MH, Benach JL, Habicht GS. Babesiosis in splenectomized adults. Review of 22 reported cases. Am J Med 1984;76:696-701.
55. Said J. AIDS-related lymphadenopathies. Semin Diagn Pathol 1988;5:365-75.
56. Sheibani K, Fritz RM, Winberg CD, Burke JS, Rappaport H. "Monocytoid" cells in reactive follicular hyperplasia with and without multifocal histiocytic reactions: an immunohistochemical study of 21 cases including suspected cases of toxoplasmic lymphadenitis. Am J Clin Pathol 1984;81:453-8.
57. Sousa Ade Q, Parise ME, Pompeu MM, et al. Bubonic leishmaniasis: a common manifestation of Leishmania (Viannia) braziliensis infection in Ceara, Brazil. Am J Trop Med Hyg 1995;53:380-5.

58. Strauchen JA. Fungal, protozoal, and filiarial lymphadenitis and other lymph node granulomas. In: Strauchen JA, ed. Diagnostic histopathology of the lymph node. New York: Oxford University Press; 1998:104-20
59. Symmers WStC. The lymphoreticular system. In: Symmers WStC, ed. Systemic pathology, 2nd ed. New York: Churchill Livingstone; 1978:507-891.
60. Symmers WStC. Lymphadenitis caused by infection and infestation. In: Henry K, Symmers WStC, eds. Systemic pathology, 3rd ed. New York: Churchill Livingstone; 1992:326-492.
61. Takaki K, Okada K, Umeno M, et al. Chronic Prototheca meningitis. Scand J Infect Dis 1996; 28:321-3.
62. Thiele D, Bergmann A. Protothecosis in human medicine. Int J Hyg Environ Health 2002;204:297-302.
63. Torres-Velez FJ, Nace EK, Won KY, Bartlett J, Eberhard M, Guarner J. Development of an immunohistochemical assay for the detection of babesiosis in formalin-fixed, paraffin-embedded tissue samples. Am J Clin Pathol 2003;120:833-8.
64. Tosoni A, Nebuloni M, Ferri A, et al. Disseminated microsporidiosis caused by Encephalitozoon cuniculi III (dog type) in an Italian AIDS patient: a retrospective study. Mod Pathol 2002;15:577-83.
65. Urban BC, Hien TT, Day NP, et al. Fatal Plasmodium falciparum malaria causes specific patterns of splenic architectural disorganization. Infect Immun 2005;73:1986-94.
66. Urdiales-Viedma M, Martos-Padilla S, Nogales-Fernandez F, Lopez-Yevenes A. Lymph node changes in echinococcosis. Arch Pathol Lab Med 1984;108:528.
67. Veress B, Omer A, Satir AA, El Hassan AM. Morphology of the spleen and lymph nodes in fatal visceral leishmaniasis. Immunology 1977;33:605-10.
68. Weissmann C, Raeber AJ, Montrasio F, Hegyi I, Frigg R, Klein MA, Aguzzi A. Prions and the lymphoreticular system. Philos Trans R Soc Lond B Biol Sci 2001;356:177-84.
69. Yagmur Y, Kara IH, Aldemir M, Buyukbayram H, Tacyildiz IH, Keles C. Spontaneous rupture of malarial spleen: two case reports and review of literature. Crit Care 2000;4:309-13.
70. Zijlstra EE, el-Hassan AM. Leishmaniasis in Sudan. Visceral leishmaniasis. Trans R Soc Trop Med Hyg 2001;95(Suppl 1):S27-58.
71. Zingman BS, Viner BL. Splenic complications in malaria: case report and review. Clin Infect Dis 1993;16:223-32.

12 SYSTEMIC AND AUTOIMMUNE ABNORMALITIES

Autoimmune conditions are characterized by dysregulation of the immune system, which leads to reactivity to self-directed antigens. Since the activation of the immune system is abnormal, abnormalities of immune organs, such as the lymph nodes and spleen, are frequent. The histologic findings are often nonspecific and include: increases in the number of plasma cells, immunoblastic proliferations, follicular hyperplasia, follicular lysis, and paracortical/interfollicular hyperplasias (92). Similar lymph node changes are present in a variety of other autoimmune disorders not specifically discussed in this section: systemic sclerosis, Sjögren syndrome, ankylosing spondylitis, primary biliary cirrhosis, and celiac disease (53,81,103,113,162).

Systemic disorders that are not autoimmune related and that cause lymph node or splenic findings are also discussed in this chapter. The histologic findings in these disorders are broad and reflect the diverse underlying etiologies and interactions with the lymph nodes and spleen. There are numerous systemic disorders that affect the lymph nodes and spleen but either are rare or not specific enough to be included as an individual entry in this chapter: uremia (splenic cysts, hypersplenism, granulomas), Crohn disease (splenic granulomas, splenic cysts) (fig. 12-1), ulcerative colitis (splenic atrophy, splenic cysts), Reiter syndrome (lymphadenopathy, splenomegaly, vasculitis) (fig. 12-2), Wilson disease (splenic rupture), Schnitzler syndrome (lymphadenopathy, splenomegaly), and Hermansky-Pudlak syndrome (splenic ceroid histiocytosis) (4,13,63,72,104,139).

IMMUNE THROMBOCYTOPENIC PURPURA

Definition. *Immune (idiopathic) thrombocytopenic purpura* (ITP) is a process of autoimmune platelet destruction. The spleen is the primary site of platelet destruction and has associated histopathologic changes.

General Features. ITP is a thrombocytopenic condition, caused by autoreactive antibodies that bind to platelets and shorten their life span (25). The antibody-coated platelets are then sequestered by tissue macrophages and destroyed (25,82). The spleen is a major site of platelet

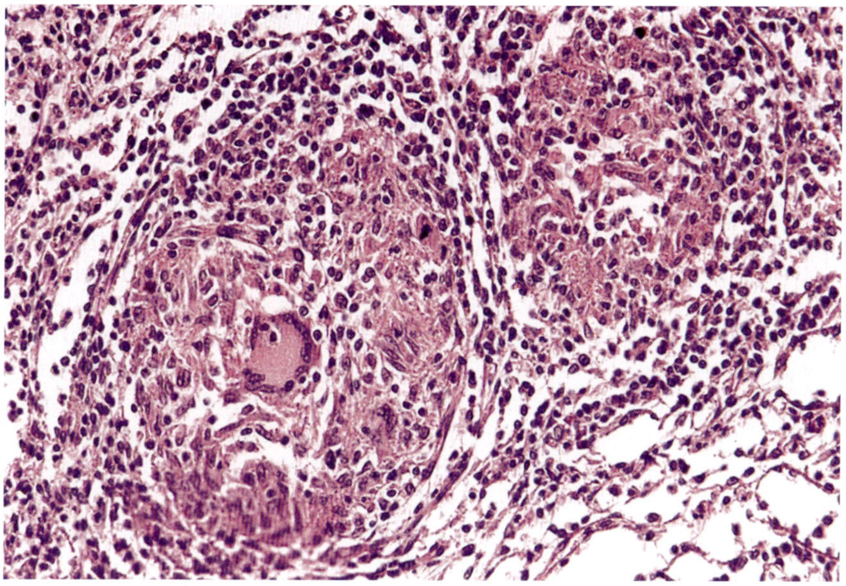

Figure 12-1

CROHN DISEASE, SPLEEN

Granulomas are present in the spleen. (Courtesy of Vito Franco, Palermo, Italy.)

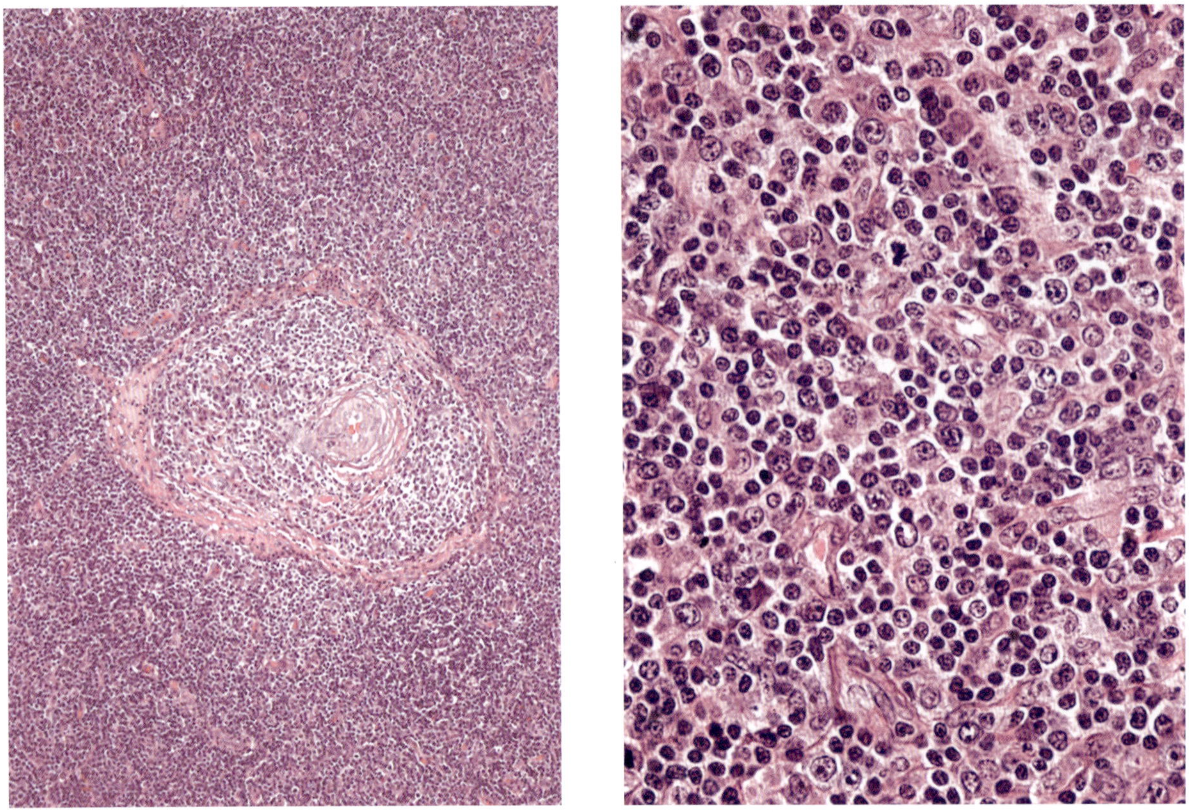

Figure 12-2

REITER SYNDROME, LYMPH NODE

Vasculitis (left) and immunoblastic proliferation (right) are seen.

clearance and of production of autoantibodies (9,32,82). Evidence has shown that the autoantibodies impair platelet production by reacting with bone marrow megakaryocytes and reducing platelet production and/or apoptotic cell death (31). As in other types of autoimmune disorders (systemic lupus erythematosis [SLE]), Sjögren syndrome) (52), clonal B-cell proliferations and clonal antiplatelet antibodies are frequently detected (143,167). The presence of B-cell clones and the production of antiplatelet antibodies in ITP may be the result of the B-cell dysfunction present in this disorder (143,167). Immunoglobulin (Ig)G and/or IgM antibodies reactive with the glycoprotein complexes of platelets have been identified on the platelets or in the plasma of most ITP patients (102,115,121).

Clinical Features. ITP is a common disorder with an incidence of approximately 1/10,000 (25). Clinically, ITP occurs as an acute or chronic disorder (25,68,124). The acute form, which is seen most commonly in children, involves in both sexes with equal frequency and is often associated with recent viral infection (31,68,98,124). It is self-limited in about 80 percent of cases. Its peak incidence is between the ages of 3 and 5 years (25,31,68,98,124).

Adult-onset ITP is a chronic illness in more than 70 percent of patients. It may occur as an isolated condition, most commonly in adult women (41–43,73,166), or, less frequently, in association with other disorders, including chronic lymphocytic leukemia (45), autoimmune hemolytic anemia (Evans syndrome) (47), or autoimmune disorders such as SLE (79), in which it may be the presenting manifestation (80). Common variable immunodeficiency (CVID) and human immunodeficiency virus (HIV) infection can also be ITP associated. A weak association with B-cell lymphoma exists, particularly in patients with chronic ITP (50,77).

Laboratory Findings. Numerous studies have characterized the pathogenic autoantibodies responsible for platelet destruction and thereby provide a way to diagnose ITP, understand its pathogenesis, and predict responsiveness to therapy. IgG antibodies that react with platelet glycoprotein (GP) IIb/IIIa and GPIb/IX have been identified in some patient serum samples and platelet eluates (66,83,116,169); however, other platelet antigens also appear to be targeted (18,39,66,69,70,134,159,163,170), and in many cases, the antibody specificity cannot be determined or even detected (25). Furthermore, there is no formal proof that any single subset of antibodies, for example, those directed at GPIIb/IIIa, is responsible for platelet destruction. Consequently, the clinical utility of measuring serum or platelet-elutable immunoglobulin is unknown and does not have a definitive role in the diagnosis or treatment of ITP or in distinguishing between the adult-onset and childhood-onset forms of the disease (58). The diagnosis of ITP remains one of exclusion and the usefulness of available platelet-antibody tests to confirm or exclude the diagnosis independent of other criteria has not been established (25).

Gross Findings. The spleen is usually only mildly enlarged and frequently weighs no more than 200 g (75,125). Grossly, it is usually unremarkable in appearance. In contrast with spleens removed from patients with autoimmune hemolytic anemia and hereditary spherocytosis, no significant congestion is observed and the organ retains its normal dark brown color. If congestion is noted, its presence suggests the possibility of Evans syndrome. The white pulp appears unremarkable or, in a proportion of the cases, displays more pronounced micronodularity than normal due to the presence of follicular lymphoid hyperplasia. The presence of significant splenomegaly suggests ITP associated with an underlying condition such as lymphoma.

Microscopic Findings. The morphology of the spleen in untreated ITP displays evidence of active antibody production and of increased platelet destruction (21,93,99,126). The white pulp shows well-developed germinal centers which are surrounded by attenuated mantle zones and hyperplastic marginal zones; the latter may contain an increased proportion of immunoblasts and plasma cells (figs. 12-3–12-5). The red pulp shows histologic evidence of phagocytosis of antibody-coated platelets, a process that predominantly occurs within cordal macrophages. The presence of platelets in varying stages of degeneration imparts a "dirty" appearance to the cords of Billroth, with granular acidophilic material both within cordal macrophages and extracellularly (9,29,65,108,110,146,160). Platelet sequestration and phagocytosis are more clearly demonstrated using touch imprints and electron microscopy (33,160).

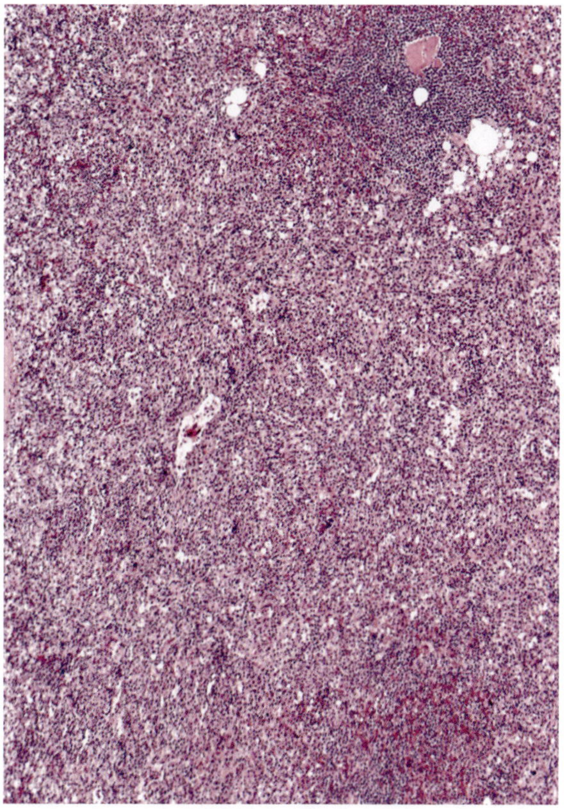

Figure 12-3

IMMUNE THROMBOCYTOPENIC PURPURA, SPLEEN

The red pulp is expanded with macrophages.

Some of the macrophages appear as single rounded cells with pale granular cytoplasm; foamy macrophages are seen in the red pulp (33,37,51,97,147,148), sometimes showing the staining characteristics of ceroid. In occasional cases, the foamy macrophages are so numerous that they mimic a storage disease such as ceroid histiocytosis or even Niemann-Pick disease. The

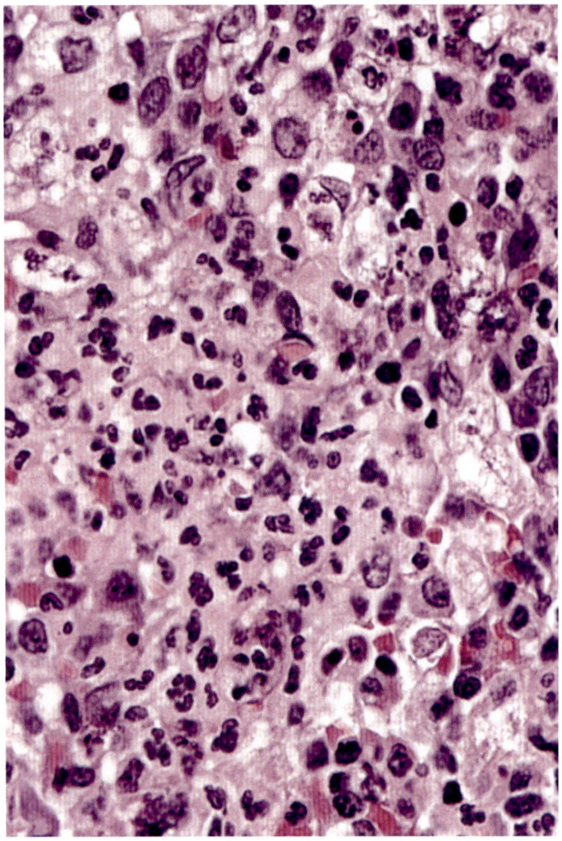

Figure 12-4

IMMUNE THROMBOCYTOPENIC PURPURA, SPLEEN

Macrophages with increased foamy cytoplasm contain fragments of destroyed platelets. These are relatively inapparent on hematoxylin and eosin (H&E)-stained sections but may be seen in touch preparations.

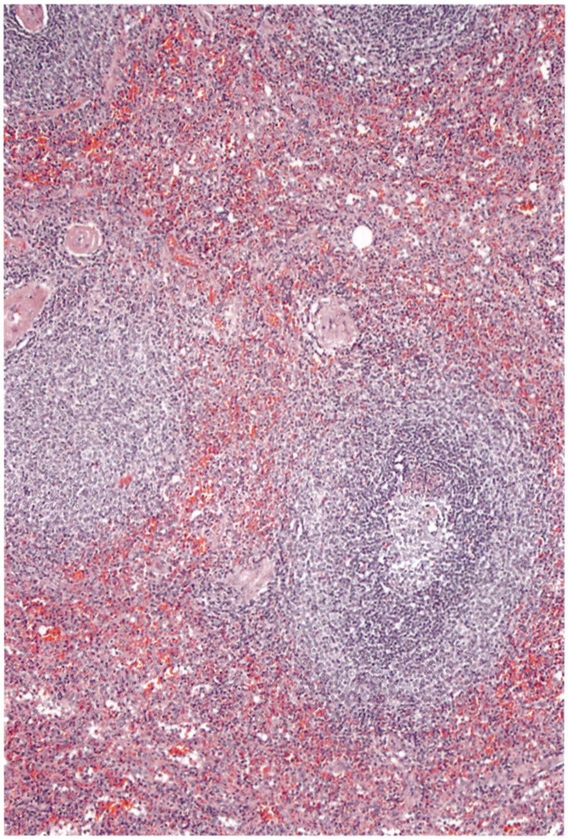

Figure 12-5

IMMUNE THROMBOCYTOPENIC PURPURA, SPLEEN

In spite of multiple therapies, or perhaps as a result of them, this spleen has expanded marginal zones, hyperplastic follicles, and red pulp congestion. (Courtesy of Cherie Dunphy, Chapel Hill, NC.)

red pulp also contains an increased number of plasma cells, neutrophilic granulocytes, and granulocytic precursors (110,147,176). Erythroblasts and megakaryocytes are less frequently seen (176). The presence of concentric periarterial fibrosis, similar to the vascular "onion skinning" that commonly occurs in the spleens of patients with SLE, has also been reported (17).

The splenic morphology may be greatly altered by previous steroid therapy (65). The white pulp in steroid-treated cases shows little or no immunologic activation, or resembles the early immune reaction with its lack of germinal center formation (see fig. 14-4). Platelet phagocytosis, however, is still demonstrated, as are foamy macrophages in some cases (65). It has been postulated that in those cases in which steroid therapy is ineffective, antibody production is curtailed but platelet phagocytosis persists, necessitating splenectomy (65).

Refractory ITP (rITP) is a chronic variant characterized by a lack of response to the common therapies (e.g., corticosteroids) or requiring unacceptably high doses of corticosteroids to maintain a safe platelet count (24). Traditionally, rITP was treated with splenectomy; however, newer therapies are now used before splenectomy, including the anti-CD20 antibodies such as rituximab. The use of rituximab in chronic ITP relies on the attempt to eliminate autoreactive B cells (158). Recent studies have shown a lack of significant histopathologic differences between ITP spleens treated with corticosteroid therapy and those treated with

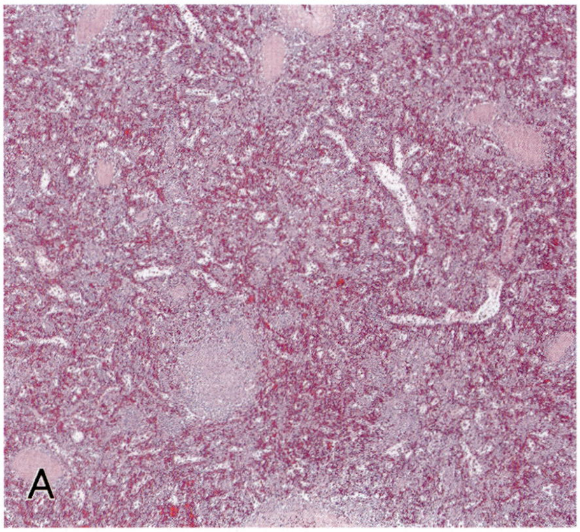

Figure 12-6

IMMUNOHISTOCHEMICAL REACTIVITY IN IMMUNE THROMBOCYTOPENIC PURPURA, SPLEEN

Rituximab therapy resulted in a decrease in white pulp cellularity (A), and absent staining for CD20 (B) and CD21 (C).

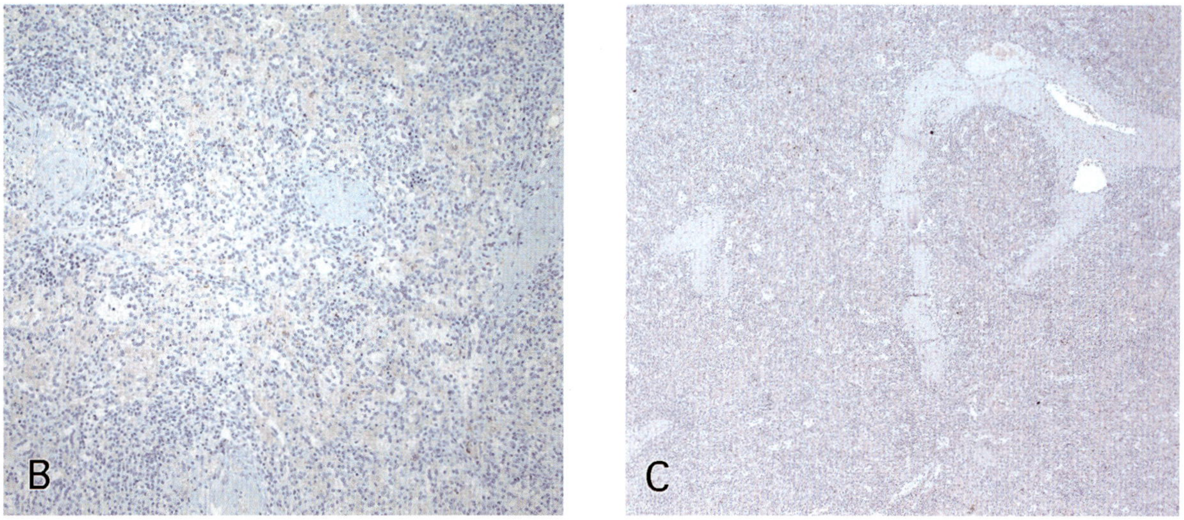

other, often multiple therapies (danazol, intravenous immunoglobulin, anti-RhD, vincristine, cyclophosphamide) (7). Rituximab markedly decreases the B cells in rITP spleens, consistent with its known effects. Changes also include a reduction in the number of follicular dendritic cells stained by CD21 and an increase in the number of macrophages (fig. 12-6).

Differential Diagnosis. Immune thrombocytopenia with both increased antiplatelet antibodies and circulating immune complexes may be observed in HIV-positive patients, especially intravenous drug users (3,78,145,152). The histologic findings in the spleen of these patients are similar to those of ITP. Marti et al. (110) compared several morphometric and morphologic features of the spleen in HIV-positive drug abusers with thrombocytopenia refractory to steroid therapy to those of spleens of ITP patients. Although several similarities were present in the two groups, the spleen from drug users showed increased weights, larger lymphoid follicles, and more abundant granulopoietic cells, with fewer macrophages and ceroid macrophages than spleens from ITP patients.

Treatment and Prognosis. Acute ITP is a self-remitting condition in most patients and often requires no treatment (109). The course of chronic ITP, however, is often characterized by multiple relapses. The initial treatment is the use of corticosteroids; however, only a minority of adult patients with chronic ITP has durable remission once the steroid treatment is tapered. Splenectomy offers a reported 70 percent rate of complete remission; in patients in whom steroid therapy had failed, splenectomy gives a 15 percent rate of stable partial response (25,34,76,82).

In the majority of cases, the antiplatelet antibody titer falls following splenectomy; in some cases, however, the antibody persists and relapse occurs, suggesting that other lymphoid organs are also involved in the pathogenesis of the disorder (155). Presently, it is impossible to accurately predict the long-term therapeutic effect of splenectomy in a given patient. Some investigators have suggested a correlation between splenic lymphoid follicle size in the excised spleen and the long-term response to splenectomy (8). Occasionally, accessory splenic tissue, either previously present or implanted at the time of splenectomy, assumes enough function to cause clinical relapse in ITP (25,48).

For splenectomy failure patients without accessory spleens, the available treatments include intravenous immunoglobulins, danazol, vinca alkaloids, azathioprine or other immunosuppressant agents, recombinant interferon, and, most recently, anti-CD20 antibodies (149). Some authors suggest that splenectomy should be performed in all cases of ITP refractory to steroids. With the new therapies, however, this stance may be somewhat extreme. Nevertheless, splenectomy should be considered in patients refractory to several treatment approaches.

AUTOIMMUNE HEMOLYTIC ANEMIA

Definition. The *autoimmune hemolytic anemias* (AIHA) are a group of disorders in which autoantibodies against antigens on the red blood cell (RBC) membrane shorten the RBC life span (10).

General Features. The spleen is important both in the production of the autoantibodies and as the site of erythrocyte destruction. In AIHA due to cold-acting antibodies, no significant splenic sequestration is observed since the hemolytic process caused by the cold agglutinin is largely extrasplenic (intravascular) (20). In contrast, in the warm type of hemolytic disorders, the antibody acts as an opsonin, facilitating splenic destruction of the antibody-coated RBCs (20). The presence of antibody on the RBC surface renders the cell less deformable, impeding passage into the splenic sinuses.

Clinical Features. AIHA is a rare disorder with an estimated incidence of 10 cases/one million population. It is more common in women than in men. Although AIHA can occur at any age, it is more common in midlife. About half of the cases are idiopathic (i.e., occurring as a primary disorder). Other cases are associated with other diseases, including other autoimmune disorders such as SLE or ITP (the latter association is known as Evans syndrome). AIHA may be associated with neoplasms such as malignant lymphoproliferative disorders (e.g., chronic lymphocytic leukemia), certain nonhematopoietic tumors such as ovarian dermoid cysts, and renal cell carcinoma; it is also induced by certain drugs (10,20,133).

AIHA shows variable clinical features including jaundice (usually mild) and symptoms and signs of anemia. The spleen is mildly to moderately enlarged in about one third of the patients, especially after several months of unremitting hemolytic anemia. The disease can present acutely, with symptoms due to rapidly developing anemia, or it can develop gradually in a relatively asymptomatic way. The blood bank may provide the diagnosis in a patient referred for transfusion therapy by discovering a positive antiglobulin (Coombs) test. The physical examination may reveal only pallor or slight jaundice, but signs of congestive heart failure are not unusual in patients with rapidly developing severe autoimmune hemolytic anemia. Lymphadenopathy, fever, hypertension, renal failure, rash, petechiae, or ecchymoses should alert the physician to the possibility of an underlying disease (153).

Laboratory Findings. The autoantibodies involved in AIHA fall into three categories, each of which has distinct serologic properties: 1) IgG warm antibodies (warm autoimmune hemolytic anemia) bind to erythrocytes at 37°C but fail to agglutinate the cells; 2) cold agglutinins (cold autoimmune hemolytic anemia), almost always IgM type, agglutinate RBCs at cold temperatures; and 3) IgG Donath-Landsteiner antibody (paroxysmal cold hemoglobinuria) fixes to RBC membranes in the cold and activates the hemolytic complement cascade when the cells are warmed to 37°C.

Gross Findings. Splenomegaly of a usually mild to moderate degree is observed (153). The organ displays a meaty, dark red appearance due to congestion of the red pulp with erythrocytes (fig. 12-7). Infarcts may be present.

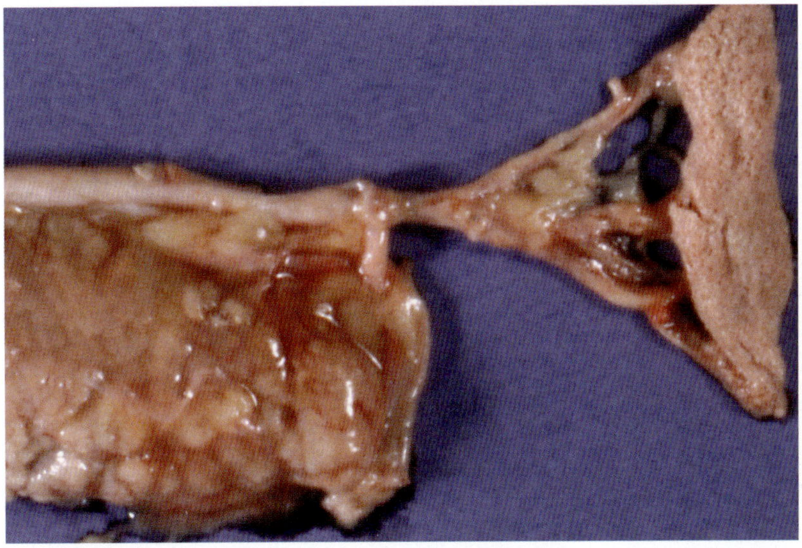

Figure 12-7

AUTOIMMUNE HEMOLYTIC ANEMIA, SPLEEN

Although the typical gross appearance of autoimmune hemolytic anemia is that of an enlarged, beefy red organ due to congestion, chronic treatment for hemolytic anemia left a shrunken, small spleen. (Courtesy of John Eble, Indianapolis, IN.)

Microscopic Findings. The white pulp in spleens of untreated patients shows reactive follicular hyperplasia with partially or fully formed tripartite germinal centers. The marginal zone often appears hyperplastic, especially in chronic cases. In contrast, the white pulp of patients treated with steroids usually does not show germinal center formation (2). The red pulp may reveal sequestration of erythrocytes in the cords, and the sinuses may appear empty, resembling hereditary spherocytosis (fig. 12-8) (2,141,172). In AIHA, however, there is a lesser degree of cordal sequestration and more evidence of erythrophagocytosis by intrasinusoidal macrophages (172). Hemosiderin deposition may be prominent and there may be a slight increase in reticulin fibrosis. Plasmacytosis is usually prominent in the red pulp, in both treated and untreated patients, and clusters of erythroid precursors may be frequent.

Treatment and Prognosis. Most cases of AIHA, particularly idiopathic and drug-induced cases, undergo spontaneous remission. In some cases, however, splenectomy is required to ameliorate the anemia (30,74). Although the immediate response to splenectomy is often favorable, the relapse rate is high, and some patients require continuing steroid therapy.

SARCOIDOSIS

Definition. *Sarcoidosis* is a systemic disease characterized by the formation of noncaseating granulomas in a variety of tissues and organs. It is thought to result from a dysregulated immune response.

General Features. A wide variety of factors interact in producing the noncaseating granulomas characteristic of sarcoidosis, making the underlying etiology unknown. Factors that underlie granuloma formation include an antigen, persistent antigenemia, macrophage presentation, T-helper cell recognition, B-cell overactivity, circulating immune complexes, and a large array of cytokines (154). Sarcoidosis may result from an exaggerated immune response to certain antigens, leading to proliferation and accumulation of CD4-positive T cells.

Infections by several bacteria, viruses, metals, and organic substances have been suggested as inciting factors for sarcoidosis. These include *Mycobacterium tuberculosis, M. avium-intracellulare, Propionibacterium* sp, *Borrelia burgdorferi,* human herpesvirus-8, Epstein-Barr virus, cytomegalovirus, Coxsackie B, beryllium, zirconium, talc, clay, and pine tree pollen (44,57). Considerable evidence suggests that *Mycobacterium* organisms are present in many cases (44).

Clinical Features. Sarcoidosis is a multisystem granulomatous disease, which often presents with bilateral hilar adenopathy on chest roentgenogram. In some, sarcoidosis is initially identified by abnormal chest radiograph; up to 50 percent of patients are asymptomatic (6).

Sarcoidosis affects all races but is more frequently seen in patients of African ancestry; both genders are equally affected. The lung is

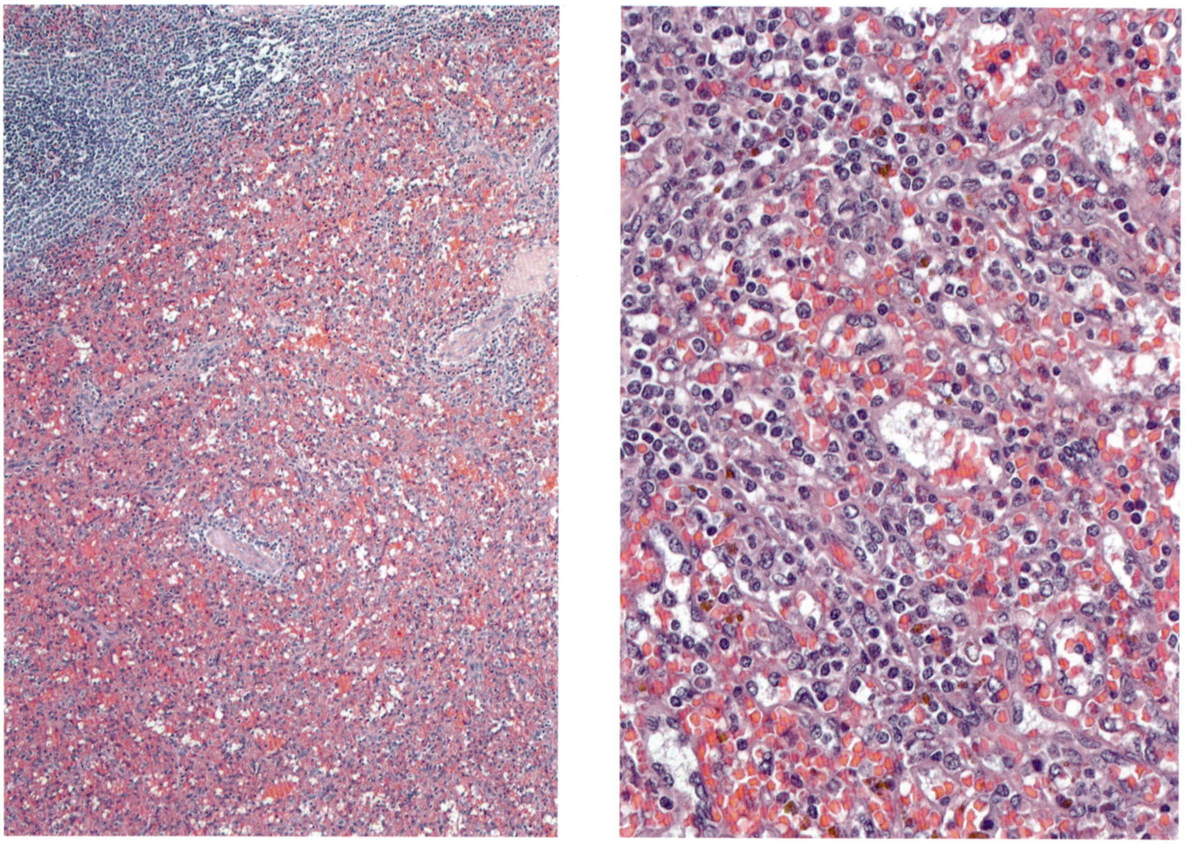

Figure 12-8

AUTOIMMUNE HEMOLYTIC ANEMIA, SPLEEN

Red pulp congestion (left) and foamy macrophages (right) are seen.

the most frequent site of involvement in sarcoidosis; other involved organs include spleen, skin, eyes, lymph nodes, liver, and nervous system (119,161). Clinical symptoms include cough, dyspnea, wheezing, and chest pain (6). Less common manifestations are hemoptysis, pleural effusions, pleural thickening, and pleural calcification. Peripheral adenopathy is seen in 20 to 30 percent of patients (6,161).

The radiologic findings should be supported by histologic evidence of noncaseating epithelioid granulomas. A variety of sites can be biopsied, and those most frequently involved by granulomas are intrathoracic sites including lung and lymph nodes (81 percent), skin (63 percent), peripheral lymph nodes (54 percent), and oropharynx (50 percent) (161).

Clinically detectable splenomegaly is seen in 5 to 10 percent of cases (135), and rarely, splenomegaly is the initial manifestation of the disease (119). The association of sarcoidosis with other autoimmune diseases is rare; however, it does occur, most commonly with SLE (154). There is also a rare association of sarcoidosis with small or large vessel vasculitis (49).

Laboratory Findings. Serum angiotensin converting enzyme (ACE) levels are abnormal in most cases of sarcoidosis. The Kveim-Siltzbach test, an intradermal injection of a sarcoid-related antigen, is usually positive, although this test is only rarely performed for confirmation.

Gross Findings. Lymph nodes involved with sarcoidosis show either focal, firm nodules (granulomas) or are diffusely replaced. The cut surface of the noncaseating granulomas is firm and white to yellow, and typically has well-circumscribed borders. In the spleen, multiple nodules are seen (fig. 12-9). These vary in size from a few millimeters to several centimeters; multiple nodules may coalesce to form large masses.

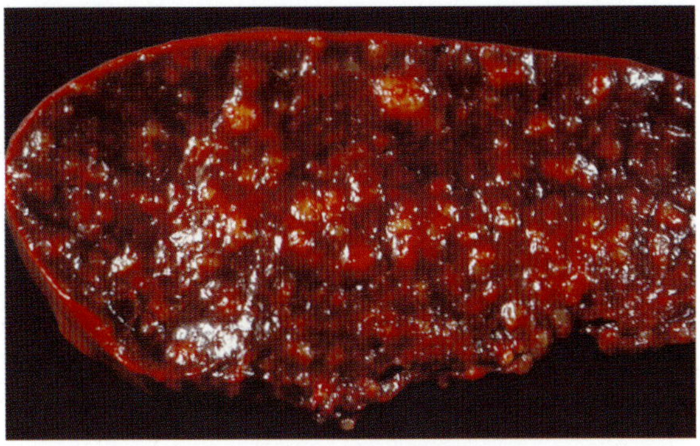

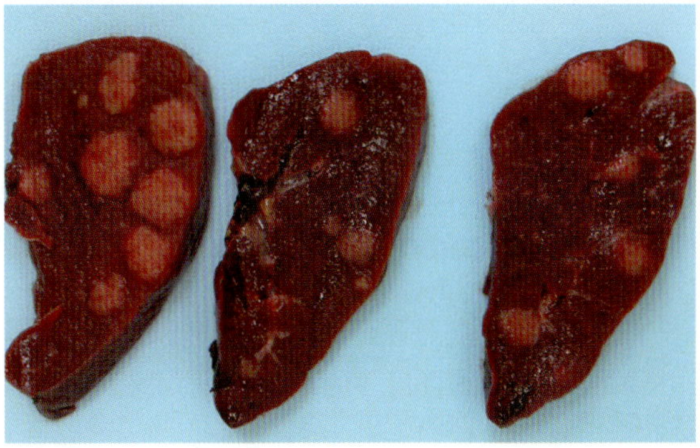

Figure 12-9

SARCOIDOSIS, SPLEEN

Discrete nodules are seen (left and right), but in some severe cases, the nodules become confluent masses. (Left courtesy of Stephen Geller, Los Angeles, CA.)

Microscopic Findings. Although the histologic features of sarcoidosis lymphadenopathy are not pathognomonic, they are highly suggestive of this disorder. The granulomas are usually well formed and better organized than those of tuberculous lymphadenitis, and most often without central necrosis (fig. 12-10). The most prominent cellular components of the granulomas are the epithelioid macrophages, which are differentiated forms of monocytes. Schaumann bodies (laminated intracellular inclusions), asteroid bodies (intracellular star-shaped crystalline inclusions), and residual bodies may be noted within the macrophages (figs. 12-11, 12-12). Multinucleated giant cells are present. Lymphocytes are a component of the granulomas. As is implied in the pathophysiology of the disorder, CD4-positive T cells are common. Splenic findings are similar to those seen in the lymph nodes (fig. 12-13) (132).

As mentioned in other sections of this book, it is prudent to evaluate any cases with granulomas for the possible presence of microorganisms. In sarcoidosis, stains for fungi and acid-fast bacilli are negative.

Differential Diagnosis. The clinical differential diagnosis is an important consideration in sarcoidosis, as these findings may determine whether to perform a tissue biopsy (e.g., lymph node). This differential includes infectious processes, pulmonary disease secondary to foreign material exposure (talc, beryllium), vasculitis, carcinomas, lymphomas, or Langerhans cell histiocytosis (6). In the spleen, the differential diagnosis includes lymphoma, granulomatous infectious processes, benign vascular tumors (such as littoral cell angioma, see chapter 18), and metastatic tumors.

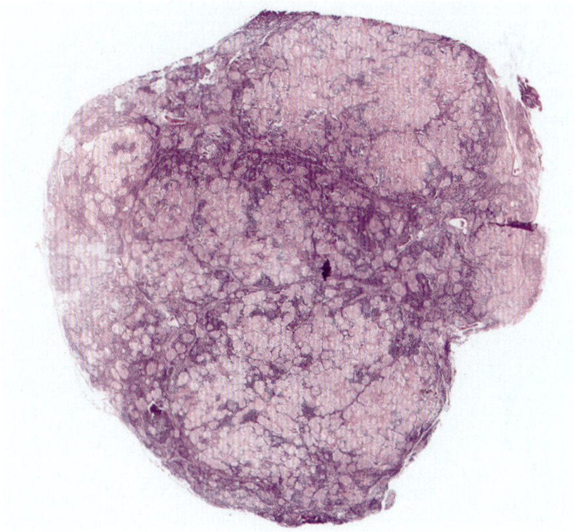

Figure 12-10

SARCOIDOSIS, LYMPH NODE

Much of this lymph node is replaced by well-circumscribed granulomas.

SYSTEMIC LUPUS ERYTHEMATOSUS

Definition. An autoimmune disorder of autoantibody production, including those directed against DNA, *systemic lupus erythematosus* (SLE), or lupus, has significant systemic symptoms as well as frequent and distinctive involvement of the lymph nodes and spleen.

Figure 12-11

SARCOIDOSIS, LYMPH NODE

A,B: Some residual lymphoid tissue is crowded into this lymph node that is only partially replaced by sarcoidal granulomas.

C: High magnification highlights the features of the epithelioid macrophages.

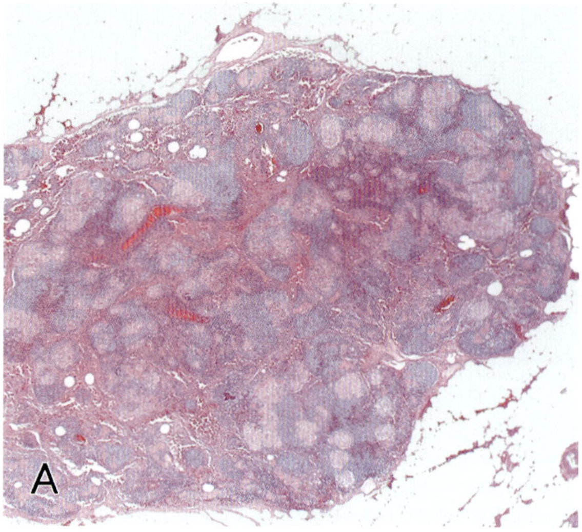

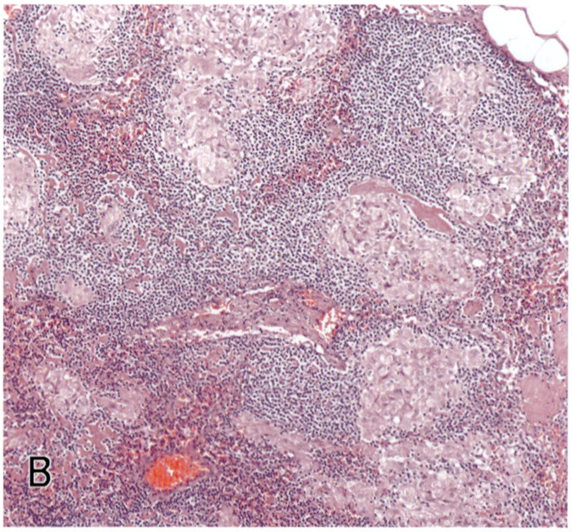

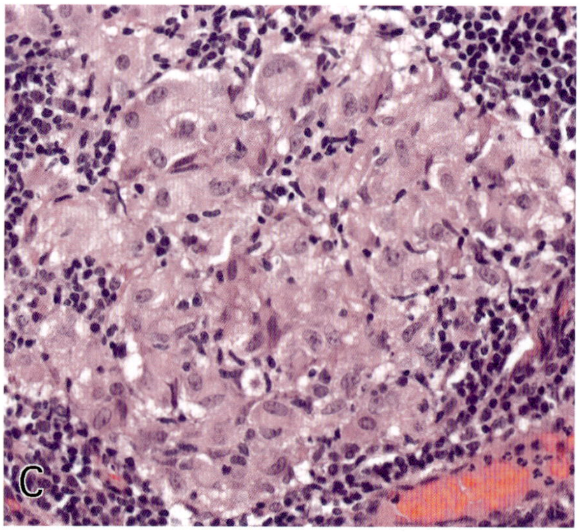

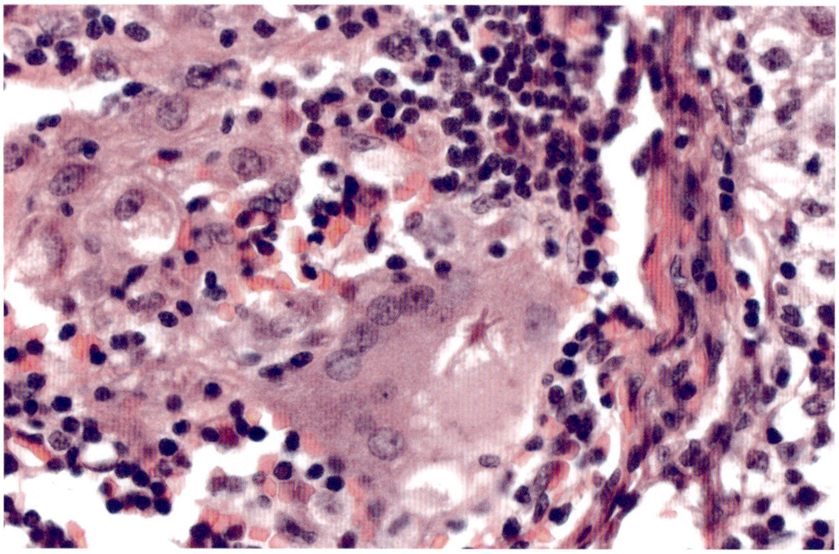

Figure 12-12

SARCOIDOSIS, LYMPH NODE

An asteroid body in a case of sarcoidosis.

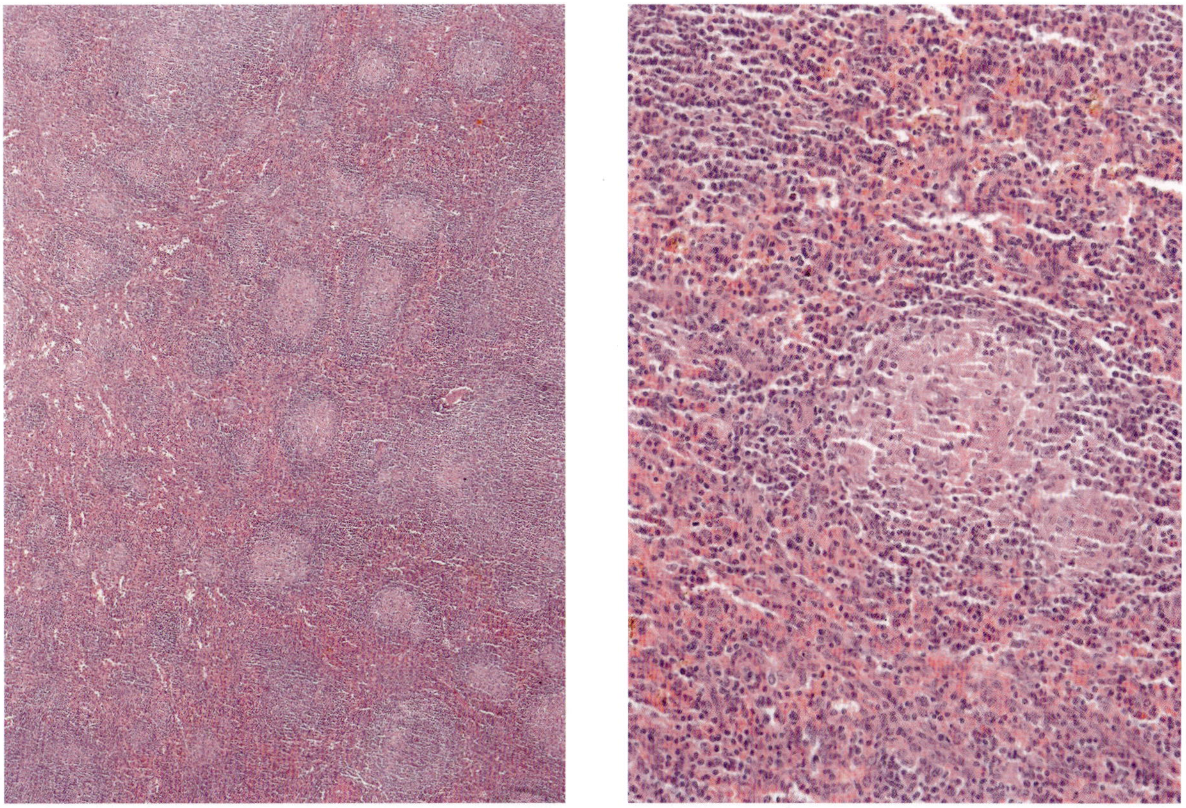

Figure 12-13

SARCOIDOSIS, SPLEEN

Splenic granulomas with intervening red pulp.

General Features. The underlying abnormality in SLE is the production of multiple autoantibodies, particularly directed against double-stranded DNA (dsDNA). It has been suggested that impaired clearance of autoantibodies by tingible body macrophages in the germinal centers is part of the process leading to SLE (14).

Clinical Features. The clinical features of SLE are protean. The diagnostic criteria are malar rash, photosensitivity, ulcers of mucous membranes, arthritis, and serositis. Other abnormalities occur in the central nervous system, renal system, and musculoskeletal system; virtually any organ or body system may be affected by SLE. Lymphadenopathy is present in 12 to 78 percent of cases (26,46,84,87). The cervical, axillary, and inguinal lymph nodes are the most commonly enlarged. Rare patients with SLE present with lymphadenopathy (84). Splenomegaly, splenic abscess and rare splenic rupture have been reported (53).

Laboratory Findings. Laboratory testing is the cornerstone for the diagnosis of SLE and includes a variety of tests for autoantibodies including antinuclear antibody (ANA). Anti-dsDNA is one of the more specific tests for SLE, as is the finding of anti-Smith antibodies. The "LE test," a method of inducing autophagocytosis of damaged white blood cells, is not considered sensitive or specific enough for the diagnosis.

Microscopic Findings. The typical findings in SLE lymph nodes are follicular hyperplasia, necrosis (sometimes large, geographic areas), and various proliferations of macrophages, immunoblasts, and plasma cells (fig. 12-14) (87,89). Striking interfollicular polyclonal plasmacytosis is occasionally seen as well as plasma cells within follicles. Involved lymph nodes show a mixed pattern of reactive lymphoid hyperplasia with areas of necrosis that is strikingly similar to that seen in Kikuchi-Fujimoto disease (fig. 12-15). This has caused some investigators to propose

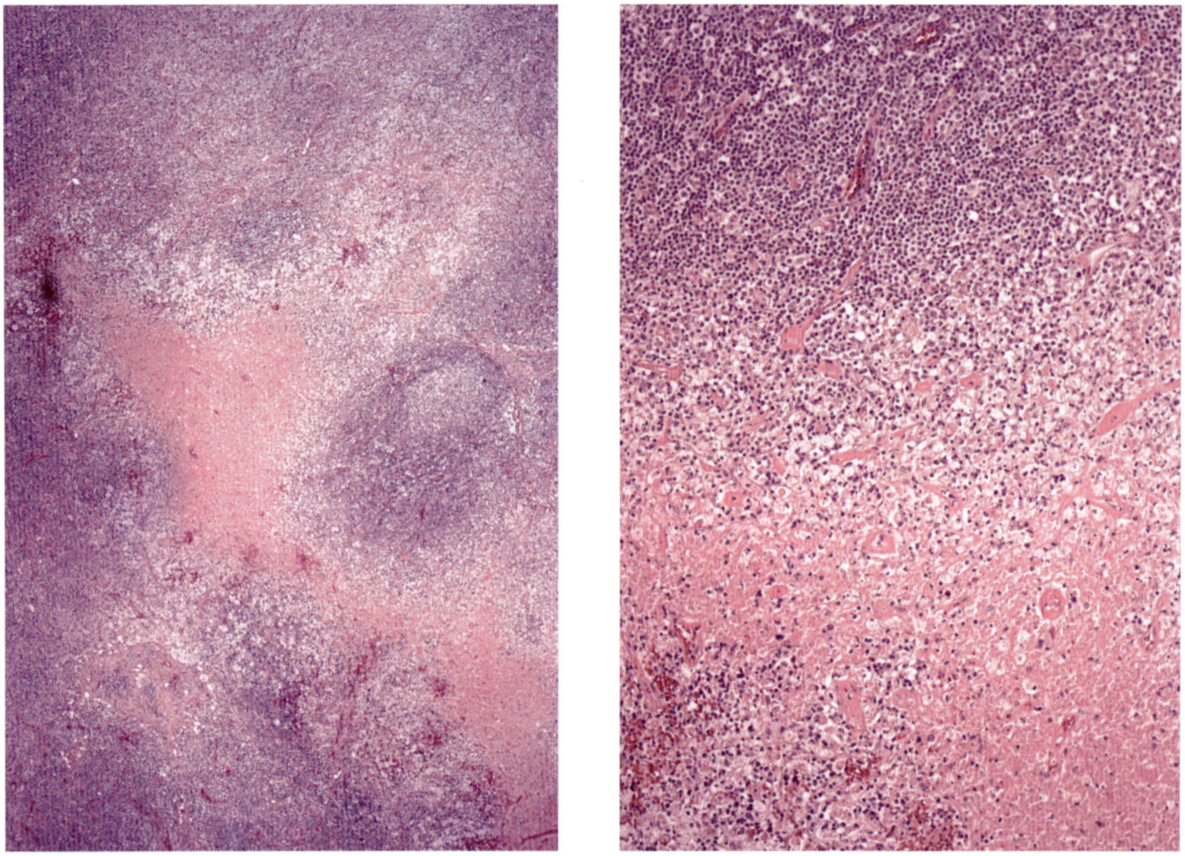

Figure 12-14

SYSTEMIC LUPUS ERYTHEMATOSUS, LYMPH NODE

Acute lupus lymphadenitis often has large areas of necrosis.

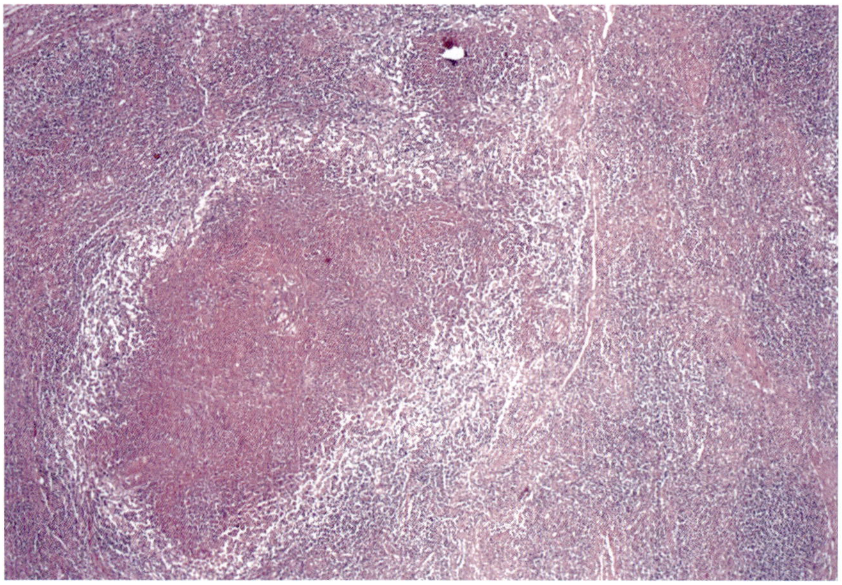

Figure 12-15

SYSTEMIC LUPUS ERYTHEMATOSUS

Acute lupus erythematosus with necrosis, which can simulate other causes of nodal necrosis.

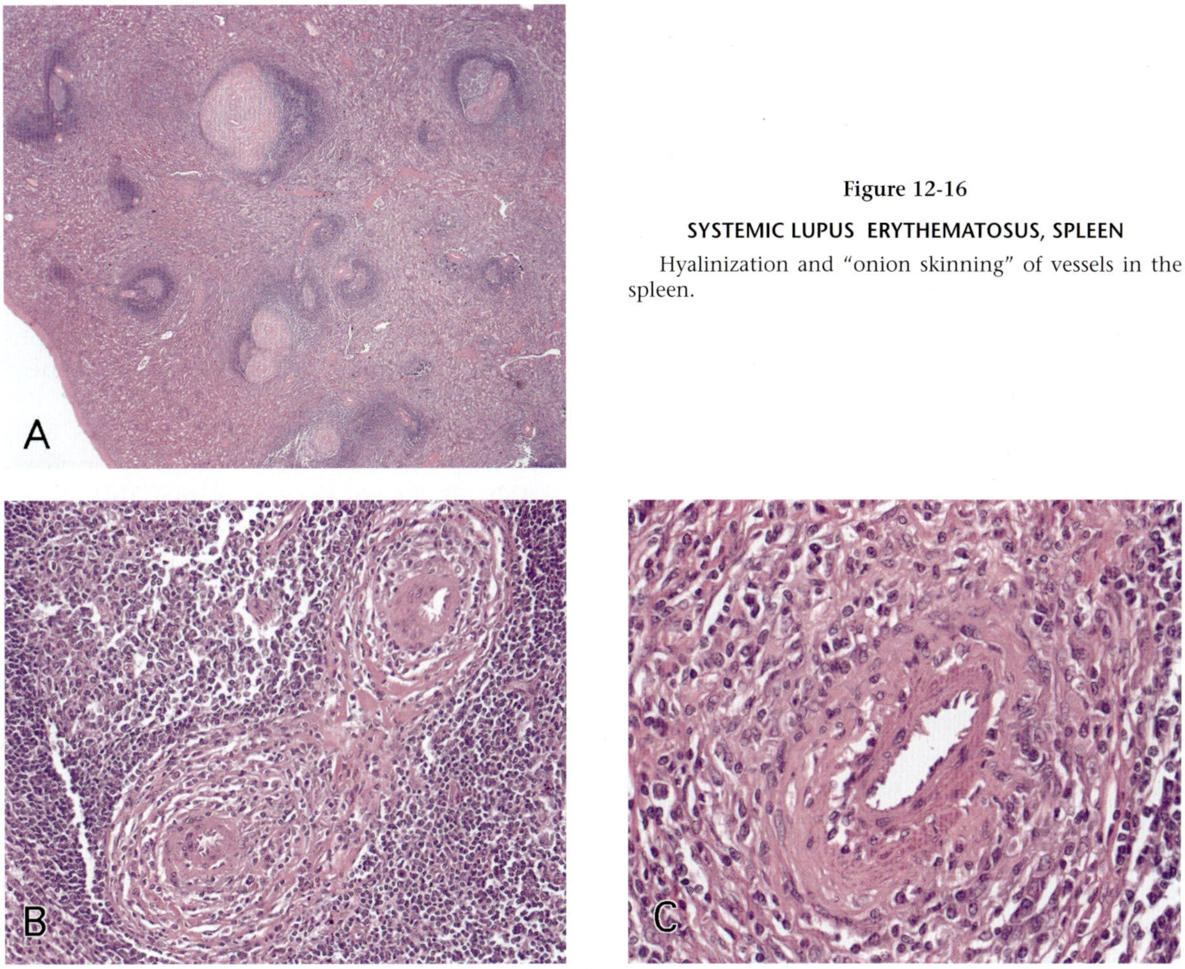

Figure 12-16

SYSTEMIC LUPUS ERYTHEMATOSUS, SPLEEN

Hyalinization and "onion skinning" of vessels in the spleen.

that Kikuchi-Fujimoto disease may represent a "forme fruste" of SLE (111,140,150). There are important differences, however, such as the variable presence of neutrophils in SLE lymphadenitis which are, by definition, absent in Kikuchi-Fujimoto disease. Although the presence of hematoxylin bodies (amorphous aggregates of deeply basophilic material, positive for periodic acid–Schiff [PAS] and Feulgen stains) in the sinuses, paracortex, or vessel walls is considered virtually diagnostic of SLE lymphadenitis, it is extremely difficult to demonstrate these in routine histologic sections.

Besides the more typical hyperplastic lymph nodes with necrosis, other patterns have been reported. There may be Castleman-like features, follicular hyperplasia with vascular proliferation, and marked interfollicular expansion by polyclonal plasma cells (19,85,87,88,91). Follicular lysis, with mantle cells intruding on the germinal centers, and proliferations of follicular dendritic cells, as illustrated by CD21, may be seen. These cases may be confused with angioimmunoblastic T-cell lymphoma or polymorphic post-transplant lymphoproliferative disease (PTLD).

Cases of SLE that resemble hyaline-vascular and plasma cell type Castleman disease have regressed follicles, with "onion-skin" mantle zones and hyalinized vessels penetrating follicles (88). Areas that resemble plasma cell Castleman disease also have areas of polyclonal plasmacytosis, including immature plasma cells and immunoblasts.

Lymphoid hyperplasia with hyperplastic and hypertrophic germinal centers is seen in the spleen. Macrophages and plasma cells are increased near arterioles. A classic histologic feature seen in spleens affected by SLE is the onion-skin fibrosis surrounding arteries (fig. 12-16). This finding is relatively specific for SLE, and is seen in over 80 percent of cases (53). Calcifications are associated with these onion-skin lesions. Rare features of capsulitis, small infarcts, and larger segmental infarcts are seen. Massive splenomegaly has been reported infrequently.

Differential Diagnosis. Bacterial infections, especially cat-scratch disease, may cause suppurative granulomas simulating either Kikuchi-Fujimoto disease (71) or SLE lymphadenitis. The invariable presence of neutrophils, the demonstration of the cat-scratch bacillus on Warthin-Starry stains, and the different clinical features, should help to distinguish cat-scratch disease from SLE or Kikuchi-Fujimoto disease. Cases with florid follicular hyperplasia may resemble HIV-related adenopathy or infectious mononucleosis, and these entities should be considered in the differential diagnosis.

Treatment and Prognosis. The treatment and outcome of patients with SLE depend on the severity of the symptoms. In some patients, the disease is mild, while in others it is serious. Combinations of steroid therapies, antiinflammatory agents, and antimetabolite chemotherapies are typically used for treatment. There is an increased risk of developing lymphoma in patients with SLE (19).

RHEUMATOID ARTHRITIS AND ADULT-ONSET JUVENILE RHEUMATOID ARTHRITIS (STILL DISEASE)

Definition. *Rheumatoid arthritis* (RA) and *adult-onset juvenile rheumatoid arthritis* (AJRA), also known as *Still disease*, are autoimmune systemic diseases with prominent rheumatologic manifestations. Both may have associated lymphadenopathy. Splenomegaly is a common feature in both as well.

General Features. RA and AJRA are inflammatory disorders. The exact cause of RA is unknown, but its primary effects are mediated by the production of excess proinflammatory cytokines by immune cells. Although considered to be an autoimmune disease, little is known about the cause of AJRA.

Clinical Features. Lymphadenopathy has been reported in 41 to 82 percent of RA patients (26). Most patients with active disease have axillary adenopathy. Generalized adenopathy is also seen, but is rare. More commonly, the adenopathy is near actively inflamed joints. Clinically detectable splenomegaly is seen in 5 to 10 percent of patients with RA (53). Studies have shown that splenic function is abnormal in these cases (53). Rarely, splenic rupture or splenic abscesses occur (53,64).

AJRA is characterized by high spiking fevers, rash, arthralgias, arthritis, polyserositis, hepatosplenomegaly, lymphadenopathy, leukocytosis, increased erythrocyte sedimentation rate, hypergammaglobulinemia, and a negative rheumatoid factor (RF) titer (75,90). Lymphadenopathy is seen in 40 to 90 percent of these patients (75,90).

Laboratory Findings. Most patients with RA have positive serologic tests for RF; approximately 50 percent have a positive ANA. There are no characteristic serologic findings in AJRA. Both ANA and RF are negative. The C-reactive protein and sedimentation rate are typically abnormal in both disorders.

Microscopic Findings. The common histologic findings in the lymph nodes of patients with RA include reactive follicular hyperplasia and interfollicular plasma cells (fig. 12-17). Deposition of eosinophilic hyaline material is frequently seen (113). The deposited material is not amyloid. Similar features are seen in patients with systemic sclerosis. The follicles may appear "burnt out": paucicellular, with hyaline material replacing the central, cellular portion of the germinal center. In exceptional cases, an atypical lymphoid proliferation consisting of a lymphoplasmacytic infiltrate, increased immunoblasts, and paracortical T-cell hyperplasia is seen (86). These findings are similar to those seen in methotrexate-associated lymphoid proliferations (see chapter 14). Ruptured spleens show dense capsular fibrosis, granulation tissue, and foamy macrophages. The changes in the white pulp are similar to those seen in the lymph nodes.

Jeon et al. (75) described four histologic patterns in the lymph nodes of patients with AJRA: follicular hyperplasia, exuberant immunoblastic proliferation, atypical paracortical/interfollicular hyperplasia, and a burnt-out histiocytic pattern (figs. 12-18, 12-19). Both the immunoblastic and atypical paracortical patterns could be confused with lymphomas, particularly large cell lymphoma and angioimmunoblastic T-cell lymphoma, respectively.

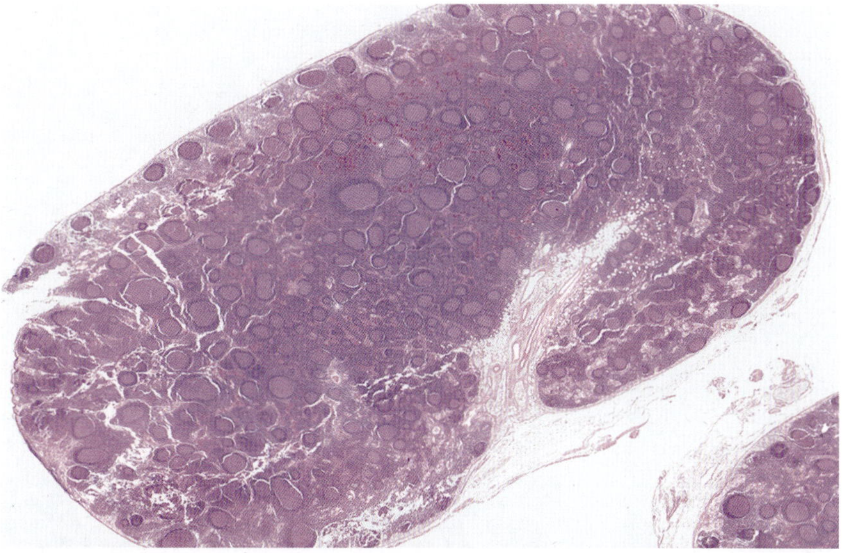

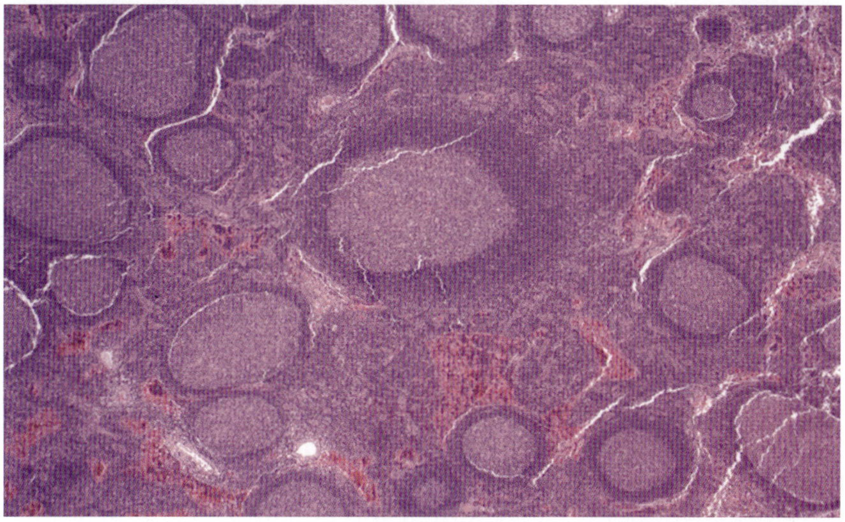

Figure 12-17

RHEUMATOID ARTHRITIS, LYMPH NODE

The follicular hyperplasia is striking.

Figure 12-18

RHEUMATOID ARTHRITIS, LYMPH NODE

Plasma cells with Russell bodies within germinal centers. Plasma cells are frequently seen in the germinal centers of patients with autoimmune lymphadenitis.

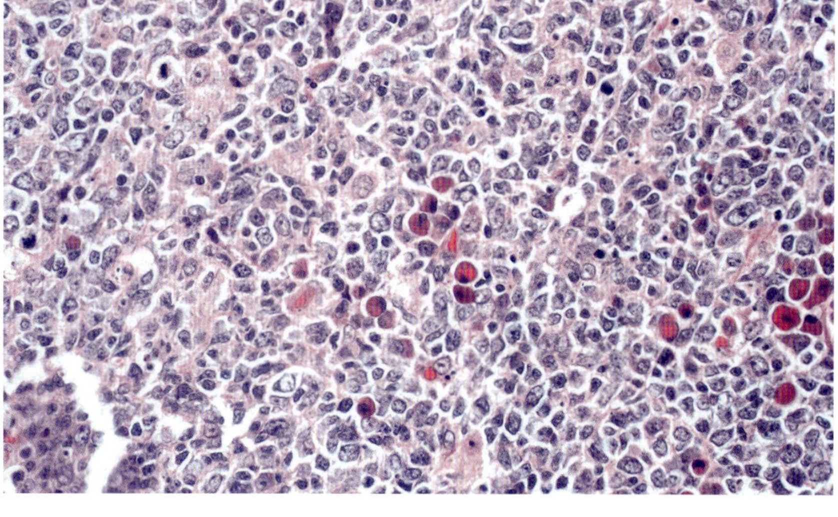

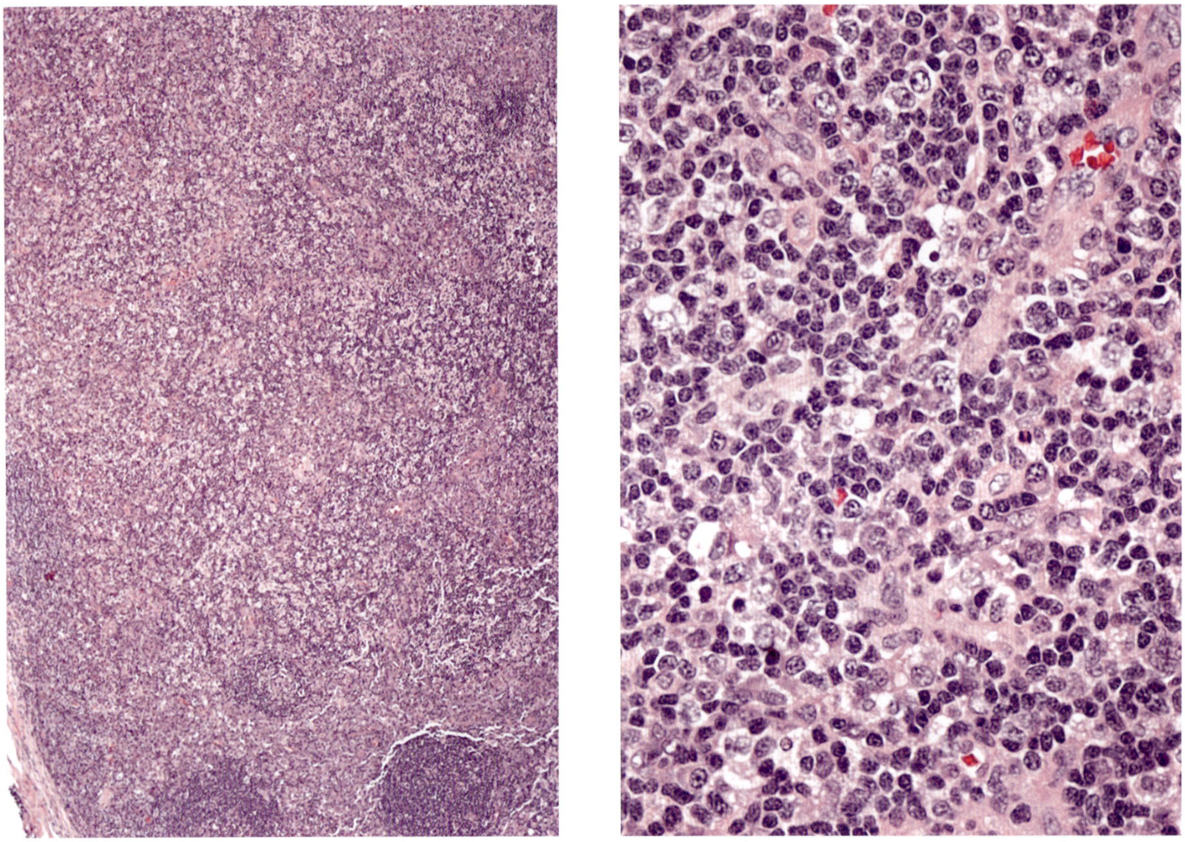

Figure 12-19

ADULT-ONSET JUVENILE RHEUMATOID ARTHRITIS, LYMPH NODE

A paracortical pattern is shown on the left and an immunoblastic pattern on the right.

The paracortical pattern is characterized by a paracortical proliferation of immunoblasts and increased density of high endothelial venules (90,165). Hyperplastic and atrophic germinal centers are seen. The interfollicular cellularity is composed of lymphocytes, immunoblasts, plasma cells, macrophages, and rare eosinophils. This is similar in appearance to interfollicular T-cell lymphoma, but is also identical to the findings in SLE, drug-induced lymphadenopathy, and other autoimmune lymphadenopathies. CD30 highlights the immunoblasts. Increased meshworks of follicular dendritic cells, as seen in angioimmunoblastic T-cell lymphoma, are not present. The burnt-out histiocytic pattern is characterized by vascular proliferation, numerous macrophages in the sinuses, and effacement of the normal follicular structures. Studies (95,129) reported findings in AJRA that mimic multicentric Castleman disease, with numerous polyclonal plasma cells and high levels of circulating interleukin (IL)-6.

Treatment and Prognosis. The prognosis of patients with RA and AJRA is variable depending on how the patient is affected by the disease. A variety of therapies are available including steroids, antiinflammatory agents, and antimetabolite chemotherapies. Newer medications that use monoclonal antibodies against specific proinflammatory cytokines (e.g., antitumor necrosis factor) are also being used.

FELTY SYNDROME

Definition. *Felty syndrome* is a complex of manifestations associated with RA, including splenomegaly. The selective splenic sequestration of granulocytes is seen.

General Features. Several mechanisms are known to play a role in the pathogenesis of the granulocytopenia in Felty syndrome (23).

Decreased neutrophil production has been reported in some cases (62). Increased suppressor T-cell activity has been implicated as well (1,11). In the majority of cases, however, the granulocytopenia is due to a shift of granulocytes from the circulating to the marginating pool (62,168,171). Previous studies have shown that in Felty syndrome the interaction of immune complexes with granulocytes leads to the peripheral sequestration of granulocytes (22,105). van Krieken et al. (168) suggested, on the basis of detailed morphologic, morphometric, and immunohistologic analyses of spleens from patients with Felty syndrome, that the spleen is the principal site of interaction between immune complexes and granulocytes. Since the level of immune complexes is not decreased after splenectomy in patients with Felty syndrome, it is unlikely that the splenic lymphoid tissue plays a significant role in the formation of immune complexes (168). Nonetheless, the fact that the spleen plays a crucial role in the cytopenias observed in Felty syndrome is also suggested by the clinical observation that corticosteroid therapy is rarely effective, but splenectomy often corrects the cytopenias (100,105,112).

Clinical Features. Felty syndrome consists of the triad of RA, splenomegaly, and neutropenia (12,36,106,138,156,157). The syndrome usually develops in less than 1 percent of patients with RA; these patients frequently have a high titer of RF and extraarticular manifestations, including refractory leg ulcers and an increased susceptibility to bacterial infection (55). Splenomegaly may result in mild anemia or thrombocytopenia, and occasionally, lymphopenia. The granulocytopenia, however, is out of proportion to the other cytopenias. Some patients also have hepatomegaly and lymphadenopathy, which correlate with a more severe degree of neutropenia.

Gross Findings. The spleens may be markedly enlarged, often with pronounced miliary nodularity.

Microscopic Findings. Granulocytes are found in T-cell areas (periarteriolar lymphoid sheath [PALS]) even in patients with severe granulocytopenia (fig. 12-20). The red pulp shows expansion of the perifollicular zones as well as sinusoidal dilatation and an increased number of macrophages. The number of red pulp plasma cells is usually not increased and perivascular fibrosis is absent (168). The white pulp follicles are usually hyperplastic with morphologic evidence of an evolving immune reaction (100,112).

Selective neutropenia occurs in association with other disorders, including other forms of arthritis, hemolytic anemia, sarcoidosis, and cirrhosis. Certain drugs also produce neutropenia (136,173). Isolated neutropenia associated with splenomegaly has been reported in the absence of an underlying disorder (94). Splenectomy is occasionally successful in increasing neutrophil counts in patients with chronic idiopathic neutropenia (38).

Treatment and Prognosis. Up to 40 percent of the patients with Felty syndrome have large granular lymphocytic leukemia (see later this chapter), and may ultimately require treatment for this disorder (96). Splenectomy results in an improvement in the number of granulocytes in 60 to 70 percent of patients (60,100,120). Perhaps paradoxically, a decreased incidence of infection has been reported in 73 percent of patients following splenectomy (100,120). Although some investigators recommend splenectomy at the time of diagnosis (142), surgical intervention is usually reserved for patients with severe neutropenia and infections (35,174). Oral methotrexate is also an effective long-term therapy in selected patients (59).

LARGE GRANULAR LYMPHOCYTOSIS

Definition. Non-neoplastic proliferations of CD8-positive cytotoxic T cells are seen in a variety of disorders, most commonly associated with autoimmune disorders. Proliferations of these *large granular lymphocytes* (LGLs) may result in splenomegaly.

General Features. Normal LGLs (e.g., CD8-positive cytotoxic T cells) function through major histocompatability (MHC)-mediated interactions with other immune function cells. They express Fas ligand (Fas-L), a member of the tumor necrosis family. Fas-L and Fas interactions on target cells initiate apoptosis. LGL proliferations are thought to be antigen-driven immune responses. It is thought that specific antigens, such as in RA, may underlie proliferations of LGLs.

Clinical Features. LGL diseases cover a heterogeneous spectrum of disorders that include reactive conditions, typically associated with

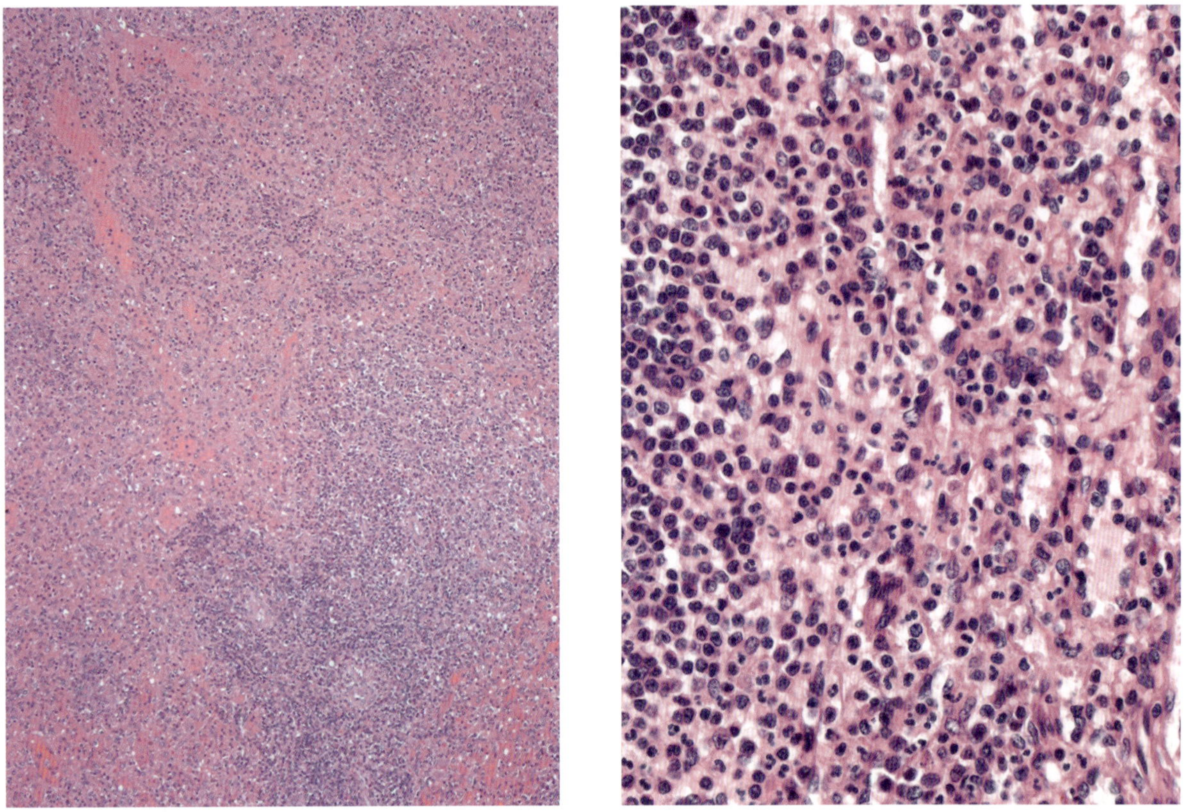

Figure 12-20

FELTY SYNDROME, SPLEEN

A neutrophilic infiltrate is seen.

autoimmune disease, to outright leukemias of LGL. Leukemias of LGL, originally described by McKenna et al. in 1977 (114), account for 2 to 3 percent of cases of small lymphocytic leukemias (28). In spite of this heterogeneity, LGL disorders have a well-defined clinical spectrum and pathologic features which help define them.

Nonleukemic LGL proliferations are either transient or chronic (16). There are undoubtedly individual cases that fall in a borderline zone between reactive and leukemic LGL disorders. Some authors have gone as far as to suggest that there is a "T-cell clonopathy of undetermined significance" ("TCUS"), analogous to monoclonal gammopathy of undetermined significance (MGUS) (40).

LGL disease and LGL leukemia are found in older individuals, of an average age of presentation of approximately 60 years, although they have been reported in all age groups including children (95,96,144). Males and females are equally affected. Median survival periods of greater than 10 years are usual with LGL leukemia (40,95,96,144).

The typical clinical symptomatology of LGL disorders includes fevers, recurrent bacterial infections, fatigue, and weight loss. Mild to moderate splenomegaly is seen in many patients (20 to 60 percent) and hepatomegaly more rarely (less than 20 percent) (67,95,96). Neutropenia, often severe, is the most uniform feature and is present in 60 to 85 percent of symptomatic patients at presentation (28,144). Lymphadenopathy is rare (40). Other associations that occur rarely are neuropathy, solid tumors, endocrinopathy, and MGUS. Serologic abnormalities are frequent in LGL leukemia (40,95,96,144).

Benign, reactive increases in LGLs are seen in association with a variety of causes: splenectomy, HIV infection, other viral infections, allogeneic stem cell transplantation, and solid organ transplantation (144,175). Persistent

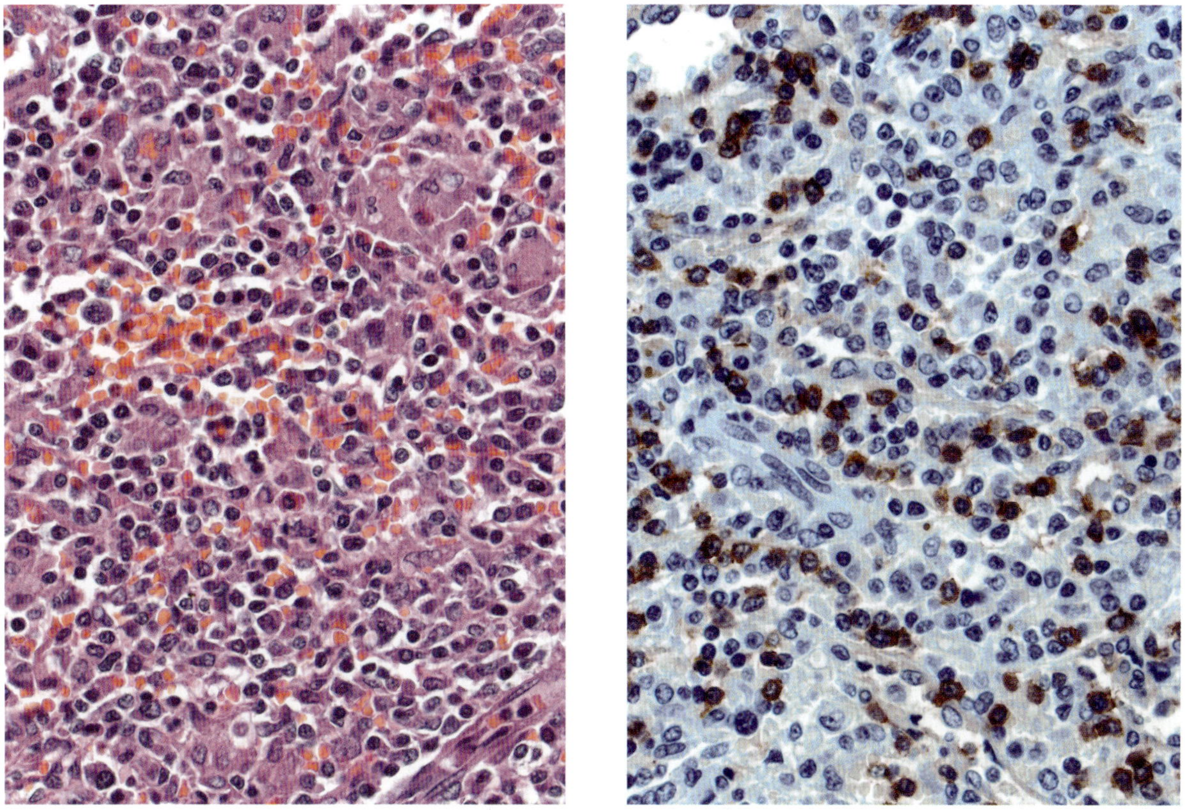

Figure 12-21

LARGE GRANULAR LYMPHOCYTOSIS, SPLEEN

Left: High magnification of a lymphoid infiltrate of large granular lymphocytes (LGL) in the red pulp. Most of these cases are clonal T-cell proliferations (e.g., LGL leukemia).

Right: CD8 reactivity in spleen with LGL disease. Numerous intrasinusoidal cytotoxic lymphocytes are highlighted.

clonal expansion of CD8-positive T-cell subsets are seen in some elderly individuals who do not develop LGL leukemia (137). The exact distinction between reactive LGL increases and LGL leukemia is difficult and both represent extreme points in a spectrum of disorders.

Many autoimmune diseases are associated both with LGL disease and LGL leukemia. LGL leukemia is associated with RA (25 percent), Felty syndrome (up to 40 percent), Evan syndrome, Sjögren syndrome, Hashimoto thyroiditis, autoimmune polyglandular syndrome, Graves disease, Cushing syndrome, hyperparathyroidism, multiple sclerosis, ulcerative colitis, recurrent uveitis, and psoriasis (40,67,95,96,127,144).

Microscopic Findings. Splenic involvement by LGL disease has a relatively characteristic appearance. In most cases, there is mild to moderate enlargement of the spleen. Typically, the red pulp expands, with only minimal changes in the white pulp. The red pulp shows increased cellularity, with a large population of small lymphocytes (fig. 12-21). In well-fixed and -prepared sections, the increased amounts of cytoplasm may be appreciated. As in other sites, LGLs in the spleen have small round nuclei with mature chromatin. They infiltrate splenic sinuses of the red pulp and distend the cords (130).

In the white pulp, germinal centers may be present, and may be hyperplastic or regressed. The PALS regions are composed predominantly of T lymphocytes. These zones are subtly expanded, often due to infiltration by the neoplastic lymphocytes of LGL disease. This infiltration is often difficult to recognize based entirely on morphologic examination, and is only apparent on immunohistochemical examination. Lymphadenopathy is a rare finding in LGL disorders.

Ancillary Studies. The immunophenotypic features are important both in the diagnosis and the pathobiology of LGL disorders. Flow cytometric analysis is the most powerful methodology for diagnosing LGL disorders, particularly LGL leukemia, by demonstrating an abnormal immunophenotype in the LGLs. Normal LGLs are CD8-positive T cells with the following immunophenotype: CD2+, cytoplasmic CD3+, CD4-, CD5+, CD7+, CD8+, CD16-, CD56-, α/β+, and γ/δ-. The neoplastic counterpart, seen in LGL leukemia, has an abnormal immunophenotype in virtually all cases (107,122). Lundell et al. (107) demonstrated that 80 percent of LGL leukemias abnormally expressed two or more pan-T-cell antigens. CD5 and CD7 are the antigens that are usually abnormally expressed; expression is dim or absent, although abnormal bright expression is also seen (61,123). Expression of natural killer (NK) cell-related antigens CD16 (about 80 percent) and CD57 (near 100 percent) is usual in LGL leukemias, although their expression is also seen in a small subset of normal cytotoxic T cells, the "NK-like T cell" (117,118,123).

Immunohistochemistry is useful for demonstrating abnormal T cells in the spleen. T cells are evaluated for a variety of T-cell antigens by tissue immunohistochemistry. Normal T-LQL would be expected to express CD2, CD3, CD5, CD7, CD8, as well as TIA-1, perforin, and granzyme B (markers of cytotoxic cells) (122).

Treatment and Prognosis. In reactive LGL proliferations, the lymphocytosis may resolve spontaneously. It may decrease in response to therapy for underlying autoimmune disorders. Many treatments are available for LGL leukemia including observation, steroids, low-dose methotrexate, cyclophosphamide, cyclosporin A, purine analogs (pentostatin, fludarabine), and alemtuzumab (Campath-1H) (95,144). The goal of therapy is improvement of the neutropenia and reduction of the infections.

BEHCET DISEASE

Definition. *Behcet disease* is a nonspecific vasculitis associated with recurrent ulcerations, relapsing vasculitis, and occasionally, splenic involvement.

Clinical Features. Behcet disease is common in the Middle East and Asia, paticularly in Japan. It is characterized by recurrent oral and genital ulcerations, ocular inflammation, pulmonary involvement, and central nervous system involvement. The etiology is unknown but the disorder is characterized by chronic, relapsing vasculitis of multiple organs and systems (15). Splenomegaly is seen in about 20 percent of patients (53).

Microscopic Findings. Histopathologic descriptions of splenic pathology are rare. Tuzun (164) describes a spleen removed for the presence of an abscess. Further examination revealed large areas of infarction surrounding a trabecular artery. An organized thrombus with recanalization and thickened vessels were also seen. Other findings include nonspecific inflammation, congestion, splenomegaly, hemosiderosis, infarction, and autosplenectomy (15).

Treatment and Prognosis. Behcet disease is a chronic multisystem disorder with a remitting relapsing course, like many other autoimmune conditions. Steroids and immunosuppressive medications are used for treatment.

THROMBOTIC THROMBOCYTOPENIC PURPURA

Definition. *Thrombotic thrombocytopenic purpura* (TTP) is a disorder of coagulation, resulting in consumptive coagulopathy and tissue damage due to the formation of small intravascular thrombi.

General Features. The pathophysiology of TTP is related to the formation and cleavage of multimers of von Willebrand factor (vWF). Ultra-large (UL) multimers of vWF are normally cleaved to form smaller molecules of vWF. The UL multimers cause inappropriate binding of platelets and the formation of small thrombi. The lack of, or lack of function of, a protease that is responsible for the cleavage of ULvWF is the cause of TTP. The lack of this protein may be inherited (very rare), but is more often due to the formation of an antibody directed against the cleavage protein. This leads to the accumulation of ULvWF and subsequent TTP.

Clinical Features. TTP is a rare condition and is most common on the 3rd to 5th decades. It is twice as common in women. Although most cases occur spontaneously, some cases are related to medications, pregnancy, infections (including HIV), autoimmune conditions (SLE), and malignancies. The manifestations of TTP are thrombocytopenia, microangiopathic

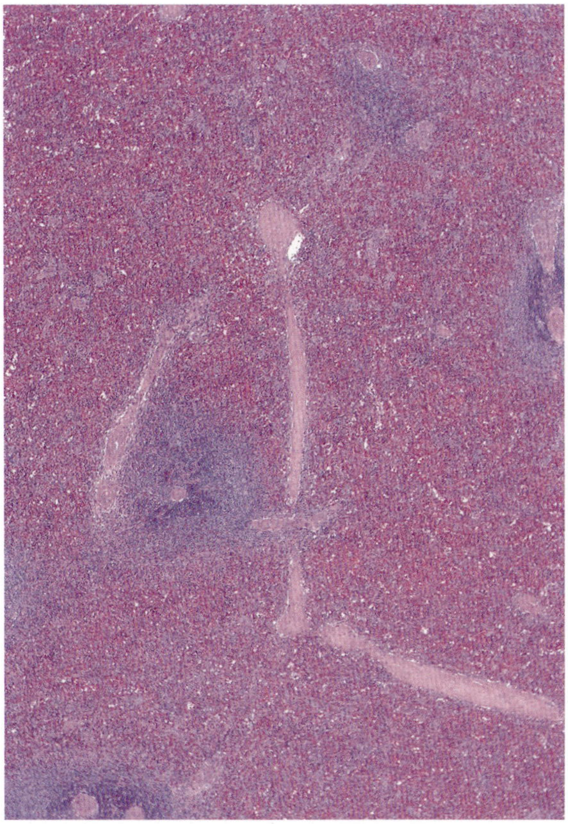

Figure 12-22

THROMBOTIC THROMBOCYTOPENIC PURPURA, SPLEEN

There are no marked abnormalities by low-magnification examination. (Figs. 12-22 and 12-23 are from the same patient.)

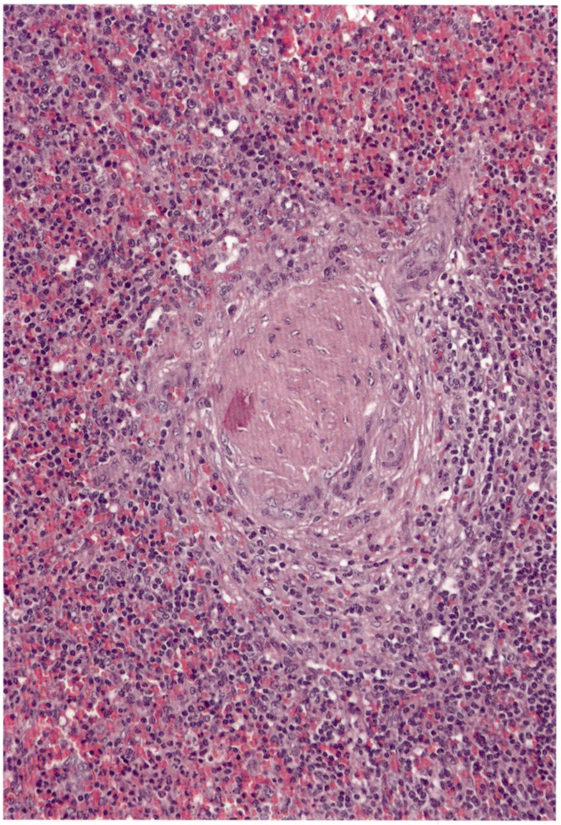

Figure 12-23

THROMBOTIC THROMBOCYTOPENIC PURPURA, SPLEEN

Vascular thrombi are present.

hemolytic anemia, neurologic abnormalities, and renal dysfunction.

Laboratory Findings. Laboratory findings are essential in the diagnosis of TTP but are not entirely specific for the diagnosis. They must be considered in the clinical context. Thrombocytopenia is present in all cases as are the features of microangiopathic hemolytic anemia, including the presence of schistocytes in the peripheral blood smear. As a consequence of hemolysis, the LDH is markedly elevated, as are the indirect bilirubin level and reticulocyte count. Prothrombin time (PT) and activated partial thromboplastin time (PTT) are normal.

Microscopic Findings. Splenomegaly and gross evidence of infarction are seen in some cases. Thrombi, composed of small clusters of platelets and fibrin, are frequently found within small, and sometimes larger, vessels (figs. 12-22–12-24). Hyaline subendothelial deposits are frequently seen, and are PAS positive and diastase sensitive. Periarteriolar concentric fibrosis (onion skinning) is seen in the majority of cases, as is moderate hemophagocytosis. Moderate to marked deposition of hemosiderin is seen in almost all cases and is highlighted by iron stains such as Prussian blue.

In most cases, PALS areas are normal in size and distribution. The follicles are often increased in size and number. Extramedullary hematopoiesis is extensive (128,151).

Differential Diagnosis. The splenic findings may suggest autoimmune disorders such as SLE, because of the onion skinning around arterioles. Cases with extensive extramedullary hematopoieses may resemble splenic involvement by neoplastic myeloid disorders (128).

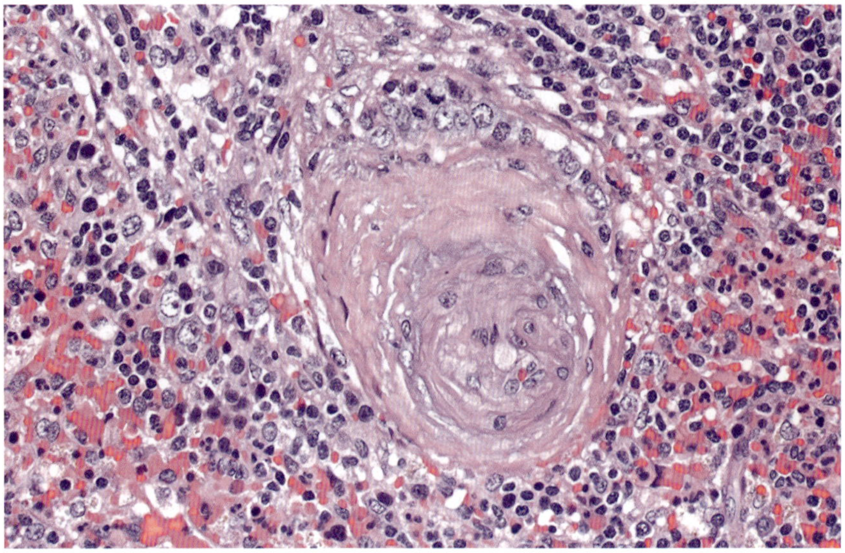

Figure 12-24

THROMBOTIC THROMBOCYTOPENIC PURPURA, SPLEEN

Perivascular fibrosis is frequently seen in splenic arteries in thrombotic thrombocytopenic purpura.

Treatment and Prognosis. Plasma exchange, to clear both the antibodies and ULvWF multimers, is effective in treating patients with TTP. The addition of immunosuppression, either by steroids or other medications, is often used in conjunction with plasmapheresis. Platelet transfusions are contraindicated, except in rare cases. In refractory disease, splenectomy is sometimes performed, with some improvement in outcome.

VASCULITIDES (WEGENER GRANULOMATOSIS, POLYARTERITIS NODOSA, CHURG-STRAUSS DISEASE, HENOCH-SCHONLEIN PURPURA)

Definition. A variety of primary inflammatory disorders of blood vessels exist; most of these have an autoimmune component. Although rare, several of these vasculitides have abnormalities of the lymph nodes or spleen.

Clinical Features. *Wegener granulomatosis* is a systemic necrotizing vasculitis of small and medium-sized arteries, with associated granulomatous inflammation. It affects middle-aged men and woman equally. Lungs, airways, and kidneys are always involved (53). The most common sites of presentation are upper airway, lung, kidney, and eye (101). It accounts for 8 percent of cases of vasculitis. The spleen is involved in 3 percent of cases. Splenomegaly, and rarely, splenic rupture, have been reported (53).

Polyarteritis nodosa (PAN) is a systemic inflammatory disease causing necrosis of medium-sized vessels with aneurysm formation. PAN represents approximately 8 percent of cases of vasculitis (101). Splenic rupture occurs rarely (54). Splenic abscess and functional hyposplenism may occur.

Churg-Strauss disease, or *allergic granulomatous angiitis*, is a vasculitis of small and medium-sized arteries. Manifestations include asthma, allergies, skin manifestations, and less commonly, involvement of the cardiovascular, renal, gastrointestinal, and nervous systems. It represents 4 percent of cases of vasculitis (101) and rarely has associated lymphadenopathy (27).

Henoch-Schonlein purpura (HSP) is an IgA-mediated immune complex vasculitis (5). Clinical findings include nonthrombocytopenic purpura, arthralgias, cutaneous leukocytoclastic vasculitis, and abdominal pain. Gastrointestinal hemorrhage and renal disease may also occur.

Laboratory Findings. Antineutrophil cytoplasmic antibody (ANCA) testing is an important serologic test for the evaluation of vasculitis, including cANCA (neutrophil serine protease PR3) and pANCA (autoantibody against myeloperoxidase). The erythrocyte sedimentation rate and C-reactive protein are typically elevated in patients with vasculitis.

Microscopic Findings. Splenic changes in Wegener granulomatosis include capsular adhesions, occasional thrombosis of splenic artery and vein, and areas of splenic necrosis and infarction. Numerous granulomas with associated necrosis are seen (53,56,101,131). These areas may be multiple small areas or large geographic

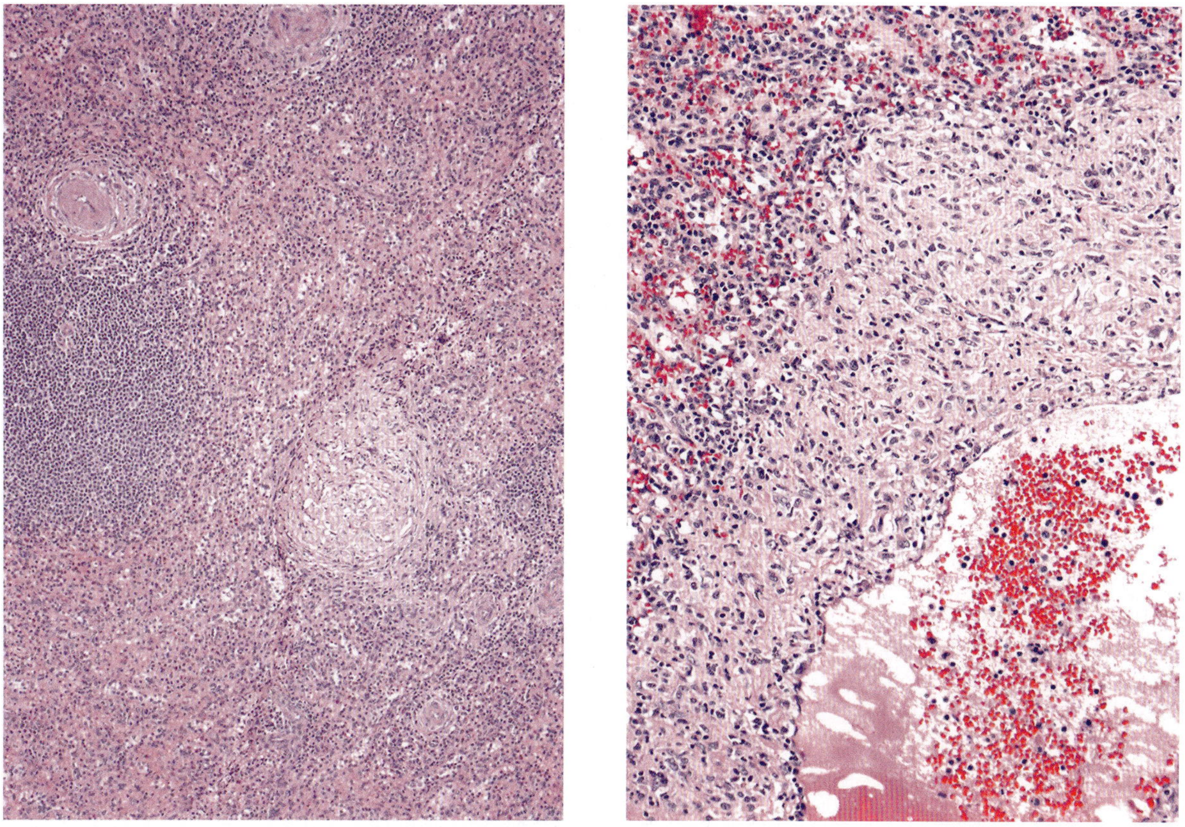

Figure 12-25

POLYARTERITIS NODOSA, SPLEEN

The vasculitis consists of thick, abnormal vessels.

areas, and are associated with arteritis, trabeculitis, and capsulitis. Necrotizing vasculitis of small and medium-sized arteries, with or without calcification, can be seen. Similar findings are less frequent in the lymph nodes.

Splenic findings in PAN include edema of sinusoidal and capillary endothelial cells. Granulocytes and plasma cells infiltrate the red pulp. In ruptured spleens associated with PAN, splenic vasculitis has been reported (fig. 12-25).

Lymph node involvement has been reported in Churg-Strauss disease. The histologic findings include large, eosinophil-rich granulomas with foci of central eosinophilic abscesses surrounded by a granulomatous macrophage reaction (fig. 12-26) (27). Charcot-Leyden crystals may be seen. General eosinophilia in the lymph nodes is associated with reactive follicles and expanded paracortical zones. The spleen is a common site of granuloma formation and vasculitis (53).

Lymph node changes in HSP include sinus histiocytosis, regressed follicles, and replacement of the follicle center by granulomas or aggregates of macrophages and dendritic cells (5). Some germinal centers contain neutrophils or microabscesses. Fibrin deposition in vessel walls and other evidence of vasculitis may be present.

Differential Diagnosis. Vasculitis is associated with lymphomas, including several types of T-cell lymphomas; occasional infectious diseases, such as Epstein-Barr virus (EBV) infection, may have a prominent component of vasculitis. Correlation of the histologic features with clinical and serologic findings is necessary in diagnosing vasculitis.

Treatment and Prognosis. Immunosuppressive drugs and steroids are the primary therapies for all types of vasculitides.

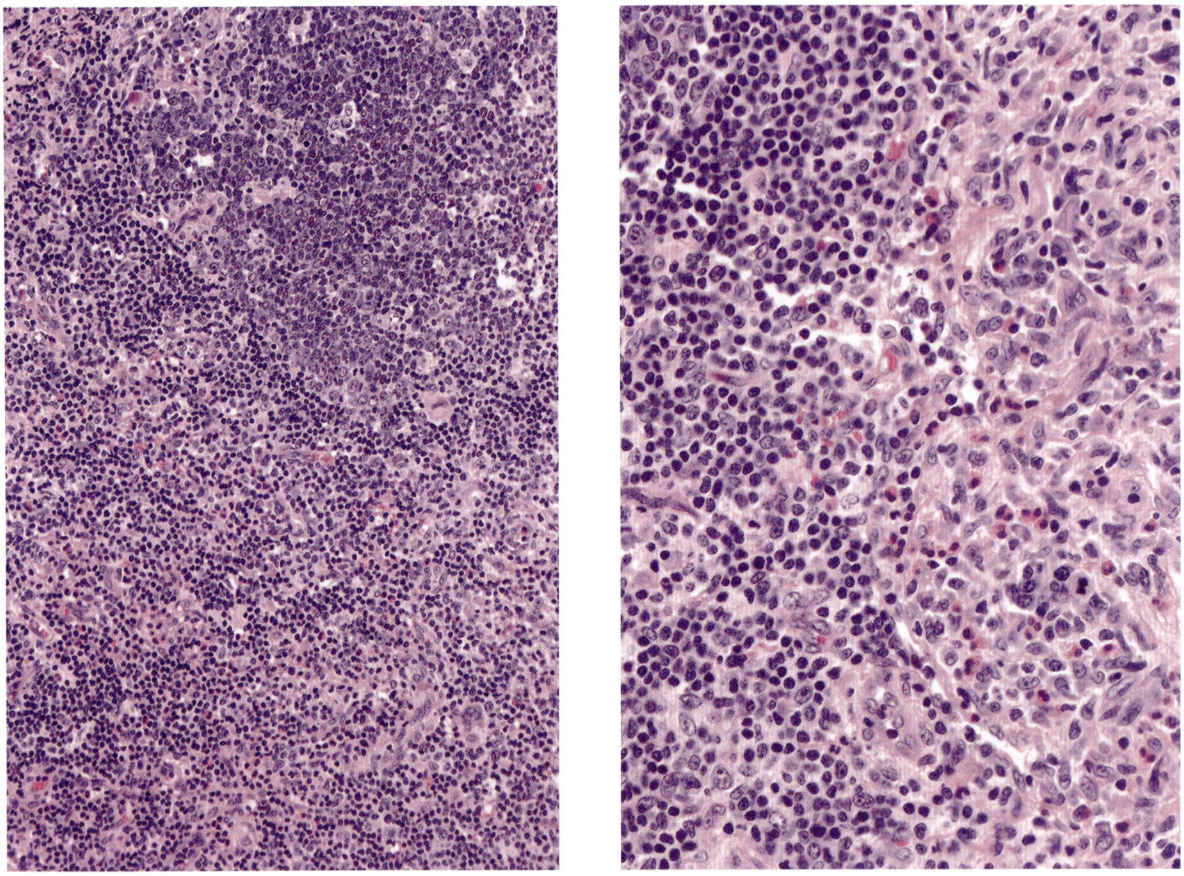

Figure 12-26

CHURG-STRAUSS DISEASE, LYMPH NODE

An immunoblastic proliferation (left) and perivascular eosinophils (right).

REFERENCES

1. Abdou NI, Napombejara C, Balentine L, Abdou NL. Suppressor cell-mediated neutropenia in Felty's syndrome. J Clin Invest 1978;61:738-43.
2. Abramson N, Lo Buglio AF, Jandl JH, Cotran RS. The interaction between human monocytes and red cells. Binding characteristics. J Exp Med 1970;132:1191-206.
3. Adams W, Rufo R, Talarico L, Silverman SL, Brauer MJ. Thrombocytopenia and intravenous heroin use. Ann Intern Med 1978;89:207.
4. Ahmed A, Feller ER. Rupture of the spleen as the initial manifestation of Wilson's disease. Am J Gastroenterol 1996;91:1454-5.
5. Akosa AB, Ali MH. Lymph node pathology in Henoch-Schonlein purpura. Histopathology 1989;15:297-301.
6. Aladesanmi OA. Sarcoidosis: an update for the primary care physician. Med Gen Med 2004;6:7.
7. Allen S, Chiu R, Orazi A, O'Malley DP. Refractory ITP: therapy-related histopathologic changes in spleens. Mod Pathol 2006;19:288A.
8. Arendt T, Nizze H, Konrad H. Prognostic significance of splenic follicle size in splenectomized idiopathic thrombocytopenic purpura patients. Blut 1988;57:347-9.
9. Aster RH, Keene WR. Sites of platelet destruction in idiopathic thrombocytopenic purpura. Br J Haematol 1969;16:61-73.
10. Axelson JA, LoBuglio AF. Immune hemolytic anemia. Med Clin North Am 1980;64:597-606.

11. Bagby GC Jr. T lymphocytes involved in inhibition of granulopoiesis in two neutrophilic patients are of the cytotoxic/suppressor (T3+T8+) subset. J Clin Invest 1981;68:1597-600.
12. Barnes CG, Turnbull AL, Vernon-Roberts B. Felty's syndrome. A clinical and pathological survey of 21 patients and their response to treatment. Ann Rheum Dis 1971;30:359-74.
13. Bauman C, Cron RQ, Sherry DD, Francis JS. Reiter syndrome initially misdiagnosed as Kawasaki disease. J Pediatr 1996;128:366-9.
14. Baumann I, Kolowos W, Voll RE, et al. Impaired uptake of apoptotic cells into tingible body macrophages in germinal centers of patients with systemic lupus erythematosus. Arthritis Rheum 2002;46:191-201.
15. Bayraktar Y, Ozaslan E, Van Thiel DH. Gastrointestinal manifestations of Behcet's disease. J Clin Gastroenterol 2000;30:144-54.
16. Beck RC, Stahl S, O'Keefe CL, Maciejewski JP, Theil KS, Hsi ED. Detection of mature T-cell leukemias by flow cytometry using anti-T-cell receptor V-beta antibodies. Am J Clin Pathol 2003;120:785-94.
17. Berendt HL, Mant MJ, Jewell LD. Periarterial fibrosis in the spleen in idiopathic thrombocytopenic purpura. Arch Pathol Lab Med 1986;110:1152-4.
18. Bierling P, Bettaieb A, Fromont P, Favrin M, Duedari N. Anti-GMP140 (CD62) autoantibody in a patient with autoimmune thrombocytopenic purpura. Br J Haematol 1994;87:631-3.
19. Blanco R, McLaren B, Davis B, Steele P, Smith R. Systemic lupus erythematosus-associated lymphoproliferative disorder: report of a case and discussion in light of the literature. Hum Pathol 1997;28:980-5.
20. Bowdler AJ. The role of the spleen and splenectomy in autoimmune hemolytic disease. Semin Hematol 1976;13:335-48.
21. Bowman HE, Pettit VD, Caldwell FT, Smith EB. Morphology of the spleen in idiopathic thrombocytopenic purpura. Lab Invest 1955;4:206-16.
22. Breedveld FC, Lafeber GJ, de Vries E, van Krieken JH, Cats A. Immune complexes and the pathogenesis of neutropenia in Felty's syndrome. Ann Rheum Dis 1986;45:696-702.
23. Breedveld FC, Lafeber GJ, Doekes G, Claas FH, Cats A. Felty's syndrome: autoimmune neutropenia or immune complex-mediated disease? Rheumatol Int 1985;5:253-8.
24. British Committee for Standards in Haematology General Haematology Task Force. Guidelines for the investigation and management of idiopathic thrombocytopenic purpura in adults, children and in pregnancy. Br J Haematol 2003;120:574-96.
25. Bussel J, Cines D. Immune thrombocytopenic purpura, neonatal alloimmune thrombocytopenia, and post-transfusion purpura. In: Hoffman R, Benz EJ Jr, Shattil S, et al, eds. Hematopathology: basic principles and practice, 3rd ed. Philadelphia: Churchill Livingston; 2000:2096-114.
26. Calguneri M, Ozturk MA, Ozbalkan Z, et al. Frequency of lymphadenopathy in rheumatoid arthritis and systemic lupus erythematosus. J Int Med Res 2003;31:345-9.
27. Casey M, Radel E, Ratech H. Lymph node manifestations of limited Churg-Strauss syndrome. J Pediatr Hematol Oncol 2000;22:468-71.
28. Chan WC, Catovsky D, Foucar K, et al. T-cell large granular lymphocyte leukemia. In: Jaffe ES, Harris NL, Stein H, Vardiman JW, eds. World Health Organization Classification of Tumours: Pathology and genetics of tumours of haematopoietic and lymphoid tissues. Lyon, France: IARC Press; 2001.
29. Chang C, Li C, Cha SS. Chronic idiopathic thrombocytopenic purpura. Splenic pathologic features and their clinical correlation. Arch Pathol Lab Med 1993;117:981-5.
30. Christensen BE, Hansen LK, Kristensen JK, Videback A. Splenectomy in haematology. Indications, results and complications in 41 cases. Scand J Haematol 1970;7:247-60.
31. Cines DB, Schreiber AD. Immune thrombocytopenia. Use of Coombs antiglobulin test to detect IgG and C3 on platelets. N Engl J Med 1979;300:106-11.
32. Clancy RL, Trent RJ. Current concepts of the pathogenesis and management of idiopathic thrombocytopenic purpura. Aust N Z J Med 1977;7:312-9.
33. Cohn J, Tygstrup J. Foamy histiocytosis of the spleen in patients with chronic thrombocytopenia. Scand J Haematol 1976;16:33-7.
34. Crosby WH. Splenectomy in hematologic disorders. N Engl J Med 1972;286:1252-4.
35. Crosby WH. What to treat in Felty's syndrome. JAMA 1973;225:1114-5.
36. Cryer PE, Kissane JM. Rheumatoid arthritis with Felty's syndrome, hyperviscosity, and immunologic hyperactivity. Am J Med 1981;70:89-100.
37. Czernobilsky B, Freedman HH, Frumin AM. Foamy histiocytes in spleens removed for chronic idiopathic thrombocytopenic purpura. Blood 1962;19:99-108.
38. Dale D, Guerry D 4th, Wewerka JR, Ball JM, Chusid MJ. Chronic neutropenia. Medicine 1979;58:128-44.
39. Deckmyn H, Zhang J, Van Houtte E, Vermylen J. Production and nucleotide sequence of an inhibitory human IgM autoantibody directed against platelet glycoprotein Ia/IIa. Blood 1994;84:1968-74.

40. Dhodapkar MV, Li CY, Lust JA, Tefferi A, Phyliky RL. Clinical spectrum of clonal proliferations of T-large granular lymphocytes: a T-cell clonopathy of undetermined significance? Blood 1994;84:1620-7.
41. DiFino SM, Lachant NA, Kirshner JJ, Gottlieb AK. Adult idiopathic thrombocytopenic purpura. Clinical findings and response to therapy. Am J Med 1980;69:430-42.
42. Dixon R, Rosse W, Ebbert L. Quantitative determination of antibody in idiopathic thrombocytopenic purpura. N Engl J Med 1975;292:230-6.
43. Doan CA, Bouroncle BA, Wiseman BK. Idiopathic and secondary thrombocytopenic purpura: clinical study and evaluation of 381 cases over a period of 28 years. Ann Intern Med 1960;53:861.
44. Drake WP, Pei Z, Pride DT, Collins RD, Cover TL, Blaser MJ. Molecular analysis of sarcoidosis tissues for mycobacterium species DNA. Emerg Infect Dis 2002;8:1334-41.
45. Ebbe S, Wittels B, Dameshek W. Autoimmune thrombocytopenic purpura ("ITP" type) with chronic lymphocytic leukemia. Blood 1962;19:23-37.
46. Eisner MD, Amory J, Mullaney B, Tierney L Jr, Browner WS. Necrotizing lymphadenitis associated with systemic lupus erythematosus. Semin Arthritis Rheum 1996;26:477-82.
47. Evans RS, Takahashi K, Duane RT, Payne R, Liu C. Primary thrombocytopenic purpura and acquired hemolytic anemia. Evidence for a common etiology. Arch Intern Med 1951;87:48-65.
48. Facon T, Caulier MT, Fenaux P, et al. Accessory spleen in recurrent chronic immune thrombocytopenic purpura. Am J Hematol 1992;41:184-9.
49. Fernandes SR, Singsen BH, Hoffman GS. Sarcoidosis and systemic vasculitis. Semin Arthritis Rheum 2000;30:33-46.
50. Fink K, Al-Mondhiry H. Idiopathic thrombocytopenic purpura in lymphoma. Cancer 1976;37:1999-2004.
51. Firkin BG, Wright R, Miller S, Stokes E. Splenic macrophages in thrombocytopenia. Blood 1969;33:240.
52. Fishleder A, Tubbs R, Hesse B, Levine H. Uniform detection of immunoglobulin-gene rearrangement in benign lymphoepithelial lesions. N Engl J Med 1987;316:1118-21.
53. Fishman D, Isenberg DA. Splenic involvement in rheumatic diseases. Semin Arthritis Rheum 1997;27:141-55.
54. Ford GA, Bradley JR, Appleton DS, Thiru S, Calne RY. Spontaneous splenic rupture in polyarteritis nodosa. Postgrad Med J 1986;62:965-6.
55. Franklin EC, Kunkel HG, Ward JR. Clinical studies of seven patients with rheumatoid arthritis and uniquely large amounts of rheumatoid factor. Arthritis Rheum 1958;1:400-9.
56. Gal AA, Masor JJ. Splenic involvement in Wegener's granulomatosis. Arch Pathol Lab Med 1996;120:974-7.
57. Gazouli M, Ikonomopoulos J, Trigidou R, Foteinou M, Kittas C, Gorgoulis V. Assessment of mycobacterial, propionibacterial, and human herpesvirus 8 DNA in tissues of Greek patients with sarcoidosis. J Clin Microbiol 2002;40:3060-3.
58. George JN, Woolf SH, Raskob GE, et al. Idiopathic thrombocytopenic purpura: a practice guideline developed by explicit methods for the American Society of Hematology. Blood 1996;88:3-40.
59. Gerster JC. Longterm effect of methotrexate in Felty's syndrome: a 12 year followup. J Rheumatol 1996;23:200.
60. Goldberg J, Pinals RS. Felty syndrome. Semin Arthritis Rheum 1980;10:52-65.
61. Gorczyca W, Weisberger J, Liu Z, et al. An approach to diagnosis of T-cell lymphoproliferative disorders by flow cytometry. Cytometry 2002;50:177-90.
62. Gupta RC, Robinson WA, Albrecht D. Granulopoietic activity in Felty's syndrome. Ann Rheum Dis 1975;34:156.
63. Guz G, Ozdemir BH, Sezer S, et al. High frequency of amyloid lymphadenopathy in uremic patients. Ren Fail 2000;22:613-21.
64. Haskard DO, Higgens CS, Temple LN, Currey HL. Spontaneous rupture of the spleen in rheumatoid arthritis. Ann Rheum Dis 1983;42:411-4.
65. Hassan NM, Neiman RS. The pathology of the spleen in steroid-treated immune thrombocytopenic purpura. Am J Clin Pathol 1985;84:433-8.
66. He R, Reid DM, Jones CE, Shulman NR. Spectrum of Ig classes, specificities, and titers of serum antiglycoproteins in chronic idiopathic thrombocytopenic purpura. Blood 1994;83:1024-32.
67. Herling M, Khoury JD, Washington LT, Duvik M, Keating MJ, Jones D. A systematic approach to diagnosis of mature T-cell leukemias reveals heterogeneity among WHO categories. Blood 2004;104:328-35.
68. Hirsh EO, Dameshek W. Idiopathic thrombocytopenia: review of eighty-nine cases with particular reference to the differentiation and treatment of acute (self-limited) and chronic types. Arch Intern Med 1951;88:701-28.
69. Honda S, Tsubakio T, Tomiyama Y, et al. Two human monoclonal antiplatelet autoantibodies established from patients with chronic idiopathic thrombocytopenic purpura. Br J Haematol 1990;75:245-9.
70. Hou M, Stockelberg D, Kutti J, Wadenvik H. Antibodies against platelet GPIb/IX, GPIIb/IIIa, and other platelet antigens in chronic idiopathic thrombocytopenic purpura. Eur J Haematol 1995;55:307-14.

71. Hu S, Kuo TT, Hong HS. Lupus lymphadenitis simulating Kikuchi's lymphadenitis in patients with systemic lupus erythematosus: a clinicopathological analysis of six cases and review of the literature. Pathol Int 2003;53:221-6.
72. Huic D, Vukovic J, Senecic-Cala I, Dodig D. Splenic atrophy as complication of ulcerative colitis diagnosed by antigranulocyte antibodies labeled with Tc-99m-pertechnetate. Croat Med J 2003;44:767-9.
73. Hymes K, Shulman S, Karpatkin S. A solid-phase radioimmunoassay for bound anti-platelet antibody: studies on 45 patients with autoimmune platelet disorders. J Lab Clin Med 1979;94:639-48.
74. Ikkala E, Kivilaakso E, Hastbacka J. Splenectomy in blood diseases. A report of 80 cases. Ann Clin Res 1974;6:290-9.
75. Jeon YK, Paik JH, Park SS, et al. Spectrum of lymph node pathology in adult onset Still's disease; analysis of 12 patients with one follow up biopsy. J Clin Pathol 2004;57:1052-6.
76. JiJi RM, Firozvi T, Spurling CL. Chronic idiopathic thrombocytopenic purpura. Treatment with steroids and splenectomy. Arch Intern Med 1973;132:380-3.
77. Kaden BR, Rosse WF, Hauch TW. Immune thrombocytopenia in lymphoproliferative diseases. Blood 1979;53:545-51.
78. Karpatkin S. Immunologic thrombocytopenic purpura in HIV-seropositive homosexuals, narcotic addicts and hemophiliacs. Semin Hematol 1988;25:219-29.
79. Karpatkin S, Siskind GW. In vitro detection of platelet antibody in patients with idiopathic thrombocytopenic purpura and systemic lupus erythematosus. Blood 1969;33:795-812.
80. Karpatkin S, Strick N, Karpatkin M, Siskind GW. Cumulative experience in the detection of antiplatelet antibody in 234 patients with idiopathic thrombocytopenic purpura, systemic lupus erythematosus and other clinical disorders. Am J Med 1976;52:776-85.
81. Keller CE, Gamboa ET, Hays AP, et al. Fatal CNS vasculopathy in a patient with refractory celiac disease and lymph node cavitation. Virchows Arch 2006;448:209-13.
82. Kelton JG, Gibbons S. Autoimmune platelet destruction: idiopathic thrombocytopenic purpura. Semin Thromb Hemost 1982;8:83-104.
83. Kiefel V, Santoso S, Kaufmann E, Mueller-Eckhardt C. Autoantibodies against platelet glycoprotein Ib/IX: a frequent finding in autoimmune thrombocytopenic purpura. Br J Haematol 1991;79:256-62.
84. Kitsanou M, Andreopoulou E, Bai MK, Elisaf M, Drosos AA. Extensive lymphadenopathy as the first clinical manifestation in systemic lupus erythematosus. Lupus 2000;9:140-3.
85. Kojima M, Matsuda H, Iijima M, Yoshida K, Masawa N, Nakamura S. Reactive hyperplasia with giant follicles in lymph node lesions from systemic lupus erythematosus patients. Report of three cases. APMIS 2005;113:558-63.
86. Kojima M, Motoori T, Hosomura Y, Tanaka H, Sakata N, Masawa N. Atypical lymphoplasmacytic and immunoblastic proliferation from rheumatoid arthritis: a case report. Pathol Res Pract 2006;202:51-4.
87. Kojima M, Motoori T, Matsuda H, Iijima M, Masawa N, Nakamura S. Atypical lymphoplasmacytic and immunoblastic proliferation from systemic lupus erythematosus. A case report. Pathol Res Pract 2005;201:531-5.
88. Kojima M, Nakamura S, Itoh H, et al. Systemic lupus erythematosus (SLE) lymphadenopathy presenting with histopathologic features of Castleman disease: a clinicopathologic study of five cases. Pathol Res Pract 1997;193:565-71.
89. Kojima M, Nakamura S, Itoh H, Yoshida K, Suchi T, Masawa N. Lymph node necrosis in systemic lupus erythematosus. A histopathological and immunohistochemical study of four cases. APMIS 2001;109:141-6.
90. Kojima M, Nakamura S, Miyawaki S, et al. Lymph node lesion in adult-onset Still's disease resembling peripheral T-cell lymphoma: a report of three cases. Int J Surg Pathol 2002;10:197-202.
91. Kojima M, Nakamura S, Morishita Y, et al. Reactive follicular hyperplasia in the lymph node lesions from systemic lupus erythematosus patients: a clinicopathological and immunohistological study of 21 cases. Pathol Int 2000;50:304-12.
92. Kojima M, Nakamura S, Oyama T, et al. Autoimmune disease-associated lymphadenopathy with histological appearance of T-zone dysplasia with hyperplastic follicles. A clinicopathological analysis of nine cases. Pathol Res Pract 2001;197:237-44.
93. Kristensen J, Jensen OM. Splenic pulp, plasma cells and foamy histiocytes in immune thrombocytopenia: combined morphometric immunohistochemical and ultrastructural studies. Scand J Haematol 1985;34:340-4.
94. Kyle RA, Linman JW. Chronic idiopathic neutropenia. A newly recognized entity? N Engl J Med 1968;279:1015-9.
95. Lamy T, Loughran TP Jr. Clinical features of large granular lymphocyte leukemia. Semin Hematol 2003;40:185-95.
96. Lamy T, Loughran TP Jr. Current concepts: large granular lymphocyte leukemia. Blood Rev 1999;13:230-40.
97. Landing BH, Strauss L, Crocker AC, et al. Thrombocytopenic purpura with histiocytosis of the spleen. N Engl J Med 1961;265:572-7.
98. Laros RK Jr, Penner JA. "Refractory" thrombocytopenic purpura treated successfully with cyclophosphamide. JAMA 1971;215:445-9.

99. Lasser A. Diffuse histiocytosis of the spleen and idiopathic thrombocytopenic purpura (ITP): histochemical and ultrastructural studies. Am J Clin Pathol 1983;80:529-33.
100. Laszlo J, Jones R, Silberman HR, Banks PM. Splenectomy for Felty's syndrome. Clinicopathologic study of 27 patients. Arch Intern Med 1978;38:597-602.
101. Lie JT. Wegener's granulomatosis: histological documentation of common and uncommon manifestations in 216 patients. Vasa 1997;26:261-70.
102. Lightsey AL Jr, McMillan R. The role of the spleen in "autoimmune" blood disorders. Am J Pediatr Hematol Oncol 1979;1:331-41.
103. Liou LB, Chen TC. Lymphadenopathy in an oriental with ankylosing spondylitis. Clin Rheumatol 1998;17:412-5.
104. Lipsker D, Veran Y, Grunenberger F, Cribier B, Heid E, Grosshans E. The Schnitzler syndrome. Four new cases and review of the literature. Medicine (Baltimore) 2001;80:37-44.
105. Logue G. Felty's syndrome: granulocyte-bound immunoglobulin G and splenectomy. Ann Intern Med 1976;85:437-42.
106. Louie JS, Pearson CM. Felty's syndrome. Semin Hematol 1971;8:216-20.
107. Lundell R, Hartung L, Hill S, Perkins SL, Bahler DW. T-cell large granular lymphocyte leukemias have multiple phenotypic abnormalities involving pan-T-cell antigens and receptors for MHC molecules. Am J Clin Pathol 2005;124:937-46.
108. Luk SC, Musclow E, Simon GT. Platelet phagocytosis in the spleen of patients with idiopathic thrombocytopenic purpura (ITP). Histopathology 1980;4:127-36.
109. Manno CS. Management of bleeding disorders in children. Hematology (Am Soc Hematol Educ Program) 2005;416-22.
110. Marti M, Feliu E, Campo E, et al. Comparative study of spleen pathology in drug abusers with Thrombocytopenia related to human immunodeficiency virus infection and in patients with idiopathic thrombocytopenic purpura. A morphometric, immunohistochemical, and ultrastructural study. Am J Clin Pathol 1993;100:633-42.
111. Martinez-Vazquez C, Hughes G, Bordon J, et al. Histiocytic necrotizing lymphadenitis, Kikuchi-Fujimoto's disease, associated with systemic lupus erythemotosus. QJM 1997;90:531-3.
112. Mason DT, Morris JJ. The variable features of Felty's syndrome. Review of the literature and report of a case with massive splenomegalyAm J Med 1964;36:463-69.
113. McCluggage WG, Bharucha H. Lymph node hyalinisation in rheumatoid arthritis and systemic sclerosis. J Clin Pathol 1994;47:138-42.
114. McKenna RW, Parkin J, Kersey JH, Gajl-Peczalska KH, Peterson L, Brunning RD. Chronic lymphoproliferative disorder with unusual clinical, morphologic, ultrastructural and membrane surface marker characteristics. Am J Med 1977;62:588-96.
115. McMillan R, Longmire RL, Yelenosky R, Donnell RL, Armstrong S. Quantitation of platelet binding IgG produced in vitro by spleens from patients with idiopathic thrombocytopenic purpura. N Engl J Med 1974;291:812-7.
116. McMillan R, Tani P, Millard F, Berchtold P, Renshaw L, Woods VL Jr. Platelet-associated and plasma anti-glycoprotein autoantibodies in chronic ITP. Blood 1987;70:1040-5.
117. Melenhorst JJ, Eniafe R, Follmann D, et al. T-cell large granular lymphocyte leukemia is characterized by massive TCRBV-restricted clonal CD8 expansion and a generalized overexpression of the effector cell marker CD57. Hematol J 2003;4:18-25.
118. Melenhorst JJ, Sorbara L, Kirby M, Hensel NF, Barret AJ. Large granular lymphocyte leukaemia is characterized by a clonal T-cell receptor rearrangement in both memory and effector CD8(+) lymphocyte populations. Br J Haematol 2001;112:189-94.
119. Mohan A, Sood R, Shariff N, Gulati MS, Gupta SD, Dutta AK. Sarcoidosis manifesting as massive splenomegaly: a rare occurrence. Am J Med Sci 2004;328:170-2.
120. Moore RA, Brunner CM, Sandusky WR, Leavell BS. Felty's syndrome: long-term follow-up after splenectomy. Ann Intern Med 1971;75:381-5.
121. Moore SB. Immune thrombocytopenias and platelet antibodies. Mayo Clin Proc 1982;57:778-80.
122. Morice WG, Kurtin PJ, Leibson PJ, Tefferi A, Hanson CA. Demonstration of aberrant T-cell and natural killer-cell antigen expression in all cases of granular lymphocytic leukaemia. Br J Haematol 2003;120:1026-36.
123. Morice WG, Leibson PJ, Tefferi A. Natural killer cells and the syndrome of chronic natural killer cell lymphocytosis. Leuk Lymphoma 2001;41:277-84.
124. Mueller-Eckhardt C. Idiopathic thrombocytopenic purpura (ITP): clinical and immunologic considerations. Semin Thromb Hemost 1977;3:125-59.
125. Myhre Jensen O, Kristensen J. Red pulp of the spleen in autoimmune haemolytic anaemia and hereditary spherocytosis: morphometric light and electron microscopy studies. Scand J Haematol 1986;36:263-6.
126. Nickerson DA, Sunderland DA. The histopathology of idiopathic thrombocytopenic purpura hemorrhagica. Am J Pathol 1937;13:463-90.
127. O'Keefe CL, Plasilova M, Wlodarski M, et al. Molecular analysis of TCR clonotypes in LGL: a clonal model for polyclonal responses. J Immunol 2004;172:1960-9.

128. O'Malley DP, Kim YS, Perkins SL, Baldridge L, Juliar BE, Orazi A. Morphologic and immunohistochemical evaluation of splenic hematopoietic proliferations in neoplastic and benign disorders. Mod Pathol 2005;18:1550-61.
129. Osone S, Morimoto A, Tsutsui J, Kano G, Todo S, Sugimoto T. Systemic juvenile idiopathic arthritis mimics multicentric Castleman's disease. Clin Rheumatol 2003;22:484-6.
130. Osuji N, Matutes E, Catovsky D, Lampert I, Wotherspoon A. Histopathology of the spleen in T-cell large granular lymphocyte leukemia and T-cell prolymphocytic leukemia: a comparative review. Am J Surg Pathol 2005;29:935-41.
131. Papo T, Huong DL, Piette JC, et al. Spleen haemorrhagic infarction and hazards of anticoagulation in Wegener's granulomatosis. Ann Rheum Dis 1999;58:654-5.
132. Payne MM, Kaimatchiev V, Loriax M. Pathologic quiz case: multiple splenic nodules. Splenic sarcoid. Arch Pathol Lab Med 2005;129:419-20.
133. Petz LD. Drug-induced immune haemolytic anaemia. Clin Haematol 1980;9:455-82.
134. Pfueller SL, David R, Firkin BG, Bilston RA, Cortizo WF, Raines G. Platelet aggregating IgG antibody to platelet surface glycoproteins associated with thrombosis and thrombocytopenia. Br J Haematol 1990;74:336-41.
135. Phatak PD, Janas JS, Sham RL, Yirinec B, Marder VJ. Disorders that resemble lymphomas. Am J Heamtol 1997;56:63-8.
136. Pisciotta AV. Drug-induced agranulocytosis. Drugs 1978;15:132-43.
137. Posnett DN, Sinha R, Kabak S, Russo C. Clonal populations of T cells in normal elderly humans: the T cell equivalent to "benign monoclonal gammapathy." J Exp Med 1994;179:609-18.
138. Price TH, Dale DC. The selective neutropenias. Clin Haematol 1978;7:501-21.
139. Puli SR, Presti ME, Alpert MA. Splenic granulomas in Crohn disease. Am J Med Sci 2003;326:141-4.
140. Quintas-Cardama A, Fraga M, Cozzi SN, Caparrini A, Maceiras F, Forteza J. Fatal Kikuchi-Fujimoto disease: the lupus connection. Ann Hematol 2003;82:186-8.
141. Rappaport H, Crosby WH. Auto-immune hemolytic anemia. II. Morphologic observations and clinicopathologic correlations. Am J Pathol 1957;33:429-57.
142. Riley SM, Aldrete JS. Role of splenectomy in Felty's syndrome. Am J Surg 1975;130:51-2.
143. Roark JH, Bussel JB, Cines DB, Siegel DL. Geneic analysis of autoantibodies in idiopathic thrombocytopenic purpura reveals evidence of clonal expansion and somatic mutations. Blood 2002;100:1388-98.
144. Rose MG, Berliner N. T-cell large granular lymphocyte leukemia and related disorders. Oncologist 2004;9:247-58.
145. Rousselet MC, Andouin J, Le Tourneau A, et al. Idiopathic thrombocytopenic purpura in patients at risk for acquired immunodeficiency syndrome. Histopathologic study, immunohistochemistry, and ultrastructural study on six spleens. Arch Pathol Lab Med 1988;112:1242-50.
146. Rubenstein JH, Sidhu GS, Schonetag R. Ultrastructural diagnosis of histologically atypical idiopathic thrombocytopenic purpura. Ultrastruct Pathol 1981;2:269-75.
147. Rywlin AM, Hernandez JA, Chastain DE, Pardo V. Ceroid histiocytosis of spleen and bone marrow in idiopathic thrombocytopenic purpura (ITP): a contribution to the understanding of the sea-blue histiocyte. Blood 1971;37:587-93.
148. Saltzstein SL. Phospholipid accumulation in histiocytes of splenic pulp associated with thrombocytopenic purpura. Blood 1961;18:73-88.
149. Sandler SG, Tutuncuoglu O. Immune thrombocytopenic purpura—current management practices. Expert Opin Pharmacother 2004;5:2515-27.
150. Santana A, Lessa B, Galrao L, Lima I, Santiago M. Kikuchi-Fujimoto's disease associated with systemic lupus erythematosus: case report and review of the literature. Clin Rheumatol 2005;24:60-3.
151. Saracco SM, Farhi DC. Splenic pathology in thrombotic thrombocytopenic purpura. Am J Surg Pathol 1990;14:223-9.
152. Savona S, Nardi M, Lennette E, Karpatkin S. Thrombocytopenic purpura in narcotics addicts. Ann Intern Med 1985;102:737-41.
153. Schwartz RS, Silberstein LE, Berkman EM. Autoimmune hemolytic anemias. In: Hoffman R, Benz EJ Jr, Shattil S, Furie B, Cohen HJ, Silberstein LE, eds. Hematology: basic principles and practice, 2nd ed. New York: Churchill Livingston; 1995:710-29.
154. Sharma OP. Sarcoidosis and other autoimmune disorders. Curr Opin Pulm Med 2002;8:452-6.
155. Shulman NR, Weinrach RS, Libre EP, Andrews HL. The role of the reticuloendothelial system in the pathogenesis of idiopathic thrombocytopenic purpura. Trans Assoc Am Phys 1965;78:374-90.
156. Sienknecht CW, Urowitz MB, Pruzanski W, Stein HB. Felty's syndrome. Clinical and serological analysis of 34 cases. Ann Rheum Dis 1977;36:500-7.
157. Spivak JL. Felty's syndrome: an analytical review. Johns Hopkins Med J 1977;141:156-62.
158. Stasi R, Pagano A, Stipa E, Amadori S. Rituximab chimeric anti-CD20 monoclonal antibody treatment for adults with chronic idiopathic thrombocytopenic purpura. Blood 2001;98:952-7.

159. Sugiyama T, Okuma M, Ushikubi F, Sensaki S, Kanaji K, Uchino H. A novel platelet aggregating factor found in a patient with defective collagen-induced platelet aggregation and autoimmune thrombocytopenia. Blood 1987;69:1712-20.
160. Tavassoli M, McMillan R. Structure of the spleen in idiopathic thrombocytopenic purpura. Am J Clin Pathol 1975;64:180-91.
161. Teirstein AS, Judson MA, Baughman RP, Rossman MD, Yeager H Jr, Moller DR. A Case Control Etiologic Study of Sarcoidosis (ACCESS) Writing Group. The spectrum of biopsy sites for the diagnosis of sarcoidosis. Sarcoidosis Vasc Diffuse Lung Dis 2005;22:139-46.
162. Terayama N, Makimoto KP, Kobayashi S, et al. Pathology of the spleen in primary biliary cirrhosis: an autopsy study. Pathol Int 1994;44:753-8.
163. Tomiyama Y, Kekomaki R, McFarland J, Kunicki TJ. Antivinculin antibodies in sera of patients with immune thrombocytopenia and in sera of normal subjects. Blood 1992;79:161-8.
164. Tuzun H, Yaman M, Gemicioglu B, Bozkurt K, Uygun N, Aktan K. Behcet's disease presenting with a pulmonary mass lesion. Chest 1993;104:1635-6.
165. Valente RM, Banks PM, Conn DL. Characterization of lymph node histology in adult onset Still's disease. J Rheumatol 1989;16:349-54.
166. Van Boxtel CJ, Oosterhof F, Engelfriet CP. Immunofluorescence microphotometry for the detection of platelet antibodies. III. Demonstration of autoantibodies against platelets. Scand J Immunol 1975;4:657-72.
167. van der Harst D, de Jong D, Limpens J, et al. Clonal B-cell populations in patients with idiopathic thrombocytopenic purpura. Blood 1990;76:2321-6.
168. van Krieken JH, Breedveld FC, te Velde J. The spleen in Felty's syndrome: a histological, morphometrical, and immunohistochemical study. Europ J Haematol 1988;40:58-64.
169. van Leeuwen EF, van der Ven JT, Engelfriet CP, von dem Borne AE. Specificity of autoantibodies in autoimmune thrombocytopenia. Blood 1982;59:23-6.
170. Varon D, Linder S, Gembom E, et al. Human monoclonal antibody derived from an autoimmune thrombocytopenic purpura patient, recognizing an intermediate filament's determinant common to vimentin and desmin. Clin Immunol Immunopathol 1990;54:454-68.
171. Vincent PC, Levi JA, MacQueen A. The mechanism of neutropenia in Felty's syndrome. Br J Haematol 1974;27:4630-75.
172. Wilkins BS, Wright DH. The spleen in hereditary blood cell abnormalities and autho-immune disorders. In: Wilkins BS, Wright DH, eds. Illustrated pathology of the spleen. Cambridge: Cambridge University Press; 2000:47-61.
173. Weitzmen SA, Stossel TP. Drug-induced immunological neutropenia. Lancet 1978;1:1068-72.
174. Welch CS, Dameshek W. Splenectomy in blood dyscrasias. N Engl J Med 1950;242:601-6.
175. Wong KF, Chan JC, Liu HS, Man C, Kwong YL. Chromosomal abnormalities in T-cell large granular lymphocyte leukaemia: report of two cases and review of the literature. Br J Haematol 2002;116:598-600.
176. Yam LT, McMillan R, Tavassoli M, Crosby WH. Splenic hemopoiesis in idiopathic thrombocytopenic purpura. Am J Clin Pathol 1974;62:830-7.

13 HEMATOLOGIC DISORDERS

The structure of the splenic red pulp provides, as part of its normal filtration function, a unique mechanism for monitoring the structural and functional status of the cellular elements of the blood. Red blood cells can be abnormally sequestered in the splenic cords of the red pulp when they lack the plasticity necessary to traverse the walls of the splenic sinuses. The lack of plasticity results from structural abnormalities of the cells themselves, from the attachment of antibodies to the cell surfaces, or from intracellular inclusions. Entrapment of blood cells in the cords of Billroth exposes them to a hypoxic, acidic environment, facilitating their lysis and/or phagocytosis by cordal macrophages.

Erythrocytes are sequestered in the spleen in a variety of congenital and acquired hematologic conditions. Three types of congenital disorders are associated with decreased erythrocyte deformability: 1) disorders of the red cell membrane, 2) hemoglobinopathies, and 3) erythrocyte enzyme deficiencies. The acquired disorders include a variety of hemolytic anemias and certain protozoal infections.

HEREDITARY SPHEROCYTOSIS/ELLIPTOCYTOSIS

Definition. *Hereditary spherocytosis* (HS) is an autosomal dominant hemolytic anemia of mild to moderate severity, characterized by the presence of spherocytosis in the peripheral blood film, and a favorable response to splenectomy. *Hereditary elliptocytosis* (*ovalocytosis*) is an uncommon disorder that is usually not associated with clinically significant hemolysis (6,15). The pathologic features in the spleen are essentially the same as those seen in HS.

General Features. HS is the prototype of congenital disorders of the erythrocyte cell membrane. The autosomal dominant condition is inherited with a variable degree of penetrance (69). The majority of the erythrocytes in the peripheral blood of patients with HS are spherocytic. They are smaller and thicker than normal erythrocytes, lack their central pallor, and have an increased mean corpuscular hemoglobin concentration (22,70). The red blood cell (RBC) abnormality is related to a deficiency or dysfunction of one of the proteins of the cell membrane, which causes destabilization of the normal lipid bilayer (14,56) and leads to surface area deficiency and the formation of spherocytes. The molecular basis of this membrane protein abnormality is heterogeneous and results in four principal HS subtypes: 1) isolated partial deficiency of spectrin; 2) combined partial deficiency of spectrin and ankyrin; 3) partial deficiency of band 3 protein; and 4) deficiency of protein 4.2 (30).

Clinical Features. The reported prevalence of HS in the Western population is 1/5,000. A typical patient with HS is often asymptomatic. Mild jaundice and splenomegaly are present in most patients. Complications include gallstones (50 percent of patients), hemolytic crisis usually triggered by an infection, the development of megaloblastic anemia (which can be the first sign of the disease and occur typically during pregnancy), and aplastic crisis due to parvovirus B19 infection. In severe cases, patients develop leg ulcers and dermatitis; both usually disappear after splenectomy.

Laboratory Findings. Spherocytes have an increased permeability to sodium (38,69) and, therefore, are more susceptible in vitro to swelling and lysis in hypotonic solutions. This forms the basis of the osmotic fragility test. They also have an increased rate of autohemolysis, which may be corrected by incubation with glucose (14,64).

Microscopic Findings. The spleen, which is moderately enlarged, shows a red pulp congested with spherocytes packing the cords (11,24,47). The sinuses appear empty and may be compressed (fig. 13-1). Hemosiderin deposition is usually minimal, except in cases in which transfusions or iron has been administered (11). Erythrophagocytosis by cordal macrophages is difficult to demonstrate by light microscopy, either in tissue sections or touch imprints. In

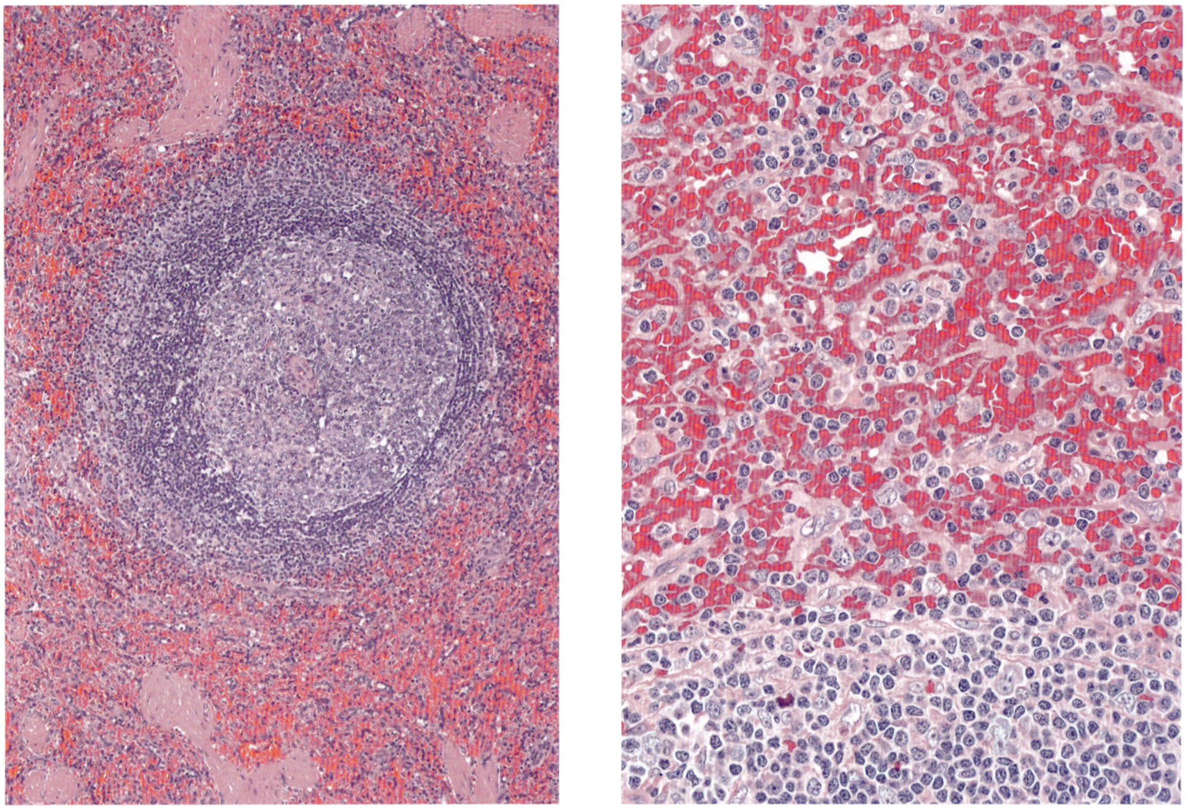

Figure 13-1

HEREDITARY SPHEROCYTOSIS, SPLEEN

Left: Hyperplastic follicles are seen, along with red pulp congestion.
Right: Higher magnification reveals red blood cells in the cords and sinuses of the spleen.

contrast to most other hemolytic conditions, extramedullary erythropoiesis or hematopoiesis is usually not noted. The majority of patients with HS have a benign course, with hemolysis compensated by erythroid hyperplasia of the bone marrow. There may be acute aplastic crises, however, usually associated with infection by parvovirus B19 (46,76), which acts by selectively inhibiting erythropoiesis (46). There may be mild to moderate thrombocytopenia (42). In common with all patients with chronic hemolysis, those with HS are vulnerable to cholelithiasis caused by bilirubin-containing stones (29).

Treatment and Prognosis. The treatment for both conditions is splenectomy. Because the spleen plays a central role in the destruction of erythrocytes in this disorder, splenectomy is almost invariably clinically curative, although the inherent membrane abnormality remains. Splenectomy is usually performed once the diagnosis is established, although it may be delayed beyond infancy in cases that manifest early in life (62). Complications include the possibility of postsplenectomy sepsis syndrome. Postsplenectomy failures are usually due to the presence of an accessory spleen that was missed during surgery or to the presence of an additional undiagnosed RBC disorder(s) (e.g., pyruvate kinase deficiency).

SICKLE CELL DISEASE

Definition. *Sickle cell disease* is an inherited, multisystem disorder due to the presence of mutant sickle cell hemoglobin (Hgb S). It is characterized by chronic hemolytic anemia associated with recurrent episodes of pain and other vasoocclusive complications.

General Features. Sickle cell disease is the most common of the hemoglobinopathies, with a prevalence among the African-American newborns

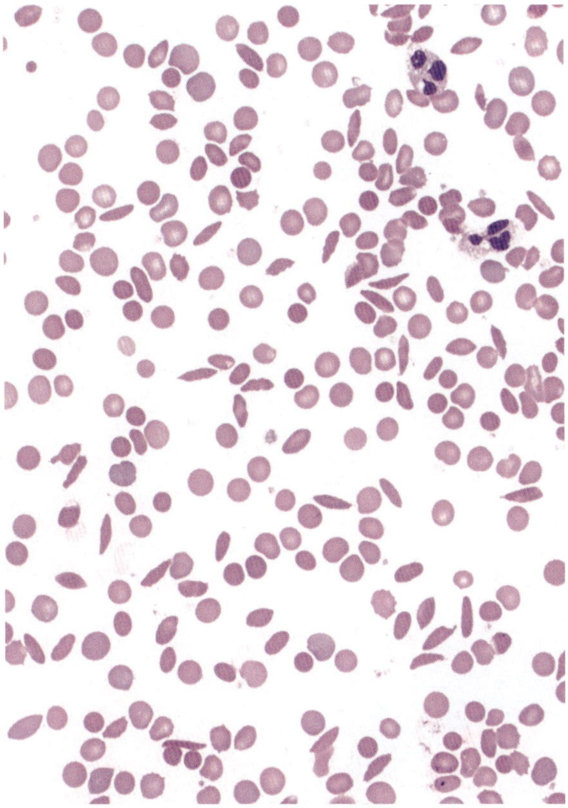

Figure 13-2

SICKLE CELL DISEASE, PERIPHERAL BLOOD

A peripheral blood smear shows the characteristic morphology of a sickle cell crisis.

of 8 to 10 percent. In western Africa the prevalence is as high as 25 to 30 percent (61).

The mutant Hgb S molecule is produced by the substitution of valine for glutamic acid at the sixth position of the hemoglobin beta chain (16,20). Hgb S molecules undergo polymerization upon deoxygenation, resulting in the characteristic sickled shape of the erythrocyte (fig. 13-2) (20). Sickling is initially a reversible phenomenon; with repeated episodes, however, membrane damage results in irreversibly sickled cells which are more adherent to endothelial cells and are more prone to cause vasoocclusion (26). Sickling also occurs in heterozygous patients with sickle cell/hemoglobin C disease and sickle cell/beta thalassemia, but these diseases tend to be milder.

Clinical Features. An acute painful episode (formerly known as sickle cell crisis), characterized by symptoms related to occlusion of small blood vessels by sickled cells, is precipitated by events such as cold, dehydration, infection, stress, excessive alcohol consumption, and reduced oxygen tension (e.g., flying at high altitudes). Repeated episodes result in chronic hypoxic multiorgan damage (16,26,40), including cerebrovascular accidents, pulmonary complications (including the acute chest syndrome), renal complications leading to chronic renal insufficiency, ocular complications, priapism, skin ulcers, and bone infarctions (including the hand-foot syndrome).

Patients homozygous for Hgb S are subject to chronic hemolytic anemia. The hypoxic environment of the cords of Billroth promotes deoxygenation and, therefore, sickling of erythrocytes in homozygous sickle cell patients. Sickle cells are rigid, lacking the plasticity to penetrate the splenic sinuses. The sickled erythrocytes then undergo phagocytosis by the cordal macrophages. This interaction between the sickled erythrocytes and the reticuloendothelial system is considered to be responsible for most of the hemolysis seen in this disorder. One third of the hemolysis is, however, intravascular, possibly due to increased RBC fragility (21).

Splenomegaly is prominent in childhood owing to the sequestration of sickled erythrocytes (48). Although the spleen is enlarged, its function is usually impaired and patients are therefore particularly susceptible to infections (53,55). The pathogenesis of the defective immune function seen in these patients is complex (10). Due to progressive atrophy from repeated infarctions, most patients do not have palpable spleens beyond 8 years of age (2,17). The presence of hyposplenism in these cases is confirmed by the finding of Howell-Jolly bodies in the circulating erythrocytes. In some patients, especially those living in areas affected by malaria, splenomegaly persists well into adulthood (2).

Aplastic crises and hemolytic crises, often associated with infection, particularly viral infection with parvovirus B19 (46), occur in patients with sickle cell disease, as well as in other patients with hemolytic anemia. Infants and young children with homozygous sickle cell disease have a 30 percent incidence of sequestration crisis due to the sudden massive pooling of erythrocytes in the spleen, resulting in rapid

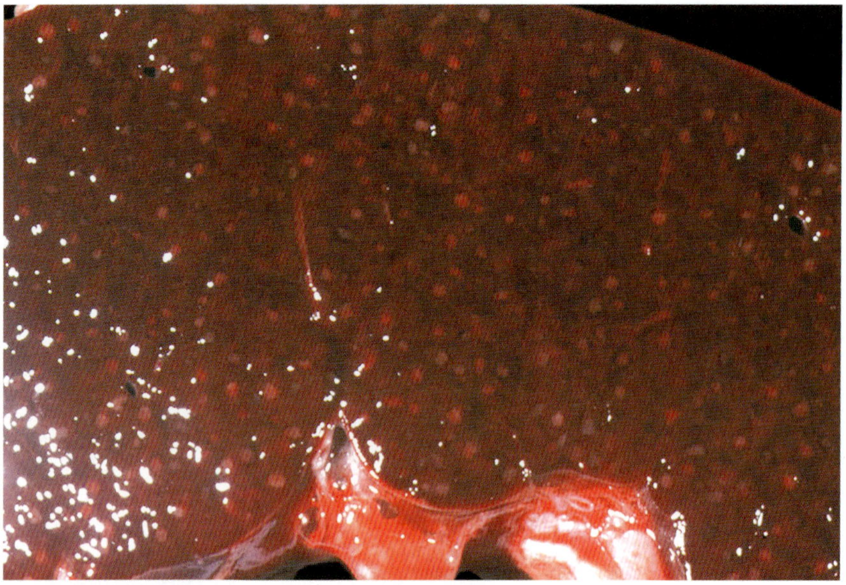

Figure 13-3

SICKLE CELL DISEASE, SPLEEN

Hemorrhagic infarction of the spleen in a patient with sickle cell disease. (Courtesy of Richard Neiman, Harpswell, ME.)

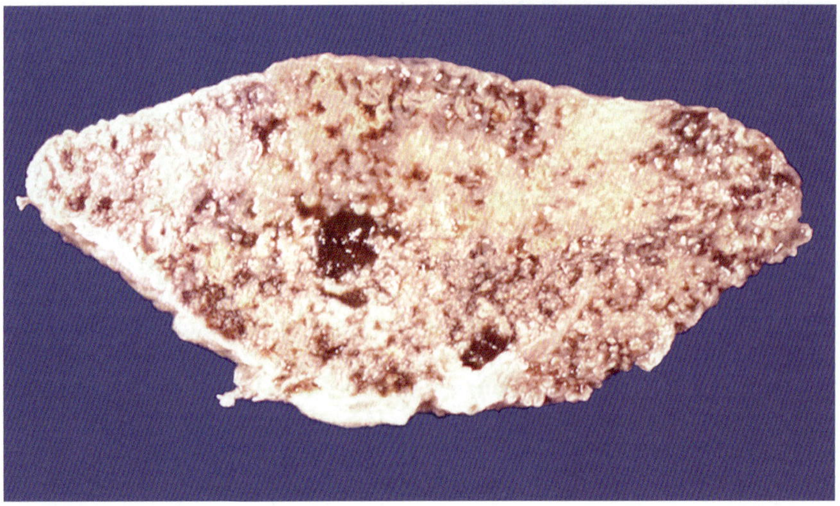

Figure 13-4

SICKLE CELL DISEASE, SPLEEN

A fibrotic, infarcted spleen in an older patient with sickle cell disease. (Courtesy of Richard Neiman, Harpswell, ME.)

enlargement of the organ. Sequestration crisis is associated with acute exacerbation of anemia, persistent reticulocytosis, and hypovolemic shock (54,66,75). Acute splenic sequestration has also been reported to occur in patients with sickle cell/hemoglobin C disease, sickle cell/thalassemia, and sickle cell trait/hereditary spherocytosis (75). Since splenic sequestration recurs in 50 percent of patients, splenectomy is recommended after the acute event remits (66). In Middle Eastern patients affected with sickle cell disease, the decrease in disease severity more commonly leads to splenic enlargement and fibrocongestive splenomegaly in contrast to splenic autoinfarction (13).

Gross Findings. Most of the spleens seen as pathology specimens are from patients with acute sequestration crisis (figs. 13-3, 13-4). Splenic infarcts are commonly present. Old fibrotic infarcts encrusted with iron and calcium, and often containing foreign body giant cells, are termed Gamna-Gandy bodies (17). In advanced stages, the spleen is small and extensively fibrotic.

Microscopic Findings. Spleens with acute sequestration show a marked degree of red pulp congestion due to the stasis of sickled erythrocytes within the splenic cords and focal hemorrhagic necrosis (figs. 13-5–13-7). In many cases, the RBCs seem to be preferentially

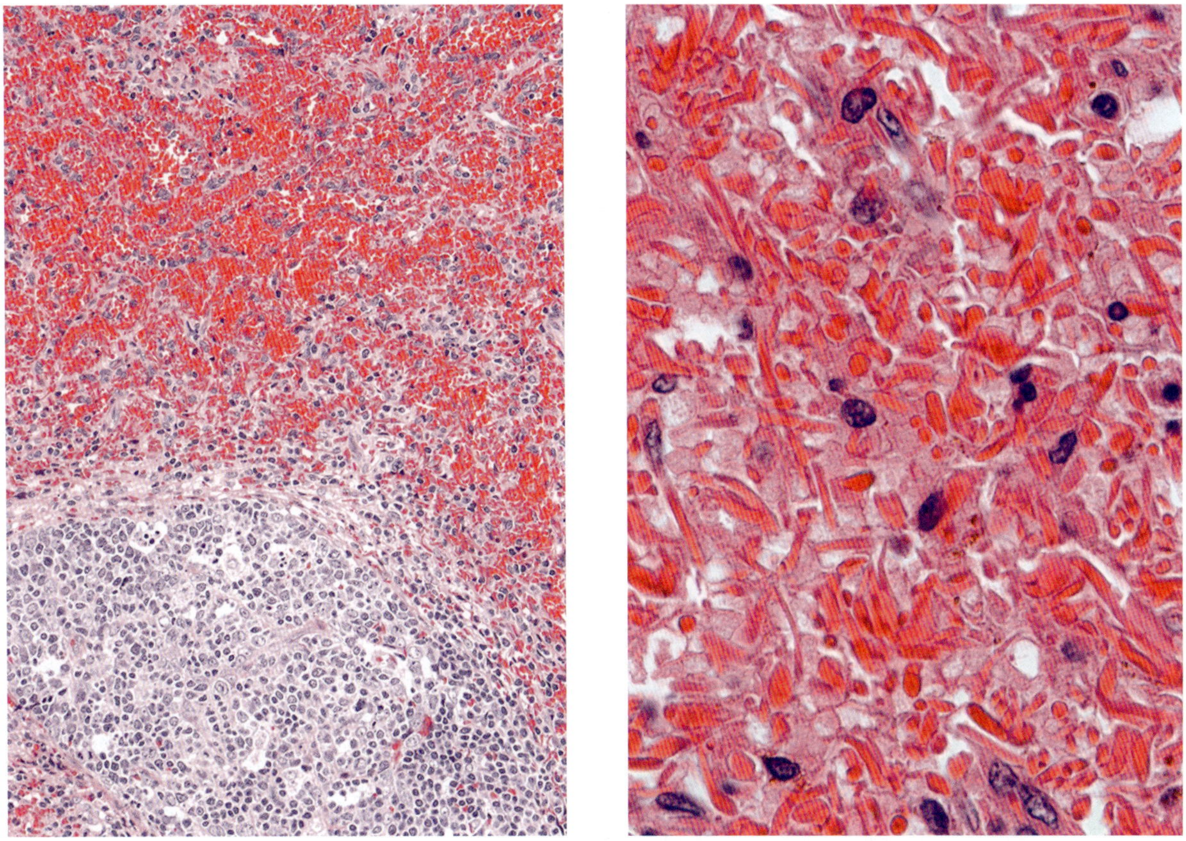

Figure 13-5

SICKLE CELL DISEASE, SPLEEN

In sequestration crisis, actively sickled cells are seen in the cords and sinuses of the spleen.

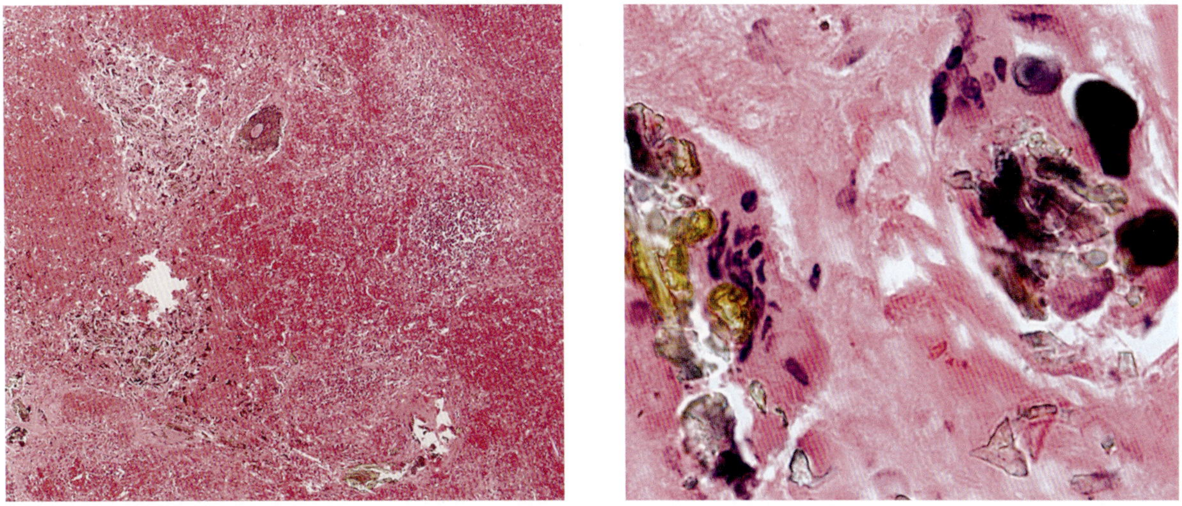

Figure 13-6

SICKLE CELL DISEASE, SPLEEN

Chronic red blood cell destruction in sickle cell disease leads to the formation of Gamma-Gandy bodies in the spleen.

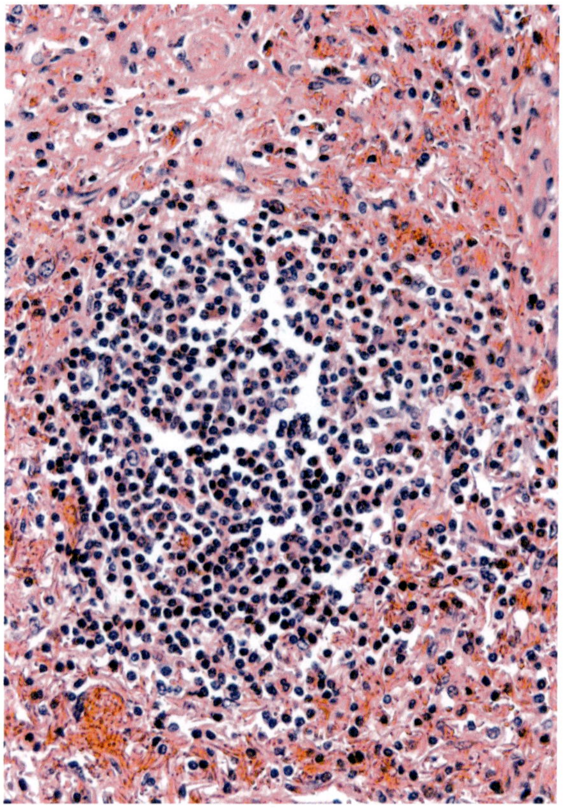

Figure 13-7

SICKLE CELL DISEASE, SPLEEN

Because of repeated vascular insult, the lymphoid components of the spleen eventually become atrophic.

sequestered in the marginal zone of the white pulp, with resultant atrophy of the follicular compartment. This phenomenon may play a role in increased susceptibility to infection in patients with sickle cell disease, even in the early splenomegalic phase.

Treatment and Prognosis. Progress in the care of patients with sickle cell anemia has significantly changed the prognosis. The mean life expectancy of patients is now above 40 years. Conventional treatment includes antibiotics and immunizations, analgesics, and blood transfusions. Reversal of the progressive decrease in spleen size and function has been reported following transfusion (8,72), bone marrow transplantation (25), and hydroxyurea administration (12). The effects of these newer therapeutic modalities are still the subject of current comparative evaluations.

In some of the other diseases associated with sickling, such as sickle cell/hemoglobin C disease and sickle cell/thalassemia, splenomegaly may persist into adult life. Splenic infarction and other thromboembolic complications have been reported in these patients (27,32), as well as the rare sequestration crisis requiring splenectomy (33).

HEMOGLOBINOPATHIES ASSOCIATED WITH UNSTABLE HEMOGLOBINS

The *hemoglobinopathies associated with unstable hemoglobin* result from the production of structurally abnormal globin chains. Almost all are associated with splenomegaly resulting from increased sequestration of RBCs in the red pulp. The unstable hemoglobin denatures and precipitates as Heinz bodies (39,57,71). These rigid inclusions are pitted out of the erythrocyte by the normal spleen and are rarely seen in the peripheral blood unless the patient has been splenectomized (57). Episodes of infection and treatment with oxidant drugs may precipitate a hemolytic crisis (39). Because of the pitting of portions of the erythrocyte, the surface area decreases, producing more spherocytic erythrocytes, which are then sequestered in the spleen, resulting in splenomegaly. Splenectomy has been useful in some patients with splenomegaly and severe hemolysis (71).

THALASSEMIA SYNDROMES

Definition. The *thalassemia syndromes* are a heterogenous group of disorders characterized by the diminished production of structurally normal globin chains resulting in an excess of one type of chain (5,58). Some rare forms of thalassemia, however, are characterized by the production of structurally abnormal globin.

General Features. *Beta thalassemia* is characterized by the deficient synthesis of the beta-globin chain, whereas *alpha thalassemia* results from deficient synthesis of the alpha-globin chain. The excess chains precipitate to form inclusion bodies. These thalassemic hemoglobinopathies share features of both thalassemia and structural hemoglobinopathies (1). Two factors contribute to the anemia that may be seen in these disorders. Erythroid precursors within the bone marrow are destroyed prior to release into the peripheral circulation, owing to the membrane damage that results from the precipitated globin chains (intramedullary hemolysis or ineffective erythropoiesis). In addition, erythrocytes containing Heinz bodies are trapped and destroyed in the spleen.

Clinical Features. Homozygous beta thalassemia may be associated with mild to marked splenomegaly (47). Cytopenias result if the bone marrow is unable to compensate for the peripheral destruction.

Clinically, thalassemia is very heterogeneous in its manifestations. In spite of seemingly identical genotypes, the severity of beta thalassemia varies greatly. The heterogeneity is the result of the nature of the beta-globin gene mutation, the alpha thalassemia gene interaction, and differences in the amount of fetal hemoglobin production which is partly associated with a specific beta-globin haplotype.

Microscopic Findings. There is prominent sequestration of RBCs in the red pulp of the spleen (fig. 13-8). Extramedullary hematopoiesis, predominantly erythropoiesis, is common (47). Foam cells resembling Gaucher cells have been described in the spleen (63). Hemosiderosis may be prominent, particularly when many transfusions have been given, and fibrosis may be seen in advanced disease (47).

Treatment and Prognosis. The standard treatment for severe thalassemia includes transfusion and iron chelation; the latter is used to prevent iron overload, which, if untreated, causes death from cardiac failure between 12 and 24 years of age. In a recent study from the United States, patients with transfusion-dependent thalassemia treated with regular subcutaneous iron chelation lived to an average of 29 years (9). The only curative treatment available at present is stem cell bone marrow transplantation (31). Splenectomy may be indicated in patients with severe anemia. The usual indication for splenectomy is the progressive shortening of the life of transfused RBCs, as evidence by an increased transfusion requirement.

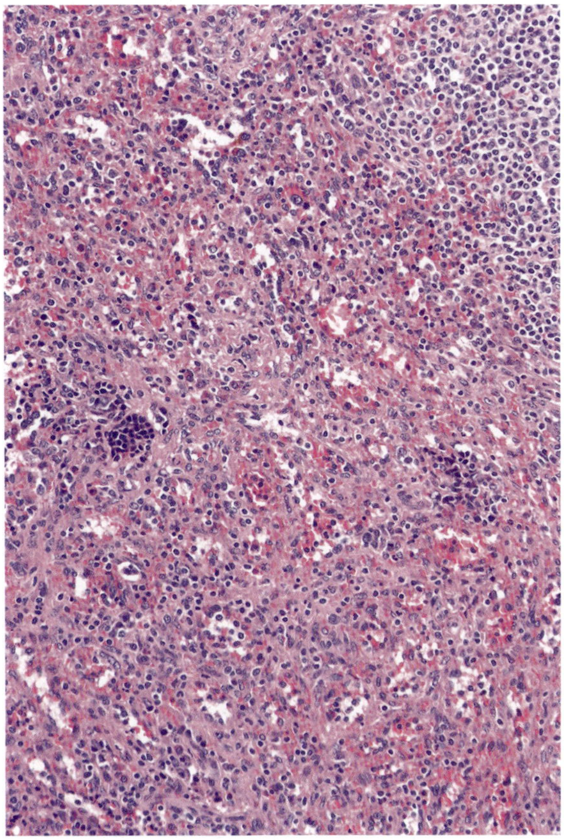

Figure 13-8

THALASSEMIA, SPLEEN

Foci of predominantly erythroid extramedullary hematopoiesis are seen in the red pulp.

ERYTHROCYTE ENZYME DEFICIENCIES

Splenomegaly is a feature of a variety of conditions associated with a congenital deficiency of an important enzyme (e.g., in the glycolytic or the hexose monophosphate shunt pathways). *Glucose-6-phosphate dehydrogenase (G6PD) deficiency*, an X-linked enzymatic deficiency disorder, is relatively common in American blacks and Mediterranean populations (43). Affected persons usually have mild anemia. Exposure to oxidizing agents, such as antimalarial drugs and sulfanilamides, causes Heinz body formation, facilitating increased erythrocyte destruction by the spleen, and possibly resulting in severe anemia (3,35). Splenectomy is only rarely helpful.

Pyruvate Kinase Deficiency

Pyruvate kinase (PK) deficiency is an inherited erythrocyte enzyme defect associated with a form of autosomal recessive, chronic nonspherocytic hemolytic anemia (45). Although PK deficiency is the most common enzymopathy, it is a rare disorder with less than 400 cases reported (34). The enzyme deficiency affects only the erythroid cell line. Patients may have splenomegaly with anemia and jaundice. The peripheral blood shows macrocytosis and reticulocytosis. Splenectomy is indicated to alleviate severe cytopenias.

The histologic findings in the spleen are not specific, and resemble those seen in other types of hemolytic anemia. Hyperplasia of cordal macrophages with a variable degree of erythrophagocytosis and increased amounts of hemosiderin may be observed (7,68). Sandoval et al. (59) described extensive erythrophagocytosis and prominent extramedullary hematopoiesis in a spleen removed from a patient with PK deficiency anemia who had failed to respond to partial splenectomy. Similar findings are associated with hexokinase deficiency and deficiencies of other enzymes of the glycolytic pathway.

EXTRAMEDULLARY HEMATOPOIESIS

Definition. *Extramedullary hematopoiesis* (EMH) is characterized by proliferations of bone marrow elements outside the expected locations. These proliferations are common in the spleen and less common in lymph nodes and other sites. EMH is due to a variety of underlying conditions, but is usually the result of hematologic disorders.

General Features. The spleen in humans does not normally function as a site of hematopoiesis and its role in fetal hematopoiesis is minimal, at best (28,49). In the normal adult spleen, there are almost always a few mature hematopoietic elements, which are derived from circulating stem cells undergoing terminal differentiation, or circulating maturing elements trapped within the spleen, or a combination of these events (28,49,73).

EMH most appropriately describes benign proliferations of bone marrow elements outside the marrow, and should not be used in reference to neoplastic myeloid proliferations found outside the marrow. It is the authors' opinion that the term myeloid metaplasia is misleading and should not be used in any circumstances. In almost all cases of underlying myeloid neoplasms, the extramedullary proliferations are clonal, and related to the bone marrow-based disorder, rather than a benign proliferation (50,51).

The circumstances under which hematopoietic elements proliferate outside the bone marrow space typically are associated with underlying hematologic disorders. EMH is often a result of conditions which disrupt the bone marrow microenvironment, facilitating the egress of progenitor and precursor cells, with an increase in circulating mature and immature bone marrow elements. EMH can be seen in a wide range of disorders of the spleen and circulation (4,11,18,19,23,36,37,41,44,52,60,65,66,74).

Clinical Features. The splenic environment is uniquely suited as a site for EMH. It is likely that the stromal microenvironment is similar enough to bone marrow to allow for near-normal development of hematopoietic cell lines (4,19). The disorders with the most significant degrees of splenic EMH include thrombotic thrombocytopenic purpura/hemolytic uremic syndrome and post-bone marrow transplantation (50). Autoimmune hemolytic anemia, thalassemia, HS, immune thrombocytopenic purpura, severe combined immunodeficiency, and fibrocongestive splenomegaly all have some degree of splenic EMH. In the lymph nodes, EMH is usually limited to pediatric patients with or without underlying hematologic disorders.

Gross Findings. Spleens with extensive red pulp involvement by EMH have the typical "beefy" red appearance of many other red pulp disorders. If the EMH is focal, it may appear as a mass lesion, possibly mimicking a focal lesion such as lymphoma or a metastasis. Lymph nodes with EMH may have a red, hemorrhagic appearance, either focally or replacing the entire node.

Microscopic Findings. In the spleen, EMH varies widely in appearance (figs. 13-9, 13-10). The most common findings are scattered megakaryocytes in the red pulp and small clusters of erythroid elements. Finding one or two of these elements per high-power field is usual in spleens without any known pathology. In cases of underlying benign hematopoietic disorders (such as congenital anemia), the proliferations may be more extensive; the degree of the proliferation often does not relate to the severity of the underlying disorder.

In some circumstances, EMH is composed of trilineage hematopoietic elements (Table 13-1). The myeloid, erythroid, and megakaryocytic elements are present in proportions that are different than those seen in the normal bone marrow. In a predominantly RBC disorder, the most numerous elements are usually erythroid precursors; however, this is not always the case.

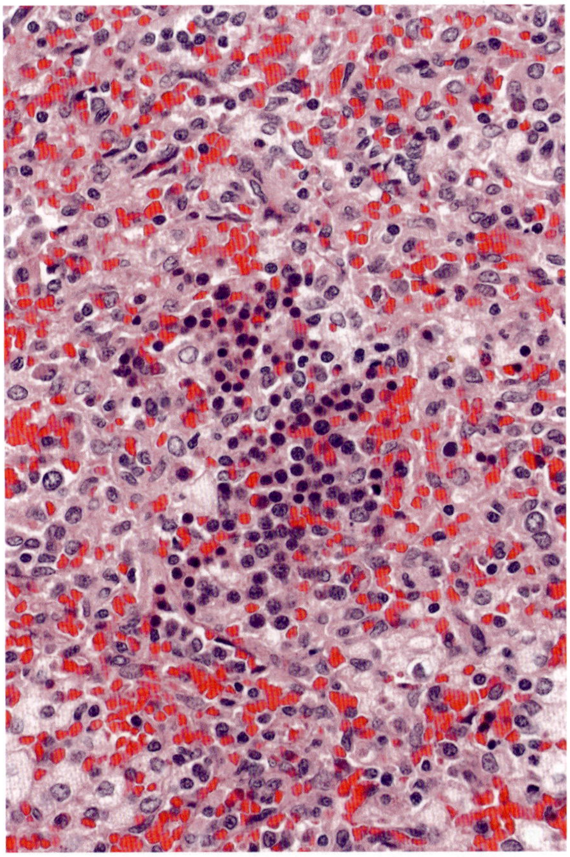

Figure 13-9

EXTRAMEDULLARY HEMATOPOIESIS, SPLEEN

A focus of maturing erythroid cells in the red pulp of a spleen.

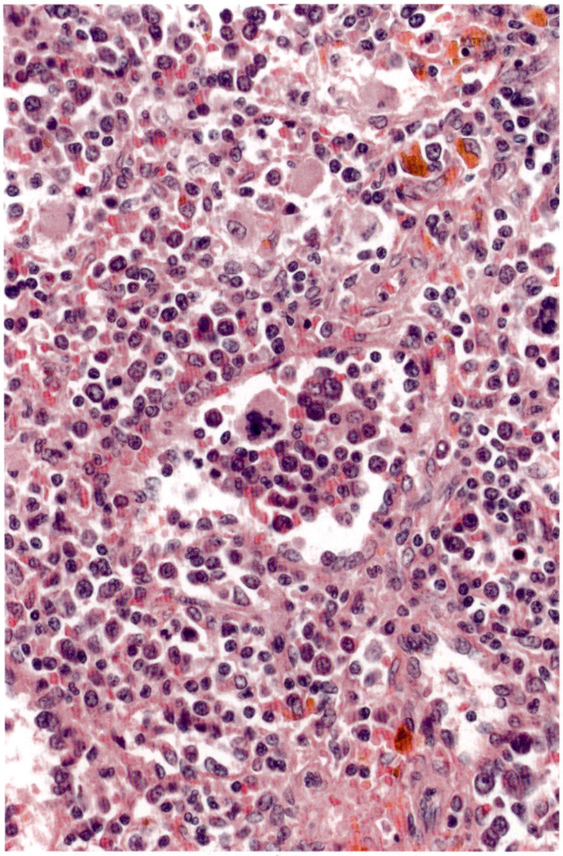

Figure 13-10

EXTRAMEDULLARY HEMATOPOIESIS, SPLEEN

An intrasinusoidal focus of extramedullary hematopoiesis includes immature myeloid cells and a megakaryocyte.

Table 13-1

HISTOLOGIC FEATURES OF SPLENIC MYELOID PROLIFERATIONS

Etiology		Hematopoiesis
Benign	Hypersplenism due to non-neoplastic etiologies	Typically trilineage hematopoiesis
	Hemolytic anemias and other anemias	Predominantly erythroid with occasional megakaryocytes
	Cytokine-induced (e.g., G-CSF)[a]	Predominantly myeloid—may simulate acute myeloid leukemia (acute myeloid leukemia or acute promyelocytic leukemia in particular)
	Lymphoma/other malignancies (carcinoma, sarcoma)	Variable degrees of trilineage hematopoiesis without atypia
Clonal	MPD	Usually trilineage—occasionally one lineage predominant; atypia seen in megakaryocytes; may represent initial site of blast transformation
	MDS/MPD	Findings overlap with both MPD and MDS
	MDS	Usually trilineage, occasionally with increased monocytes/macrophages; dysplasia seen in megakaryocytes; increased immature myeloid/blasts may herald blast transformation

[a]G-CSF = granulocyte-colony stimulating factor; MPD = myeloproliferative disorder; MDS = myelodysplastic syndrome.

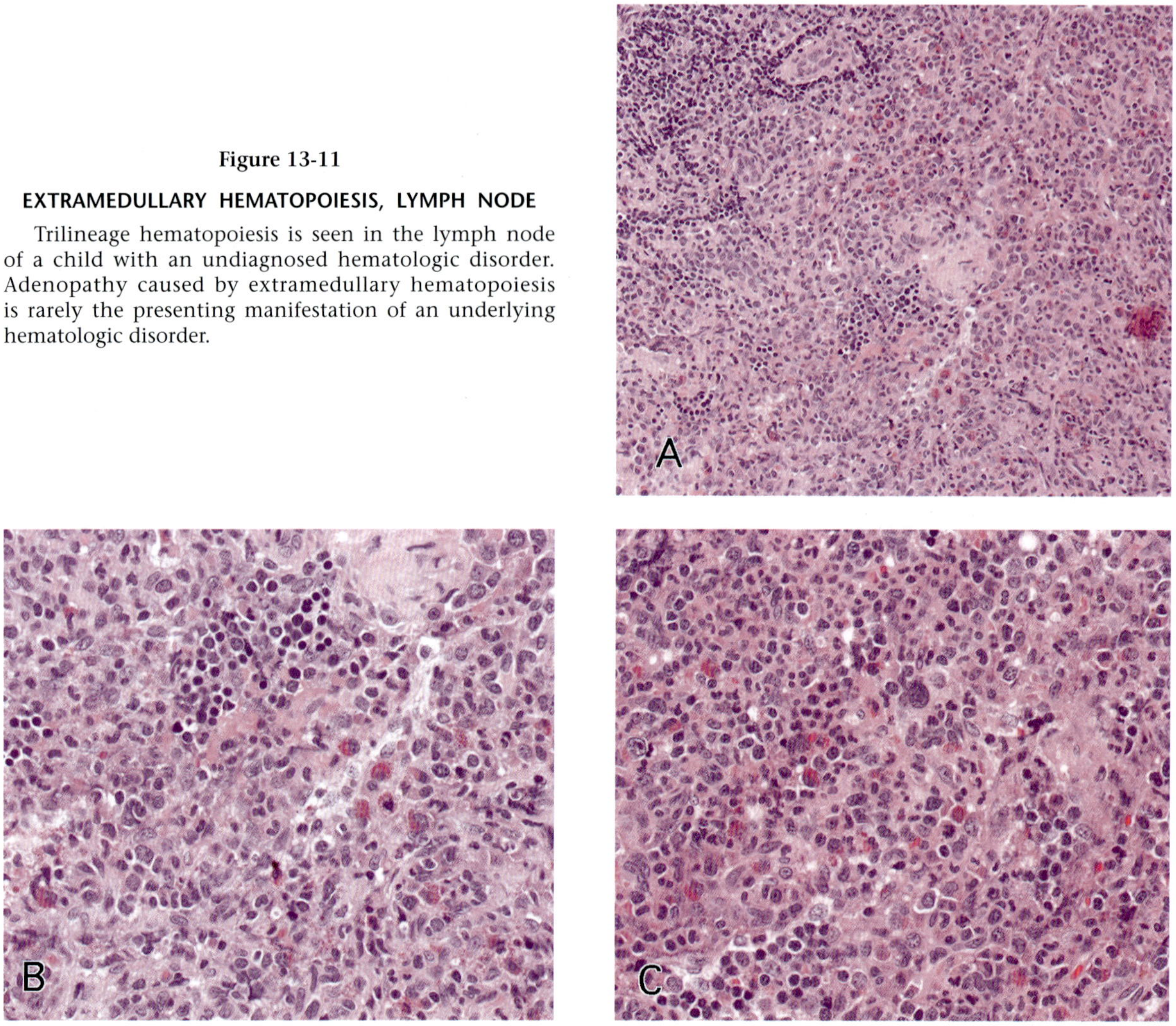

Figure 13-11

EXTRAMEDULLARY HEMATOPOIESIS, LYMPH NODE

Trilineage hematopoiesis is seen in the lymph node of a child with an undiagnosed hematologic disorder. Adenopathy caused by extramedullary hematopoiesis is rarely the presenting manifestation of an underlying hematologic disorder.

Morphologically, the individual hematopoietic elements appear fairly normal. Significant dysplasia in the form of immature-appearing myeloid elements (high nuclear to cytoplasmic ratio, scant cytoplasm) or abnormal megakaryocytes (unilobate, small size, bizarre chromatin or nuclei) should raise the possibility of an underlying neoplastic myeloid disorder. EMH in the lymph nodes is similar morphologically to that of the spleen (fig. 13-11).

Ancillary Studies. Immunohistochemical stains may be necessary to evaluate the nature, extent, and composition of EMH (50). Appropriate stains include myeloperoxidase or lysozyme (to identify granulocytic/monocytic elements), hemoglobin or glycophorin (to identify erythroid elements), CD41/CD42/CD61 or factor VIII (to identify megakaryocytic elements), and, most importantly, CD34 and CD117 (to identify the presence of immature hematopoietic precursor cells). The presence of even moderate numbers of precursor cells should suggest a neoplastic myeloid disorder rather than benign EMH.

Differential Diagnosis. The differentiation of neoplastic myeloid proliferations, such as those seen commonly in chronic myeloproliferative disorders, from EMH associated with benign conditions is difficult in some cases (48). In most cases, the degree of EMH seen in spleens with non-neoplastic conditions or in association with nonhematopoietic neoplasms is inconspicuous enough to not raise concern for possible involvement by a myeloid disease. Occasionally, however, the EMH is extensive enough to suggest a myeloid neoplasm.

Treatment and Prognosis. In most circumstances, EMH has little clinical significance in either the spleen or lymph nodes, although enlargement of these structures may cause concern for malignancy. In benign hematologic disorders, significant enlargement is rare, but may cause symptoms due to compression of other organs. In any case, management of the underlying hematologic disorder is the primary treatment.

REFERENCES

1. Adams JG 3rd, Coleman MB. Structural hemoglobin variants that produce the phenotype of thalassemia. Semin Hematol 1990;27:229-38.
2. Adekile AD, McKie KM, Adeodu OO, et al. Spleen in sickle cell anemia: comparative studies of Nigerian and U.S. patients. Am J Hematol 1993;42:316-21
3. Allen DW, Jandl JH. Oxidative hemolysis and precipitation of hemoglobin. II. J Clin Invest 1961;40:454-75.
4. Arnold R, Calvo W, Heymer B, Schmeiser T, Heimpel H, Kubanek B. Extramedullary hematopoiesis after bone marrow transplantation. Scan J Haematol 1985;34:9-12.
5. Benz EJ Jr, Forget BG. The thalassemia syndromes: models for molecular analysis of human disease. Ann Rev Med 1982;33:363-73.
6. Blackburn EK, Jordan A, Lytle WJ, Swan HT, Tudhope GR. Hereditary elliptocytic haemolytic anaemia. J Clin Pathol 1958;11:316-20.
7. Bowman HS, Oski FA. Splenic macrophage interaction with red cells in pyruvate kinase deficiency and hereditary spherocytosis. Vox Sang 1970;19:168-75.
8. Buchanan GR, McKie V, Jackson EA, Vedro DA, Hamner S, Holtkamp CA. Splenic phagocytic function in children with sickle cell anemia receiving long-term hypertransfusion. J Pediatr 1989;115:568-72.
9. Calleja EM, Shen JY, Lesser M, Grady RW, New MI, Giardina PJ. Survival and morbidity in transfusion-dependent thalassemic patients on subcutaneous desferrioxamine chelation. Nearly two decades of experience. Ann N Y Acad Sci 1998;850:469-70.
10. Cetiner S, Akoglu TF, Kilinc Y, Akoglu E, Kumi M. Immunological studies in sickle cell disease: comparison of homozygote mild and severe variants. Clin Immunol Immunopathol 1989:53:32-9.
11. Chang C, Li C, Liang Y, Cha SS. Clinical features and splenic pathologic changes in patients with autoimmune hemolytic anemia and congenital hemolytic anemia. Mayo Clin Proc 1993;68:757-62.
12. Charache S, Dover GJ, Moore RD, et al. Hydroxyurea: effects on hemoglobin F production in patients with sickle cell anemia. Blood 1992;79:2555-65.
13. Chopra R, Al-Mulhim AR, Al-Baharani AT. Fibrocongestive splenomegaly in sickle cell disease: a distinct clinicopathological entity in the Eastern province of Saudi Arabia. Am J Hematol 2005;79:180-6.
14. Cooper RA, Jandl JH. The selective and conjoint loss of red cell lipids. J Clin Invest 1969;48:906-14.
15. Cutting HO, McHugh WJ, Conrad FG, Marlow AA. Autosomal dominant hemolytic anemia characterized by ovalocytosis. A family study of seven involved members. Am J Med 1965;39:21-34.
16. Dean J, Schechter AN. Sickle-cell anemia: molecular and cellular bases of therapeutic approaches. N Engl J Med 1978;299:752-63.
17. Diggs LW. Siderofibrosis of the spleen in sickle cell anemia. J Am Med Assoc 1935;104:538-541.
18. Dilly SA, Sloane JP. Cellular composition of the spleen after human allogeneic bone marrow transplantation. J Pathol 1988;155:151-60.
19. Douay L, Laporte JP, Lefrancois G, et al. Blood and spleen haematopoiesis in patients with myelofibrosis. Leuk Res 1987;11:725-30.
20. Eaton JW, Hebbel RP. Pathogenesis of sickle cell disease. Pathobiol Annu 1981;11:31-52.
21. Ebbel RP, Miller WJ. Phagocytosis of sickle erythrocytes: immunologic and oxidative determinants of hemolytic anemia. Blood 1984;64:733-41.
22. Erslev AJ, Atwater J. Effect of mean corpuscular hemoglobin concentration on viscosity. J Lab Clin Med 1963;62:401-6.
23. Farhi DC, Ashfaq R. Splenic pathology after traumatic injury. Am J Clin Pathol 1996;105:474-8.
24. Ferreira JA, Feliu E, Rozman C, et al. Morphologic and morphometric light and electron microscopic PIC studies of the spleen in patients with hereditary spherocytosis and autoimmune haemolytic anaemia. Br J Haematol 1989;72:246-53.

25. Ferster A, Bryan W, Corazza F, et al. Bone marrow transplantation corrects the splenic reticuloendothelial dysfunction in sickle cell anemia. Blood 1993;81:1102-5.
26. Finch CA. Pathophysiologic aspects of sickle cell anemia. Am J Med 1972;53:1-6.
27. Fishbone G, Nunez D Jr, Leon R, Paz G, Isturiz P, McLaughlin C. Massive splenic infarction in sickle cell hemoglobin C disease: angiographic findings. AJR Am J Roentgenol 1977;129:927-8.
28. Freedman MH, Saunders EF. Hematopoiesis in the human spleen. Am J Hematol 1981;11:271-5.
29. Gairdner D. The association of gallstones with acholuric jaundice in children. Arch Dis Child 1939;14:109-20.
30. Gallagher PG, Ferriera JD. Molecular basis of erythrocyte membrane disorders. Curr Opin Hematol 1997;4:128-35.
31. Gaziev J, Lucarelli G. Stem cell transplantation and gene therapy for hemoglobinopathies. Curr Hematol Rep 2005;4:126-31.
32. Geola F, Kukreja SC, Schade SG. Splenic sequestration with sickle cell-C disease. Arch Intern Med 1978;138:307-8.
33. Girot R, Begue P. [Sickle cell disease in childhood in 2004]. Bull Acad Natl Med 2004;188:491-505. [French]
34. Gregg XT, Prchal JT. Red blood cell enzymopathies. In: Hoffman R, Benz EJ Jr, Shattil SJ, eds. Hematology. Basic principles and practice, 4th ed. New York: Elsevier Churchill Livingstone; 2005;605-44.
35. Harley JD, Mauer AM. Studies on the formation of Heinz bodies. I. Methemoglobin production and oxyhemoglobin destruction. Blood 1960;16:1722-35.
36. Hassan NM, Neiman RS. The pathology of the spleen in steroid-treated immune thrombocytopenic purpura. Am J Clin Pathol 1985;84:433-8.
37. Horny H-P, Ruck M, Kaiserling E. Immunohistology of the human spleen after bone marrow transplantation for leukemia with special reference to the early post-transplantation period. Path Res Pract 1990;186:775-83.
38. Jacob HS, Ruby A, Overland ES, et al. Abnormal membrane protein of red blood cells in hereditary spherocytosis. J Clin Invest 1971;50:1800.
39. Jandl JH, Engle LK, Allen DW. Oxidative hemolysis and precipitation of hemoglobin. I. Heinz body anemias as an acceleration of aging. J Clin Invest 1960;39:1818-36.
40. Jensen M, Shohet SB, Nathan DG. The role of red cell energy metabolism in the generation of irreversibly sickled cells in vitro. Blood 1973;42:835-42.
41. Kraus MD, Bartlett NL, Fleming MD, Dorfman DM. Splenic pathology in myelodysplasia. A report of 13 cases with clinical correlation. Am J Surg Pathol 1998;22:1255-66.
42. Krueger HC, Burgert EO. Hereditary spherocytosis in 100 children. Mayo Clin Proc 1966;41:281-30.
43. Marks PA, Gross RT. Erythrocyte glucose-6-phosphate dehydrogenase deficiency: Evidence of differences between Negroes and Caucasians with respect to this genetically determined trait. J Clin Invest 1959;38:2253-62.
44. Mathew A, Raviglione MC, Niranjan U, Sabatini MT, Distenfeld A. Splenectomy in patients with AIDS. Am J Hematol 1989;32:184-9.
45. Miwa S, Kanno H, Fujii H. Concise review: pyruvate kinase deficiency: historical perspective and recent progress of molecular genetics. Am J Hematol 1993;42:31-5.
46. Mortimer PP, Humphries RK, Moore JG, Parcell RH, Young NS. A human parvovirus-like virus inhibits haematopoietic colony formation in vitro. Nature 1983;302:426-9.
47. Myhre Jensen O, Kristensen J. Red pulp of the spleen in autoimmune haemolytic anaemia and hereditary spherocytosis: morphometric light and electron microscopy studies. Scand J Haematol 1986;36:263-6.
48. Neiman RS, Orazi A. Myeloproliferative Disorders. In: Neiman RS, Orazi A, eds. Disorders of the Spleen, 2nd ed. Philadelphia: W.B. Saunders; 1999;220-36.
49. O'Keane JC, Wolf BC, Neiman RS. The pathogenesis of splenic extramedullary hematopoiesis in metastatic carcinoma. Cancer 1989;15;63:1539-43.
50. O'Malley DP, Kim YS, Perkins S, Baldridge LA, Juliar BE, Orazi A. Comparison of splenic extramedullary hematopoiesis in benign and neoplastic hematopoietic disorders. Mod Pathol 2005;18:1550-61.
51. O'Malley DP, Orazi A, Wang M, Cheng L. Analysis of loss of heterozygosity and X-chromosome inactivation in spleens with myeloproliferative disorders and acute myeloid leukemia. Mod Pathol 2005;18:1562-8.
52. Palitzsch KD, Falk S, Muller H, Stutte HJ. Splenic haematopoiesis in patients with cirrhosis of the liver. Virchows Arch A Pathol Anat Histopathol 1987;411:179-83.
53. Pearson HA, McIntosh S, Ritchey AK, Lobel JS, Rooks Y, Johnston D. Developmental aspects of splenic function in sickle cell diseases. Blood 1979;53:358-65.
54. Pearson HA, Spencer RP, Cornelius EA. Functional asplenia in sickle-cell anemia. N Engl J Med 1969;281:923-6.
55. Pekrun A, Linne S, Schroter W. [Fatal course of a sequestration crisis in hemoglobin SC disease.] Monatsschr Kinderheilkd 1993;141:573-5. [German]

56. Reed CF, Swisher SN. Erythrocyte lipid loss in the pathogenesis of hereditary spherocytosis. J Clin Invest 1966;45:777-81.
57. Rifkind RA. Heinz body anemia: an ultrastructural study. II. Red cell sequestration and destruction. Blood 1965;26:433-48.
58. Rund D, Rachmilewitz E. Beta thalassemia. N Engl J Med 2005; 353:1135-46.
59. Sandoval C, Stringel G, Weisberger J, Jayabose S. Failure of Partial splenectomy to ameliorate the anemia of pyruvate kinase deficiency. J Pediatr Surg 1997;132:641-2.
60. Saracco SM, Farhi DC. Splenic pathology in thrombotic thrombocytopenic purpura. Am J Surg Pathol 1990;14:223-9.
61. Saunthararajah Y, Vichinsky E, Embury SH. Sickle cell disease. In: Hoffman R, Benz EJ Jr, Shattil SJ, eds. Hematology. Basic principles and practice, 4th ed. New York: Elsevier Churchill Livingstone; 2005:605-44.
62. Schwartz SI, Bernard RP, Adams JT, Bauman AW. Splenectomy for hematologic disorders. Arch Surg 1970;101:338-47.
63. Sen Gupta PC, Chatterjea JB, Mukherjee AM, Chatterji A. Observations on the foam cell in thalassemia. Blood 1960;16:1039-44.
64. Simon ER. Expanded autohemolysis as an investigative and diagnostic tool in hemolytic disorders. Clin Res 1963;11:200.
65. Snover DC, Frizzera G, Spector BD, Perry GS 3rd, Kersey JH. Wiskott-Aldrich syndrome: histopathologic findings in the lymph nodes and spleens of 15 patients. Hum Pathol 1981;12:821-31.
66. Solanki DL, Kletter GG, Castro O. Acute splenic sequestration crises in adults with sickle cell disease. Am J Med 1986;80:985-90.
67. Steensma DP, Tefferi A, Li C. Splenic histopathological patterns in chronic myelomonocytic leukemia with clinical correlations: reinforcement of the heterogeneity of the syndrome. Leuk Res 2003;27:775-82.
68. Tanaka KR, Paglia DE. Pyruvate kinase deficiency. Semin Hematol 1971;8:367-96.
69. Tse WT, Lux SE. Red blood cell membrane disorders. Br J Haematol 1999:104:2-13.
70. Valentine WN. Hereditary spherocytosis revisited. West J Med 1978;128:35-45.
71. Vichinsky EP, Lubin BH. Unstable hemoglobins, hemoglobins with altered oxygen affinity, and M-hemoglobins. Pediatr Clin North Am 1980;27:421-8.
72. Wethers DL, Grover R. Reversibility of splenic function by transfusion in two young adults with sickle cell anemia. Am J Pediatr Hematol Oncol 1987;9:209-11.
73. Wilkins BS, Green A, Wild AE, Jones DB. Extramedullary haemopoiesis in fetal and adult human spleen: a quantitative immunohistological study. Histopathology 1994;24:241-7.
74. Wolf BC, Banks PM, Mann RB, Neiman RS. Splenic hematopoiesis in polycythemia vera. A morphologic and immunohistologic study. Am J Clin Pathol 1988;89:69-75.
75. Yang YM, Donnell C, Wilborn W, et al. Splenic sequestration associated with sickle cell trait and hereditary spherocytosis. Am J Hematol 1992;40:110-6.
76. Young N. Hematologic and hematopoietic consequences of B19 parvovirus infection. Semin Hematol 1988;25:159-72.

14 MEDICATION AND TREATMENT EFFECTS

Although not commonly seen or recognized, significant changes may be induced in the lymph nodes and spleen in association with specific types of therapy and medications. These changes may lead to significant morphologic features that mimic other reactive, infectious, or neoplastic processes.

Recognition of these changes can be difficult, if not impossible, without a clinical history of medication use. In many circumstances, the effects of a treatment or medication are difficult to separate from the underlying pathologic process. In rheumatoid arthritis, the morphologic effects of treatment with methotrexate, gold, and other medications, are similar to those of the underlying disease. It is impossible to distinguish which changes are due to the disease, the medications, and most importantly, the interaction of the disease and medication.

A hypersensitivity drug reaction may cause lymphadenopathy with diffuse atypical paracortical immunoblastic hyperplasia, which is difficult to distinguish from viral-associated lymphadenopathy or angioimmunoblastic lymphadenopathy/angioimmunoblastic T-cell lymphoma (fig. 14-1) (see chapter 6). Cytoreductive chemotherapy is associated with a reduction of the cellularity and lymphoid depletion of lymph nodes and splenic white pulp. The splenic red pulp may be congested or normal. These changes are dependent on the type and duration of chemotherapy as well as the underlying disorder. In certain circumstances, follicular hyperplasia or immunoblastic hyperplasia is seen. The morphologic changes that are attributed specifically to medications and therapies are outlined in the sections that follow.

RITUXIMAB THERAPY AND OTHER MONOCLONAL ANTIBODY THERAPIES FOR LYMPHOMA

Definition. *Rituximab* is a monoclonal anti-CD20 antibody used for the treatment of B-cell lymphomas, as well as a variety of other disorders, typically immune related. Anti-CD20 antibodies may have significant morphologic effects on lymphoid tissues, including those that are not necessarily involved by a B-cell neoplastic process.

General Features. Rituximab is a chimeric murine/human monoclonal antibody directed against the CD20 molecule. It causes cell death

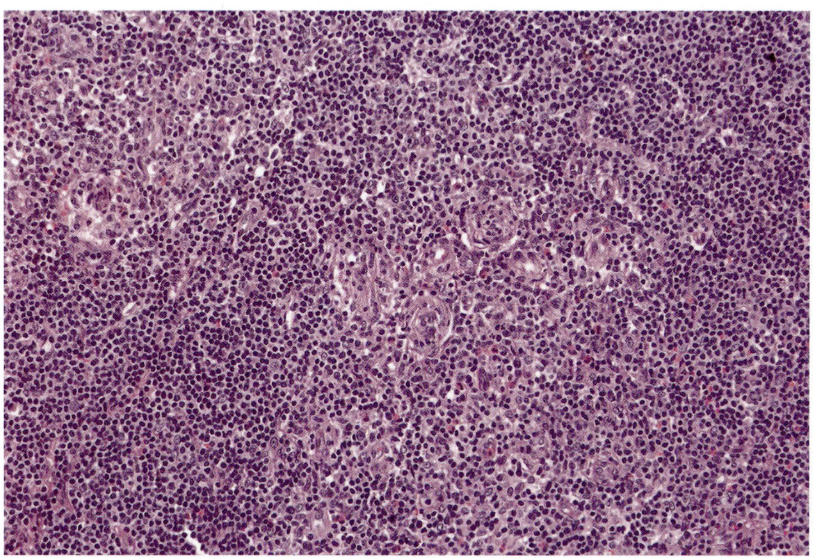

Figure 14-1

HYPERSENSITIVITY REACTION, LYMPH NODE

Increases in vasculature, inflammatory cells such as eosinophils, and large, transformed lymphocytes can simulate the appearance of T-cell lymphoma.

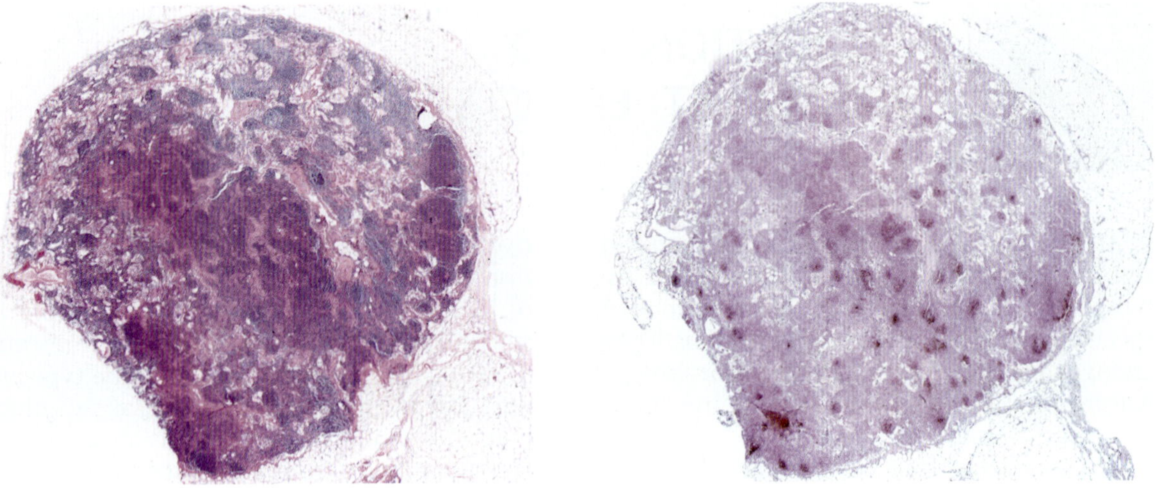

Figure 14-2

RITUXIMAB THERAPY, LYMPH NODE

Left: A hematoxylin and eosin (H&E)-stained lymph node in a patient treated with rituximab (anti-CD20) for lymphoma shows a retained architecture.

Right: Immunohistochemistry shows a greatly reduced number of CD20-positive cells.

by inducing apoptosis, antibody-dependent cytotoxicity, and complement-mediated cytotoxicity. The immune modulation effects of rituximab are used in the treatment of immune thrombocytopenic purpura, thrombotic thrombocytopenic purpura, autoimmune hemolytic anemia, pure red cell aplasia, and a variety of other autoimmune phenomena (33). The incidence monoclonal antibody therapy will steadily increase as experience with this approach and the number of available antibodies increase.

A similar antibody, *I^{131}-tositumomab*, is a radiolabeled anti-CD20 monoclonal antibody. The CD20 molecule is not required for B-cell survival, as shown in knockout mouse studies (15,38).

Laboratory Findings. Flow cytometric analysis of the peripheral blood in patients treated with anti-CD20 antibodies may reveal a decrease in circulating B cells. Ultimately, the B cells return to normal on cessation of therapy. If therapy is extended (as in rituximab maintenance therapy), a significant portion of the circulating B cells may lack CD20 expression.

Microscopic Findings. The microscopic changes in normal lymph nodes or spleen treated with anti-CD20 antibodies have not been extensively reported, but are somewhat predictable. The lymph nodes decrease in size, with decreased size and frequency of germinal centers (fig. 14-2). Most follicles are primary follicles, consisting of small, mantle type lymphocytes. The sinuses and T-cell zones increase in size.

Anti-CD20 antibodies are used for a variety of non-neoplastic disorders, including immune thrombocytopenic purpura (50). Only small studies of spleen specimens after rituxan treatment for immune thrombocytopenic purpura or other non-neoplastic hematologic disorders have been published (3). Spleens show depleted numbers, or even absence, of B cells, with a particular reduction of follicles (fig. 14-3) (33). Downregulation of CD20 on the surface of B cells may be seen, with other CD19-positive B cells still present. Follicular dendritic cells are reduced in number.

Ancillary Studies. As anticipated, CD20 staining is significantly decreased, along with the overall reduction of B cells. Staining for other compartments, such as T cells, is usually unaffected.

Differential Diagnosis. A clinical history is of paramount importance in identifying the changes associated with monoclonal antibodies, particularly in lymph nodes unaffected by the disorder that the therapy was intended for. The morphologic changes associated with monoclonal antibody therapy can vary.

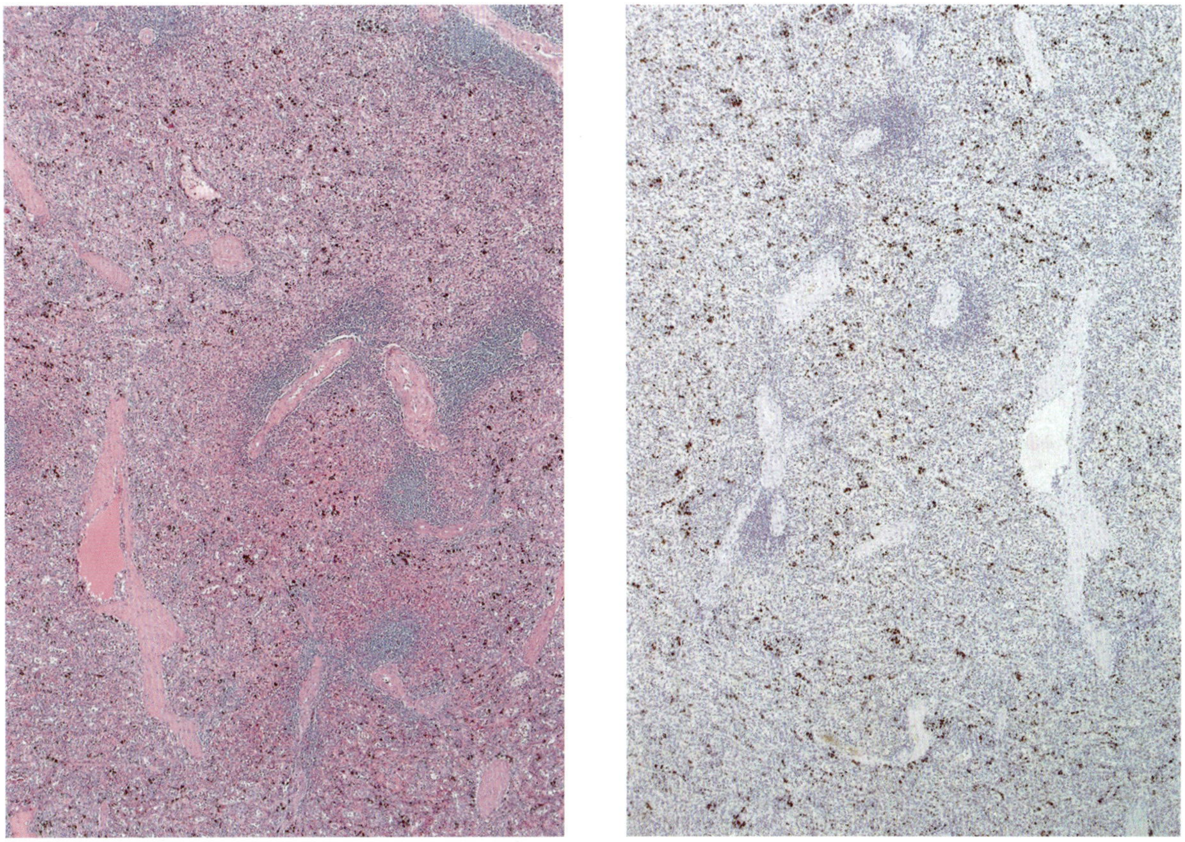

Figure 14-3

RITUXIMAB THERAPY, SPLEEN

Left: The white pulp is depleted in a spleen treated with rituximab for immune thrombocytopenic purpura (ITP).

Right: Immunohistochemical reactivity for CD20 is almost absent. The focal brown staining is hemosiderin pigment, which is also seen in the H&E section (left figure). Contrast these findings with those seen in figure 14-4, which is a spleen treated with corticosteroids for ITP.

Anti-CD20 antibodies, in particular, can cause morphologic changes that suggest a primary or secondary immunodeficiency disorder.

Treatment and Prognosis. When anti-CD20 is used for the treatment of lymphoma, it is important to evaluate for possible recurrence. Anti-idiotype antibodies may select for clones that are no longer recognized by the therapeutic antibody (15,22,24,32,38). The morphologic findings associated with recurrence are not likely to be affected by the use of anti-CD20 antibodies; however, changes in the immunophenotype may make recurrences more difficult to identify.

CORTICOSTEROID THERAPY

Definition. *Corticosteroids* are used to treat a wide array of medical conditions, including immune thrombocytopenic purpura (ITP) (see chapter 12). The use of corticosteroid therapy causes significant morphologic changes in the spleen.

General Features. Corticosteroids are potent hormones that have a variety of effects, including a reduction of inflammation and suppression of the innate immune responses. These hormones are normally produced by the body, but are given in much higher doses in therapeutic situations.

Clinical Features. The splenic changes associated with corticosteroid therapy use are seen commonly. However, it is difficult to separate the features of treated ITP spleens (the most commonly encountered disease treated with corticosteroids) from those of spleens treated with steroid therapy for other causes (5,11,23).

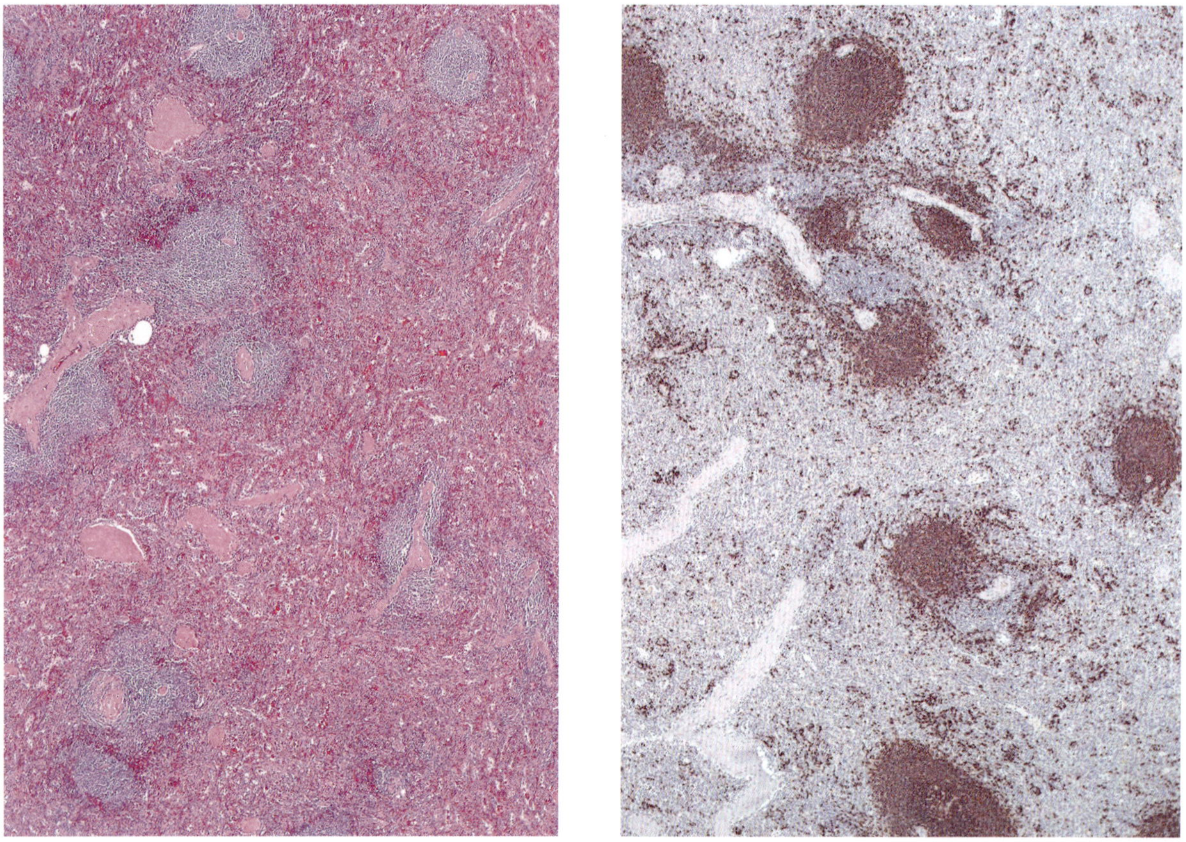

Figure 14-4

CORTICOSTEROID THERAPY, SPLEEN

Left: Secondary follicles are absent, but the PALS regions are maintained.
Right: Immunohistochemical reactivity for CD20 highlights B cells in primary follicles.

Microscopic Findings. The most frequent morphologic changes associated with corticosteroid treatment are reduction and shrinkage of the B-cell regions of the splenic white pulp. In untreated cases of ITP, there is frequent follicular hyperplasia. After corticosteroid treatment, germinal centers are reduced in size and number, or are absent (fig. 14-4). B-cell areas are often limited to primary follicles, which can be smaller than usual. The T-cell zones (e.g., periarteriolar lymphoid sheath [PALS]) are typically unaffected. Red pulp congestion with foamy macrophages is seen in untreated ITP; it is often reduced after continued treatment with corticosteroids.

METHOTREXATE

Definition. *Methotrexate* is an antimetabolite chemotherapy agent that is used in the treatment of a variety of neoplastic diseases, rheumatoid arthritis, and other disorders. Its use is associated with a spectrum of lymphoid proliferations.

General Features. Methotrexate is a folic acid derivative and acts as an antagonist of folic acid. It competes with folic acid, which is essential for DNA synthesis in the cells. This is the basis for its use in cancer treatment, and this is also the mechanism by which it can alter the course of autoimmune disorders, such as rheumatoid arthritis.

Clinical Features. The frequency of lymphoid proliferations, which range from typical hyperplasia to frank lymphoma, associated with methotrexate therapy is not known (28,29,34,60,62,63). At the extreme ends of this spectrum, the evaluation and treatment are straightforward. Cases with features of "atypical lymphoid hyperplasia" are problematic. It may also be difficult to separate the effects of methotrexate therapy from the disorders that

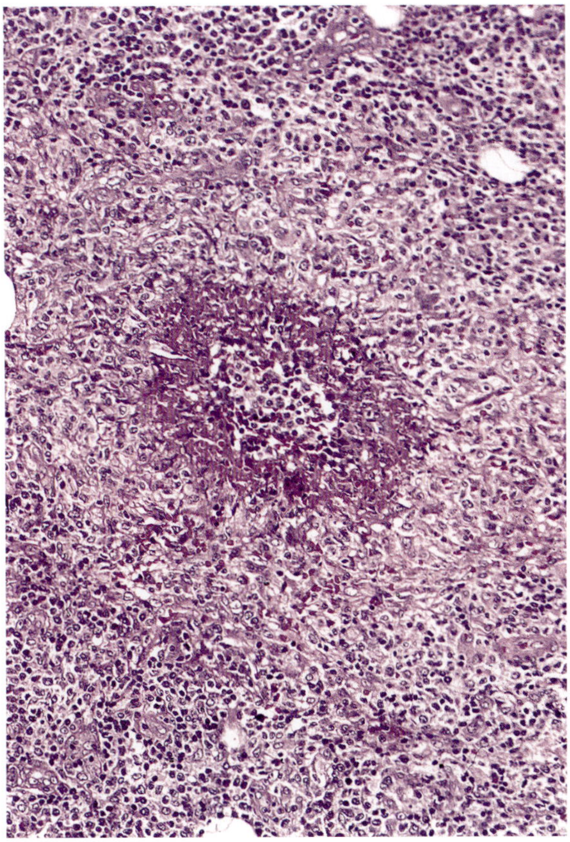

Figure 14-5

METHOTREXATE-ASSOCIATED LYMPHOID PROLIFERATION, LYMPH NODE

Granulomas with central necrosis are a manifestation of methotrexate-associated lymphoid proliferation.

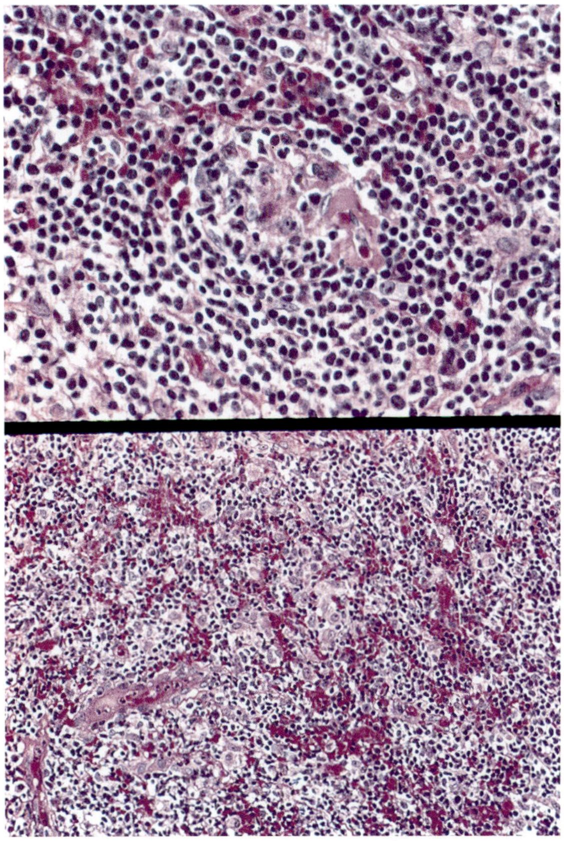

Figure 14-6

METHOTREXATE-ASSOCIATED LYMPHOID PROLIFERATION, LYMPH NODE

Regressed follicles (top) and vascular proliferation are seen in some methotrexate-associated lymphoid proliferations.

are being treated, especially in the case of rheumatoid arthritis (see chapter 12).

Microscopic Findings. The histologic features of methotrexate treatment are variable (figs. 14-5–14-7) (27,29). In some cases, there is a polymorphic proliferation of cells in the interfollicular spaces. These cells include plasmacytoid lymphocytes, small lymphocytes, large transformed lymphocytes, and Hodgkin- and Reed-Sternberg–like cells. There may be partial effacement of the normal lymph node architecture by this process. In other cases, the proliferations more closely resemble nodular lymphocyte-predominant Hodgkin lymphoma or the proliferations are composed of predominantly large, transformed lymphocytes, resembling diffuse large B-cell lymphoma.

Ancillary Studies. In most cases, it is recommended that immunoglobulin (Ig) gene rearrangement studies for IgH be performed, to evaluate for the presence of a clonal population of B cells. Particularly in cases with a morphology that is reminiscent of diffuse large B-cell lymphoma, a clonal population may be seen. Immunohistochemical or in situ studies for Epstein-Barr virus (EBV) may be positive. Unlike typical Reed-Sternberg cells, the large reactive cells are CD15 negative.

Treatment and Prognosis. Discontinuation of methotrexate therapy often reverses the morphologic changes and atypical appearance. If a frank lymphoma or lymphoid proliferation has developed, however, then conventional chemotherapy is required.

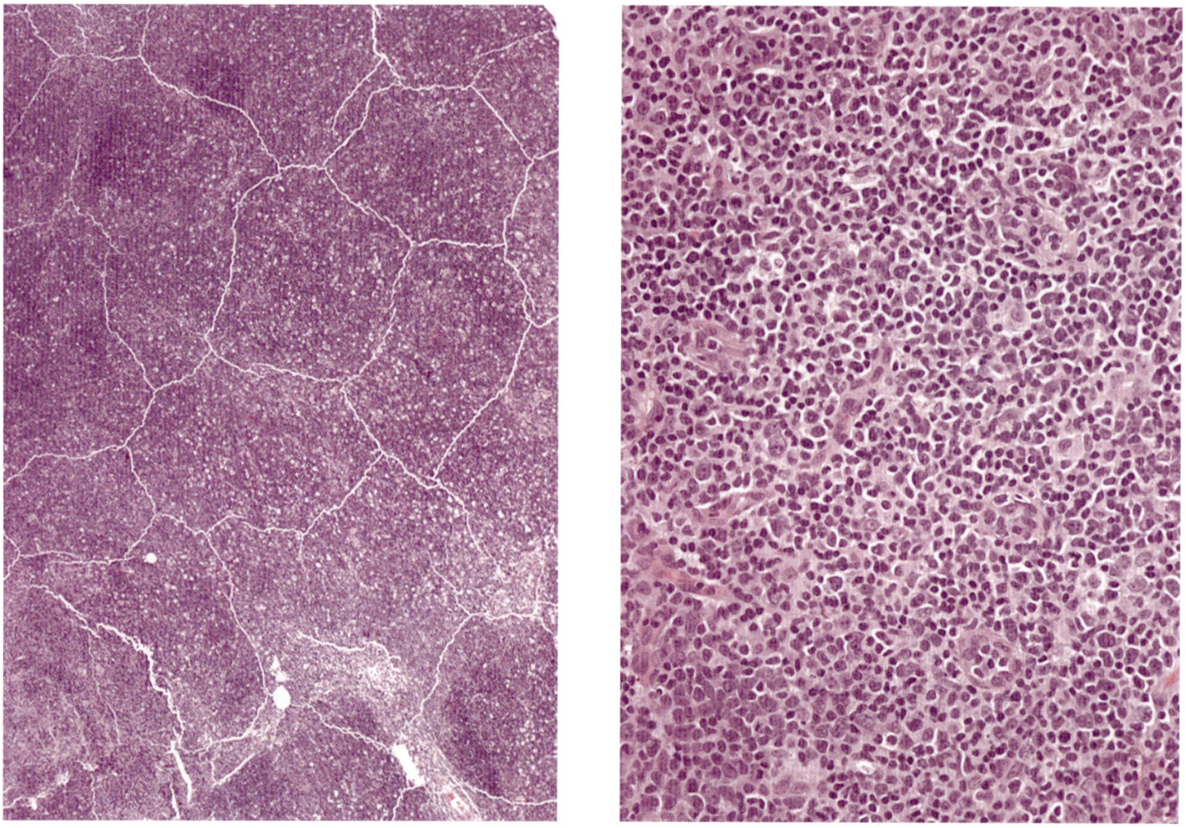

Figure 14-7

METHOTREXATE-ASSOCIATED LYMPHOID PROLIFERATION, LYMPH NODE

Highly proliferative lymph nodes (left) and large atypical cells (right) are features of this case of methotrexate-associated lymphoid proliferation.

ANTICONVULSANT MEDICATIONS

Definition. Lymphoid abnormalities, typically florid hyperplasia, are associated with acute or chronic administration of *anticonvulsants*. Although phenytoin (Dilantin) is most commonly implicated, other anticonvulsant drugs also result in abnormalities. Anticonvulsant drug-related lymphadenopathy may simulate malignant processes such as lymphoma.

General Features. It is difficult to definitively determine whether the histologic changes in the lymph nodes of patients on anticonvulsant medications are a result of the drug itself or an incidental unrelated finding. If the classic clinicopathologic features of a hypersensitivity syndrome are present at the time of excisional lymph node biopsy (i.e., rash, eosinophilia, rapid onset following drug intake), it is more likely that drug intake is related to the lymphadenopathy.

Clinical Features. Histologic descriptions of anticonvulsant-associated lymphadenopathy first appeared in the literature approximately 20 years after the initial use of phenytoin (53). Many cases of lymphadenopathy associated with anticonvulsants were diagnosed as "pseudolymphoma" because of their confusing and worrisome histologic features (12,13,54). This was especially true of cases associated with phenytoin (1), first used for the treatment of seizure disorders in 1938 (40). Other anticonvulsant drugs, including *ethosuximide, carbamazepine,* and *mesantoin,* have been reported to cause lymphadenopathy (31,43,52).

Microscopic Findings. The lymph nodes of patients being treated with the antiseizure medications, including phenytoin, show a spectrum of histopathologic features. These include varying degrees of architectural effacement by

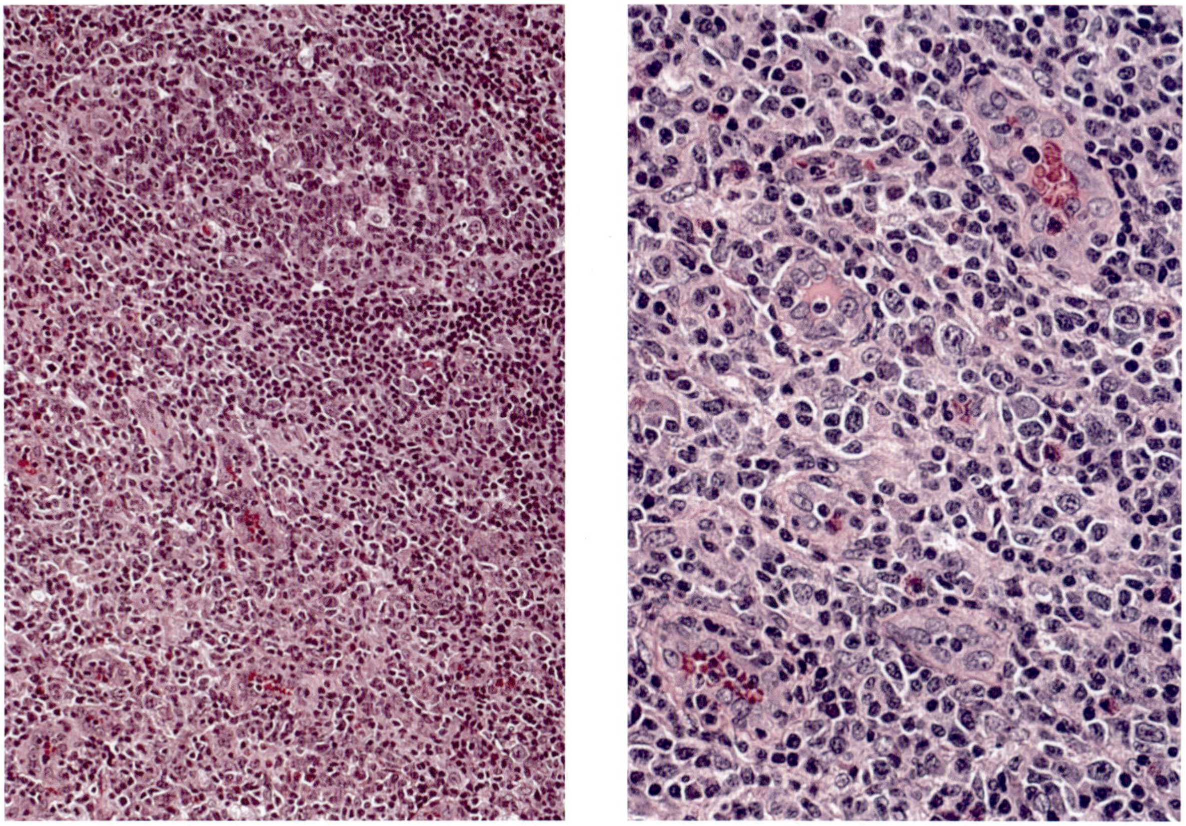

Figure 14-8

ANTICONVULSANT-ASSOCIATED LYMPHOID PROLIFERATION, LYMPH NODE

Phenytoin-associated lymphadenopathy with diffuse paracortical hyperplasia (left), accentuated vascularity, eosinophilia, and scattered immunoblasts (right).

a mixed inflammatory cell infiltrate (especially eosinophils, plasma cells, lymphocytes, and immunoblasts) and focal, small vessel vasculitis (figs. 14-8–14-10) (1). The histologic patterns in cases of phenytoin-associated lymphadenopathy are divided into three groups: 1) prominent immunoblastic hyperplasia with germinal center hyperplasia and disruption, with or without focal obliteration; 2) prominent immunoblastic hyperplasia with germinal center atrophy; and 3) miscellaneous nonimmunoblastic lesions.

The atypical reactive lymphoid hyperplasia associated with phenytoin therapy characteristically shows expansion of the paracortex by a polymorphous population of cells including immunoblasts and eosinophils. Vascularity is increased. Nonspecific reactive follicular hyperplasia may also be present (13). Immunoblastic hyperplasia in the presence of "dissolved" germinal centers, foci of necrosis, and obliterative endarteritis has been described and may simulate a malignant lymphoma (1). The atypical paracortical immunoblastic hyperplasia and the disrupted or dissolved germinal centers may be difficult to distinguish from a malignant lymphoma. A review of the literature suggests that these features most likely represent the challenging histopathologic changes that were diagnosed originally as pseudolymphoma. Pseudolymphoma is a confusing and potentially misleading diagnostic term that should be replaced with a detailed description of the histologic features.

The splenic changes associated with anticonvulsant therapy are similar to those seen in the lymph nodes. In addition, T-cell hyperplasia, with expansion of the PALS region by CD4-positive T lymphocytes, may be seen (fig. 14-11).

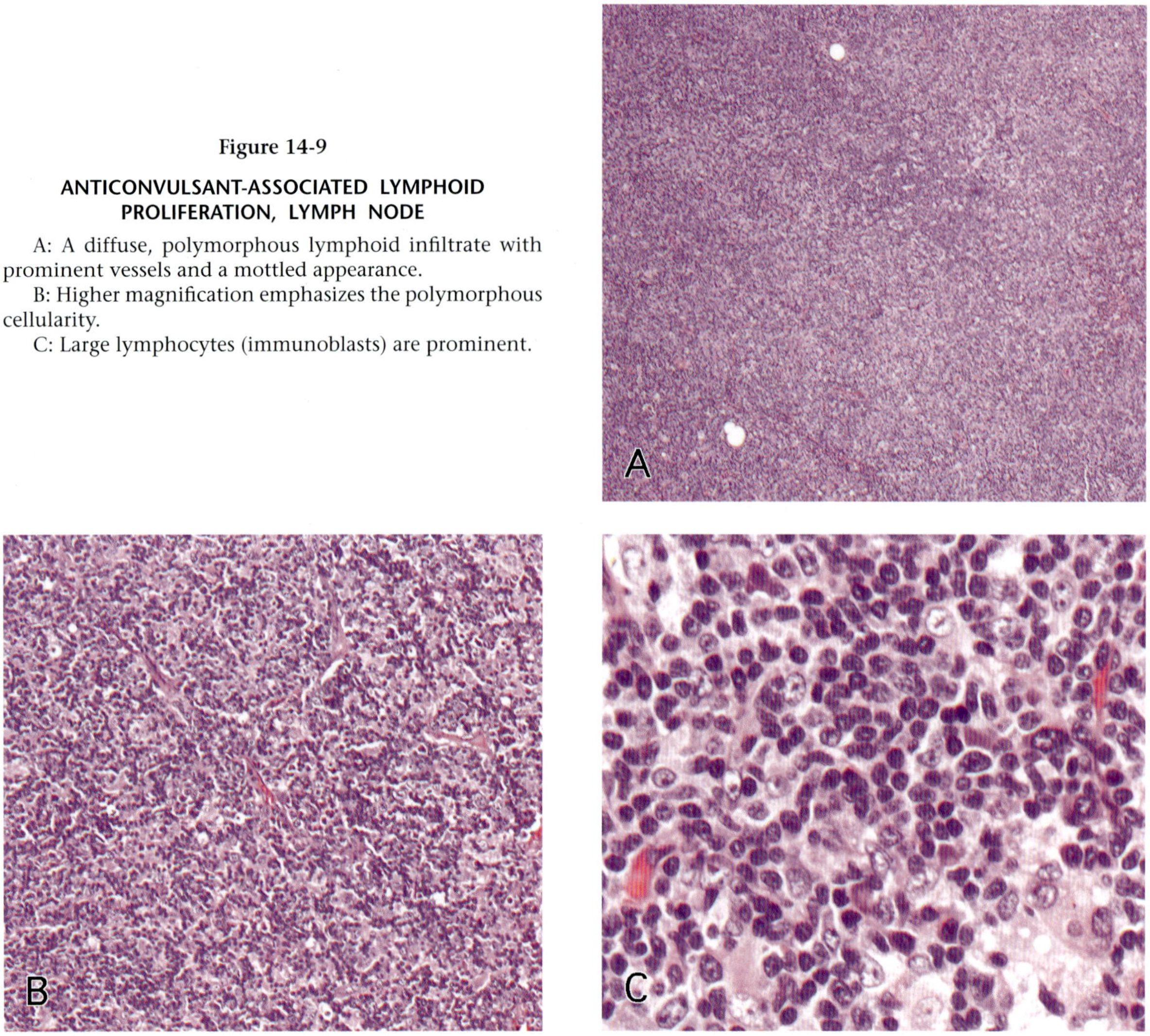

Figure 14-9

ANTICONVULSANT-ASSOCIATED LYMPHOID PROLIFERATION, LYMPH NODE

A: A diffuse, polymorphous lymphoid infiltrate with prominent vessels and a mottled appearance.

B: Higher magnification emphasizes the polymorphous cellularity.

C: Large lymphocytes (immunoblasts) are prominent.

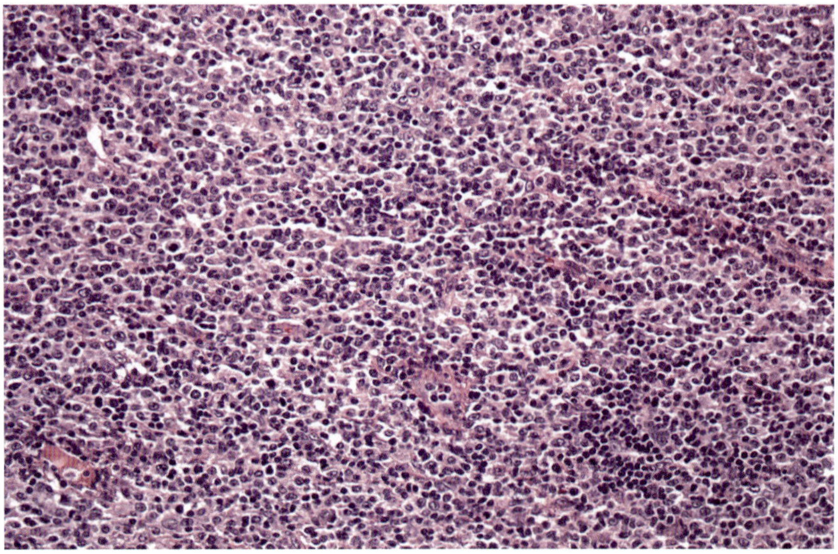

Figure 14-10

TEGRETOL (ANTICONVULSANT)-ASSOCIATED LYMPHOID PROLIFERATION, LYMPH NODE

A polymorphous interfollicular proliferation accompanies lymphadenopathy associated with the use of an anticonvulsant.

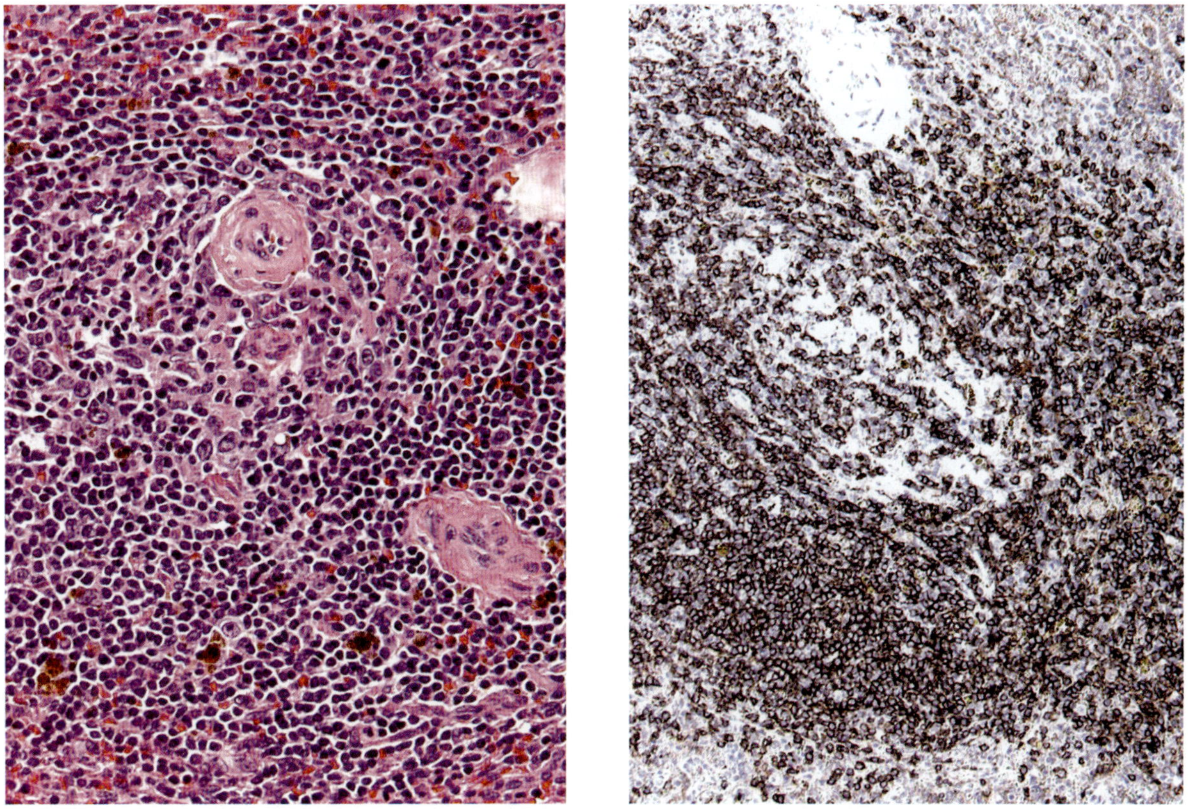

Figure 14-11

PHENYTOIN-ASSOCIATED LYMPHOID PROLIFERATION, SPLEEN

Left: Hyperplasia of T cells in spleen in response to phenytoin therapy.
Right: CD4 reactivity in the same case.

Differential Diagnosis. The differential diagnosis depends on the morphologic findings. When increased immunoblasts are seen, the main diagnoses are viral infections, inflammatory pseudotumor, diffuse large B-cell lymphoma with mixed small cells, or T-cell lymphoma. Careful histologic examination, correlation with medication history, and, in selected cases, the use of polymerase chain reaction (PCR) for T- or B-cell gene rearrangements help to distinguish difficult cases from lymphoma.

Treatment and Prognosis. The importance of obtaining a good clinical history, including the type and duration of any medications, and pertinent laboratory data cannot be overemphasized. Anticonvulsant-associated lymphadenopathy may develop shortly after starting the drug or over a longer period of time. Anticonvulsant-related lymphadenopathy usually occurs as localized disease and regresses after excisional lymph node biopsy and cessation of the drug. Close clinical follow-up of the patient, however, with alternate drug therapy to treat the seizure disorder, may also be recommended. The most recent studies did not find any association between phenytoin therapy and the subsequent development of malignant lymphoma, in contrast to previous reports in the literature (6,9).

GRANULOCYTE-COLONY STIMULATING FACTOR AND OTHER CYTOKINES

Definition. The use of colony stimulating factors, including *granulocyte-colony stimulating factor* (G-CSF), for a variety of disorders, is now common. G-CSF is used to increase the number of circulating white blood cells. G-CSF therapy may be associated with splenic pathology, and less commonly, lymph node pathology. Other cytokine therapies based on increasing or modifying a number of cell types or immune responses are commonly used.

General Features. G-CSF is a hematopoietic cytokine, with multiple effects on normal hematopoiesis. Most of these effects are primarily on neutrophils and include regulation of production, release, proliferation, and state of activation of progenitor cells (4). Recombinant G-CSF is used in a variety of clinical settings including chemotherapy-induced myelosuppression, recovery from bone marrow aplasia due to bone marrow transplantation, mobilization of stem cells, and other causes of neutropenia.

Clinical Features. Splenic rupture is a rare, but well-documented consequence of G-CSF administration (7,8,18,21,30,42). In a study by Platzbecker et al. (46), splenic length and diameter were calculated in normal, healthy donors after 5 days of G-CSF administration. Splenic volume increased by 30 percent. The authors suggest that this volume change increases capsular tension, and predisposes the spleen to rupture. Other studies have confirmed these results (45,56).

The clinical features associated with G-CSF administration are typically short-term and dose related. These include bone pain, fatigue, headache, and nausea (4,45,56).

Laboratory Findings. The most striking changes associated with G-CSF therapy are seen in the peripheral blood. Peripheral white blood cell counts are often elevated, although this depends on the baseline white blood cell count. Other peripheral blood changes are left shift with occasional blasts and toxic granulation or vacuoles in granulocytes. Mild changes may be seen in coagulation tests, including increased levels of factor VIII and thrombin (4,46). Increased levels of liver enzymes (alanine aminotransferase [ALT], aspartate aminotransferase [AST], lactate dehydrogenase [LDH]) may also be seen.

Gross Findings. Although not extensively described, the gross pathologic features associated with G-CSF therapy reflect the general pathologic process. Variable degrees of enlargement of spleen are expected, depending on the dose, duration, and disorder for which the therapy is being used. As in other disorders with predominant red pulp involvement, the spleen has a beefy red appearance (36). Splenic infarction, hemorrhage, and rupture are associated with G-CSF therapy. These changes are nonspecific and are seen with other disorders of the spleen.

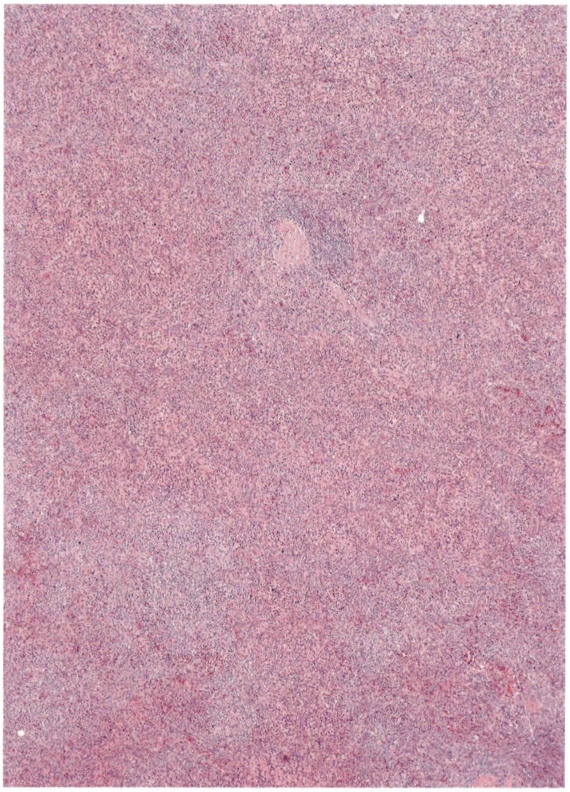

Figure 14-12

GRANULOCYTE-COLONY STIMULATING FACTOR (G-CSF) EFFECTS, SPLEEN

The spleen was removed after sudden enlargement in a patient taking G-CSF. The red pulp is distended by masses of granulocytes and precursors.

Microscopic Findings. The microscopic appearance of the spleen varies somewhat, depending on the underlying condition of the patient. If splenectomy is performed because of sudden onset of symptoms, hemorrhage, or rupture, it is likely that the microscopic findings are more pronounced than a spleen removed incidentally. In the most extreme cases, the red pulp is expanded by a large population of granulocytic elements. These myeloid elements may be predominantly mature, a mixture of mature and immature elements, predominantly immature. In extreme cases, the proliferation of granulocytic precursors is so monotonous as to simulate involvement by acute leukemia (figs. 14-12, 14-13) (42). Variable amounts of monocytic, erythroid, and megakaryocytic elements

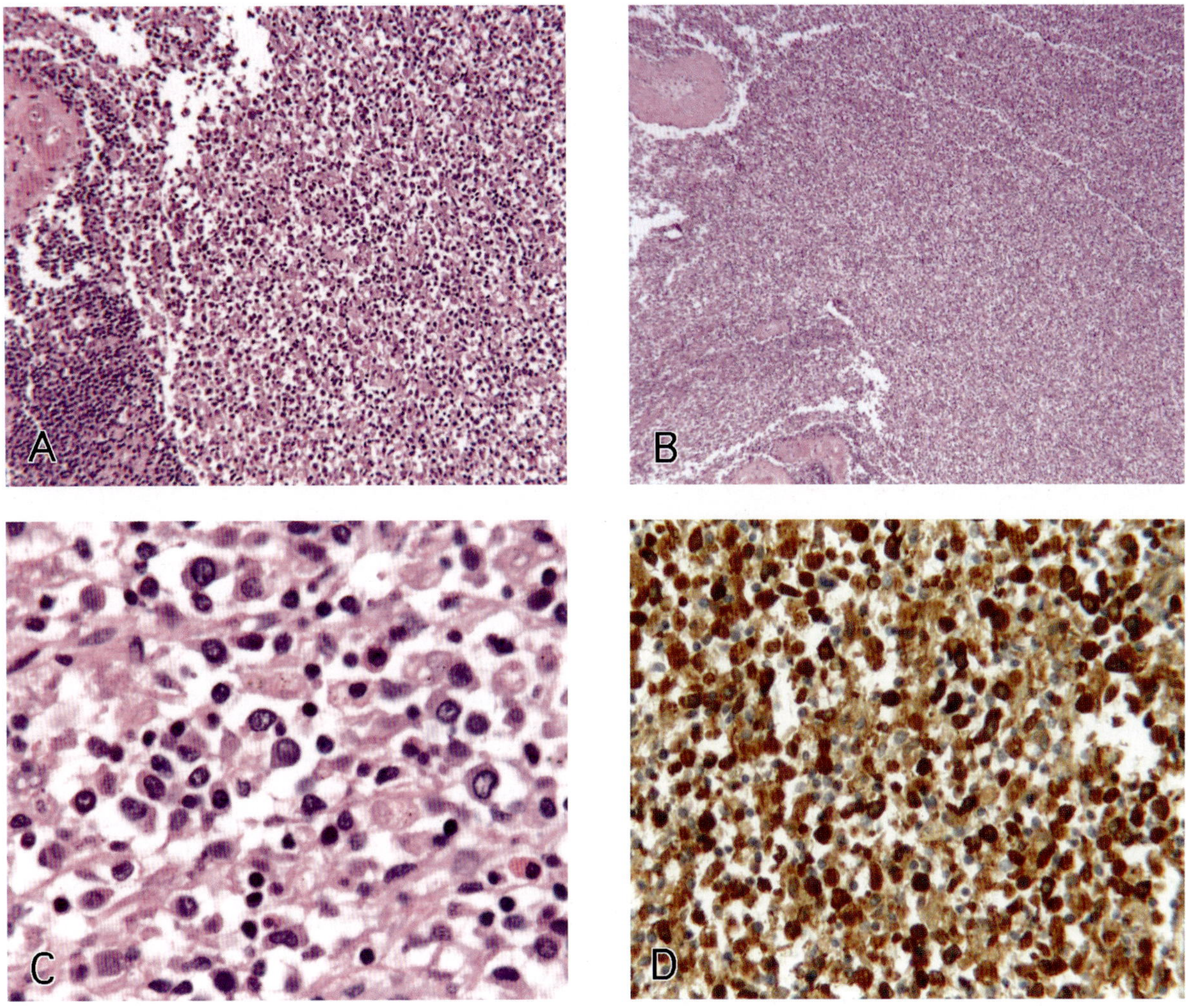

Figure 14-13

GRANULOCYTE-COLONY STIMULATING FACTOR EFFECTS, SPLEEN

Rupture of the spleen necessitated an emergency splenectomy. Numerous granulocytes and precursors (A-C) are seen. Immunohistochemical staining with myeloperoxidase reveals diffuse positivity (D).

may also be seen proliferating in the red pulp (36); however, these components typically make up only a minor component of the red pulp infiltrate. Other changes include hemorrhage, focal necrosis, hemosiderin deposition, and clusters of macrophages. The white pulp is often present, but is usually compressed by the expanding red pulp elements. Although the white pulp is usually unaffected, occasionally, proliferation of myeloid elements can be seen within the structure of the PALS.

Rarely, G-CSF treatment is associated with lymphadenopathy (47). Extramedullary proliferations of myeloid elements are seen. Although granulocytic proliferation predominates, other elements, including erythroid precursors and megakaryocytes, are present, similar to the appearance of the splenic red pulp.

Ancillary Studies. Immunohistochemical stains are an important adjunct in the evaluation of myeloid proliferations in the spleen. If acute leukemia is being considered in the differential diagnosis, stains that highlight immature hematopoietic elements are useful. It is unlikely that large numbers of blasts are present in a G-CSF–stimulated proliferation. The presence of large numbers of cells positive for CD34, CD117, or terminal deoxynucleotidyltransferase

Table 14-1

COMPARISON OF SPLENIC CHANGES ASSOCIATED WITH GRANULOCYTE-COLONY STIMULATING FACTOR (G-CSF) AND ACUTE MYELOID LEUKEMIA (AML) INVOLVING THE SPLEEN

Feature	G-CSF Proliferation	AML
Cytology	Variable; may be monotonous	Monotonous
Myeloid elements	Often mixture of mature and immature; rarely, only immature elements	Immature
Other bone marrow elements (erythroid, megakaryocytic)	Only rare nonmyeloid elements present	May be present in leukemias derived from MPD[a]; typically absent in de novo AML
Distribution	Red pulp	Red pulp
CD34 staining	Only rare blasts stain	Variably positive in numerous blasts
CD117 staining	Only rare blasts seen; rare mast cells	If positive, is seen in numerous cells
Lysozyme, myeloperoxidase staining	Most cells positive	Frequently positive

[a]MPD = myeloproliferative disorder.

(TdT) suggests a diagnosis of acute leukemia, rather than a G-CSF stimulated proliferation. Stains to identify granulocytes, such as myeloperoxidase or lysozyme, help delineate the extent of the myeloid proliferation.

Differential Diagnosis. Because of the proliferation of myeloid elements, these lesions often have an unexpected, monotonous appearance, and as mentioned above, simulate malignancy. Since the morphologic changes most commonly simulate myeloid leukemias, it is important to determine the underlying condition that is being treated with G-CSF (Table 14-1). If there is an underlying hematologic disorder or previous chemotherapy that could induce a hematologic disorder, then the possibility of acute leukemia presenting in the spleen must be considered. Correlation with bone marrow and peripheral blood findings is critical in determining the underlying disorder.

Treatment and Prognosis. Except in cases of splenic hemorrhage or rupture, no specific therapy is required for splenic enlargement due to G-CSF therapy. When G-CSF therapy is withdrawn, the spleen gradually returns to normal size within about 10 days, but increased size may persist up to several months in some patients (46,57). It is during this time that the risk of splenic rupture is highest.

IONIZING RADIATION EFFECTS

Definition. *Ionizing radiation effects* are changes seen in lymph nodes or spleen due to the effects of intentional or unintentional ionizing radiation.

General Features. Lymphocytes are among the most radioresponsive cells in humans, and the effects of radiation are more prominent on proliferating cells; nonproliferating cells are more radioresistant (19). The effects of radiation on lymph nodes or spleen depend on the radiation dose and the amount of time since exposure. Most of the effects are chronic changes associated with treatment-related exposure. The radiation dose is measured in gray units (Gy), which is a measure of absorbed energy per unit mass at a specific point.

Clinical Features. Most changes associated with irradiation are due to radiation given as medical treatment, although less common, similar effects are the result of accidental or intentional exposure to radiation. Acute total body exposure to radiation, as in the case of intentional exposure, has profound effects on the body. The most manifest signs of illness are seen in the gastrointestinal system, the hematopoietic system, the central nervous system, and the skin (14).

Lymphocytes are profoundly affected by ionizing radiation. The changes in the lymphocytes can be used as biomarkers for the degree of radiation exposure. These include chromosomal damage such as breakage and the formation of dicentric and ring chromosomes.

Gross Findings. The lymph nodes are typically smaller than normal in size (less than 1 cm) and firm due to extensive fibrosis (26).

Microscopic Findings. Irradiation initially affects the lymphocytes, sparing the

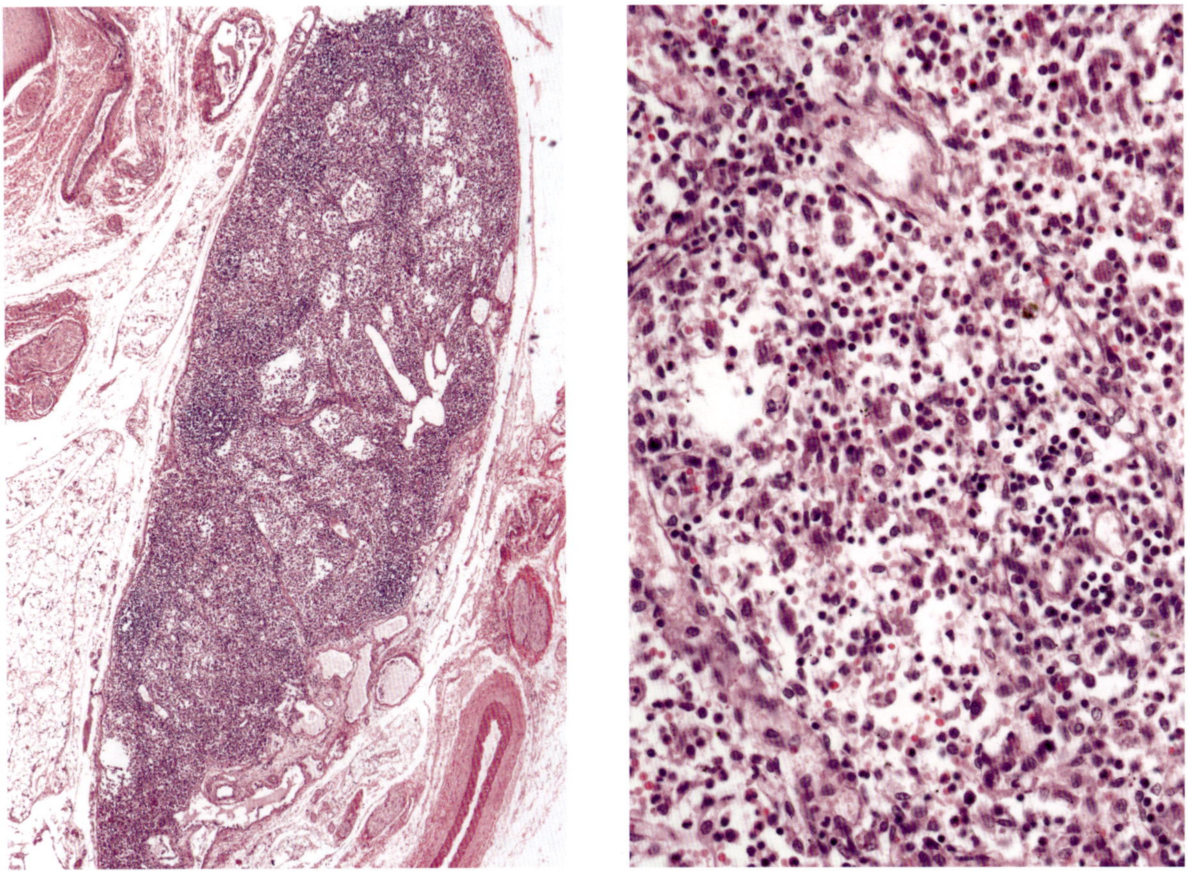

Figure 14-14

IONIZING RADIATION EFFECTS, LYMPH NODE

Left: Radiation injury in a lymph node of a 7-year-old boy, after 9 Gy of exposure for acute lymphoblastic leukemia (ALL) therapy. The sinus architecture is intact, and there is overall lymphocyte depletion.

Right: Higher magnification shows an increase in macrophages and patent sinuses.

reticuloendothelial tissues. Early effects include marked necrosis of lymphocytes, with the loss of lymphocytes in the germinal centers; prominent vasculature; and sinuses and frequent red blood cell congestion (figs. 14-14, 14-15) (10,19,26). In later stages or at higher doses, irradiated lymph nodes become atrophic and often develop fibrosis (59). Although radiation dosage effects may not be accurately predicted by the histologic changes in humans, animal studies have shown that doses of over 20 Gy result in significantly more severe changes, including hyalinization and fibrosis. In humans, increasing doses are associated with an increase in the extent of atrophy and fibrosis (10).

The spleen is generally reduced in size after radiation, and the capsule is thickened (figs. 14-16, 14-17) (20). The red pulp is variably fibrotic. The sinuses may be obliterated by fibrosis. Marked vascular proliferation may be seen. The sites of previous tumor may be seen as fibrous or collagenous nodules.

Ancillary Studies. Immunohistochemical analysis of irradiated lymph nodes shows severe depletion of B cells. The remaining lymphocytes are typically small T cells or plasma cells. Dendritic cells and other stromal elements are highlighted by appropriate stains (e.g., CD21, CD31, CD68) and are relatively more radioresistant than lymphocytes (19).

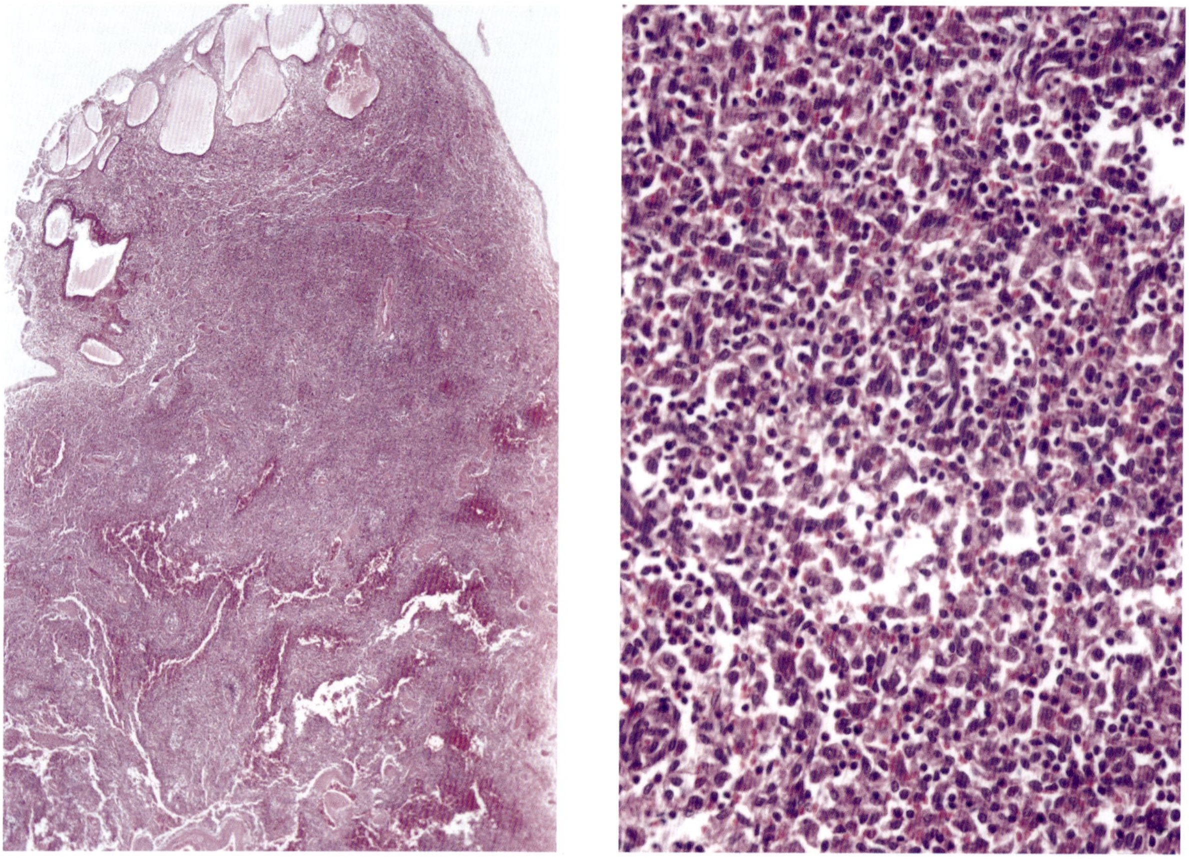

Figure 14-15

IONIZING RADIATION EFFECTS, LYMPH NODE

Left: Radiation injury in lymph node after accidental industrial exposure to plutonium in a 38-year-old male. Overall exposure estimated to be 4.9 Gy. Widely patent sinuses, loss of normal architecture, and hemorrhage, as well as the beginnings of fibrosis are noted.

Right: Higher magnification shows mostly small lymphocytes with a prominence of dendritic cells and macrophages.

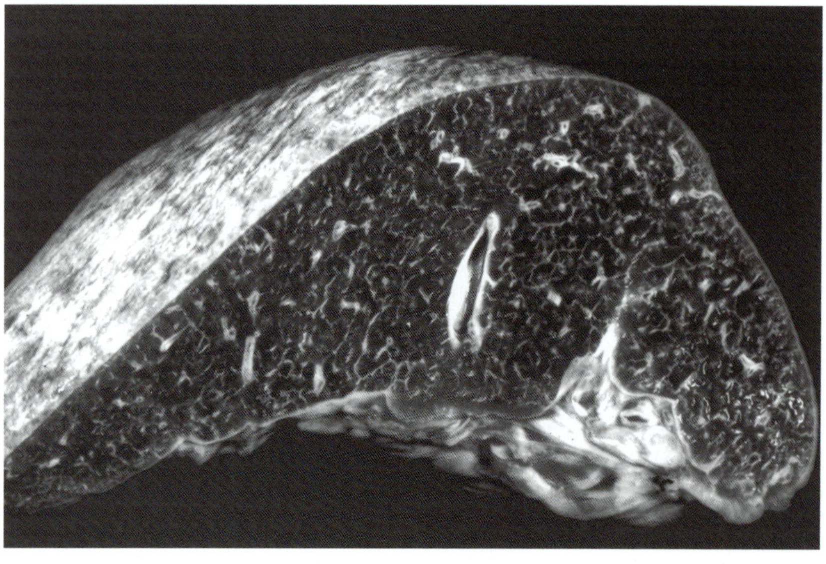

Figure 14-16

IONIZING RADIATION EFFECTS, SPLEEN

A 58-g spleen from a patient who received 4,485 rad 8 years previously. The fibrous trabeculae are prominent. (Fig. 11-8 from Fajardo LG. Pathology of radiation injury. New York: Masson Pub.; 1982:154.)

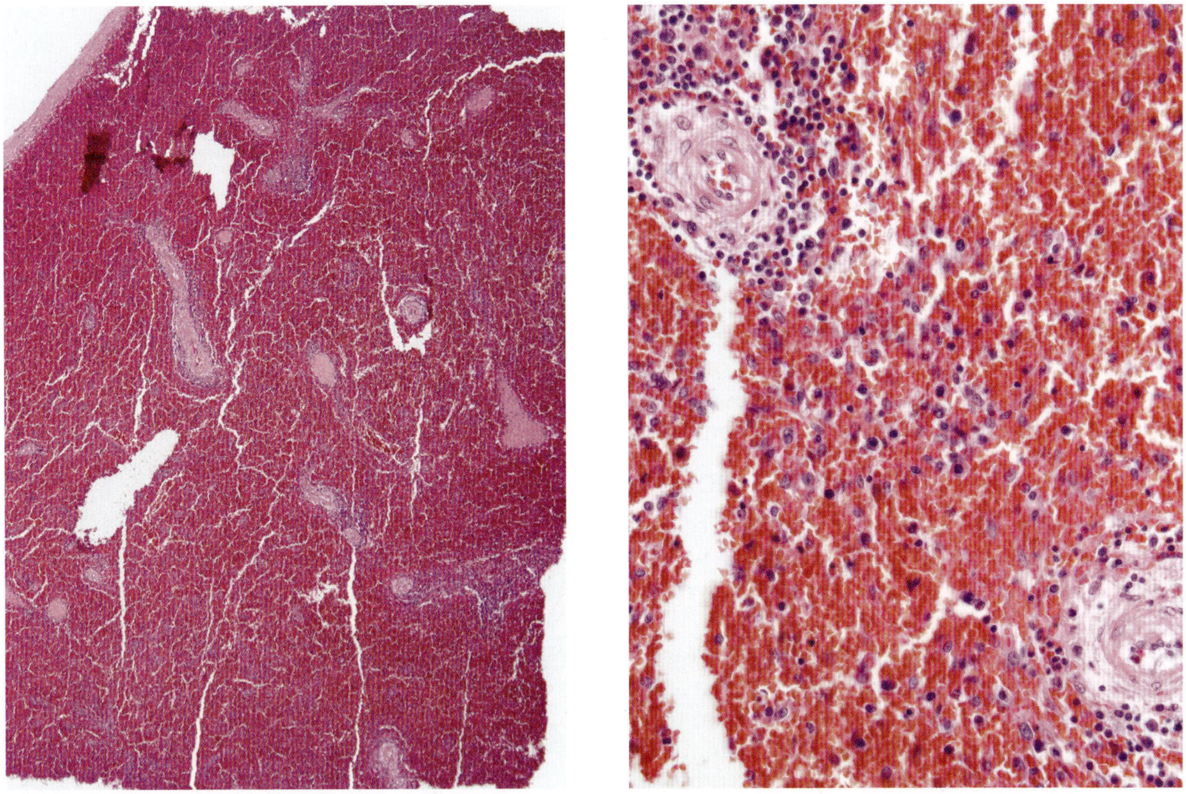

Figure 14-17

IONIZING RADIATION EFFECTS, SPLEEN

Left: Radiation injury in a spleen in a 32-year-old male with accidental industrial exposure to radiation of 20 Gy. Sample is from 9 days after exposure. Note the marked congestion of the red pulp, depletion of lymphoid cells, and beginnings of vascular and perivascular fibrosis.

Right: Higher magnification shows depleted lymphocytes in red pulp and early perivascular concentric fibrosis.

SULFASALAZINE

Definition. Lymph node changes are associated with the drug *sulfasalazine*.

General Features. Sulfasalazine has antiinflammatory, antibacterial, and immunosuppressive properties. When metabolized, it is cleaved into two main components: 5-aminosalicylic acid and sulfapyridine. Sulfasalazine is most commonly used to treat inflammatory bowel disease.

Clinical Features. Sulfasalazine administration is associated with rare severe clinical manifestations, termed the "3-week sulfasalazine syndrome." After approximately 2 to 3 weeks on the drug, patients present with severe systemic signs and symptoms: fever, rash, arthralgias, polyarteritis, nephrotoxicity, lymphadenopathy, eosinophilia, and lymphocytosis or agranulocytosis (35).

Fulminant hepatic necrosis is probably the most severe of the adverse outcomes, and is potentially fatal. Necrotizing pancreatitis can also be seen. These features indicate that the drug reaction is idiosyncratic.

Microscopic Findings. Affected lymph nodes are typically enlarged. Architectural disruption or effacement, necrosis, increased immunoblasts, and vascular proliferation are often seen. Small lymphocytes and plasma cells are increased in number. The term "angioimmunoblastic lymphadenopathy" has been used in this condition, but should be avoided so as not to be confused with angioimmunoblastic T-cell lymphoma (44). Increased numbers of eosinophils and erythrophagocytosis may also be identified. The features of lymphoma or specific infections are not identified.

Ancillary Studies. Because this benign condition could potentially mimic both T- and B-cell lymphomas, ancillary studies are helpful in evaluating the process. Flow cytometric analysis of an affected lymph node does not yield an aberrant immunophenotype. Gene rearrangement studies for both T-cell receptors and immunoglobulin heavy chain receptors are negative.

Treatment and Prognosis. The management of the clinical symptoms is most important in the resolution of the adverse effects of sulfasalazine administration. Symptoms usually abate on cessation of the drug. The adenopathy resolves without specific treatment, in contrast to lymphoma.

CLOFAZIMINE CRYSTAL DEPOSITION

Definition. Deposition of crystals of the drug *clofazimine* in the histiocytes of lymph nodes leads to a distinctive-appearing lymphadenopathy.

General Features. Clofazimine is an antileprotic drug that is routinely prescribed in areas endemic for leprosy (25). It has also been used in the treatment of discoid lupus erythematosus (37). Clofazimine has a high tissue distribution throughout the body and crystalline forms of the drug may be deposited in various anatomic sites, especially the reticuloendothelial organs (58). Clofazimine crystal deposits in the lymph nodes and spleen of treated rats and mice have been reported (39,61).

Microscopic Findings. The lymph nodes of patients treated with this medication show characteristic histologic features such as histiocytic hyperplasia and reddish orange crystal deposits in macrophages (58). The crystals may be visualized by light microscopy on hematoxylin and eosin (H&E)-stained slides (figs. 14-18, 14-19).

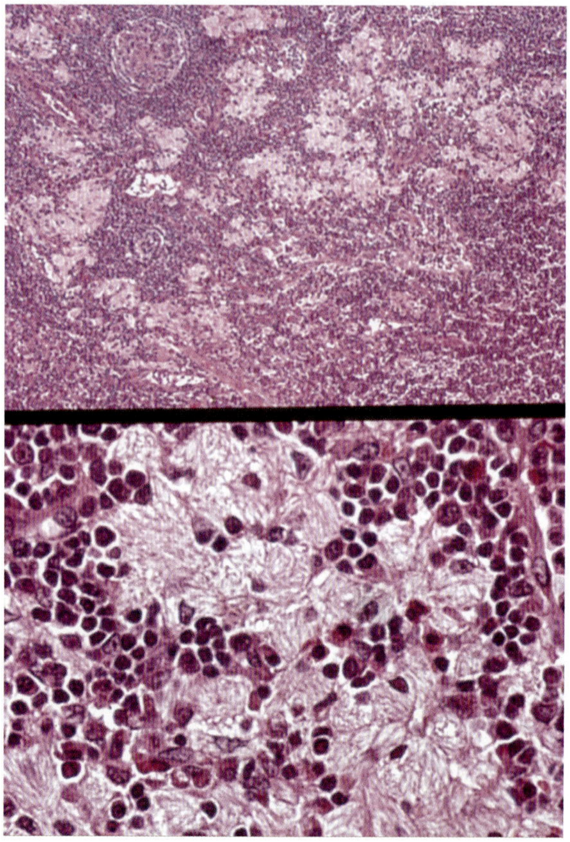

Figure 14-18

CLOFAZIMINE, LYMPH NODE

Clofazimine-associated lymphadenopathy with macrophage hyperplasia (top) and fibrillary crystalline structures within macrophages (bottom).

BONE MARROW TRANSPLANTATION AND GRAFT-VERSUS-HOST DISEASE

Definition. Allogeneic bone marrow transplantation requires significant pretransplant conditioning. This includes significant depletion of the lymphoid organs (spleen, lymph nodes) in preparation for the immune challenges of transplantation of an allogeneic graft. *Graft-versus-host disease (GVHD) lymphadenopathy* consists of morphologic changes in the lymph node (and possibly spleen) due to a transplantation-induced reaction to donor leukocytes.

General Features. Pretransplant conditioning regimens typically include irradiation or combination chemotherapy. The rationale for conditioning is to eliminate the underlying disease and to suppress the patient's natural immunity. In GVHD, donor lymphocytes initiate a cascade of proliferation in host cells. The donor T cells also proliferate, leading to transient clonal expansion of both populations.

Clinical Features. Bone marrow transplantation has become standard therapy for a wide variety of neoplastic and non-neoplastic hematologic disorders. In addition, it is an adjunctive therapy in the treatment of nonhematologic disorders. Although a wide variety of symptoms and secondary changes are seen, few reports have commented on changes in lymph node and splenic histology (16,17,26,41).

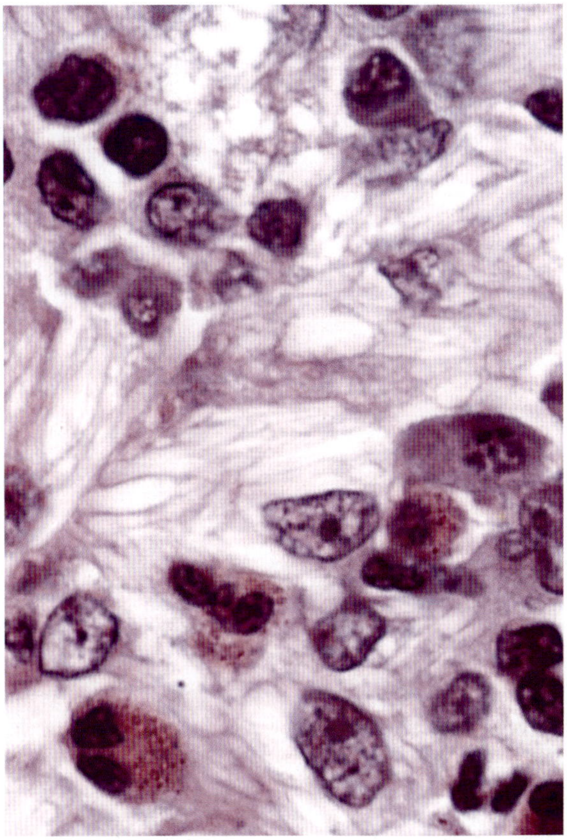

Figure 14-19

CLOFAZIMINE, LYMPH NODE

High magnification of pale crystalline material within macrophages.

The mixed lymphocyte reaction is an early immunologic response by host tissues to passenger donor leukocytes. The clinical manifestations of this reaction include lymphadenopathy, splenomegaly, and intestinal lymphoid hyperplasia without destruction of host tissues (41). Unlike typical GVHD, this reaction is not associated with tissue destruction. This process is also distinct from post-transplant lymphoproliferative disorder, and notably is not due to EBV infection.

GVHD is commonly recognized in skin, gastrointestinal tract, liver, and bone marrow. It is only rarely evaluated in lymph nodes or spleen. Manifestations in other organs may be more prominent, and other tissue biopsies may be more informative regarding the presence and degree of GVHD.

Microscopic Findings. After transplant conditioning, there is marked depletion of lymphocytes and loss of normal architectural features in the lymph nodes (17). Follicles are not seen. The remaining structures are composed of predominantly stromal elements, with collections of lymphocytes, macrophages, and plasma cells. Blood vessels are prominent. Erythrophagocytosis and foamy macrophages are present in some cases. When collections of lymphocytes are seen, they appear to be primary follicles. After transplantation, there is marked depletion of the white pulp of the spleen (16). The number of lymphocytes in the PALS is reduced, and follicles or germinal centers are not seen. The red pulp varies in appearance, but may show congestion, hemosiderin deposition, and focal extramedullary hematopoiesis.

The mixed lymphocyte reaction associated with GVHD shows lymph nodal architecture that is partially or completely effaced. The cellularity is composed of a mixture of B immunoblasts, small lymphocytes, macrophages, and plasma cells. Follicles are inapparent, but residual follicular dendritic cell networks are present. The interdigitating dendritic cells may be hyperplastic. Necrosis is not seen.

Differential Diagnosis. In cases of transplant-related depleted lymph nodes or GVHD, the possibility of recurrence of the original (hematologic) disease or the presence of a post-transplant lymphoproliferative disorder must be considered. In addition, infections associated with immunosuppression, especially those caused by EBV (see chapter 9), need to be considered.

Treatment and Prognosis. The depletion seen after transplant conditioning eventually resolves. However, the composition of the lymph nodes may not return to normal for months or even years. The mixed lymphocyte GVHD reaction is also transient. In contrast to post-transplant lymphoproliferative disorders, this reaction resolves with decreases in immunosuppression.

GOLD THERAPY (CHRYSOTHERAPY)

Definition. Although considered in other chapters as well (chapter 15), the changes in the lymph nodes from gold exposure are virtually always due to the use of gold as a therapeutic substance, also known as *chrysotherapy*.

General Features. Injection of gold sodium thiomalate, or chrysotherapy, is used almost

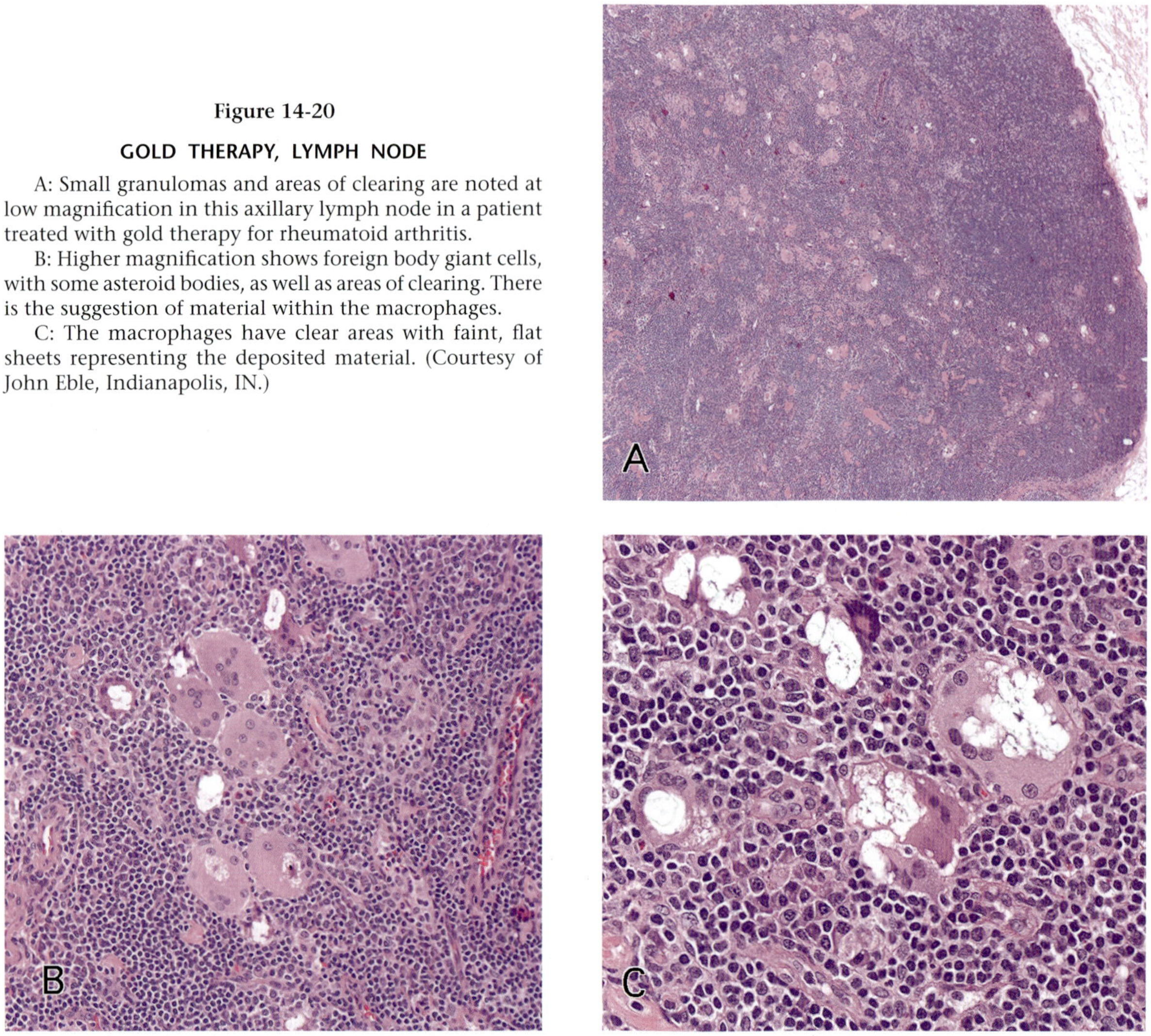

Figure 14-20

GOLD THERAPY, LYMPH NODE

A: Small granulomas and areas of clearing are noted at low magnification in this axillary lymph node in a patient treated with gold therapy for rheumatoid arthritis.

B: Higher magnification shows foreign body giant cells, with some asteroid bodies, as well as areas of clearing. There is the suggestion of material within the macrophages.

C: The macrophages have clear areas with faint, flat sheets representing the deposited material. (Courtesy of John Eble, Indianapolis, IN.)

exclusively in the treatment of rheumatoid arthritis. Gold salts can also be taken orally (49).

Clinical Features. Rheumatoid arthritis is associated with lymphadenopathy in approximately 50 to 75 percent of patients. The histologic features, as discussed in chapter 12, most often include follicular hyperplasia and interfollicular polyclonal plasmacytosis. The toxicity associated with chrysotherapy includes hepatic damage, bone marrow suppression, and rash. Lymphadenopathy is rare and difficult to distinguish from the background lymphadenopathy of the rheumatoid arthritis.

Microscopic Findings. Follicular hyperplasia and sinus histiocytosis are the main histologic findings in lymph nodes draining gold injection sites (2,48,49,51,55). Foreign body giant cells may be seen. Crystalline structures (round, oval, or plate-like) are seen in various compartments of the lymph node, usually within the cytoplasm of macrophages or giant cells (fig. 14-20) (49). These may take the form of asteroid bodies, similar to those seen in sarcoidosis. These crystals of gold salts do not polarize. Isolated gold particles may be found in the cords and sinuses of the lymph nodes (51). In other cases, partial or complete lymph node infarction is seen. Splenomegaly may be a result of gold therapy.

Ancillary Studies. Although not generally available, energy-dispersive X-ray microanalysis confirms the presence of elemental gold (49). The lack of polarization of the crystalline material distinguishes gold crystals from other materials.

REFERENCES

1. Abbondanzo SL, Irey NS, Frizzera G. Dilantin-associated lymphadenopathy: spectrum of histologic patterns. Am J Surg Pathol 1995;9:675-86.
2. Abraham JL. Silicone in gold-associated lymphadenopathy (Letter). Arch Pathol Lab Med 1991;115:862.
3. Allen S, Chiu R, Orazi A, O'Malley DP. Refractory ITP: therapy-related histopathologic changes in spleens. Mod Pathol 2006;19:288A.
4. Anderlini P, Przepiorka D, Champlin R, Korbling M. Biologic and clinical effects of granulocyte colony-stimulating factor in normal individuals. Blood 1996;88:2819-25.
5. Andres E, Zimmer J, Noel E, Kaltenbach G, Koumarianou A, Maloisel F. Idiopathic thrombocytopenic purpura: a retrospective analysis in 139 patients of the influence of age on the response to corticosteroids, splenectomy and danazol. Drugs Aging 2003;20:841-6.
6. Anthony JJ. Malignant lymphoma associated with hydantoin drugs. Arch Neurol 1970;22:450-4.
7. Balaguer H, Galmes A, Ventayol G, Bargay J, Besalduch J. Splenic rupture after granulocyte-colony-stimulating factor mobilization in a peripheral blood progenitor cell donor. Transfusion 2004;44:1260-1.
8. Becker PS, Wagle M, Matous S, et al. Spontaneous splenic rupture following administration of granulocyte colony-stimulating factor (G-CSF): occurrence in an allogeneic donor of peripheral blood stem cells. Biol Blood Marrow Transplant 1997;3:45-9.
9. Bichel J. Hydantoin derivatives and malignancies of the haemopoietic system. Acta Med Scand 1975;198:327-8.
10. Burge JS. Histological changes in cervical lymph nodes following clinical irradiation. Proc R Soc Med 1975;68:77-9.
11. Bussel JB. Fc receptor blockade and immune thrombocytopenic purpura. Semin Hematol 2000;37:261-6.
12. Cacatian AA, Rando J. Diphenylhydantoin-induced pseudolymphoma syndrome with severe thrombocytopenia. NY State J Med 1981;81:1085-7.
13. Charlesworth EN. Phenytoin-induced pseudolymphoma syndrome: an immunologic syndrome. Arch Dermatol 1977;113:477-80.
14. Dainiak N. Hematologic consequences of exposure to ionizing radiation. Exp Hematol 2002;30:513-28.
15. Davis TA, Czerwinski DK, Levy R. Therapy of B-cell lymphoma with anti-CD20 antibodies can result in the loss of CD20 antigen expression. Clin Cancer Res 1999;5:611-5.
16. Dilly SA, Sloane JP. Cellular composition of the spleen after human allogeneic bone marrow transplantation. J Pathol 1988;155:151-60.
17. Dilly SA, Sloane JP, Psalti IS. The cellular composition of human lymph nodes after allogenic bone marrow transplantation: an immunohistological study. J Pathol 1986;150:213-21.
18. Dincer AP, Gottschall J, Margolis DA. Splenic rupture in a parental donor undergoing peripheral blood progenitor cell mobilization. J Pediatr Hematol Oncol 2004;26:761-3.
19. Fajardo LF. Effects of ionizing radiation on lymph nodes. A review. In: The Lymphatic system and cancer. front radiat ther oncol 1994;28:37-45.
20. Fajardo LF. Pathology of radiation injury. New York: Masson Pub.; 1982:147-65.
21. Falzetti F, Aversa F, Minelli O, Tabilio A. Spontaneous rupture of spleen during peripheral blood stem-cell mobilisation in a healthy donor. Lancet 1999;353:555.
22. Foran JM, Norton AJ, Micallef IN, et al. Loss of CD20 expression following treatment with rituximab (chimaeric monoclonal anti-CD20): a retrospective cohort analysis. Br J Haematol 2001;114:881-3.
23. Gernsheimer T. Pathophysiology and thrombokinetics in autoimmune thrombocytopenia. Blood Rev 2002;16:7-8
24. Haidar JH, Shamseddine A, Salem Z, et al. Loss of CD20 expression in relapsed lymphomas after rituximab therapy. Eur J Haematol 2003;70:330-2.
25. Holdiness MR. Clinical pharmacokinetics of clofazimine: a review. Clin Pharmacokinet 1989;16:74-85.
26. Horny HP, Horst HA, Ehninger G, Kaiserling E. Lymph node morphology after allogeneic bone marrow transplantation for chronic myeloid leukemia: a histological and immunohistological study focusing on the phenotype of the recovering lymphoid cells. Blut 1988;57:31-40.
27. Ioachim HL, Ratech H. Ioachim's lymph node pathology, 3rd edition. Philadelphia: Lippincott Williams & Wilkins; 2002.
28. Kamel OW, Weiss LM, van de Rijn M, Colby TV, Kingma DW, Jaffe ES. Hodgkin's disease and lymphoproliferations resembling Hodgkin's disease in patients receiving long-term low-dose methotrexate therapy. Am J Surg Pathol 1996;20:1279-87.
29. Kamel OW. Iatrogenic lymphoproliferative disorders in nontransplantation settings. Semin Diagn Pathol 1997;14:27-34.
30. Kasper C, Jones L, Fujita Y, Morgenstern GR, Scarffe JH, Chang J. Splenic rupture in a patient with acute myeloid leukemia undergoing peripheral blood stem cell transplantation. Ann Hematol 1999;78:91-2.
31. Katzin WE, Julius CJ, Tubbs RR, McHenry MC. Lymphoproliferative disorders associated with carbamazepine. Arch Pathol Lab Med 1990;114:1244-8.

32. Kennedy GA, Tey S, Cobcroft R, et al. Incidence and nature of CD20-negative relapses following rituximab therapy in aggressive B-cell non-Hodgkin's lymphoma: a retrospective review. Br J Haematol 2002;119:412-6.
33. Kneitz C, Wilhelm M, Tony HP. Effective B cell depletion with rituximab in the treatment of autoimmune diseases. Immunobiology 2002;206:519-27.
34. Kremer IM, Phelps CT. Long-term prospective study of the use of methotrexate in the treatment of rheumatoid arthritis: update after a mean of 90 months. Arthritis Rheum 1992;35:138-45.
35. Lau G, Kwan C, Chong SM. The 3-week sulphasalazine syndrome strikes again. Forensic Sci Int 2001;122:79-84.
36. Litam PP, Friedman HD, Loughran TP Jr. Splenic extramedullary hematopoiesis in a patient receiving intermittently administered granulocyte colony-stimulating factor. Ann Intern Med 1993;118:954-5.
37. Mackey JP, Barnes J. Clofazimine in the treatment of discoid lupus erythematosus. Br J Dermatol 1974;91:93-6.
38. Maloney DG, Grillo-Lopez AJ, White CA, et al. IDEC-C2B8 (Rituximab) anti-CD20 monoclonal antibody therapy in patients with relapsed low-grade non-Hodgkin's lymphoma. Blood 1997;90:2188-95.
39. Mamidi NV, Rajasekhar A, Prabhakar MC, Krishna DR. Tissue distribution and deposition of clofazimine in rat following subchronic treatment with or without rifampicin. Arzneimittelforschung 1995;45:1029-31.
40. Merritt HH, Putnam TJ. Sodium diphenyl hydantoinate in the treatment of seizure disorders. JAMA 1938;111:1068-73.
41. Nodit L, Murase N, Reyes JD, Mazariegos GV, Sindhi R, Jaffe R. Transient posttransplant graft-versus-host lymphadenopathy. Pediatr Dev Pathol 2004;7:533-7.
42. O'Malley DP, Whalen M, Banks PM. Spontaneous splenic rupture with fatal outcome following G-CSF administration for myelodysplastic syndrome. Am J Hematol 2003;73:294-5.
43. Ojinnaka NC, Iloeje SO. Ethosuximide induced lymphadenopathy—a case report. Cent Afr J Med 2001;47:18-9.
44. Pay S, Dinc A, Simsek I, Can C, Erdem H. Sulfasalazine-induced angioimmunoblastic lymphadenopathy developing in a patient with juvenile chronic arthritis. Rheumatol Int 2000;20:25-7.
45. Picardi M, De Rosa G, Selleri C, et al. Spleen enlargement following recombinant human granulocyte colony-stimulating factor administration for peripheral blood stem cell mobilization. Haematologica 2003;88:794-800.
46. Platzbecker U, Prange-Krex G, Bornhauser M, et al. Spleen enlargement in healthy donors during G-CSF mobilization of PBPCs. Transfusion 2001;41:184-9.
47. Redmond J 3rd, Kantor RS, Auerbach HE, Spiritos MD, Moore JT. Extramedullary hematopoiesis during therapy with granulocyte colony-stimulating factor. Arch Pathol Lab Med 1994;118:1014-5.
48. Roberts C, Batstone PJ, Goodlad JR. Lymphadenopathy and lymph node infarction as a result of gold injections. J Clin Pathol 2001;54:562-4.
49. Rollins SD, Craig JP. Gold-associated lymphadenopathy in a patient with rheumatoid arthritis: histologic and scanning electron microscopic features. Arch Pathol Lab Med 1991;115:175-7.
50. Ross JS, Schenkein DP, Pietrusko R, et al. Targeted therapies for cancer 2004. Am J Clin Pathol 2004;122:598-609.
51. Rothschild B, Marshall H. Lymphadenopathy and lymph node infarction in the course of gold therapy. Am J Med 1986;80:537-40.
52. Saeki H, Etoh T, Toda K, Mihm MC Jr. Pseudolymphoma syndrome due to carbamazepine. J Dermatol 1999;26:329-31.
53. Saltzstein SL, Ackerman LV. Lymphadenopathy induced by anticonvulsant drugs and mimicking clinically and pathologically malignant lymphomas. Cancer 1959;12:164-82.
54. Schreiber MM, McGregor JG. Pseudolymphoma syndrome. A sensitivity to anticonvulsant drugs. Arch Dermatol 1968;97:297-300.
55. Spark RP. Gold-associated lymphadenopathy in a patient with rheumatoid arthritis. Arch Pathol Lab Med 1991;115:861-2.56. Stroncek D, Shawker T, Follmann D, Leitman SF. G-CSF-induced spleen size changes in peripheral blood progenitor cell donors. Transfusion 2003;43:609-13.
57. Stroncek DF, Dittmar K, Shawker T, Heatherman A, Leitman SF. Transient spleen enlargement in peripheral blood progenitor cell donors given G-CSF. J Transl Med 2004;2:25.
58. Sukpanichnant S, Hargrove NS, Kachintorn U, et al. Clofazamine-induced crystal storing histiocytosis producing chronic abdominal pain in a leprosy patient. Am J Surg Pathol 2000;24:129-35.
59. Symmers WStC. The lymphoreticular system. In: Symmers WStC, ed. Systemic pathology, 2nd ed. New York: Churchill Livingstone, Edinburgh; 1978;507-891.
60. Thomason WR, Craig FE, Banks PM, Sears DL, Myerson GE, Gulley ML. Epstein-Barr virus and lymphoproliferation in methotrexate-treated rheumatoid arthritis. Mod Pathol 1996:9:261-6.
61. Vandeputte D, Jacob W, Van Grieken R, Boddingius J. Study of intracellular deposition of the anti-leprosy drug clofazimine in mouse spleen using laser microprobe mass analysis. Biol Mass Spectrom 1993;22:221-5.
62. Weinblatt ME, Weissman BN, Holdsworth DE, et al. Long-term prospective study of methotrexate in the treatment of rheumatoid arthritis: 84 month update. Athritis Rheum 1992:35:129-37.
63. Weinstein A, Marlowe S, Korn J, Farouhar F. Low-dose methotrexate treatment of rheumatoid arthritis. Long-term observations. Am J Med 1985:79:331-7.

15 FOREIGN BODIES AND CHEMICALS

The lymph nodes may show the characteristic histopathologic changes associated with the presence of noninfectious endogenous and exogenous materials such as proteins, lipids, and foreign bodies. These deposits are found intracellularly or extracellularly. Some nonhematopoietic elements are incidental findings with little or no clinical significance except that they result in lymphadenopathy. Pathologically, however, it is important to recognize the nature of the changes associated with such elements, and to differentiate them from a metastatic process, infectious disease, or metabolic disorder. Ultrastructural analysis may be necessary to identify many of the exogenous particles discussed in this chapter. The characteristic histologic features and cytochemical reactivity in conjunction with the clinical history, however, are often sufficient to make the correct diagnosis.

PROTEINACEOUS LYMPHADENOPATHY

Definition. *Proteinaceous lymphadenopathy,* or *angiocentric sclerosing lymphadenopathy,* is a clinicopathologic entity characterized by extensive deposition of eosinophilic extracellular material in the lymph nodes and other organs, not due to amyloid or immunoglobulin deposition, and not associated with lymphoma.

General Features. This rare entity was initially described in 1979 by Osborne et al. (70) as a distinctive "sclerosis" of lymph nodes detected in three patients who presented with polyclonal hypergammaglobulinemia and lymphadenopathy. Such sclerosis has also been shown to be present in other organs and it appears to now be a systemic disorder of disseminated angiocentric sclerosis characterized by dense concentric bundles of reticulin fibers involving vessels walls (59).

While deposition of the eosinophilic extracellular material raises a differential diagnosis of amyloidosis, ultrastructural features do not show the typical fibrillar appearance of amyloid and Congo red stain is negative. There is no evidence of lymphoma or plasma cell dyscrasia in these patients. While some reports of proteinaceous lymphadenopathy refer to patients with light chain deposition disease or multiple myeloma (4,76), we prefer to distinguish those patients separately, as this latter group of patients shows different clinical and immunophenotypic features (discussed later in this chapter).

The etiology of proteinaceous lymphadenopathy is unknown, although it is postulated that the disorder may reflect a hyperimmune response to an infectious or inflammatory trigger. There is no evidence that there is excessive production of a polyclonal globulin and some authors have speculated that a systemic host defect may render individuals susceptible to deposition of the eosinophilic extracellular material (59).

Clinical Features. Proteinaceous lymphadenopathy has been described in relatively few, but well-documented, patients in the literature (1,56,59,70). The patient age ranges from 30 to 77 years, with a female predominance. The progressive systemic symptoms include fever, weight loss, anorexia, pruritus, and weakness, and physical findings of generalized lymphadenopathy. A history of rheumatoid arthritis has been described in the majority of patients and similar findings were seen in a patient with systemic sclerosis (1,56). Angiocentric sclerosis has been found in the lymph nodes, liver, heart, spleen, gastrointestinal tract, and kidney of patients with proteinaceous lymphadenopathy.

Laboratory Findings. Transient hypergammaglobulinemia and liver function abnormalities are associated with proteinaceous lymphadenopathy. Patients with rheumatoid arthritis have a positive rheumatoid factor and elevated erythrocyte sedimentation rate (ESR). Hypocomplementemia, cryoglobulinemia, and decreased T-helper/T-suppressor cell ratios have also been described (59).

Gross Findings. The lymph nodes are enlarged, firm, and gray-white, with a homogenous consistency. Lymph nodes enlarged to 7 cm have been described (59).

Microscopic Findings. Lymph node biopsies show extensive replacement and obliteration of the normal architecture by acellular eosinophilic material with a concentric pattern of deposition (figs. 15-1, 15-2). The amorphous eosinophilic material is concentrically arranged around blood vessels, resulting in an onion-skin appearance. Vessel walls are replaced by sclerotic material. Residual small lymphocytes, macrophages, and plasma cells may remain within the hyalinized material, especially at the edge of the lymph node. A few residual atrophic follicles remain and foreign body type giant cells may surround the eosinophilic extracellular material.

In patients with rheumatoid arthritis, reactive follicular hyperplasia with interfollicular plasma cells, sarcoid-like granulomas, and caseating granulomas have been described in lymph node (56). Focal calcification has also been described in patients with rheumatoid arthritis. This pattern of angiocentric sclerosis has also been described in biopsies and autopsy findings of other organs including heart, spleen, liver, and gastrointestinal tract.

Ancillary Testing. Given the similar morphologic appearance of proteinaceous lymphadenopathy to amyloid deposition, a Congo red stain is necessary to exclude amyloidosis. Ultrastructural studies may also be necessary. A reticulin stain documents the deposition of fine reticulin fibers. Periodic acid–Schiff (PAS) positivity has been described in the cases of proteinaceous lymphadenopathy associated with rheumatoid arthritis (56). Immunohistochemical stains to exclude lymphomas and plasma cell dyscrasias may prove useful depending on the clinical and histologic features. There should be no evidence of light chain or heavy chain deposition.

Electron micrograph studies show irregular clumps of eosinophilic material that tend to become confluent. Cells are randomly and sparsely distributed throughout the material and include lymphocytes and plasma cells. Remnants of collagen fibrils are found, and while the material is predominantly amorphous, some areas show a fine fibrillar composition.

Differential Diagnosis. The differential diagnosis of proteinaceous lymphadenopathy includes amyloidosis, monoclonal nonamyloid immunoglobulin deposition disease, and sclerosis associated with lymphoma. Sclerosis can be seen in follicular lymphoma, as well as in diffuse large B-cell lymphoma and Waldenstrom macroglobulinemia. In follicular lymphoma, the nodules consist of varying proportions of large and small cleaved cells associated with abundant amorphous PAS-positive eosinophilic material, often in the center of neoplastic follicles. Ultrastructural studies have shown this material to consist of membranous structures, membrane-bound vesicles, and electron-dense bodies (15).

The sclerosis associated with diffuse large B-cell lymphoma, such as in the variant of primary mediastinal large B-cell lymphoma, segregates clusters of large lymphoid cells. In contrast to proteinaceous lymphadenopathy, a monoclonal B-cell population is present in both types of lymphoma. The pathologic correlate of Waldenstrom macroglobulinemia, lymphoplasmacytic lymphoma, contains monoclonal B cells and monoclonal plasma cells.

Amyloidosis, as discussed below, shows a typical ultrastructure and is eosinophilic on Congo red stain with apple-green birefringence under polarized light. Monoclonal nonamyloid immunoglobulin deposition disease may also show similar light microscopic findings to proteinaceous lymphadenopathy, but is formed by the deposition of light chains, heavy chains, or both. Monoclonal antibodies specific for light and heavy chains aid in the evaluation of this entity.

Treatment and Prognosis. Proteinaceous lymphadenopathy responds to corticosteroid therapy in some patients, with the disappearance of peripheral lymphadenopathy, improvement of liver function, and resolution of hypergammaglobulinemia.

EXTRACELLULAR IMMUNOGLOBULIN DEPOSITS

Definition. *Extracellular immunoglobulin deposits* are deposits formed of monotypic immunoglobulin light chains, heavy chains, or both, without evidence of an amyloid component. The tissue deposition diseases resulting from such deposits are designated *nonamyloid monoclonal immunoglobulin deposition disease*, recognizing that amyloid has a different ultrastructure and different mechanism governing tissue deposition, as discussed later in this chapter.

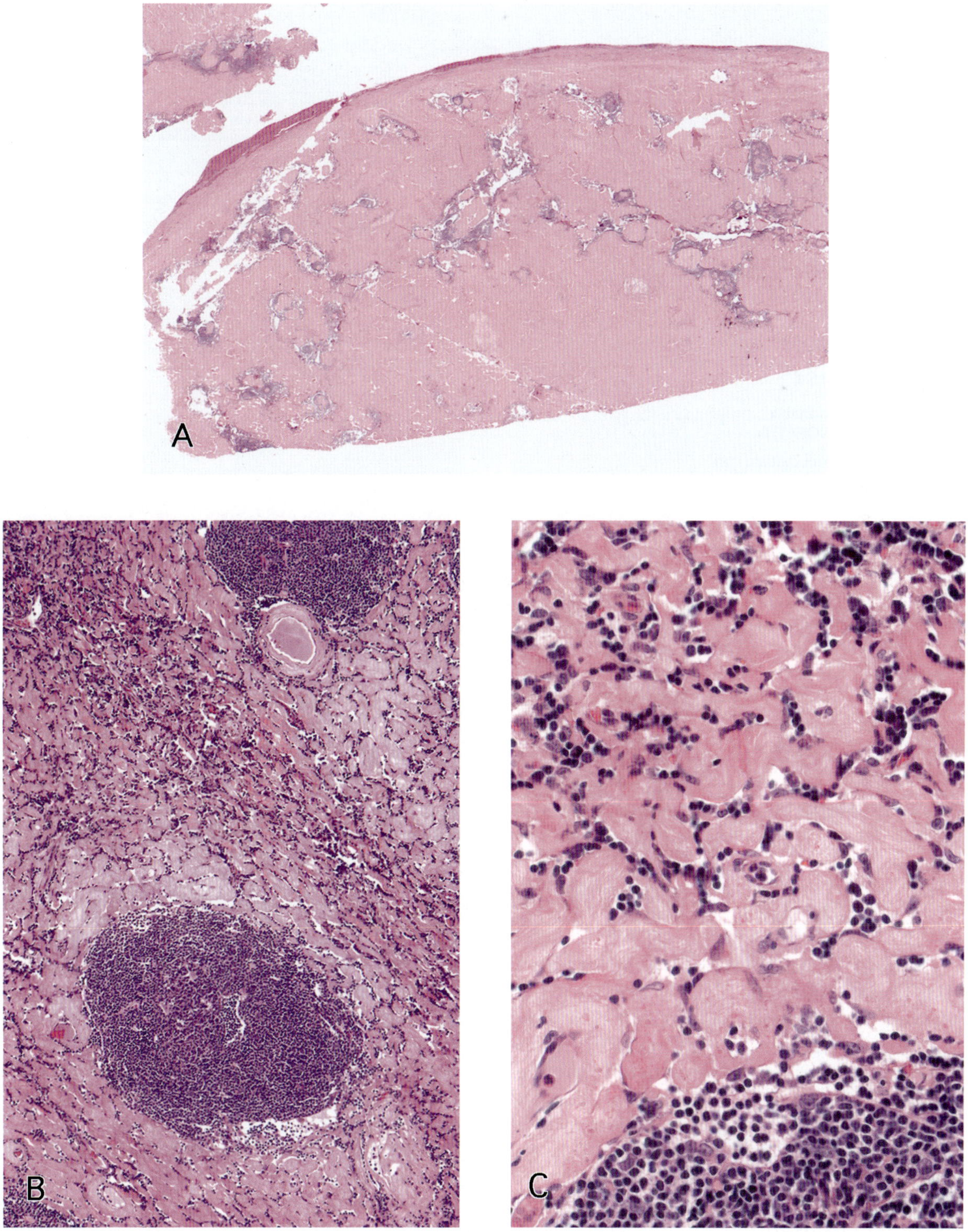

Figure 15-1

PROTEINACEOUS LYMPHADENOPATHY

Massive (A) and partial (B,C) replacement of lymph nodes by glassy hyaline protein that is not amyloid.

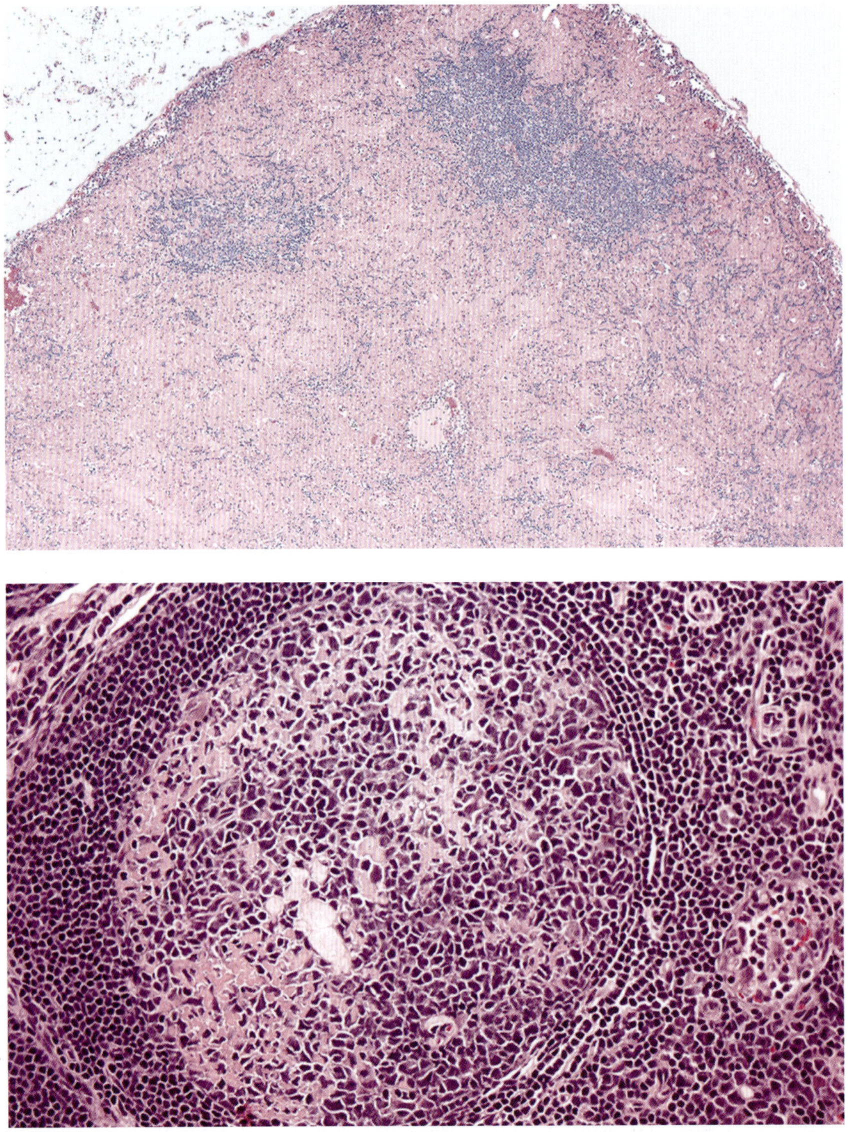

Figure 15-2

PROTEINACEOUS LYMPHADENOPATHY

While protein deposition can be diffuse (top), it is occasionally found only in germinal centers. (Bottom figure courtesy of Young Kim, Duarte, CA.)

General Features. Nonamyloid extracellular immunoglobulin deposits occur with or without an associated plasma cell dyscrasia. Immunoglobulins can cause direct tissue damage or immune complex–mediated damage. When immunoglobulin deposits are formed from only light chains, this is known as *light chain deposition disease*; when these deposits are formed from heavy chains only, this is termed *heavy chain deposition disease;* and if both light and heavy chains are present, this is called *light and heavy chain deposition disease*. While kappa light chain deposition disease is recognized as the most common form of nonamyloid monoclonal immunoglobulin deposition disease presenting with primarily renal involvement (13), only light and heavy chain deposition disease has been described in the small number of patients presenting with nonamyloid immunoglobulin deposits in lymph nodes. In this latter group of patients, all have had an associated plasma cell dyscrasia or lymphoplasmacytic lymphoma.

Clinical Features. Nonamyloid extracellular immunoglobulin deposits have been described in many organs (kidney, bone marrow, lung), but their presence in lymph nodes is extremely infrequent. Four well-documented cases have been described in the literature (4,61,76). The patients ranged in age from 37 to 62 years, with a male to female ratio of 3 to 1. Two patients had no remarkable past medical history, one patient presented with hypertension and an isolated 2-cm supraclavicular lymph node, and the last complained of a viral-like illness with left inguinal lymph node enlargement. Further work-up revealed mediastinal and abdominal lymphadenopathy in the first patient, with a computerized tomography (CT) scan reporting multiple "calcified" lymph nodes (76); the second patient had multiple lytic rib lesions and ascites (4); the third patient had a long history of vasculitis, recurrent joint pain, rash, and recent episodes of cellulitis and pneumococcal sepsis with persistent cervical and inguinal lymphadenopathy (4); and the fourth patient, a 54-year-old Japanese woman, presented with a left lung mass on chest radiograph, ultimately found to be an extramedullary plasmacytoma of the lung associated with nodular deposits of immunoglobulin-producing tumor and deposits in the regional lymph nodes (61). All biopsies showed large amorphous eosinophilic light and heavy chain deposits without evidence of amyloid. The first patient was also diagnosed with lymphoplasmacytic lymphoma on lymph node biopsy and found to have extracellular immunoglobulin deposits on renal biopsy as well. The second and third patients had no evidence of significant renal disease, but multiple myeloma was found in the second patient and the lymph node also contained evidence of myeloma. A lymphoplasmacytic infiltrate was found in the lymph node of the third patient.

A rare variant of immunoglobulin deposition diseases is *crystal storing histiocytosis* (36,47). This disorder is characterized by the deposition of crystallized immunoglobulin in macrophages in many tissues (fig. 15-3). Patients have a variety of plasma cell neoplasms and the deposition occurs in many sites including lymph nodes and spleen.

Laboratory Findings. Immunoglobulin levels are elevated, with an associated M-protein present in two of three patients (immunoglobulin [Ig]G kappa, IgG lambda) (4,61,76). In the patient with renal disease, elevated creatinine, uric acid, potassium, and gamma globulins were three noted with proteinuria of 1.0 g/dL; however, no M-protein component was found in this patient. The third patient described above, a 37-year-old man with a long history of hypocomplementemic vasculitis, had laboratory findings characteristic of that disease including low total complement, C3, and C4; hypergammaglobulinemia; impaired leukocyte adhesion; positive antinuclear antibody (speckled pattern); and a rheumatoid factor of 1:1280. In this patient, M-protein was present in the serum 1 year prior to diagnosis, with free light chains in the urine at time of biopsy. The absolute lymphocyte count was 3.9×10^9/L and platelets were 638×10^9/L.

Microscopic Findings. The histopathologic features include nodules or sheets of amorphous eosinophilic material which is negative by Congo red staining but positive with immunohistochemical stains for immunoglobulin light and/or heavy chains. The extracellular deposits are located within the blood vessel walls or in the lymph node parenchyma itself, scattered in interstitial and perivascular areas (figs. 15-4, 15-5). Multinucleated foreign body type giant cells, asteroid bodies, and Russell bodies may also be seen, as well as intranuclear inclusions (Dutcher bodies) (4). A diffuse lymphocytic/plasmacytic infiltrate has been described in association with deposits located primarily in the cortex of the node. Perivascular neutrophils and eosinophils may be found. Focal ossification of deposits has been described in an intrapulmonary lymph node (61).

Ancillary Testing. Exclusion of an amyloid origin of these deposits is essential, and supported by a lack of congophilic properties with Congo red stain, including no birefringence under polarized microscopy. Monoclonal antibodies directed against light and heavy chains reveal light and heavy chain restriction of both amorphous deposits and associated plasmacytic/lymphoplasmacytic proliferations. Other techniques to document clonality, including the protein A-gold technique and Western blotting, may not be necessary with the current repertoire of monoclonal antibodies available with immunohistochemical techniques.

Electron micrography of these deposits reveals the lack of the typical fibrillar structure of amyloid. Instead, the extracellular material is granular, with outer deposits more opaque than central deposits (4). The deposits are described ultrastructurally as amorphous and situated between plasma cells and around collagen fibers (61).

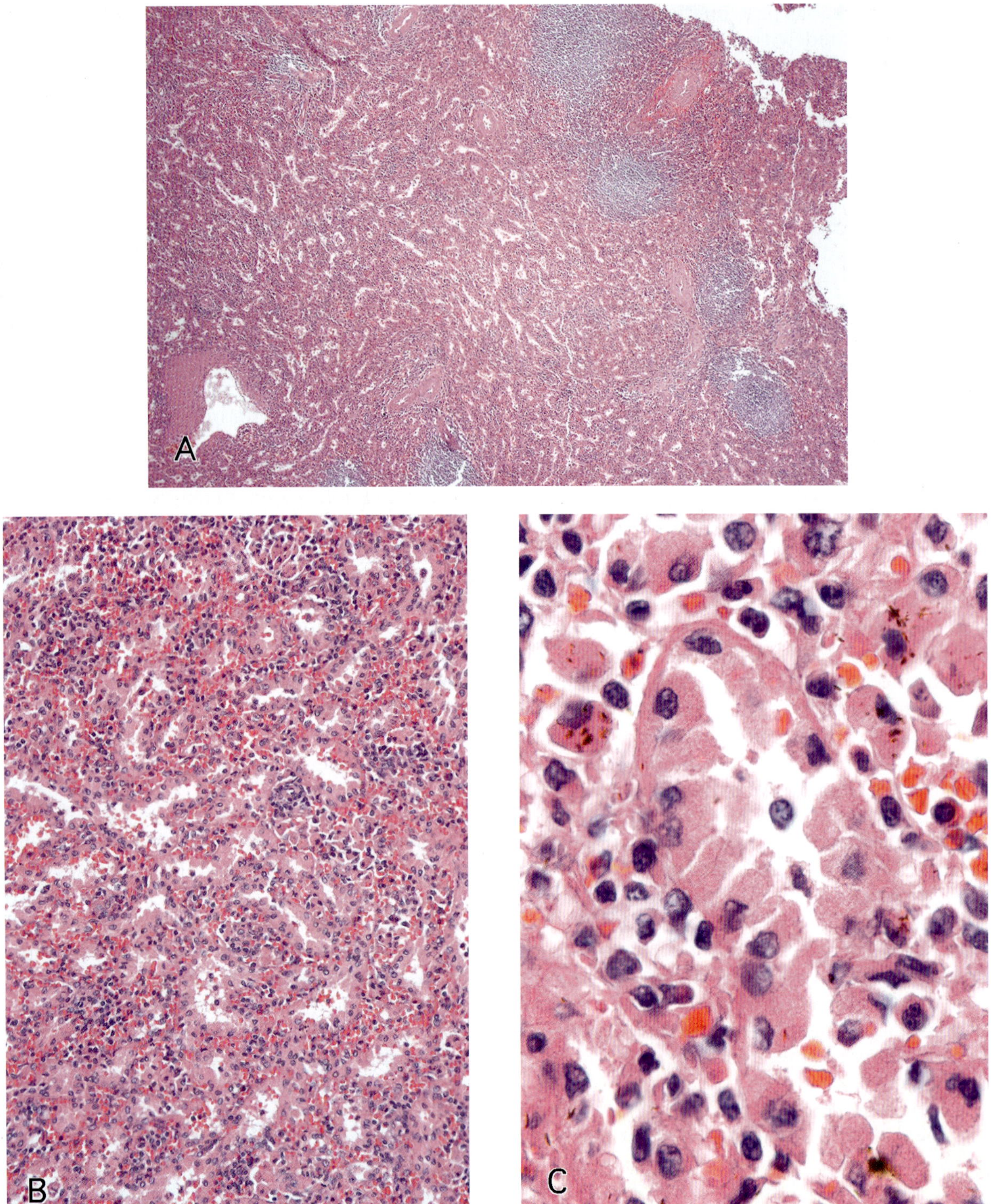

Figure 15-3

CRYSTAL STORING HISTIOCYTOSIS

In this low-magnification image, there is no apparent abnormality (A), but higher magnification (B,C) reveals deposition of crystalline material in the littoral cells of the spleen. The patient had a known history of myeloma, and crystalline immunoglobulin was deposited in the spleen. (Courtesy of Craig Zuppan, Loma Linda, CA.)

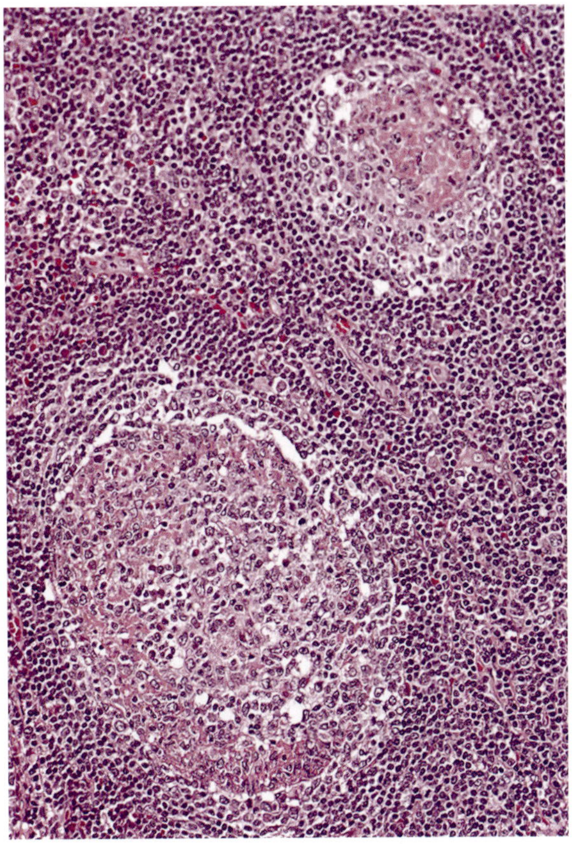

Figure 15-4

EXTRACELLULAR IMMUNOGLOBULIN DEPOSITION

Proteinaceous deposits in the germinal centers of reactive follicular hyperplasia.

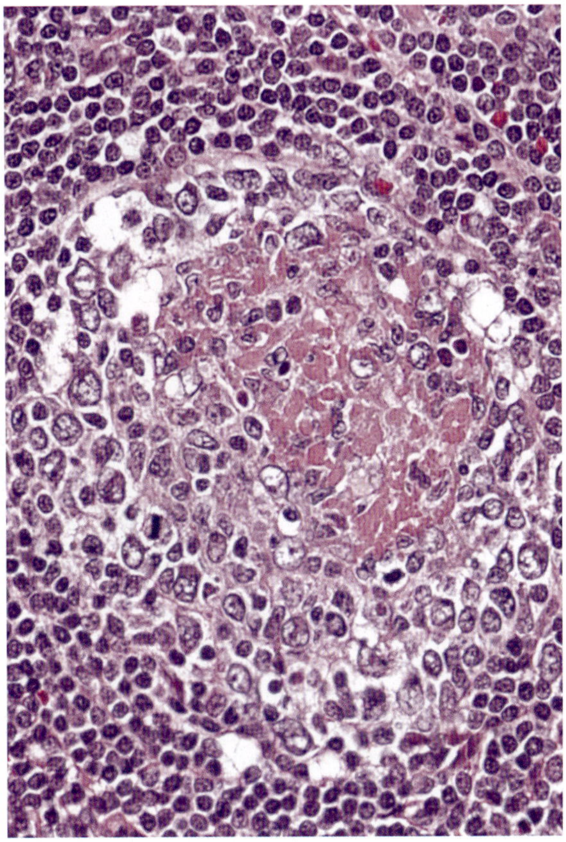

Figure 15-5

EXTRACELLULAR IMMUNOGLOBULIN DEPOSITION

Immunoglobulin deposits within a reactive germinal center.

Differential Diagnosis. In contrast to proteinaceous lymphadenopathy (70), these deposits are light chain and heavy chain restricted. Lymphocytes and/or plasma cells show a similar immunoglobulin restriction. While morphologically resembling amyloid, these deposits lack the typical histochemical behavior of amyloid as seen with Congo red staining and lack its fibrillar ultrastructure.

Treatment and Prognosis. At present, the treatment and prognosis of the patients presenting with primary lymph node disease are not documented, but intuitively should be driven by the associated hematologic disorder (i.e., multiple myeloma [1 case] or lymphoplasmacytic lymphoma [2 cases]) (4,76). The previously described fourth patient with the extramedullary plasmacytoma of lung and associated deposits of immunoglobulin underwent left lower lobe resection, but multiple disseminated tumor nodules remained on the visceral and parietal pleura (61).

AMYLOID DEPOSITS/AMYLOIDOSIS

Definition. *Amyloid deposition* or *amyloidosis* is characterized by the extracellular deposition of insoluble fibrils composed of protein subunits in a beta-pleated sheet configuration.

General Features. Amyloid deposition in a lymph node may occur in association with neoplasia, systemic amyloidosis, or localized amyloidosis (40,53). The lymph node is involved in 37 percent of patients with amyloidosis at autopsy (37) and in 22 percent of uremic patients (29). However, lymphadenopathy as the presenting symptom of amyloidosis is rare (37,40,45,64,65,87,93). Neoplastic disorders associated with amyloidosis include plasma cell dyscrasia and non-Hodgkin lymphoma.

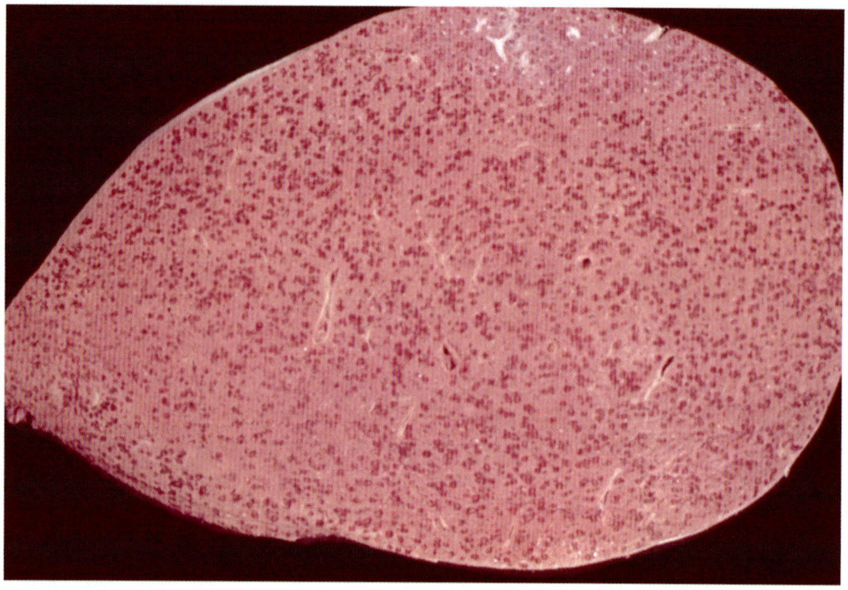

Figure 15-6

AMYLOID "SAGO" SPLEEN

Sago spleen is a description taken from the sago palm, indicating nodular deposition of amyloid in the white pulp. (Fig. 80 from Enriquez P, Neiman RN. The pathology of the spleen: a functional approach. Chicago: ASCP Press; 1976:37.)

Several forms of amyloidosis exist and are identified by analyzing the amyloid protein fibrils. The two main types of amyloid are AA and AL types, although other types have been reported, including beta-2-microglobulin–associated amyloid in hemodialysis patients. AA type amyloid is found with inflammatory, immune, infectious, hereditary, and neoplastic conditions, whereas immunoglobulin-derived fibrils (AL) are found in association with plasma cell dyscrasia and in patients with no underlying disease (primary amyloidosis).

Clinical Features. Only a handful of cases of localized primary amyloidosis of lymph nodes are documented in the literature (37,40,45,64,65, 74,84,87,93). Patient age ranges from 41 to 76 years, with a male predominance. A single lymph node is involved in two thirds of cases (inguinal, axillary, cervical, and rarely, mediastinal); in other patients, multiple bilateral lymph nodes are involved. Patients with localized primary amyloidosis have no associated diseases and the lymph nodes commonly are diffusely replaced by amyloid. Primary amyloidosis presenting with massive generalized lymphadenopathy and associated plasma cell dyscrasia (AL type) is reported, but is unusual (44).

Laboratory Findings. Laboratory findings in patients with localized primary amyloidosis include normal serum and urine electrophoresis results, with only a subset of patients showing a small M-protein component. For the patient with massive generalized lymphadenopathy, free light chains were present in the urine and an associated plasma cell dyscrasia was identified (44).

Gross Findings. In the spleen, the gross findings of amyloidosis have been recognized and have acquired descriptive names. Partial, nodular involvement has been described as "sago" spleen (fig. 15-6). Within the red pulp parenchyma of the spleen, there are firm yellow or tan nodules, similar to the appearance of the cut surface of the sago palm. "Lardaceous" spleen refers to more diffuse involvement of the spleen, giving it a gross, waxy appearance, similar to lard (fig. 15-7). If lymph nodes are diffusely affected, they have a similar gross appearance.

Microscopic Findings. The characteristic histologic features include amorphous eosinophilic deposits in a follicular, diffuse or mixed pattern of distribution throughout the lymph node and splenic parenchyma, or within the blood vessel walls (fig. 15-8). Foreign body giant cells are often present as well as abundant plasma cells. Areas of bone metaplasia have been described (87).

Ancillary Testing. The presence of amyloid is confirmed by Congo red staining (fig. 15-9) (which imparts a characteristic apple-green birefringence when viewed under polarized light), immunohistochemical analysis with

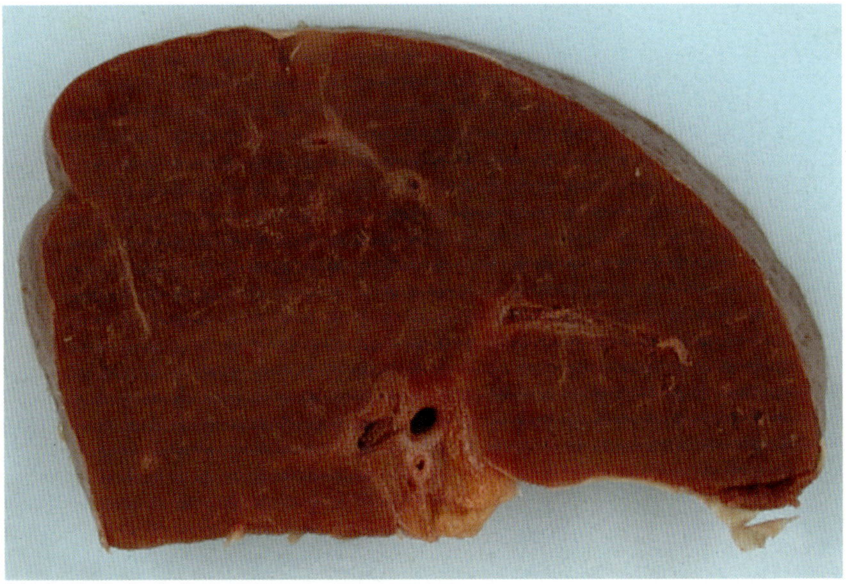

Figure 15-7

AMYLOID "LARDACEOUS" SPLEEN

Amyloid is diffusely deposited in the spleen, giving it an overall waxy or "greasy" appearance. (Courtesy of Terrance Katona, Indianapolis, IN.)

amyloid type–specific antiserum, and electron microscopy showing a fibrillar structure that is a cross-pleated configuration on X-ray diffraction (fig. 15-10) (65). Immunohistochemically, localized primary amyloidosis consists of AL type amyloid (87). Amyloid is also metachromatic with crystal violet or methyl violet and shows secondary fluorescence in ultraviolet light with thioflavine T and S. On trichrome stain, amyloid appears gray.

Differential Diagnosis. The differential diagnosis of amyloidosis of the lymph node includes proteinaceous lymphadenopathy and extracellular immunoglobulin deposits (71). These latter disorders, while morphologically resembling amyloidosis, lack the histochemical and ultrastructural features typical of amyloid. Extracellular immunoglobulin deposits, furthermore, demonstrate light and heavy chain restriction with accompanying plasma cell dyscrasia or lymphoplasmacytic lymphoma. Proteinaceous lymphadenopathy, by definition, shows no evidence of amyloid or lymphoma/plasma cell dyscrasia.

Treatment and Prognosis. Patients with localized primary amyloidosis may remain asymptomatic, without progression to systemic amyloidosis or plasma cell dyscrasia (87). Patients with systemic amyloidosis typically have associated heart disease and renal failure, and die within several years of diagnosis.

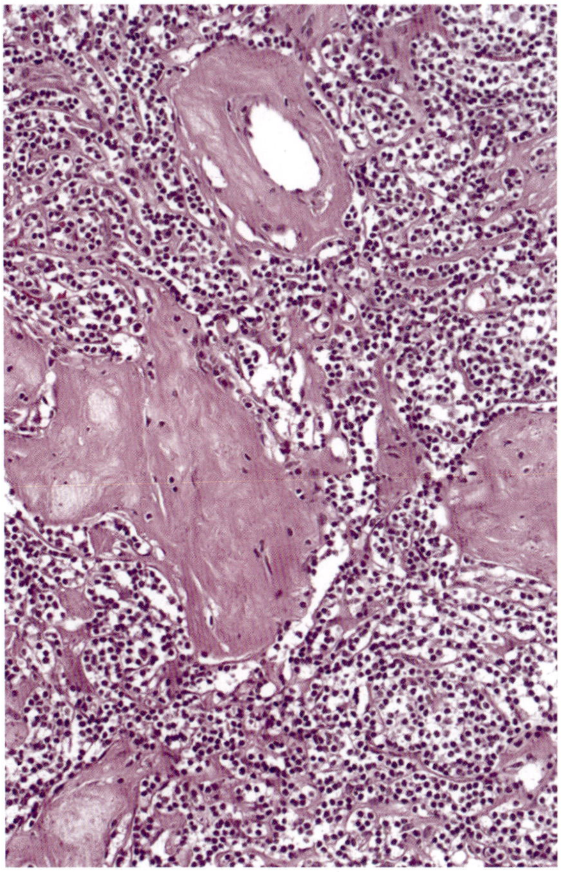

Figure 15-8

AMYLOID

In the earliest stages, amyloid is deposited in vessel walls.

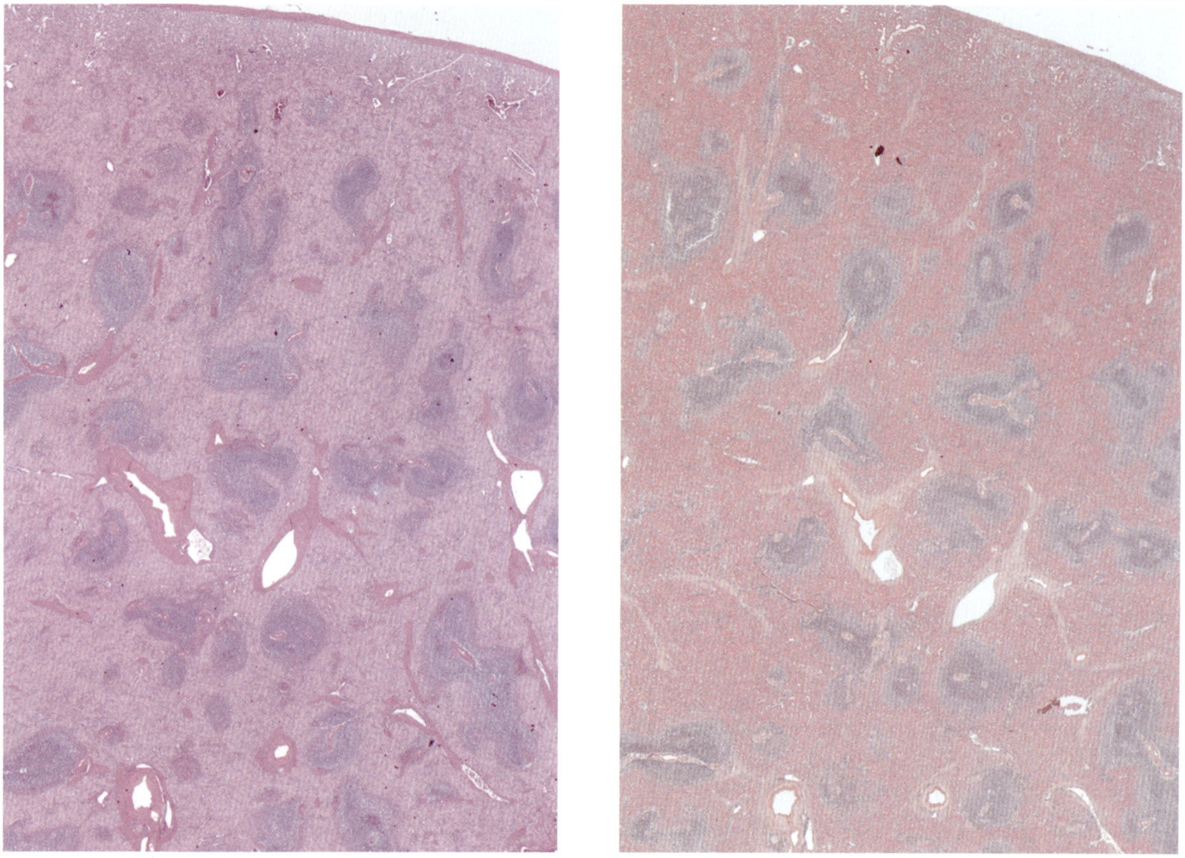

Figure 15-9

AMYLOID, SPLEEN

Left: Extensive amyloid deposition.

Right: A Congo red stain shows diffuse, brick red positivity of the amyloid. The amyloid would have apple-green birefringence when polarized. (Courtesy of the California Tumor Tissue Registry, Loma Linda, CA.)

Figure 15-10

AMYLOID

An example of the classic "pick-up sticks" appearance of amyloid by electron microscopy.

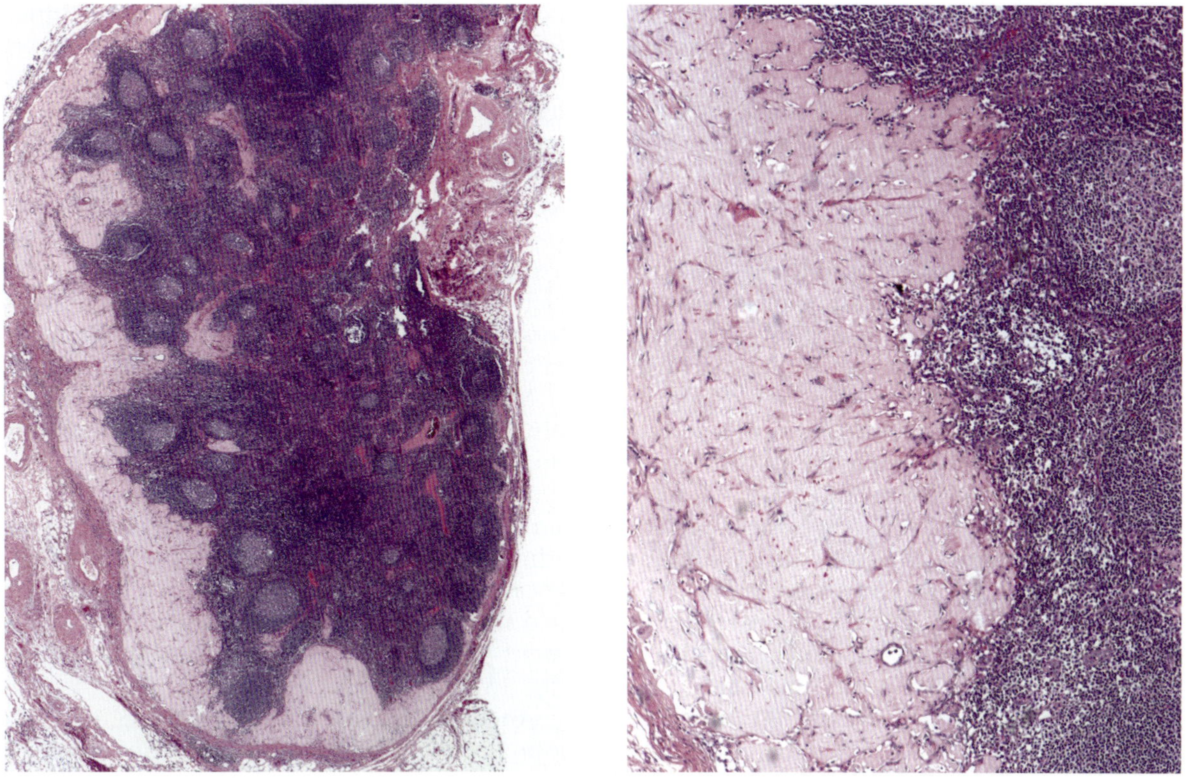

Figure 15-11

TAMM-HORSFALL PROTEIN

Deposition of Tamm-Horsfall protein in lymph node.

TAMM-HORSFALL PROTEIN DEPOSITS

Definition. *Tamm-Horsfall protein* is produced from damaged renal tubules and has been described in the sinuses of lymph nodes removed with nephrectomy specimens.

General Features. Tamm-Horsfall protein is deposited interstitially in the pararenal lymph nodes in a variety of kidney diseases, including in kidneys with tumors and in non-neoplastic kidneys (101,110). Presumably, Tamm-Horsfall protein escapes from the kidney tubules, produces a localized inflammatory cell reaction in the renal interstitium, and gains access to intrarenal lymphatics and regional lymph nodes (108).

Clinical Features. Initially described in 1981, Tamm-Horsfall protein was reported in lymph nodes removed with a Wilms tumor (108). Zanetti (110) then described six cases of both non-neoplastic and neoplastic kidneys with lymph nodes containing sinusoidal deposits of Tamm-Horsfall protein and admixed benign epithelial cells. A series of metastatic mimics, including 29 cases containing Tamm-Horsfall protein, was then described in a report from the National Wilms Tumor Study Pathology Center (101). This series included 18 boys, 10 girls, and one of gender not known, and an age range from 13 to 134 months. More recently, a single case report of Tamm-Horsfall protein in the lymph node sinuses, lymphatic vessels, renal sinus, and in kidney not affected by tumor was reported in a 16-month-old girl with nephroblastoma (11).

Microscopic Findings. Histologically, Tamm-Horsfall protein appears as waxy, amorphous masses in the lymphatic vessels, peripheral sinuses, and germinal centers of lymph nodes (fig. 15-11). These masses are often admixed with benign epithelial cells, presumably derived from damaged renal tubules. The benign epithelial cells present as small tubular structures, singly or in clusters.

Ancillary Testing. Tamm-Horsfall deposits are PAS positive, with and without diastase digestion, and Congo red negative.

Differential Diagnosis. The differential diagnosis includes amyloid deposition and metastatic tumors such as nephroblastoma (11). Tamm-Horsfall protein lacks the congophilic properties of amyloid and does not have a fibrillar ultrastructure. Mixtures of epithelial cells and Tamm-Horsfall protein within lymph node sinuses have been mistaken for metastatic tumor in pediatric specimens. Antibodies for cytokeratin stain the epithelial cells. Antisera against Tamm-Horsfall protein can be used to highlight the protein. Perhaps most helpful is comparing the primary renal neoplasm with the lymph node lesion in question wherein the epithelial cells associated with Tamm-Horsfall protein show benign features including small size and bland nuclei.

Treatment and Prognosis. The presence of Tamm-Horsfall protein itself has no bearing on prognosis; rather, it is the accompanying renal disease that dictates treatment and prognosis.

LIPID DEPOSITS

Definition. *Mineral oil lipidosis*, also known as *follicular lipidosis*, refers to deposits of mineral oil and its metabolic products in tissues.

General Features. Mineral oil lipidosis is a common incidental finding, documented in more than 50 percent of lymph nodes (mesenteric, porta hepatis, mediastinum) and 76 percent of spleens in one large autopsy series (19). This lipidosis is not restricted only to these nodal sites, but may also be found in paraaortic and internal iliac lymph nodes, suggesting a differential diagnosis that includes lymphangiogram effect and Whipple disease.

Clinical Features. Routine autopsy studies have documented the high incidence of mineral oil lipidosis in spleen, lymph nodes, liver, and bone marrow (19). The association of lipidosis and mineral oil was documented early in the literature with the observation that 7 of 11 patients with mesenteric lymph node lipogranulomas used mineral oil medicinally, suggesting that deposition of lipid first occurs in mesenteric lymph nodes (91). Other authors have demonstrated the common finding of lipogranulomas in lymph nodes removed at cholecystectomy and in lymph nodes from the porta hepatis (9,99,105). The anatomic distribution of lipogranulomas in lymph nodes shows its greatest to least incidence as follows: porta hepatis, superior mesenteric/celiac, mediastinal, inferior mesenteric, para-aortic, cervical, internal iliac, with only trace involvement of axillary lymph nodes (19).

Lipogranulomas have been described in the axillary lymph nodes of a 13-year-old boy with Netherton syndrome, a congenital ichthyosiform erythroderma, who used large amounts of emollients on his skin (17).

Microscopic Findings. Lipid droplets are distributed throughout the nodal tissue, with no preference for sinusoids (fig. 15-12). The droplets are usually less than 1 mm and are surrounded by large vacuolated macrophages admixed with lymphocytes and plasma cells. Focal fibrosis accompanies the lipogranulomas in a small subset of cases (19). Splenic involvement shows predominantly lipogranulomas (fig. 15-13).

Ancillary Testing. Mineral oil and its metabolic products in tissues are positive with a combined osmic acid-oil red O stain. They contain saturated hydrocarbons with chemical extraction and mass spectrometry (9,10).

Differential Diagnosis. Mineral oil lipidosis in lymph nodes may be mimicked morphologically by Whipple disease and lymphangiogram effect involving oil-based radiopaque substances (Table 15-1). In Whipple disease, the stroma and sinusoids of the lymph nodes contain collections of foamy, PAS-positive granules. Lymphangiogram effect typically shows a sinusoidal distribution of macrophages. These macrophages are typically larger than those found in mineral oil lipidosis and less vaculated, with eosinophilic cytoplasm.

Treatment and Prognosis. Mineral oil lipidosis is usually an incidental finding requiring no treatment.

LYMPHANGIOGRAM EFFECT

Definition. *Lymphangiogram effect* consists of the lymph node changes that result from the injection of oil-based radiopaque substances used in lymphangiography.

General Features. Since the inception of lymphangiography in 1952 as an important radiologic technique for the clinical staging of

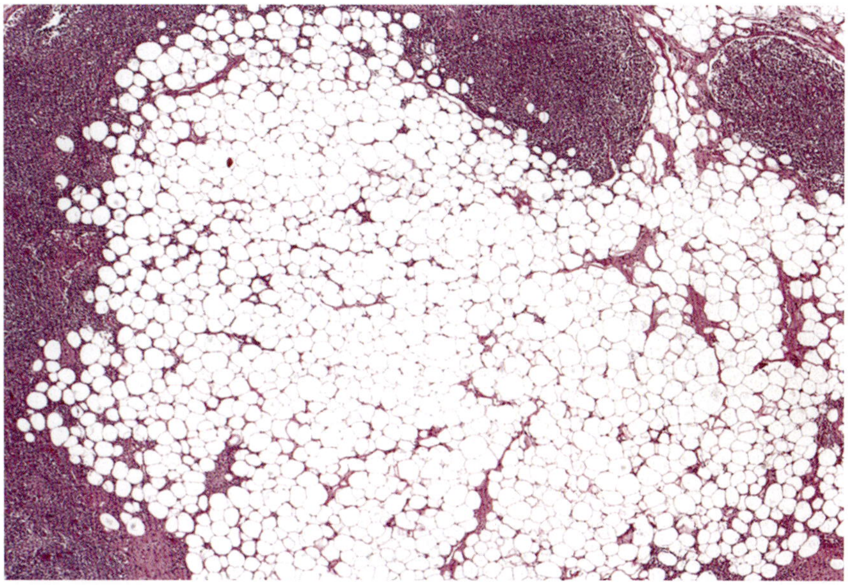

Figure 15-12

LIPIDOSIS, LYMPH NODE

Arising from the hilum, fatty deposition has replaced much of the nodal parenchyma.

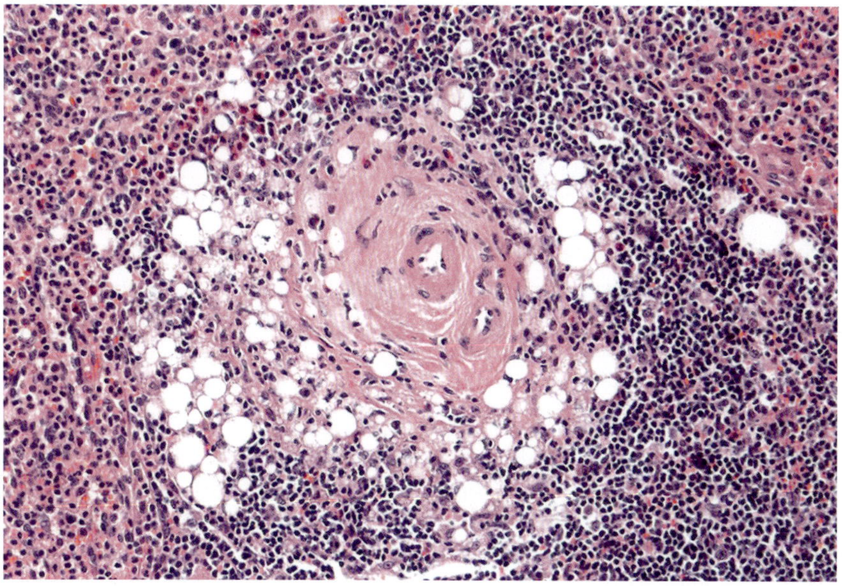

Figure 15-13

LIPOGRANULOMA, SPLEEN

Lipogranulomas are typically seen in a perivascular location in the spleen. Because of possible mimics, "fat" vacuoles should be polarized to rule out deposition of foreign substances.

Table 15-1

DIFFERENTIAL DIAGNOSIS OF LYMPH NODE DISORDERS WITH AMORPHOUS EOSINOPHILIC DEPOSITS AND SELECT CLINICAL, IMMUNOPHENOTYPIC, HISTOCHEMICAL, AND ULTRASTRUCTURAL FEATURES

Disorder	Congophilic Properties[a]	Ultrastructural Fibrils	Associated Neoplasms	Immunoglobulin Restricted
Proteinaceous lymphadenopathy	No	No	No	No
Amyloidosis	Yes	Yes	Variable	Yes, light chain
Extracellular immunoglobulin deposits	No	No	Yes	Yes
Tamm-Horsfall protein	No	No	Renal, may be benign	No

[a]Congophilic properties refers to eosinophilic staining of amorphous material with Congo red stain and apple-green birefringence under polarized light.

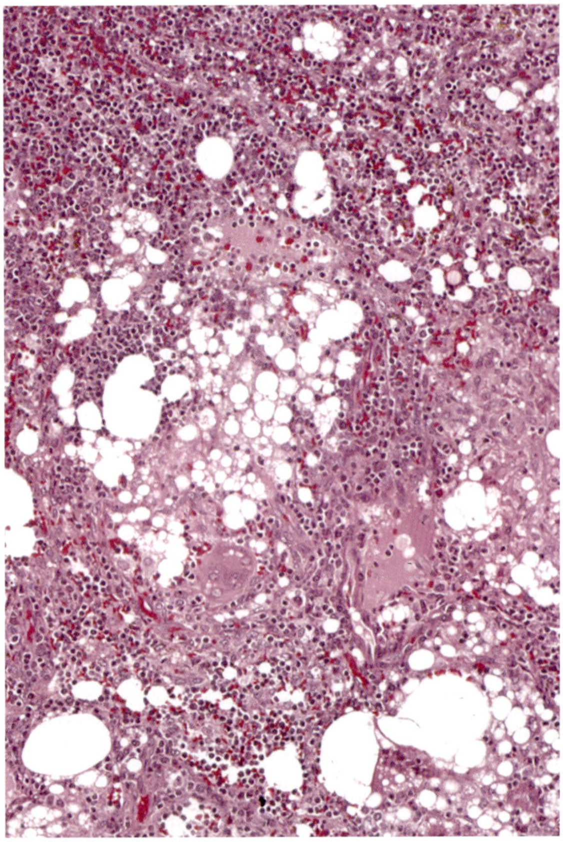

Figure 15-14

LYMPHANGIOGRAM EFFECT, LYMPH NODE

Vacuolated macrophages, granulomas, and a foreign body reaction are characteristic of lymphangiogram effect.

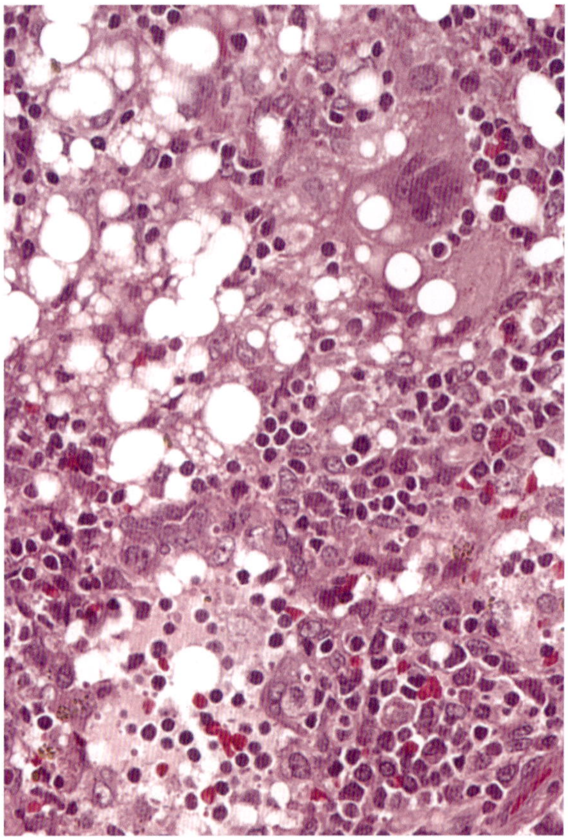

Figure 15-15

LYMPHANGIOGRAM EFFECT, LYMPH NODE

Following lymphangiography, multinucleated giant cells surround the oil droplets.

lymphoma (especially Hodgkin lymphoma), characteristic reactive lymphangiogram changes in lymph nodes have been reported (31,77). The contrast material used in the procedure is iodized oil, which is injected into the lymphatics of the foot and travels to the pelvic and retroperitoneal lymph nodes. The oily base of the contrast material results in a granulomatous reaction in the lymph node sinuses and the accumulation of multinucleated giant cells surrounding the large droplets of oil.

Although CT and magnetic resonance imaging (MRI) have replaced lymphangiography as the main staging procedures in most cases of lymphoma, lymphangiography is still occasionally used in the work-up of Hodgkin lymphoma and testicular germ cell neoplasms (90).

Clinical Features. Oil-based radiopaque substances have been used in lymphangiography, primarily in the past, for the work-up of malignancies. These substances may persist for up to 30 months after the procedure (77).

Microscopic Findings. The lymph node sinuses are distended by the contrast material within macrophages. Fine droplets of oil may be present and are responsible for the vacuolated appearance of the cytoplasm of the macrophages and giant cells (figs. 15-14–15-16). Lipid deposition may be noted in the hypoplastic germinal centers as well. Eosinophils, neutrophils, and plasma cells are present in the first few weeks after the procedure has taken place (92). When vacuoles are present in the cytoplasm, they are frequently large, greater than 1 mm (19). The presence of fibrosis has been described by some authors (24), but others did not find increased fibrosis when compared to control subjects (77).

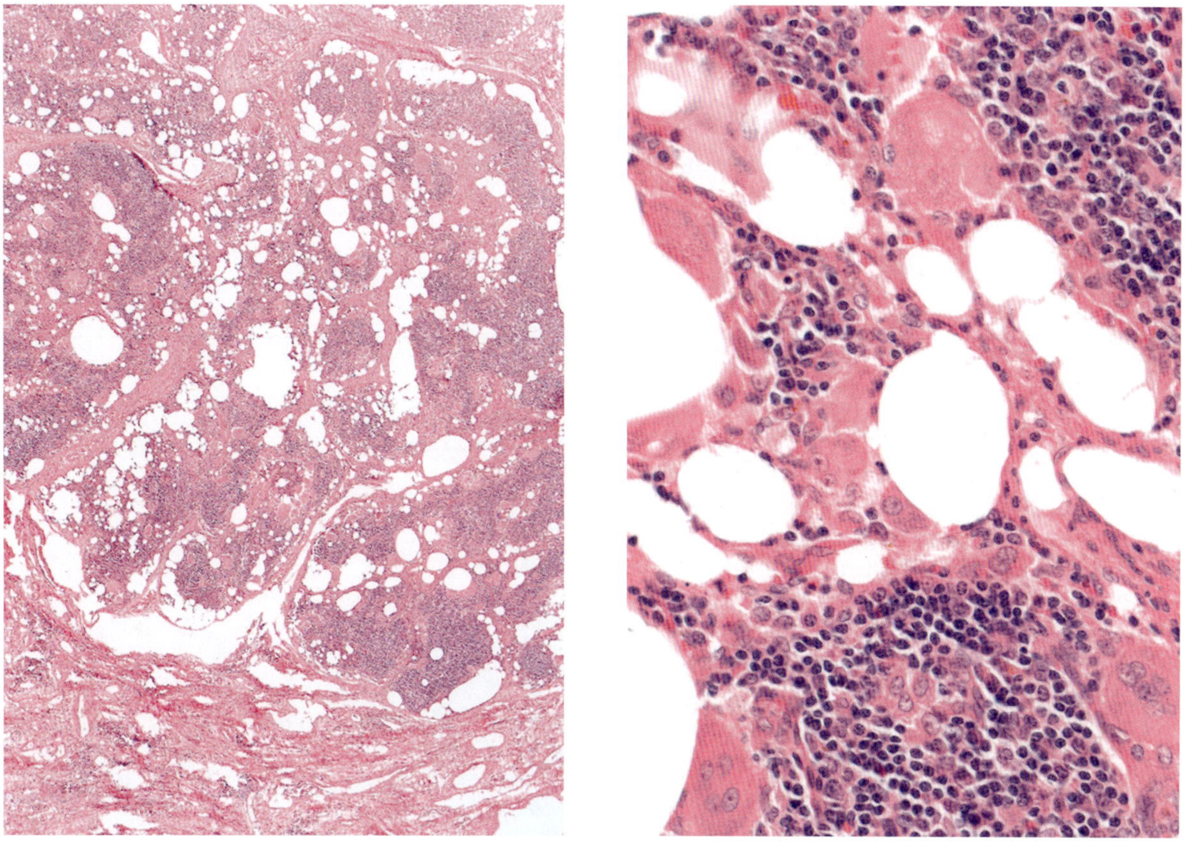

Figure 15-16

LYMPHANGIOGRAM EFFECT, LYMPH NODE

A striking example of the disruption of the lymph node architecture as a result of lymphangiogram. (Courtesy of the California Tumor Tissue Registry, Loma Linda, CA.)

Ancillary Testing. Ancillary testing, including special stains for atypical acid-fast bacilli or fungal organisms, helps exclude other disorders that can mimic lymphangiogram effect.

Differential Diagnosis. The differential diagnosis of lymphangiogram lymphadenopathy (Table 15-2) includes infections caused by fungi or atypical mycobacteria which result in macrophages or giant cells with intracytoplasmic vacuoles. Special stains for organisms and an appropriate clinical history should help in this distinction. Any process that causes a lipogranulomatous reaction in the lymph nodes, such as the intravenous injection of drugs that use oily substances as their base, may also result in changes that are reminiscent of lymphangiogram effect.

Whipple disease shows histologic features that are similar to those of lymphangiogram lymphadenitis. In Whipple disease, however, there is a characteristic "Swiss cheese" appearance on low-power microscopy due to sinusoidal dilatation and foamy macrophages in the interstitial region that are filled with PAS-positive material and causative organisms (21). Silicone lymphadenopathy is also in the differential diagnosis from a histologic point of view but a good clinical history helps differentiate the two conditions. The histologic changes in lymph nodes associated with cystic pneumatosis of the gastrointestinal tract may simulate those seen in lymphangiogram effect (92). Malignant lymphoma may be simulated by the pronounced follicular hyperplasia seen in the lymph nodes of patients who have undergone repeated lymphangiography procedures even though the changes associated with this procedure are benign and reactive (14).

Table 15-2

DIFFERENTIAL DIAGNOSIS OF LYMPH NODE DISORDERS RESULTING IN LARGE VACUOLES WITH DISCRIMINATING HISTOLOGIC AND HISTOCHEMICAL FEATURES

Disorder	Vacuole Location	Vacuole Size	PAS[a] Reaction in Macrophages	Acid-Fast Stain	Fibrosis
Mineral oil lipidosis	Diffuse	< 1 mm	Neg	Neg	Typically not present
Lymphangiogram effect	Sinusoidal	Often >1 mm	Neg	Neg	Variable
Whipple disease	Stroma, sinusoids	< 1 mm	Pos	Neg	Present in later stages
Silicone deposition	Cortex or medulla, multifocal	Average 130 µm	Neg	Neg	Absent

[a]PAS = Periodic acid–Schiff stain.

SILICONE DEPOSITS

Definition. Lymphadenopathy may develop in regional lymph nodes as a reaction to the leakage of *silicone* from bag-gel implants, direct injection, or after small joint arthroplasty.

General Features. Silicone consists of dimethylsiloxane polymers and may appear in liquid, gel, or solid form. Silicone is commonly used in implants.

Clinical Features. Silicone lymphadenopathy is associated with augmentation and reconstruction mammoplasty and with the insertion of joint prostheses (26,94). The subsequent lymphadenopathy is believed to result from either the migration of liquid silicone following injection or leakage from a bag-gel through lymphatic channels to regional lymph nodes (92). Following large joint replacement surgery, fragments of polyester or polyethylene derived from the articulating surfaces of the joint prosthesis may similarly travel to regional lymph nodes via the lymphatic channels (26). Silicone lymphadenopathy also occurs after small joint replacement surgery (57,72). In one study of silastic arthroplasty, silicone lymphadenopathy occurred in 13 percent of patients (46).

Microscopic Findings. An important histologic feature of silicone lymphadenopathy is subtotal effacement of the normal nodal architecture by large and small vacuoles, which represent either empty "spaces" from which the silicone has been washed away, or residual silicone deposits (figs. 15-17, 15-18). Foreign body giant cells and granulomas may be seen in the sinuses and parenchyma of the lymph node. In most cases, sinus histiocytosis is present and prominent follicular hyperplasia is not (38). Foamy macrophages are present within the nodal tissue, from small collections to confluent sheets, replacing on average one fourth of the lymph node in one study of 96 patients (38).

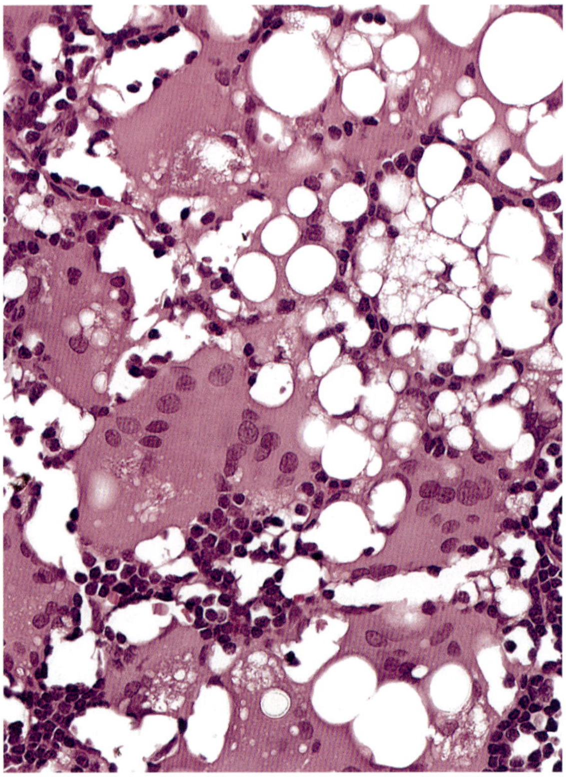

Figure 15-17

SILICONE DEPOSITION, LYMPH NODE

Silicone-related axillary lymphadenopathy in a patient with a ruptured silicone gel breast implant. Multinucleated giant cells surround empty cystic spaces containing thin, refractile strands of residual silicone.

The clinical significance of silicone lymphadenopathy is unclear, but the clinical presentation of lymphadenopathy in a patient with

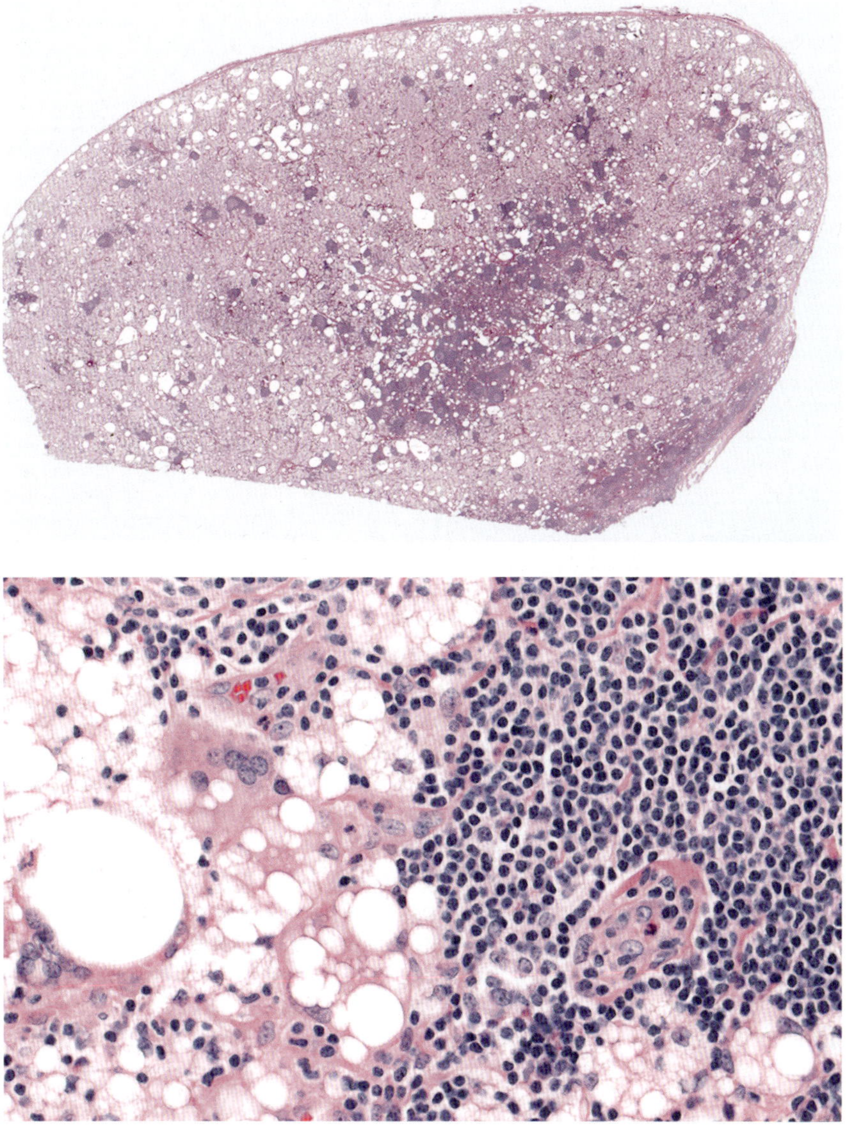

Figure 15-18

SILICONE DEPOSITION, LYMPH NODE

Marked architectural distortion is seen in this lymph node with massive silicone deposition.

a silicone breast implant raises an important differential diagnosis of metastatic breast cancer and silicone lymphadenopathy. Case reports have documented the presence of silicone lymphadenopathy and lymphoma in the same lymph node, but the etiology of lymphoma is not clear in these cases (5).

Ancillary Testing. The lymph nodes usually demonstrate a variable amount of unstained, nonbirefringent refractile material that can be shown to contain elemental silicon by energy-dispersive X-ray analysis (94). This technique serves as an adjunct to light and polarization microscopy, which are often sufficient to make the diagnosis of silicone lymphadenopathy. Other methods of identification include infrared imaging spectroscopy or Fourier transform infrared spectroscopy (30,38,39). Oil red O stains may also highlight silicone deposits (fig. 15-19), although not consistently.

Differential Diagnosis. A thorough clinical history is important for identifying the presence of a silicone implant or silicone injections. A number of conditions that present with foamy macrophages containing vacuoles may mimic silicone lymphadenopathy (Table 15-2). These include infectious diseases, such as Whipple disease and *Mycobacterium avium-intracellulare*, in which PAS and acid-fast stains are positive, respectively. Mineral oil lipidosis also mimics

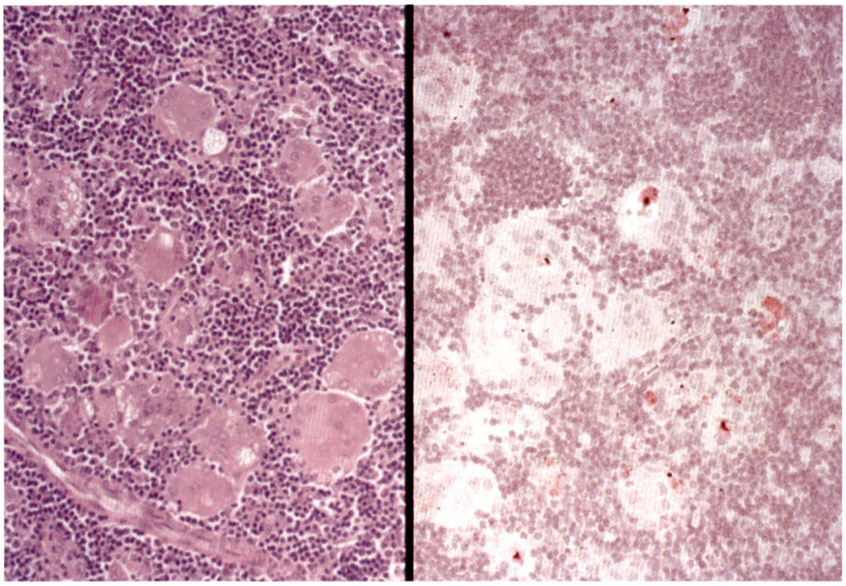

Figure 15-19

SILICONE DEPOSITION, LYMPH NODE

Multinucleated giant cells with silicone (left) are highlighted by an oil red O stain (right).

silicone lymphadenopathy and is commonly seen in mesenteric lymph nodes as a diffuse distribution of small vacuoles containing lipid. Lymphangiogram effect, another mimic, commonly shows a sinus pattern with very large vacuoles. Careful examination of the lymph nodes involved by silicone will show a variable amount of unstained, nonbirefringent, refractile material characteristic of silicone. Histiocytic lymphadenitis associated with large joint prostheses may mimic silicone lymphadenitis. These macrophages are PAS positive, in contrast to silicone lymphadenopathy, and contain birefringent particles of polyethylene.

HISTIOCYTIC LYMPHADENOPATHY AFTER JOINT PROSTHESIS

Definition. *Histiocytosis of regional lymph nodes after large joint prosthesis*, or *postarthroplasty histiocytic lymphadenopathy*, has been documented in multiple patients. The foreign body response characterized by benign histiocytosis is a reaction to polyethylene and metal wear particles.

General Features. Florid sinus histiocytosis was initially reported in the regional lymph nodes draining the sites of large joint prostheses (26). The sinuses of these lymph nodes were dilated by macrophages containing abundant granular material, revealing needle-like particles under polarized light (26). The foreign material was characterized as polyethylene particles, and cobalt-chromium and titanium microparticles using ultrastructural and X-ray microanalysis studies (2). This is an important phenomenon to recognize and to distinguish from other benign histiocytic sinusoidal proliferations and metastatic processes.

Clinical Features. Large joint prostheses wear over time and shed particles of metal, polyethylene, and cement into tissues surrounding them (23). Wear particles can migrate to regional lymph nodes that drain these sites and cause clinically significant lymphadenopathy (26). Histiocytic lymphadenitis associated with large joint prostheses has been described in pelvic lymph nodes in men undergoing prostatectomy (12,20,26), in gynecologic oncology patients who have undergone large joint replacements (109), following total hip arthroplasty (2,6,8,18,20,26,33,62), after knee replacement (6,18,89), and in axillary lymph nodes removed during modified radical mastectomy in a patient with total shoulder joint replacement (68).

Wear particles have also been found in the liver, spleen, and abdominal lymph nodes of patients after total joint replacement; the presence of these particles in liver or spleen is more prevalent in patients with a failed hip arthroplasty rather than a primary joint replacement (102). Lymphatic vessels are the likely route of dissemination to these organs.

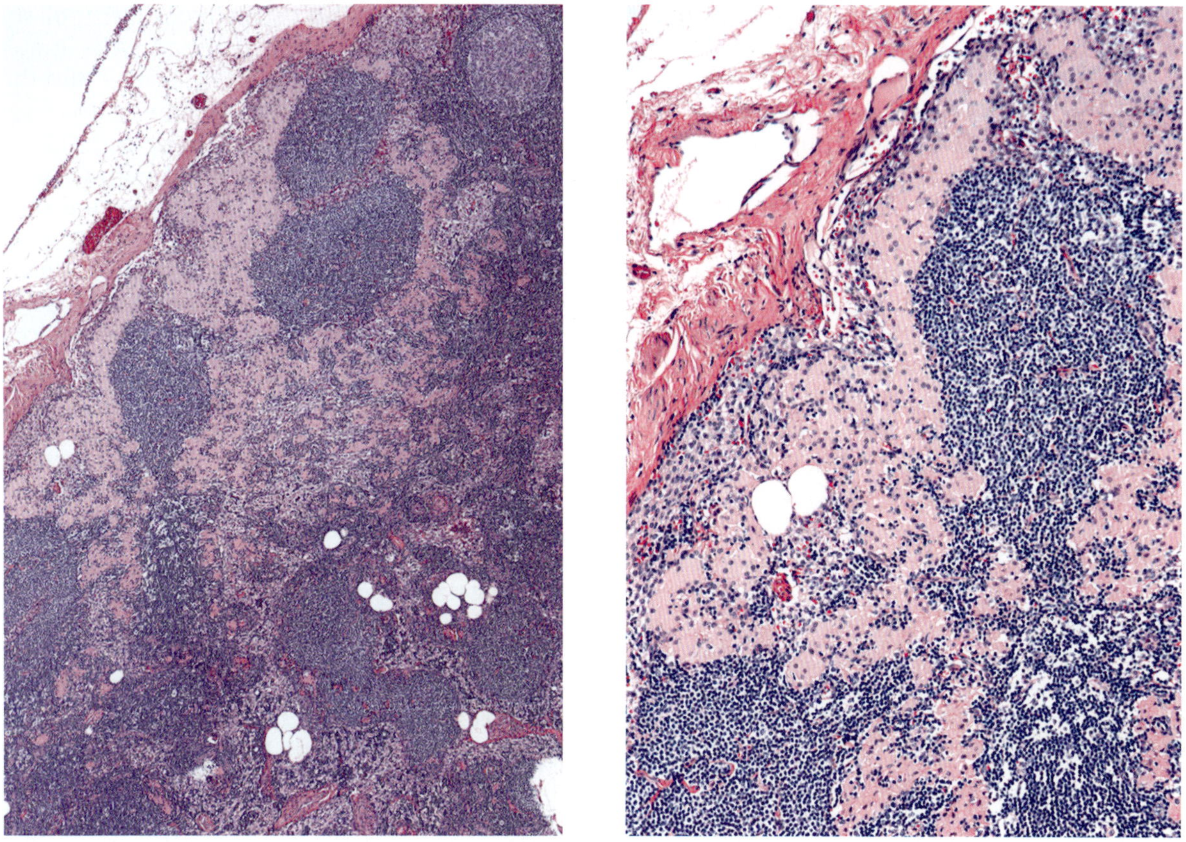

Figure 15-20

HISTIOCYTOSIS, FOLLOWING ORTHOPEDIC PROCEDURE, LYMPH NODE

The paracortex of the lymph node is expanded (left) by macrophages with abundant pink cytoplasm (right).

Gross Findings. Lymph nodes are typically enlarged, up to 35 cm in one report (12), and soft to firm in consistency. While most lymph nodes are unremarkable, a dark brown or black color has been noted both focally and diffusely in some patients (2,95). No areas of hemorrhage have been described, but necrosis was described in one patient with a revised hip replacement and paraaortic lymphadenopathy (95).

Microscopic Findings. A prominent histiocytic infiltrate is present in both enlarged and unenlarged lymph nodes (fig. 15-20). While a sinusoidal pattern has been described most often (26), paracortical and medullary aggregates of macrophages are also seen and may compress uninvolved sinuses (109). Medullary and subcapsular sinuses are often involved by macrophages, which fill and distend these sinuses and may coalesce to focally efface parts of the lymph node. Expansion beyond the lymph node capsule has also been described (109). Otherwise, the surrounding lymphoid tissue is unremarkable.

The macrophages are enlarged and polygonal, with abundant pale and foamy cytoplasm containing coarsely granular eosinophilic material. Small black particles are present within the cytoplasm. The macrophages contain round to oval nuclei with dispersed nuclear chromatin and unremarkable nuclear cytology. Multinucleated macrophages are also seen. Focal granuloma-like lesions composed of epithelioid macrophages and multinucleated giant cells have been described (109), as well fibrosis (33,95).

Fine needle aspiration of lymph nodes with histiocytic lymphadenopathy after hip replacement shows consistent cytologic features including numerous foamy macrophages, unremarkable nuclei, and birefringent particles within the foamy cytoplasm (62). In the spleen, infiltrates of foamy macrophages are present near the splenic trabeculae; wear particles are located within the cytoplasm of these macrophages (95).

Ancillary Testing. The macrophages of postarthroplasty histiocytic lymphadenopathy contain abundant eosinophilic PAS-positive granular material resistant to diastase digestion. Examination under polarized light typically reveals abundant needle-like and particulate birefringent particles within the cytoplasm of macrophages and multinucleated giant cells, consistent with polyethylene. Polarized light has limitations, however, as shown by one study which found birefringent particulate debris in lymph nodes from patients after a total joint replacement as well as in lymph nodes from patients prior to total joint replacement (83). Small irregular, polygonal and needle-shaped black particles which do not polarize may also be present. A modified oil red O procedure can be used to highlight the cytoplasm of macrophages (diffuse orange-red staining), consistent with the presence of polyethylene particles (8). The macrophages show immunoreactivity typical of benign macrophages: positive for lysozyme, alpha-1-antitrypsin, alpha-1-antichymotrypsin, cathepsin D, CD68, and CD163; negative for cytokeratin and S-100 protein.

Ultrastructural analysis shows irregular electron-dense microparticles (less than 2 µm in largest diameter) within macrophages, some within vacuoles, and electron-lucent round or oval structures bound by an electron-dense rim (12,62). Detailed ultrastructural studies show bone cement and polyethylene wear particles in all cases, with metallic wear particles in 90 percent of analyzed cases (12). Energy-dispersive X-ray microanalysis, Fourier transform infrared spectroscopy, and hot-stage thermal analysis also identify specific metals (2,95).

Differential Diagnosis. The differential diagnosis includes other histiocytic processes or mimickers with a sinus pattern in the lymph node or focal involvement/obliteration of lymph node architecture. Metastatic melanoma and metastatic adenocarcinoma may have similar material histologically, but the immunohistochemical markers of melanoma (S-100 protein, HMB45, melan A, MART1) are positive in the former and epithelial markers (cytokeratins) are positive in the latter. The changes described in silicone lymphadenopathy are also similar to those seen in postarthroplasty histiocytic lymphadenopathy, but the material in the macrophage is PAS negative and the macrophage of silicone lymphadenopathy contains fine vacuoles, often showing translucent refractile material. A history of a lymphangiogram distinguishes the histologic features seen in lymphangiogram effect. Leprosy, Whipple disease, and *Mycobacterium avium-intracellulare* are infectious diseases that show foamy macrophages in lymph nodes, and appropriate special stains and history should help distinguish these entities. Storage diseases, such as Gaucher disease, can cause the accumulation of foamy macrophages. Rosai-Dorfman disease (sinus histiocytosis with massive lymphadenopathy) shows similar features, but lacks the refractile material within macrophages, while demonstrating the emperipolesis and atypical cytologic features typical of that disorder. Lastly, reactive sinus histiocytosis is typically seen in lymph nodes draining malignancy or inflammation, but lacks the birefringent particles seen in postarthroplasty histiocytic lymphadenopathy.

Treatment and Prognosis. Lymph nodes are removed for staging procedures for prostatic carcinoma or because of enlargement. The recognition of this benign process is important in distinguishing it from malignancy. By itself, postarthroplasty histiocytic lymphadenopathy has no prognostic significance, but the presence of wear particles not just in lymph nodes, but in liver and spleen has unknown effects. Case reports have documented malignant tumors arising next to joint prostheses, but no clear evidence exists of an increased risk of malignancy (95).

BERYLLIOSIS

Definition. *Berylliosis* may involve the lymph nodes when beryllium deposits (salts) are disseminated through the body from either a primary inoculation site or a pulmonary focus.

General Features. Inhalation is the typical route that results in beryllium disease. The disease may be acute (chemical pneumonitis) or more typically chronic (granulomatous pneumonitis or the more serious pulmonary complication of pulmonary fibrosis). Local implantation is followed usually by granulomatous skin nodules. Sarcoid-like granulomas can be seen in the lungs and other organs in chronic beryllium disease.

Clinical Features. Chronic beryllium disease is a rare granulomatous lung disease clinically resembling sarcoidosis, with which it is occupationally related. Insoluble beryllium dust is inhaled, inducing chronic disease in a small subset of exposed individuals (82). Genetic susceptibility is thought to determine an individual's immune response to beryllium (67). It is estimated that as many as 134,000 workers, most of whom worked in beryllium-manufacturing plants, have been exposed to beryllium in the United States (32). The smaller number of European and Israeli patients worked in metal-processing occupations. The clinical features of patients with chronic beryllium disease include occupational beryllium exposure and pulmonary manifestations resembling sarcoidosis, such as noncaseating granulomas in transbronchial biopsies (58).

Laboratory Findings. Berylliosis is confirmed by a beryllium lymphocyte proliferation test on blood or bronchoalveolar lavage fluid (66).

Microscopic Findings. In acute pulmonary disease, the associated lymphadenitis is characterized by sinus histiocytosis with prominent phagocytosis, without granuloma formation that is commonly seen in the chronic form. In chronic disease, the granulomas may be well formed and discrete, resembling sarcoidosis, or show central necrosis, as in tuberculosis.

Ancillary Testing. The distinction between berylliosis and either sarcoidosis or tuberculosis relies upon clinicopathologic correlation and demonstration of beryllium in the tissue by spectrographic studies (92). Formalin-fixed tissues can be analyzed for beryllium using atomic absorption spectrophotometry (98).

Differential Diagnosis. The chronic form of berylliosis suggests diseases of granulomatous formation, both caseating and noncaseating forms. Special stains to exclude infectious organisms such as acid-fast bacilli and fungi are recommended. Tissue should be examined under polarized light to exclude foreign material. Granulomatous reactions can also be seen secondary to lymph nodes draining malignancies or inflammatory lesions or in patients with autoimmune diseases such as sarcoidosis. Clinical correlation is essential.

Treatment and Prognosis. Chronic beryllium disease is treated with corticosteroids. The response to corticosteroids is variable. Lung function improves when exposure to beryllium terminates (88).

ASBESTOS DEPOSITS

Definition. Pulmonary hilar lymph nodes from patients with *asbestos-related diseases* can contain asbestos or the more generic term, *ferruginous bodies*.

General Features. Patients with asbestos-related diseases are known to contain asbestos bodies within their lungs (16). Asbestos fibers are thought to migrate to pulmonary hilar lymph nodes where they are located within macrophages.

Clinical Features. Exposure to asbestos is linked to the development of benign and malignant lung diseases. The size, shape, and concentration of the different forms of asbestos fibers determines whether an individual will get an asbestos-related disease. Asbestos bodies in the lung parenchyma have been linked to an elevated tissue asbestos burden (79). Asbestos bodies may also be observed in pulmonary hilar lymph nodes and are indicative of a heavy asbestos body burden in the lung (78). In one large study, patients with asbestos bodies in lymph nodes ranged in age from 46 to 76 years and were all men with occupations related to airborne asbestos exposure of duration from as little as 4 years to 40 years (78). The vast majority of patients had diagnoses of asbestosis as well as lung carcinoma, pleural plaques, and/or mesothelioma.

Microscopic Findings. Asbestos bodies are dumbbell-, beaded-, or javelin-shaped and yellow-brown, and are usually found in association with clusters of macrophages (figs. 15-21, 15-22). Pigment-laden macrophages may partially obscure these bodies.

Ancillary Testing. Iron staining of tissue helps highlight asbestos bodies. Scanning electron micrography can identify asbestos fibers from lymph node digests (78). Energy-dispersive X-ray microanalysis chemically characterizes the particles (73). Specific methods for asbestos quantification have been described in the literature (79).

Differential Diagnosis. Asbestos is not the only inorganic particulate that may be coated by iron-protein complexes, which is why the generic term of "ferruginous body" is used. Once an asbestos core is demonstrated, the more specific term of asbestos body can be used.

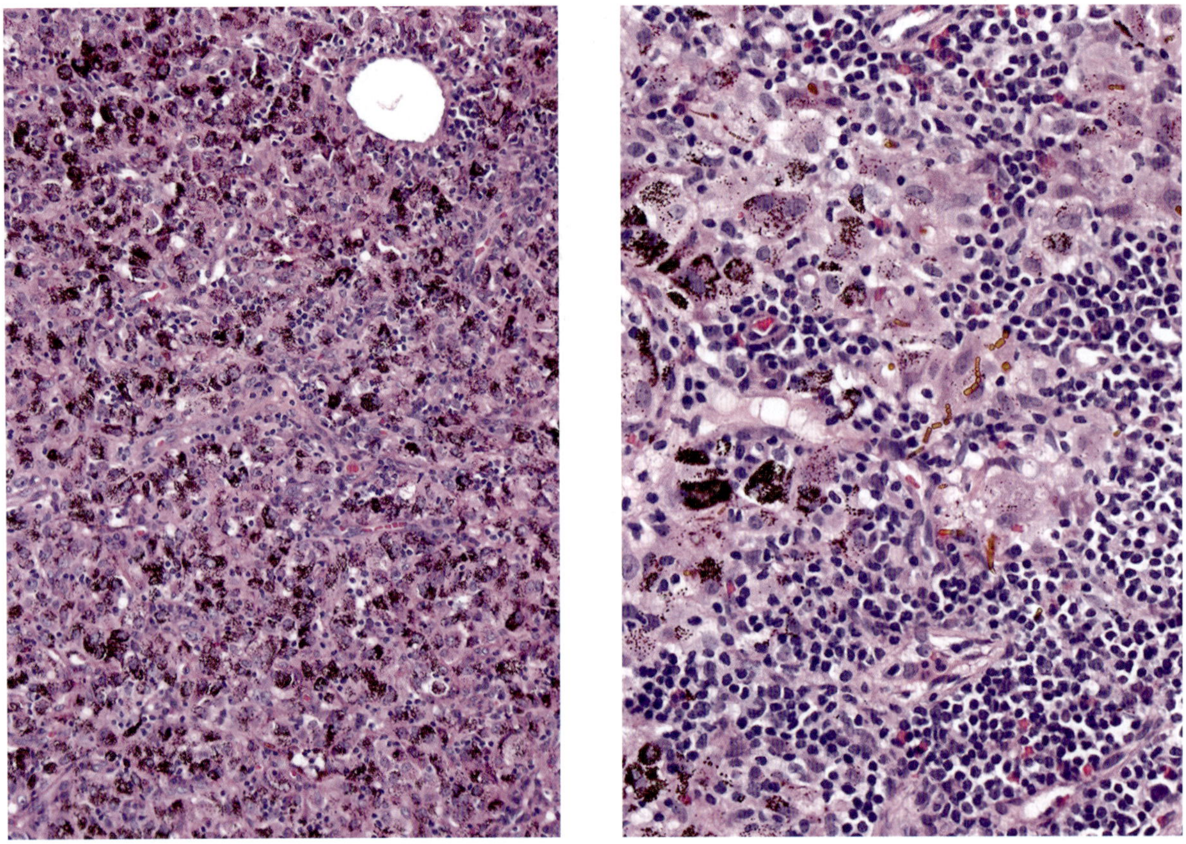

Figure 15-21

ASBESTOS DEPOSITION, LYMPH NODE

An anthracotic lymph node (left) harbors small, geometric fragments of asbestos (right). (Courtesy of Victor Roggli, Durham, NC.)

Treatment and Prognosis. While individuals from the general population may have small numbers of asbestos bodies, the highest levels are seen in asbestos workers with occupational exposure (16). While the presence of asbestos bodies does not equate with asbestosis, high levels of asbestos bodies in pulmonary hilar lymph nodes suggest a high lung burden of asbestos bodies (78). Histologic sections of lung showing greater than or equal to 0.5 asbestos bodies/cm^2 confirm an asbestos-related mesothelioma (100). Individual prognosis ultimately relates to the asbestos-related disease the patient has, if any.

SILICOSIS

Definition. Pulmonary silicosis can spread *silicotic lesions* to the liver, spleen, bone marrow, and lymph nodes via hematogenous and lymphatic channels (86).

General Features. Inhalation of silica (crystalline silicon dioxide) causes silicosis, an occupational lung disease characterized by progressive, nodular fibrosing pneumoconiosis, which develops after many years of exposure. Silica occurs in crystalline and amorphous forms, with the former being more fibrogenic, especially quartz. After silica particles are inhaled, they interact with macrophages and epithelial cells to cause pulmonary fibrosis. Silica causes macrophages to activate and release cell mediators which cause more damage. The fibrotic lesions typical of silicosis in the lung are also seen in the pleura and hilar lymph nodes. Calcification in lymph nodes gives an "eggshell" appearance on radiographs. Extrathoracic silicosis is rare.

Clinical Features. Silicosis is one of the most common chronic occupational lung diseases, typically described in coal miners or in

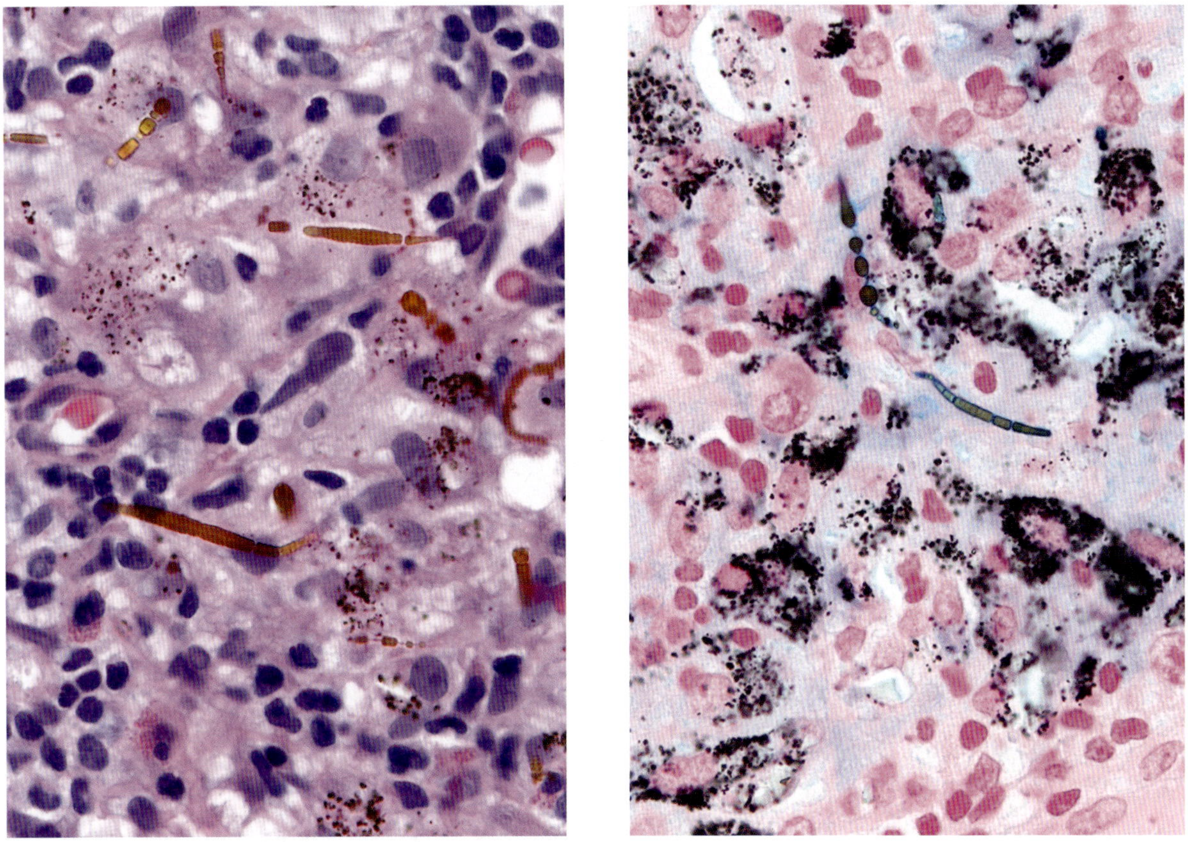

Figure 15-22

ASBESTOS DEPOSITION, LYMPH NODE

Left: Higher magnification of figure 15-21 shows the unusual shapes of the deposited asbestos. Right: Iron stain is positive (Prussian blue stain). (Courtesy of Victor Roggli, Durham, NC.)

other occupations associated with silica dust. In asymptomatic patients, disease is detected on routine chest radiograph, which shows fine nodularity in the upper zones of the lung. Shortness of breath is a late feature of this slowly progressive disease.

Extrathoracic silicosis has been described infrequently in the European and English language literature, but is nicely summarized by Slavin et al. (86). Patients ranged from 25 to 72 years in age, with a male predominance. All had occupations, where stated, that exposed them to silica (e.g., miners, sand blasters). Exposure to silica varied from 0.2 years in a patient who inhaled cleanser as a child to 30 years in a sandblaster. The majority of patients had spleen, liver, and multiple lymph node sites involved by disease. Peripheral adenopathy attributable to silicosis was also present.

Microscopic Findings. Under polarized microscopy, silicotic nodules are composed of concentric layers of hyalinized collagen with birefringent particles. Three stages have been described in the formation of silicotic nodules in lymph nodes (86). The initial silicotic nodules are collections of macrophages admixed with a few plasma cells, lymphocytes, and occasional giant cells. Necrosis may be seen. Intracytoplasmic silica particles, needle-shaped white crystals 1 to 2 μm in length, are present. The second stage shows nodules with a mixture of fibroblasts and macrophages; focal necrosis may be present. The final stage consists of large, relatively acellular sclerohyaline nodules. The centers of these lesions appear acellular, with more normal-appearing fibroblasts at the edges of the nodule. Apoptotic lymphocytes may be present.

The spleen also contains silicotic nodules, located typically between the mantle zone of the white pulp and the central artery. Large sclerohyaline nodules can be seen scattered diffusely throughout the spleen, grossly in some cases. Mixed dust nodules containing silica and other minerals are histologically similar to silicotic nodules.

Ancillary Testing. Transmission and scanning electron microscopy and particle analysis confirm the presence of silica particles. These particles are incorporated into the lysosomes of macrophages (86). The ultrastructural findings show collagen broken down into short and long fragments.

Differential Diagnosis. At extrathoracic sites, silicotic nodules raise a differential diagnosis that includes fibrous histiocytoma (104). The presence of crystals consistent with silica under polarized light, coupled with the appropriate clinical history, should distinguish these two entities.

Treatment and Prognosis. Silicosis is slowly progressive, limiting pulmonary function. The interval from cessation of silica exposure to death in patients with extrathoracic silicosis varies widely from 1 to 34 years (52,75).

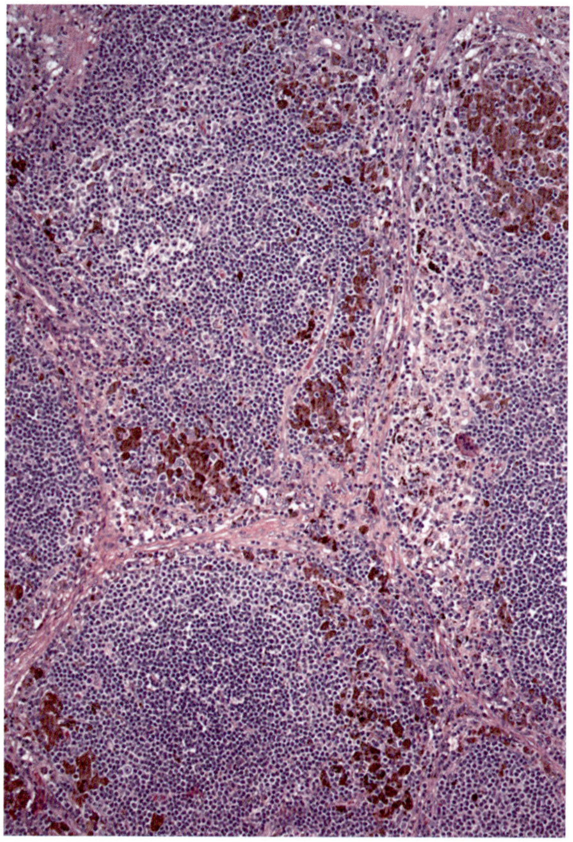

Figure 15-23

HEMOCHROMATOSIS, LYMPH NODE

Deposition of hemosiderin is golden brown.

HEMOCHROMATOSIS

Definition. *Hemochromatosis* is a disease in which increased iron storage causes pathologic changes.

General Features. Hemochromatosis is divided into primary hemochromatosis and secondary hemochromatosis. Primary or hereditary hemochromatosis is most commonly due to mutations in the human leukocyte antigen (HLA)-linked *HFE* gene. Secondary hemochromatosis is the result of transfusion for various disorders that cause anemia. Hemochromatosis of the spleen and lymph nodes has been most commonly reported in patients with thalassemia, due to the transfusion requirements of these patients. One milliliter of red blood cells carries with it 1 mg of iron.

Clinical Features. Increased transfusions result in secondary hemochromatosis, which is due to increased exogenous iron absorption and subsequent iron deposition in multiple organs. In particular, children with beta-thalassemia major require repeated blood transfusions to prevent the associated morbidity and mortality of the disease. Iron deposits within macrophages in multiple organs, including liver, spleen, bowel, adrenal gland, and pancreas (51). Drainage to adjacent lymph nodes causes lymphatic iron deposition (60). CT of organs involved by hemochromatosis shows increased density of tissue (51,60). Increased splenic hemosiderosis correlates with increased splenic weight (69).

Microscopic Findings. The lymph nodes involved by hemochromatosis are enlarged, with expansion of cortical and medullary sinusoids by macrophages containing iron pigment (figs. 15-23, 15-24). Iron pigment is typically brown-green on hematoxylin and eosin (H&E)-stained slides.

Iron deposition in the spleen concentrates in the red pulp with sparing of the white pulp. The sinusoids of the red pulp are highlighted by iron-containing littoral cells.

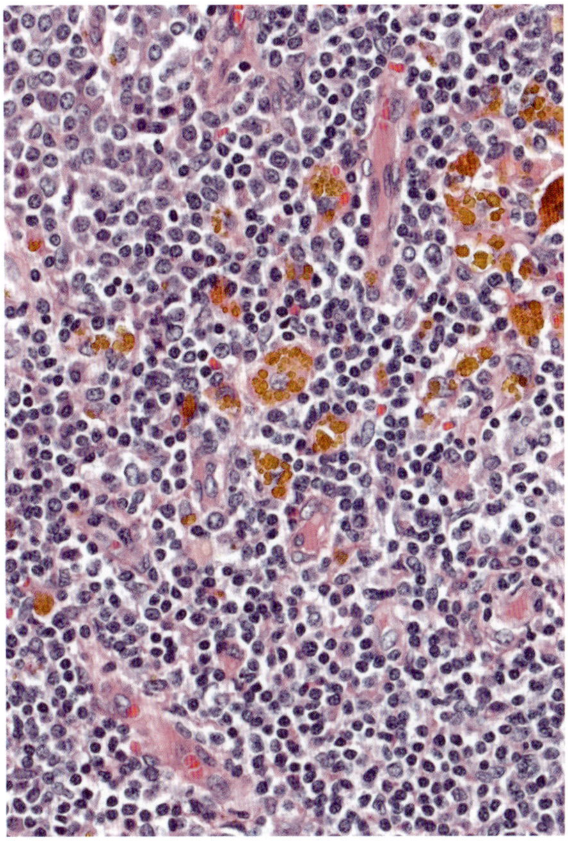

Figure 15-24

HEMOCHROMATOSIS, LYMPH NODE

Iron deposition in lymph node.

Ancillary Testing. A Prussian blue stain confirms the presence of iron, although the clinical history and microscopic appearance are most helpful.

Differential Diagnosis. Heavy pigmentation of lymph nodes from tattoo pigment or metastatic malignant melanoma may mimic hemochromatosis. Tattoo pigment, in general, is black and coarse, and predominantly extracellular. Heavy melanin pigment may obscure accompanying malignant melanoma, although careful examination should reveal the atypical cytologic features. A bleaching procedure and Fontana-Masson stain confirm the presence of melanin pigment.

Treatment and Prognosis. Chelation therapy alleviates the chronic iron overloading of patients (50). New orally active iron chelators, which are easier to use than the typical parenteral deferoxamine, are now in clinical trials (7).

THOROTRAST DEPOSITION

Definition. *Thorotrast*, which contains ^{232}thorium, was used as a contrast medium in the 1930s and 1940s to identify vascular abnormalities in radiology.

General Features. Thorotrast, injected intravascularly, preferentially deposits in liver, spleen, bone marrow, and lymph nodes (103). The effect of thorotrast accumulation in these organs, along with the concomitant radiation to these organs, results in an increased incidence of liver tumors, thorotrastomas, rare splenic vascular lesions, and fibrosis in liver, spleen, and lymph nodes. A long period of latency is observed between the time of thorotrast injection and subsequent pathology (24 to 30 years) (102).

Clinical Features. Thorotrast accumulation in lymph nodes and spleen is now largely a historical finding from a time when intravascular injections of this radioactive medium were used to map the vascular abnormalities of aneurysms, brain tumors, arteriovenous fistulae, and other vascular anomalies. Given the extremely long latency period (20 to 40 years) between injection and subsequent complications, including death, recognition of the effects of thorotrast exposure was delayed (63). Subsequent autopsy and pathologic studies identified the accumulation of large amounts of this radioactive medium surrounded by fibrous tissue located in the area of the original site of injection (thorotrastomas), as well as accumulation of thorotrast in the reticuloendothelial system (102,103).

Microscopic Findings. Thorotrast deposits within the medullary sinuses of lymph nodes and is predominantly extracellular (fig. 15-25). Follicles and germinal structures contain little thorotrast. Hilar lymph nodes show a similar deposition of thorotrast as seen with anthracotic pigment. In lymph nodes containing greater amounts of this contrast medium (periportal and peripancreatic lymph nodes), however, there is both intercellular and intracellular deposition. This is often accompanied by marked fibrosis, which may proceed to complete obliteration of the lymph node, with minimal lymphoid tissue remaining (103). Malignancy of lymph nodes is rare.

In the spleen, thorotrast accumulates within the red pulp. Aggregates of thorotrast accumulate around the trabeculae, and may be associated

Figure 15-25

THOROTRAST DEPOSITION

A: The dark granular material is thorotrast.

B: The spleen is extensively fibrotic due to thorotrast deposition.

C: Intracellularly, thorotrast is associated with perivascular fibrosis (trichrome stain). (Courtesy of Kurt Wegener, Heidelberg, Germany.)

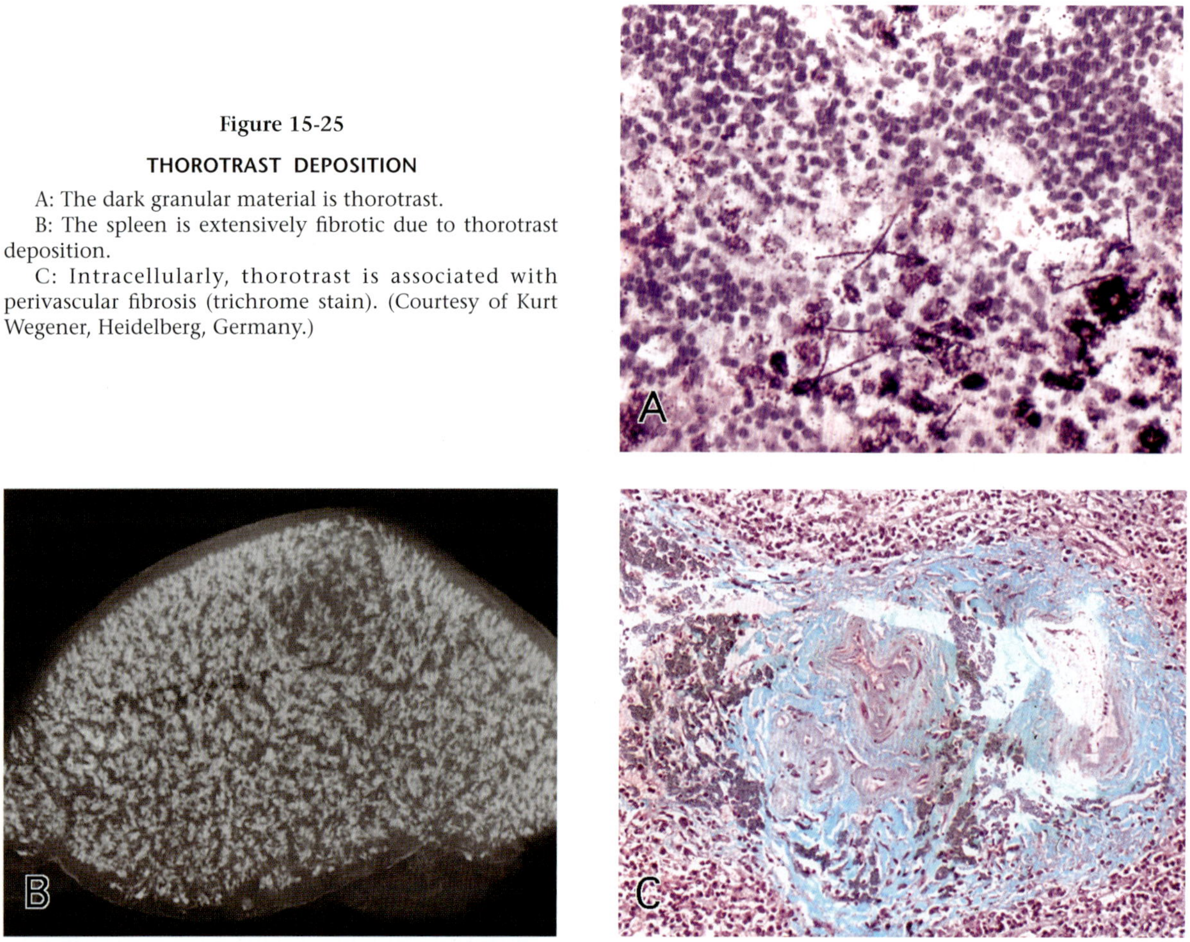

with fibrosis and intimal thickening of arteries. This leads to splenic atrophy, with organ weights of 20 to 30 g (102). Rarely, primary vascular tumors are described in the spleen, including a hemangioendothelioma (102).

Ancillary Testing. While increased fibrosis is readily identified on H&E-stained specimens, additional stains to highlight fibrosis, such as reticulin and trichrome stains, are useful. Specialized methods of detecting thorotrast include autoradiography and neutron activating analysis (103).

Differential Diagnosis. Other foreign materials may accumulate in lymph nodes, including talc and anthracotic material, but these have a different morphologic appearance when compared to thorotrast.

Treatment and Prognosis. Given the widespread deposition of thorotrast within the body, there is no specific treatment.

TALC DEPOSITION

Definition. *Disseminated talc granulomatosis* is the deposition of talc crystals in multiple organs, including lymph nodes and spleen, and found in intravenous drug users.

General Features. Intravenous drug users who may or may not be immunocompromised, inject suspensions of tablets intended for oral use which contain insoluble fillers such as talc, potato starch, maize starch, microcrystalline cellulose, magnesium stearate, siliciumoxid, and cotton fibers (42). These insoluble particles are disseminated intravenously and lodge in various organs listed from highest to lowest frequency: lung, spleen, lymph nodes, liver, bone marrow, heart, and kidney (42). Birefringent material is found more frequently in portal lymph nodes than in hilar lymph nodes. Birefringent crystals are often present in microscopic emboli throughout the body and a granulomatous reaction may be seen.

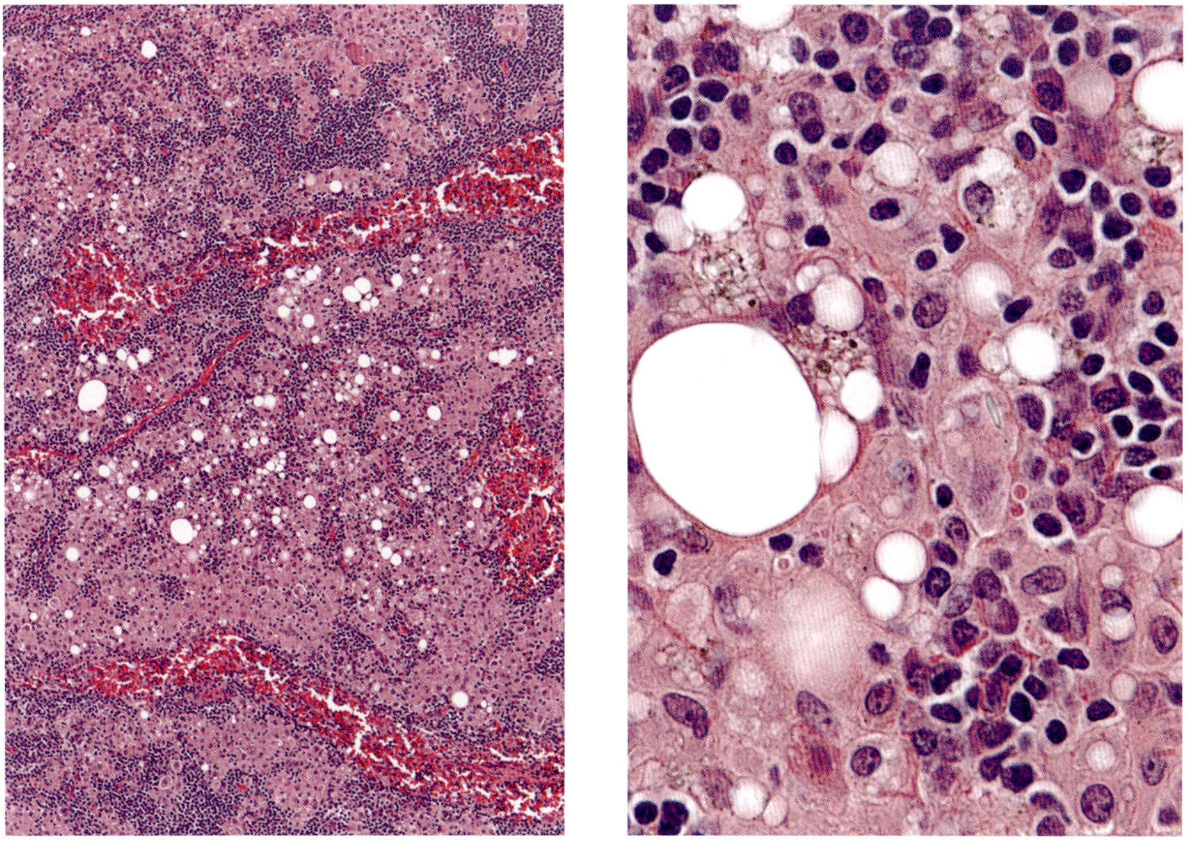

Figure 15-26

TALC DEPOSITION, LYMPH NODE

Left: In this lymph node from an intravenous drug user, low magnification shows extensive granulomas.

Right: High magnification shows epithelioid macrophages, some with ingested crystals, presumably talc, a common contaminant of street drugs.

Clinical Features. Intravenous drug users are at high risk for human immunodeficiency virus (HIV) and infectious diseases such as tuberculosis (50,55). Patients may present with constitutional symptoms including fever, dyspnea, weakness, night sweats, lymphadenopathy, and weight loss.

Laboratory Findings. In immunocompromised patients, laboratory findings typical of a specific disease may be found. Similarly, patients with concurrent infections may or may not show positive microbiology cultures. One patient with miliary tuberculosis was anergic when PPD (purified protein derivative) was administered and had multiple negative cultures for mycobacteria, but at autopsy caseating granulomas with *Mycobacterium tuberculosis* were found (55).

Microscopic Findings. Granulomas consisting of macrophages, foreign body giant cells, lymphocytes, and plasma cells are typically seen in the lungs in reaction to talc and other injected foreign materials. Colorless needle-shaped and flat birefringent crystals may be seen individually and in clusters within macrophages and giant cells (fig. 15-26). Talc (magnesium silicate) crystals are usually 5 to 15 µm in length and white under polarized light (42). Intracellular crystals may be seen in organs without an accompanying granulomatous reaction in spleen and lymph nodes (42). Caseous necrosis and areas of dense fibrosis were described in a patient with concomitant tuberculosis (55). Fine needle aspiration of a peripheral lymph node involved by talc granulomatosis revealed granulomas features, including epithelioid macrophages, lymphocytes, giant cells, and multiple birefringent crystals under polarized light (34).

Ancillary Testing. Examination of tissue under polarized light is essential, even in the absence of granulomas. Polarized light highlights the birefringent crystals of talc, which are irregular and needle-like. Other foreign material, such as starch, may also be present. PAS staining is negative in the majority of filler materials, including talc, except for potato starch, maize starch, and microcrystalline cellulose (42). Scanning electron microscopy and energy dispersive X-ray analysis demonstrate the crystal structure and the crystal composition, respectively (55).

Differential Diagnosis. The differential diagnosis of granulomatous reactions is large and includes acid-fast and fungal infections, reactions to foreign materials, and granulomatous reactions secondary to malignancies and autoimmune diseases. Examination of tissue under polarized light is critical in identifying the crystalline foreign material.

Treatment and Prognosis. The prognosis of intravenous drug users with systemic talc granulomatosis is poor, and complicated by multiple factors including concurrent infections, malnourishment, and recidivism.

SYNTHETIC POLYMER DEPOSITION

Definition. *Synthetic polymers*, most notably polyvinylpyrrolidone (PVP), may deposit within macrophages in lymph nodes.

General Features. PVP is a synthetic polymer that was widely used as both a plasma expander and a vehicle for parenteral drug administration. Deposition of PVP in macrophages of the lymphoreticular system is a well-recognized, albeit rare, phenomenon. Teflon© (polytetrafluoroethylene) was briefly used as an injectable material for larynx and vocal cords. Although "chemically inert," the material does induce a striking foreign body reaction in regional tissues and lymph nodes (fig. 15-27).

Microscopic Findings. The sinuses and interfollicular regions of involved lymph nodes show a proliferation of macrophages that contain basophilic, homogeneous globules (fig. 15-28) (90).

Ancillary Testing. The presence of PVP in tissue sections is supported by intense positivity for mucicarmine (mucicarmine histiocytosis) and Congo red (fig. 15-29). Immunohistochemical and histochemical studies directed at macrophages (CD68, CD163, lysozyme) help in excluding metastatic carcinoma and confirming the presence of macrophages. Mucicarminophilic histiocytosis with signet ring cell morphology was reported in Taiwan in association with PVP deposition, secondary to intravenous fluids containing PVP (43).

Differential Diagnosis. Sinusoidal infiltration by PVP-containing macrophages simulates storage diseases such as Gaucher or Niemann-Pick disease, as well as metastatic carcinoma. Although the storage disorders rarely present with lymphadenopathy, incidental lymph node involvement may be noted (90). The macrophages in Gaucher disease are large, with abundant pale cytoplasm, and show the characteristic striations that resemble wrinkled tissue paper. They are weakly positive with iron and PAS stains. Clinicopathologic correlation is essential for the diagnosis of Gaucher disease. These patients usually present with splenomegaly and hematologic abnormalities and may have associated dysproteinemias (85).

The macrophages in Niemann-Pick disease have foamy or bubbly appearing cytoplasm without striations. These cells are characteristically positive for oil red O and Sudan B black stains. The oxidation of sphingomyelin results in a brownish yellow ceroid protein that is PAS and acid-fast positive (90). Niemann-Pick disease is diagnosed by the documentation of sphingomyelinase deficiency in peripheral blood leukocytes (25).

PVP involvement in lymph nodes can also simulate signet ring adenocarcinoma. In one case, a supraclavicular lymph node with mesothelial inclusions and mucicarmine-positive material, consistent with PVP, was reported as a simulator of metastatic carcinoma (28).

Treatment and Prognosis. PVP is an incidental finding requiring no treatment.

TATTOO PIGMENT/ ANTHRACOSIS/LIPOFUSCIN DEPOSITION

Definition. Reactive lymph nodes can contain pigment from a variety of sources, including, but not limited to *tattoos, anthracosis*, and *lipofuscin deposition. Anthracosilicosis* (silica and coal dust) has been described in the spleen (3,48).

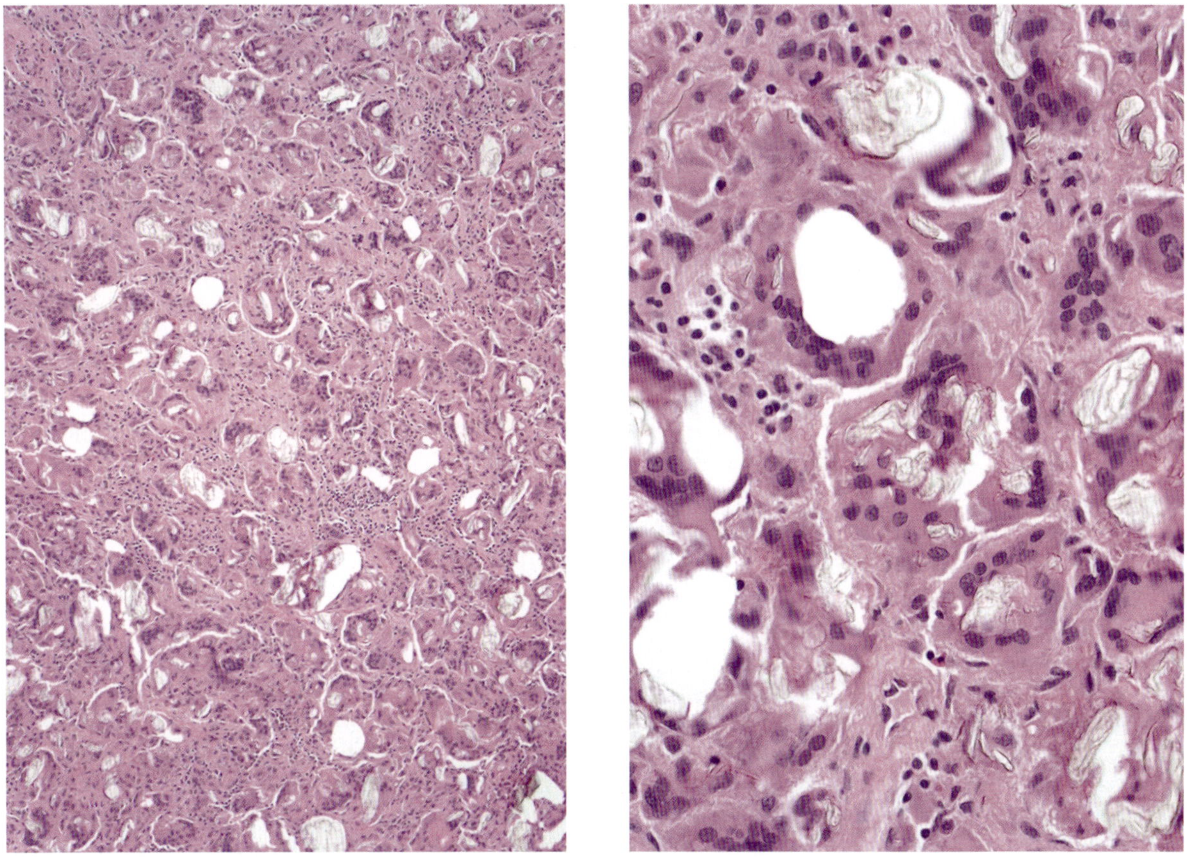

Figure 15-27

REACTION TO TEFLON©, LYMPH NODE

Left: A remarkable foreign body reaction is seen in this cervical lymph node of a patient who had vocal cord injection of Teflon.

Right: The offending material is seen within macrophages.

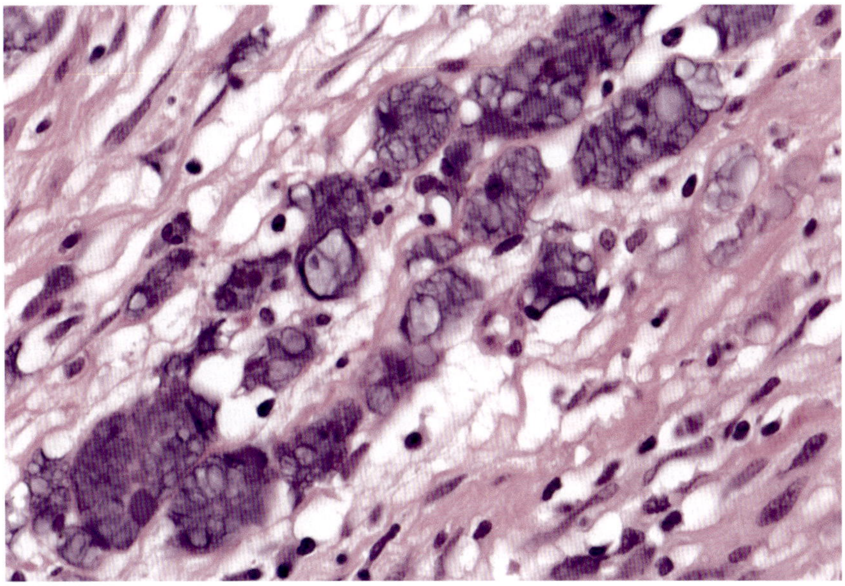

Figure 15-28

POLYVINYLPYRROLIDONE (PVP) DEPOSITION, LYMPH NODE

PVP-containing macrophages in a lymph node sinus.

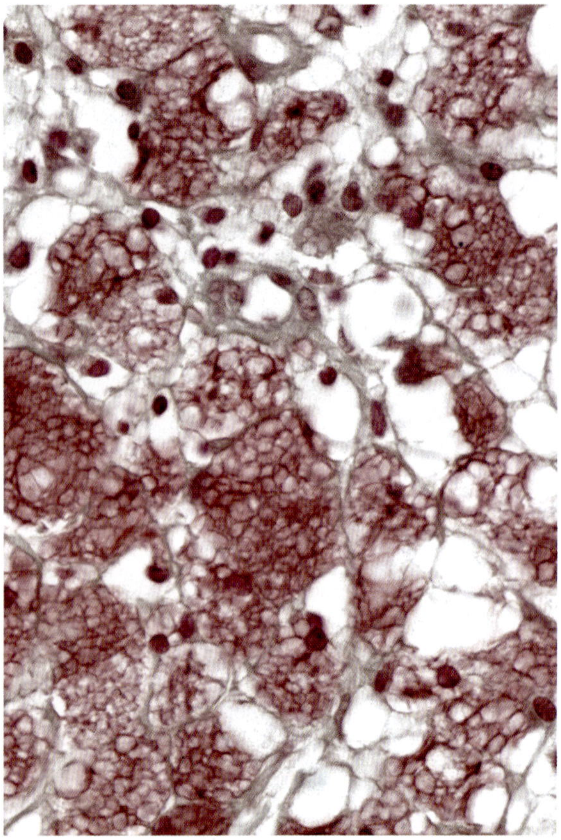

Figure 15-29

POLYVINYLPYRROLIDONE (PVP) DEPOSITION, CONGO RED

Congo red stains PVP-containing macrophages.

General Features. Pigment in lymph nodes may mimic metastatic malignancies, especially malignant melanoma. Thus, it is important to recognize reactive lymphadenopathies that may also show pigment. This includes tattoo pigment in sentinel lymph nodes (21,81), anthracosis (41), unusual anthracotic and anthracosilicotic pseudotumors of lymph nodes (3), lipofuscin pigment (35), and pigmented granulomatous reaction to arthroplastic joints (107). This latter phenomenon, also known as postarthroplasty histiocytic lymphadenopathy, is discussed earlier in this chapter. Anthracotic pigment has been described in the liver and spleen of coal workers (48).

Clinical Features. A common theme in all of these disorders is pigment migration through the lymphatic system to regional lymph nodes and, in some cases, liver and spleen. This results in macroscopic gray-black lymph nodes, which may or may not be enlarged. Thus, the gross appearance of a pigmented lymph node is not pathognomonic for metastatic melanoma.

Patients with primary melanoma and tattoo pigment in sentinel lymph nodes have decorative tattoos in the vicinity of the melanoma (22,81). Dynamic dermatolymphoscintigraphy identifies deeply pigmented lymph nodes. The presence of pigment is suspicious for metastatic melanoma, but the morphologic features of melanoma should not be present.

In patients with anthracosis, intrapulmonary lymph nodes are rare, but when detected clinically and biopsied show prominent anthracosis and often silicosis. A constant clinical feature in patients with lymph node anthracosis is cigarette smoking (41). Many patients also have a history of asbestos exposure or other work-related exposure to inorganic dust. The deposition of black anthracotic pigment in coal miners' lungs has been well described in the literature (27). This pigment may also be seen in the liver (10 percent) and spleen (about 20 percent) of coal workers (48). Increased tissue pigmentation shows a positive correlation with age at death, years underground, and severity of pneumoconiosis, suggesting that the cumulative exposure to coal mine dust is the most important factor in extrapulmonary pigment deposition (48). Interestingly, in an autopsy study of 108 coal workers, cigarette smoking negatively correlated with pigmentation in liver and spleen (48).

Reactive mediastinal spindle cell lesions associated with anthracosis and anthrasilicosis have been described (3). These unusual lesions are present in men aged 43 to 68 years, and are associated with a mediastinal mass, bulky lymphadenopathy, a large perihilar mass found on chest radiograph, and mediastinal nodules identified during coronary bypass graft surgery. Anthracotic pigment was found within the thoracic cavity in three of the five patients studied; interestingly, only two had a history of exposure to silica dusts.

Patients with chronic cholestatic liver disease can develop portal lymphadenopathy associated with the presence of lipofuscin pigment (35).

Gross Findings. Lymph nodes that contain dark pigment from tattoos are usually of normal size, soft, and diffusely pigmented throughout (81). This differs from lymph nodes with metastatic melanoma which range from unremarkable in size and appearance to markedly enlarged, firm, and diffusely discolored. Small black nodules may also be present on the lymph node surface in metastatic melanoma.

Intrapulmonary lymph nodes with anthracosis are typically detected by radiographic techniques as small, noncalcified pulmonary nodules, for which the differential diagnosis includes metastatic malignancy (41). Anthrasilicotic nodules tend to be subpleural and are round, ovoid, or angular. Grossly, the lesions are black nodules less than 1.5 cm in size (41). Anthrasilicotic lesions in the spleen may show multiple calcifications, including eggshell calcifications in adjacent abdominal lymph nodes (96).

Microscopic Findings. Dark carbon pigment may be noted in the macrophages of lymph nodes that are proximal to tattoos (fig. 15-30). The macrophages are bland and lack cytologic atypia.

Anthracotic intrapulmonary lymph nodes show prominent sinus histiocytosis, with macrophages containing anthracotic pigment. Polarized light reveals the presence of silica, which are needle-shaped and birefringent crystals 2 to 4 µm in length (41). The crystals may be extracellular and intracellular; hyalinized silicotic nodules may also have concentric rings of fibrosis. These nodules may extend into adjacent lung, causing mild interstitial pulmonary fibrosis. In coal workers, anthracotic pigment accumulates within macrophages around the trabeculae and marginal zones of the spleen; amorphous masses may form when abundant pigment is present (48). The pigment is uniformly dense and black, but on higher microscopic resolution, multiple individual particles are present ranging from black and round to yellow-brown and angulated. Brightly birefringent needle-shaped particles of silicate may also be seen.

Anthracosilicotic spindle cell pseudotumors of mediastinal lymph nodes have a storiform pattern of spindle cells, and may show perineural involvement and extend through the lymph node capsule (3). These lesions lack cytologic atypia and mitoses, but contain anthracotic pigment within macrophages. Polarizable material consistent with silica can be identified intracellularly and extracellularly. Nodular hyaline scars, typical of silica exposure, are also seen. Fine needle aspiration of these lesions shows bland polygonal and spindle cells containing anthracotic pigment and particles, similar to silica under polarized light (97).

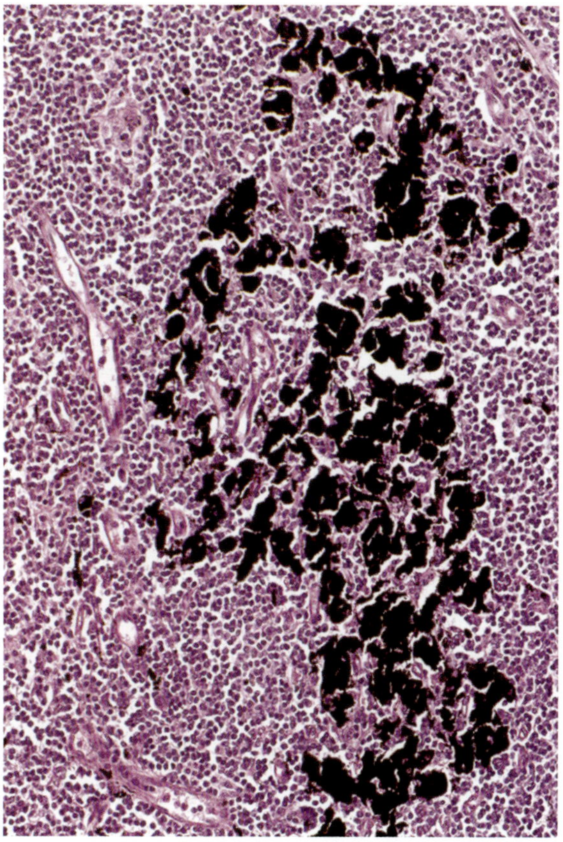

Figure 15-30

TATTOO PIGMENT, LYMPH NODE

Exogenous pigment deposition in the macrophages of a proximal lymph node.

Lipofuscin pigment deposition in lymph nodes features sinus histiocytosis in which brown pigment is noted within the macrophages. Follicular hyperplasia is common. Lipogranulomas in the medullary sinus, as well as epithelioid cell granulomas, may be seen.

Other substances that may be present in the lymph nodes of patients with chronic liver disease include ceroid pigment (Hamazaki-Wesenberg bodies), hemosiderin, and copper-associated protein (35). Hamazaki-Wesenberg bodies are characteristically associated with sarcoid lymphadenopathy (80), but are also

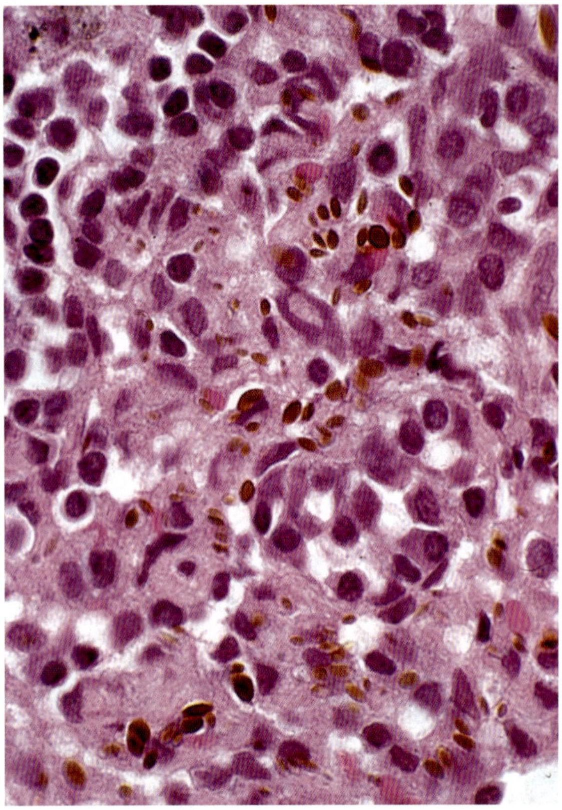

Figure 15-31

HAMAZAKI-WESENBERG BODIES

Brown yeast-like structures in a hilar lymph node of a patient with lung carcinoma.

seen in reactive lymph nodes that are adjacent to tumors. They represent giant extracellular lysosomes and appear as pigmented, budding "yeast-like" structures that are located near the peripheral sinuses (fig. 15-31).

Ancillary Testing. The carbon pigment associated with tattoos is not highlighted by silver stains and resists bleaching. Polarized light microscopy of intrapulmonary anthracotic lymph nodes shows the birefringent crystals characteristic of silica; similar crystals are seen in anthracosis of the spleen in coal workers as well as in anthracosilicotic spindle cell pseudotumors of mediastinal lymph nodes. These spindle cells mark with antibodies against CD68 and a subset of cells stain for smooth and common muscle actin; S-100 protein staining is limited to occasional cells with the appearance of dendritic cells.

Differential Diagnosis. The differential diagnosis of pigment in lymph nodes (Table 15-3) should always include metastatic malignant melanoma and trigger a pavlovian response of a search for atypical cytology and frequent mitoses. Melanin granules of melanoma are usually finely granular and dark brown in melanoma cells, but may be coarser in macrophages. Melanin granules are highlighted by silver stains and decolorized by bleaching agents. Immunohistochemical stains such as S-100 protein, HMB45, and melan A highlight the atypical melanocytes of melanoma. For some pigmented lymph node lesions, including anthracotic and anthracosilicotic lesions, polarized birefringent needle-shaped crystals of silica are present. The clinical history may or may not elicit a history of industrial exposure. Patients with lipofuscin pigment deposition in lymph nodes have a history of liver disease and the deposition occurs in the portal lymph nodes; the pigment is also brown. Pigmented postarthroplasty histiocytic lymphadenopathy typically shows foamy macrophages in a sinus pattern containing wear particles of metal, polyethylene, and cement origin; a history of total joint arthroplasty is present. Metal particles are small, less than 1 µm, and seen as refractile, black, irregular particles present in the cytoplasm of macrophages. Hemosiderin deposition also causes dark pigment, but a Prussian blue stain for iron should distinguish this readily if the histology is not clear.

The anthracotic and anthracosilicotic spindle cell pseudotumors of mediastinal lymph nodes mimic a different spectrum of disorders due to the spindled nature of these lesions (3). The lack of cytologic atypia, lack of mitoses, and presence of foreign material should distinguish this disorder from spindle cell neoplasms such as follicular dendritic cell tumor, intranodal hemorrhagic spindle cell tumor with amianthoid fibers, spindle cell metastatic melanoma, spindle cell carcinoma, Kaposi sarcoma, fibrosing mediastinitis, and inflammatory pseudotumor. Infectious diseases, including leprosy and atypical mycobacteria, can also mimic a spindle cell appearance of macrophages (54,106).

Treatment and Prognosis. There is no effective treatment to reverse the pigment deposition of these various disorders. It is the prognosis of

Table 15-3

DIFFERENTIAL DIAGNOSIS OF PIGMENTED LYMPH NODES WITH DISCRIMINATING HISTOLOGIC, HISTOCHEMICAL, AND IMMUNOHISTOCHEMICAL FEATURES

Disorder	Pigment	Atypical Cytology	Polarization	Special Stains
Metastatic melanoma	Melanin	Yes	No	S-100 protein, HMB45, Melan A
Tattoo pigment deposition	Carbon	No	No	None
Anthracosis	Carbon	No	Yes[a]	None
Lipofuscin deposition	Lipofuscin	No	No	None
Postarthroplasty lymphadenopathy	Metal, polyethylene, cement	No	Yes[b]	Modified oil red O
Hemochromatosis	Iron	No	No	Prussian blue

[a]Polarization of anthracotic lymph nodes may reveal birefringent, needle-shaped particles consistent with silica.
[b]Polarization of postarthroplasty lymph nodes typically shows needle-like or thread-like birefringent shapes of 10 or 20 μm consistent with polyethylene particles.

any associated disorder, such as coexistent pulmonary disease in patients with intrapulmonary anthracotic lymph nodes or anthracosis due to coal miners' dust, that is important. The spindle cell pseudotumors of mediastinal lymph nodes associated with anthracosis and anthracosilicosis appear benign, with no progression of disease during follow-up.

REFERENCES

1. Al Rikabi AC, Naddaf HO, al Balla SR, al Sohaibani MO. Proteinaceous lymphadenopathy in a patient with known rheumatoid arthritis—case report and review of the literature. Br J Rheumatol 1995;34:1087-9.
2. Albores-Saavedra J, Vuitch F, Delgado R, Wiley E, Hagler H. Sinus histiocytosis of pelvic lymph nodes after hip replacement. A histiocytic proliferation induced by cobalt-chromium and titanium. Am J Surg Pathol 1994;18:83-90.
3. Argani P, Ghossein R, Rosai J. Anthracotic and anthracosilicotic spindle cell pseudotumors of mediastinal lymph nodes: report of five cases of a reactive lesion that simulates malignancy. Hum Pathol 1998;29:851-5.
4. Banerjee D, Mills DM, Hearn SA, Meek M, Turner KL. Proteinaceous lymphadenopathy due to monoclonal nonamyloid immunoglobulin deposit disease. Arch Pathol Lab Med 1990;114:34-9.
5. Benjamin E, Ahmed A, Rashid AT, Wright DH. Silicone lymphadenopathy: a report of two cases, one with concomitant malignant lymphoma. Diagn Histopathol 1982;5:133-41.
6. Benz EB, Sherburne B, Hayek J, Falchuk KH, Sledge CV, Spector M. Lymphadenopathy associated with total joint prostheses. A report of two cases and a review of the literature. J Bone Joint Surg 1996;78:588-93.
7. Beutler E, Hoffbrand AV, Cook JD. Iron deficiency and overload. Hematology Am Soc Heamatol Educ Program 2003:40-61.
8. Bjornsson BL, Truong LD, Cartwright J Jr, Abrams J, Rutledge ML, Wheeler TM. Pelvic lymph node histiocytosis mimicking metastatic prostatic adenocarcinoma: association with hip prostheses. J Urol 1995;154:470-3.
9. Boitnott JK, Margolis S. Mineral oil in human tissues. II. Oil droplets in lymph nodes of the porta hepatis. Bull Johns Hopkins Hosp 1966;118:414-22.
10. Boitnott JK, Margolis S. Saturated hydrocarbons in human tissues: 3. Oil droplets in the liver and spleen. Johns Hopkins Med J 1970;127:65-78.
11. Boman F, Boccon-Gibod L. Benign epithelial cells and Tamm-Horsfall protein in lymph nodes from nephrectomy specimens with nephroblastoma: a diagnostic pitfall. Ann Pathol 2004;24:632-6.
12. Bos I, Johannisson R. Foreign body reactions in lymph nodes of oncology patients with joint prostheses—light-, electron microscopic and immunohistological investigations. Path Res Pract 2004;200:189-96.

13. Buxbaum J, Gallo G. Nonamyloidotic monoclonal immunoglobulin deposition disease. Light-chain, heavy-chain, and light- and heavy-chain deposition diseases. Hematol Oncol Clin North Am 1999;13:1235-48.
14. Castellino RA. Observations on the "reactive (follicular) hyperplasia" as encountered in repeat lymphography in the lymphomas. Cancer 1974;34:2042-50.
15. Chittal SM, Caveriviere P, Voigt JJ, et al. Follicular lymphoma with abundant PAS-positive extracellular material. Immunohistochemical and ultrastructural observations. Am J Surg Pathol 1987;11:618-24.
16. Churg AM, Warnock ML. Asbestos and other ferruginous bodies: their formation and clinical significance. Am J Pathol 1981;102:447-56.
17. Cockayne SE, Lee JA, Harrington CI. Oleogranulomatous response in lymph nodes associated with emollient use in Netherton's syndrome. Br J Dermatol 1999;141:562-4.
18. Cooper CS, Donovan JF, Terrell RB, Cohen MB, Winfield HN. Hip and knee replacement as a relative contraindication to laparascopic pelvic lymph node dissection. J Urol 1997;158:128-30.
19. Cruickshank B, Thomas MJ. Mineral oil (follicular) lipidosis: II. Histologic studies of spleen, liver, lymph nodes, and bone marrow. Hum Pathol 1984;15:731-7.
20. Dudorkinova D, Povysil C, Tomanova R. Histiocytosis of regional lymph nodes associated with hip replacement. Gen Diagn Pathol 1997;143:197-201.
21. Enzinger FM, Helwig EB. Whipples's disease: a review of the literature and report of fifteen patients. Virchows Arch Pathol Anat Physiol Klin Med 1963;336:238-69.
22. Friedman T, Westreich M, Mozes SN, Dorenbaum A, Herman O. Tattoo pigment in lymph nodes mimicking metastatic malignant melanoma. Plast Reconstr Surg 2003;111:2120-2.
23. Forest M, Carlioz A, Vacher Lavenu MC, et al. Histological patterns of bone and articular tissues after orthopaedic reconstructive surgery (artificial joint implants). Pathol Res Pract 1991;187:963-77.
24. Frischbier HJ. Studies on the effect on the tissues of oily contrast media. In: Ruttimann A, ed. Progress in lymphology: proceedings of the international symposium on lymphology, Zurich, Switzerland, July 19-23, 1966. Stuttgart, George Thieme Verlag; 1967:331.
25. Gal AE, Brady RO, Hibbert SR, Pentchev PG. A practical chromogenic procedure for the detection of homozygotes and heterozygous carriers of Niemann-Pick disease. N Engl J Med 1975;293:632-6.
26. Gray MH, Talbert ML, Talbert WM, Bansal M, Hsu A. Changes seen in lymph nodes draining the sites of large joint prostheses. Am J Surg Pathol 1989;13:1050-6.
27. Green FH, Laquer WA. Coal workers' pneumoconiosis. Pathol Annu 1980;15:333-410.
28. Groisman GM, Amar M, Weiner P, Zamir D. Mucicarminophilic histiocytosis (benign signet-ring cells) and hyperplastic mesothelial cells: two mimics of metastatic carcinoma within a single lymph node. Arch Pathol Lab Med 1998;122:282-4.
29. Guz G, Ozdemir BH, Sezer S, et al. High frequency of amyloid lymphadenopathy in uremic patients. Ren Fail 2000;22:613-21.
30. Hardt NS, Yu LT, La Torre G, Steinbach B. Fourier transform microspectroscopy used to identify foreign materials related to breast implants. Mod Pathol 1994;7:669-76.
31. Harrison CV. Lymph nodes after lymphangiography. In: Harrison CV, ed. Recent advances in pathology, ed 8. London: J & A Churchill, Ltd; 1966:221-3.
32. Henneberger PK, Goe SK, Miller WE, Doney B, Groce DW. Industries in the United States with airborne beryllium exposure and estimates of the number of current workers potentially exposed. J Occup Environ Hyg 2004;1:648-59.
33. Hicks DG, Judkins AR, Sickel JZ, Rosier RN, Puzas JE, O'Keefe RJ. Granular histiocytosis of pelvic lymph nodes following total hip arthroplasty. The presence of wear debris, cytokine production, and immunologically activated macrophages. J Bone Joint Surg 1996;78:482-96.
34. Housini I, Dabbs DJ, Coyne L. Fine needle aspiration cytology of talc granulomatosis in a peripheral lymph node in a case of suspected intravenous drug abuse. Acta Cytologica 1989;34:342-4.
35. Hübscher SG, Harrison RF. Portal lymphadenopathy associated with lipofuscin in chronic cholestatic liver disease. J Clin Pathol 1989;42:1160-5.
36. Jones D, Bhatia VK, Krausz T, Pinkus GS. Crystal-storing histiocytosis: a disorder occurring in plasmacytic tumors expressing immunoglobulin kappa light chain. Hum Pathol 1999;30:1441-8.
37. Kahn H, Strauchen JA, Gilbert HS, Fuchs A. Immunoglobulin-related amyloidosis presenting as recurrent isolated lymph node involvement. Arch Pathol Lab Med 1991;115:948-50.
38. Katzin WE, Centeno JA, Feng LJ, Kiley M, Mullick FG. Pathology of lymph nodes from patients with breast implants: a histologic and spectroscopic evaluation. Am J Surg Pathol 2005;29:506-11.
39. Kidder LH, Kalasinsky VF, Luke JL, Levin IW, Lewis EN. Visualization of silicone gel in human breast tissue using new infrared imaging spectroscopy. Nat Med 1997;3:235-7.

40. Ko HS, Davidson JW, Pruzanski W. Amyloid lymphadenopathy. Ann Intern Med 1976;85:763-4.
41. Kradin RL, Spirn PW, Mark EJ. Intrapulmonary lymph nodes: clinical, radiologic, and pathologic features. Chest 1985;87:662-7.
42. Kringsholm B, Christoffersen P. The nature and the occurrence of birefringent material in different organs in fatal drug addiction. Forensic Sci Int 1987;34:53-62.
43. Kuo TT, Hsueh S. Mucicarminophilic histiocytosis: a polyvinylpyrrolidone (PVP) storage disease simulating signet-ring cell carcinoma. Am J Surg Pathol 1984;8:419-28.
44. Kutlay S, Hasan T, Keven K, Nergizoglu G, Ates K, Karatan O. Primary amyloidosis presenting with massive generalized lymphadenopathy. Leuk Lymphoma 2002; 43:1501-3.
45. Lanzafame S, Magro G, Buffone N, Emmanuele C, Cirino E. Localized primary amyloidosis of axillary lymph nodes. Histopathology 1996;28:369-71.
46. Lazaro MA, Garcia-Morteo D, de Benyacar MA, et al. Lymphadenopathy secondary to silicone hand joint prosthese. Clin Exp Rheumatol 1990;8:17-22.
47. Lebeau A, Zeindl-Eberhart E, Muller EC, et al. Generalized crystal-storing histiocytosis associated with monoclonal gammopathy: molecular analysis of a disorder with rapid clinical course and review of the literature. Blood 2002;100:1817-27.
48. LeFevre ME, Green FH, Joel DD, Laqueur W. Frequency of black pigment in livers and spleens of coal workers: correlation with pulmonary pathology and occupational information. Hum Pathol 1982;13:1121-6.
49. Leon MB, Jeffrey SB, Bacharach SL, et al. Detection of early cardiac dysfunction in patients with severe beta-thalassemia and chronic iron overload. N Engl J Med 1979;301:1143-8.
50. Lewis JH, Sundeen JT, Simon GL, et al. Disseminated talc granulomatosis. An unusual finding in a patient with acquired immunodeficiency syndrome and fatal cytomegalovirus infection. Arch Pathol Lab Med 1985;109:147-50.
51. Long JA Jr, Doppman JL, Nienhus AW, Mills SR. Computed tomographic analysis of beta-thalassemic syndromes with hemochromatosis: pathologic findings with clinical and laboratory correlations. J Comput Assist Tomogr 1980:4:159-65.
52. Lynch KM. Silicosis of systemic distribution. Am J Pathol 1942;18:313-21.
53. MacKenzie DH. Amyloidosis presenting as lymphadenopathy. Br Med J 1963;2:1449-50.
54. Mansfield RE. Histoid leprosy. Arch Pathol 1969;87:580-5.
55. Mariani-Costantini R, Jannotta FS, Johnson FB. Systemic visceraltalc granulomatosis associated with military tuberculosis in a drug addict. Am J Clin Pathol 1982;78:785-9.
56. McCluggage WG, Bharucha H. Lymph node hyalinization in rheumatoid arthritis and systemic sclerosis. J Clin Pathol 1994;47:138-42.
57. McNearney T, Haque A, Wen J, Lisse J. Inguinal lymph node foreign body granulomas after placement of a silicone rubber (Silflex) implant of the first metatarsophalangeal joint. J Rheumatol 1996;23:1449-52.
58. Meyer KC. Beryllium and lung disease. Chest 1994;106:942-6.
59. Michaeli J, Niesvizky R, Siegel D, Ladanyi M, Lieberman PH, Filippa DA. Proteinaceous (angiocentric sclerosing) lymphadenopathy: a polyclonal systemic, nonamyloid deposition disorder. Blood 1995;86:1159-62.
60. Mitnick JS, Bosniak MA, Megibow AJ, et al. CT in B-thalassemia: iron deposition in the liver, spleen, and lymph nodes. AJR Am J Roentgenol 1981:136:1191-4.
61. Morinaga S, Watanabe H, Gemma A, et al. Plasmacytoma of the lung associated with nodular depositions of immunoglobulin. Am J Surg Pathol 1987;11:989-95.
62. Munichor M, Cohen H, Volpin G, Kerner H, Iancu TC. Chromium-induced lymph node histiocytic proliferation after hip replacement Acta Cytol 2003:47:270-4.
63. Muth H, Heyer J, van Kaick G, et al. Results of biophysical and clinical examination of thorotrast patients and their importance for better knowledge about radiation late effects: 4, U.N. international conference peaceful use of atomic energy, Geneva 1971;6-16.
64. Naschitz JE, Yeshururn D, Kuknreich E, Pick AI, Boss J. Isolated amyloid lymphadenopathy. Acta Haematol 1984;72:274-9.
65. Newland JR, Linke RP, Lennert K. Amyloid deposits in lymph nodes: a morphologic and immunohistochemical study. Hum Pathol 1986;17:1245-9.
66. Newman LS. Beryllium disease and sarcoidosis: clinical and laboratory links. Sarcoidosis 1995;12:7-19.
67. Newman LS, Kreiss K, King TE Jr, Seay S, Campbell PA. Pathologic and immunologic alterations in early stages of beryllium disease. Re-examination of disease definition and natural history. Am Rev Respir Dis 1989;139:1479-86.
68. O'Connell JX, Rosenberg AE. Histiocytic lymphadenitis associated with a large joint prosthesis. Am J Clin Pathol 1993;99:314-6.
69. Okon E, Levij IS, Rachmilewitz EA. Splenectomy, iron overload and liver cirrhosis in beta-thalassemia major. Acta Haematol 1976;56:142-50.

70. Osborne BM, Butler JJ, Mackay B. Proteinaceous lymphadenopathy with hypergammagllbulinema. Am J Surg Pathol 1979;3:137-45.
71. Oyaizu N, Shikata N, Tsubura A, Morii S, Taniguchi N, Miura K. Systemic amyloidosis with a mesenteric mass which had the appearance of proteinaceous lymphadenopathy. Acta Pathol Jpn 1987;37:133-9.
72. Peoc'h M, Duprez D, Grice G, Fabre-Bocquentin B, Gressin R, Pasquier B. Silicone lymphadenopathy mimicking a lymphoma in a patient with a metatarsophalangeal joint prosthesis. J Clin Pathol 2000;53:549-51.
73. Philippou S, Mandelartz H. [Detection of asbestos in thoracic lymph nodes in patients with asbestosis.] Pneumologie 1993;47:409-13. [German]
74. Plockinger B, Muller MR, Eckersberger F. [Isolated amyloidosis of hilar lymph nodes.] Langernbecks Arch Chir 1993;378:167-70. [German]
75. Polachek AA, Pijanowski WJ. Extrathoracic eggshell calcifications in silicosis. Am Rev Respir Dis 1960;82:714-20.
76. Ramos FJ, Gomez-Martino JR, Fernandez-Rojo FP, Suarez D. Proteinaceous lymphadenopathy and the kidney. Arch Pathol Lab Med 1992;116:8-9.
77. Ravel R. Histopathology of lymph nodes after lymphangiography. Am J Clin Pathol 1966;46:335-40.
78. Roggli VL, Benning TL. Asbestos bodies in pulmonary hilar lymph nodes. Mod Pathol 1990;3:513-7.
79. Roggli VL, Pratt PC. Numbers of asbestos bodies on iron-stained tissue sections in relation to asbestos body counts in lung tissue digests. Hum Pathol 1983;14:355-61.
80. Rosen Y, Vuletin JC, Pertschuk LP, Silverstein E. Sarcoidosis: from the pathologist's vantage point. Pathol Annu 1979;14:405-39.
81. Rozen S, Nahabedian MY. Melanoma and decorative tattoos: is a black sentinel lymph node unequivocally metastatic? Plast Reconstr Surg 2004;113:1304-5.
82. Saltini C, Markham TN, Jones Williams W. Beryl-liosis. In: James DG, Zumla A, eds. The granulomatous disorders. Cambridge: Cambridge Univ. Press; 1999:336-51.
83. Shea KG, Bloebaum RD, Avent JM, Birk T, Samuelson KA. Analysis of lymph nodes for polyethylene particles in patients who have had a primary joint replacement. J Bone Joint Surg 1996;78:497-504.
84. Shi Q, Fan K, Chen H. Localized amyloidosis of cervical lymph nodes. Chin Med J 2000;113:184-5.
85. Shoenfeld Y, Berliner S, Pinkhas J, Beutler E. The association of Gaucher's disease and dysproteinemias. Acta Haematol 1980;64:241-3.
86. Slavin RE, Swedo JL, Brandes D, Gonzalez-Vitale JC, Osornio-Vargas A. Extrapulmonary silicosis: a clinical, morphologic, and ultrastructural study. Hum Pathol 1985;16:393-412.
87. Spitale LS, Jimenez DB, Montenegro RB. Localised primary amyloidosis of inguinal lymph node with superimposed bone metaplasia. Pathology 1998;30:321-2.
88. Sood A, Beckett WS, Cullen MR. Variable response to long-term corticosteroid therapy in chronic beryllium disease. Chest 2004;126:2000-7.
89. Stewart AJ, Southcott BM, Raweily E. Lymphadenopathy after joint replacement for osteoclastoma. J R Soc Med 2003;96:404-6.
90. Strauchen JA. Storage and deposition disorders. In: Strauchen JA, ed. Diagnostic histopathology of the lymph node. New York: Oxford University Press; 1998:321-8.
91. Stryker WA. Absorption of liquid petrolaturm ("mineral oil") from the intestine: a histologic and chemical study. Arch Pathol (Chic) 1941;31:670-92.
92. Symmers W StC. The lymphoreticular system. In: Symmers W St C, ed. Systemic pathology, Vol. 2. Edinburgh: Churchill Livingstone; 1978:504-891.
93. Takeshita K, Yamada S, Sato N, et al. An unusual case of mediastinal lymphadenopathy caused by amyloidosis. Intern Med 2000;39:839-42.
94. Truong LD, Cartwright J, Goodman MD, Woznicki D. Silicone lymphadenopathy associated with augmentation mammaplasty: morphologic features of nine cases. Am J Surg Pathol 1988;12:484-91.
95. Urban RM, Jacobs JJ, Tomlinson, MJ, Gavrilovic J, Black J, Peoc'h M. Dissemination of wear particles to the liver, spleen and abdominal lymph nodes of patients with hip or knee replacement. J Bone Joint Surg Am 2000;82:457-77.
96. Vanhoenacker FM, Van den Brande P, De Schepper AM. Hepatosplenic antracosilicosis: a rare cause of splenic calcifications. Eur Radiol 2001;11:1184-6.
97. Varghese LR, Stanley MW, Wakely PE Jr, Lucido ML, Mallery S, Bardales RH. A case report of anthrasilicotic spindle-cell pseudotumor of mediastinal lymph node: cytologic diagnosis by endoscopic ultrasound-guided fine-needle aspiration. Diagn Cytopathol 2005;33:268-72.
98. Verma DK, Ritchie AC, Shaw ML. Measurement of beryllium in lung tissue of a chronic beryllium disease case and cases with sarcoidosis. Occup Med 2003;53:223-7.
99. Warner NE, Friedman NB. Lipogranulomatous pseudosarcoid. Ann Intern Med 1956;45:662-73.
100. Warnock ML. Lung asbestos burden in shipyard and construction workers with mesothelioma: comparison with burdens in subjects with asbestosis or lung cancer. Environ Res 1989;50:68-85.

101. Weeks DA, Beckwith JB, Mierau GW. Benign nodal lesions mimicking metastases from pediatric renal neoplasms: a report of the national Wilms' tumor study pathology center. Hum Pathol 1990;21:1239-44.
102. Wegener K, Wesch H, Kampmann H, Zahnert R. Pathological findings in the RES (liver, spleen, lymph nodes, bone marrow) of thorotrast patients (histological and autoradiographic investigations. RISO Rep 1973;294:248-58.
103. Wegener K, Wesch H. Pathological changes of lymph nodes in thorotrast patients: pathoanatomical, autoradiographical, and quantitative investigations. Environ Res 1979;18:245-55.
104. Weiss SW, Enzinger FM, Johnson FB. Silica reaction simulating fibrous histiocytoma. Cancer 1978;42:2738-43.
105. Williams G, Whittaker JS. Diagnostic problems in biliary duct lymph nodes. J Clin Pathol 1965;18:43-6.
106. Wood C, Nickoloff BJ, Todes-Taylor NR. Pseudotumor resulting from atypical mycobacterial infection: a "histoid" variety of mycobacterium avium-intracellulare complex infection. Am J Clin Pathol 1985;83:524-7.
107. Xin W, Davenport RD, Chang AE, Michael CW. Exaggerated pigmented granulomatous reaction to the artificial joint implant mimics metastatic melanoma. Diagn Cytopathol 2004;30:198-200.
108. Yunis EJ, Jaffe R. Tamm-Horsfall protein in lymph nodes. Hum Pathol 1981;12:179-83.
109. Zaloudek C, Treseler PA, Powell CB. Postarthroplasty histiocytic lymphadenopathy in gynecologic oncology patients. A benign reactive process that clinically may be mistaken for cancer. Cancer 1996;78:834-44.
110. Zanetti G. Epithelial inclusions and Tamm-Horsfall protein in paranephric lymph nodes. A light microscopy and immunocytochemical study. Virchows Arch A Pathol Anat Histopathol 1986;408:593-601.

16 METABOLIC DISEASES

OVERVIEW

A subset of metabolic diseases, known as storage diseases, results in visceromegaly; those that typically result in splenic enlargement are listed in Table 16-1. These diseases generally do not manifest as lymphadenopathies, with the exceptions of *Wolman disease, Tangier disease,* and *Niemann-Pick disease*. The storage diseases are often lysosomal disorders and present in infancy or childhood. The clinical signs of storage disease include facial dysmorphism, ascites, macroglossia, bone changes, macular cherry red spots, vacuolated lymphocytes, and hydrops fetalis. Infants and children with these disorders may or may not have accompanying chronic diarrhea and failure to thrive (26).

Disorders that present in the neonatal and early infancy periods with coarse facies and bone changes include GM1 gangliosidosis, sialidosis type II, and I-cell disease. *GM1 gangliosidosis* is a rare autosomal recessive disease resulting in a deficiency of β-galactosides and an accumulation of ganglioside GM1 in brain and viscera. Foam cells, or macrophages with enlarged cytoplasm containing inclusions, representing the ganglioside GM1, are found in spleen or other viscera (31).

The glycoprotein storage diseases, *sialidosis type II, alpha* (α)*-mannosidosis*, and *fucosidosis*, result from specific enzyme deficiencies in the degradation of glycoprotein. *Sialidosis type II* is the dysmorphic form of sialidosis, and the majority of patients present with coarse facies and developmental delay; 50 percent have splenomegaly (fig. 16-1). The infantile form of *α-mannosidosis* presents with progressive mental retardation, hepatosplenomegaly, severe dysostosis multiplex, hearing loss, and early death. *Fucosidosis* presents with mental retardation and neurologic deterioration as primary features, with 30 percent of patients showing visceromegaly. The cellular accumulation of metabolites resulting from partial degradation of oligosaccharides results in vacuolated cells in multiple organs (32).

I-cell disease, or *inclusion-cell disease (mucolipidosis II),* is a disorder of lysosomal enzyme phosphorylation in which enzymes are secreted into the extracellular medium instead of directed to lysosomes. Affected cells contain dense inclusions and patients have elevated levels of lysosomal enzymes in the serum and body fluids. Patients with I-cell disease have severe progressive psychomotor retardation and minimal splenomegaly; death occurs in the first decade of life (13).

Disorders with progressive neurologic dysfunction, presenting at age 1 to 2 years, include select *mucopolysaccharidoses*, the glycoprotein storage diseases *fucosidosis* and *α-mannosidosis, galactosialidosis,* and *multiple sulfatase deficiency*. The *mucopolysaccharidoses* (MPS) are lysosomal storage disorders with enzyme deficiencies involving the degradation of mucopolysaccharides, resulting in the accumulation of glycosaminoglycans in tissues. Affected cells are vacuolated; the vacuoles are clear or contain fine granular material on ultrastructural studies. Infants with *Hurler syndrome* (*MPS type I*) develop coarse facies during the first year of life, with hepatosplenomegaly, skeletal abnormalities, developmental delay, mental retardation, and cardiac abnormalities. Children with *Maroteaux-Lamy syndrome* (*MPS VI*) show normal mental development, with skeletal abnormalities, growth deformities, variable coarse facies, and splenomegaly in fifty percent. *Sly syndrome* (*MPS VII*) presents with variable clinical features: mild or absent mental retardation, soft tissue and skeletal abnormalities, and hydrops fetalis (21).

Galactosialidosis is a combined deficiency of beta (β)-galactosidase and neuraminidase, resulting in the accumulation of sialyloligosaccharides within lysosomes. Hepatosplenomegaly may be seen in the early or late infantile forms of the disease. The late infantile form shows more marked hepatosplenomegaly, coarse facies, growth retardation, and fetal hydrops (8).

Table 16-1

METABOLIC DISEASES RESULTING IN SPLENOMEGALY, ORGANIZED BY AGE OF ONSET, AND INCLUDING KEY CLINICAL FEATURES

Disease	Onset	Main Manifestations	Other Manifestations
Wolman disease	First week of life	Vomiting, diarrhea	Hepatosplenomegaly, steatorrhea, FTT[a], adrenal gland calcifications, lymphadenopathy
GM1 gangliosidosis	0-3 months	Coarse facies, bone changes	Arrested development, neurologic deterioration, HSM, bony dysplasia
I-cell disease	0-18 months	Severe psychomotor retardation	Coarse facies, bone abnormalities, FTT, joint stiffness, hepatomegaly, minimal splenomegaly
Sialidosis type II	1 month-20 years	Coarse facies	Mental retardation, cherry red spot, developmental delay
Acid ceramidase deficiency (Farber disease)	1st weeks of life	Deformed joints	Skin nodules, hoarseness, HSM
Gaucher disease, type II	1-6 months	Acute neurologic dysfunction	HSM
Niemann-Pick disease, type IA	6-12 months	HSM	Neurologic deterioration, FTT, cherry red spots, vacuolated lymphocytes
Multiple sulfatase deficiency (Austin disease)	1-2 years	Neurologic dysfunction	Variable coarse facies, growth retardation, skeletal anomalies, stiff joints, HSM
Fucosidosis	6-12 months	Psychomotor retardation, mental retardation	Coarse facies, HSM, vacuolated lymphocytes, neurologic dysfunction
α-Mannosidosis	varied	Mental retardation	HSM, dysostosis multiplex, vacuolated lymphocytes, hearing loss, bacterial infections
Galactosialidosis	varied	Coarse facies	Growth retardation, cardiac involvement, HSM, fetal hydrops
MPS, type I (Hurler syndrome)	6-12 months	Mental retardation	Dysostosis multiplex, HSM, coarse facies, cardiac disease
MPS, type VI (Maroteaux-Lamy syndrome)	1-3 years	Skeletal abnormalities	Coarse facies, respiratory disease, joint abnormalities, normal intelligence
MPS, type VII (Sly syndrome)	0-6 months	Soft tissue and skeletal retardation	Hydrops fetalis, mild/absent mental retardation
Lysinuric protein intolerance	1-2 years[b]	Vomiting, diarrhea	Hyperammonemic attacks, FTT, aversion to protein, HSM, osteoporosis, muscle hypotonia, pancytopenia
Gaucher, type I	1-6 years	Splenomegaly	Bone/bone marrow disease, cytopenias
Niemann-Pick, type B	2-6 years	Splenomegaly	Short stature, cherry red spot, interstitial pneumonia
Niemann-Pick, type C	Late infancy/childhood	Progressive neurologic dysfunction	Variable HSM
Tangier disease	Childhood	HSM	Premature coronary disease, peripheral neuropathy
Gaucher, type III	Childhood/adolescence	Splenomegaly	Subacute neurologic dysfunction

[a]FTT = failure to thrive, HSM = hepatosplenomegaly, MPS = mucopolysaccharidosis.
[b]Symptoms develop after infants are weaned from being breast-fed.

Multiple sulfatase deficiency (*Austin disease*) is a storage disorder in which at least seven sulfatases are deficient. The clinical features include metachromatic leukodystrophy with signs of mucopolysaccharidosis (including hepatosplenomegaly) and ichthyosis. In the infantile variant of the disease, development is normal until approximately 2 years of age, when spasticity, blindness, hearing loss, and convulsions occur along with the variable features of mucopolysaccharidosis (34).

Diseases with splenomegaly and failure to thrive present in early infancy and include acid ceramidase deficiency, Wolman disease, lysinuric protein intolerance, Niemann-Pick disease type IA, and Gaucher disease type II. *Acid*

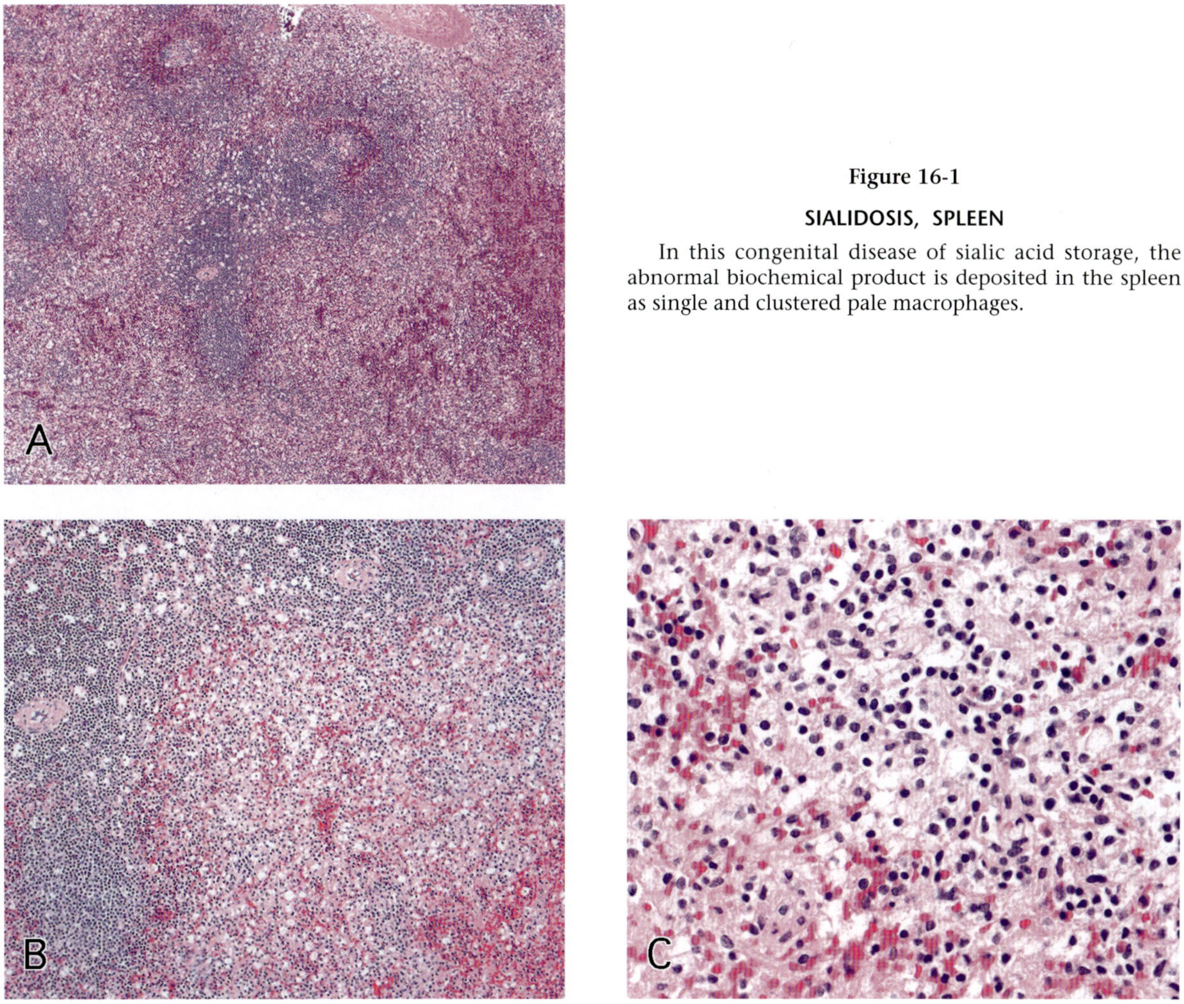

Figure 16-1

SIALIDOSIS, SPLEEN

In this congenital disease of sialic acid storage, the abnormal biochemical product is deposited in the spleen as single and clustered pale macrophages.

ceramidase deficiency (*Farber lipogranulomatosis*) is a disorder of lipid metabolism defined by a deficiency of lysosomal acid ceramidase, resulting in the accumulation of ceramide in lysosomes. Early in infancy, patients have deformed joints, subcutaneous nodules, and hoarseness. This disorder is characterized by multiple granulomas with lipid-laden macrophages involving spleen, liver, lung, heart, and nervous system. A rapidly fatal neonatal form presents with massive hepatosplenomegaly (19).

Wolman disease is the severe form of *acid lipase deficiency*, with the accumulation of cholesterol esters and triglycerides in most tissues of the body. Infants present within the first week of life with vomiting, diarrhea, steatorrhea, and abdominal distension. They develop hepatosplenomegaly, fail to thrive, and generally die of disease before 1 year of age. A characteristic of the disease is adrenal calcifications. The spleen is often greater than 200 g and firm, with compressed follicles and a massive accumulation of foam cells. Swelling and vacuolization of endothelial cells occurs. Lymphadenopathy is present, with firm, enlarged yellow lymph nodes showing features similar to those found in the spleen (1).

Lysinuric protein intolerance (*hyperdibasic aminoaciduria type II, familial protein intolerance*) results from the abnormal membrane transport of the cationic amino acids lysine, arginine, and ornithine. Subsequently, urinary excretion and clearance of these amino acids are increased, since they are poorly absorbed from the intestine, resulting in depletion of body stores of these amino acids. Patients develop periods of hyperammonemia, nausea and vomiting, an aversion to protein-rich foods, and failure to

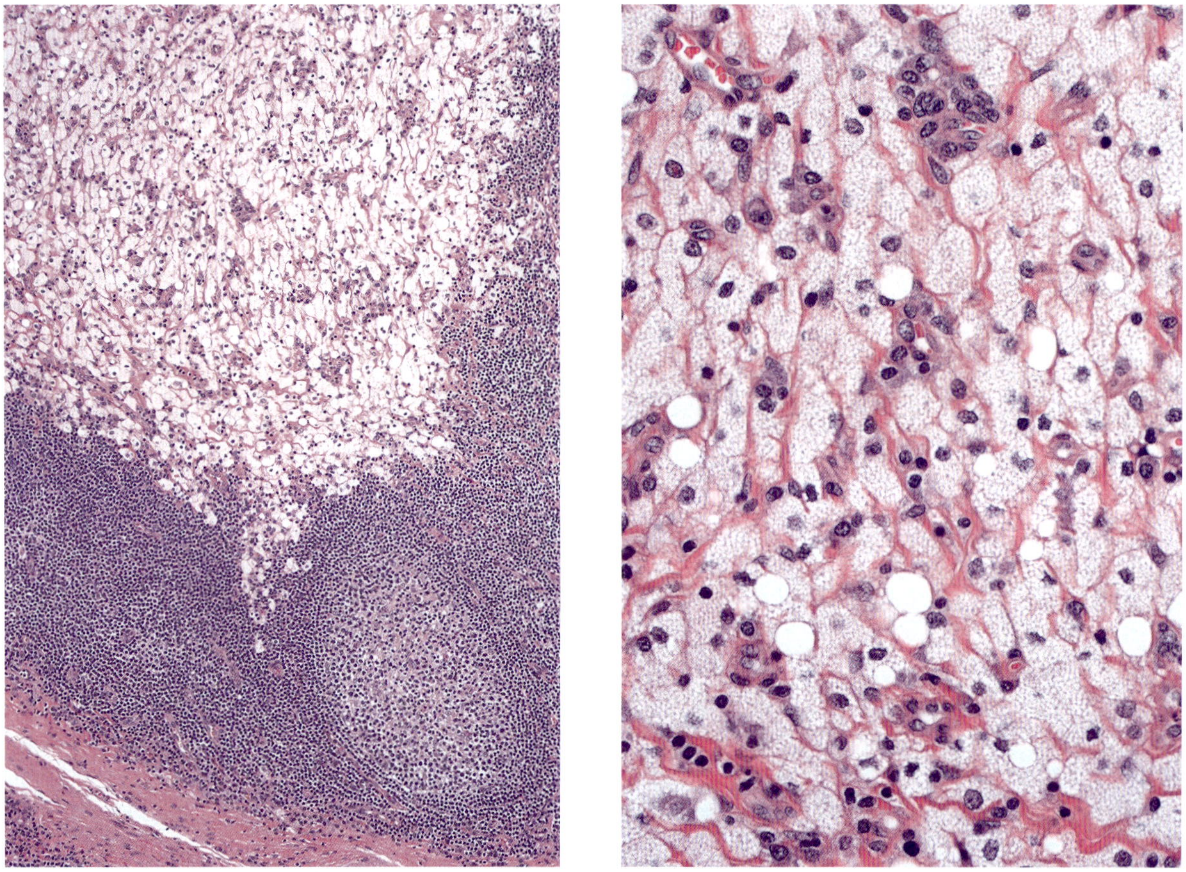

Figure 16-2

TANGIER DISEASE, TONSIL

Left: There are large collections of macrophages.
Right: The foamy cytoplasm is apparent on high magnification.

thrive. When breast-fed, infants are symptom free, but develop vomiting and diarrhea after weaning. Following infancy, failure to thrive persists with hepatosplenomegaly, muscle hypotonia, osteoporosis and fractures, and sparse hair. Generally, affected individuals are pancytopenic and may develop pulmonary alveolar proteinosis (30).

Tangier disease is one of the hereditary peripheral neuropathies that typically develop in childhood, but the disease's main manifestations are hepatosplenomegaly and premature coronary artery disease, resulting from impaired cholesterol efflux from macrophages (2). Foam cells are found throughout the body, with cholesterol ester deposition in tonsils, spleen, liver, lymph nodes, bone marrow, gastrointestinal tract, and Schwann cells (fig. 16-2). Caused by mutations in the gene encoding adenosine triphosphate (ATP)-binding cassette transporter 1 (24), Tangier disease is an autosomal codominant disease. There is absent high density lipoprotein (HDL) cholesterol in plasma in the homozygous state and 50 percent of normal HDL cholesterol in the heterozygous state (1,33).

The storage diseases presenting with isolated splenomegaly in late infancy to childhood are most familiar to the pathologist, including Niemann-Pick disease type B and Gaucher disease type I. Niemann-Pick disease type C and Gaucher disease type III present with splenomegaly, a variety of neurologic signs, and deterioration. The remainder of this chapter describes splenic findings in Gaucher disease, Niemann-Pick disease, and ceroid (sea-blue) histiocytosis.

Table 16-2

CLINICAL TYPES OF GAUCHER DISEASE

Type	Age of Onset	Neuronopathic	Bone Disease	Ethnic Groups
I	Childhood/adult	No	Yes	Ashkenazi Jews
II	Neonatal/infantile	Acute	No	Panethnic
III	Childhood/adolescents	Subacute	Yes	Norrbottnian Swedes

NOTES: All clinical types of Gaucher disease have hepatosplenomegaly, ranging from mild to severe.

Type I disease involves the liver, spleen, bone, bone marrow, and hematologic and pulmonary systems. Analysis of the age of onset in a large group of patients followed by the International Collaborative Gaucher Group Registry (6), shows two major subgroups: one group with median age of onset before 20 years (average, 10 years; majority of patients), and a second group after 20 years (average, 30 years). The spleen volumes average 14X normal, with younger patients (<18 years) showing greater spleen volumes (about 19X normal) compared to adult patients (>18 years) with spleen volumes of about 10X normal. Specific defined genotypes cluster within certain age ranges and show differences in spleen and liver volumes, although this is outside the realm of this discussion. Bone disease (i.e., Erlenmeyer flask deformities, lytic lesions, osteopenia) is present in virtually all patients.

The rare type II disease includes the classic infantile presentation between 3 and 6 months of age and a perinatal lethal variant. Children display distended abdomen due to hepatosplenomegaly, with developmental delay, bulbar signs, poor motor development, and acute neuronopathic deterioration with death before 2 years of age. Features of the perinatal variant include prematurity, nonimmune hydrops fetalis, in utero death, hepatosplenomegaly, ichthyosis, and facial dysmorphy.

Type III disease shows similar neurologic involvement as type II, but a subacute course and a more heterogeneous phenotype. Three subtypes of type III Gaucher disease have been described: type IIIa—progressive dementia, ataxia, and myoclonus first recognized in Norrbottnian Swedes; type IIIb—CNS involvement including only supranuclear gaze palsy and extensive visceral and bone involvement; and type IIIc—supranuclear gaze palsy, corneal opacities, and cardiovascular calcification, with little visceral involvement.

GAUCHER DISEASE

Definition. *Gaucher disease* is the most common of the lysosomal storage diseases. It results from a deficiency of glucocerebrosidase (β-glucosidase), an enzyme necessary for the recycling of glycolipids. Deficiency of this key enzyme results in the accumulation of glucocerebroside (glycosylceramide) within the lysosomes of macrophages.

General Features. Gaucher disease is an autosomal recessive disorder. Three clinical types of disease have been described, all showing hepatosplenomegaly (Table 16-2). The gene for glucocerebrosidase is located on chromosome 1q21 and over 180 mutations have been detected. Certain recurrent mutant alleles are present in the majority of patients. The N370S allele leads to type I Gaucher disease and is the most common allele (about 50 percent of mutant alleles); the L444P allele is typical of type III disease, which occurs in northern Sweden (about 20 percent of mutant alleles); and the 84GG allele (about 7 percent of mutant alleles) causes no protein to be synthesized (6). These three mutations account for the majority of alleles in Ashkenazi patients (greater than 90 percent).

Clinical Features. Gaucher disease occurs in about 1/75,000 births worldwide, with type I Gaucher disease having a higher prevalence in Ashkenazi Jews (18) and the rarer type III disease more common in northern Sweden (9).

While three clinical types of Gaucher disease are classically described (Table 16-2), it is now recognized that this disease shows a spectrum of clinical phenotypes and natural history. All share hepatosplenomegaly, usually bone and bone marrow involvement, and involvement of lungs and other visceral organs. Type I lacks central nervous system (CNS) involvement, present in both types II and III. Type II Gaucher disease is an acute form of the disease with early CNS involvement resulting in death by 2 years of age. Type III Gaucher disease is a subacute neuronopathic form of the disease with a later onset and chronic course.

The overall risk of cancer in type I patients with Gaucher disease is not increased. However, the relative risk of hematologic malignancies is significantly increased, and the incidence of multiple myeloma is six-fold greater than expected (5). An association of Gaucher disease and monoclonal gammopathy has been described, and yearly screening for monoclonal gammopathy is now recommended.

Laboratory Findings. The laboratory findings are best described in type I Gaucher disease,

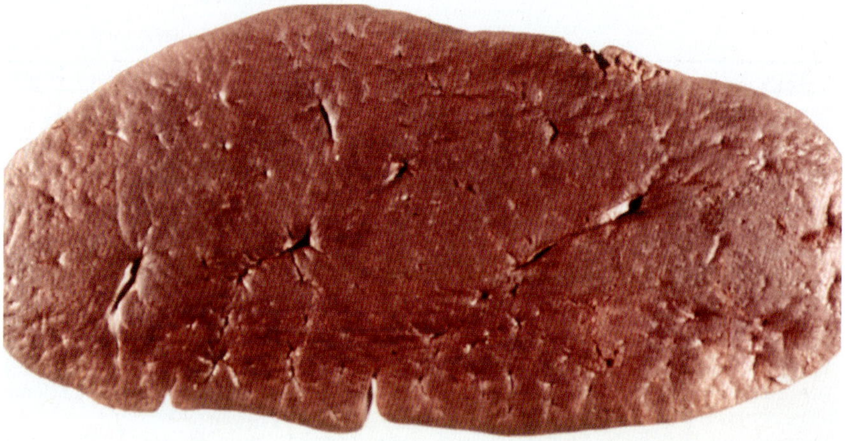

Figure 16-3

GAUCHER DISEASE, SPLEEN

Loss of the normal red and white pulp is seen. (Courtesy of Richard Neiman, Harpswell, ME.)

the most common type. Approximately 20 to 30 percent of patients have anemia and the majority of patients have thrombocytopenia (5). Deficiency in coagulation factor XI is described, as well as abnormalities in factor IX, vWF antigen, and factor VIII. Serum angiotensin converting enzyme may be increased, as well as liver enzymes (16). Plasma chitotriosidase activity, a marker of macrophage activation, is now used to indicate clinical response to enzyme replacement therapy (12).

Gross Findings. The volume of the spleen and liver is increased in all types of Gaucher disease. Average spleen volumes in type I disease are 14 times normal, and in patients less than 18 years of age can be 18 times normal. The spleen may contain nodules, representing infarcts, resolving infarcts, or collections of Gaucher cells. The spleen is red to yellow (infarcts) to purple (extramedullary hematopoiesis), with areas of fibrosis (fig. 16-3).

Microscopic Findings. Gaucher disease results in the accumulation of glycolipid glucocerebrosidase within macrophages in the reticuloendothelial system. On light microscopy, the Gaucher cell shows a recognizable appearance, akin to "wrinkled tissue paper" (figs. 16-4, 16-5). Cells are 20 to 100 µm in size, with low nuclear to cytoplasmic ratios, and one or more nuclei. The cytoplasm is abundant and striated, fibrillar, or tubular. It is blue-gray with the Romanowsky stain and pink with the hematoxylin and eosin (H&E) stain. Erythrophagocytosis may be present.

Ancillary Studies. Gaucher cells show activity for nonspecific esterase, tartrate-resistant acid phosphatase, and periodic acid–Schiff (PAS), and are variably positive with iron stains. Ultrastructural analysis of Gaucher cells shows that the cytoplasm is irregular due to arrays of twisted tubules (15). The twisted tubules are contained within dilated membrane-bound vesicles, which on X-ray diffraction analysis show bilayers of 10 to 12 fibrils twisted into a right-handed helix representing a tubule (5). The tubules are thought to represent the polymerization of glucocerebrosidase. By immunoelectron study, glucocerebrosidase protein and stored lipid material are in irregular vacuoles, which contain other lysosomal enzymes as well (34).

The diagnosis of Gaucher disease depends on finding reduced glucocerebrosidase activity in peripheral blood leukocytes or measuring enzyme activity in cultured skin fibroblasts (11). Mutation analysis to detect common mutations is recommended for classification and prediction of clinical involvement. Prenatal diagnosis is achieved by analyzing fetal cells for enzyme activity via amniocentesis or chorionic villus sampling.

Differential Diagnosis. The differential diagnosis of splenomegaly, anemia, and thrombocytopenia (features of the more common type I Gaucher disease) includes hematologic malignancies, autoimmune diseases such as rheumatoid arthritis, and Niemann-Pick disease. Other storage diseases can also be considered (see Table 16-1), but show clinical symptoms that allow them to be distinguished from Gaucher disease. The work-up of the cytopenias often includes bone marrow aspiration and biopsy; these show the presence of Gaucher cells.

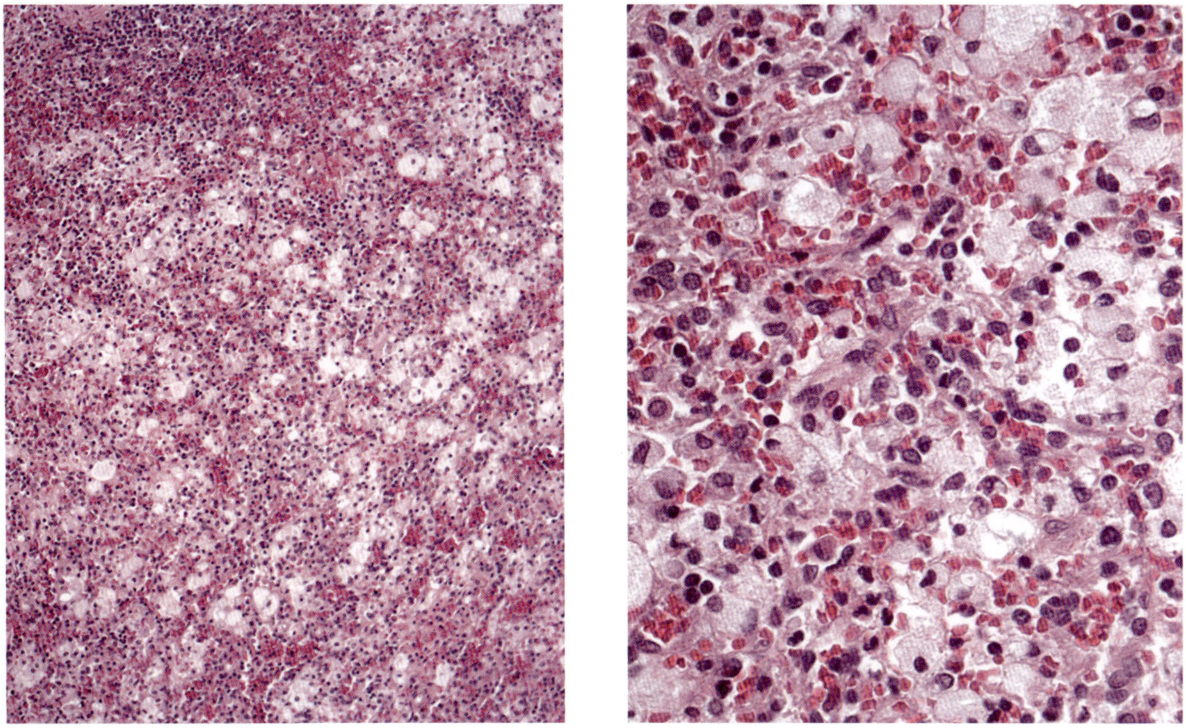

Figure 16-4

GAUCHER DISEASE, SPLEEN

Pale macrophages are deposited in the red and white pulp.

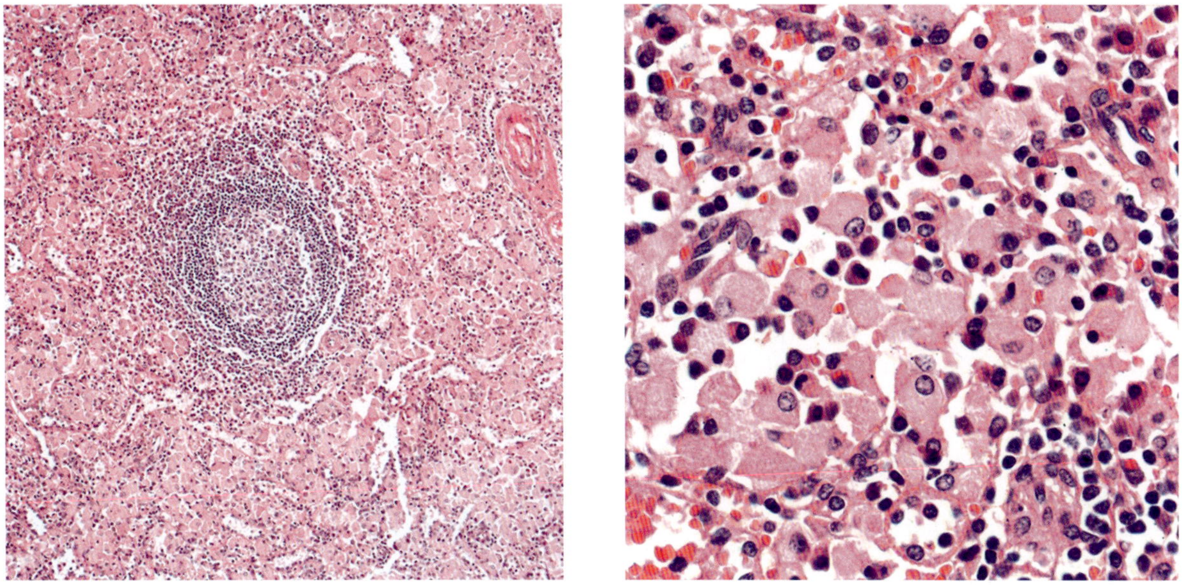

Figure 16-5

GAUCHER DISEASE, SPLEEN

Left: Red pulp is expanded by large macrophages.
Right: Closer examination reveals a faint granular or irregular appearance of the material filling these cells.

Table 16-3

DISTINGUISHING CYTOLOGIC, HISTOCHEMICAL, AND ULTRASTRUCTURAL FEATURES OF GAUCHER DISEASE AND NIEMANN-PICK DISEASE

	Gaucher Disease	Niemann-Pick Disease
Cytology	Abundant striated cytoplasm	Foam cells with uniform vacuolated cytoplasm
Histochemical reactions	Strong PAS +[a], NSE +, Iron +/–, TRAP –/+	PAS +/–, Sudan black B +, Oil red O +, TRAP –/+
Ultrastructural findings	Twisted fibrils, distended lysosomes	Lamellar bodies, zebra bodies

[a]PAS = periodic acid–Schiff; NSE = nonspecific esterase; TRAP = tartrate-resistant acid phosphatase.

Table 16-4

CLASSIFICATION OF NIEMANN-PICK DISEASE BY MOLECULAR, BIOCHEMICAL, AND KEY CLINICAL FEATURES

Type	Gene Defect	Enzyme Deficiency	Age of Onset	Clinical Findings
IA[a]	Sphingomyelin phosphodiesterase I	Acid sphingomyelinase, <5% activity	Neonatal/early infancy	HSM[b], rapid loss of neurologic function, peripheral neuropathy, macular cherry red spot
IS	Sphingomyelin phosphodiesterase I	Acid sphingomyelinase, <10% activity	Infancy/childhood	HSM, short stature, macular cherry red spot
IC			Adult	HSM, variable neurologic signs
IIS	Niemann-Pick C1 Niemann-Pick C2	NPC1 and 2[c] protein	Infancy/ childhood	Vertical supranuclear ophthalmoplegia, seizures, dystonia
IIC			Adult	Dementia, variable organomegaly

[a]A = acute, S = subacute, C = chronic.
[b]HSM=hepatosplenomegaly.
[c]NPC1= Niemann-Pick C1, NPC2 = Niemann-Pick C2.

Features distinguishing Gaucher cells from the foam cells of Niemann-Pick disease are listed in Table 16-3.

Treatment and Prognosis. Enzyme replacement therapy exists for Gaucher disease using a recombinant enzyme; this prevents complications of the disease (3).

NIEMANN-PICK DISEASE

Definition. *Niemann-Pick disease (sphingomyelin-cholesterol lipidosis)* is a group of lysosomal storage disorders resulting from deficiencies of acid sphingomyelinase (types A and B) or Niemann-Pick C1 or C2 protein (types C and D). These deficiencies result in the accumulation of either sphingomyelin or unesterified cholesterol, respectively, within foam cells throughout the reticuloendothelial system.

General Features. The disorders included in Niemann-Pick disease present with splenomegaly and variable neurologic defects. These diseases are divided into two classes based on molecular defects and further subtyped according to severity and age of onset (Table 16-4) (7). Types A and B disease, now reclassified as type IA and IS disease, respectively, result from mutations in the sphingomyelin phosphodiesterase 1 gene, leading to deficiencies in sphingomyelinase and the subsequent accumulation of sphingomyelin within macrophages (27). Type C disease, now reclassified as type IIS, is a separate disorder, a lipidosis resulting from mutations in the Niemann-Pick C1 gene (about 95 percent of cases) or Niemann-Pick C2 gene (about 5 percent of cases). This lipidosis causes defects in cells transporting exogenous cholesterol, with excess unesterified cholesterol, sphingomyelin, phospholipids, and glycolipids accumulating in macrophages. Type D disease is now known to be a variant phenotype of type C disease (23).

Clinical Features. Type IA (previously type A) represents the acute neuronopathic form of Niemann-Pick disease, with a high incidence in Ashkenazi Jews. Occurring in early infancy, there is hepatosplenomegaly with failure to thrive and a rapid and progressive loss of neurologic function, including peripheral neuropathy (hypotonia) and death in the first few years of life.

Type IS (previously type B) is a chronic non-neuronopathic form of Niemann-Pick disease with a variable phenotype. Hepatosplenomegaly occurs in infancy or childhood, often associated with delayed skeletal growth and macular cherry red spots. These children generally survive into adulthood, with progressive splenomegaly and deterioration of lung function. Neurologic involvement is minimal.

Type IC disease (previously type E), is a rare subtype occurring in adults, with hepatosplenomegaly and variable neurologic involvement (7). A rare case report describes a case of Niemann-Pick disease type IC disease occurring with glycogen storage disease and multiple hepatic adenomas (20).

Type IIS disease, a lipidosis, includes the former classification types C and D Niemann-Pick disease. It is now thought to have a prevalence of 1/150,000, rendering it more common than either types IA or IS Niemann-Pick disease. Type IIS disease includes a severe infantile form of the disease and a late infantile/childhood form of the disease, with normal early development followed by dystonia, vertical supranuclear ophthalmoplegia, and seizures. Hepatosplenomegaly is variable. These patients have shortened life spans with death before age 15 years. Type D disease represents an allelic variant of type C disease with a later age of onset and minimal deterioration of neurologic function in young adults. Type IIC Niemann-Pick disease occurs in adults as dementia, extrapyramidal signs, and variable organomegaly (7).

Laboratory Findings. In types IA and IS disease, there are abnormalities in lipids, including decreased HDL cholesterol, increased low density lipoprotein (LDL) cholesterol, and hypertriglyceridemia. Liver dysfunction is also present in type IS disease.

Gross Findings. In types IA and IS disease, the spleen is the most extensively involved organ and is as large as 10 times normal size. The red pulp is infiltrated by foam cells, giving it a firm and pale gross appearance. Lymph node involvement is variable, with mesenteric lymph nodes and hilar lymph nodes of lung, liver, and spleen typically involved. These lymph nodes are gray-yellow and firm. Peripheral lymph nodes are usually not enlarged. Visceromegaly may be absent in type IIS disease.

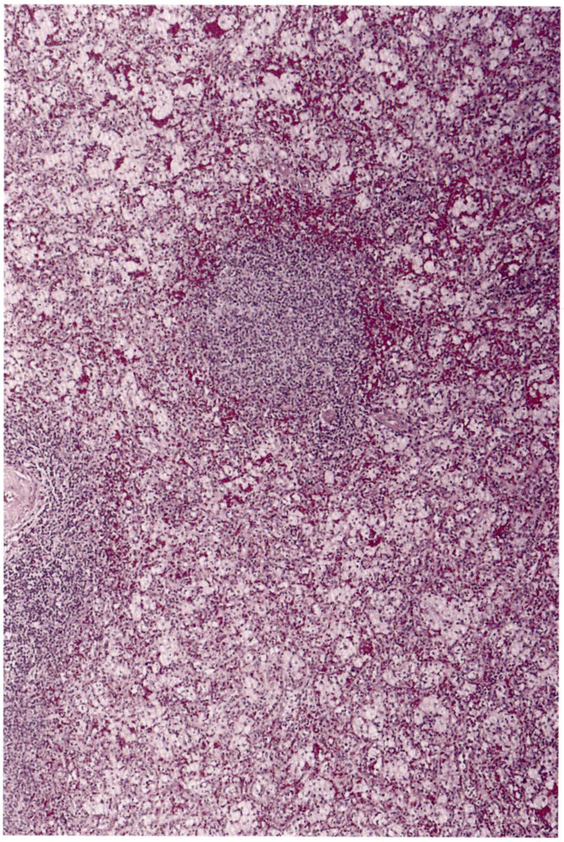

Figure 16-6

NEIMANN-PICK DISEASE, SPLEEN

As in other storage diseases, the deposition is more prominent in the red pulp.

Microscopic Findings. In type IA disease, lipid-laden foam cells expand the organs of the reticuloendothelial system (spleen, bone marrow, lymph nodes), blood vessels, and Schwann cells in the peripheral and central nervous systems and retina. These foam cells are present most often in spleen, liver, and bone marrow (figs. 16-6, 16-7). Foam cells are 25 to 75 µm in size, typically with one nucleus and expanded cytoplasm containing multiple uniform lipid droplets. Foam cells and sea-blue histiocytes (macrophages) are also found in many tissues in type IIS disease, but can be absent in cases lacking visceromegaly (23).

Ancillary Studies. Foam cells are birefringent under polarized light and strongly positive for the lipid stains Sudan black B and oil red O. They are also positive for the Schultz reaction

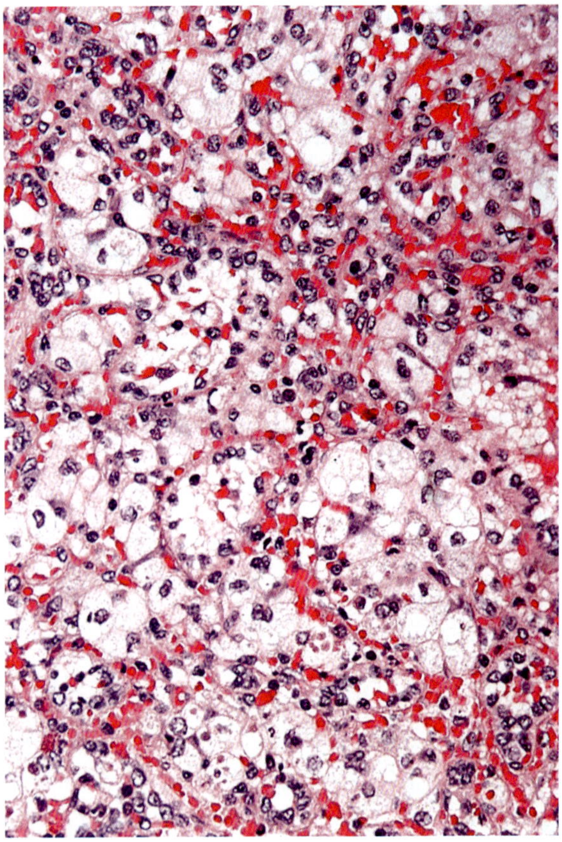

Figure 16-7

NEIMANN-PICK DISEASE, SPLEEN

The foamy macrophages of Niemann-Pick disease are seen.

for cholesterol and acid phosphatase, and show weak PAS and acid phosphatase reactivity. The cytoplasm may appear bluish and resemble sea-blue macrophages.

Ultrastructural studies show inclusions within lysosomes and myelin within peripheral nerves, which represent the accumulation of sphingomyelin and related proteins. The cytoplasm of foam cells contains numerous lamellar lipid inclusions ranging in size from 0.5 to 50.0 µm, with an average periodicity of 50Å (27). In one study of fetal type IIS disease, crystalline structures resembling cholesterol crystals were also found (10). Ultrastructural studies in type IIS disease show that the histiocytic cytoplasmic inclusions within macrophages are polymorphic structures of varying electron density. A biopsy of skin or conjunctiva in patients with type IIS disease shows typical lamellar inclusions. Neuronal cells contain polymorphous cytoplasmic bodies (23).

In the spleen, enzyme analysis shows accumulations of sphingomyelin and bis (monacylglycero) phosphate in types IA, IS, and IIS Niemann-Pick disease. There is markedly deficient sphingomyelinase activity in type IA spleens, and some residual activity in type IS (4).

Niemann-Pick disease is diagnosed by finding abnormal cholesterol metabolism on fibroblast cell culture. Genetic testing is available, as well as prenatal testing using amniocentesis or chorionic villus sampling.

Differential Diagnosis. The differential diagnosis of the Niemann-Pick cell, or foam cell, includes the Gaucher cell, but the morphologic and histochemical findings differ between the two cell types (Table 16-3). Foam cells are not unique to Niemann-Pick disease, however, and may be seen in Wolman disease, cholesterol ester storage disease, lipoprotein lipase deficiency, and GM1 gangliosidosis. The Niemann-Pick foam cell also resembles cells seen in sea-blue histiocytosis. The underlying defect in sea-blue histiocytosis is unknown and many of those originally described cases are thought to have been Niemann-Pick disease (17).

Treatment and Prognosis. Currently, no treatment prevents the onset or neurologic progression of this disease, or alters the lifespan of affected individuals. Rare reports of successful hematopoietic stem cell transplants have been described in patients with type IS disease, but neurologic disease has not been prevented by hematopoietic stem cell transplants in patients with types IA or IIS Niemann-Pick disease (23,27).

SEA-BLUE (CEROID) HISTIOCYTOSIS

Definition. *Sea-blue,* or *ceroid, histiocytosis* is splenomegaly with numerous sea-blue macrophages.

General Features. Sea-blue macrophages may be seen in numerous conditions including Niemann-Pick disease, Gaucher disease, cholesterol ester storage disease, Tangier disease, apolipoprotein E mutation, hypertriglyceridemia, and lecithin-cholesterol acyltransferase deficiency. They are increased in number in disorders with a high cell turnover, such as chronic myeloid leukemia, idiopathic thrombocytopenic purpura, or other hematologic disorders (22,25,28,29).

Clinical Features. Originally described in 1970 (29), sea-blue histiocytosis is now recognized as a finding present in multiple conditions. A variant of Niemann-Pick disease features sea-blue macrophages (14). The exact etiology of sea-blue histiocytosis is unknown, although it has been hypothesized that there may be abnormalities in the lipid pathway (28). Sea-blue macrophages are most commonly described in spleen, bone marrow, and liver.

Microscopic Findings. Sea-blue macrophages take their name from their staining quality with Romanowsky stains, staining a distinct blue-green color (figs. 16-8, 16-9). On unstained films, these macrophages are brown; on H&E-stained sections, they are brown-yellow.

Ancillary Studies. Sea-blue macrophages are positive for PAS and Sudan black B, with variable positivity for iron stains. Under ultraviolet light, the macrophages show a yellow-green fluorescence.

Differential Diagnosis. The presence of numerous sea-blue macrophages in the spleen should prompt an investigation into any underlying storage disorders, especially Niemann-Pick disease, or conditions with increased cellular turnover.

Treatment and Prognosis. There is no treatment, for sea-blue histiocytosis. It is important to identify the underlying condition and treat that condition accordingly.

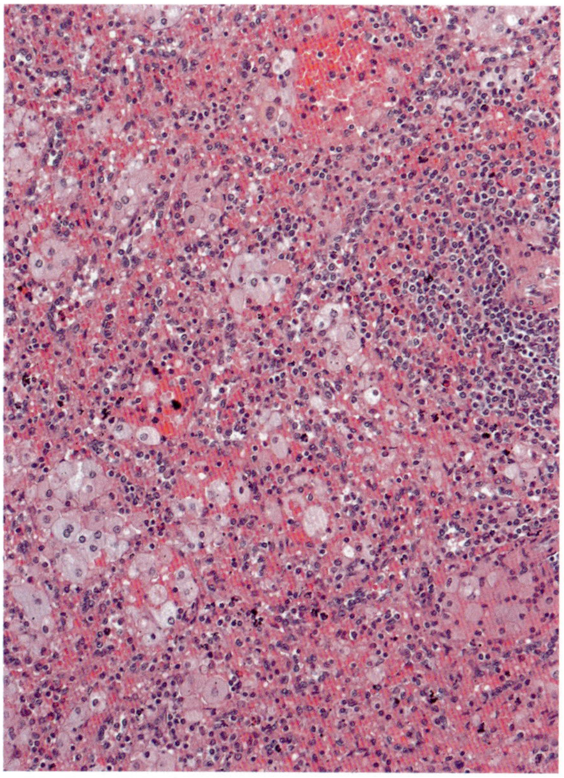

Figure 16-8

SEA-BLUE HISTIOCYTOSIS

Sea-blue macrophages appear as pale or slightly brown large macrophages on initial examination. (Courtesy of the California Tumor Tissue Registry, Loma Linda, CA.)

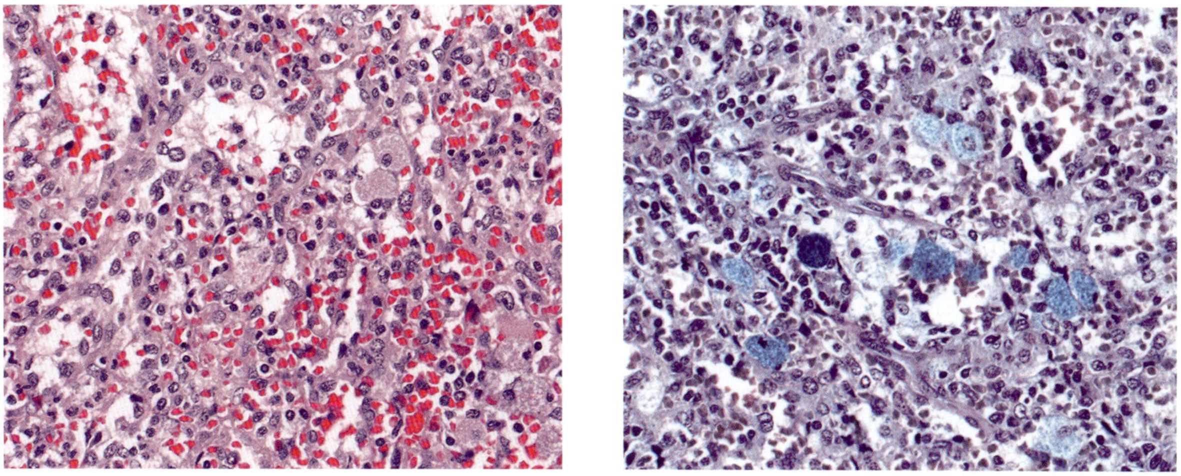

Figure 16-9

SEA-BLUE HISTIOCYTOSIS

Left: The ceroid-filled macrophages have granular, faintly brown cytoplasm when stained with hematoxylin and eosin (H&E).

Right: Giemsa staining reveals the origin of the name "sea-blue" histiocytosis.

REFERENCES

1. Assman G, Seedorf U. Acid lipase deficiency: Wolman disease and cholesteryl ester storage disease. In: Scriver CR, Beaudet AL, Sly WS, et al, eds. The metabolic and molecular bases of inherited disease, 8th ed, vol 3. New York: McGraw-Hill; 2001:3551-72.
2. Assmann G, von Eckardstein A, Brewer HB Jr. Familial analphalipoproteinemia: Tangier disease. In: Scriver CR, Beaudet AL, Sly WS, et al, eds. The metabolic and molecular bases of inherited disease, 8th ed, vol 2. New York: McGraw-Hill; 2001:2937-60.
3. Baldellou A, Andria G, Campbell PE, et al. Paediatric non-neuronopathic Gaucher disease: recommendations for treatment and monitoring. Eur J Pediatr 2004;163:67-75.
4. Besley GT, Elleder M. Enzyme activities and phospholipids storage patterns in brain and spleen samples from Niemann-Pick disease variants: a comparison of neuropathic and non-neuropathic forms. J Inherit Metab Dis 1986;9:59-71.
5. Beutler E, Grabowski GA. Gaucher disease. In: Scriver CR, Beaudet AL, Sly WS, et al, eds. The metabolic and molecular bases of inherited disease, 8th ed, vol 3. New York: McGraw-Hill; 2001:3635-68.
6. Charrow J, Andersson HC, Kaplan P, et al. The Gaucher registry: demographics and disease characteristics of 1698 patients with Gaucher disease. Arch Intern Med 2000;160:2835-43.
7. Cruse RP. Overview of Niemann-Pick disease. In: Rose BD, ed. UpToDate Wellesley: BDR-UptoDate, Inc; 2006.
8. D'Azzo A, Andria G, Strisciuglio P, Galjaard H. Galactosialidosis. In: Scriver CR, Beaudet AL, Sly WS, et al, eds. The metabolic and molecular bases of inherited disease, 8th ed, vol 3. New York: McGraw-Hill; 2001:3811-26.
9. Dahl N, Lagerstrom M, Erikson A, Pettersson U. Gaucher disease type III (Norrbottnian type) is caused by a single mutation in exon 10 of the glucocerebrosidase gene. Am J Hum Genet 1990;47:275-8.
10. Dumontel C, Girod C, Dijoud F, Dumez Y, Vanier MT. Fetal Niemann-Pick disease type C: ultrastructural and lipid findings in liver and spleen. Virchows Arch A Pathol Anat Histopathol 1993;422:253-9.
11. Grabowski GA, Andria G, Baldellou A, et al. Pediatric non-neuronopathic Gaucher disease: presentation, diagnosis and assessment. Consensus statements. Eur J Pediatr 2004;163:58-66.
12. Hollak CE, Maas M, Aerts JM. Clinically relevant therapeutic endpoints in type I Gaucher disease. J Inherit Metab Dis 2001;24(Suppl 2):97-105.
13. Kornfeld S, Sly WS. I-cell diseae and pseudo-Hurler polydystrophy: disorders of lysosomal enzyme phosphorylation and localization. In: Scriver CR, Beaudet AL, Sly WS, et al, eds. The metabolic and molecular bases of inherited disease, 8th ed, vol 3. New York: McGraw-Hill; 2001:3469-82.
14. Landas S, Foucar K, Sando GN, Ellefson R, Hamilton HE. Adult Niemann-Pick disease masquerading as seal blue histiocyte syndrome: report of a case confirmed by lipid analysis and enzyme assays. Am J Hematol 1985;20:391-400.
15. Lee RE. The fine structure of the cerebroside occurring in Gaucher's disease. Proc Natl Acad Sci U S A 1968;61:484-9.
16. Lieberman J, Beutler E. Elevation of serum angiotensin-converting enzyme in Gaucher's disease. N Engl J Med 1976;294:1442-4.
17. Long RG, Lake BD, Pettit JE, Scheuer PJ, Sherlock S. Adult Niemann-Pick disease: its relationship to the syndrome of the sea-blue histiocyte. Am J Med 1977;62:627-35.
18. Meikle PJ, Hopwood JJ, Clague AE, Carey WF. Prevalence of lysosomal storage disorders. JAMA 1999;281:249-54.
19. Moser HW, Linke T, Fensom AH, Levade T, Sandhoff K. Acid ceramidase deficiency: Farber lipogranulomatosis. In: Scriver CR, Beaudet AL, Sly WS, et al, eds. The metabolic and molecular bases of inherited disease, 8th ed, vol 3. New York: McGraw-Hill; 2001:3573-88.
20. Narita T, Hakazawa H, Hizawa Y, Kudo H. Glycogen storage disease associated with Niemann-Pick disease: histochemical, enzymatic, and lipid analyses. Mod Pathol 1994;7:416-21.
21. Neufeld EF, Muenzer J. The mucopolysaccharidoses. In: Scriver CR, Beaudet AL, Sly WS, et al, eds. The metabolic and molecular bases of inherited disease, 8th ed, vol 3. New York: McGraw-Hill; 2001:3421-52.
22. Nguyen TT, Kruckeberg KE, O'Brien JF, et al. Familial splenomegaly: macrophage hypercatabolism of lipoproteins associated with apolipoprotein E mutation [apolipoprotein E (delta 149 leu)]. 2000;85:4354-8.
23. Patterson MC, Vanier MT, Suzuki K, et al. Niemann-Pick disease type C: a lipid trafficking disorder. In: Scriver CR, Beaudet AL, Sly WS, et al, eds. The metabolic and molecular bases of inherited disease, 8th ed, vol 3. New York: McGraw-Hill; 2001:3611-33.

24. Rust S, Rosier M, Funke H, et al. Tangier disease is caused by mutations in the gene encoding ATP-binding cassette transporter 1. Nat Genet 1999;22:352-5.
25. Rywlin AM, Hernandez JA, Chastain DE, Pardo V. Ceroid histiocytosis of spleen and bone marrow in idiopathic thrombocytopenic purpura (ITP): a contribution to the understanding of the sea-blue histiocyte. Blood 1971;37:587-93.
26. Saudubray JM, Charpentier C. Clinical phenotypes: diagnosis/algorithms. In: Scriver CR, Beaudet AL, Sly WS, Valle D, Childs B, eds. The metabolic and molecular bases of inherited disease, 8th ed, vol 1. New York: McGraw-Hill; 2001:1327-403.
27. Schuchman EH, Desnick RJ. Niemann-Pick disease types A and B: Acid sphingomyelinase deficiencies. In: Scriver CR, Beaudet AL, Sly WS, et al, eds. The metabolic and molecular bases of inherited disease, 8th ed, vol 3. New York: McGraw-Hill; 2001:3589-610.
28. Silverstein MN, Ellefson RD. The syndrome of the sea-blue histiocyte. Semin Hematol 1972;9:293-307.
29. Silverstein MN, Ellefson RD, Ahern EJ. The syndrome of the sea-blue histiocyte. N Engl J Med 1970;282:1-4.
30. Simell O. Lysinuric protein intolerance and other cationic aminoacidurias. In: Scriver CR, Beaudet AL, Sly WS, et al B, eds. The metabolic and molecular bases of inherited disease, 8th ed, vol 3. New York: McGraw-Hill; 2001:4933-56.
31. Suzuki Y, Oshima A, Nanba E. b-Galactosidase deficiency (b-Galactosidosis): G_{M1} gangliosidosis and morquio B disease. In: Scriver CR, Beaudet AL, Sly WS, et al, eds. The metabolic and molecular bases of inherited disease, 8th ed, vol 3. New York: McGraw-Hill; 2001:3775-809.
32. Thomas GH. Disorders of glycoprotein degradation: a-mannosidosis, b-mannosidosis, fucosidosis and sialidosis. In: Scriver CR, Beaudet AL, Sly WS, et al, eds. The metabolic and molecular bases of inherited disease, 8th ed, vol 3. New York: McGraw-Hill; 2001:3507-33.
33. von Figura K, Gieselmann V, Jaeken J. Metachromatic leukodystrophy. In: Scriver CR, Beaudet AL, Sly WS, et al, eds. The metabolic and molecular bases of inherited disease, 8th ed, vol 3. New York: McGraw-Hill; 2001:3695-724.
34. Willemsen R, van Dongen JM, Aerts JM, et al. An immunoelectron microscopic study of glucocerebrosidase in type 1 Gaucher's disease spleen. Ultrastruct Pathol 1988;12:471-8.

17 PHYSICAL INJURY AND VASCULAR ABNORMALITIES

Physical injury, particularly associated with trauma, is a relatively frequent occurrence in the spleen. It is one of the most common reasons for splenectomy. The evaluation of spleens that are removed incidentally or for trauma should be as thorough as those removed for specific pathologies.

Vascular abnormalities may induce striking changes in both lymph nodes and spleen. The changes associated with congestion may lead to chronic changes in the stroma and vascular elements of both spleen and lymph nodes, leading to architectural distortion. Furthermore, vascular changes may become prominent enough to mimic a vascular neoplasm. Chronic changes in the vascular system may even predispose to the development of vascular neoplasms.

SPLENIC RUPTURE (TRAUMATIC AND ATRAUMATIC)

Definition. *Rupture of the spleen* is defined as a tear in the capsule or vasculature of the spleen, typically resulting in hemorrhage and hemoperitoneum.

Clinical Features. Rupture of the spleen is seen in a variety of circumstances. Symptoms associated with splenic rupture include left upper quadrant pain and tenderness and signs associated with hemorrhagic shock. The pain is often referred to the left shoulder and arm. Aside from presentation as an "acute abdomen," splenic rupture can mimic several specific clinical conditions including angina, myocardial infarction, pulmonary embolus, ectopic pregnancy, acute appendicitis, and acute diverticulitis.

Traumatic rupture of the spleen is far more common than atraumatic rupture. Because of the location in the left upper quadrant, the spleen is relatively protected by the overlying rib cage. However, it is estimated that the spleen is ruptured in up to 30 percent of cases of significant blunt abdominal trauma (35). In a study by Farhi and Ashfaq (17), splenic trauma was associated with motor vehicle injury (45 percent), gunshot wounds (14 percent), and other causes (41 percent). Rupture of the splenic capsule is caused by deceleration and torsional injuries at the splenic hilum, as well as direct impact and laceration by bone fragments, such as broken ribs. Abnormal mobility of the spleen may be a contributing factor to rupture.

In contrast to traumatic rupture, pathologic rupture of the spleen also occurs. Pathologic rupture is typically spontaneous or associated with trivial trauma or actions such as sneezing or coughing. Traditionally referred to as "spontaneous" rupture, pathologic rupture is virtually always associated with some systemic disorder or underlying pathology of the spleen (12). The literature reports extraordinary cases of splenic rupture with no associated trauma or underlying pathology, which are most appropriately termed "idiopathic" splenic rupture. There are four criteria that must be met to qualify as idiopathic rupture: 1) absence of a history of trauma; 2) absence of adhesions, suggesting previous trauma; 3) absence of preexisting splenic disease; and 4) normal microscopic and macroscopic spleen.

Pathologic rupture can be due to a variety of conditions, both reactive and neoplastic. These are summarized in Table 17-1. Rupture of the spleen should always prompt pathologic evaluation of the splenic tissue since various infectious etiologies, infectious mononucleosis in particular, have pathologic findings that are distinctive enough to make a presumptive diagnosis, or suggest further studies. Splenic rupture is the most common fatal complication of infectious mononucleosis and occurs in 0.1 to 0.5 percent of patients with the disease (54). Rupture occurs 2 to 4 weeks after onset. Infectious mononucleosis–associated splenic rupture is the archetype of splenic rupture due to infiltration and weakening of capsular, stromal, and vascular structures by infiltrating inflammatory cells.

Vascular damage is likely the underlying mechanism of rupture associated with the use of thrombolytic and anticoagulant medications,

Table 17-1

ETIOLOGIES ASSOCIATED WITH PATHOLOGIC SPLENIC RUPTURE

Infectious	Viral	Epstein-Barr virus CMV[a] Hepatitis A Hepatitis B Dengue Mumps Rubella Influenza Varicella-zoster virus HIV
	Bacterial	*Actinomyces* sp. *Borrelia recurrentis* *Brucella* sp. *Campylobacter jejuni* *Clostridium* sp. *Coxiella burnetii* (Q fever) *Enterobacter cloacae* *Francisella tularensis* (tularemia) *Haemophilus* sp. *Legionella pneumophila* *Leptospira* sp. *Mycobacterium tuberculosis* *Neisseria meningitidis* *Pseudomonas* sp. *Rickettsia typhi* (typhus) *Salmonella* sp. *Staphylococcus* sp. *Streptococcus* sp. Syphilis
	Fungal	*Aspergillus* sp. *Candida* sp.
	Parasitic/ protozoal	Malaria (*Plasmodium* sp.) *Echinococcus* sp. *Leishmania* sp.
Medication Related	Anticoagulant/ thrombolytic	Heparin Low molecular weight heparin Warfarin Dicumarol Ticlopidine Streptokinase Urokinase Tissue plasminogen activator
	Cytokines	G-CSF GM-CSF
Hematologic	Non-neoplastic	Hemophilia Congenital afibrinogenemia Factor XIII deficiency Protein S deficiency Immune thrombocytopenic purpura Hemolytic anemia
	Neoplastic	Acute leukemia Chronic myeloproliferative disorders Lymphoma Myeloma
Systemic Disorders	Storage/ metabolic disorders	Amyloidosis Gaucher disease Niemann-Pick disease Sea-blue (ceroid) histiocytosis Wilson disease
	Connective tissue diseases	Rheumatoid arthritis Systemic lupus erythematosus Polyarteritis nodosa Wegener granulomatosis Ehlers-Danlos syndrome
	Other	Uremia Acute pancreatitis Chronic pancreatitis Infective endocarditis Pregnancy Crohn disease Sarcoidosis Cirrhosis
Vascular	Non-neoplastic	Infarct Peliosis
	Neoplastic	Angiosarcoma
Iatrogenic		Extracorporeal shock wave lithotripsy Colonoscopy Transesophageal echocardiography Electroconvulsive shock therapy Implantation of automatic defibrillators Hysterectomy Other surgeries
Physical		Vomiting/retching
Neoplastic	Nonhematologic	Renal cell carcinoma Teratoma Esophageal carcinoma Pancreatic carcinoma Pheochromocytoma Hepatocellular carcinoma Choriocarcinoma Melanoma
Other		Cyst

[a]CMV = cytomegalovirus; HIV = human immunodeficiency virus; G-CSF = granulocyte-colony stimulating factor; GM-CSF = granulocyte/monocyte-colony stimulating factor.

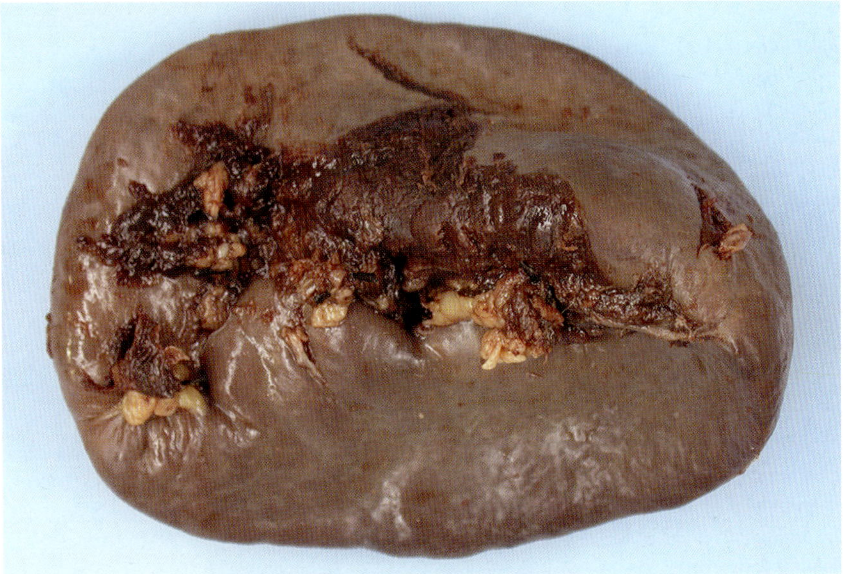

Figure 17-1

INCIDENTAL SPLENIC RUPTURE

The capsule of this spleen is disrupted in the region of the splenic hilum. Adherent blood clot is often present, but was removed in this case to make the site of rupture more apparent.

as well as vasculitides. Subcapsular hematomas also form due to anticoagulant medications and in uremia. Splenic rupture associated with pregnancy is multifactorial and may be due to combinations of the following factors: hypervolemia, splenic enlargement, decreased peritoneal cavity volume, muscular contractions associated with labor, and the exceedingly rare splenic pregnancy (implantation of the fertilized ovum on the spleen surface). Vomiting and retching are associated with rare splenic rupture and are likely due to diaphragmatic contraction and a tractional tear of either the splenic capsule or hilar vessels.

Splenic rupture as a primary presentation of hematologic malignancy is quite rare, but has been reported with both low-grade and high-grade lymphoid malignancies. Nonhematopoietic lesions are also associated with splenic rupture, including cysts, infarctions, vascular lesions/neoplasms, and metastatic malignancies.

Gross Findings. The gross pathologic features of splenic rupture are variable (fig. 17-1). Most often, there is evidence of one or more capsular tears, often with adherent blood clot. In trauma, lacerations are found most commonly at the superior pole (38 percent) and hilum (23 percent), and can vary from 1.0 to 11.5 cm in length (17). Depending on the underlying condition, there may be splenomegaly. In some conditions, the capsule is weakened focally or diffusely.

Subcapsular hemorrhage, infarction, or focal pathology such as cysts or tumors may be found, depending on the underlying etiology. Diffuse pathology of the spleen is more frequently associated with splenic rupture, so zonal or diffuse gross abnormalities may be identified.

Microscopic Findings. The microscopic features of splenic rupture depend on the underlying etiology. Features that are common to most ruptured spleens are hemorrhage and focal red pulp congestion at the rupture site (fig. 17-2). Many ruptures occur at the site of a previous subcapsular hemorrhage. As such, there may be evidence of old hemorrhage or organizing thrombus associated with a rupture site. In addition, infarctions are associated with rupture.

Mild subcapsular neutrophilic infiltrates may be seen in traumatic rupture. Most cases (68 percent) have widely patent sinuses and hemorrhage, often in a perifollicular location (17). Follicular hyperplasia, mantle zone hyperplasia, marginal zone hyperplasia, and lipogranulomas are frequent findings. The T-cell zones (periarterial lymphatic sheath [PALS] areas) are typically normal in spleens removed for trauma.

Other etiologies, such as storage diseases, often present with characteristic histologic findings as well, which may clarify the etiology of the rupture.

Treatment and Prognosis. Because of the presentation of splenic rupture, immediate

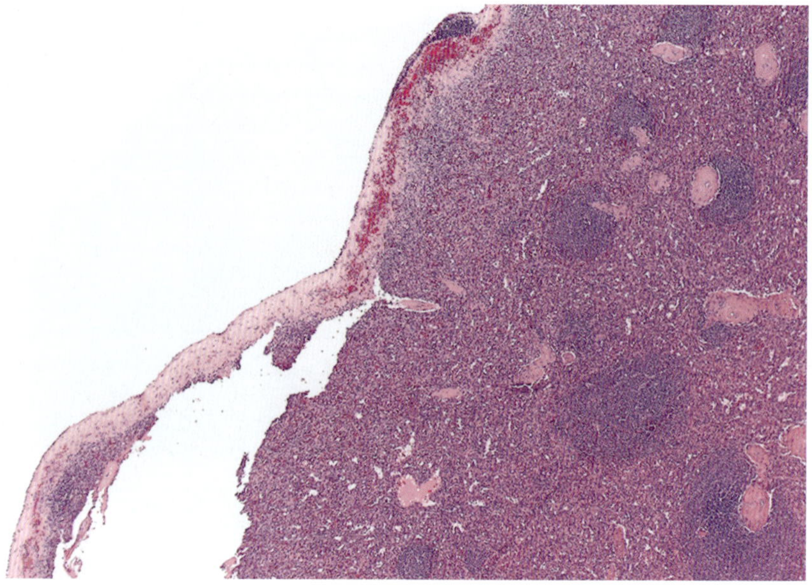

Figure 17-2

SPONTANEOUS SPLENIC RUPTURE

Focal hemorrhage within the capsule suggests weakening of the capsule at this site.

surgical intervention is usually required. Rarely, rupture is managed conservatively, with careful radiologic evaluation and medical support. Typically, however, an open or laparoscopic evaluation and intervention are required. Traditionally, splenectomy has been the treatment of choice. However, because of the subsequent immunologic deficit in dealing with encapsulated bacterial infections, other spleen-sparing surgeries (splenorrhaphy, partial splenectomy) are being attempted more frequently.

Because of the spleen's role in immunologic protection against encapsulated bacteria (*Pneumococcus, Haemophilus, Neisseria*) it is recommended that patients are immunized against these organisms to avoid postsplenectomy sepsis. Postsplenectomy sepsis is an often fatal consequence of these infections.

FIBROCONGESTIVE SPLENOMEGALY (INCLUDING PORTAL HYPERTENSION)

Definition. *Fibrocongestive splenomegaly* is chronic local or regional venous congestion leading to permanent vascular and stromal changes in the spleen. *Banti syndrome* is idiopathic portal hypertension resulting in splenomegaly.

Pathogenesis. A variety of etiologies may cause splenic congestion, including any disorder that causes right-sided heart failure. Most commonly, chronic congestion is due to localized effects in the portal venous system, usually as a result of liver cirrhosis (40). Budd-Chiari syndrome and schistosomiasis may cause portal hypertension, leading to fibrocongestive splenomegaly.

Gross Findings. Spleens with fibrocongestive splenomegaly are often moderately enlarged (up to 1,000 g) and often have a thickened capsule (fig. 17-3). The cut surface is firm, due to increases in the stromal elements. The white pulp may be less conspicuous than usual, due to expansion and widening of the red pulp. Increased firmness of the parenchyma may be due to expanded stroma, and infarcts may be evident.

Microscopic Findings. The sinuses are normal in size but increased in number, with decreases in cordal tissue and capillaries. Sinus lining cells (e.g., littoral cells) may be enlarged and activated (fig. 17-4). Vessels may be thickened (fig. 17-5). There is an increase in reticulin fibers. Hemosiderin deposition and Gamna-Gandy bodies (iron and calcium in fibrotic nodules) may be seen.

Ancillary Studies. Smooth muscle actin shows increased staining in reticulum cells, suggesting a phenotypic change in response to the chronic vascular/pressure changes (fig. 17-6). Smooth muscle actin stains also show increased numbers of myofibroblastic cells, especially in the red pulp. Staining with low-affinity nerve growth factor receptor (LNGFR) is markedly increased in the reticulum cells of the red pulp. Reticulin fibers are increased surrounding the sinuses and in the cords.

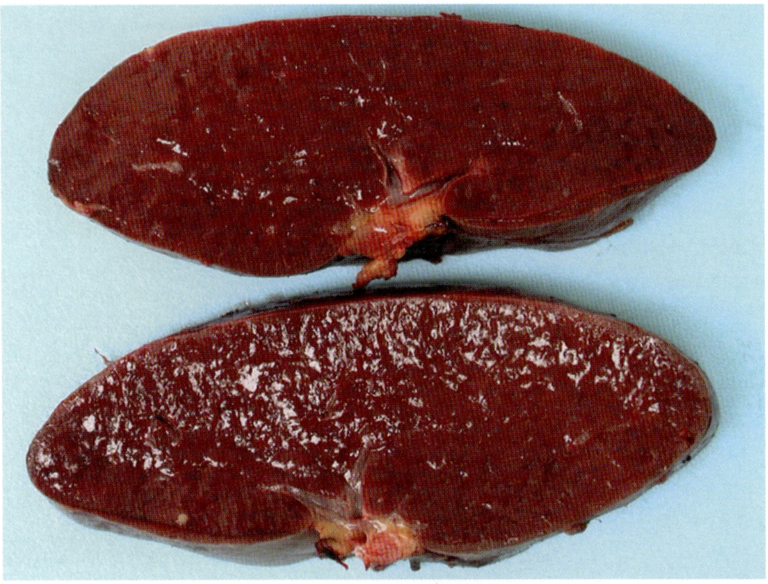

Figure 17-3

FIBROCONGESTIVE SPLENOMEGALY

There are no focal abnormalities seen, although the red pulp appears more hemorrhagic than usual. Splenic enlargement may be moderate or severe, but lacks specific gross findings unless another process, such as infarction, supervenes.

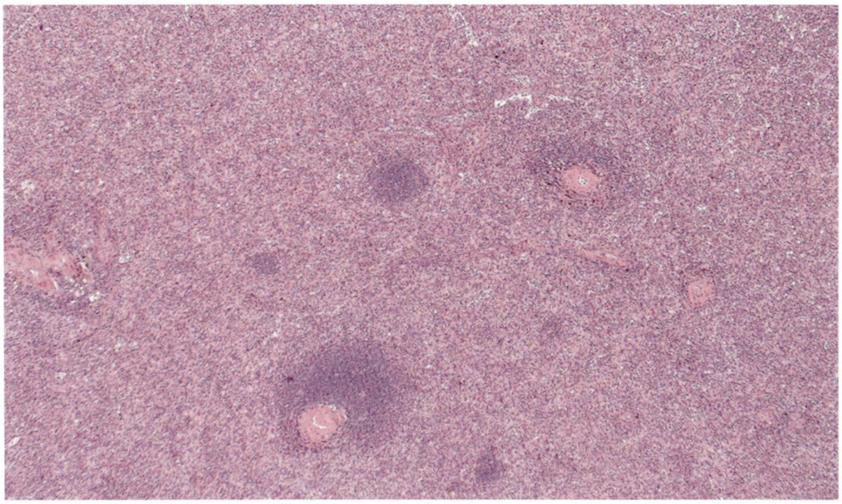

Figure 17-4

FIBROCONGESTIVE SPLENOMEGALY

Unremarkable white pulp is paired with massive expansion of the red pulp.

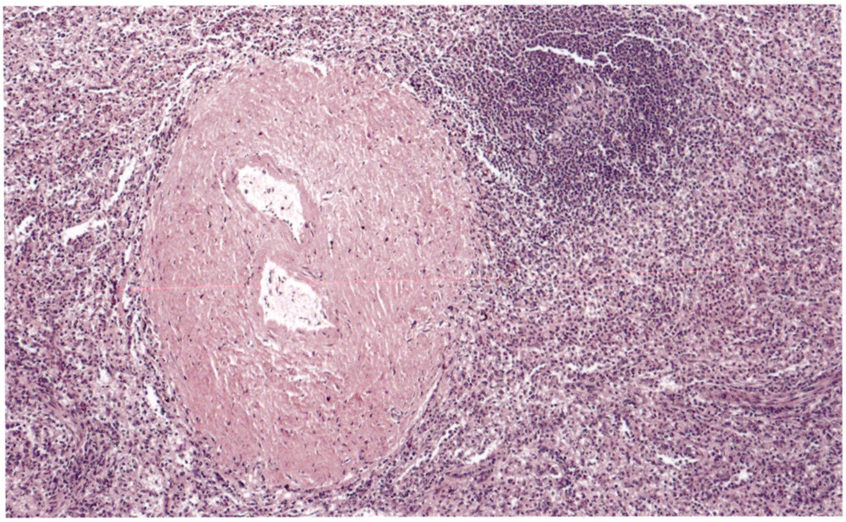

Figure 17-5

FIBROCONGESTIVE SPLENOMEGALY

Vessels are thickened.

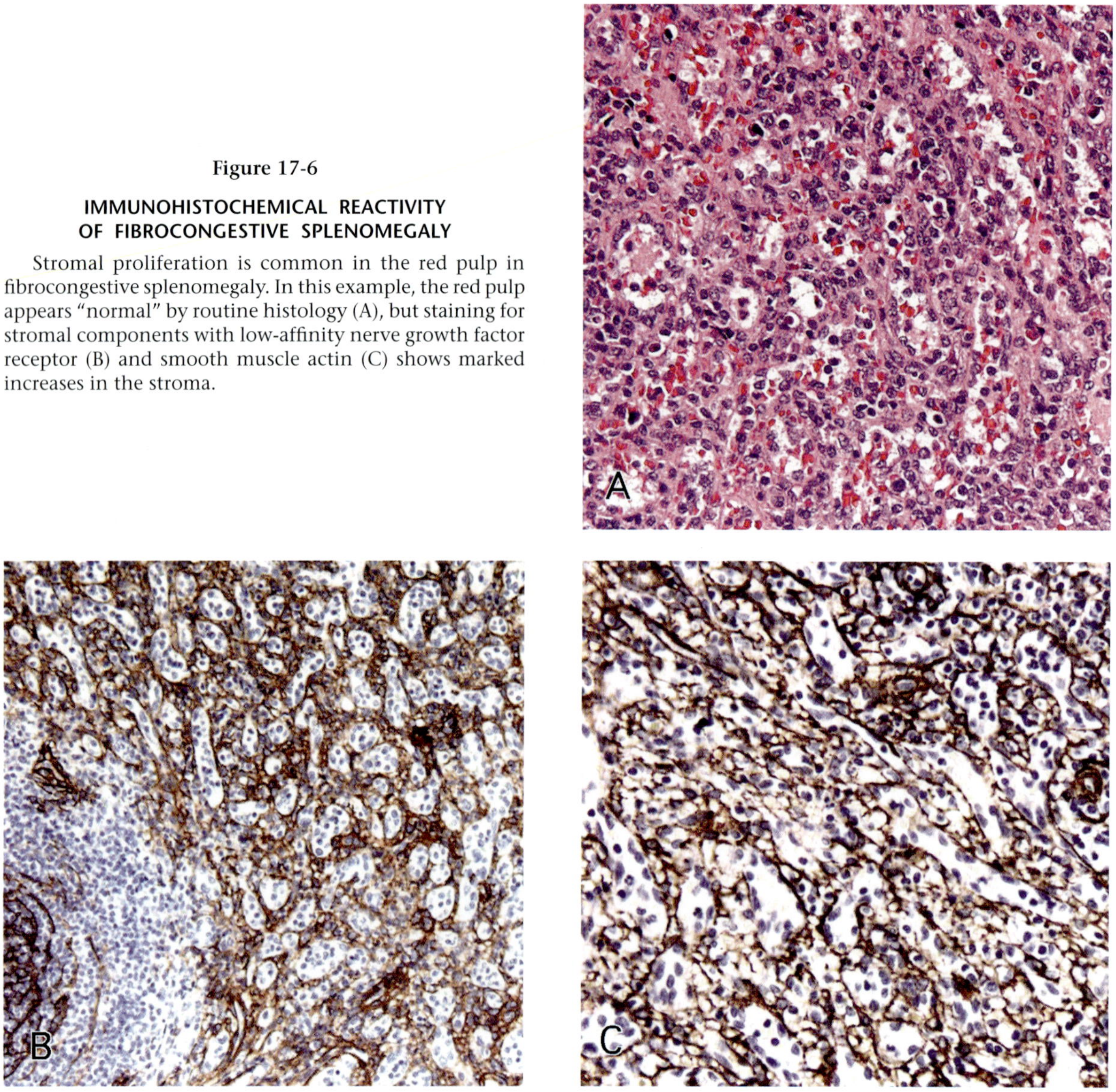

Figure 17-6

IMMUNOHISTOCHEMICAL REACTIVITY OF FIBROCONGESTIVE SPLENOMEGALY

Stromal proliferation is common in the red pulp in fibrocongestive splenomegaly. In this example, the red pulp appears "normal" by routine histology (A), but staining for stromal components with low-affinity nerve growth factor receptor (B) and smooth muscle actin (C) shows marked increases in the stroma.

Differential Diagnosis. Any cause of red pulp expansion and congestion can mimic fibrocongestive splenomegaly. Careful gross examination should be performed and any focal lesions sampled for microscopic examination. Processes that are primarily based in the red pulp should be evaluated in the context of the clinical history. Many of the neoplastic hematologic disorders with red pulp expansion have blood and bone marrow abnormalities. A peripheral blood smear should be examined for abnormalities, if possible. Other disorders with increases in macrophages and red pulp congestion include: immune thrombocytopenic purpura, thrombotic thrombocytopenic purpura, hemolytic anemias, and possibly, storage diseases. Chronicity, clinical findings, and correlation with blood findings help distinguish these entities from fibrocongestive splenomegaly.

Treatment and Prognosis. It is unclear whether the architectural changes in the spleen revert to normal after the correction of vascular congestion. Although possible, the stromal changes would take a considerable amount of time to revert to normal, if ever. Regardless, the underlying causes of vascular congestion should be addressed to have any impact on fibrocongestive splenomegaly.

INFARCTION OF LYMPH NODE AND SPLEEN

Definition. *Infarction of lymph node or spleen* is defined as parenchymal ischemia and necrosis caused by vascular compromise, often the result of embolization.

General Features. Because of the vascular nature of lymph nodes and spleen, infarction is a rare event. When present, it is typically due to underlying causes such as thrombosis, vascular disorders, or malignancies.

Clinical Features. Primary infarction of lymph nodes is rare, and is usually due to regional thrombotic events (25). More frequently, lymph nodes are involved by metastatic tumor or lymphoma (37). Lymph node necrosis is secondary to lymphoma in 32 to 89 percent of cases following fine needle aspiration biopsy, and also due to metastatic malignancies (such as breast carcinoma, small cell carcinoma, melanoma) (54). Other rare causes of lymph nodal infarction include: granulocytic sarcoma (28), infectious mononucleosis (29), and gold injections (45).

Splenic infarcts may be clinically silent or cause significant manifestations, including splenic rupture and acute abdomen. Clinical features of splenic infarction include left upper quadrant pain, fever, pleuritic chest pain, back pain, left shoulder pain, and increased abdominal girth. As in lymph nodes, thromboembolic conditions are a common cause of splenic infarction (40,62). Splenic embolization is associated with atherosclerosis, myocardial infarction, atrial fibrillation, and bacterial endocarditis, and as a complication of cardiac catheterization. Chronic myeloproliferative disorders with splenic involvement also frequently cause splenic infarction (40). Systemic vasculitis, malarial infections, and rarely, vascular compromise caused by hematologic or nonhematologic malignancy may result in splenic infarction.

The process of splenic infarction can be seen in sickle cell anemia (see also chapter 12). In homozygotes for sickle type hemoglobin (hemoglobin SS), the spleen undergoes repeated vascular infarction due to occlusion of small vessels by red blood cells, which become sickle shaped in the acidotic, hypoxic environment of the spleen. Eventually, the repeated infarction and necrosis lead to complete loss of all functional splenic tissue, leaving a tiny fibrotic husk remaining.

Computerized tomography (CT) scans reveal splenic infarcts as hypodense areas, which do not enhance with contrast. Ultrasonography shows the difference between recent infarcts (hypoechoic) and older infarcts (hyperechoic).

A splenic condition that may clinically mimic splenic infarction, or ultimately result in infarction of the spleen, is torsion of the spleen. Torsion of the spleen is secondary to "wandering spleen"; the latter rare condition is due to a congenital or acquired weakness or absence of the ligaments (lienogastric, lienorenal, and phrenocolic) that support the spleen in its usual left upper quadrant position (40,52). Other factors that may contribute to a wandering spleen are splenomegaly of any cause, trauma, abdominal laxity, gastric distension, and possibly, the hormonal effects of pregnancy. Clinically, torsion of the spleen may be mistaken for appendicitis or ovarian torsion, with pain in the midabdomen or left lower quadrant.

Gross Findings. A completely infarcted lymph node does not appear grossly normal. The appearance varies according to the time elapsed since the necrotic event. In general, the lymph node is soft, with a white-yellow appearance. Gross suppuration or grumous tissue may be seen.

Infarcts are wedge shaped in the spleen (figs. 17-7, 17-8). Segmental splenic vasculature that radiates outward from the hilum is responsible for this pattern. Initially, splenic infarcts are hemorrhagic and red-black, but with resolution, they become firm and yellow-tan. Torsion of the spleen may result in a tortuous splenic pedicle, with marked vascular congestion.

Microscopic Findings. Infarction of a lymph node may be partial or complete (figs. 17-9, 17-10). When the node is mostly involved, there is typically sparing of a small rim of tissue in a subcapsular location. The infarcted tissue consists of eosinophilic material, sometimes with the ghost-like outlines of cells. Depending on the date of onset of the necrosis, inflammatory elements are variably present: recent infarcts often have neutrophils and their cellular debris within the necrotic tissue; later, chronic inflammatory elements predominate; and finally, granulation tissue forms.

As with lymph nodes, the appearance of splenic infarction depends on the age of the infarct. Recent infarcts typically have regions

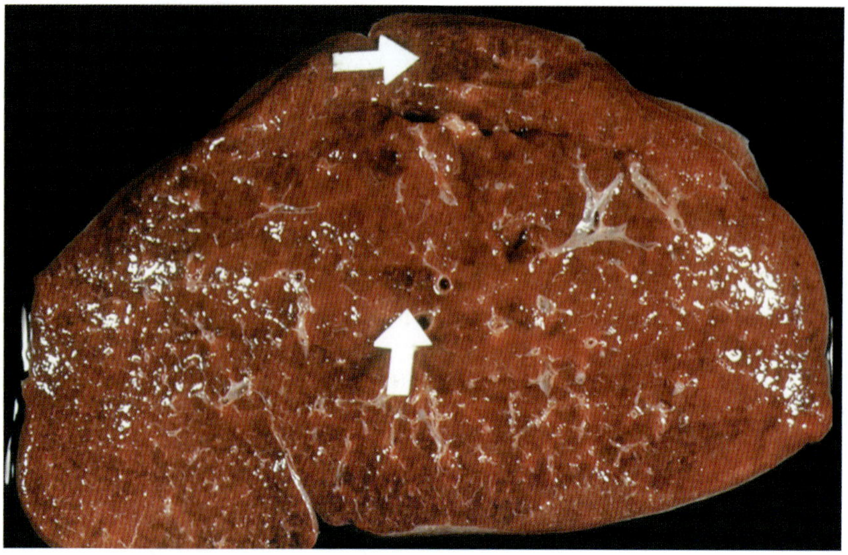

Figure 17-7

SPLENIC INFARCT, RECENT

Arrows point to areas of infarct. Early infarction of the spleen may be seen as areas of slight darkening, irregularity, or hemorrhage. (Courtesy of Richard Neiman, Harpswell, ME.)

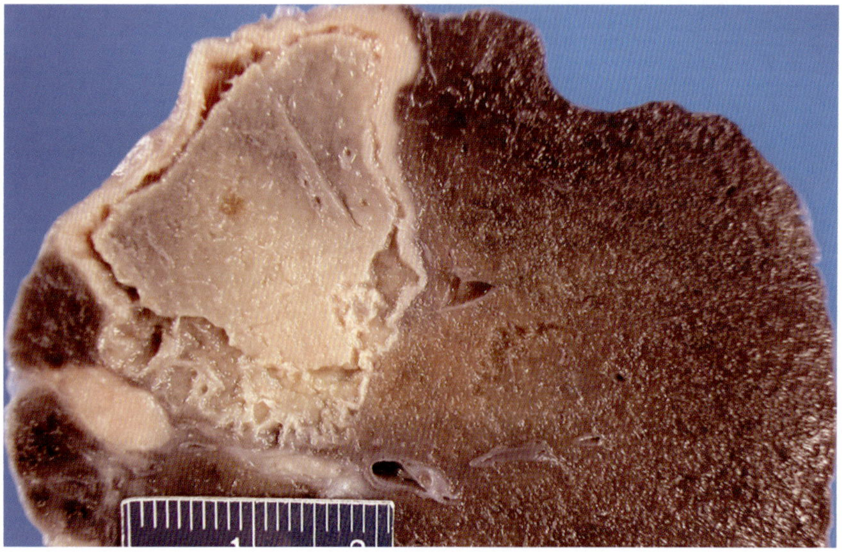

Figure 17-8

SPLENIC INFARCT, REMOTE

The infarct is subcapsular, firm, and tan. The border of the infarct is well circumscribed from the surrounding intact spleen.

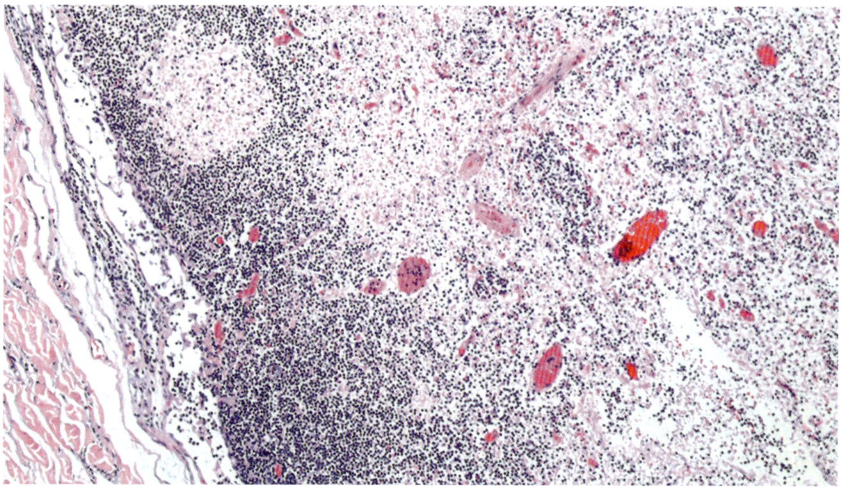

Figure 17-9

INFARCT, LYMPH NODE

Portions of this lymph node are viable, while the more central portion is completely necrotic.

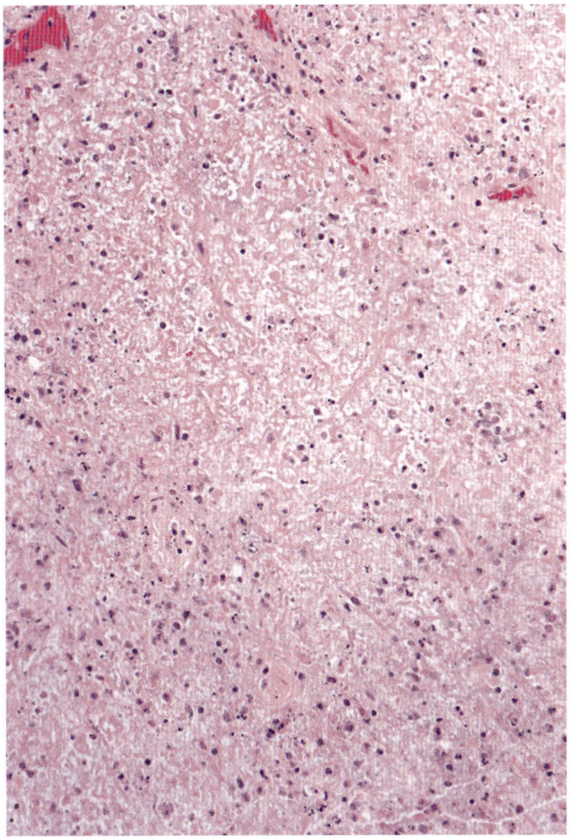

Figure 17-10

INFARCT, LYMPH NODE

Necrosis is almost complete and the etiology is not apparent.

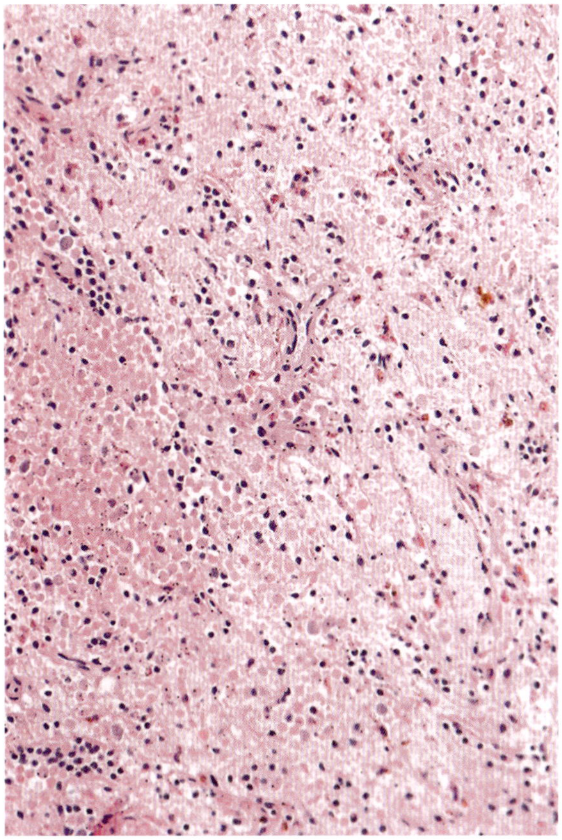

Figure 17-11

INFARCT, SPLEEN

Faint outlines of splenic sinuses are appreciated in this example.

of individual necrotic cells with preserved cell outlines (i.e., coagulative necrosis), often with extensive parenchymal hemorrhage (fig. 17-11). As time progresses from the original insult, there is infiltration by acute inflammatory elements, including granulocytes and monocytes. Monocytes differentiate into macrophages, which often become laden with the debris of tissue breakdown. Still later, there are denser infiltrates of macrophages, followed by loose stromal proliferations. Eventually, organized fibrotic regions with neovascularization form (fig. 17-12).

Ancillary Studies. Studies have shown that despite necrosis, immunohistochemical reactivity is maintained for some antigens (fig. 17-13) (29,30,41,54,60). Staining for CD79a, CD3, CD43, and CD45RO is well preserved in necrotic tissue; CD20 is less well preserved, and cytokeratins and epithelial membrane antigen (EMA) are variably preserved. Gene rearrangement analysis (Southern blot, polymerase chain reaction [PCR]) has been successful in selected cases (34,60). Angiography of duplex Doppler color flow studies of the spleen may be helpful in determining the vascular integrity and extent of the splenic infarction (52).

Differential Diagnosis. In lymph nodes, distinguishing benign lymph node infarction from infarction of an underlying neoplasm is difficult, and occasionally impossible. As outlined above, immunohistochemical stains may be of benefit in determining the nature of the infarcted cells. However, it is prudent to evaluate the patient thoroughly for other evidence of adenopathy or disease. If possible, additional tissue should be obtained. In the authors' experience, repeated biopsies are sometimes necessary to obtain viable, diagnostic tissue.

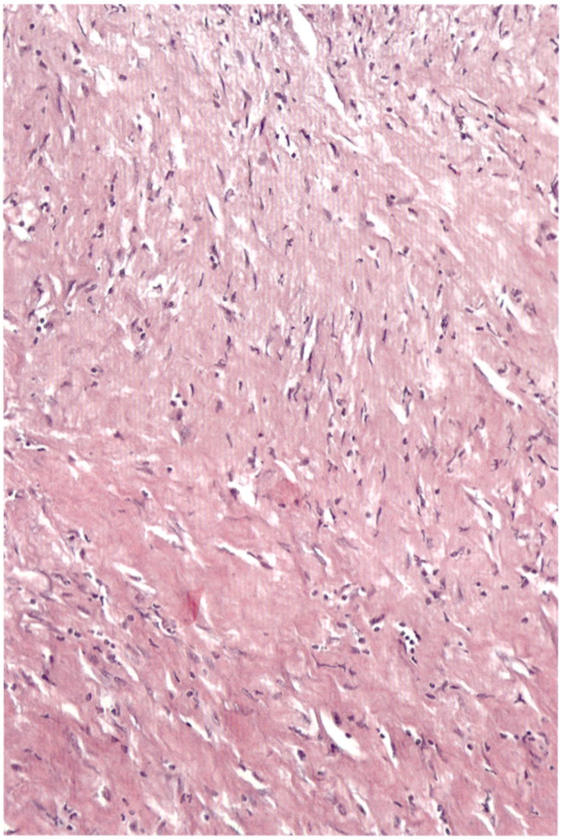

Figure 17-12

INFARCT, LYMPH NODE

In final stages of an infarct, the infarcted area may be totally replaced by fibrosis and neovascularization, as in this lymph node.

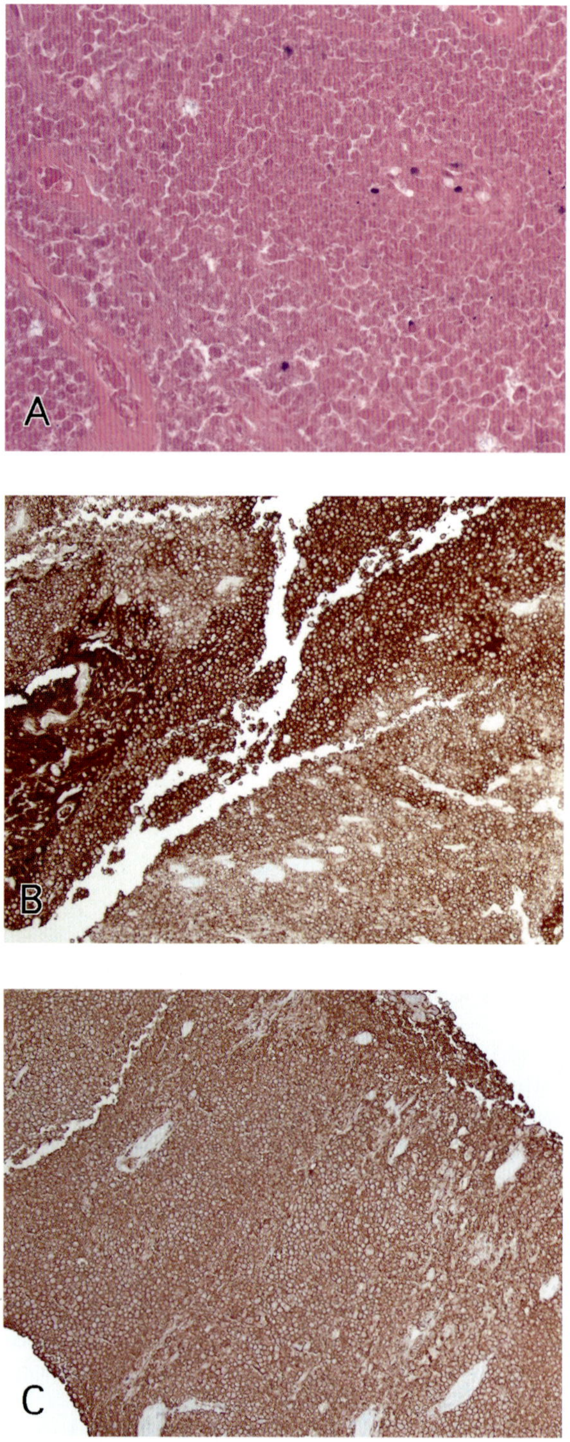

Figure 17-13

IMMUNOHISTOCHEMICAL REACTIVITY IN INFARCTED LYMPHOID TISSUE

The hematoxylin and eosin (H&E)-stained section appears completely infarcted (A), while immunohistochemical reactivity for CD45RB (B) and CD20 (C) is positive.

Splenic infarction typically presents fewer diagnostic difficulties than infarction of the lymph node. In spite of this, it is important to critically evaluate the areas of splenic infarction for potential significant underlying pathology.

Treatment and Prognosis. Infarcted lymph nodes are typically painful and surgical removal is important both for control of symptoms and diagnostic purposes. The prognosis is entirely dependent on the underlying etiology of the necrosis. Since there is a significant association with underlying malignancy, the diagnosis of a completely necrotic lymph node should prompt a thorough evaluation for underlying pathology.

The complications of splenic infarction are quite broad. Gangrene, abscess formation, peritonitis, intestinal obstruction, necrosis of the pancreatic tail, and rupture are all possible outcomes,

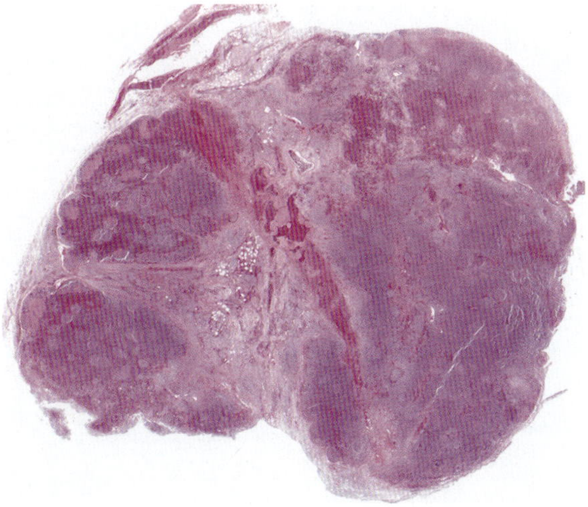

Figure 17-14

CHANGES ASSOCIATED WITH FINE NEEDLE ASPIRATION/BIOPSY, LYMPH NODE

The needle track and the associated damage to the lymph node architecture are seen.

although many patients with splenic infarcts have no significant morbidity. A 5 percent mortality rate is associated with splenic infarction.

CHANGES ASSOCIATED WITH FINE NEEDLE ASPIRATION/BIOPSY

Definition. Morphologic changes are associated with the performance of fine needle aspiration biopsy (FNAB) in lymph nodes, spleen, and other lymphoid tissues.

General Features. FNAB is a common diagnostic procedure. In the lymph node, histologic alterations caused by the procedure that may affect diagnostic interpretation of the excised node have been reported in 1.4 to 85.0 percent of cases (39); a study by Tsang and Chan (56) reported an incidence of 4.3 percent of cases. There is great room for interpretation within this wide range.

The spleen is not amenable to partial excision or excisional biopsy (31). FNAB of spleen is a rare technique in the North America, although it is performed more often in Europe (11). Complications occur in approximately 5 percent of patients and include hemoperitoneum, pneumothorax, pseudoaneurysm, intrasplenic hemorrhage, and hematoma formation (11,33).

Microscopic Findings. Three patterns of histologic alteration due to FNAB are described: focal hemorrhage with or without organization, segmental necrosis with organization, and complete coagulative necrosis (fig. 17-14) (56). A needle track may be visible both grossly and microscopically in some cases, and makes the evaluation of these lesions easier (fig. 17-15). Sclerosis, vascular and spindle cell proliferations, and areas of infarction and necrosis are common. In complete necrosis, only eosinophilic necrotic "ghost" cells are present (39,56).

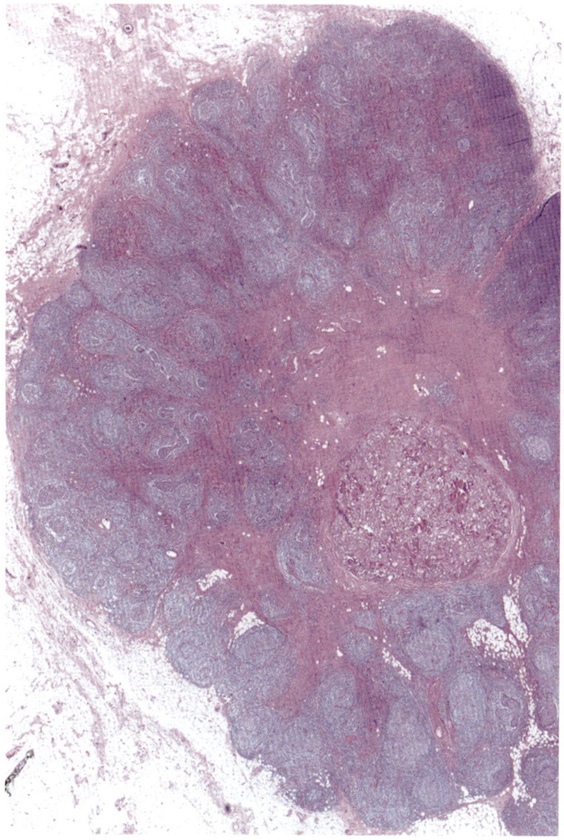

Figure 17-15

CHANGES ASSOCIATED WITH FINE NEEDLE ASPIRATION BIOPSY, LYMPH NODE

A needle track is filled with necrotic debris, and a massive fibrous proliferation surrounds the site of damage.

Ancillary Studies. In partially affected lymph nodes, standard evaluations usually suffice for diagnosis. Immunohistochemical stains may be of benefit in the evaluation of completely necrotic nodes. Some immunohistochemical stains continue to be convincingly reactive in necrotic cells, including keratin and CD79a (39,54). A specimen for flow cytometric analysis should

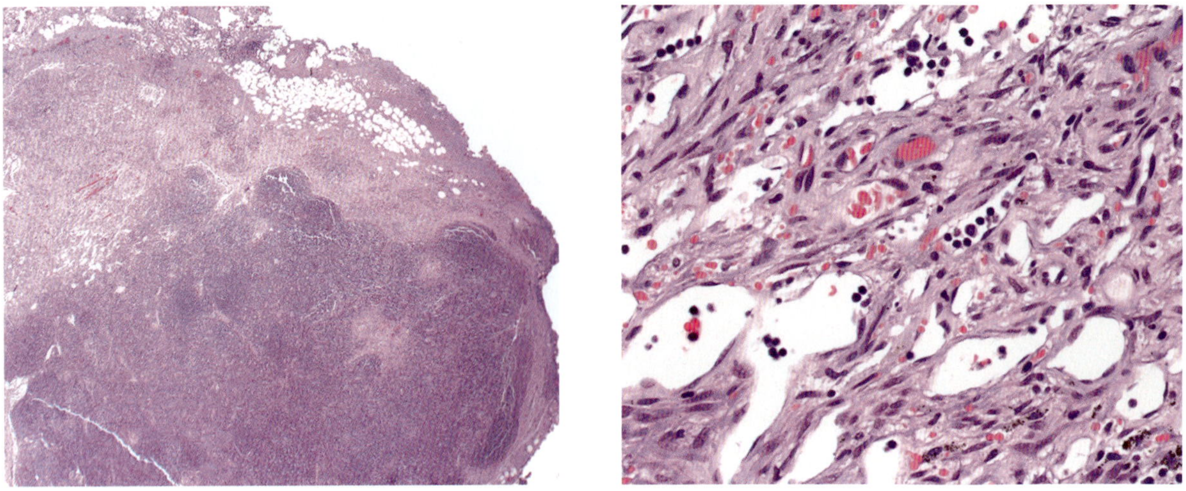

Figure 17-16

VASCULAR TRANSFORMATION OF SINUSES, LYMPH NODE

Left: The upper left portion of the lymph node is undergoing vascular transformation.
Right: At higher magnification, the vascular spaces are lined by bland endothelial cells.

be obtained in all lymph nodes where a lymphoproliferative disorder is being considered and in essentially all cases of splenic FNAB.

Differential Diagnosis. Areas of fibrosis and reorganization sometimes suggest a vascular tumor, especially early nodal involvement by Kaposi sarcoma. Careful evaluation of the clinical history, and possibly, use of immunohistochemical stains for human herpesvirus (HHV)-8 are of benefit. Complete nodal infarction can be seen in a variety of conditions (see chapter 5). In cases where a diagnosis is not possible, excisional biopsy of nodes that have not undergone FNAB procedures may be necessary.

In spleen, false positive and false negative diagnoses of conditions may occur, albeit rarely (11,33). In any case where the diagnosis is not straightforward (i.e., large cell lymphoma, carcinoma), or is not strongly supported by ancillary studies (cytogenetics, flow cytometry), a splenectomy should be performed for a definitive diagnosis.

VASCULAR TRANSFORMATION OF LYMPH NODE SINUSES (NODAL ANGIOMATOSIS)

Definition. *Vascular transformation of lymph node sinuses* (VTS), sometimes referred to as *nodal angiomatosis*, is a rare change of the subcapsular and medullary lymph node sinuses from simple vascular channels to an anastomosing network of smaller vascular channels. It is often associated with vascular occlusion and subsequent proliferation of sinus endothelial elements, but may also be related to other angiogenic factors.

Clinical Features. VTS is uncommon and has no gender or age predilection. It occurs most commonly in abdominal nodes, followed by roughly equal occurrence in cervical, supraclavicular, axillary, and inguinal locations. In many cases, VTS is an incidental finding, usually associated with staging lymph node dissection for a malignancy. Less frequently, VTS presents as isolated lymphadenopathy. Although most common in single nodes, nodal groups, multiple individual nodes, and bilaterality can be seen (9,24).

In 70 percent of cases, vascular obstruction is reported (9). The mechanisms involved with VTS are adjacent or nodal tumor, thrombosis, congestive heart failure, constrictive pericarditis, or previous surgery or radiation to the area.

Gross Findings. Lymph nodes affected by VTS typically appear normal on gross examination.

Microscopic Findings. The main histologic feature is the formation of small endothelium-lined channels in the lymph node sinuses (figs. 17-16–17-18). Several microscopic patterns have been described, alone or in combination: cleft-like spaces (about 70 percent), rounded vascular spaces (60 percent), solid areas (40 percent), and plexiform pattern (rare). Fibrosis may also be

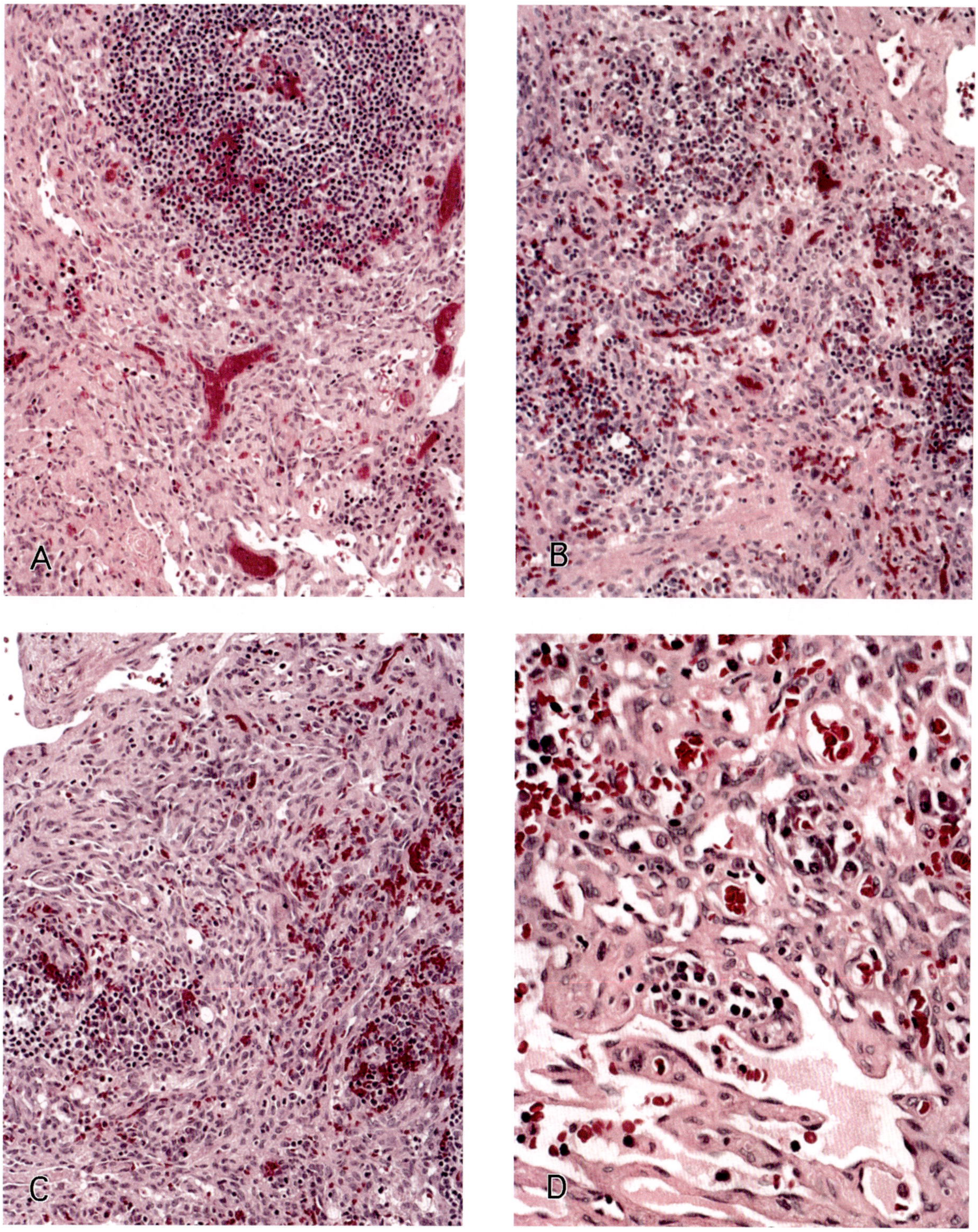

Figure 17-17

VASCULAR TRANSFORMATION OF SINUSES, LYMPH NODE

Parafollicular spaces are expanded with spindle-shaped endothelial cells (A), some of which are filled with red blood cells (B). These vascular elements are bland (C) and can simulate Kaposi sarcoma or other benign vascular neoplasms (D).

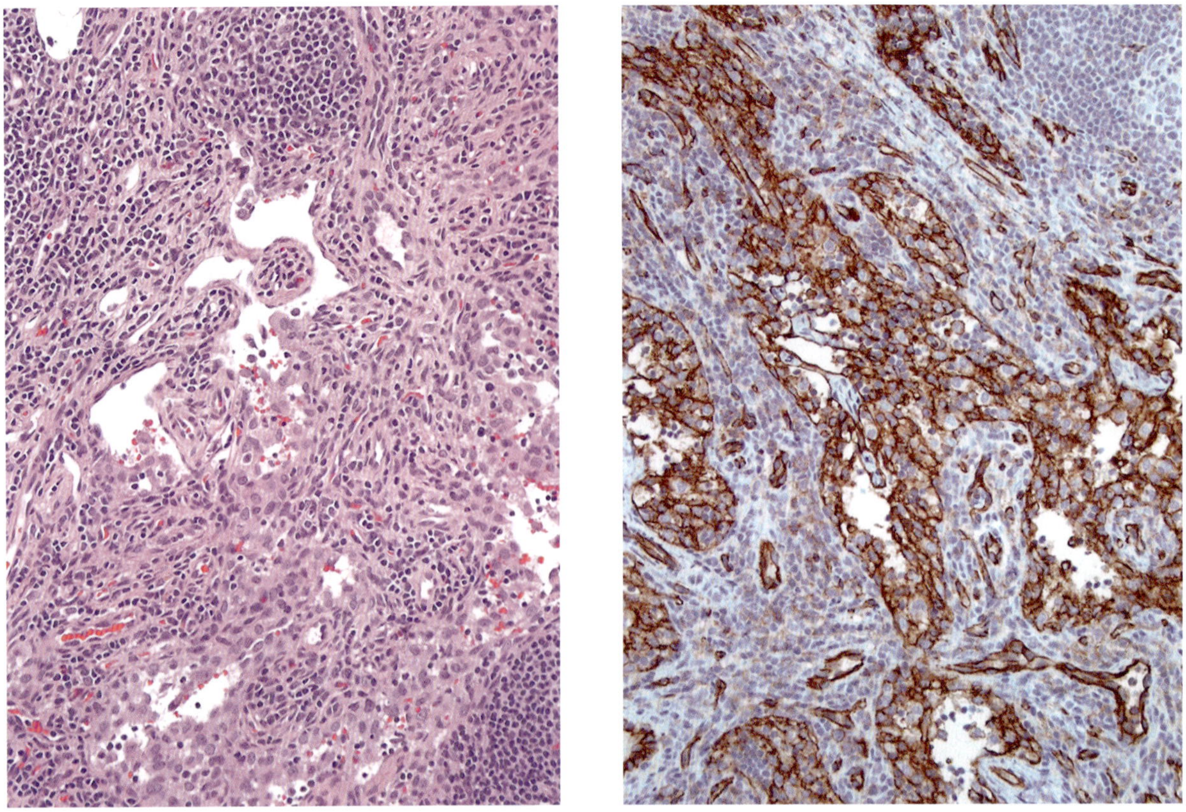

Figure 17-18

VASCULAR TRANSFORMATION OF SINUSES, LYMPH NODE

H&E (left) and CD31 (right) staining in vascular transformation of lymph node sinuses. The plump endothelial cells are highlighted by the CD31 stain.

present. Extravasation of red blood cells is seen and rarely, hyaline globules, similar to those of Kaposi sarcoma, are observed (9). The lymph node capsule is not involved in VTS, in contrast to Kaposi sarcoma.

The bland cytologic appearance of the cells and the absence of mitoses in VTS distinguish it from primary vascular tumors that occur in lymph nodes (8). Kaposi sarcoma characteristically shows slit-like vessels with cytologic atypia, extravasated red blood cells, and eosinophilic globules, features that are not characteristically seen in VTS (Table 17-2).

Ancillary Studies. Immunohistochemical stains highlight the vascular nature of the proliferation, especially in areas that are solid. Stains such as CD31, CD34, factor VIII antigen, *Ulex europaeus* lectin, and Fli-1 confirm the vascular nature of the neoplasm. Interestingly, a recent report has shown VTS to be positive for D2-40, a marker of lymphatic differentiation (19). Ki-67 has a low to absent proliferation rate in VTS. Immunohistochemical or in situ stains for HHV-8 are negative in VTS, in contrast to Kaposi sarcoma.

Differential Diagnosis. In a general sense, the differential diagnosis of VTS includes all possible vascular proliferations that can be seen in a lymph node. However, in a practical evaluation, only a few need be considered (Kaposi sarcoma, hemangioma, angiosarcoma, or other vascular proliferations). Features that favor a diagnosis of Kaposi sarcoma versus VTS include nuclear atypia, capsular involvement, hyaline globules, and predominance of short slit-like vascular spaces (Table 17-2).

Treatment and Prognosis. No specific treatment is required for VTS. It is unlikely to cause specific problems other than enlarged lymph nodes.

Table 17-2

DISTINCTION OF VASCULAR TRANSFORMATION OF LYMPH NODE SINUSES (VTS) FROM KAPOSI SARCOMA

Features	VTS	Kaposi Sarcoma
Slit-like vascular spaces	Some	Predominant
Spindle shaped cells	Yes	Yes
Extravasated RBC[a]	Occasional	Frequent
Capsular involvement	Not seen	Frequently seen
Cytologic atypia	Not seen	Occasionally seen
Hyaline globules	Rare	Occasionally seen

[a]RBC = red blood cell.

LYMPHANGIECTASIA AND PELIOSIS

Definition. *Lymphangiectasia* is an abnormal dilatation of preexisting sinuses and lymphatic channels in a lymph node. *Peliosis* is a rare, presumably non-neoplastic, proliferation of blood-filled cavities in the liver, spleen, or other organs (including lymph node).

Clinical Features. Lymphangiectasis is a reactive process that is usually associated with proximal soft tissue obstruction involving preexisting structures as compared to a nodal lymphangioma that has a hamartomatous or neoplastic origin (63). The dilated channels in lymphangiectasis are filled with proteinaceous fluid that surrounds islands of residual lymphoid tissue.

Peliosis occurs most frequently in the liver. Less commonly, it occurs in both liver and spleen, but isolated splenic peliosis has been reported, as have rare cases in lymph node. Other rare sites include bone marrow, lung, kidney, and parathyroid gland. Conditions associated with peliosis are tuberculosis, cirrhosis, hematologic neoplasms, intravenous drug abuse, chronic alcoholism, chemotherapy, and steroid treatment (58). The exact etiology is unknown but the pathogenesis of peliosis is speculated to be underlying vascular malformations that are made apparent by local alterations of vascular pressure.

Gross Findings. Sectioning of the spleen in peliosis reveals multiple round to oval, blood-filled cavities (fig. 17-19). Their distribution in the spleen is in clusters or distributed throughout the parenchyma. The blood is liquid or clotted, or forms thrombi.

Microscopic Findings. The microscopic features of lymphangiectasia are those of a dilated lymphatic vessel filled with proteinaceous fluid (fig. 17-20). The lining cells are typically flattened and have bland cytology. They are most typically filled with eosinophilic, proteinaceous fluid. Occasional lymphocytes and red blood cells are present as well.

Peliotic lesions are well demarcated from the surrounding normal spleen (figs. 17-21, 17-22). Ectatic sinusoids and blood-filled cysts are present throughout the organ. They are limited to the red pulp, and are most often located adjacent to the PALS and in the perifollicular zones. These blood-filled spaces are focally lined by attenuated, cytologically normal endothelial cells, but may also lack an endothelial lining.

Ancillary Studies. Immunohistochemical staining for lymphatic vessels has improved recently. In the past, staining of lymphatic

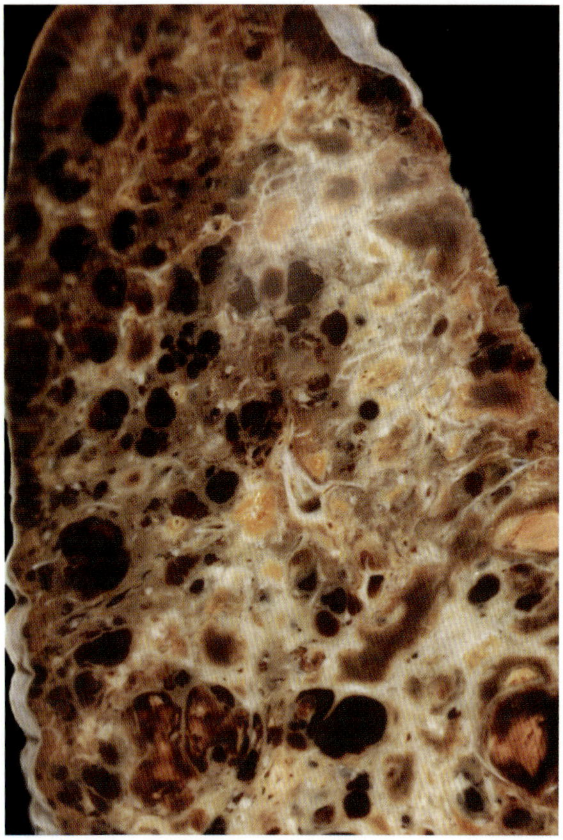

Figure 17-19

PELIOSIS, SPLEEN

There are numerous blood-filled spaces. (Courtesy of Richard Neiman, Harpswell, ME.)

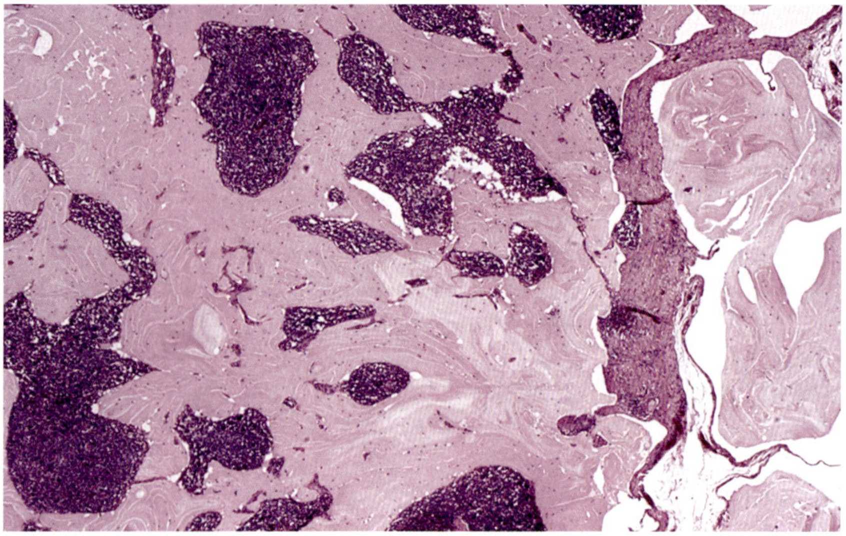

Figure 17-20

LYMPHANGIECTASIA

Dilated lymphatics are filled with proteinaceous fluid.

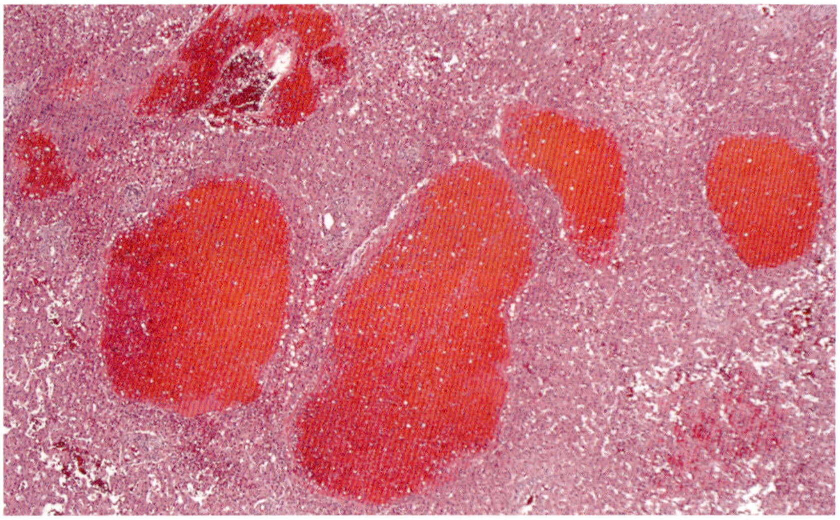

Figure 17-21

PELIOSIS, SPLEEN

Well-demarcated blood-filled spaces are in the spleen.

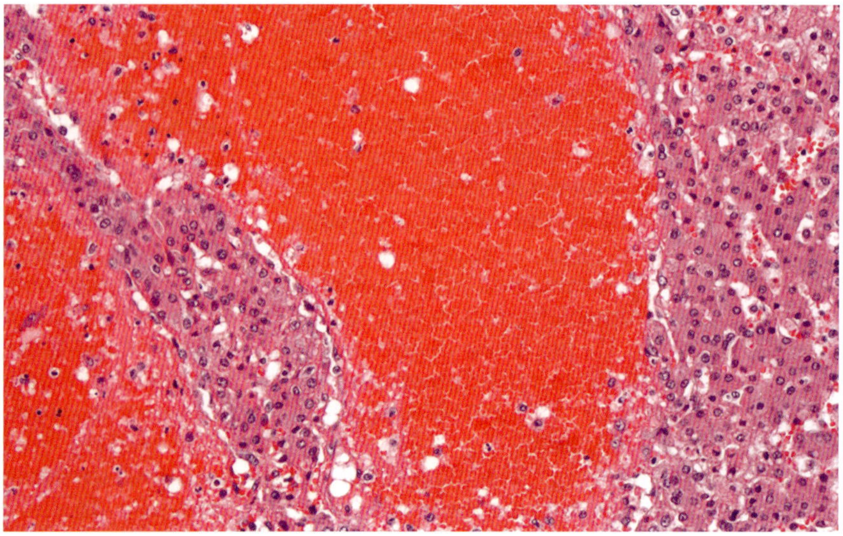

Figure 17-22

PELIOSIS, SPLEEN

The vascular lining of ectatic, blood-filled spaces is inapparent.

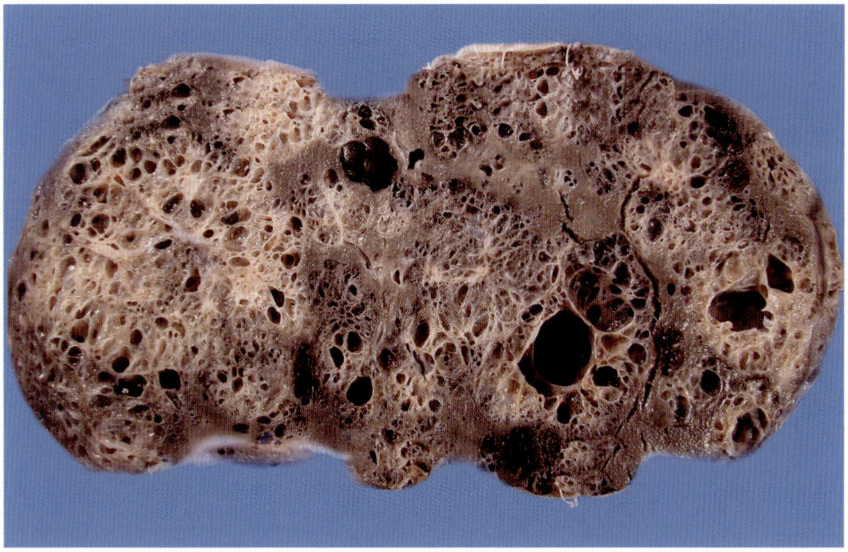

Figure 17-23

LYMPHANGIOMATOSIS

Numerous, varying-sized, smooth-walled cystic spaces of congenital lymphangiomatosis. These would be filled with clear fluid (lymph), although hemorrhage could lead to bloody or brownish fluid.

components was accomplished by using endothelial markers. Currently, new antibodies that are specific for lymphatic endothelium are more commonly available (e.g., podoplanin, D2-40, lymphatic vessel endothelial hyaluronan receptor [LYVE]-1). These stains allow the distinction of lymphatic processes from other vascular-derived processes.

In peliosis, because of the association with infectious etiologies, stains for organisms (e.g., acid-fast bacillus [AFB], Gomori methenamine silver [GMS]) should be evaluated.

Differential Diagnosis. The features of lymphangiectasia overlap with those of vascular transformation of sinuses (see previous section). Lymphangiectasia also may be confused with isolated lymphangioma and systemic lymphangiomatosis. The morphologic similarities are considerable and clinical factors, extent of disease, and possible underlying etiologies (such as stasis) should be considered.

The important entities in the differential diagnosis of peliosis are vascular lesions and neoplasms and hairy cell leukemia. In vascular neoplasms, typically there is a proliferation of vascular elements rather than dilation and cyst formation of preformed elements. In addition, significant cytologic atypia is frequently seen in angiosarcoma, but is lacking in peliosis. Hairy cell leukemia has formation of blood lakes and other vascular dilatations, but has a proliferation of neoplastic, intermediate-sized B lymphocytes, which are not present in peliosis.

Treatment and Prognosis. Lymphangiectasia is typically only an incidental finding, without significant clinical consequences. The clinical importance of peliosis lies in its association with spontaneous splenic rupture, due to a combination of spleen enlargement and fragility of the dilated, cystic sinusoids. When rupture occurs it causes hemoperitoneum and rarely, death (58,59).

LYMPHANGIOMA AND LYMPHANGIOMATOSIS

Definition. *Splenic* and *nodal lymphangiomas* are proliferations of lymph vessel–derived, thin-walled cystic structures filled with pink, watery proteinaceous fluid. *Lymphangiomatosis* is a rare disease of diffuse and/or multifocal involvement of tissues with lymphangioma.

Clinical Features. Lymphangiomas are rare as isolated findings in both lymph node and spleen (20). Lymphangiomatosis is rare and is usually seen in infants.

Gross Findings. Lymphangioma has either a variably sized multicystic appearance, or less commonly, a solid appearance (fig. 17-23).

Microscopic Findings. In the spleen, lymphangiomas are often subcapsular or trabecular in location. In both lymph node and spleen, cystic spaces are lined with flat, bland endothelium (figs. 17-24, 17-25). Papillary tufts of lining cells are found in most cases. These cystic spaces are separated by collagenous stroma, sometimes with bundles of smooth muscle. The cysts are

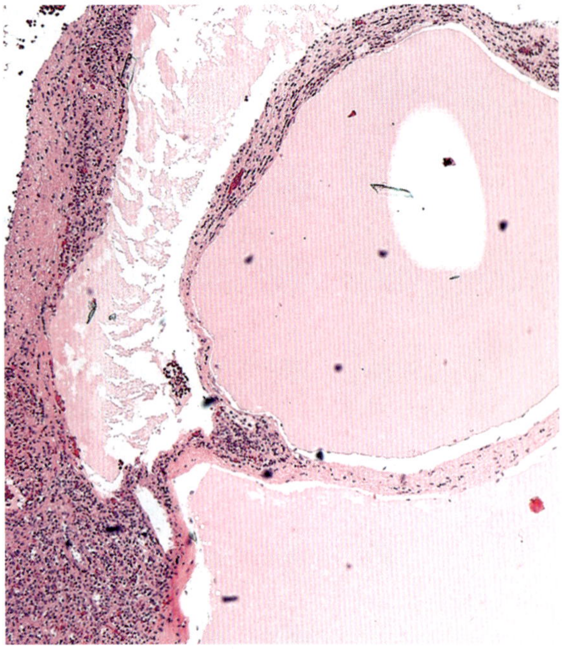

Figure 17-24

LYMPHANGIOMA, SPLEEN

Smooth-walled cystic spaces are filled with clear lymphatic fluid.

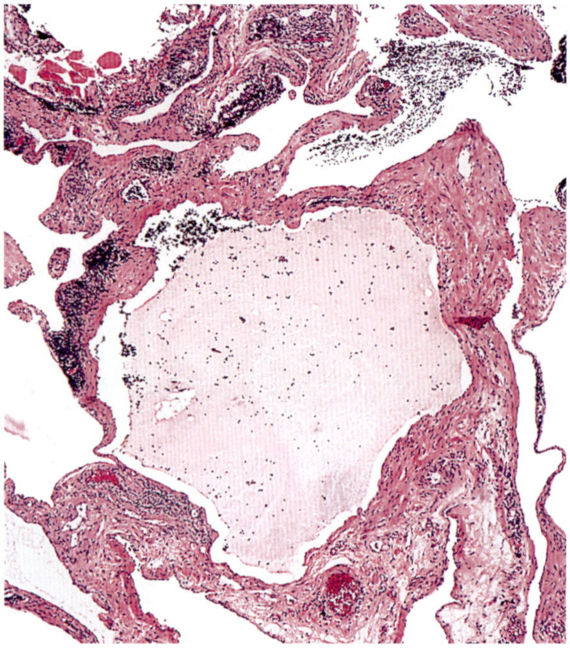

Figure 17-25

LYMPHANGIOMA, LYMPH NODE

Large lymph-filled cystic spaces replace the nodal parenchyma. (Fig. 21-44 from Fascicle 14, Third Series.)

filled with watery, pink proteinaceous fluid. Occasionally, foamy macrophages or cholesterol deposits are present within the cysts.

Ancillary Studies. Immunohistochemical staining confirms the lymphatic derivation of the lining cells, and distinguishes these lesions from other, similar appearing processes (see below). Vascular-related antigens (CD34, CD31, factor VIII-related antigen, *Ulex europaeus* lectin) are variably positive (fig. 17-26). More specific markers of lymphatic derivation are typically positive in lymphangiomas (D2-40, LYVE-1, vascular endothelial growth factor [VEGF]-related stains).

Differential Diagnosis. Isolated lymphangiomas of the spleen may be easily mistaken for mesothelial cysts (4). If the lining is keratin positive, then it is more likely a mesothelial cyst rather than a lymphangioma (5).

Treatment and Prognosis. Incompletely excised lymphangiomas may recur.

OTHER VASCULAR TUMORS

A variety of vascular proliferations, both neoplastic and non-neoplastic, occur in the lymph nodes and spleen (2,8,32,51). The spleen has increased numbers of vascular tumors because of its highly vascular nature. Complete coverage of this topic is beyond the scope of this text, and is best reviewed in a more specialized pathology text (61). Several entities, including *hemangioma*, *littoral cell angioma* (LCA), *lymphangioma*, *Kaposi sarcoma* (KS), and *angiosarcoma* are covered briefly (Table 17-3).

General Features. Other than those seen in congenital syndromes, benign vascular proliferations have no identified specific etiologic factors or cytogenetic abnormalities. There are, however, specific factors associated with malignant vascular tumors. KS is mostly commonly associated with human immunodeficiency virus (HIV) infection. HHV-8 appears to be associated with the pathogenesis of KS. Angiosarcomas are associated with chronic lymphedema, radiation, thorium dioxide (Thorotrast), arsenic-containing insecticides, and vinyl chloride.

Clinical Features. Capillary and cavernous hemangiomas occurring in the spleen are solitary, or less commonly, multiple (5,32). Hemangiomas also occur as isolated lesions of the lymph node (3,22,27). Diffuse hemangiomatosis is a congenital

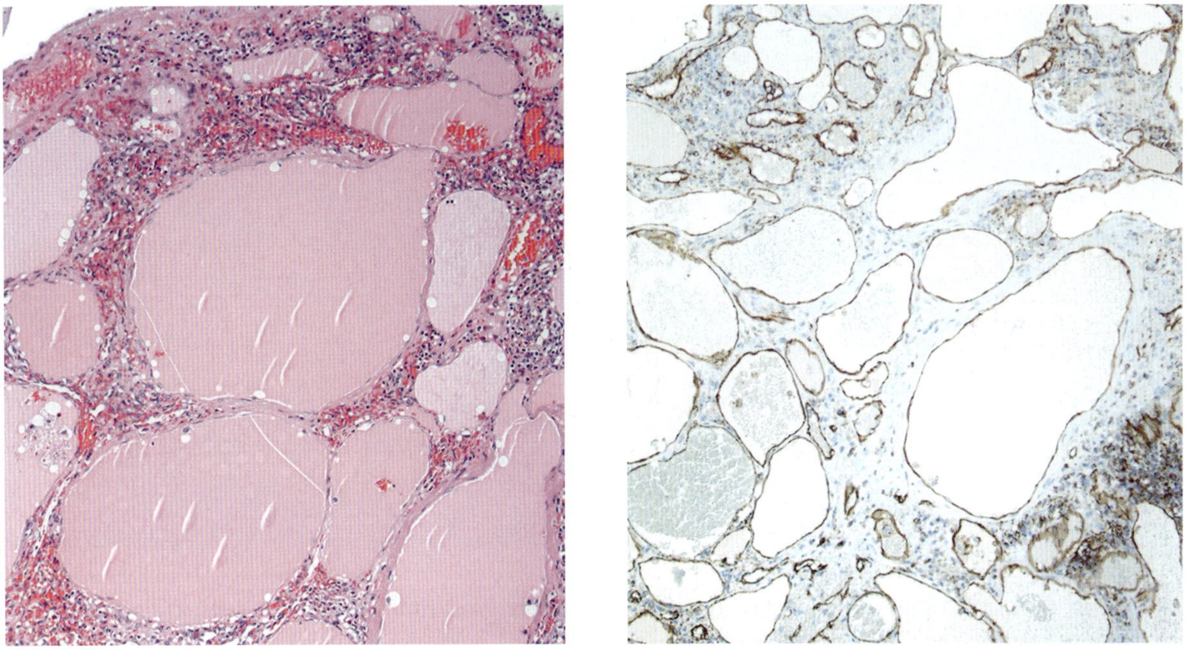

Figure 17-26

CD31 REACTIVITY IN LYMPHANGIOMA

A histologic section of lymphangioma (left) is reactive for CD31 (right).

Table 17-3

FEATURES OF VASCULAR NEOPLASMS OF THE SPLEEN

Diagnosis		Features	Immunostain/Special Studies
Non-neoplastic neoplasms	Peliosis	Rare, unknown etiology, ectatic sinusoids and blood-filled spaces	Endothelial lining positive for CD31/FVIII/Ulex[a]
	Hamartoma	Red pulp, little or no white pulp	CD31+, FVIII+, CD8+
Benign neoplasms	Angiomyolipoma	Very rare; combination of adipose tissue, abnormal blood vessels, and smooth muscle	HMB45+
	Hemangioma	Most common vascular neoplasm of spleen, cavernous or capillary, single or multiple, similar features to other body sites	CD31+, FVIII+, CD34+
	Lymphangioma[b]	Flattened lining cells, filled with cyst proteinaceous fluid, rarely single, more often part of multisystem lymphangiomatosis	Must rule out mesothelial cyst which is keratin+; lined by CD31+, FVIII+, D2-40+, CD34- cells
	Littoral cell angioma	Neoplasm of sinus lining cells; larger, plump cells; may have papillary features and form cystic spaces; focal hemophagocytosis	CD31+, FVIII+, CD34-, CD68+, CD21+ CD8 usually -
Neoplasms with potentially aggressive behavior	Kaposi sarcoma	Vascular neoplasm, typically seen in HIV/AIDS patients; small slit-like vascular spaces, with spindled endothelial cells	CD31+, FVIII+, CD34+, most HHV8+
Malignant neoplasms	Littoral cell angiosarcoma	Very rare, malignant vascular tumor with similar histologic or immunohistologic features of LCA	CD31/FVIII/Ulex variably positive, CD68+
	Angiosarcoma	Vascular malignancy, may have solid areas; anaplasia, mitoses, necrosis not uncommon	CD31/FVIII/Ulex variably positive, CD34+ in 50%, CD8 variable

[a]FVIII = factor VIII-related antigen; Ulex = *Ulex europaeus* lectin; HHV = human herpesvirus; HIV = human immunodeficiency virus; AIDS = acquired immunodeficiency syndrome.

[b]Many "lymphangiomas" are actually thin-walled mesothelial-derived cysts, which stain for cytokeratin.

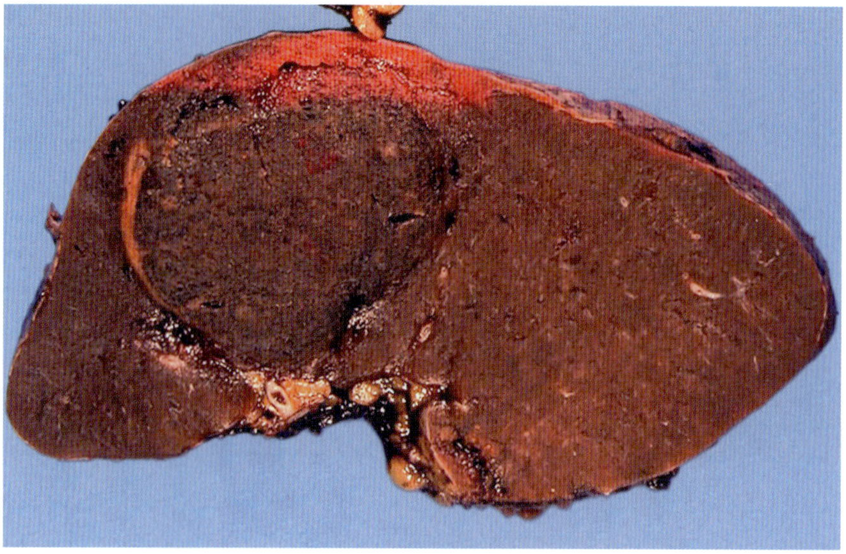

Figure 17-27

HEMANGIOMA, SPLEEN

This vascular tumor appears relatively well circumscribed and spongy. (Courtesy of Jess Savala Jr., Irvine, CA.)

condition with multiple organ involvement by hemangiomas. Besides the spleen, involvement often includes the liver, bone marrow, and less commonly, skin. These "diffuse" benign conditions need to be distinguished from the highly malignant angiosarcoma of the spleen. Large hemangiomas may be associated with Kasabach-Merritt syndrome, a coagulopathy due to platelet and coagulation factor consumption in hemangiomas (13,21,42,48).

LCA is a vascular neoplasm unique to the spleen, with no counterpart in soft tissue (4,16, 32). LCA is most often found incidentally during a radiologic evaluation. There is a well-documented but poorly understood association between LCA and second malignancies including lymphomas and carcinomas. The histogenesis of LCA is likely related to cells that line the red pulp sinuses (e.g., littoral cells).

KS is a vascular tumor of intermediate malignancy (4,8,32). It has locally aggressive behavior and can recur and metastasize. Involvement in lymph nodes is common. Often, KS of lymph node arises from or adjacent to the lymph node capsule, trabeculae, or nodal medulla. The cellular proliferation is composed of spindle cells, which form slit-like vascular spaces. Extravasated red blood cells and intracellular and extracellular hyaline globules can be seen. The spleen is not commonly involved. The majority of these tumors are seen in patients with HIV/acquired immunodeficiency syndrome (AIDS), and there is often evidence of HHV-8 infection.

Angiosarcomas of the spleen are rare, usually multifocal proliferations and heterogeneous in morphology and clinical behavior (4,8,15,32). They are usually symptomatic, as compared to the benign splenic vascular lesions. Patients often present with splenomegaly, and rarely, with spontaneous rupture. Low-grade lesions may resemble LCA, but they contain areas of unequivocal malignancy (15). A recent study suggests that a neoplasm termed *littoral cell hemangioendothelioma* is intermediate between LCA and angiosarcoma (6). This tumor is purported to have more aggressive clinical behavior than its benign counterpart. It is reasonable to assume that there is a spectrum of clinical behavior in these neoplasms, but that LCA is by far the most common, and is benign. The malignant features that distinguish a more aggressive neoplasm from LCA include cellular atypia, higher mitotic activity, and an arborizing, highly anastomotic or solid pattern of growth. Rare cases of malignant littoral cell tumors (termed *littoral cell angiosarcoma*) have been reported (47); they are characterized by distinctly malignant features including necrosis, severe cytologic atypia, and more than rare mitoses.

Gross Findings. Hemangioma is a nonencapsulated, hemorrhagic and spongy mass with irregular borders (fig. 17-27). Prominent cystic changes may occur, as can thrombosis and infarction. Grossly, LCA most often appears as multiple spongy, cystic nodules (fig. 17-28). Lymphangioma is typically multicystic in appearance and most

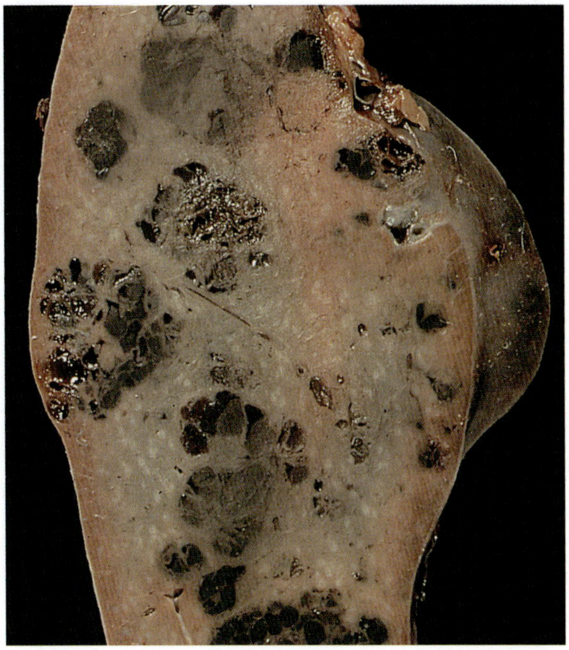

Figure 17-28

LITTORAL CELL ANGIOMA, SPLEEN

Multiple blood-filled nodules are scattered throughout the spleen. (Fig. 21-98 from Fascicle 14, Third Series.)

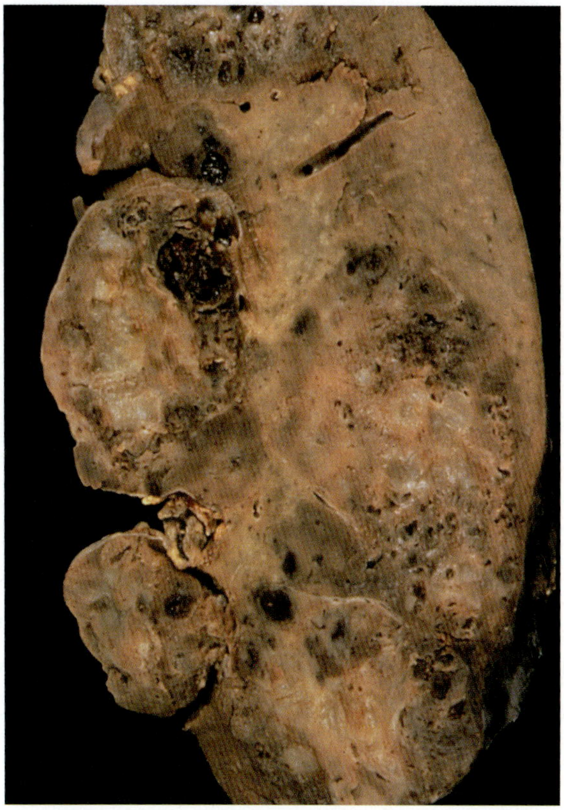

Figure 17-29

ANGIOSARCOMA, SPLEEN

Most of the spleen is replaced by tumor, which is hemorrhagic and necrotic. (Fig. 21-106 from Fascicle 14, Third Series.)

often subcapsular or paratrabecular. Angiosarcomas often involve much of the spleen and vary from hemorrhagic and necrotic to solid masses (fig. 17-29).

Microscopic Findings. The histologic features of hemangiomas in lymph node and spleen are similar to those observed elsewhere (fig. 17-30). The endothelial cells of LCA are usually plump and cuboidal (figs. 17-31–17-33). A distinctive feature is focal aggregates of intracytoplasmic eosinophilic globules (32). Papillary projections of LCA cells may protrude into the vascular spaces. Vascular lumens also contain abundant desquamated littoral cells and macrophages (sometimes exhibiting erythrophagocytosis). Mild cytologic atypia may be present.

KS, which is often multifocal in the spleen, is localized to the trabeculae and/or red pulp (fig. 17-34). The histologic findings are similar to those of KS in other body sites: slit-like vascular spaces formed by spindle-shaped endothelial cells.

High-grade angiosarcomas in the spleen usually contain solid areas with a spindle cell morphology and little evidence of vascular differentiation (figs. 17-35–17-37). In these cases, the differential diagnosis includes other spindle cell sarcomas; most of these have been regarded as examples of malignant fibrous histiocytoma in older publications.

Ancillary Studies. There are a large number of immunohistochemical stains available to characterize vascular lesions (Table 17-4) (7,14,18,26, 38,43,44,46,50). Often, the choices of specific stains are driven by the usefulness of the particular stain for other uses, such as CD34 and Fli-1.

Hemangiomas are positive for vascular markers (CD31, vWF, *Ulex europaeus*) and for CD34 and negative for CD8. Problems in the differential diagnosis are occasionally encountered in cases of diffuse angiomatosis and LCA. Some capillary hemangiomas have a large degree of sclerosis. When this occurs, they can closely resemble inflammatory pseudotumor (see chapter 18) (36).

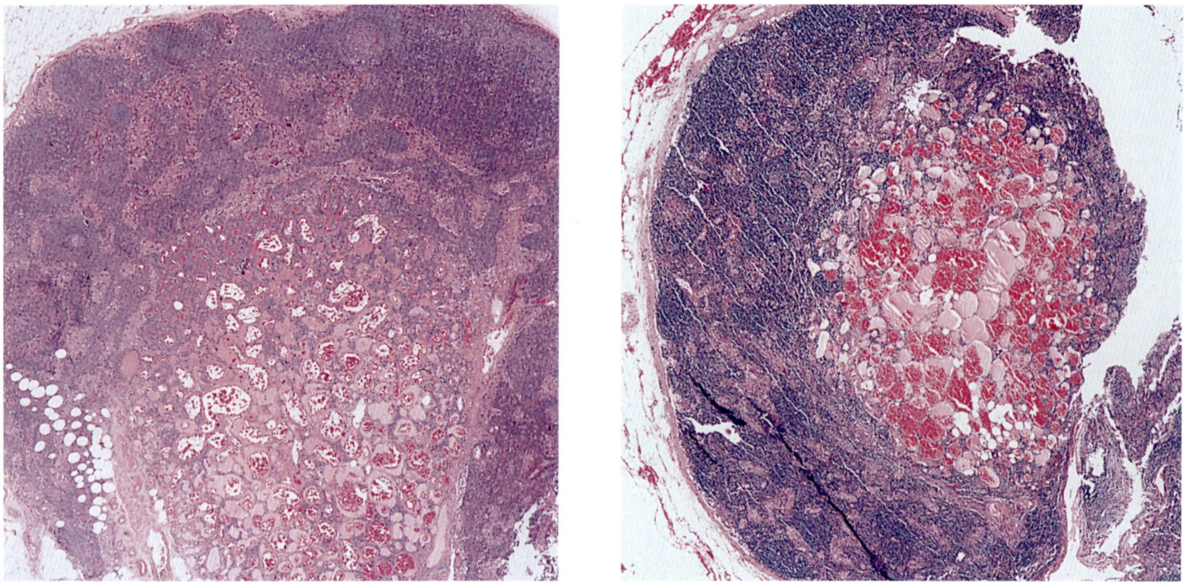

Figure 17-30

HEMANGIOMA, LYMPH NODE

Left: This capillary/cavernous hemangioma is characterized by a localized collection of vascular channels.

Right: This capillary/cavernous hemangioma mainly involves the medulla and hilum of the lymph node. (Fig. 21-31 from Fascicle 14, Third Series.)

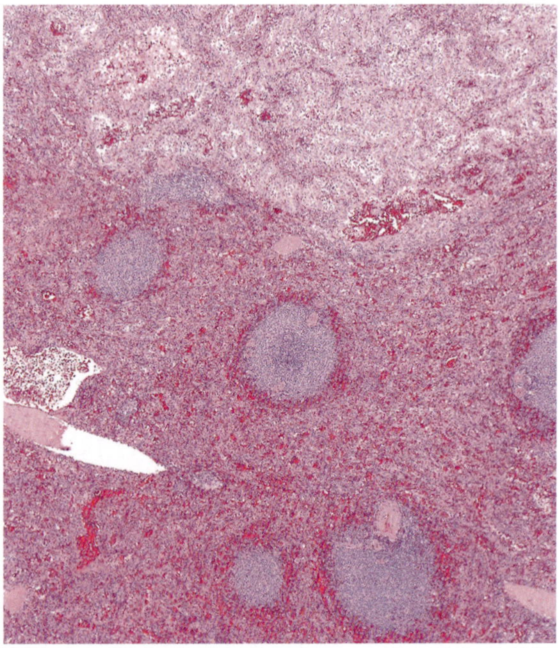

Figure 17-31

LITTORAL CELL ANGIOMA, SPLEEN

Uninvolved spleen is in the lower portion and littoral cell angioma in the upper. The border is somewhat ill-defined and there is no capsule seen.

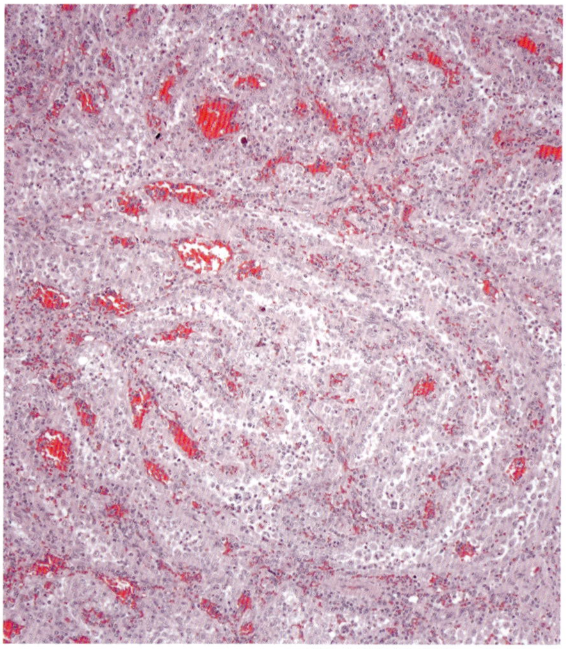

Figure 17-32

LITTORAL CELL ANGIOMA, SPLEEN

Numerous channel-like vascular spaces are lined by littoral type cells. These cells are plump and surround fibrovascular cores. In the vascular spaces are a mixture of cell types.

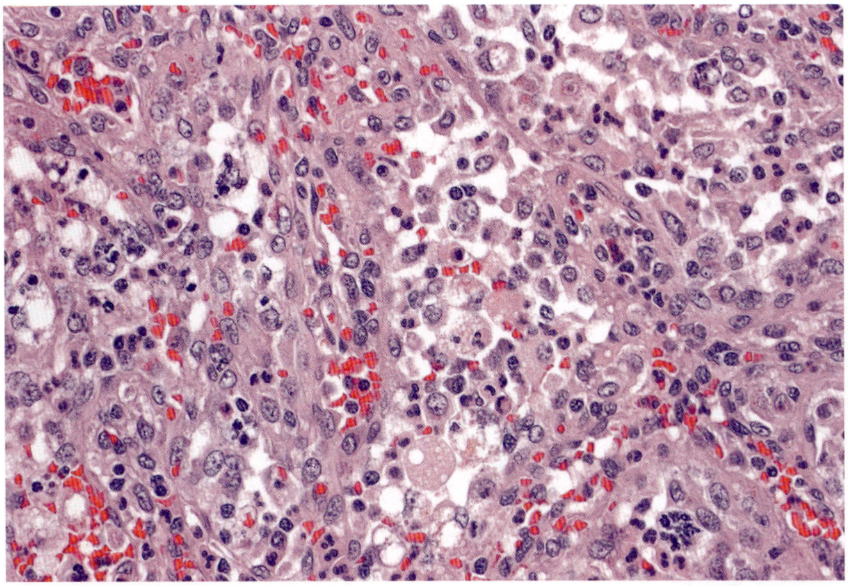

Figure 17-33

LITTORAL CELL ANGIOMA, SPLEEN

The neoplastic cells have a plump, "tombstone" appearance. Although the cells are large, there is no cytologic atypia. The cells in the vascular lumens are desquamated littoral cells and macrophages.

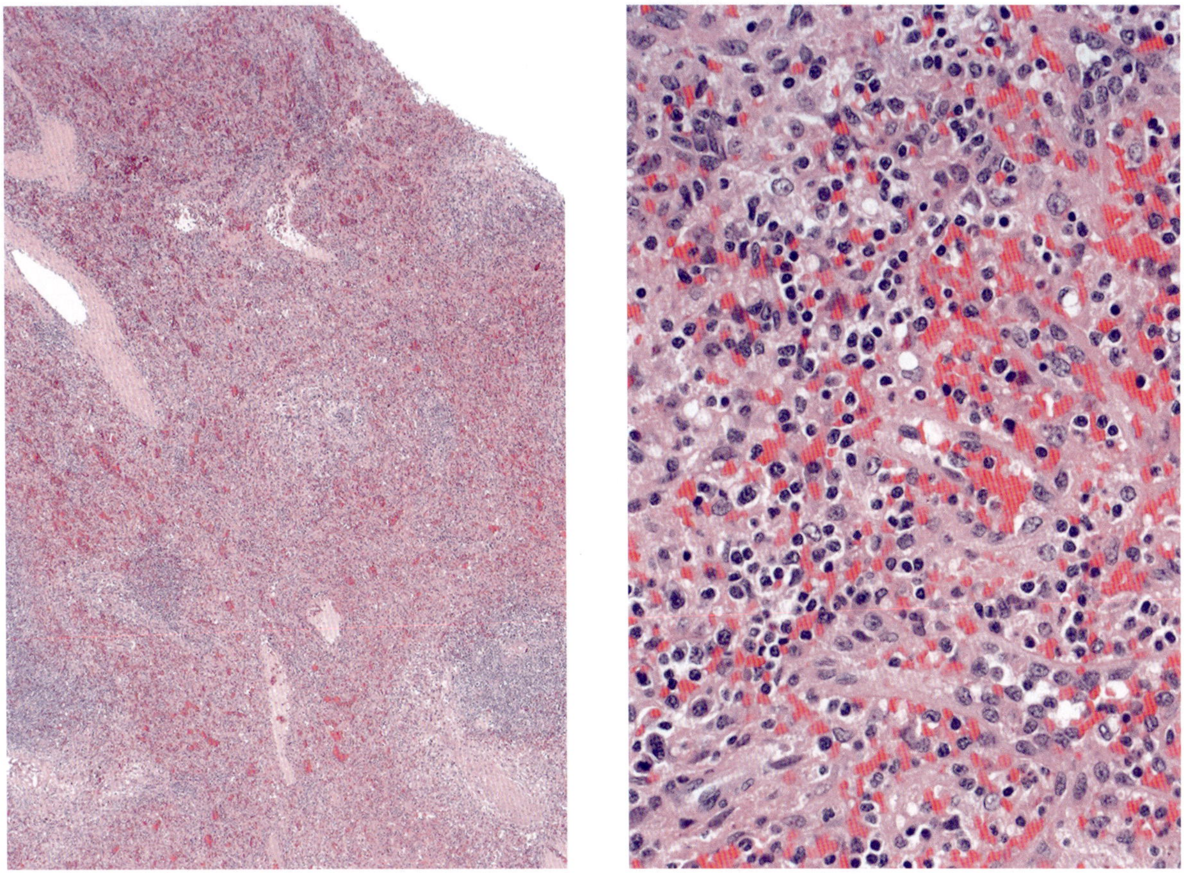

Figure 17-34

KAPOSI SARCOMA, SPLEEN

Low (left) and high (right) magnification. Kaposi sarcoma typically involves the red pulp. It is composed of spindle cells, which are atypical on close examination. Poorly formed vascular spaces may contain lymphocytes or red blood cells.

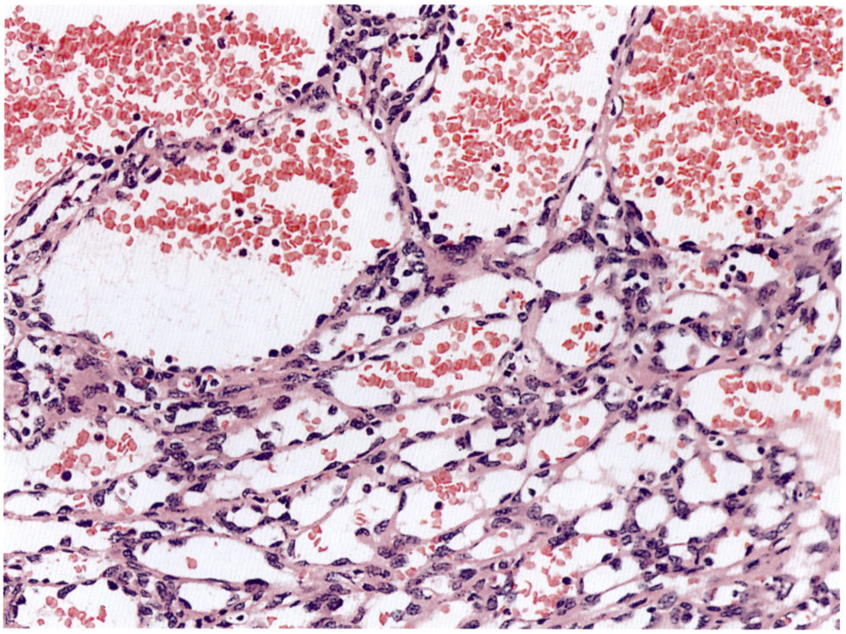

Figure 17-35

ANGIOSARCOMA, SPLEEN

Deceptively benign appearance of angiosarcoma. The illustrated focus appears similar to hemangioma, but the nuclei of the endothelial cells are plump and hyperchromatic, making the lesion suspicious. In other foci, there was evidence of definitive malignancy. (Fig. 21-108 from Fascicle 14, Third Series.)

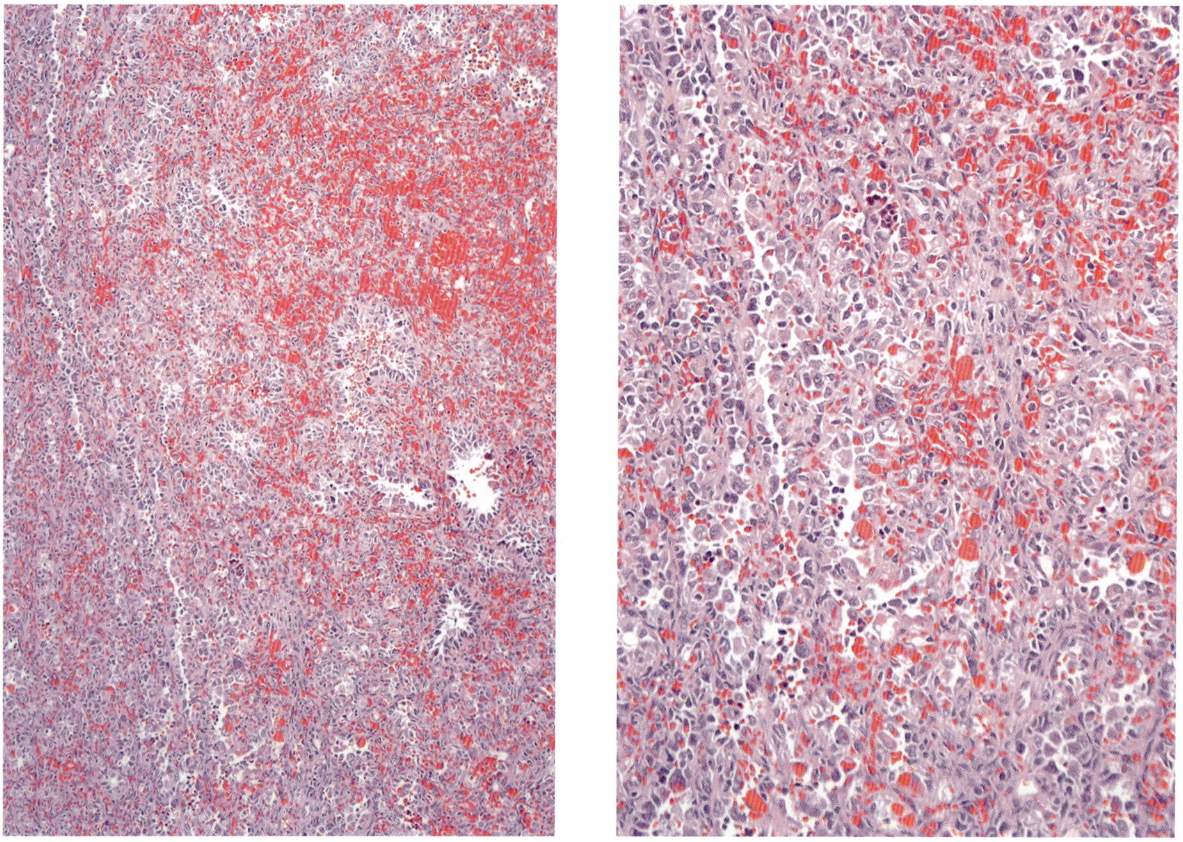

Figure 17-36

ANGIOSARCOMA, SPLEEN

Examples of the cellular atypia seen in angiosarcoma of the spleen.

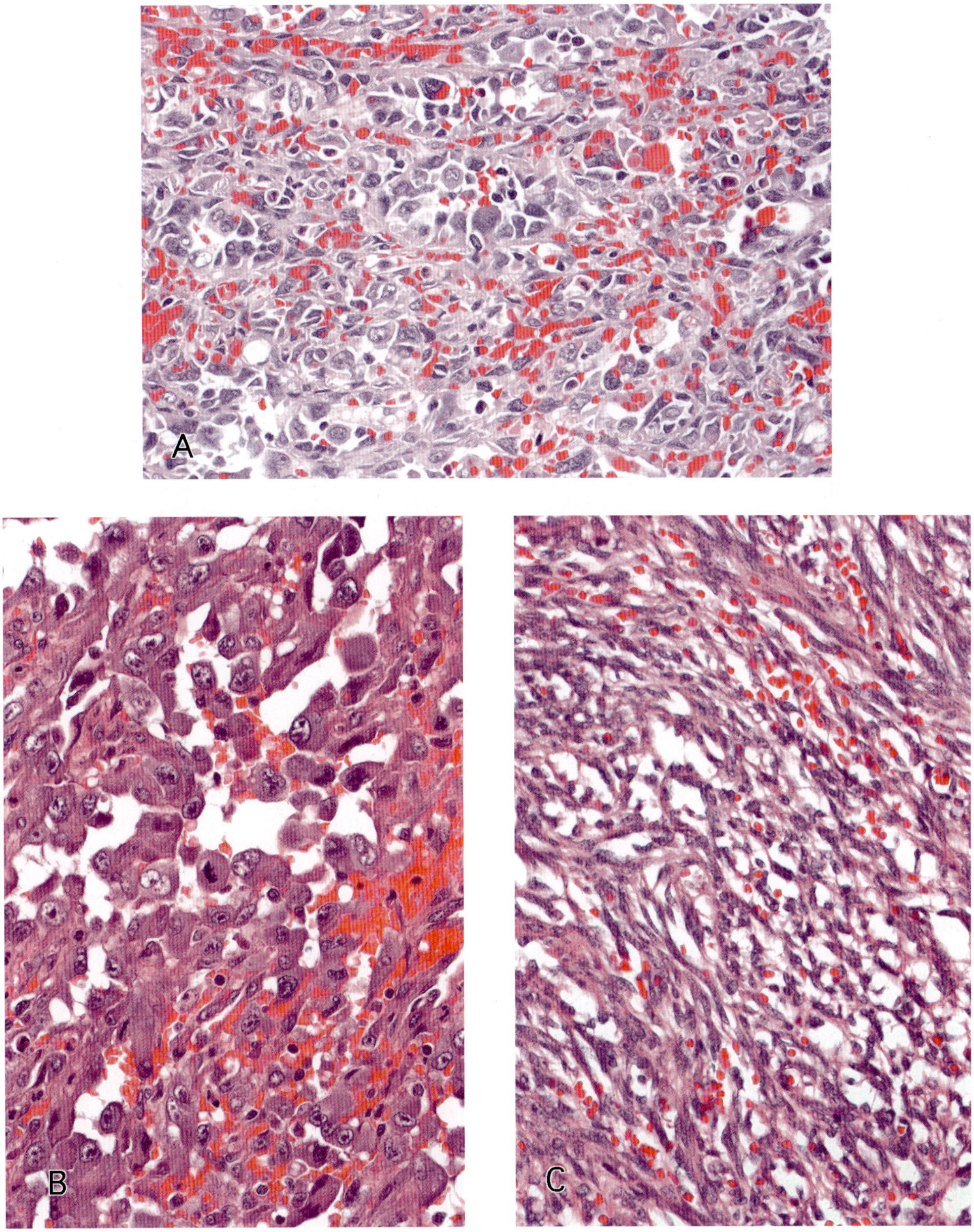

Figure 17-37

ANGIOSARCOMA, SPLEEN

The variety of histologic appearances of splenic angiosarcoma includes highly pleomorphic (A), epithelioid (B), and spindled (C).

Table 17-4

IMMUNOHISTOCHEMICAL STAINS FOR VASCULAR/LYMPHATIC-DERIVED CELLS

Stain/Antibody	Specificity	Notes
CD31 (platelet endothelial cell adhesion molecule-1 [PECAM-1])	Endothelial-derived cells, including lymphatic	Highly sensitive and specific, also stains macrophages
CD34	Endothelial-derived cells, including lymphatic	Highly sensitive, but less specific than CD31
CD105 (endoglin)	Endothelial-derived cells, including lymphatic	
CD146 (MUC18, MCAM, S-Endo, A32 antigen)	Endothelial-derived cells, including lymphatic	Member of immunoglobulin gene superfamily
Von Willebrand factor antigen/factor VIII-related antigen	Endothelial-derived cells, including lymphatic	Typically expressed only in well-differentiated vascular neoplasms
Duffy antigen receptor for chemokines (DARC)	Venules	Chemokine binding protein
MECA-79	Venules	Associated with L-selectin counter-receptors
Ulex europaeus[a]	Endothelial-derived cells, including lymphatic	
Fli-1	Endothelial-derived cells, including lymphatic	Nuclear staining of endothelial nuclei
VEGF-B,[b] VEGF-C, VEGF-D, VEGF-D, VEGF-3	Endothelial-derived cells, including lymphatic	Some VEGF-related proteins are more exclusively expressed on lymphatic endothelium
Podoplanin/ D2-40	Lymphatic[c]	
Prox-1	Lymphatic	
LYVE-1	Lymphatic	

[a]*Ulex europaeus* is not an immunohistochemical stain but a lectin.
[b]VEGF = vascular endothelial growth factor; LYVE = lymphatic vessel endothelial hyaluronan receptor.
[c]Expression may be seen in vascular neoplasms that are not strictly lymphatic in origin.

The most useful vascular markers in LCA are CD31, vWF, and *Ulex europaeus*, which stain the majority of cases (fig. 17-38). CD34 is uniformly negative. LCAs are also variably positive for CD68 and CD21. LCA may rarely express CD8, typical of splenic sinusoidal endothelium, although more recent publications suggest that they are more often negative (4).

The most useful marker for confirmation of the vascular nature of a poorly differentiated angiosarcoma is CD31. CD8 or CD68 positivity in some of these tumors supports the concept that a subset of angiosarcomas arises from splenic sinusoidal endothelium. Many angiosarcomas and KS stain either partially or strongly for lymphatic-related antigens, such as D2-40 or podoplanin. This finding may suggest lymphatic derivation of some of these neoplasms; however, the lack of differentiation may also account for aberrant expression.

Treatment and Prognosis. Hemangioma is a benign lesion, and when present in isolated lymph nodes, is treated simply by resection. In the spleen, however, a risk of rupture and subsequent hemoperitoneum is present, albeit rare. When part of a congenital syndrome (e.g., hemangiomatosis), the prognosis is dependent on impingement and dysfunction of involved organs.

The prognosis for patients with LCA is excellent. It is typically a benign lesion and is best treated by resection. Occasional cases of LCA have atypical cytologic and histologic features and have a more variable course. The clinical course of KS depends greatly on the clinical findings in the patient. In the context of advanced AIDS with disseminated KS, the prognosis is poor. Angiosarcoma is a clinically aggressive disease with an associated poor prognosis. Surgery is combined with radiation and possibly chemotherapy for treatment.

SPLENIC ARTERY ANEURYSMS

Definition. *Splenic artery aneurysms* (SAAs) are rare vascular anomalies, usually found in females. They rarely cause symptoms, but may rupture, leading to hemoperitoneum.

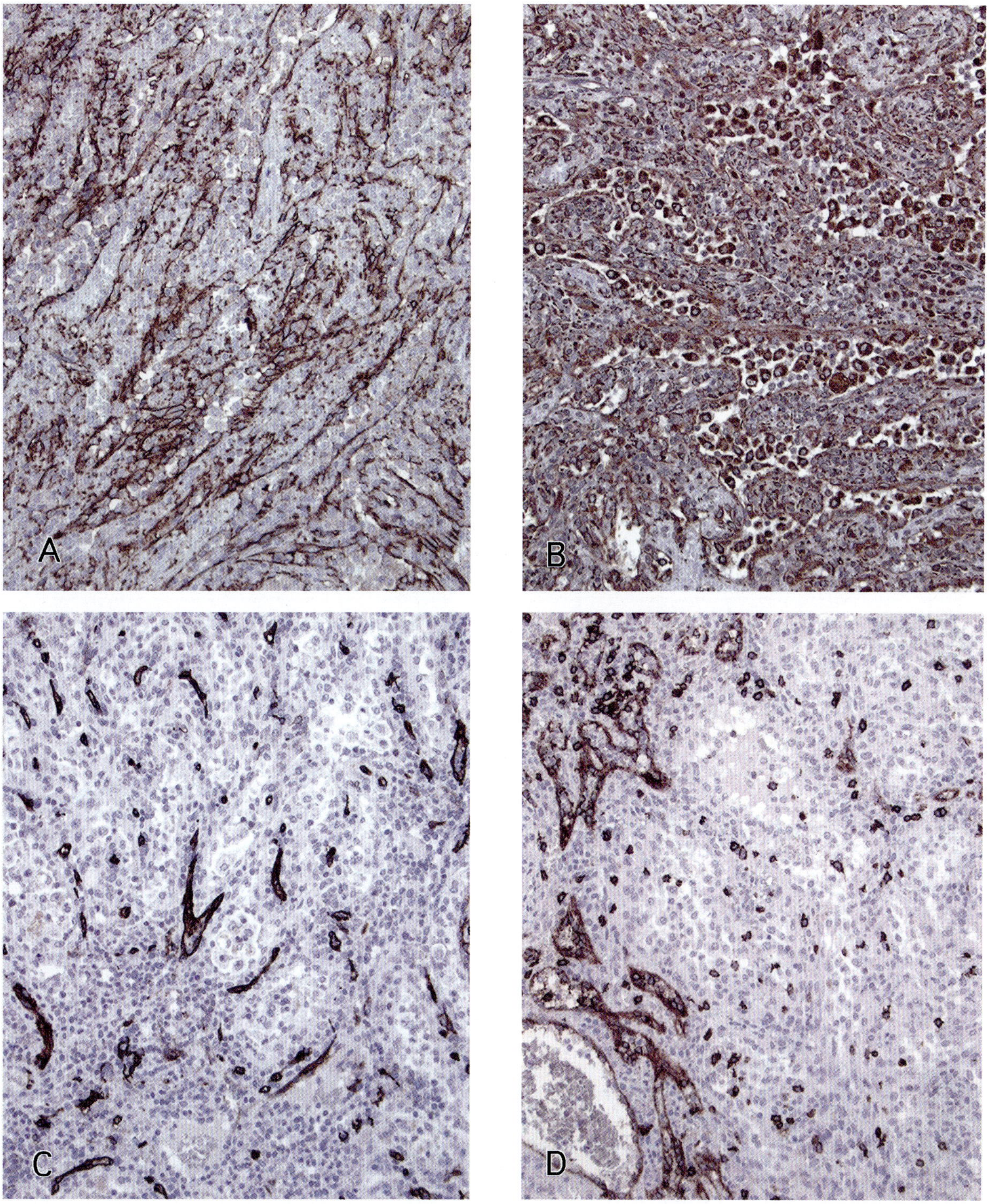

Figure 17-38

IMMUNOHISTOCHEMICAL REACTIVITY IN LITTORAL CELL ANGIOMA, SPLEEN

A,B: CD31 (A) and CD68 (B) are positive, highlighting the vascular and macrophage characteristics of littoral cell angioma.

C: CD34 is not immunoreactive in littoral cell angioma, although small feeder vessels are positive.

D: CD8 highlights the lack of reactivity in littoral cell angioma (upper portion), but normal splenic sinuses (lower portion) are positive.

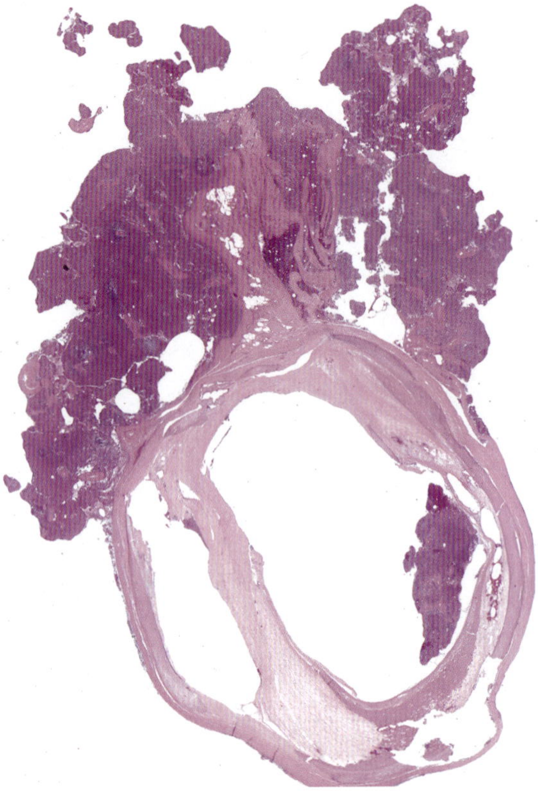

Figure 17-39

SPLENIC ARTERY ANEURYSM

Some fragments of splenic tissue are attached (top).

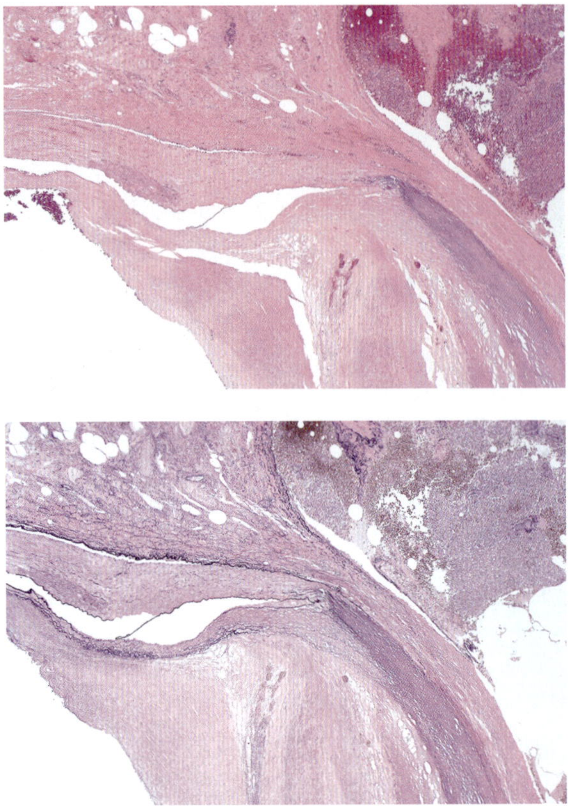

Figure 17-40

SPLENIC ARTERY ANEURYSM

H&E (top) and elastic stain (bottom) of the same splenic artery aneurysm seen in figure 17-39 show the loss of the elastic layers in the wall of the aneurysm (right).

Clinical Features. The incidence of SAA is low, estimated to be between 0.01-0.98 percent, based on autopsy series (49,57). It is much more common in women than men. It has a strong association with pregnancy, possibly due to medial weakening of the artery by pregnancy-related hormonal changes or parturient strain (23,49). Rupture in pregnancy is most common in the third trimester, followed by during labor and delivery.

SAA is also associated with hypertension, obesity, coronary artery disease, hypercholesterolemia, peptic ulcer disease/gastritis, collagen vascular disease, alpha-1-antitrypsin deficiency, infectious disorders, and portal hypertension with splenomegaly (1). Other associations include congenital laxity of the arterial wall, arteriosclerosis, diffuse elastica deficiency, and fibromuscular dysplasia (23).

Splenic artery pseudoaneurysm is rarer than SAA (56). It is usually the result of erosion of the outer linings of the vessel by acute or chronic pancreatitis. Many of the patients have a significant alcohol history.

Gross Findings. SAAs are typically saccular outpouchings of the splenic artery (fig. 17-39). They vary in size, averaging 2.2 cm (unruptured diameter) (1). Calcification is present in 90 percent of ruptured aneurysms (1). Intraluminal thrombus and attached blood clot are often seen.

Microscopic Findings. Cross sections of SAA often reveal abnormalities in the vessel wall. Sites of disruption of the internal elastic lamina, myxoid degeneration, and periarterial fibrosis may be seen (fig. 17-40) (49). Abnormalities of the media, including hyperplasia of the muscular layers, are often present. Trichrome or elastic stains may show disruption of the elastic layers of the vessel.

Ancillary Studies. Radiologic examinations are frequently used to diagnose and monitor

SAA. CT scans, ultrasound, and other techniques have been used.

Treatment and Prognosis. When SAA ruptures, immediate surgical intervention is critical. Splenectomy, ligation or embolization of the bleeding artery, and blood component replacement are usual therapies. Hemoperitoneum, shock, and death often follow shortly after rupture. In pregnancy, rupture of SAA results in maternal mortality of up to 75 percent and fetal mortality of up to 90 percent (23). Management of unruptured SAA is somewhat controversial; some authors recommend surgical repair in all aneurysms over 2.0 cm or in any aneurysm discovered during pregnancy (1,10).

REFERENCES

1. Abbas MA, Stone WM, Fowl RJ, et al. Splenic artery aneurysms: two decades experience at Mayo clinic. Ann Vasc Surg 2002;16:442-9.
2. Abbott RM, Levy AD, Aguilera NS, Gorospe L, Thompson WM. From the archives of the AFIP: primary vascular neoplasms of the spleen: radiologic-pathologic correlation. Radiographics 2004;24:1137-63.
3. Almagro UA, Choi H, Rouse TM. Hemangioma in a lymph node. Arch Pathol Lab Med 1985;109:576-8.
4. Arber DA, Strickler JG, Chen YY, Weiss LM. Splenic vascular tumors: a histologic, immunophenotypic, and virologic study. Am J Surg Pathol 1997;21:827-35.
5. Arber DA, Strickler JG, Weiss LM. Splenic mesothelial cysts mimicking lymphangiomas. Am J Surg Pathol 1997;21:334-8.
6. Ben-Izhak O, Bejar J, Ben-Eliezer S, Vlodavsky E. Splenic littoral cell haemangioendothelioma: a new low-grade variant of malignant littoral cell tumour. Histopathology 2001;39:469-75.
7. Breiteneder-Geleff S, Soleiman A, Kowalski H, et al. Angiosarcomas express mixed endothelial phenotypes of blood and lymphatic capillaries: podoplanin as a specific marker for lymphatic endothelium. Am J Pathol 1999;154:385-94.
8. Chan JK, Frizzera G, Fletcher CD, Rosai J. Primary vascular tumors of lymph nodes other than Kaposi's sarcoma. Analysis of 39 cases and delineation of two new entities. Am J Surg Pathol 1992;16:335-50.
9. Chan JK, Warnke RA, Dorfman R. Vascular transformation of sinuses in lymph nodes. A study of its morphological spectrum and distinction from Kaposi's sarcoma. Am J Surg Pathol 1991;15:732-43.
10. Chiesa R, Astore D, Guzzo G, et al. Visceral artery aneurysms. Ann Vasc Surg 2005;19:42-8.
11. Civardi G, Vallisa D, Berte R, et al. Ultrasound-guided fine needle biopsy of the spleen: high clinical efficacy and low risk in a multicenter Italian study. Am J Hematol 2001;67:93-9.
12. Debnath D, Valerio D. Atraumatic rupture of the spleen in adults. J R Coll Surg Edinb 2002;47:437-45.
13. Dufau JP, le Tourneau A, Audouin J, Delmer A, Diebold J. Isolated diffuse hemangiomatosis of the spleen with Kasabach-Merritt-like syndrome. Histopathology 1999;35:337-44.
14. Evangelou E, Kyzas PA, Trikalinos TA. Comparison of the diagnostic accuracy of lymphatic endothelium markers: Bayesian approach. Mod Pathol 2005;18:1490-7.
15. Falk S, Krishnan J, Meis JM. Primary angiosarcoma of the spleen. A clinicopathologic study of 40 cases. Am J Surg Pathol 1993;17:959-70.
16. Falk S, Stutte HJ, Frizzera G. Littoral cell angioma. A novel splenic vascular lesion demonstrating histiocytic differentiation. Am J Surg Pathol 1991;15:1023-33.
17. Farhi DC, Ashfaq R. Splenic pathology after traumatic injury. Am J Clin Pathol 1996;105:474-8.
18. Folpe AL, Chand EM, Goldblum JR, Weiss SW. Expression of Fli-1, a nuclear transcription factor, distinguishes vascular neoplasms from potential mimics. Am J Surg Pathol 2001;25:1061-6.
19. Fukunaga M. Expression of D2-40 in lymphatic endothelium of normal tissues and in vascular tumors. Histopathology 2005;46:396-402.
20. Goh BK, Tan YM, Ong HS, et al. Intra-abdominal and retroperitoneal lymphangiomas in pediatric and adult patients. World J Surg 2005;29:837-40.
21. Goyal A, Babu SN, Kim V, Katariya S, Rao KL. Hemangioendothelioma of liver and spleen: trauma-induced consumptive coagulopathy. J Pediatr Surg 2002;37:E29.
22. Har-El G, Heffner DK, Ruffy M. Haemangioma in a cervical lymph node. J Laryngol Otol 1990;104:513-5.
23. Hunsaker DM, Turner S, Hunsacker JC 3rd. Sudden and unexpected death resulting from splenic artery aneurysm rupture: two cases reports of pregnancy-related fatal rupture of splenic artery aneurysm. Am J Forensic Med Pathol 2005;23:338-41.

24. Ide F, Shimoyama T, Horie N. Vascular transformation of sinuses in bilateral cervical lymph nodes. Head Neck 1999;21:366-9.
25. Ioachim HL, Ratech H. Ioachim's lymph node pathology. Philadelphia: Lippincott William & Wilkins; 2002.
26. Kahn HJ, Bailey D, Marks A. Monoclonal antibody D2-40, a new marker of lymphatic endothelium, reacts with Kaposi's sarcoma and a subset of angiosarcomas. Mod Pathol 2002;15:434-40.
27. Kasznica J, Sideli RV, Collins MH. Lymph node hemangioma. Arch Pathol Lab Med 1989;113:804-7.
28. Kojima M, Nakamura S, Shimizu K, Yamane Y, Itoh H, Masawa N. Granulocytic sarcoma presenting with lymph node infarction at disease onset. APMIS 2003;111:1133-6.
29. Kojima M, Nakamura S, Sugihara S, Sakata N, Masawa N. Lymph node infarction associated with infectious mononucleosis: report of a case resembling lymph node infarction associated with malignant lymphoma. Int J Surg Pathol 2002;10:223-6.
30. Kojima M, Nakamura S, Yamane Y, et al. Antigen preservation in infarcted nodal B-cell lymphoma, with special reference to follicular center cell markers. Int J Surg Pathol 2004;12:251-5.
31. Kraus MD, Fleming MD, Vonderheide RH. The spleen as a diagnostic specimen: a review of 10 years' experience at two tertiary care institutions. Cancer 2001;91:2001-9.
32. Kutok JL, Fletcher CD. Splenic vascular tumors. Semin Diagn Pathol 2003;20:128-39.
33. Lal A, Ariga R, Gattuso P, Nemcek AA, Nayar R. Splenic fine needle aspiration and core biopsy. A review of 49 cases. Acta Cytologica 2003;47:951-9.
34. Laszewski MJ, Belding PJ, Feddersen RM, et al. Clonal immunoglobulin gene rearrangement in the infarcted lymph node syndrome. Am J Clin Pathol 1991;96:116-20.
35. Lieberman ME, Levitt MA. Spontaneous rupture of the spleen: a case report and literature review. Am J Emerg Med 1989;7:28-31.
36. Martel M, Cheuk W, Lombardi L, Lifschitz-Mercer B, Chan JK, Rosai J. Sclerosing angiomatoid nodular transformation (SANT): report of 25 cases of a distinctive benign splenic lesion. Am J Surg Pathol 2004;28:1268-79.
37. Maurer R, Schmid U, Davies JD, Mahy NJ, Stansfeld AG, Lukes RJ. Lymph-node infarction and malignant lymphoma: a multicentre survey of European, English and American cases. Histopathology 1986;10:571-88.
38. Middleton J, Americh L, Gayon R, et al. A comparative study of endothelial cell markers expressed in chronically inflamed human tissues: MECA-79, Duffy antigen receptor for chemokines, von Willebrand factor, CD31, CD34, CD105 and CD146. J Pathol 2005;206:260-8.
39. Nasuti JF, Gupta PK, Baloch ZW. Clinical implications and immunohistochemical staining in the evaluation of lymph node infarction after fine-needle aspiration. Diagn Cytopathol 2001;25:104-7.
40. Neiman RS, Orazi A. Disorders of the spleen, 2nd ed. Philadelphia: Saunders; 1999.
41. Norton AJ, Ramsay AD, Isaacson PG. Antigen preservation in infarcted lymphoid tissue. A novel approach to the infarcted lymph node using monoclonal antibodies effective in routinely processed tissues. Am J Surg Pathol 1988;12:759-67.
42. Pampin C, Devillers A, Treguier C, et al. Intratumoral consumption of indium-111-labeled platelets in a child with splenic hemangioma and thrombocytopenia. J Pediatr Hematol Oncol 2000;22:256-8.
43. Partanen TA, Paavonen K. Lymphatic versus blood vascular endothelial growth factors and receptors in humans. Microsc Res Tech 2001;55:108-21.
44. Poblet E, Gonzalez-Palacios F, Jimenez FJ. Different immunoreactivity of endothelial markers in well and poorly differentiated areas of angiosarcomas. Virchows Arch 1996;428:217-21.
45. Roberts C, Batstone PJ, Goodlad JR. Lymphadenopathy and lymph node infarction as a result of gold injections. J Clin Pathol 2001;54:562-4.
46. Rossi S, Orvieto E, Furlanetto A, Laurino L, Ninfo V, Dei Tos AP. Utility of the immunohistochemical detection of FLI-1 expression in round cell and vascular neoplasm using a monoclonal antibody. Mod Pathol 2004;17:547-52.
47. Rosso R, Paulli M, Gianelli U, Boveri E, Stella G, Magrini U. Littoral cell angiosarcoma of the spleen. Case report with immunohistochemical and ultrastructural analysis. Am J Surg Pathol 1995;19:1203-8.
48. Schulz AS, Urban J, Gessler P, Behnisch W, Kohne E, Heymer B. Anaemia, thrombocytopenia and coagulopathy due to occult diffuse infantile haemangiomatosis of spleen and pancreas. Eur J Pediatr 1999;158:379-83.
49. Selo-Ojeme DO, Welch CC. Review: spontaneous rupture of splenic artery aneurysm in pregnancy. Eur J Obstet Gynecol Reprod Biol 2003;109:124-7.
50. Sharma S, Sharma MC, Sarkar C. Morphology of angiogenesis in human cancer: a conceptual overview, histoprognostic perspective and significance of neoangiogenesis. Histopathology 2005;46:481-9.
51. Silva EG, Phillips MJ, Langer B, Ordonez NG. Spindle and histiocytoid (epithelioid) hemangioendothelioma. Primary in lymph node. Am J Clin Pathol 1986;85:731-5.

52. Sodhi KS, Saggar K, Sood BP, Sandhu P. Torsion of a wandering spleen: acute abdominal presentation. J Emerg Med 2003;25:133-7.
53. Stockinger ZT. Infectious mononucleosis presenting as spontaneous splenic rupture without other symptoms. Mil Med 2003;168:722-4.
54. Strauchen JA, Miller LK. Lymph node infarction. An immunohistochemical study of 11 cases. Arch Pathol Lab Med 2003;127:60-3.
55. Tessier DJ, Stone WM, Fowl RJ, et al. Clinical features and management of splenic artery pseudoaneurysm: Case series and cumulative review of the literature. J Vasc Surg 2003;38:969-74.
56. Tsang WY, Chan JK. Spectrum of morphologic changes in lymph nodes attributable to fine needle aspiration. Hum Pathol 1992;23:562-5.
57. Tsokos M, Erbersdobler A. Pathology of peliosis. Forensic Sci Int 2005;149:25-33.
58. Tsokos M, Nolting R, Lockemann U. Sudden, unexpected death due to splenic artery aneurysm rupture. Am J Forensic Med Pathol 2005;26:83-5.
59. Tsokos M, Puschel K. Isolated peliosis of the spleen. Report of 2 autopsy cases. Am J Forensic Med Pathol 2004;25:251-4.
60. Vega F, Lozano MD, Alcalde J, Pardo-Mindan FJ. Utility of immunophenotypic and immunogenotypic analysis in the study of necrotic lymph nodes. Virchows Arch 1999;434:245-8.
61. Weiss SW, Goldblum JR. Benign tumors and tumor-like lesions of blood vessels. In: Weiss SW, Goldblum JR, eds. Enzinger and Weiss's soft tissue tumors, 4th ed. St. Louis: Mosby; 2001;837-90.
62. Wilkins BS, Wright DH. Illustrated pathology of the spleen. Cambridge: Cambridge University Press; 2000.
63. Williams HB. Hemangiomas and lymphangiomas. Adv Surg 1981;15:317-49.

18 BENIGN DISORDERS OF UNCLEAR ETIOLOGY AND NEOPLASMS

This chapter contains descriptions of conditions of lymph nodes and spleen that are not easily classified within other sections of this book. These benign and neoplastic conditions are unified by their lack of known splenic etiologies. Many are mesenchymal in origin, and are more thoroughly discussed in specialized texts of soft tissue tumors. Others have significant histologic similarity to benign lesions and merit discussion. In addition, tumors metastatic to spleen (a rare occurrence) and to lymph node are discussed briefly.

SPLENIC HAMARTOMA

Definition. *Splenic hamartoma*, sometimes referred to as a *splenoma*, is a rare, benign lesion composed predominantly of red pulp components. Other names used historically include splenoadenoma, spleen-in-spleen, splenic splenunculus, and fibrosplenoma. It is typically well circumscribed from surrounding, normal spleen.

General Features. It is unlikely that splenic hamartomas are truly hamartomatous lesions. There is speculation that hamartomas may be vascular neoplasms, but the varied components of hamartomas tend to argue against this (41). In any case, the origin of these rare lesions is still debatable.

Clinical Features. Splenic hamartoma occurs in all age groups (11 months to 86 years) (41), although the average age at presentation is 40 to 50 years (3). The incidence is 0.13 to 0.20 percent of the general population (4,16), with both genders affected equally.

Approximately 15 percent of hamartomas present symptomatically (41). Fever, malaise, and weight loss may be present (30). Splenic hamartomas occasionally result in hypersplenism, although they are more commonly incidental findings at autopsy or in spleens removed for unrelated causes. Systemic manifestations are rare but occur. The most common manifestations are hematologic and include anemia, thrombocytopenia, or pancytopenia (3,60,70). Benign hematologic disorders associated with hamartomas include aplastic anemia, hereditary spherocytosis, sickle cell disorders, hemolytic anemia, and congenital dyserythroblastic anemia.

Hamartomas are associated with several malignancies: hairy cell leukemia, Hodgkin lymphoma, chronic lymphocytic leukemia, chronic myelogenous leukemia (CML), non-CML myeloproliferative disorders, lymphoma, breast carcinoma, gastric carcinoma, lung carcinoma, transitional cell carcinoma, sarcomas, and thymoma (60). Other diseases associated with hamartomas are tuberous sclerosis, congestive heart failure, stroke, hypertension, myocardial infarction, myocarditis, cirrhosis, and portal hypertension. An unusual case of splenic hamartoma was associated with multiple capillary hemangiomas, membranoproliferative glomerulonephritis, and anemia, which resolved upon resection of the splenic lesion (34).

Gross Findings. Splenic hamartomas are typically well-circumscribed, but not encapsulated, masses within the spleen (figs. 18-1–18-3).

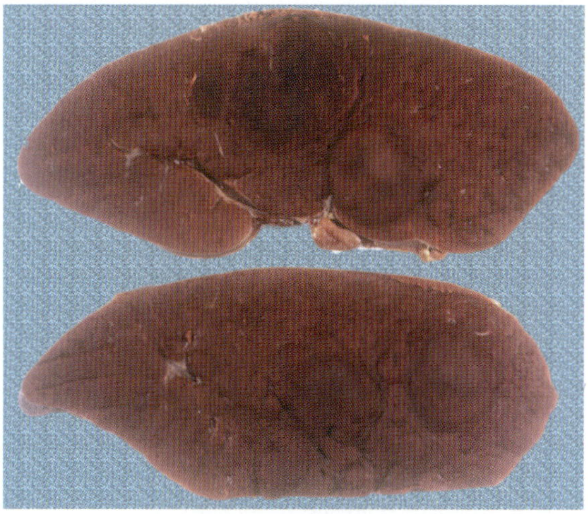

Figure 18-1

HAMARTOMA, SPLEEN

Two relatively well-circumscribed masses are seen. (Courtesy of Richard Neiman, Harpswell, ME.)

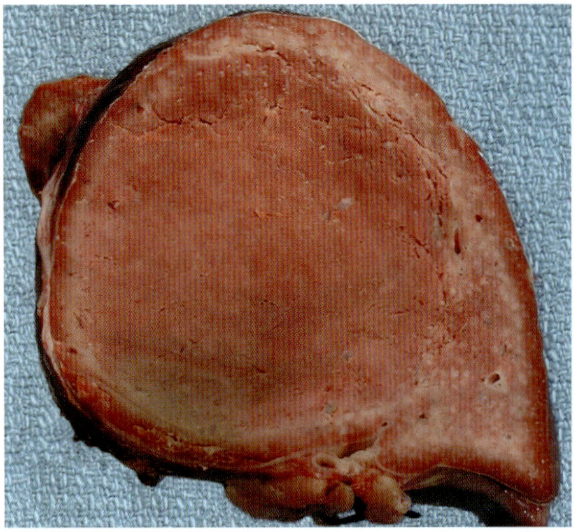

Figure 18-2

HAMARTOMA, SPLEEN

Although fixed, the surrounding rim shows white pulp. (Courtesy of Jess Savala Jr, Irvine, CA.)

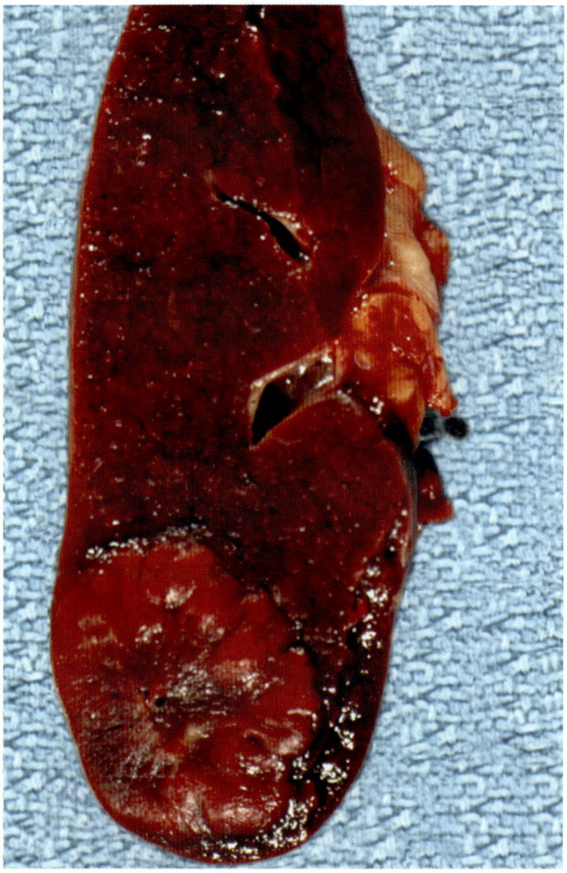

Figure 18-3

HAMARTOMA, SPLEEN

This hamartoma appears hemorrhagic and bulges from the cut surface of the spleen.

Although most often single, they may be multiple. Size varies from less than 1 to 20 cm. Very large hamartomas distort the normal architecture of the spleen. On cut surface, hamartomas often bulge outward from the surface of the surrounding spleen.

Microscopic Findings. Splenic hamartomas are usually well-circumscribed nodules that resemble normal red pulp histologically. Tortuous, slit-like vascular spaces are lined by plump endothelial cells of littoral cell derivation (i.e., CD8 positive). The vascular spaces are of a similar width to those of the normal red pulp (figs. 18-4–18-6) and are separated by disorganized stroma. Capillaries may be seen within the cordal areas. White pulp structures are only rarely seen in hamartomas, although scattered lymphocytes are common (28,41). Variable numbers of inflammatory cells are present, including macrophages, lymphocytes, and plasma cells. Eosinophils and neutrophils are less common. Foci of macrophages with granular or lipid-filled cytoplasm may be seen. Fibrosis, hemorrhage, and calcification are present in varying degrees.

Rarely, large, bizarre stromal cells are seen in splenic hamartomas (16). These cells appear to represent altered stromal cells. They have a very low mitotic rate and lack the immunohistochemical features of megakaryocytes, lymphocytes, macrophages, endothelial cells, or epithelial cells. The presence of these cells should not be interpreted as a sign of malignancy. Extramedullary hematopoiesis is frequent within hamartomas.

Krishnan and Frizzera (41) have proposed four subtypes of splenic hamartoma: classic hamartoma, cord capillary hemangioma, myoid angioendothelioma, and macrophage-rich type hamartoma. Each subtype presents with a dominant expression of one or more components of the splenic red pulp. The cord capillary type differs from classic hamartoma by its striking lobularity, bands of fibrosis, abundant plasma cells, and CD34-positive/CD8-negative phenotype of the vascular lining cells (fig. 18-7). This lesion may overlap with splenic capillary hemangioma

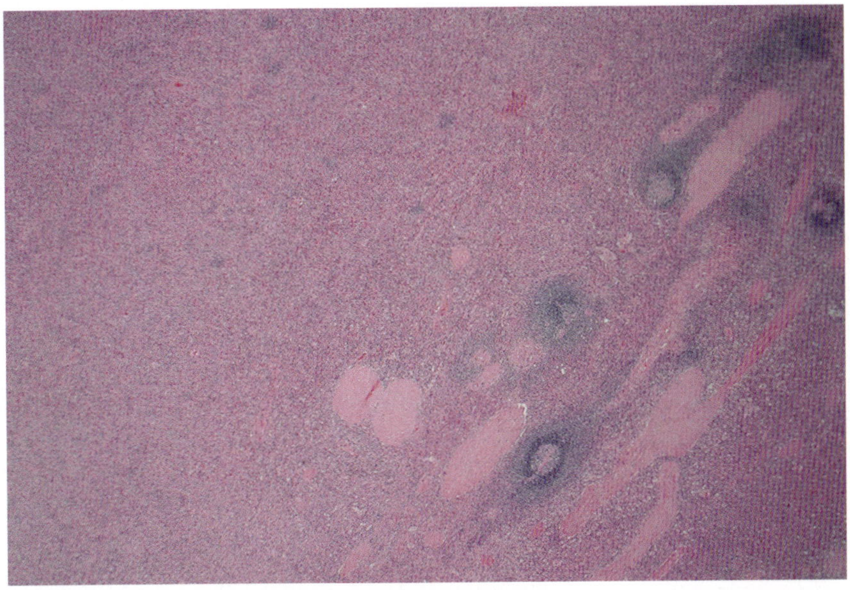

Figure 18-4

HAMARTOMA, SPLEEN

Normal spleen with white pulp is seen in the lower right. The border between uninvolved spleen and hamartoma is vague.

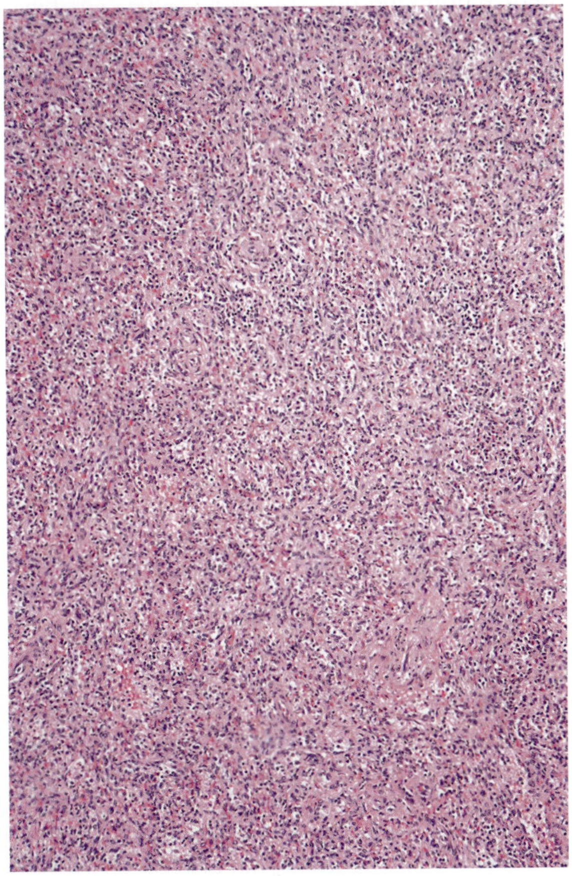

Figure 18-5

HAMARTOMA, SPLEEN

At intermediate magnification, bland splenic red pulp structures (sinuses, cords) are seen.

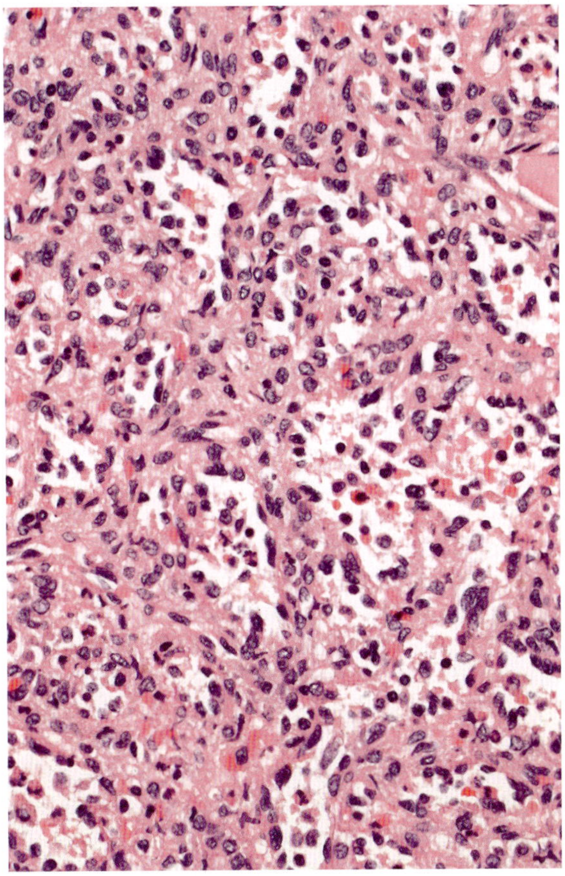

Figure 18-6

HAMARTOMA, SPLEEN

At high magnification, bland splenic red pulp structures (sinuses, cords) are seen.

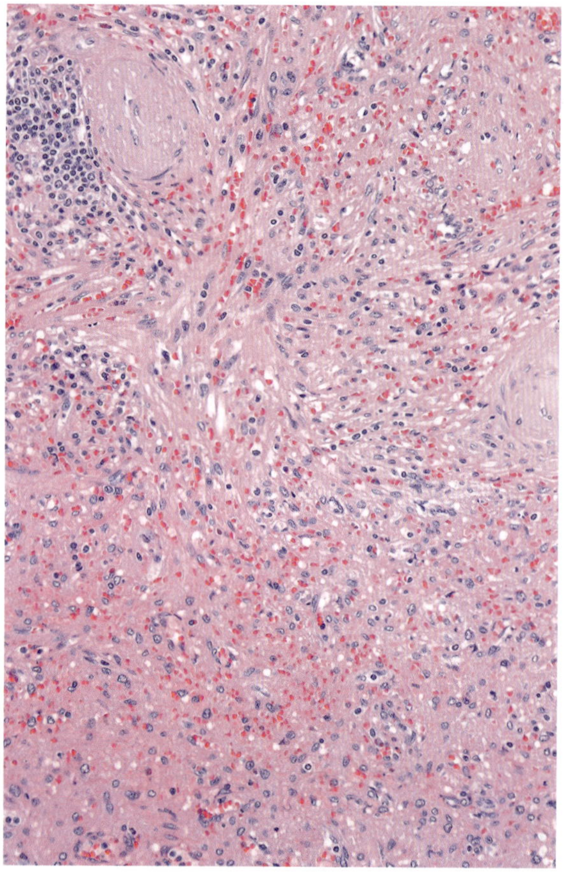

Figure 18-7

SCLEROSING HEMANGIOMA, SPLEEN

Sclerosing hemangioma, or sclerosing angiomatoid nodular transformation (SANT), is composed of a lobulated mass of inconspicuous vascular spaces with fibrosis.

with sclerosis and the SANT (sclerosing angiomatoid nodular transformation) hemangioma described by Martel et al. (fig. 18-8) (47). The myoid angioendothelioma (originally described as "benign vascular neoplasm of the spleen with myoid and angioendotheliomatous features" by Kraus and Dehner [39]), is a vascular lesion lined by CD34-positive cells and prominent stromal cells positive for smooth muscle actin and muscle-specific actin. The macrophage-rich type has a predominance of macrophages, including pseudosinuses lined by CD68-positive macrophages, not endothelial cells (fig. 18-9). The latter two lesions are exceptionally rare. It is unclear whether the division into these subgroups has any clinical significance.

Ancillary Studies. Classic hamartomas are easily distinguished from capillary hemangioma by their typical immunohistochemical reactivity with CD8 and CD68 and lack of expression of CD34 (fig. 18-9) (72). The red pulp components are strongly positive for CD31, factor VIII, and vimentin, similar to normal red pulp. A complex network of reticulin fibers is seen in virtually all cases of hamartoma. In contrast to littoral cell angioma, a relatively common splenic neoplasm with a similar clinical presentation, hamartomas are negative for CD21. Proliferation within hamartomas, as assessed by Ki-67 staining, is very low (less than 5 percent), although proliferative areas may be seen in extramedullary hematopoiesis within the hamartoma (3,54).

Ultrastructural analysis of hamartomas shows well-developed endothelial cells resting on a basement membrane (4). The endothelial cells have typical features including Weibel-Palade bodies, pinocytotic vessels, mitochondria, and sparse rough endoplasmic reticulum. Fibrous long-spacing collagen, present in some cases, does not appear to be present in other splenic lesions.

The diagnosis of hamartoma can be made by a variety of radiologic techniques including computerized tomography (CT), ultrasound, and technetium-99m scintigraphy (41).

Differential Diagnosis. In classic hamartoma, the diagnosis is often straightforward. As mentioned, however, there are several morphologic variants that closely mimic other splenic lesions including inflammatory pseudotumor, inflammatory myofibroblastic tumor, sclerosing hemangioma or SANT, and inflammatory pseudotumor-like follicular dendritic cell tumor (Table 18-1).

Treatment and Prognosis. Splenic hamartomas are benign lesions. Their clinical significance typically lies in their mimicry of other splenic processes such as infections or neoplasms, including vascular neoplasms (6). No specific treatment is required although typically they are resected for diagnostic purposes. Associated hematologic abnormalities may return to normal after resection of the hamartoma (18,34). Rarely, hamartomas rupture and present as hemoperitoneum; as with other causes of splenic rupture, this is a serious medical emergency and may result in death.

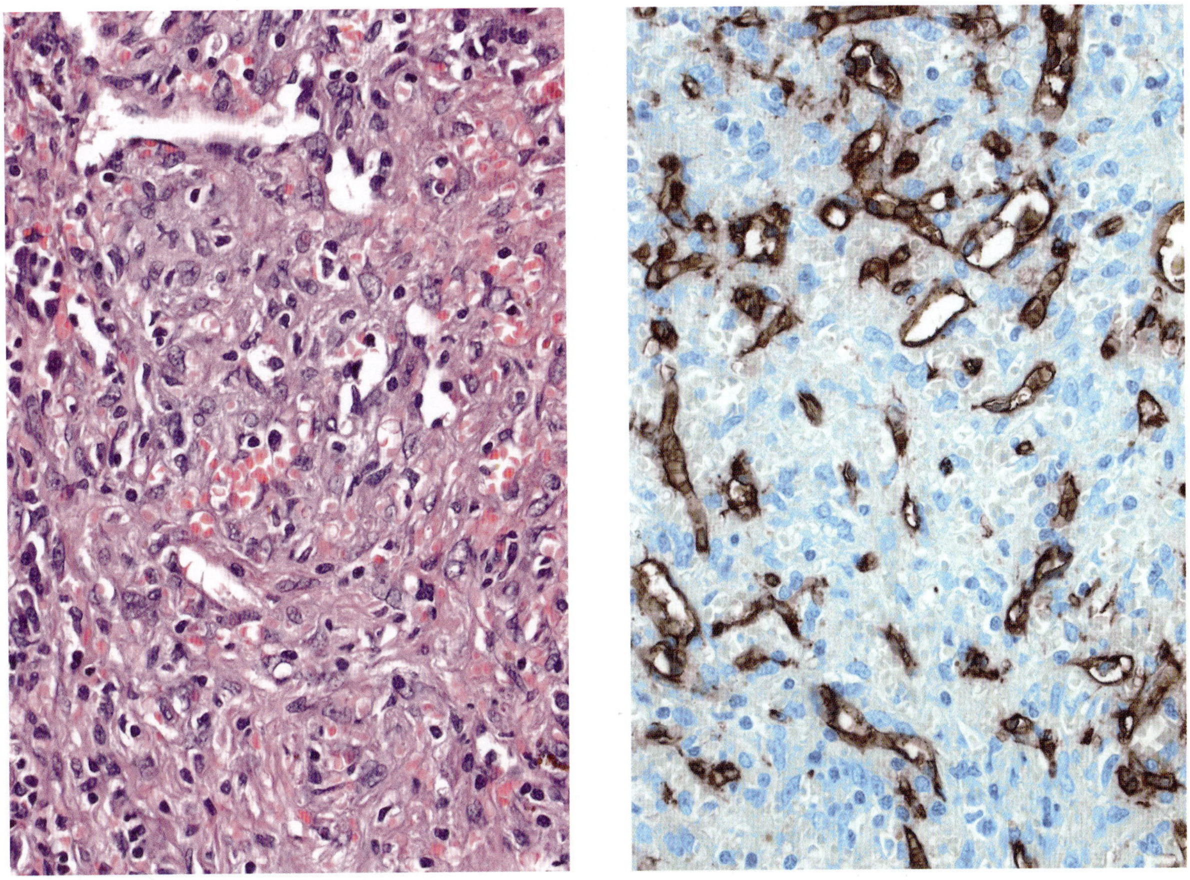

Figure 18-8

SCLEROSING HEMANGIOMA, SPLEEN: CD34 REACTIVITY

Sclerosing hemangioma has extensive CD34 reactivity, while the classic hamartoma lacks such expression.

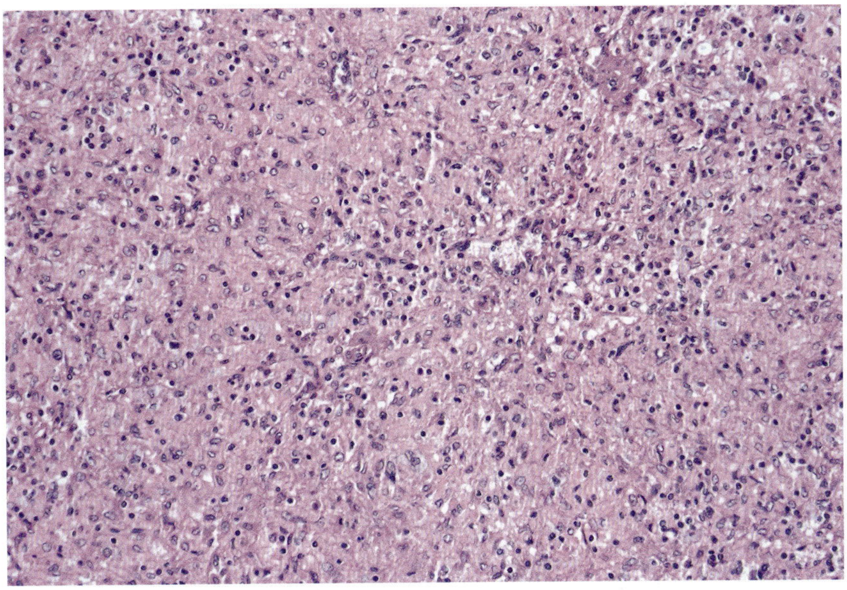

Figure 18-9

HAMARTOMA, SPLEEN

An example of the macrophage-rich variant of hamartoma.

Table 18-1

DIFFERENTIAL DIAGNOSIS OF INFLAMMATORY PSEUDOTUMOR OF SPLEEN

	Etiology	Distinguishing Features
Hamartoma	Non-neoplastic proliferation of stromal components, simulating red pulp	Red pulp appearance with slit-like vascular sinuses, little or no white pulp
Inflammatory pseudotumor	Reactive, most probably secondary to infectious causes	Prominence of inflammatory and/or sclerotic changes, clinical history
Inflammatory pseudotumor-like follicular dendritic cell tumor	Neoplasm of follicular dendritic cells; EBV[a]-associated	Spindle cells are CD21/CD35 positive, EBV positive
Inflammatory myofibroblastic tumor	Neoplasm of myofibroblastic cells	Numerous actin-positive spindle cells, occasionally ALK positive, cytogenetic abnormalities frequent
Capillary hemangioma with prominent sclerosis/SANT	Benign neoplasm of vascular components	Simulates IPT but with prominent vasculature, lobular nature of involvement is a diagnostic clue, vascular markers highlight prominent capillaries

[a]EBV = Epstein-Barr virus; SANT = sclerosing angiomatoid nodular transformation; ALK = anaplastic lymphoma kinase; IPT = inflammatory pseudotumor.

INFLAMMATORY PSEUDOTUMOR (LYMPH NODE AND SPLEEN)

Definition. The rare *inflammatory pseudotumor of lymph node* (IPT-LN) and *inflammatory pseudotumor of spleen* (IPT-S) include a broad range of similar lesions of varied etiologies. They predominantly consist of proliferations of spindle cells with a mixed inflammatory infiltrate. As the name implies, the majority of these lesions have a benign clinical course.

General Features. The etiology and pathogenesis of inflammatory pseudotumor have not been fully elucidated. Using strict definitions, these are rare lesions. Several recently described lesions that have considerable overlap with IPT-LN and IPT-S are distinct neoplasms. These include inflammatory myofibroblastic tumor, inflammatory pseudotumor-like follicular dendritic cell tumor, and other tumors of dendritic/immune accessory cells. When these true tumors of neoplastic etiology are considered, the number of true "pseudotumors" of unknown etiology is greatly reduced. Because of the clinical and histologic overlap, these entities continue to cause considerable diagnostic confusion. Some studies suggest that "true" IPT-LN may represent an evolving, dynamic process with different histologic features depending on the stage of evolution (23,27). Some investigators have demonstrated the presence of Epstein-Barr virus (EBV) RNA by in situ hybridization in these lesions, suggesting a possible etiologic role for this infectious agent (5,45). An unusual tissue response to injury or infection has also been postulated as a potential cause of these pseudotumors (56).

Clinical Features. IPT-LN is a distinctive benign lesion that occurs at any age. Similar lesions have been previously referred to as plasma cell granulomas in other anatomic sites, especially lung and bronchus (8,10), skin (33), and gastrointestinal tract (52). Rarely, IPT-LN presents with multiple sites of involvement or as disseminated disease (36,50). Recent reports have included inflammatory pseudotumors in the spectrum of idiopathic fibrosclerotic disorders (24) or inflammatory myofibroblastic tumor (17).

IPT-LN was first reported by Perrone and colleagues (56) in seven patients in 1988. The clinical presentations included lymphadenopathy and systemic symptoms such as fever, fatigue, and night sweats. The histologic features of the involved lymph nodes were similar in each case.

Historically, IPT-S has been used as a catch-all term for identifying distinct entities that occur in the spleen, some of which are clonal rather than pseudotumor (5,21,41,42,53,57,63). These entities are biologically distinct but have considerable morphologic overlap, and include clonal neoplasms of myofibroblastic cells (inflammatory myofibroblastic tumor), clonal neoplasms of follicular dendritic cells that are associated with EBV infection (inflammatory pseudotumor-like follicular dendritic cell tumor), and polyclonal entities that are truly inflammatory and likely infection related (Table 18-1). Any of these lesions can mimic a malignant process of the spleen clinically, radiologically, and grossly. IPT-S is often asymptomatic; occasional patients have abdominal pain or a sense of fullness. Review of the clinical history may reveal an infectious etiology, but typically studies for specific organisms are negative in the splenic tissues.

Gross Findings. Lymph nodes may be enlarged up to 3 cm. The findings depend on the degree of nodal involvement (fig. 18-10). Smaller lesions are often firm and pale, with variably circumscribed borders. Larger lesions entirely replace the lymph node with firm, fibrous tissue. IPT-S is usually a solitary, circumscribed, pale whitish nodule (fig. 18-11). The borders can be well circumscribed or vague and indefinite.

Microscopic Findings. Histologically, IPT-LN demonstrates hyperplasia of the stromovascular lymph node compartment (5,23,27,51,56). There is a proliferation of spindle cells with a storiform pattern primarily involving the connective tissue framework of the node, marked vascularity, and a mixed inflammatory cell infiltrate, including numerous plasma cells, in a collagenous background (fig. 18-12). The process occasionally extends into the perinodal soft tissue. The mixed inflammatory cell infiltrate consists of neutrophils, plasma cells, macrophages, lymphocytes, and eosinophils.

Small vessel proliferation with occasional lumen obliteration is an important feature of IPT-LN. Although necrosis and infarction have been reported in one series of cases (23), these are not considered to be characteristic features of IPT-LN. Moran and colleagues (51), in a study from the Armed Forces Institute of Pathology, studied 25 cases of IPT-LN that showed histologic and immunophenotypic findings similar to those previously described for this lesion. These include the typical features of the lesion: a mixed inflammatory and myofibroblastic cell infiltrate (fig. 18-13) with a prominent plasma cell component (fig. 18-14) involving the connective tissue framework of the lymph node. Moran and colleagues, however, noted variability in the histologic findings and broadly divided the lesions into three groups or stages based on the degree of cellularity and fibrosis, the overall

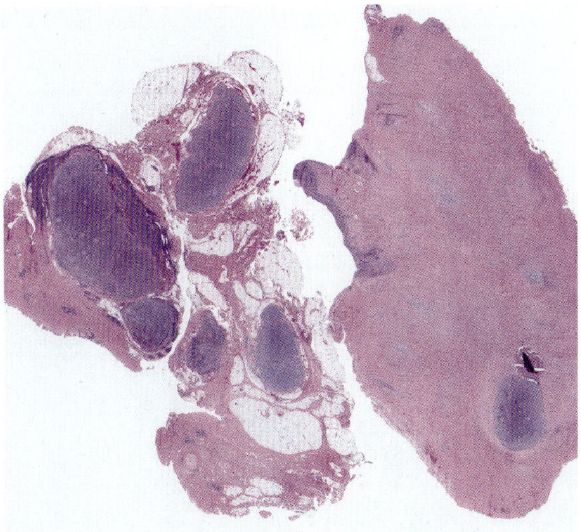

Figure 18-10

INFLAMMATORY PSEUDOTUMOR, LYMPH NODE

A single node is almost completely involved by the inflammatory process, while adjacent nodes are spared.

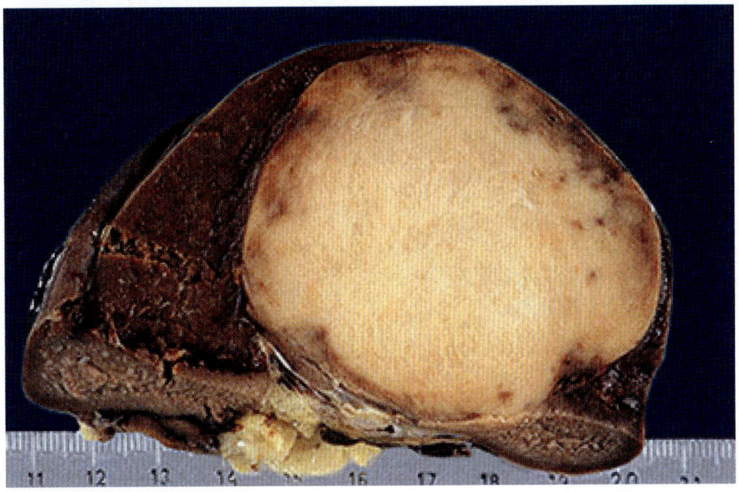

Figure 18-11

INFLAMMATORY PSEUDOTUMOR, SPLEEN

The lesion is circumscribed and firm, with hemorrhagic foci.

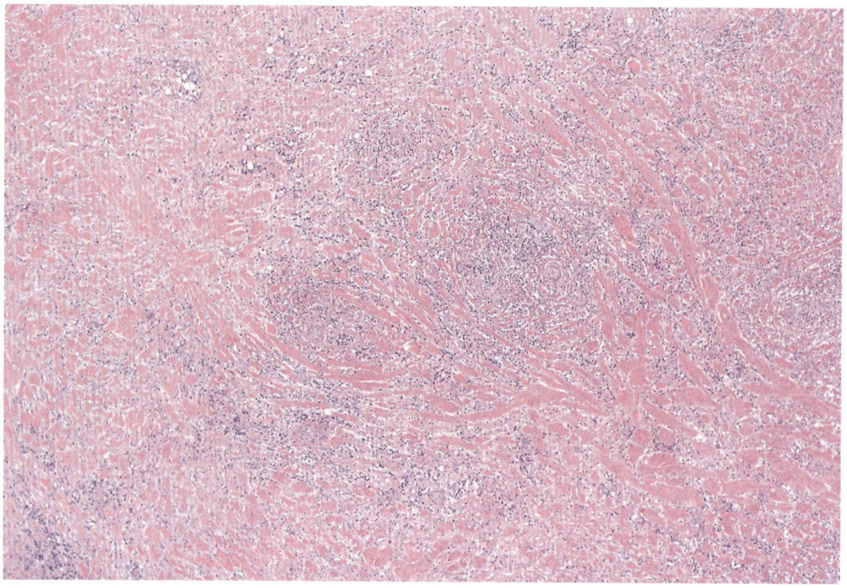

Figure 18-12

INFLAMMATORY PSEUDOTUMOR, LYMPH NODE

Hypocellularity, fibrosis, sclerosis, and scattered inflammatory elements are seen.

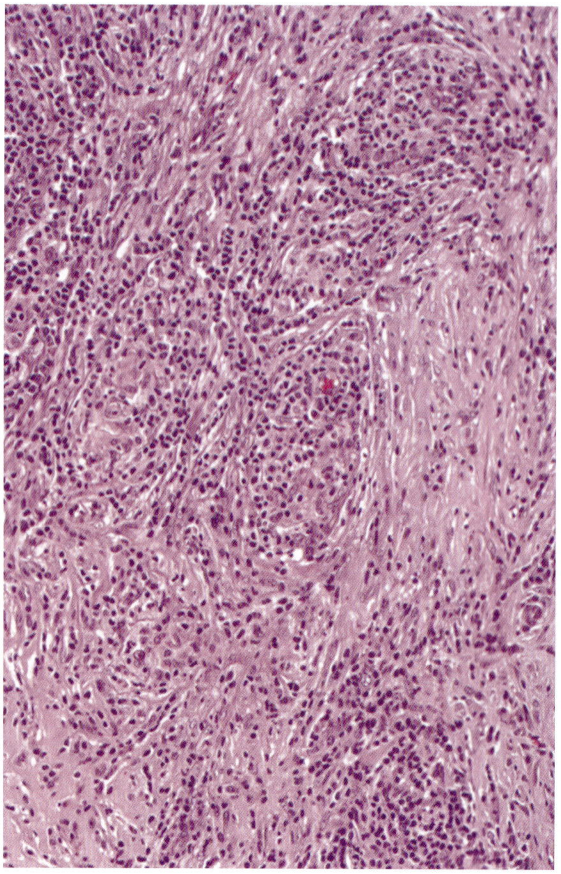

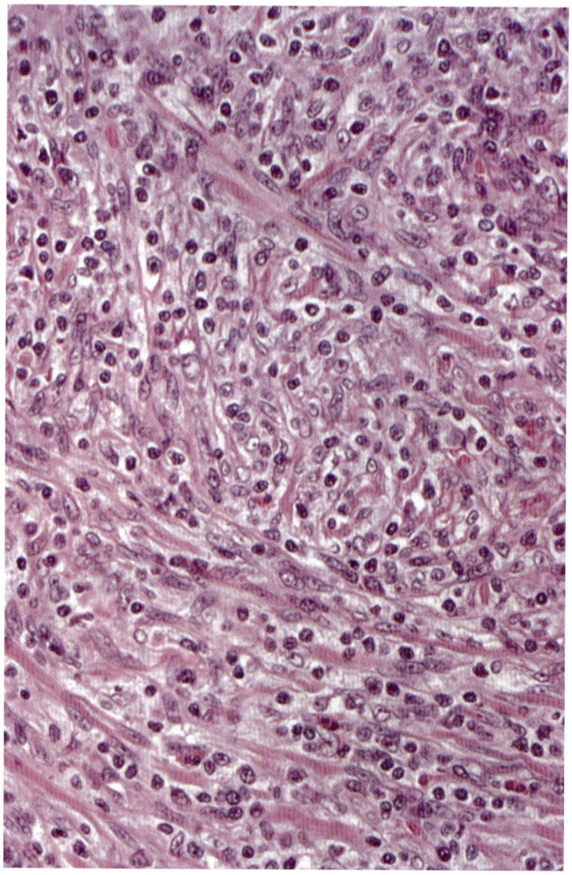

Figure 18-13

INFLAMMATORY PSEUDOTUMOR, LYMPH NODE

Left: There is a vague storiform pattern and mixed inflammatory cell component.
Right: Interspersed lymphocytes and macrophages are within a fibroblastic proliferation.

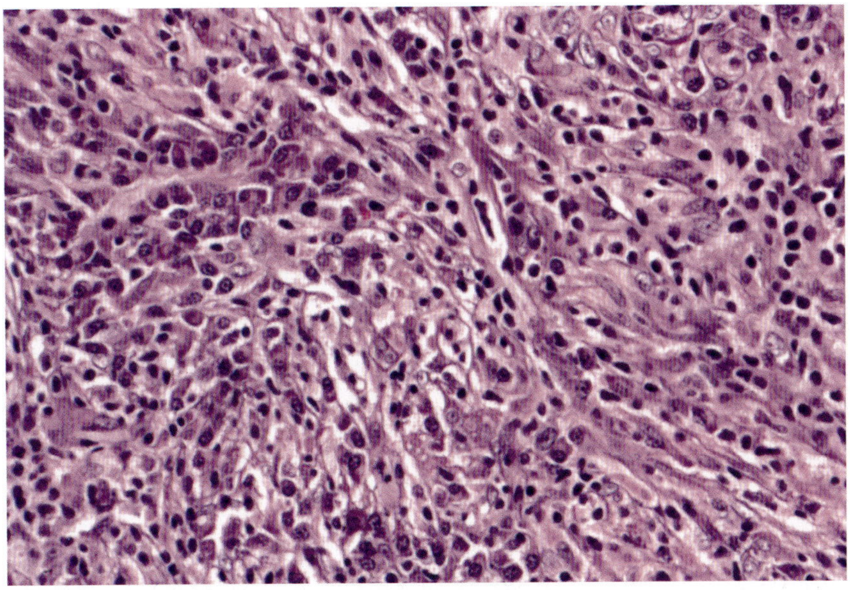

Figure 18-14

INFLAMMATORY PSEUDOTUMOR, LYMPH NODE

There is a prominent reactive plasma cell component.

Table 18-2

HISTOPATHOLOGIC GRADING SYSTEM FOR INFLAMMATORY PSEUDOTUMOR OF LYMPH NODE[a]

	Histologic Findings
Stage I	Small, localized nodules; preservation of normal nodal architecture
Stage II	Disruption/distortion of lymph node architecture; replacement of node by mixture of mixed inflammatory infiltrate and myofibroblastic spindle cell proliferation
Stage III	Total or near-total replacement of lymph node; dense sclerosis with minimal inflammatory infiltrate; only small island of residual lymphoid tissue

[a]Table 2 from Moran CA, Suster S, Albondanzo SL. Inflammatory pseudotumor of lymph nodes: a study of 25 cases with emphasis on morphological heterogeneity. Hum Pathol 1997;28:333.

Table 18-3

IMMUNOHISTOCHEMICAL FINDINGS IN SPINDLE CELLS OF INFLAMMATORY PSEUDOTUMOR

Stain	Result
CD68	+/–
Smooth muscle actin	+/–
Vimentin	+
Desmin	–
CD21	–
CD35	–
Keratin	–
HMB45	–
S-100 protein	–

architectural pattern, and the extent of the lesion (Table 18-2). The identification of focal areas in which these histologic features overlap supports the possibility that the changes observed in IPT-LN represent a dynamic, evolving process.

The common histologic findings observed in IPT-S include a proliferation of bland-looking spindle-shaped cells and a polymorphic background of monocytes, lymphocytes, granulocytes, and polyclonal plasma cells (fig. 18-15). Collagenous stroma is a universal feature, with extensive sclerotic changes commonly observed.

Ancillary Studies. The characteristic spindle cells are reactive with vimentin, and variably reactive for CD68 or smooth-muscle actin, supporting a fibroblastic/myofibroblastic origin (Table 18-3). The vague storiform pattern can be highlighted with immunohistochemical markers for vimentin and actin (figs. 18-16, 18-17). Anaplastic lymphoma kinase (ALK) is not expressed and thus eliminates an alternate diagnosis, such as inflammatory myofibroblastic tumor. Immunohistochemical staining of the inflammatory cells shows a mixture of B and T cells, polytypic plasma cells, and rare CD30-positive transformed lymphocytes.

Because of the inflammatory appearance of these lesions, stains for microorganisms, such as acid-fast bacillus (AFB), Gomori methenamine silver (GMS), and periodic acid–Schiff (PAS),

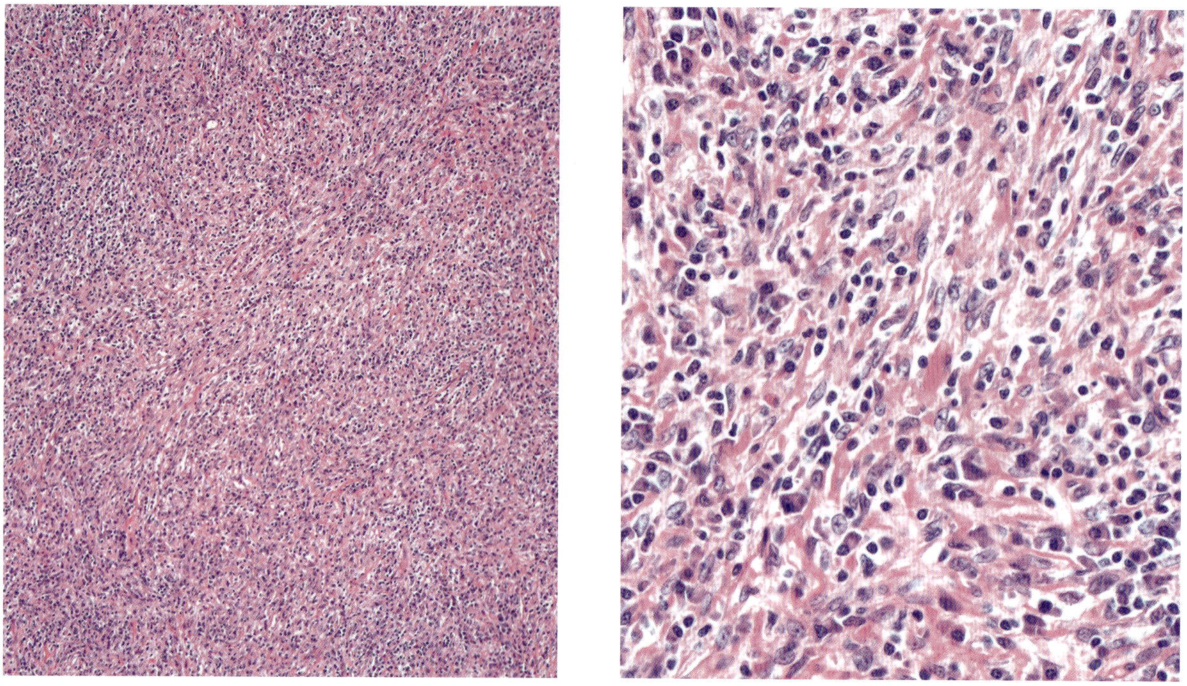

Figure 18-15

INFLAMMATORY PSEUDOTUMOR, SPLEEN

A proliferation of mixed inflammatory elements and spindle cells is seen. (Courtesy of Milton Drachenberg, Long Beach, CA.)

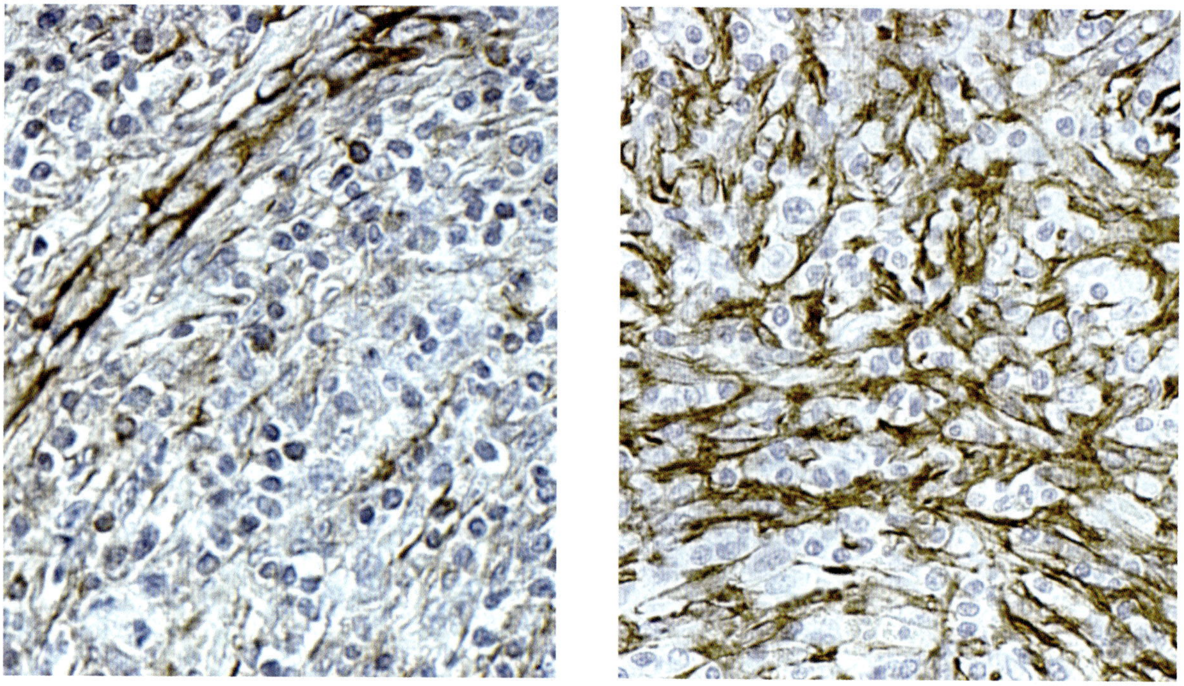

Figure 18-16

IMMUNOHISTOCHEMICAL REACTIVITY IN INFLAMMATORY PSEUDOTUMOR, LYMPH NODE

Vimentin (left) and smooth muscle actin (right) immunoreactivity are seen.

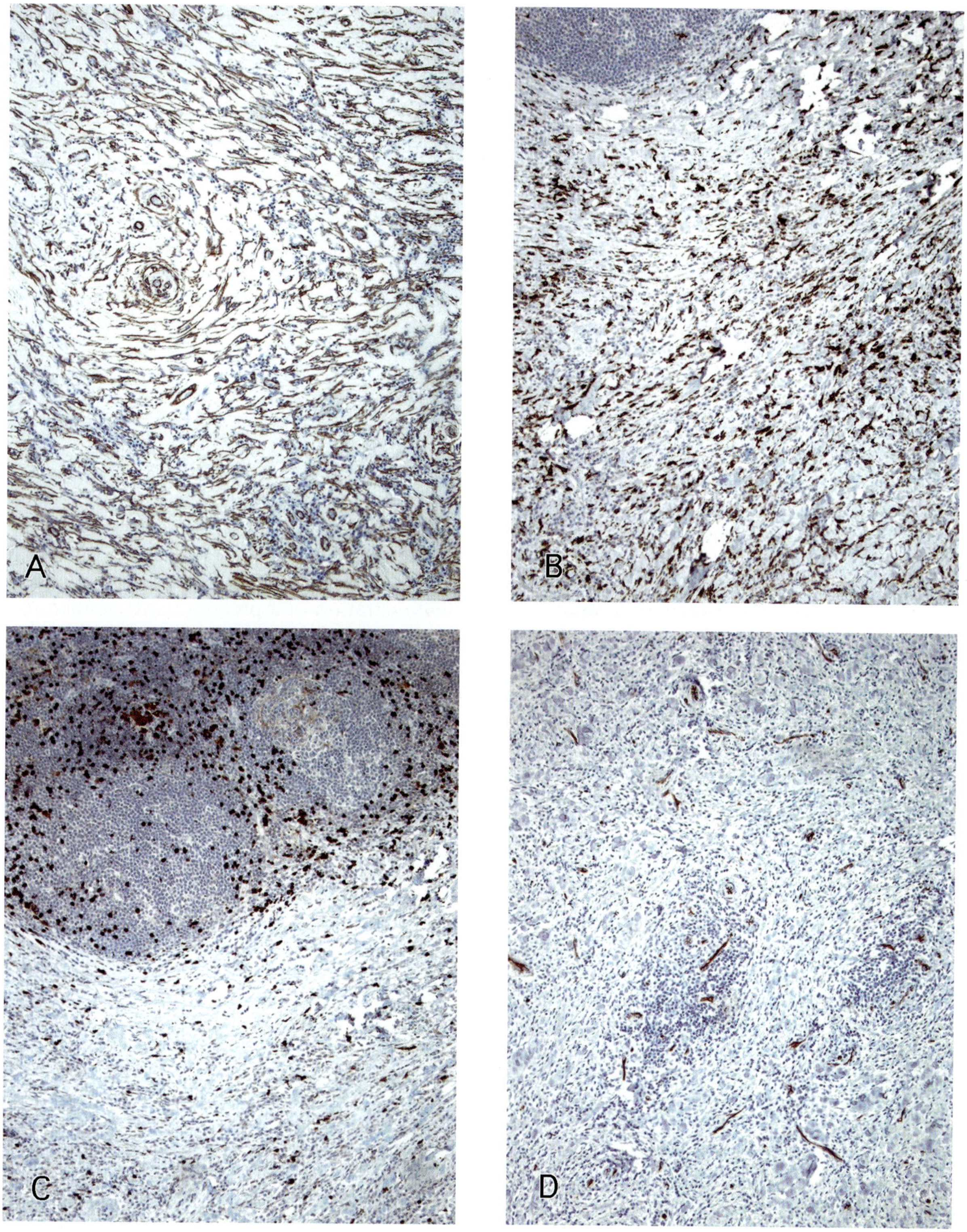

Figure 18-17

IMMUNOHISTOCHEMICAL REACTIVITY IN INFLAMMATORY PSEUDOTUMOR, SPLEEN

Smooth muscle actin (A) and CD163 (B) are positive, but there is little reactivity for S-100 protein (C) or CD34 (D).

may be warranted in select cases. These stains are negative in IPT. Evaluation of lesions for the presence of EBV infection may also be useful. Some cases express EBV encoded RNA (EBER) by in situ techniques, and rare cases express EBV-latent membrane protein (LMP). If cytogenetic abnormalities are identified, the lesion more likely represents one of the many neoplastic morphologic mimics (see below), rather than a true IPT.

Differential Diagnosis. The differential diagnosis of IPT-LN includes both benign and malignant lesions. Some of the more common entities that have similar histologic features are Castleman disease (29), drug (Dilantin)-related lymphadenopathy (1), Langerhans cell histiocytosis, dendritic cell neoplasms, peripheral T-cell lymphoma, and Hodgkin lymphoma.

Two features that Castleman disease and IPT-LN have in common are prominent interfollicular vascularity and polyclonal plasmacytosis (29,40). An important distinguishing feature, however, characteristic of lymph nodes associated with Castleman disease, is regressive transformation of germinal centers with "onion-skinning" of the mantle zone. Prominent fibrosis and a storiform proliferation of spindle cells are not typically seen in Castleman disease.

The lymph nodes of patients being treated with the antiseizure medication, phenytoin, may show a spectrum of histopathologic features including architectural effacement by a mixed inflammatory cell infiltrate (especially eosinophils, plasma cells, lymphocytes, and immunoblasts) and focal small vessel vasculitis (1). Spindle cell proliferation and hyalinization, however, are not characteristically seen in Dilantin-related lymphadenopathy (1) and should help to distinguish this lesion from IPT-LN. A good clinical history is also important in the diagnosis of Dilantin-related lymphadenopathy.

Langerhans cell histiocytosis may be confused with IPT-LN when the histiocytic proliferation occurs in a paracortical or interfollicular location. Langerhans cell histiocytosis, however, is not characterized by a storiform pattern of spindle cells. The presence of nuclear grooves and immunoreactivity for S-100 protein and CD1a are characteristic features of Langerhans cells. In addition, the demonstration of Birbeck granules by electron microscopy offers definitive proof of this entity.

Other spindle cell lesions in the differential diagnosis of IPT-LN are follicular dendritic or interdigitating dendritic cell neoplasms. Unlike IPT-LN, the spindle cells in a follicular dendritic cell tumor show nuclear atypia and are reactive for the follicular dendritic cell markers, CD21 and CD35 (fig. 18-18) (11). An interdigitating reticulum cell neoplasm similarly shows a storiform pattern of spindle cells, which may totally efface the normal nodal architecture (35). The cells, however, characteristically express S-100 protein, demonstrate nuclear atypia, and have an increased mitotic rate (fig. 18-19).

Peripheral T-cell lymphoma is an important entity to consider in the differential diagnosis of IPT-LN. Distinguishing features of this neoplasm include cytologic atypia, increased mitoses, accentuated vascularity, and diffuse effacement of the normal nodal architecture. Inflammatory cells (especially eosinophils) may be seen in T-cell lymphomas; these neoplasms, however, characteristically lack a spindle cell proliferation or storiform pattern. The immunohistochemical demonstration of a predominant, or aberrant, T-cell population is another useful finding.

Hodgkin lymphoma (especially the fibroblastic variant of nodular sclerosis type) may be confused with IPT-LN if classic Reed-Sternberg cells or mononuclear cell variants are sparse. Adequate and extensive sampling of the tissue may be necessary to identify the neoplastic cells of Hodgkin lymphoma. Immunoreactivity with CD15 and CD30 and lack of reactivity with CD45 help to confirm a diagnosis of classic Hodgkin lymphoma.

Other entities such as Kaposi sarcoma, intranodal hemorrhagic spindle cell tumor with amianthoid fibers (palisaded myofibroblastoma) (61,67), amyloidosis, and proteinaceous lymphadenopathy, are also in the differential diagnosis of IPT-LN. Kaposi sarcoma may be differentiated from IPT-LN by its cytologic atypia, increased mitotic rate, and extravasated red blood cells. Palisaded myofibroblastoma, an extremely rare entity, typically shows almost total effacement of the nodal architecture by a spindle cell proliferation, with only a thin rim of residual lymph node tissue displaced toward the periphery. Amyloidosis or proteinaceous lymphadenopathy may be diagnosed by the use of special stains or immunohistochemical

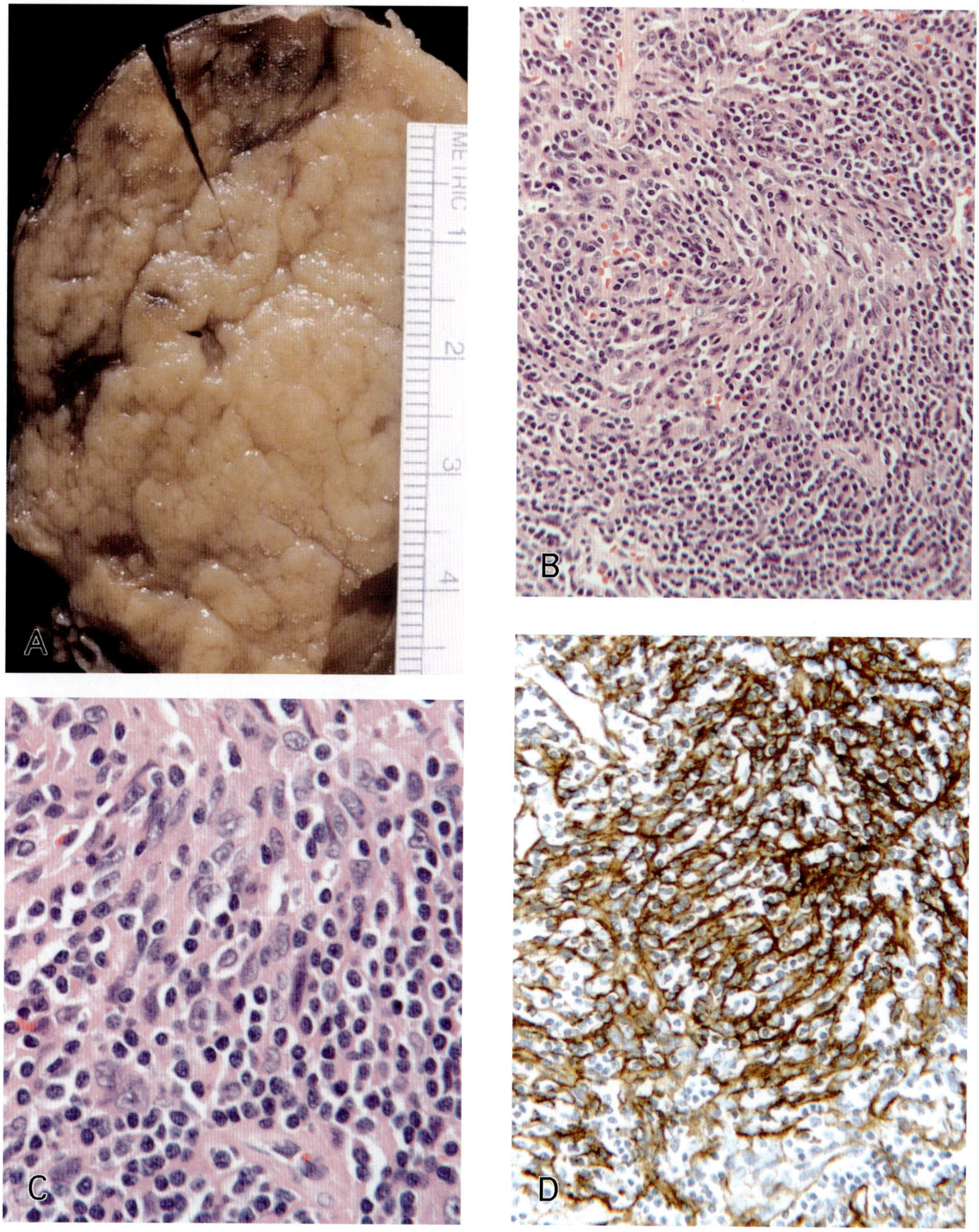

Figure 18-18

FOLLICULAR DENDRITIC CELL TUMOR, LYMPH NODE

The cut surface is fleshy and nodular (A). A storiform pattern (B) of plump spindle cells (C) can be seen. Immunoreactivity for CD21 is diagnostic for this neoplasm.

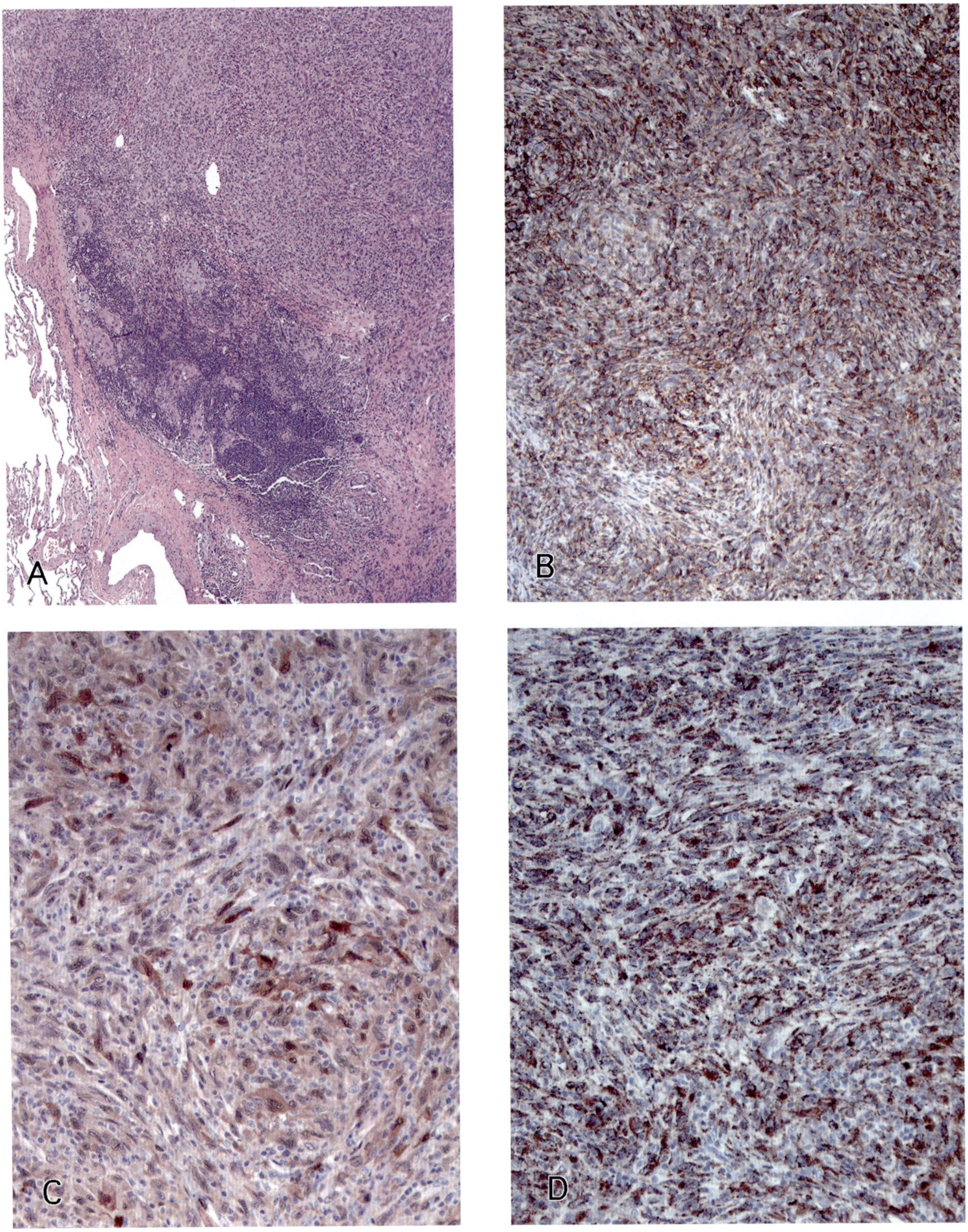

Figure 18-19

INTERDIGITATING DENDRITIC CELL TUMOR, LYMPH NODE

In this spindle cell proliferation (A), interdigitating dendritic cells are positive for CD45 (B), S-100 protein (C), and CD68 (D).

analysis, which demonstrates the characteristic features of amyloid or paraamyloid material.

Distinction of IPT-S from diffuse large cell lymphoma with prominent sclerosis is greatly facilitated by immunohistochemistry or molecular techniques. In addition to splenic lymphoma, the differential diagnosis of IPT-S includes splenic hamartoma and hemangioma. Splenic hamartomas are typically surrounded by a rim of compressed red pulp, usually without associated fibrosis. In addition, the sinus or cord-like spaces characteristically observed in splenic hamartoma are not observed in IPT-S. Splenic capillary hemangiomas with sclerosis may occasionally resemble IPT-S. These tend to have a predominant component of small vessels with increased numbers of macrophages. Their histologic pattern is often lobular in appearance. They can be differentiated by immunohistochemistry, which highlights the vascular nature of lesion. This entity may correspond to the "cord capillary hemangioma" described by Krishnan and Frizzera (41).

Inflammatory myofibroblastic tumor (IMT) is a true neoplasm of spindle cells of myofibroblastic lineage (53). The clinical findings show a female predominance and a wide age range of presentation, associated with rare recurrences and even metastatic spread. Immunohistochemical staining by smooth muscle actin reveals uniform positivity in the spindle cell population. Occasional cases of IMT are positive for ALK and p80, a result that confirms their neoplastic nature. IMT shows genetic abnormalities in almost 50 percent of cases, including translocations or duplications involving the ALK receptor at 2p23 (42,55).

Another close mimic of IPT-S is the inflammatory pseudotumor-like follicular dendritic cell tumor (IPTLFDC) (16). Unlike conventional follicular dendritic cell tumors (see above), IPTLFDC has a marked female predominance. The clinical behavior is typically indolent. As the name implies, IPTLFDC shows an IPT-like background which contains bland spindle cells positive for dendritic cell markers (CD21, CD35). Essentially all cases are positive for EBV.

Treatment and Prognosis. For virtually all cases of IPT, either splenic or nodal, resection is typically curative. Cases with associated clinical symptomatology may resolve after complete resection of the lesion. Local recurrence is rare; however, it should prompt consideration of the many histologically similar disorders that may be clinically more aggressive (20).

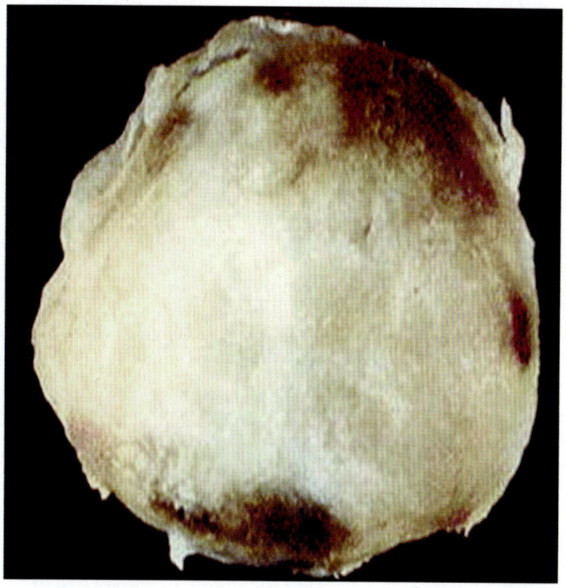

Figure 18-20

PALISADED MYOFIBROBLASTOMA, LYMPH NODE

The cut surface shows a firm mass with foci of hemorrhage. (Courtesy of California Tumor Tissue Registry, Loma Linda, CA.)

PALISADED MYOFIBROBLASTOMA

Definition. *Palisaded myofibroblastoma,* occasionally called *intranodal hemorrhagic spindle cell tumor with amianthoid fibers,* is a rare, benign lymph node lesion that closely resembles a schwannoma but is derived from myofibroblastic cells.

Clinical Features. There is a slight male predominance with a wide age range. The lymphadenopathy is localized and may be painful. Inguinal lymph nodes are the most common site although it has also been reported in submandibular and cervical lymph nodes. The etiology of these tumors is unknown.

Gross Findings. The tumors are firm and gray-white, with focal hemorrhage (fig. 18-20). A residual compressed lymph node may be visible, depending on the extent of nodal involvement.

Microscopic Findings. The salient histologic feature of this lesion is a storiform pattern of palisaded, intersecting spindle cells surrounding

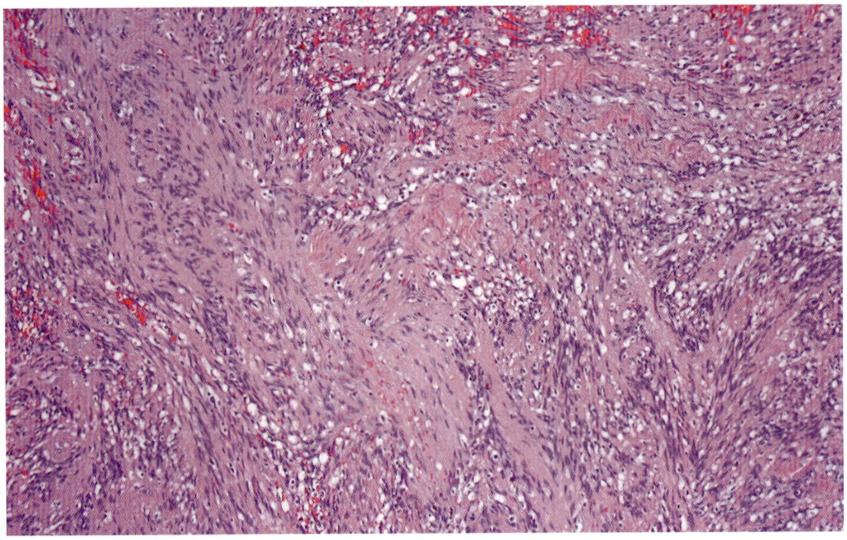

Figure 18-21

PALISADED MYOFIBROBLASTOMA, LYMPH NODE

A diffuse proliferation of spindle cells, with some evidence of palisading of nuclei. (Courtesy of the California Tumor Tissue Registry, Loma Linda, CA.)

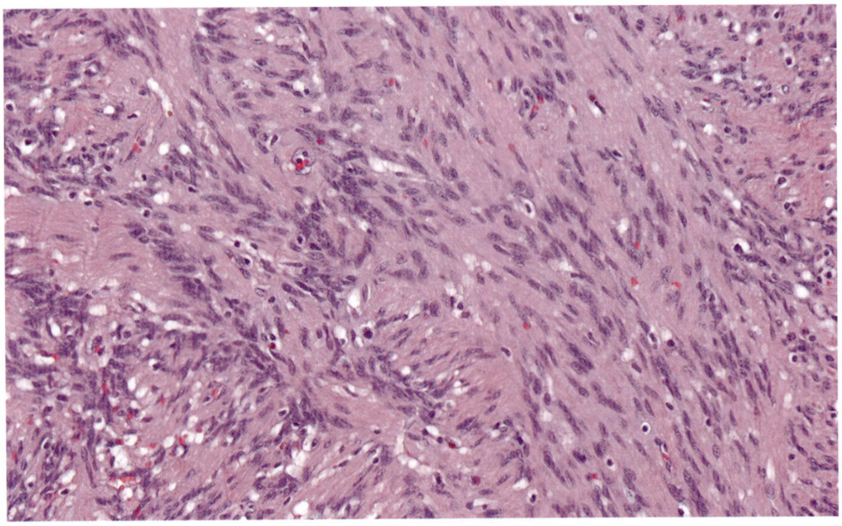

Figure 18-22

PALISADED MYOFIBROBLASTOMA, LYMPH NODE

Higher magnification of figure 18-21 reveals intersecting bundles of bland spindle cells. (Courtesy of the California Tumor Tissue Registry, Loma Linda, CA.)

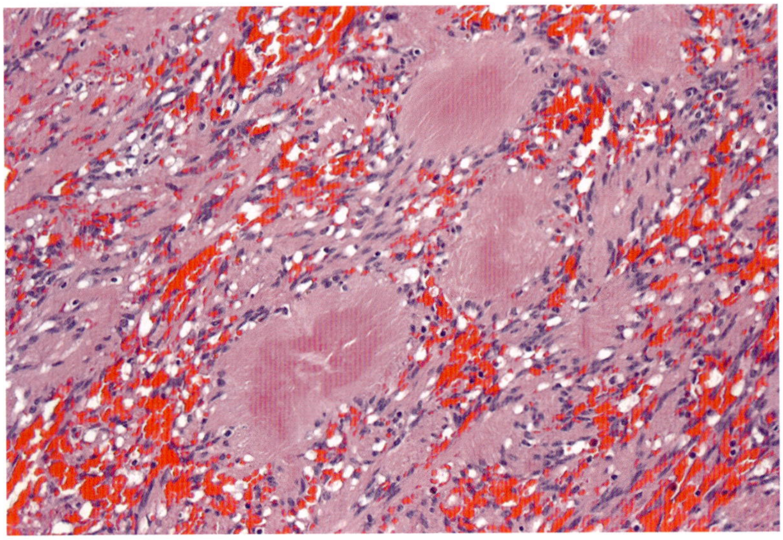

Figure 18-23

PALISADED MYOFIBROBLASTOMA, LYMPH NODE

Foci of hemorrhage are seen in association with amianthoid fibers. (Courtesy of the California Tumor Tissue Registry, Loma Linda, CA.)

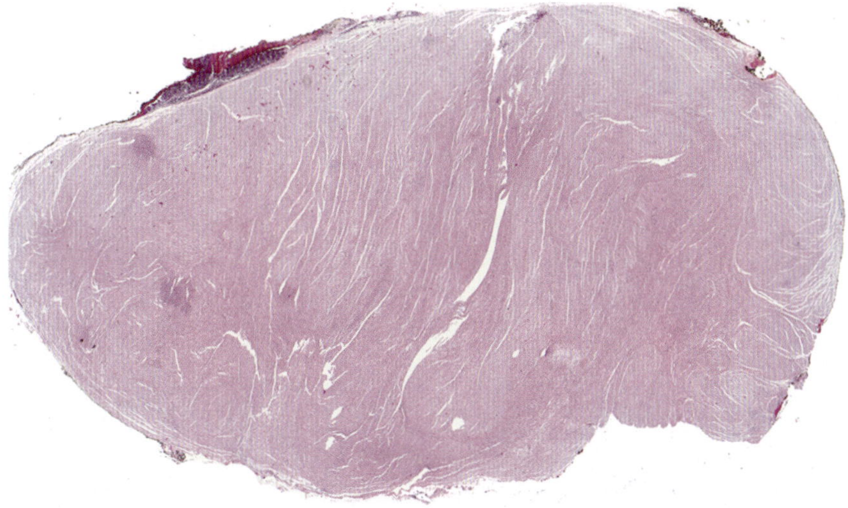

Figure 18-24

METASTATIC LEIOMYOSARCOMA

In contrast to palisaded myofibroblastoma, this example of metastatic leiomyosarcoma lacks hemorrhage and amianthoid fibers.

eosinophilic collagenous areas (figs. 18-21–18-23). The distinctive, so-called amianthoid fibers are stellate areas of collagen deposits that may be calcified. The spindle cells do not show atypia and mitotic figures are rare. The residual normal lymph node is compressed and surrounds areas of hemorrhage with hemosiderin deposits. Variable amounts of fibrosis or granulation tissue may be present.

Ancillary Studies. The spindle cells in palisaded myofibroblastoma are reactive with vimentin and smooth muscle actin, variably positive for factor XIIIa, and negative for desmin, S-100 protein, and factor VIII–related antigen. The proliferation rate is less than 5 percent by Ki-67 staining. A single case has been reported with cyclin D1 overexpression, although no evidence of genetic abnormalities associated with the *CCNDD1* gene was reported (38). There is no evidence of an association with EBV. The amianthoid-like fibers are positive for collagen types I and III.

Electron microscopic examination shows the spindle cells to have pinocytotic vescicles, well-developed endoplasmic reticulum, and aggregates of actin filaments, similar to myofibroblastic cells (38).

Differential Diagnosis. The immunophenotypic findings help to distinguish this lesion from benign or malignant simulators, such as inflammatory pseudotumor of lymph node, Kaposi (or other) sarcoma, metastatic carcinoma, metastatic melanoma, intranodal schwannoma, follicular dendritic cell tumors, and benign metastasizing leiomyoma. There are histologic and immunophenotypic differences that should help in the distinction of palisaded myofibroblastoma from these entities. Sarcomas show nuclear pleomorphism and an increased mitotic rate. Follicular dendritic cell tumors are CD21, CD23, and CD35 positive. The characteristic PAS-positive globules of Kaposi sarcoma are absent in palisaded myofibroblastoma. Intranodal schwannomas are S-100 protein positive and show characteristic Antoni A and B areas that can be distinguished from palisaded myofibroblastoma. Since the description of palisaded myofibroblastoma, the existence of intranodal schwannoma has come into question. Although palisaded myofibroblastoma may simulate a benign metastasizing leiomyoma, the latter does not show areas of interstitial hemorrhage or amianthoid fibers (fig. 18-24).

Treatment and Prognosis. These are benign lesions and resection is typically curative, even incomplete resection. Rare cases have recurred (22,46).

LIPOMATOSIS, LIPOMA, AND FATTY REPLACEMENT OF LYMPH NODE

Definition. *Lipomatosis* is a non-neoplastic process of fatty infiltration or "transformation" of a lymph node. *Lipoma* is a localized, benign tumor of fat cells. It has been reported in the spleen.

Clinical Features. Lipomatosis of lymph node is a common cause of lymphadenopathy, especially in axillary lymph nodes. It is usually an incidental finding that is clinically insignificant (66). Lipomatosis is a common finding and

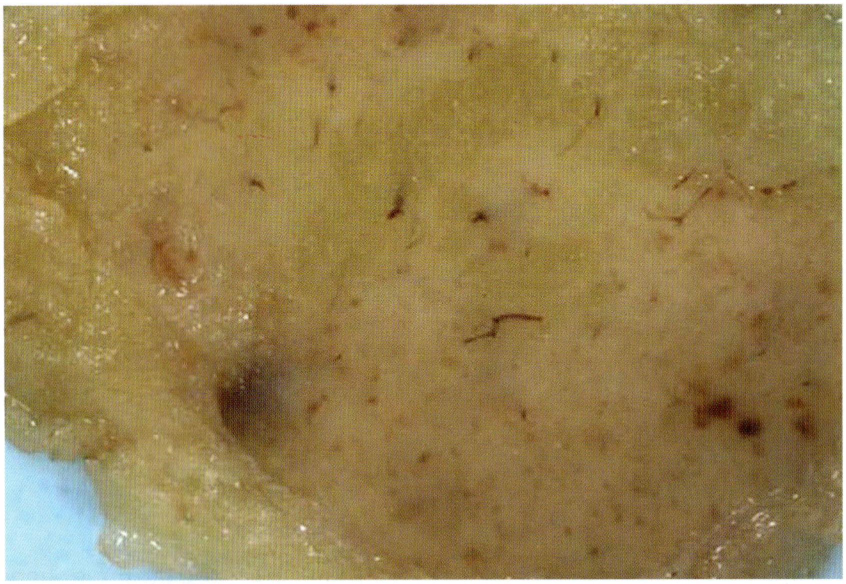

Figure 18-25

LIPOMATOSIS, LYMPH NODE

Lipomatosis of lymph nodes grossly appears as fatty nodules. Residual lymphoid tissue is difficult to distinguish from fat.

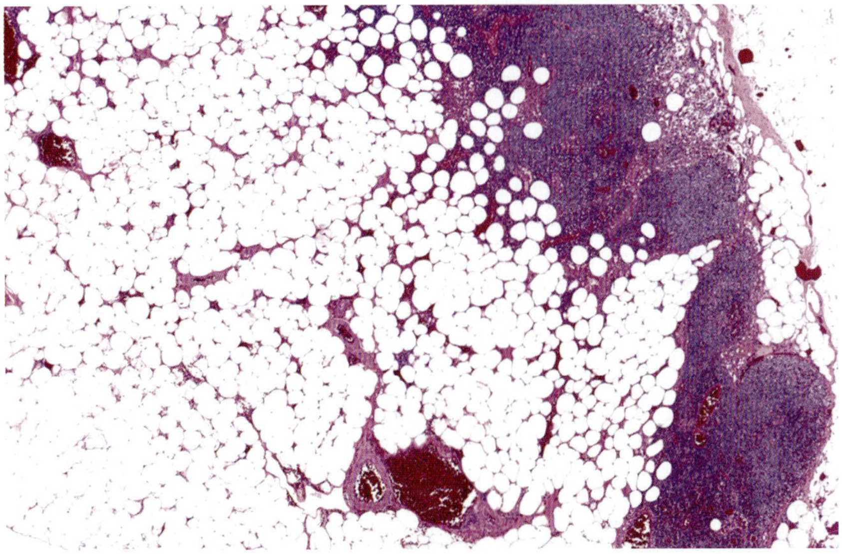

Figure 18-26

LIPOMATOSIS, LYMPH NODE

A large portion of the hilum and parenchyma is replaced by mature adipose tissue.

does not present a diagnostic difficulty except in cases where the lymph node, usually from the pelvis or abdomen, is very large. It may be mistaken for a lipoma if the surrounding identifiable lymphoid tissue is not evident. Lipoma of spleen is an exceedingly rare tumor (26).

Gross Findings. The lymph nodes are soft, greasy, and often bright yellow (fig. 18-25). Their size depends on the site and duration of the lesion. In some cases, the distinct borders of the node are difficult to distinguish from perinodal fat. Occasionally, a thin rim of residual lymph node may be seen at the periphery of the lipoma near the typically thin capsule.

Microscopic Findings. Lipomatosis is a nodular/lobular proliferation of mature fat. It is important to note that adipose tissue is not a normal finding in spleen, and is always associated with a pathologic process. The histologic features of lipomatosis include subtotal or total effacement of the normal nodal architecture (especially the hilum) by mature adipose cells. A compressed, thin rim of residual normal lymphoid tissue may be seen (fig. 18-26). Distinction of lipoma and lipomatosis is essentially impossible by histologic means, and is of little clinical consequence.

Ancillary Studies. Although rarely evaluated, the cytoplasm of fat cells is reactive for S-100 protein. Cytogenetics performed on lipomas show chromosomal abnormalities in 50 to 80 percent of cases. These include translocations involving 12q13-15, deletions of 13q, and rearrangements involving 6p21-23 (68).

Differential Diagnosis. In lymph node and spleen, lipomas may need to be distinguished from angiomyolipoma with a predominance of mature fat. The diagnosis of angiomyolipoma is discussed below.

Treatment and Prognosis. Lipomatosis is a benign lesion, and no treatment beyond excision is required.

ANGIOMYOLIPOMA

Definition. *Angiomyolipomas* are well-described hamartomatous lesions that typically involve the kidney and rarely the retroperitoneal lymph nodes and spleen. The lesions are characterized by a proliferation of smooth muscle cells, thick-walled blood vessels, and adipose cells.

General Features. Angiomyolipomas are clonal mesenchymal neoplasms that appear to be derived from perivascular epithelioid cells (PEC) (48). The vascular, myomatous, and lipomatous components are all monoclonal, but may arise from independent, abnormal clones (15). Although most angiomyolipomas are sporadic, many are associated with tuberous sclerosis. Sporadic cases appear to be approximately four times as common as those associated with tuberous sclerosis. Tuberous sclerosis is an inherited neurocutaneous disorder characterized by multiple benign neoplasms primarily involving the kidney, skin, and brain, but not limited to these organs (see chapter 7).

Clinical Features. The mean age of patients with angiomyolipoma is 25 to 35 years for those with TS and 45 to 55 years for those without. There is a 4 to 1 female predominance in sporadic cases and no apparent sex predilection in patients with tuberous sclerosis.

Angiomyolipoma involving regional lymph nodes is rare; metastases of angiomyolipoma to perirenal lymph nodes, however, may be not be as rare as reported but may simply be an issue of tissue sampling. Angiomyolipoma is rare in the spleen, and usually as part of involvement by multifocal disease (2,7,32); there has been a single case report of primary splenic angiomyolipoma (62).

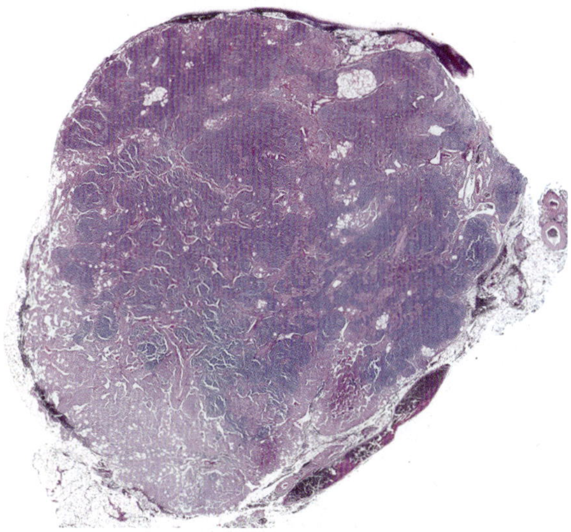

Figure 18-27

ANGIOMYOLIPOMA, LYMPH NODE

Partial involvement of a lymph node by angiomyolipoma.

Microscopic Findings. Angiomyolipomas contain variable mixtures of mature adipose tissue, thick-walled abnormal vessels, and smooth muscle (figs. 18-27–18-29). The smooth muscle cells often have a radial arrangement around the blood vessels. When all three components are present, the diagnosis is straightforward. In rare cases, however, one or two components predominate. Severe nuclear pleomorphism and significant mitotic activity and necrosis in the spindle cell (myomatous) component also occur rarely.

Ancillary Studies. Angiomyolipomas are positive for smooth muscle actin in the smooth muscle component, and for HMB45 (fig. 18-30) (2,7,37,48). The cells also express melanoma-associated markers such as Mart1/Melan A, tyrosinase, and microophthalmia transcription factor.

Differential Diagnosis. The spindled nature of the cellular component of angiomyolipoma may be confused with a primary vascular neoplasm, most notably Kaposi sarcoma. Correlation with clinical findings is of paramount importance, but immunohistochemical reactivity for vascular markers in the spindled component is not seen in angiomyolipoma.

Metastatic well-differentiated leiomyosarcoma may also mimic angiomyolipoma, particularly if a smooth muscle component

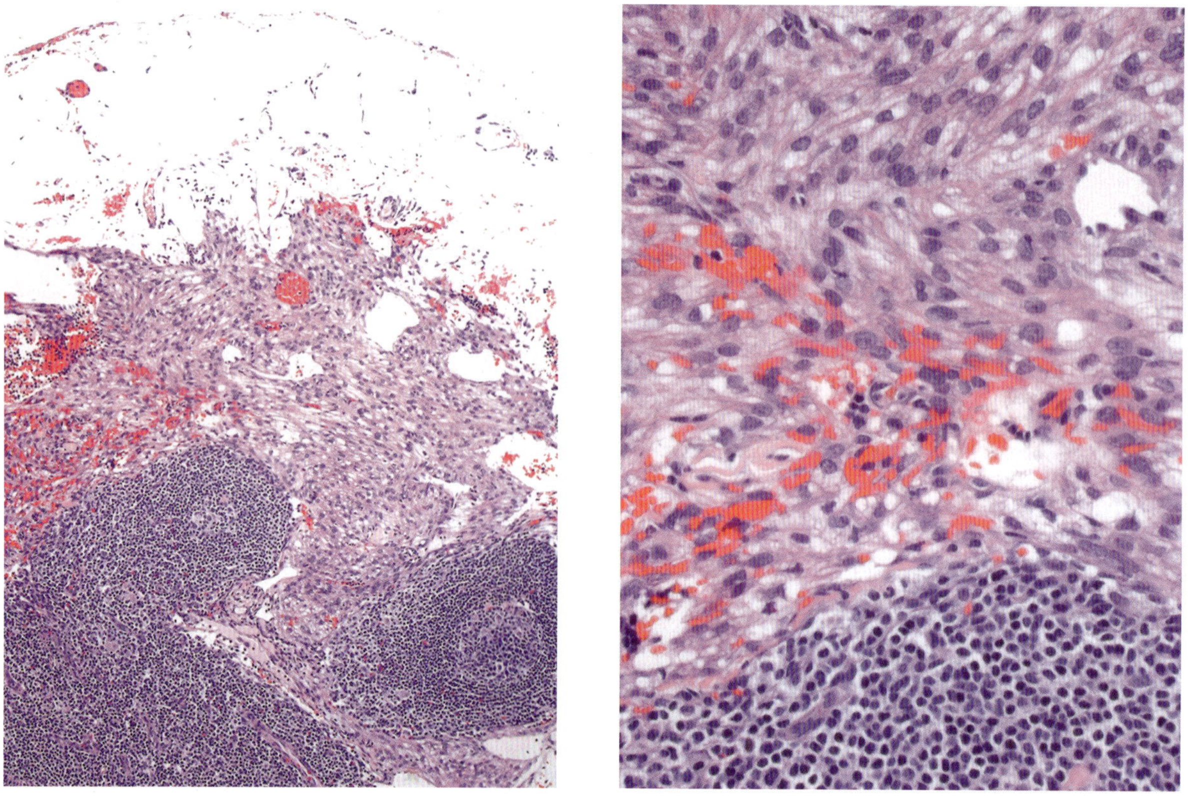

Figure 18-28

ANGIOMYOLIPOMA, LYMPH NODE

The smooth muscle and fatty components are seen. (Courtesy of Mahul Amin, Los Angeles, CA.)

predominates, but spleen and lymph nodes are not usual sites of metastasis for leiomyosarcoma. Similarly, vascular tumors of the spleen should be investigated for smooth muscle and adipose components to exclude angiomyolipoma.

Treatment and Prognosis. Angiomyolipomas are benign in virtually all cases and resection alone is sufficient treatment.

ANGIOMYOMATOUS HAMARTOMA, LYMPHANGIOMYOMA, LEIOMYOMATOSIS, AND LEIOMYOMA

Definition. There are many types of smooth muscle or vasoproliferative lesions of both hyperplastic and neoplastic origins described in the lymph node and spleen (65,66). These include nonspecific smooth muscle proliferations in the hilar region: *angiomyomatous hamartoma, lymphangiomyoma* (or *lymphangiomyomatosis*), *leiomyomatosis*, and *intranodal/intrasplenic leiomyoma.*

Clinical Features. Angiomyomatous hamartoma is an extensive smooth muscle proliferation that occurs in the hilum, medulla, and cortex of inguinal lymph nodes (12). It predominantly affects males of a wide age range.

Lymphangiomyoma (71) is a hamartomatous proliferation of lymphatic channels and smooth muscle that occurs exclusively in females in the child-bearing years (see fig. 6-18). There is a generalized, progressive form of the disease (lymphangiomyomatosis [13,64]) that may have extensive organ involvement and result in death from respiratory insufficiency (19). Lymphangiomyoma is a localized, solitary lesion that may be an incidental finding in the abdomen. Many cases are associated with TS, while others are sporadic (58). A study of loss of heterozygosity in lymphangiomyomatosis showed abnormalities in the *TSC2* gene locus in several cases (58).

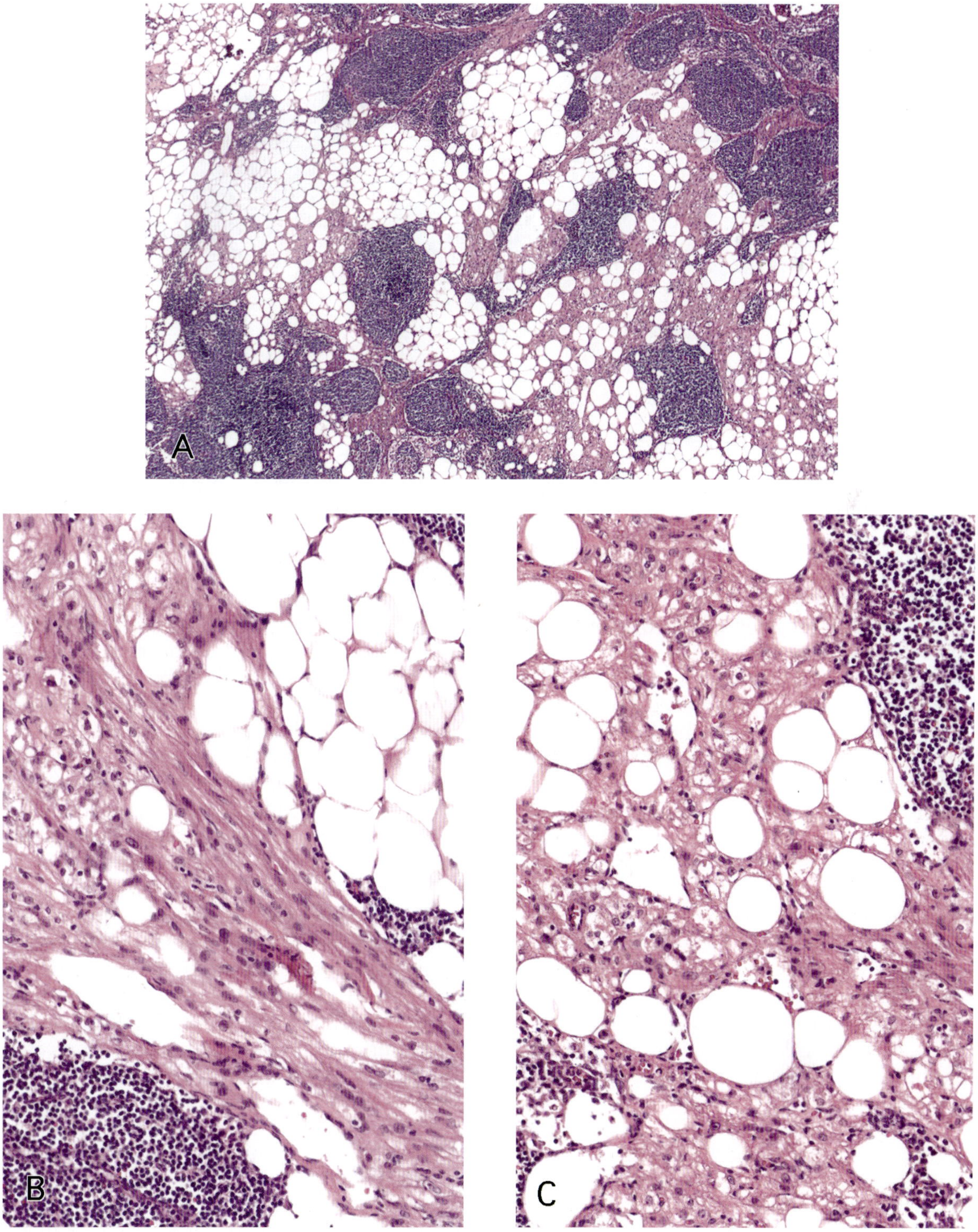

Figure 18-29

ANGIOMYOLIPOMA, LYMPH NODE

In a lymph node extensively involved with angiomyolipoma (A), the fatty and smooth muscle components are prominent (B,C). (Courtesy of David Grignon, Detroit, MI).

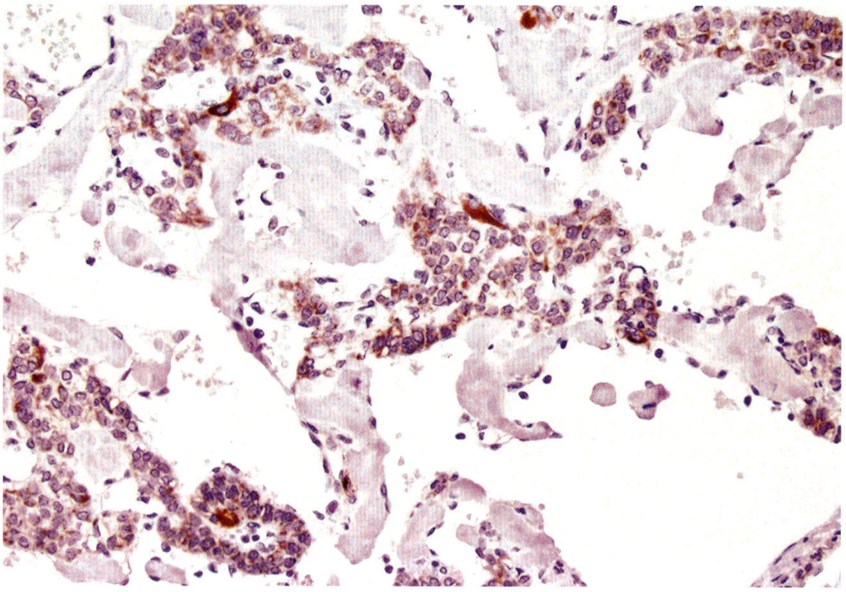

Figure 18-30

ANGIOMYOLIPOMA, LYMPH NODE: HMB45 REACTIVITY

Reactivity for HMB45 is focal.

Leiomyomatosis of lymph node is an exceedingly rare lesion of unknown etiology that occurs in intraabdominal or pelvic lymph nodes (49). This intriguing lesion may represent involvement by either a metastasizing uterine leiomyoma or leiomyomatosis peritonealis disseminate (31), or it may be derived directly from subcoelomic mesenchyme. Another possibility is that it arises through the organization of intranodal decidua or endometriosis by smooth muscle cells. It may be confused with an intranodal leiomyoma (59), which is a rare primary smooth muscle tumor of lymph node that has similar histologic features to leiomyomas in other anatomic sites. In the era of immunohistochemistry, it is likely that most cases historically recognized as leiomyoma of lymph node are more likely lymphangiomyoma. Leiomyomas of the spleen, arising from vascular elements, have been described in association with leiomyomas in other sites, bilateral microlithiasis, and empty sella turcica (25).

Gross Findings. Lymph nodes involved by angiomyomatous hamartoma are firm and fibrotic. The typical firm, white-tan, whorled appearance of leiomyoma is anticipated in most lesions derived from smooth muscle cells (fig. 18-31).

Microscopic Findings. Angiomyomatous hamartoma shows fibrosis of the hilar region that extends into the lymph node parenchyma. Proliferation of medium-sized thick-walled vessels is also seen (fig. 18-32). Smooth muscle bundles are irregularly arranged in the fibrotic stroma, closely associated with blood vessels. Congestion and thrombosis of the vessels may be present. This lesion can be distinguished from hilar smooth muscle proliferations by its extensive intranodal component (fig. 18-33).

In leiomyoma or leiomyomatosis of lymph node, there is a proliferation of bland-appearing smooth muscle cells that may partially or totally involve the lymph node. These lesions are histologically identical to leiomyomas of the uterus.

Histologic features of lymphangiomyoma include sinusoidal involvement by a proliferation of smooth muscle cells around an anastomosing network of endothelium-lined spaces. In contrast to leiomyoma, the smooth muscle cells are plump, without nuclear atypia or increased mitoses, and with clear or pale cytoplasm and more open nuclear chromatin (64).

Ancillary Studies. In all of the lesions discussed, the smooth muscle cells are reactive for actin (fig. 18-34). In addition, there is variable, but frequently weak, expression of desmin and other muscle-related antigens. Characteristic of lymphangiomyoma and lymphangiomyomatosis is reactivity for HMB45 and other melanocytic markers, which is seen in other PEC-derived tumors (13).

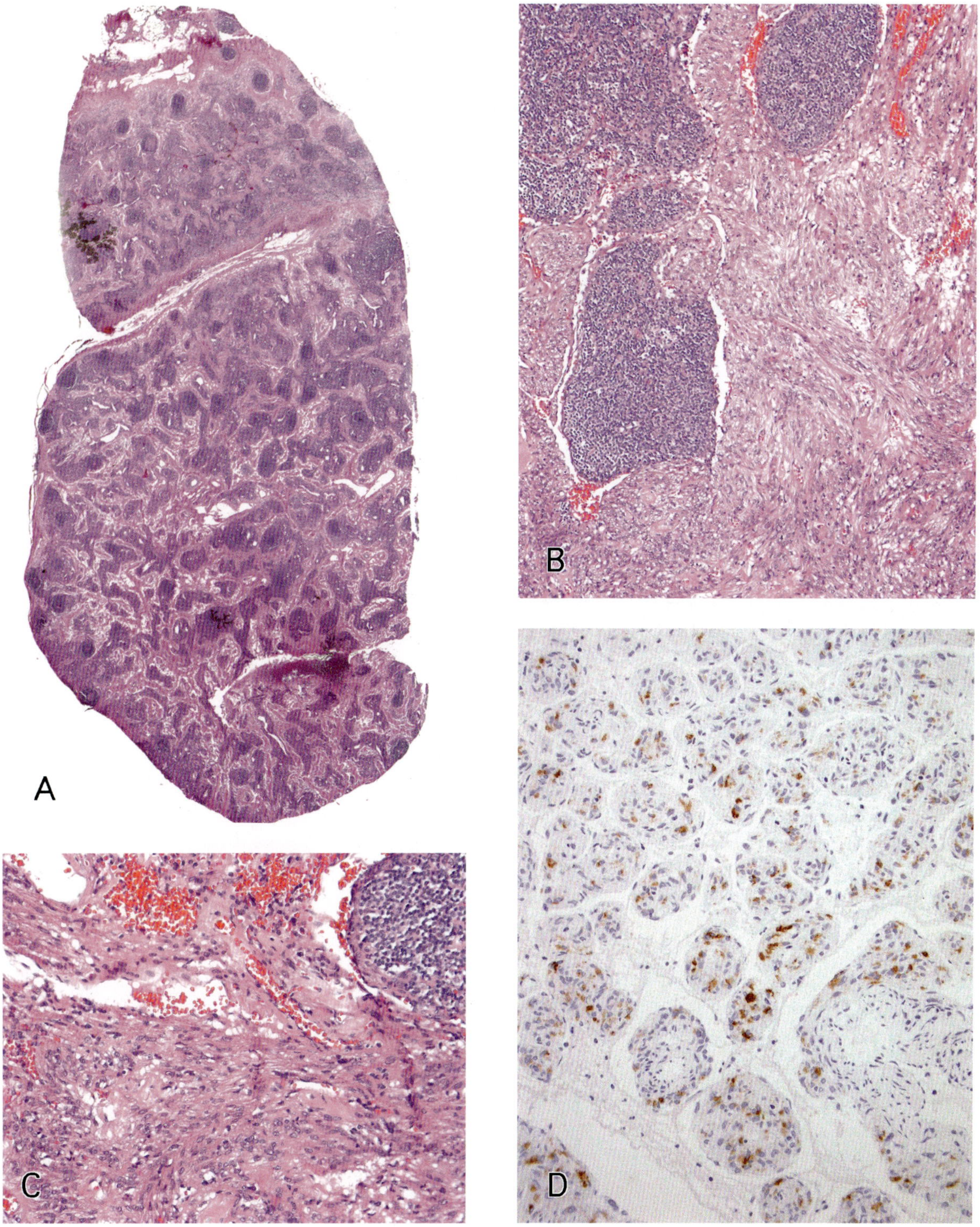

Figure 18-31

LYMPHANGIOMYOMA, LYMPH NODE

Low (A) and high (B,C) magnification show spindle cell proliferations that are reactive for HMB45. (A: Courtesy of the California Tumor Tissue Registry, Loma Linda, CA; B–D courtesy of Christopher Fletcher, Boston, MA.)

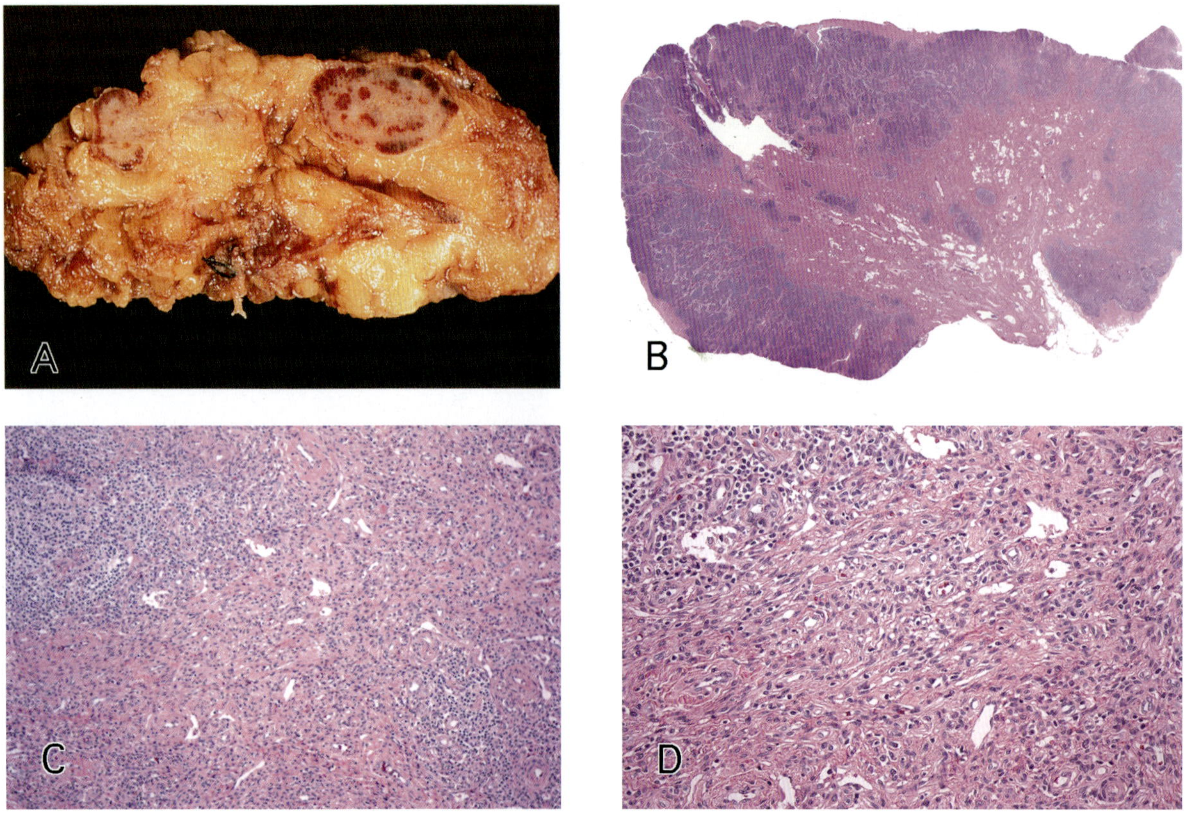

Figure 18-32

ANGIOMYOMATOUS HAMARTOMA, LYMPH NODE

In a groin dissection, the abnormal lymph nodes are embedded in fat (A). The nodes are extensively replaced by tan, firm tissue (B–D). (A: Figure 21-7 Fascicle 14, Third Series; B–D courtesy of Christopher Fletcher, Boston, MA.)

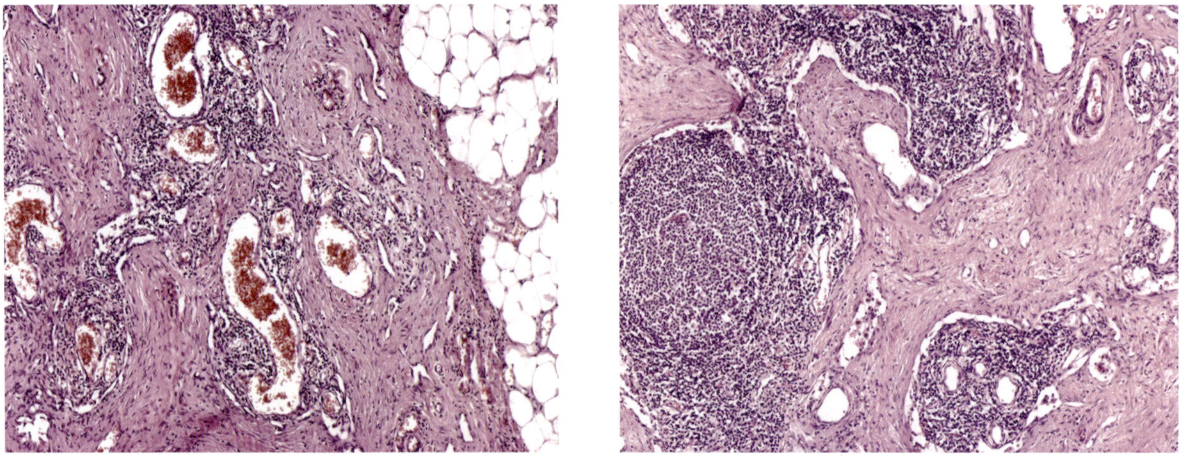

Figure 18-33

ANGIOMYOMATOUS HAMARTOMA, LYMPH NODE

Left: Extensive smooth muscle proliferation in the hilar and medullary regions of an inguinal lymph node with medium- to large-sized vessels.

Right: The intranodal component of angiomyomatous hamartoma shows a residual lymph node with germinal centers.

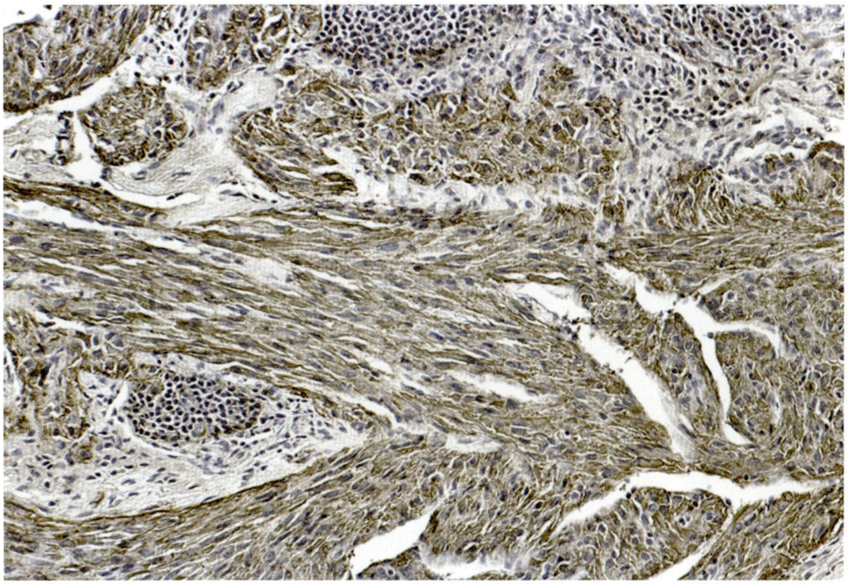

Figure 18-34

IMMUNOHISTOCHEMICAL REACTIVITY IN ANGIOMYOMATOUS HAMARTOMA

Smooth muscle actin reactivity in angiomyomatous hamartoma of lymph node.

Differential Diagnosis. Angiomyomatous hamartoma, lymphangiomyoma (or lymphangiomyomatosis), leiomyomatosis, and leiomyomas have broad differential diagnoses. Any bland spindle cell proliferation, either benign or malignant, may mimic these lesions. Furthermore, it is possible that infectious etiologies could have similar appearances. In all cases, a combination of histologic, clinical, and immunohistochemical findings help differentiate these entities. Lymphangiomyoma may be distinguished from a well-differentiated leiomyosarcoma by its bland cytologic features and HMB45 reactivity.

METASTATIC TUMORS OF SPLEEN

Definition. The presence of tumor cells in the spleen at a distance from the primary site is an uncommon finding. When present, they usually represent late, disseminated disease.

Clinical Features. Metastatic tumors are uncommon in the spleen, partly because of the absence of splenic afferent lymphatics, although hematogenous metastases are also rare, probably due to the hypoxic, inhospitable environment of the spleen. Splenic metastases are seen in 2.3 to 7.1 percent of patients (14,44) and a wide variety of types of carcinomas, melanoma, and more rarely, germ cell tumors and sarcomas, have been reported (69). Patients are often asymptomatic (43).

Adenocarcinomas are the most common type of metastasis reported (43,44), with breast and lung primaries the most frequent. The most common subtype of sarcoma is malignant fibrous histiocytoma.

Gross Findings. Splenic metastases are usually single tumor masses; less commonly, multiple masses; and rarely, diffuse infiltrates (figs. 18-35, 18-36).

Microscopic Findings. The appearance of metastatic tumors in spleen is similar to metastases in other sites (figs. 18-37, 18-38). One notable exception is choriocarcinoma (fig. 18-39); these metastases have a distinctive appearance with hemorrhage and necrosis, and can simulate a primary vascular neoplasm of the spleen.

Differential Diagnosis. Metastases may clinically, radiologically, and grossly mimic a variety of other splenic processes, notably splenic lymphomas. In most cases, the clinical history and microscopic examination resolve most diagnoses. Occasionally, batteries of immunohistochemical stains must be performed to accurately identify the primary site of the metastasis.

Treatment and Prognosis. As mentioned previously, most splenic metastases occur in the setting of disseminated, high clinical stage disease. Thus, the associated prognosis is poor. Very rarely, spontaneous rupture of the spleen occurs in association with splenic metastases.

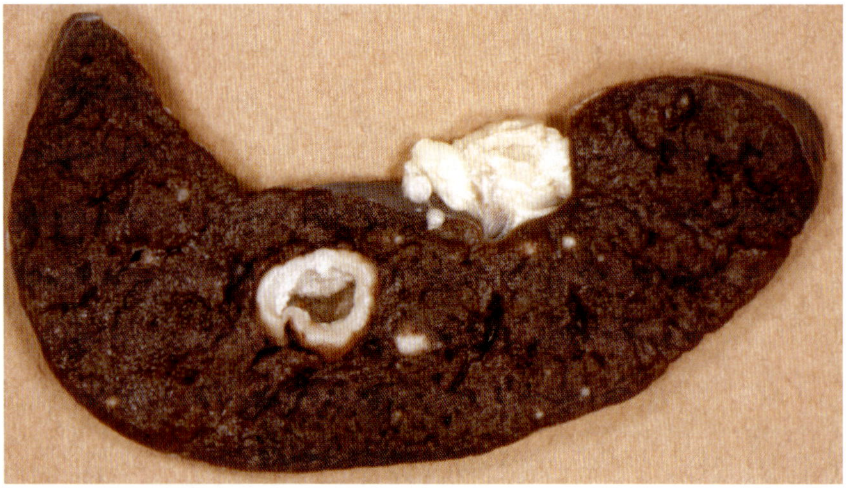

Figure 18-35

METASTASIS, SPLEEN

Several firm, white nodules of metastatic carcinoma are in the parenchyma of the spleen. (Courtesy of John Eble, Indianapolis, IN.)

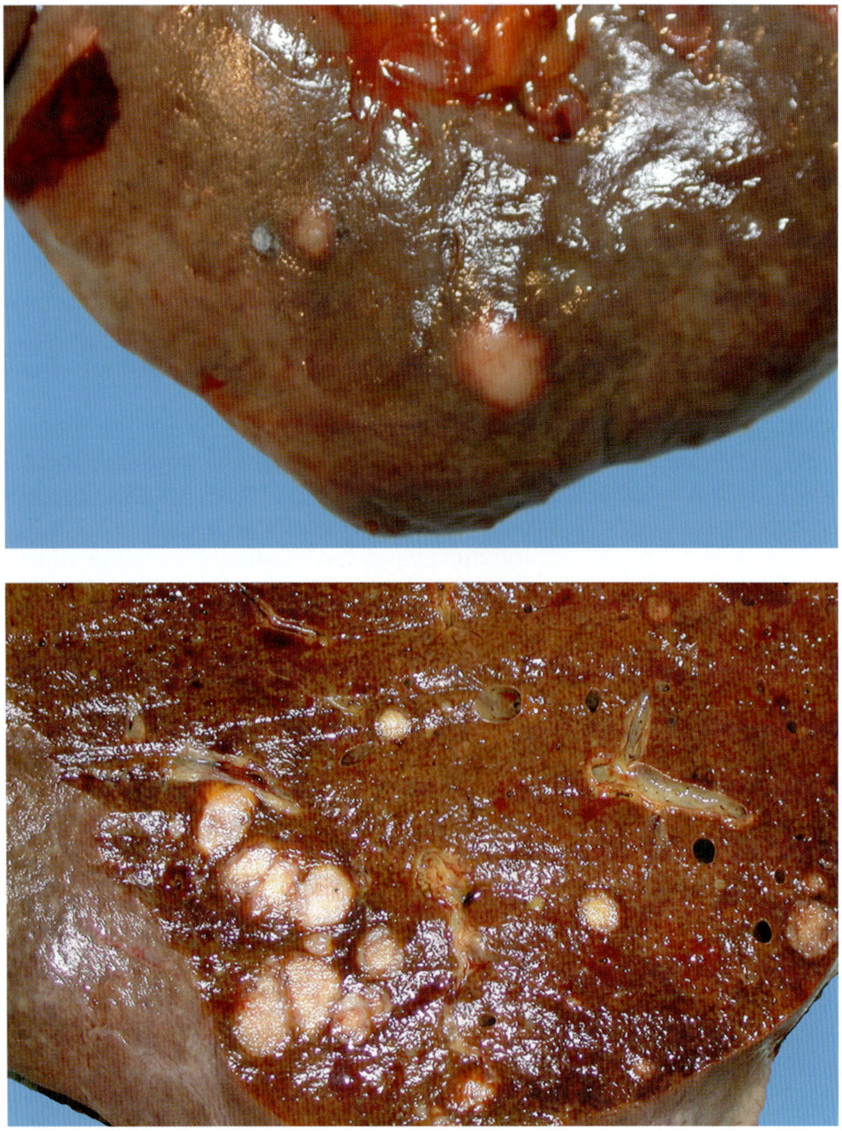

Figure 18-36

METASTASIS, SPLEEN

This metastatic adenocarcinoma is composed of tan nodules that abut the capsule (top) and are present throughout the parenchyma (bottom). (Courtesy of Dean Hawley, Indianapolis, IN.)

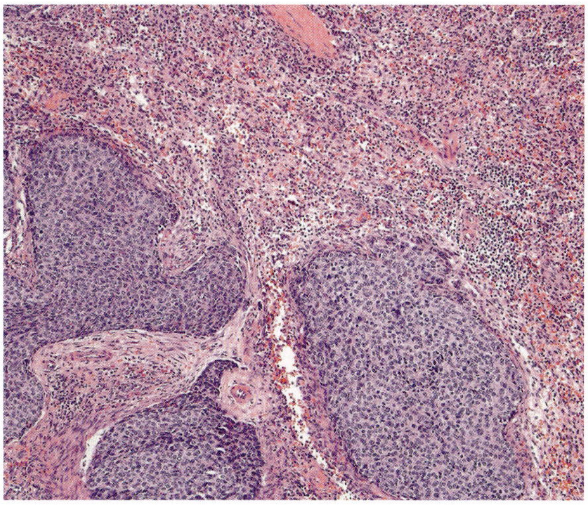

Figure 18-37

METASTASIS, SPLEEN

Transitional cell carcinoma, metastatic to the spleen.

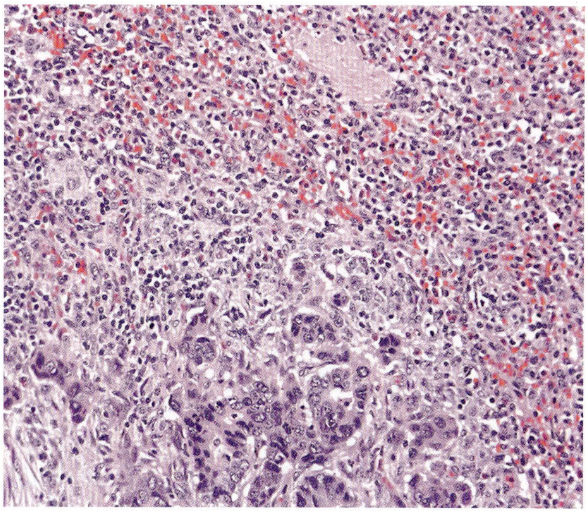

Figure 18-38

METASTASIS, SPLEEN

Cholangiocarcinoma may represent a true metastasis or direct extension.

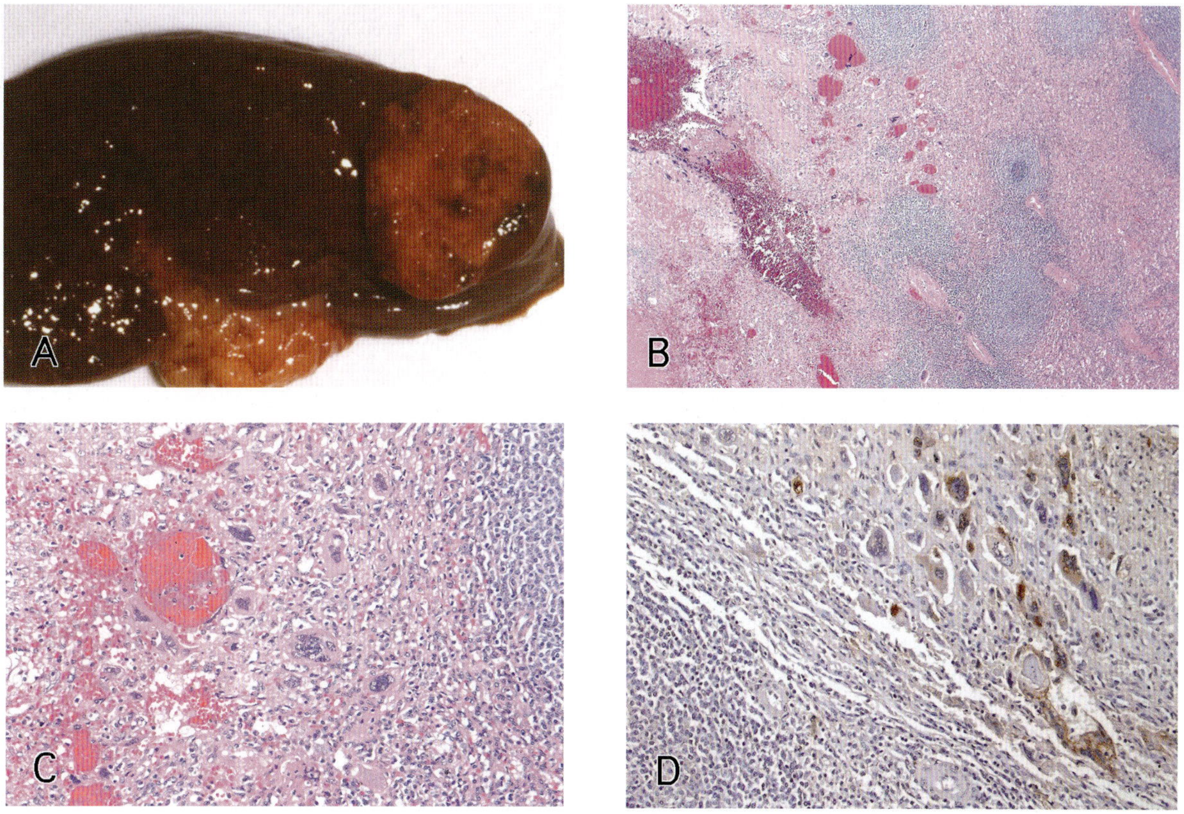

Figure 18-39

CHORIOCARCINOMA METASTATIC TO SPLEEN

Hemorrhagic masses are often seen (A), and are distinct from the normal spleen (B,C). Beta-human chorionic gonadotropin (β-HCG) immunoreactivity is seen in syncytiotrophoblast cells (D).

REFERENCES

1. Abbondazo SL, Irey NS, Frizzera G. Dilantin-associated lymphadenopathy. Spectrum of histopathologic patterns. Am J Surg Pathol 1995;19:675-86.
2. Abdulla M, Bui HX, del Rosario AD, Wolf BC, Ross JS. Renal angiomyolipoma. DNA content and immunohistochemical study of classic and multicentric variants. Arch Pathol Lab Med 1994;118:735-9.
3. Abramowsky C, Alvarado C, Wyly JB, Ricketts R. "Hamartoma" of the spleen (splenoma) in children. Pediatr Dev Pathol 2004;7:231-6.
4. Ali TZ, Beyer G, Taylor M, Volpe C, Papadimitriou JC. Splenic hamartoma: immunohistochemical and ultrastrtructural profile of two cases. Int J Surg Pathol 2005;13:103-11.
5. Arber DA, Kamel OW, van de Rijn M, et al. Frequent presence of the Epstein-Barr virus in inflammatory pseudotumor. Hum Pathol 1995;26:1093-8.
6. Arber DA, Strickler JG, Chen YY, Weiss LM. Splenic vascular tumors: a histologic, immunophenotypic and virologic study. Am J Surg Pathol 1997;21:827-35.
7. Asayama Y, Fukuya T, Honda H, et al. Chronic expanding hematoma of the spleen caused by angiomyolipoma in a patient with tuberous sclerosis. Abdom Imaging 1998;23:527-30.
8. Bahadori M, Liebow AA. Plasma cell granulomas of the lung. Cancer 1973;31:191-208.
9. Ben-Izhak O, Bejan J, Ben-Eliezer S, Vlodavsky E. Splenic littoral cell haemangioendothelioma: a new low-grade variant of malignant littoral cell tumour. Histopathology 2001;39:469-75.
10. Buell R, Wang NS, Seemayer TA, Ahmed MN. Endobronchial plasma cell granuloma (xanthomatous pseudotumor); a light and electron microscopic study. Hum Pathol 1976;7:411-26.
11. Chan JK, Fletcher CD, Nayler SJ, Cooper K. Follicular dendritic cell sarcoma. Clinicopathologic analysis of 17 cases suggesting a malignant potential higher than currently recognized. Cancer 1997;79:294-313.
12. Chan JK, Frizzera G, Fletcher CD, Rosai J. Primary vascular tumors of lymph nodes other than Kaposi's sarcoma. Analysis of 39 cases and delineation of two new entities. Am J Surg Pathol 1992;16:335-50.
13. Chan JK, Tsang WY, Pau MY, Tang MC, Pang SW, Fletcher CD. Lymphangiomyomatosis and angiomyolipoma: closely related entities characterized by hamartomatous proliferation of HMB-45-positive smooth muscle. Histopathology 1993;22:445-55.
14. Chen LW, Chien RN, Yen CL, Chang LC. Splenic tumour: a clinicopathological study. Int J Clin Pract 2004;58:924-7.
15. Cheng L, Gu J, Eble JN, et al. Molecular genetic evidence for different clonal origin of components of human renal angiomyolipomas. Am J Surg Pathol 2001;25:1231-6.
16. Cheuk W, Chan JK, Shek TW, et al. Inflammatory pseudotumor-like follicular dendritic cell tumor: distinctive low-grade malignant intra-abdominal neoplasm with consistent Epstein-Barr virus association. Am J Surg Pathol 2001;6:721-31.
17. Coffin CM, Dehner LP, Meis-Kindblom JM. Inflammatory myofibroblastic tumor, inflammatory fibrosarcoma, and related lesions: an histrorical review with differential diagnostic considerations. Semin Diagn Pathol 1998;15:161-73.
18. Compton CN, McHenry CR, Aijazi M, Chung-Park M. Thrombocytopenia caused by splenic hamartoma: resolution after splenectomy. South Med J 2001;94:542-4.
19. Corrin B, Liebow AA, Friedman PJ. Pulmonary lymphangiomyomatosis. A review. Am J Pathol 1975;79:348-82.
20. Cossu A, Lissia A, Dedola MF, et al. Classic follicular dendritic reticulum cell tumor of the lymph node developing in a patient with a previous inflammatory pseudotumor-like proliferation. Hum Pathol 2005;36:207-11.
21. Cotelingam JD, Jaffe ES. Inflammatory pseudotumor of the spleen. Am J Surg Pathol 1984;8:375-80.
22. Creager AJ, Garwachi CP. Recurrent intranodal palisaded myofibroblastoma with meatplastic bone formation. Arch Pathol Lab Med 1999;123:433-6.
23. Davis RE, Warnke RA, Dorfman RF. Inflammatory pseudotumor of lymph nodes. Additional observations and evidence for an inflammatory etiology. Am J Surg Pathol 1991;15:744-56.
24. Dehner LP, Coffin CM. Idiopathic fibrosclerotic disorders and other inflammatory pseudotumors. Semin Diagn Pathol 1998;15:161-73.
25. Demirel S, Erk O, Akkaya V, et al. Multiple vascular leiomyomas involving bilateral adrenal glands, spleen, and epicardium, associated with bilateral testicular microlithiasis and empty sella turcica. J Pediatr Surg 1997;32:1365-7.
26. Easler RE, Dowlin WM. Primary lipoma of the spleen. Report of a case. Arch Pathol 1969;88:557-9.
27. Facchetti F, De Wolf Peeters C, De Wever I, Frizzera G. Inflammatory pseduotumor of lymph nodes. Immunohistochemical evidence for its fibrohistiocytic nature. Am J Pathol 1990;137:281-9.

28. Falk S, Stutte HJ. Hamartomas of the spleen: a study of 20 biopsy cases. Histopathology 1989;14:603-12.
29. Frizzera G. Castleman's disease and related disorders. Semin Diagn Pathol 1988;5:346-64.
30. Hayes TC, Britton HA, Mewborne EB, Troyer DA, Saldivar VA, Ratner IA. Symptomatic splenic hamartoma: case report and literature review. Pediatrics 1998;101:E10.
31. Hsu YK, Rosenshein NB, Parmley TH, Woodruff JD, Elberfeld HT. Leiomyomatosis in pelvic lymph nodes. Obstet Gynecol 1981;57:91s-93s.
32. Hulbert JC, Graf R. Involvement of the spleen by renal angiomyolipoma: metastasis or multicentricity? J Urol 1983;130:328-9.
33. Hurt MA, Santa Cruz DJ. Cutaneous inflammatory pseudotumor. Lesions resembling "inflammatory pseudotumors" or "plasma cell granulomas" of extracutaneous sites. Am J Surg Pathol 1990;14:764-73.
34. Kassarjian A, Patenaude YG, Bernard C, Bell L. Symptomatic splenic hamartoma with renal, cutaneous, and hematological abnormalities. Pediatr Radiol 2001;31:111-4.
35. Kawachi K, Nakatani Y, Inayama Y, Kawano N, Toda N, Misugi K. Interdigitating dendritic cell sarcoma of the spleen: report of a case with a review of the literature. Am J Surg Pathol 2002; 26:530-7.
36. Kemper CA, Davis RE, Deresinski SC, Dorfmann RF. Inflammatory pseudotumor of intra-abdominal lymph nodes manifesting as recurrent fever of unknown origin: a case report. Am J Med 1991;90:519-23.
37. Kimura N, Watanabe M, Date F, et al. HMB-45 and tuberin in hamartomas associated with tuberous sclerosis. Mod Pathol 1997;10:952-9.
38. Kleist B, Poetsch M, Schmoll J. Intranodal palisaded myofibroblastoma with overexpression of cyclin D1. Arch Pathol Lab Med 2003;127:1040-3.
39. Kraus MD, Dehner LP. Benign vascular neoplasms of the spleen with myoid and angioendotheliomatous features. Histopathology 1999;35:328-36.
40. Krishnan J, Danon AD, Frizzera G. Reactive lymphadenopathies and atypical lymphoproliferative disorders. Am J Clin Pathol 1993;99:385-96.
41. Krishnan J, Frizzera G. Two splenic lesions in need of clarification: hamartoma and inflammatory pseudotumor. Semin Diagn Pathol 2003;20:94-104.
42. Kutok JL, Pinkus GS, Dorfman DM, Fletcher CD. Inflammatory pseudotumor of lymph node and spleen: an entity biologically distinct from inflammatory myofibroblastic tumor. Hum Pathol 2001;32:1382-7.
43. Lam KY, Tang V. Metastatic tumors to the spleen: a 25-year clinicopathologic study. Arch Pathol Lab Med 2000;124:526-30.
44. Lee SS, Morgenstern L, Phillips EH, Hiatt JR, Margulies DR. Splenectomy for splenic metastases: a changing clinical spectrum. Am Surg 2000;66:837-40.
45. Lewis JT, Gaffney RL, Casey MB, Farrell MA, Morice WG, Macon WR. Inflammatory pseudotumor of the spleen associated with a clonal Epstein-Barr virus genome. Case report and review of the literature. Am J Clin Pathol 2003;120:56-61.
46. Lioe TF, Allen DC, Bell JC. A case of multicentric intranodal palisaded myofibroblastoma. Histopathology 1994;24:173-5.
47. Martel M, Cheuk W, Lombardi L, Lifschitz-Mercer B, Chan JK, Rosai J. Sclerosing angiomatoid nodular transformation (SANT): report of 25 cases of a distinctive benign splenic lesion. Am J Surg Pathol 2004;28:1268-79.
48. Martignoni G, Amin MB. Angiomyolipoma. In: World Health Organization Classification of Tumours. Pathology and genetics of tumours of the urinary system and male genital organs. Eble JN, ed. Oxford: IARC Press; 2004:65-7.
49. Mazzoleni G, Salerno A, Santini D, Marabini A, Martinelli G. Leiomyomatosis in pelvic lymph nodes. Histopathology 1992;21:588-9.
50. Miras-Parra FJ, Parra-Ruiz J, Gomez-Morales M, Gomez-Jimenez FJ, de la Higuera-Torres-Puchol J. Inflammatory pseudotumor of lymph nodes with focal infiltration in liver and spleen. Dig Dis Sci 2003;48:2003-4.
51. Moran CA, Suster S, Abbondanzo SL. Inflammatory pseudotumor of lymph nodes: a study of 25 cases with emphasis on morphological heterogeneity. Hum Pathol 1997;28:332-8.
52. Myint MA, Medeiros LJ, Sulaiman RA, Aswad BI, Glantz L. Inflammatory pseudotumor of the ileum. A report of a multifocal, transmural lesion with regional lymph node involment. Arch Pathol Lab Med 1994;118:1138-42.
53. Neuhauser TS, Derringer GA, Thompson LD, et al. Splenic inflammatory myofibroblastic tumor (inflammatory pseudotumor): a clinicopathologic and immunophenotypic study of 12 cases. Arch Pathol Lab Med 2001;125:379-85.
54. O'Malley DP, Poulos C, Czader MB, Sanger W, Orazi A. Intraocular inflammatory myofibroblastic tumor with ALK overexpression. Arch Pathol Lab Med 2004;128:e5-7.
55. O'Malley DP, Sen J, Orazi A. Ki-67 staining patterns in benign and malignant disorders of the spleen. Am J Clin Pathol 2004;122:654.
56. Perrone T, De Wolf-Peeters C, Frizzera G. Inflammatory pseudotumor of lymph nodes. A distinctive pattern of nodal reaction. Am J Surg Pathol 1988;12:351-61.

57. Sarker A, An C, Davis M, Praprotnik D, McCarthy LJ, Orazi A. Inflammatory pseudotumor of the spleen in a 6-year-old child: a clinicopathologic study. Arch Pathol Lab Med 2003;127:e127-30.
58. Smolarek TA, Wessner LL, McCormack FX, Mylet JC, Menon AG, Henske EP. Evidence that lymphangiomyomatosis is caused by TSC2 mutations: chromosome 16p13 loss of heterozygosity in angiomyolipomas and lymph nodes from women with lymphangiomyomatosis. Am J Hum Genet 1998;62:810-5.
59. Starasoler L, Vuitch F, Albores-Saavedra J. Intranodal leiomyoma: another distinctive primary spindle cell neoplasm of lymph node. Am J Clin Pathol 1991;95:858-62.
60 Steinberg JJ, Suhrland M, Valensi Q. The spleen in the spleen syndrome: the association of splenoma with hematopoietic and neoplastic disease—compendium of cases since 1864. J Surg Oncol 1991;47:193-202.
61. Suster S, Rosai J. Intranodal hemorrhagic spindle-cell tumor with "amianthoid" fibers. Report of six cases of a distinctive mesenchymal neoplasm of the inguinal region that simulates Kaposi's sarcoma. Am J Surg Pathol 1989;13:347-57.
62. Tang P, Alhindawi R, Farmer P. Case report: primary isolated angiomyolipoma of the spleen. Ann Clin Lab Sci 2001;31:405-10.
63. Thomas RM, Jaffe ES, Zarate-Osorno A, Medeiros LJ. Inflammatory pseudotumor of the spleen. A clinicopathologic and immunophenotypic study of eight cases. Arch Pathol Lab Med 1993;117:921-6.
64. Tsang WY, Chan JK. Primary leiomyomatosis of lymph node or nodal lymphangiomyoma? Histopathology 1993;23:393-4.
65. Tsang WY, Chan JK, Dorfman RF, Rosai J. Vasoproliferative lesions of the lymph node. Pathol Annu 1994;29(Pt 1):63-133.
66. Warnke RA, Weiss LM, Chan JKC, Cleary ML, Dorfman RF. Nonhematolymphoid tumors and tumor-like lesions of lymph node and spleen. In: Rosai J, Sobin LH, eds. Tumors of the lymph node and spleen. Atlas of Tumor Pathology, Third Series, Fascicle 14. Washington D.C.: American Registry of Pathology; 1995:435-526.
67. Weiss SW, Gnepp DR, Bratthauer GL. Palisaded myofibroblastoma. A benign mesenchymal tumor of lymph node. Am J Surg Pathol 1989;13:341-6.
68. Weiss SW, Goldblum JR. Benign lipomatous tumors. In: Enzinger and Weiss' soft tissue tumors, 4th ed. Philadelphia: Mosby; 2001:571-640.
69. Wick MR, Scheitauer BW, Smith SL, Beart RW Jr. Primary nonlymphoreticular malignant neoplasms of the spleen. Am J Surg Pathol 1982;6:229-42.
70. Wirbel RJ, Uhlig U, Futterer KM. Case report: splenic hamartoma with hematologic disorders. Am J Med Sci 1996;311:243-6.
71. Wolff M. Lymphangiomyoma: clinicopathologic study and ultrastructural confirmation of its histogenesis. Cancer 1973;31:988-1007.
72. Zukerberg LR, Kaynor BL, Silverman ML, Harris NL. Splenic hamartoma and capillary hemangioma are distinct entities: immunohistochemical analysis of CD8 expression by endothelial cells. Hum Pathol 1991;22:1258-61.

19 SPLENIC CYSTS

Splenic cysts are usually classified as nonparasitic or parasitic, based on their etiology, and true cysts (primary) or pseudocysts (false, secondary) based on the presence or absence of a lining epithelium. Cystic lesions of the spleen are rare (6,7,14,15,16,28,37,38,40). Parasitic cysts involving the spleen, such as hydatid cysts, although rare in the United States and western Europe, are common in countries where the zoonoses are endemic (27). Abdominal ultrasound and computerized tomography (CT) are useful in the identification of cystic lesions of the spleen, as is angiography, which often delineates an avascular mass (6,8,21).

NONPARASITIC CYSTS

Pseudocysts

Definition. *Pseudocyst* is a non-neoplastic lesion that is the result of the lack of resorption or organization of a post-traumatic splenic hematoma (16,37–40,46). A history of previous trauma is often not obtained. Other possible etiologies include cystic degeneration of a splenic infarct, hamartoma, or angioma.

General Features. Pseudocyst is the most common nonparasitic splenic cyst, constituting 80 percent of the total. Most pseudocysts are incidental findings, but some are large and cause symptoms.

Gross Findings. Although most pseudocysts are unilocular, rare cases of multiloculated pseudocysts have been reported (1). Pseudocysts differ from epithelial cysts in that the luminal surface in the former is shaggy and hemorrhagic rather than shiny with coarse fibrous trabeculations (fig. 19-1). Pseudocysts are often filled with opaque or cloudy fluid.

Microscopic Findings. The wall of the pseudocyst is formed by fibrous tissue, which may contain areas of calcification and cholesterol crystals. Hemosiderin is often present in the fibrous wall. By definition, an epithelial lining is absent (fig. 19-2). Pseudocysts must be differentiated from true cysts and cystic lymphangioma. Immunostaining for cytokeratin or vascular markers confirms the lack of an epithelial or endothelial lining, respectively.

Treatment and Prognosis. Once diagnosed, splenic pseudocyst should be treated if it is

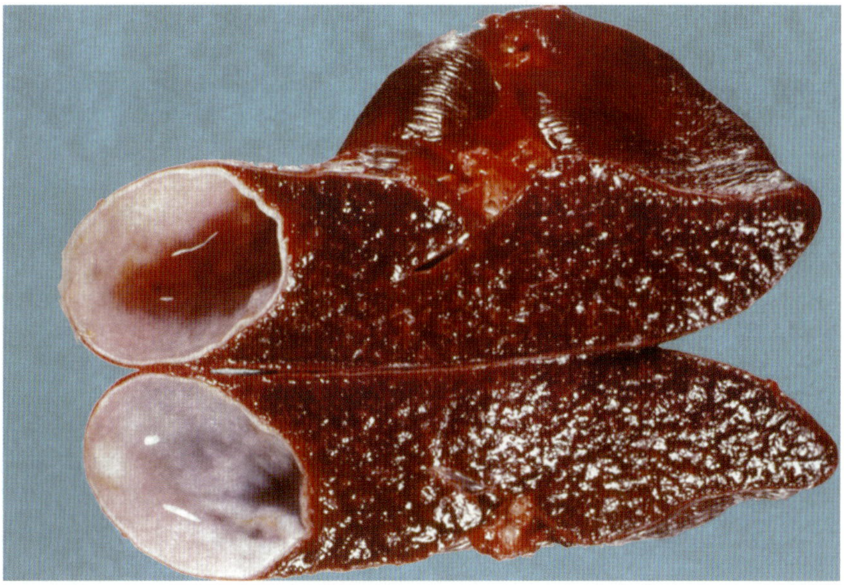

Figure 19-1

PSEUDOCYST, SPLEEN

The inner lining of the cyst often appears smooth. (Courtesy of John Eble, Indianapolis, IN.)

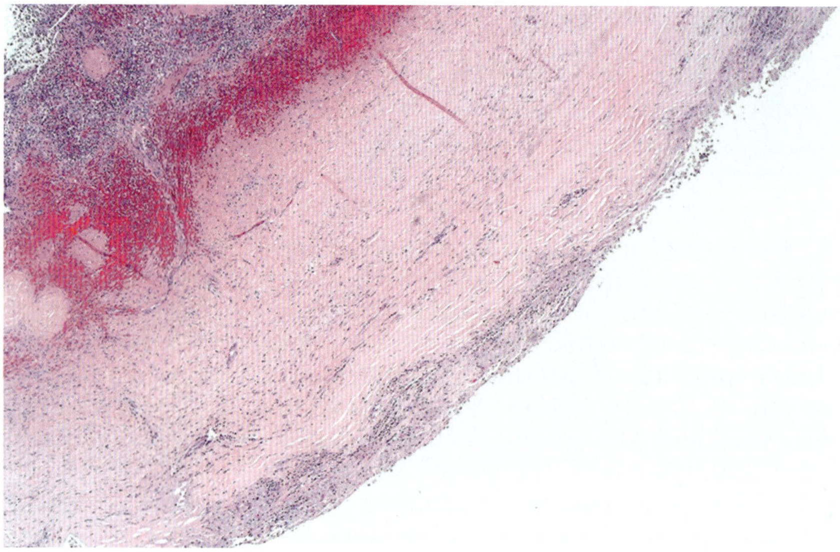

Figure 19-2

PSEUDOCYST, SPLEEN

A distinct epithelial lining is lacking. Typically, the cyst wall is composed of macrophages and fibrous tissue.

symptomatic or larger than 10 cm (46). Risks of unremoved splenic pseudocysts include spontaneous rupture with hemoperitoneum and infection with abscess formation. Traditionally, splenectomy has been the treatment of choice. Currently, many authors advocate splenic preservation mainly to reduce morbidity and mortality since infections are often associated with the postsplenectomy state (25,29,45). This is particularly important in children and in tropical countries where post-traumatic cysts are common and splenectomy may be fatal in patients with malaria (29). Spleen-sparing procedures include cyst excision and splenorrhaphy or, alternatively, partial cyst excision and marsupialization (25,28,41,45). Despite a high incidence of recurrences, radiographically assisted percutaneous drainage can be successfully employed in selected cases (41).

True Cysts: Splenic Mesothelial, Epidermoid, and Epithelial

Definition. *True splenic cysts*, also referred to as *mesothelial, epidermoid,* or *epithelial cysts*, are non-neoplastic cystic lesions lined with squamous, transitional, flat, or cuboidal epithelium or mesothelial cells.

General Features. True cysts account for approximately 20 percent of splenic nonparasitic cysts (2,6,18,32,42). They are usually found in children or young adults, and most series report no sex predominance (32). A few familial cases have been reported (17,19). They are believed by most authors to be congenital in origin, derived from inclusions of splenic capsular mesothelium into the splenic parenchyma (9,22,34). Electron microscopic studies have provided supportive evidence of this hypothesis (9). Others, however, have postulated various alternatives such as derivation from mesodermic tissue (10) or a teratomatous origin (23). An acquired pathogenetic mechanism has also been suggested, at least for some cases. True cysts have been reported in patients with a history of abdominal trauma, raising the possibility that a subclinical tear in the splenic capsule, with subsequent mesothelial displacement and intrasplenic entrapment, may be the etiologic factor in some "spontaneous" cases as well. True cysts have been described in accessory spleens (1,43).

Clinical Features. True cysts usually do not cause symptoms but pressure symptoms may result from a mass effect, adherence to adjacent viscera, or adherence to the diaphragm; less commonly, they are responsible for poorly localized abdominal pain.

Gross Findings. True cysts are mostly single, large (average size in one series of 10 cm), and unilocular, although occasionally there are satellites in the wall of the main cyst (fig. 19-3) (16). Multiple as well as multilocular cysts have been reported (8,16,17,19,21). The lining of a true cyst is usually whitish and shiny, and displays characteristic coarse fibrous trabeculations (30). The fluid content may be either thin and serous, or turbid and viscous (30). The fluid varies from clear to yellow, green, or brown (30).

Microscopic Findings. Histologically, the cyst wall is composed of fibrous tissue with an interior epithelial lining (figs. 19-4, 19-5) (5,6,20,30). Since the epithelial lining is often partially denuded, numerous histologic sections may be required to identify it (5,6). The cyst is most commonly lined by stratified squamous epithelium which may show keratinization. Rete ridges and skin appendages are absent. Transitional epithelium has been reported (38); this may be associated with foci of intraepithelial cyst-like structures containing mucin and may closely resemble cystitis cystica. The cyst lining is occasionally composed partially or wholly of columnar, cuboidal, or flattened epithelium, a finding generally interpreted as evidence of mesothelial differentiation. Immunohistochemical studies have also generally confirmed a mesothelial origin by showing reactivity with keratin and vimentin as well as the mesothelial-associated marker HBME-1 (3,22).

Differential Diagnosis. The main entity in the differential diagnosis of true splenic cyst is splenic pseudocyst. Immunohistology confirms the presence of an epithelial layer in the former. Immunostaining with vascular endothelial markers confirms the diagnosis in cases mimicking lymphangioma. The extremely rare splenic dermoid cyst should also be considered in the differential diagnosis (see next section) (7). Primary splenic lymphoma may occasionally simulate, radiologically, a splenic cyst (33). Obviously, the histologic findings are remarkably different.

Treatment and Prognosis. The main complications of true splenic cysts include hemorrhage, rupture, and secondary bacterial infections (5, 24,30). Rarely, rupture of a cyst causes symptoms of an acute abdomen (12). Although cysts may lead to marked splenomegaly, signs of hypersplenism are uncommon. Patients with true cysts

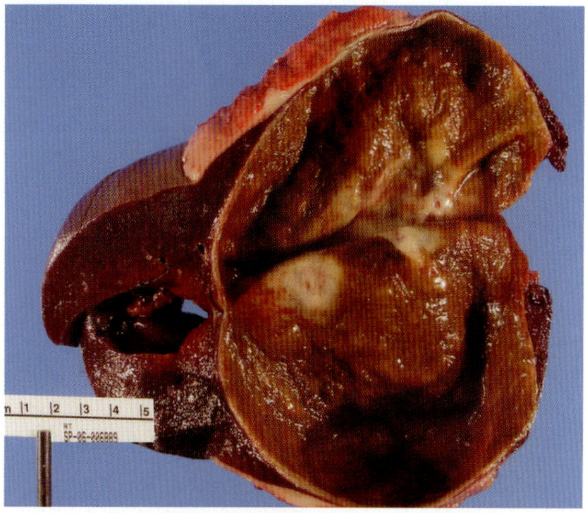

Figure 19-3

SPLENIC EPITHELIAL CYST

In contrast to the splenic pseudocyst, this epithelial cyst has a somewhat roughened inner surface. The cyst is distinct from the adjacent, uninvolved spleen. (Courtesy of Milton Drachenberg, Long Beach, CA.)

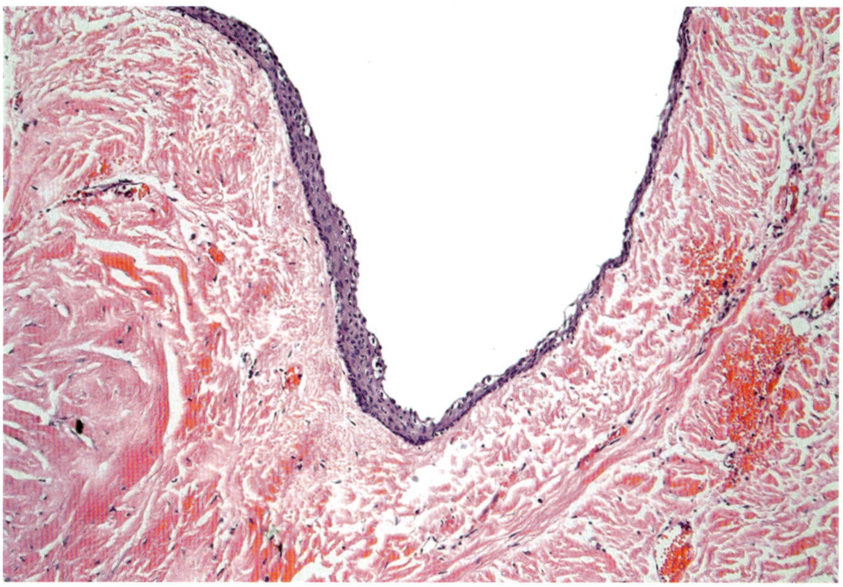

Figure 19-4

SPLENIC EPITHELIAL CYST

The epithelial lining is bland.

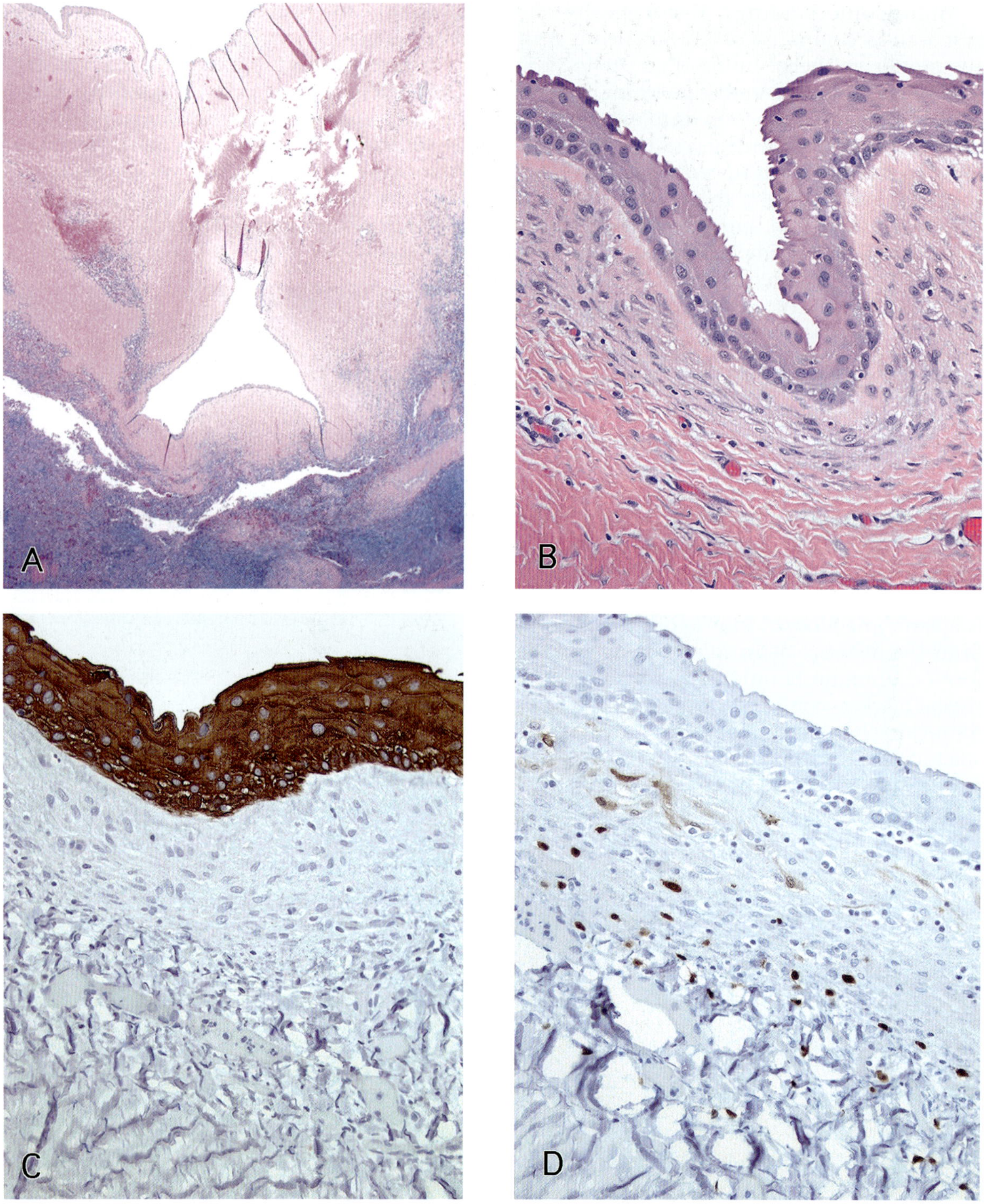

Figure 19-5

SPLENIC EPITHELIAL CYST

Although of little clinical importance, distinguishing splenic epithelial and mesothelial cysts may be difficult. These images represent an epithelial cyst (low magnification [A]; high magnification [B]), which is positive for cytokeratin (C), but lacks reactivity for calretinin (D), while a mesothelial cyst is reactive for both keratin and calretinin. (A,B: hematoxylin and eosin [H&E]; C: cytokeratin; D: calretinin.)

are treated in the same way as patients with false cysts. Complete excision of the cyst wall and its lining in its entirety is the only treatment that protects the patient from recurrence (30).

An exceptionally rare complication is the possibility of malignant transformation. Elit and Aylward (13) reported a case of squamous cell carcinoma arising from a true splenic cyst in a pregnant woman, and Morinaga et al. (31) described a case of splenic low-grade mucinous cystadenocarcinoma in a 69-year-old man. Carcinosarcoma of the spleen was reported by Westra et al. (44) in a 55-year-old woman; the authors suggested a derivation from entrapped mesothelium that underwent mullerian differentiation as a pathogenetic mechanism. A case of malignant splenic teratoma was reported by Daftary and Barnett (11) in a 69-year-old woman. It is conceivable that this case represented malignant transformation of a splenic dermoid cyst.

True Cysts: Splenic Dermoid

True dermoid cysts, similar to benign cystic teratomas of the ovary, with hair follicles and sebaceous glands, are rare in the spleen (7). Skin appendages are only present in dermoid cysts, making them easy to distinguish from other splenic cysts (fig. 19-6).

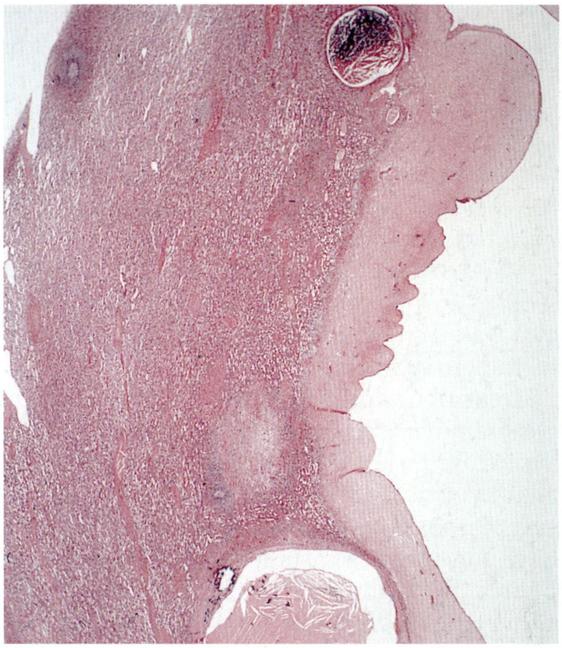

Figure 19-6

SPLENIC EPIDERMOID CYST

The luminal wall is rugged. A few cystic inclusions are seen in the fibrous wall. (Fig. 21-117 from Fascicle 14, Third Series.)

PARASITIC CYSTS

Definition. The most common *parasitic cyst* is caused by the larvae of the tapeworm of the genus *Echinococcus*, resulting from the ingestion of tapeworm eggs (4,7,26,27,35,37).

General Features. Two thirds of *echinococcal (hydatid) cysts* are found in the liver. The larvae invade the tributaries of the portal vein and encyst in the organ. Whenever echinococcal cysts form, the larvae incite an inflammatory response. The most prevalent species is *Echinococcus granulosus*, which forms unilocular cysts. Infection is worldwide, but most common in the western United States, New Zealand, Australia, and Near East. Dogs and sheep are the definitive hosts. *E. multilocularis* is also found in central and eastern Europe, and *E. vogeli* is found in northern Latin America. The latter species forms multilocular cysts. Echinococcal cysts of the spleen are rare in the United States. The reported prevalence of splenic involvement varies from 0.9 to 8.0 percent.

Splenic echinococcal cysts generally develop by means of systemic dissemination or intraperitoneal spread from a ruptured liver cyst. Isolated splenic involvement is uncommon (37). Splenic hydatid cysts are usually solitary, and their imaging characteristics are similar to those of hepatic hydatid cysts.

Sonography is usually diagnostic without requiring other investigations (36). On CT scans, an echinococcal cyst appears as a well-defined hypoattenuating lesion with a distinguishable wall; coarse wall calcifications occur in 50 percent of cases and daughter cysts in 75 percent (36). Serologic testing is more specific, but less sensitive, than most imaging modalities.

Clinical Features. Clinically, most patients are asymptomatic. Large cysts, however, may cause pressure symptoms owing to compression of other viscera. Severe complications are the result of secondary infection, rupture of the cyst into adjacent structures, or rupture intraperitoneally with anaphylaxis.

Gross Findings. The outer cyst is composed of a laminated fibrous layer, which is lined by an inner germinative layer made up of daughter cysts, termed "brood capsules" (fig. 19-7) (4,36). The cyst may be surrounded by inflammatory cells, predominantly mononuclear cells and eosinophils. Scolices develop on the inner aspect of the brood capsules, which separate from the cyst wall and form sand-like material. This becomes suspended in the cyst fluid.

Microscopic Findings. The echinococcal scolices can be recognized in imprints of the cyst wall using the acid-fast stain and standard histologic stains (fig. 19-8) (16).

Treatment and Prognosis. Treatment is surgical removal of the cyst. Care must be taken to avoid rupture at surgery, which may result in an anaphylactic reaction or the spread of multiple cysts throughout the abdomen. Recent studies have suggested that surgery (with albendazole pretreatment) should be reserved for those with either curable disease or complications and that all other patients should be managed, at least initially, with albendazole alone (26,35).

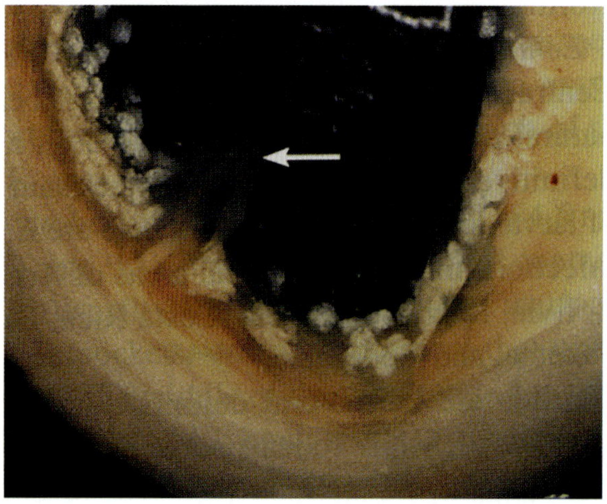

Figure 19-7

ECHINOCOCCAL CYST, SPLEEN

"Brood capsules" line the inner wall of the cyst. (Fig. 9.5 from Meyers WM, Neafie RC, Marty AM, Wear DJ. Pathology of infectious diseases: helminthiases, Vol. 1. Washington DC: American Registry of Pathology; 2000:147.)

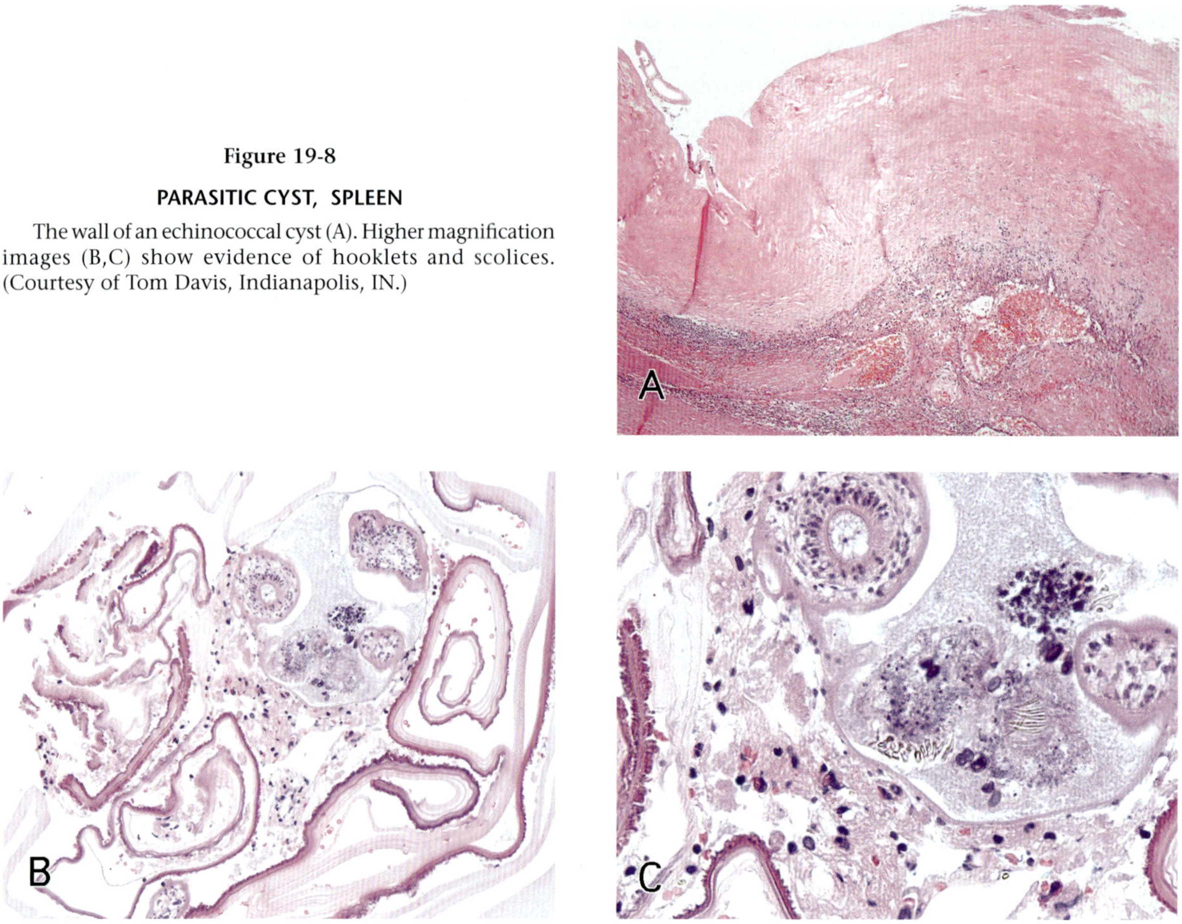

Figure 19-8

PARASITIC CYST, SPLEEN

The wall of an echinococcal cyst (A). Higher magnification images (B,C) show evidence of hooklets and scolices. (Courtesy of Tom Davis, Indianapolis, IN.)

REFERENCES

1. Adsay NV, Hasteh F, Cheng JD, Klimstra DS. Squamous-lined cysts of the pancreas: lymphoepithelial cysts, dermoid cysts (teratomas), and accessory-splenic epidermoid cysts. Semin Diagn Pathol 2000;17:56-65.
2. Allen RP, Condon VR. Epidermoid cysts of the spleen in children. Am J Roentgenol Radium Ther Nucl Med 1961;86:534-9.
3. Arber DA, Strickler JG, Weiss LM. Splenic mesothelial cysts mimicking lymphangiomas. Am J Surg Pathol 1997;21:334-8.
4. Binford CH, Connor DH, eds. Pathology of tropical and extraordinary diseases, Washington DC: Armed Forces Institute of Pathology; 1976.
5. Bisceglia M, Nirchio V, Di Mattia A, Scaramuzzi G, Tardio B. [Primary splenic cysts. Report of 5 cases, 4 of which unpublished and review of the literature.] Pathologica 1994;86:638-44. [Italian]
6. Blank E, Campbell JR. Epidermoid cysts of the spleen. Pediatrics 1973;51:75-84.
7. Bostick WL, Lucia SP. Nonparasitic noncancerous cystic tumors of the spleen. Arch Pathol (Chic) 1949;47:215-22.
8. Bron KM, Hoffman WJ. Preoperative diagnosis of splenic cysts. Arch Surg 1971;102:459-461.
9. Burrig KF. Epithelial (true) splenic cysts. Pathogenesis of the mesothelial and so-called epidermoid cyst of the spleen. Am J Surg Pathol 1988;12:275-81.
10. Cave RH, Garvin DF, Doohen DJ. Metaplastic mesodermal cyst of the spleen. Am Surg 1971;37:97-102.
11. Daftary M, Barnett RN. Malignant teratoma of the spleen. Yale J Biol Med 1971;43:283-7.
12. Dibble JB, Weigent CE. Epidermoid cyst of the spleen presenting as an abdominal emergency. Report of a case. JAMA 1965;194:1144-6.
13. Elit L, Aylward B. Splenic cyst carcinoma presenting in pregnancy. Am J Hematol 1989;32:57-60.
14. Fowler RH. Cystic tumors of the spleen. Int Abstr Surg 1940;70:213-23.
15. Fowler RH. Nonparasitic benign cystic tumors of the spleen. Int Abstr Surg 1953;26:209-27.
16. Garvin DF, King FM. Cysts and nonlymphomatous tumors of the spleen. Pathol Ann 1981;16:61-80.
17. Gilmartin D. Familial multiple epidermoid cysts of the spleen. Conn Med 1978;42:297-300.
18. Griscom NT. Huge splenic cysts. Am J Dis Child 1965;109:224-7.
19. Iwanaka T, Nakanishi H, Tsuchida Y, Oka T, Honna T, Shimizu K. Familial multiple mesothelial cysts of the spleen. J Pediatr Surg. 1995;30:1743-5.
20. Jameson EM, Smith OF. Calcified cyst of the spleen. U S Naval Med Bull 1945;45:537-41.
21. King MC, Glick BW, Freed A. The diagnosis of splenic cysts. Surg Gynecol Obstet 1968;127:509-12.
22. Lee YS, Teh M. Histogenesis of true splenic cysts: a histological and immunohistochemical study. Ann Acad Med Singapore 1993;22:372-6.
23. Lifschitz-Mercer B, Open M, Kushnir I, Czernobilsky B. Epidermoid cyst of the spleen: a cytokeratin profile with comparison to other squamous epithelia. Virchows Arch 1994;424:213-6.
24. Lippitt WH, Akhavan T, Caplan GE. Epidermoid cyst of the spleen with rupture and inflammation. Arch Surg 1967;95:74-8.
25. Liu KK, Lee KH, Ku KW, Yeung CK. Decapsulation of symptomatic splenic pseudocyst—a further use for laparoscopic surgery in children. Eur J Surg 1996;162:921-3.
26. Lynch AC, Stubbs RS. Hydatid disease in New Zealand. What remains and how should we treat it? N Z Med J 1999;112:131-4.
27. Manterola C, Vial M, Losada H, et al. Uncommon locations of abdominal hydatid disease. Trop Doct 2003;33:179-80.
28. Martin JW. Congenital splenic cysts. Am J Surg 1958;96:302-8.
29. Millar JS. Partial excision and drainage of posttraumatic splenic cysts. Br J Surg 1982;69:477-8.
30. Morgestern L. Nonparasitic splenic cysts: pathogenesis, classification, and treatment. J Am Coll Surg 2002;194:306-14.
31. Morinaga S, Ohyama R, Koizumi J. Low-grade mucinous cystadenocarcinoma in the spleen. Am J Surg Pathol 1992;16:903-8.
32. Musy PA, Roche B, Belli D, Bugmann P, Nussle D, Le Coultre C. Splenic cysts in pediatric patients—a report on 8 cases and review of the literature. Eur J Pediatr Surg 1992;3:137-40.
33. Nakashima A, Nakashima K, Seto H, Kamei T, Kakishita M, Kitagawa M. Primary splenic lymphoma presenting as a large cyst. Radiat Med 1994;12:42-5.
34. Ough YD, Nash HR, Wood DA. Mesothelial cysts of the spleen with squamous metaplasia. Am J Clin Pathol 1981;76:666-9.
35. Polat P, Kantarci M, Alper F, Suma S, Koruyucu MB, Okur A. Hydatid disease from head to toe. Radiographics 2003;23:475-94.
36. Poole JB, Marcial-Rojas RA. Echinococcosis. In: Marcial-Rojas RA, ed. Pathology of protozoal and helminthic diseases. Baltimore: Williams & Wilkins; 1971:635-57.

37. Qureshi MA, Hafner CD. Clinical manifestations of splenic cysts: study of 75 cases. Am Surg 1965;31:605-8.
38. Shousha S. Splenic cysts. A report of six cases and brief review. Post Grad Med J 1978;54:265-9.
39. Simmons TC. Traumatic pseudocyst of the spleen. J Natl Med Assoc 1990;82:727-9.
40. Sirinek KR, Evans WE. Nonparasitic splenic cysts. Case report of epidermoid cyst with review of the literature. Am J Surg 1973;126:8-13.
41. Smith GW. Tumors, cysts, and abscesses of the spleen. In: Cameron JL, ed. Current surgical therapy, 5th ed. St. Louis: Mosby; 1995:474-7.
42. Talerman A, Hart S. Epithelial cysts of the spleen. Br J Surg 1970;57:201-4.
43. Tateyama H, Tada T, Murase T, Fujitake S, Eimoto T. Lymphoepithelial cyst and epidermoid cyst of the accessory spleen in the pancreas. Mod Pathol 1998;11:1171-7.
44. Westra WH, Anderson BO, Klimstra DS. Carcinosarcoma of the spleen. An extragenital malignant mixed mullerian tumor? Am J Surg Pathol 1994;18:309-15.
45. Williams RJ, Glazer G. Splenic cysts: changes in diagnosis, treatment and aetiological concepts. Ann R Coll Surg Engl 1993;75:87-9.
46. Woody JD, Craft PR, Fabian TS, Somberg LB. Traumatic pseudocyst of the spleen. Tenn Med 1996;89:372-3.

Index*

*In a series of numbers, those in boldface indicate the main discussion of the entity.

D

E

F

G

H

I

J

K

L

R

S

T

U